NURSING OF ADULTS

NURSING
OF ADULTS

Dorothy W. Smith, R.N., Ed.D.

Professor of Nursing and Chairman,
Department of Medical-Surgical Nursing,
College of Nursing, Rutgers University

Carol P. Hanley Germain, R.N., B.S.N., M.S.

Lecturer and Consultant in Clinical Nursing;
formerly Assistant Professor, Continuing Education
Program for Nurses, Rutgers University

Edited by

Patricia Heenan, R.N., M.A.

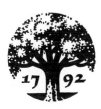

J. B. Lippincott Company

Philadelphia   Toronto

Copyright © 1972 by J. B. Lippincott Company

This book is fully protected by copyright and, with the exception of brief excerpts for review, no part of it may be reproduced in any form, by print, photoprint, microfilm, or any other means, without the written permission of the publisher.

Distributed in Great Britain by
Blackwell Scientific Publications
Oxford, London and Edinburgh

ISBN 0-397-54015-9

Library of Congress Catalog Card Number 78-37297

Printed in The United States of America

3   5   6   4   2

Library of Congress Cataloging in Publication Data

Smith, Dorothy W.
　　Nursing of adults.

　　"Adapted from Care of the adult patient, third edition."

　　Includes bibliographies.

　　1. Nurses and nursing. I. Germain, Carol P. Hanley, joint author. II. Title. [DNLM: 1. Nursing care. WY 156 S645n 1972]

RT41.S579　　　　　　　610.73　　　　　　78-37297

ISBN 0-397-54015-9

Consultants

The following nurses, physicians and health care specialists contributed to the revision of a number of chapters for the third edition of *Care of the Adult Patient*. Their material was adapted for inclusion in *Nursing of Adults*.

Robert R. Abel, M.D., Assistant Clinical Professor of Dermatology, Cornell University Medical College and Assistant Attending Physician, The New York Hospital, contributed to the material concerning dermatologic conditions.

Stephen M. Ayers, M.D., Director, Cardiopulmonary Laboratory, St. Vincent's Hospital and Medical Center, New York, N.Y., and Associate Professor of Clinical Medicine, New York University School of Medicine, served as consultant for the material concerning respiratory insufficiency and failure, acidosis and alkalosis.

Charles W. Clarke, Jr., M.D., Associate Attending in Medicine, Overlook Hospital, Summit, N.J.; formerly Assistant, Peripheral Vascular Clinic, St. Luke's Hospital, New York, contributed to the material concerning peripheral vascular disease.

Armand F. Cortese, M.D., Assistant Professor of Surgery, New York Hospital, Cornell Medical Center, contributed to the chapter on disorders of the liver, gallbladder and pancreas.

Maximilian Fabrykant, M.D., Assistant Professor of Clinical Medicine, New York University School of Medicine, and Chief of Metabolism, New York Infirmary, contributed to the chapter on diabetes mellitus.

Agnes Fahy, National Tuberculosis and Respiratory Disease Association, assisted in the preparation of the chapter on pulmonary tuberculosis.

Kathleen S. Felix, R.N., Nurse Consultant, Transplant-Dialysis-Biochemistry Team, New York Hospital, Cornell University Medical Center, New York, contributed to the material concerning the patient in renal failure.

Donald J. Fishman, M.D., Associate Professor of Medicine (Neurology), and Associate Professor of Pediatrics, Hahnemann Medical College and Hospital, Philadelphia, contributed to the chapters concerning the patient with neurologic disturbance.

Solomon Garb, M.D., F.A.C.P., Scientific Director, American Medical Center at Denver, Colorado.

Timothy S. Gee, M.D., Clinical Assistant, Memorial Hospital for Cancer and Allied Diseases, Research Associate, Sloan-Kettering Institute for Cancer Research, and Instructor, Cornell Medical College, contributed to the material concerning blood and lymph disorders.

Mario P. Grasso, M.D., Medical Director, New Jersey Hospital for Chest Diseases, Glen Gardner, New Jersey, contributed to the chapter on pulmonary tuberculosis.

Frances Gutowski, R.N., Supervisor-Instructor, Memorial-Sloan Kettering Cancer Center, contributed to the chapters concerning care of the patient with cancer and nursing management in radiotherapy.

Harold T. Hansen, M.D., F.A.C.S., A.A.O.S., Attending Orthopaedist, New Jersey Orthopaedic Hospital, Orange, New Jersey, contributed to the chapter concerning fractures.

Raymond Harrison, M.D., F.A.C.S., Attending Surgeon, Manhattan Eye, Ear and Throat Hospital, and Attending Ophthalmologist, The New York Hospital, contributed to the material concerning visual impairment.

Sister Mary Louise Hoeller, R.N., Specialist in Surgical Nursing, University of Wisconsin-Milwaukee, and Administrative Assistant, St. Mary's Hospital, Milwaukee, contributed to the material on the surgical patient.

John S. Johnson, M.D., Senior Investigator, The National Institute of Allergy and Infectious Diseases, National Institutes of Health, contributed to the material dealing with allergy.

Elizabeth Agnes Katona, R.N., M.A., Staff Development Coordinator, Community General Hospital, Assistant Professor of Nursing, Syracuse University, Syracuse, N.Y.; and Formerly Clinical Assistant Professor of Nursing, State University Hospital, Downstate Medical Center, Brooklyn, N.Y., contributed to the chapter on the patient with an ileostomy or colostomy.

Eugene R. Kelly, M.D., Associate Attending in Medicine and Cardiology, Overlook Hospital, Summit, N.J., contributed to the chapters concerning fundamental processes of illness and shock.

John G. Keuhnelian, M.D., Clinical Assistant Professor of surgery (Urology), Cornell University Medical College; Associate Attending Surgeon, New York Hospital, Cornell Medical Center; and Associate Urologist, Lenox Hill Hospital, New York, contributed to the chapters concerning urology and the male reproductive system.

Robert L. Kozam, M.D., Clinical Assistant Professor of Medicine, State University of New York, Downstate Medical Center, Brooklyn, and Chief of Cardiology and Cardiopulmonary Laboratory, Methodist Hospital of Brooklyn, New York, contributed to the chapters concerning respiratory disorders.

Ronald W. Lamont-Havers, M.D., Associate Director for Extramural Research and Training, National Institutes of Health, Bethesda, Maryland, contributed to the chapter concerning diseases of bones and joints.

Ferdinand La Venuta, M.D., Research Fellow and Instructor in Otolaryngology, New York Hospital, Cornell University Medical Center, contributed to the chapters concerning hearing impairment and diseases of the nose and throat.

Irving M. Levitas, M.D., Director of Rehabilitation Medicine, Hackensack Hospital, and Medical Director, Bergen County Heart Association Cardiac Work Evaluation Unit, Hackensack, N.J., contributed to the material concerning rehabilitation of patients with heart disease.

C. Walton Lillehei, Ph.D., M.D., Professor and Chairman, Department of Surgery, Cornell University Medical Center, New York, N.Y., contributed to the material concerning cardiac surgery.

Alvin Mancusi-Ungaro, M.D., Attending Plastic Surgeon, St. Barnabas Hospital, Livingston, N.J., Clara Maas Hospital, Belleville, N.J. and Presbyterian Hospital, Newark, N.J., contributed to the material concerning plastic surgery.

Henry Mannix, Jr., M.D., Clinical Associate Professor of Surgery, Cornell University Medical College, contributed to the material concerning endocrine disorders.

Irwin R. Merkatz, M.D., Associate Professor of Obstetrics and Gynecology, Cornell University Medical School, contributed to the chapters concerning the female reproductive system.

Warren B. Nestler, M.D., Clinical Assistant Professor (Medicine), New Jersey College of Medicine and Dentistry, Newark, N.J., and Medical Coordinator, Overlook Hospital, Summit, N.J., contributed to the material concerning rheumatic fever and heart disease, bacterial endocarditis, and hypertension.

Sanford M. Reiss, M.D., Visiting Physician, Gastrointestinal Clinic, New York Hospital, Cornell Medical Center; Instructor, Department of Medicine, Cornell University Medical College; and Attending Physician in Medicine, Overlook Hospital, Summit, N.J., contributed to the chapters concerning diagnosis of gastrointestinal disorders, ulcerative colitis, peptic ulcer, gastrointestinal cancer, disorders of the mouth, intestinal disorders, rectal surgery, and disorders of the liver, gallbladder and pancreas.

Guy F. Robbins, M.D., Associate Attending Surgeon, Breast Service, Department of Surgery, Memorial Hospital for Cancer and Allied Diseases, New York, contributed to the chapter concerning breast disease.

Morton J. Rodman, Ph.D., Professor of Pharmacology, Rutgers University, contributed to the chapter concerning dependence on alcohol, drugs, and tobacco dependence.

Barbara Rogoz, R.N., M.S.N., Cardio-Surgical Clinical Nurse Specialist, Cornell University Medical Center, New York, contributed to the material concerning cardiac surgical nursing.

Allen S. Russek, M.D., Associate Professor of Rehabilitation Medicine, Institute of Rehabilitation Medicine, New York University Medical Center, New York, contributed to the material concerning the patient with an amputation.

Jules Saltman, National Tuberculosis and Respiratory Disease Association, assisted in the preparation of the chapter on pulmonary tuberculosis.

Alan C. Scheer, M.D., Associate Professor of Radiology and Chief, Division of Radiation Therapy, Wayne State University School of Medicine, Detroit, assisted in the preparation of the material concerning radiotherapy.

Owen A. Shteir, M.D., formerly Coordinator, Venereal Disease Program, State of New Jersey, Department of Health, contributed to the material concerning venereal infection.

Gertrud B. Ujhely, R.N., Ph.D., Associate Professor and Director, Graduate Program in Psychiatric Nursing, Adelphi University, New York, contributed to the concepts expressed in the chapter on nurse-patient relationships.

Dabney R. Yarbrough, III, M.D., F.A.C.S., Assistant Professor of Surgery, Medical College of South Carolina, Charleston, contributed to the material concerning the burned patient.

Preface

This book has been adapted from *Care of the Adult Patient,* third edition, in response to requests from those who wish a more concise text which emphasizes some of the most common and fundamental aspects in the nursing care of medical-surgical patients.

Our decisions in selecting content have been guided by a concern to include material which we consider fundamental to the direct nursing care of medical-surgical patients. We have shortened or deleted detailed information which may be burdensome or distracting to the reader who is not actually involved in and responsible for aspects of nursing care requiring this information.

The early chapters of *Care of the Adult Patient* have been retained with very little change, in the belief that the concepts presented in those chapters concerning development over the adult life span, nurse-patient relationships and care of the dying patient constitute material fundamental to the care of medical-surgical patients. We have made considerable change in some of the later chapters. For example, in relation to care of patients during acute physiological crises such as myocardial infarction, we have selected material which we believe will be useful to the student who may participate in care of these acutely ill patients but who is not prepared to assume major responsibility for planning and giving their nursing care. The chapter on care of patients with allergies provides another illustration of the changes we have made. The description of overall concepts concerning the allergic reaction was retained, while material dealing with detailed biochemical processes was deleted. We have in some instances rearranged material, consolidating it and using new chapter headings.

Many of the contributions of the consultants for the third edition of *Care of the Adult Patient* have been incorporated in this shorter book. This has been carried out with their consent, and in some instances, with their participation in development of the shorter version of the material. Their contributions have meant a great deal in presenting material which is up to date and accurate in the wide variety of nursing situations which are discussed.

It is not our intent (nor it is within our scope as individual nurse educators) to attempt a delineation of various levels of nursing education in relation to care of medical-surgical patients. Such decisions must be made by the profession as a whole. Nor do we view it as a mark of inferiority to consult a shorter book. Thus, the nurse whose major clinical interest lies in care of mothers and infants may wish to use a concise chapter dealing with care of seriously ill patients in intensive care units, without wading through detailed descriptions of abnormal ECG tracings. We view the two versions of our text as a realistic acknowledgment that nurses have different skills and varying levels of competence in working with particular types of patients and that they will choose reading materials which best suit their purposes at a particular time in their nursing careers.

Dorothy W. Smith
Carol Hanley Germain
Patricia Heenan

Contents

UNIT ONE: CONCEPTS BASIC TO THE CARE OF PATIENTS

1. Adult Development and Developmental Tasks 1
2. Caring for the Young Adult 5
3. Caring for the Patient Who is in Middle Life 12
4. Caring for the Elderly Patient 20
5. Nurse-Patient Relationships 36
6. Fundamental Processes of Health and Illness 56
7. The Interaction of Body and Mind ... 77
8. The Patient in Pain 84
9. Dependence on and Abuse of Alcohol and Drugs and Tobacco 90
10. Care of the Dying Patient 107
11. Nursing in Emergencies 111
12. The Surgical Patient 123

UNIT TWO: ONCOLOGIC NURSING

13. Care of the Patient with Cancer 143
14. Nursing Management in Radiotherapy 154

UNIT THREE: DISTURBANCES OF BODY SUPPORTIVE STRUCTURES AND LOCOMOTION

15. The Patient with a Fracture 161
16. The Patient with Disease of Bones and Joints 181
17. The Patient with an Amputation 195

UNIT FOUR: DISORDERS OF COGNITIVE, SENSORY OR PSYCHOMOTOR FUNCTION

18. The Patient with Neurologic Disturbance 205
19. The Patient with Cerebral Vascular Disease 228
20. The Patient with Spinal Cord Impairment 242
21. Visual and Hearing Impairment 255

UNIT FIVE: THREATS TO ADEQUATE RESPIRATION

22. The Patient with Disease of the Nose or the Throat 280
23. The Patient with Acute Respiratory Disorder 292
24. The Patient with Chronic Respiratory Disorder 305
25. The Patient with Pulmonary Tuberculosis 324

UNIT SIX: INSULTS TO CARDIOVASCULAR INTEGRITY

26. The Patient with a Blood or Lymph Disorder 335
27. The Patient with Heart Disease: Anatomy; Diagnostic Tests 349
28. The Patient with Heart Disease 357
29. The Patient with Inflammatory or Valvular Disease of the Heart 368
30. The Patient with Heart Disease: Coronary Heart Disease; Functional Heart Disease 380
31. The Patient with Hypertension 386

32. The Patient with Peripheral Vascular Disease: Thrombosis and Embolism ... 391

33. Rehabilitation of Patients with Heart Disease 409

UNIT SEVEN: DISTURBANCES OF INGESTION, DIGESTION, ABSORPTION AND ELIMINATION

34. Introduction: Diagnostic Tests, Functional Disorders 415

35. The Patient with Ulcerative Colitis or a Peptic Ulcer 428

36. The Patient with Cancer of the Gastrointestinal Tract 432

37. The Patient with an Ileostomy or a Colostomy 446

38. The Patient with an Intestinal or Rectal Disorder 461

39. Care of the Patient with Disorder of the Liver, Gallbladder, or Pancreas ... 473

40. The Urologic Patient 488

UNIT EIGHT: PROBLEMS RESULTING FROM ENDOCRINE IMBALANCE

41. The Patient with an Endocrine Disorder 519

42. The Patient with Diabetes Mellitus 533

UNIT NINE: DISTURBANCES OF SEXUAL STRUCTURES OR REPRODUCTIVE FUNCTION

43. Introduction: The Female Reproductive Pattern 545

44. The Woman Patient with a Disorder of the Reproductive System 556

45. The Male Patient with a Disorder of the Reproductive System 575

46. The Patient with Breast Disease 584

47. The Patient with Venereal Infection .. 596

UNIT TEN: COMMON PROBLEMS INVOLVING DISFIGUREMENT

48. The Patient with a Dermatologic Condition 603

49. The Patient Undergoing Plastic Surgery 620

UNIT ELEVEN: ACUTE LIFE-THREATENING PHYSIOLOGIC CRISES

50. Intensive Care Nursing 625

51. The Patient in Shock 627

52. Respiratory Insufficiency and Failure .. 634

53. The Patient with Heart Disease: Cardiac Arrhythmias 643

54. The Patient with Acute Myocardial Infarction 660

55. Cardiac Surgical Nursing 672

56. The Patient in Renal Failure 683

57. The Burned Patient 692

58. The Patient with Neurologic Disease .. 701

Index 711

Adult Development and Developmental Tasks

1

The Developmental Process • Developmental Tasks of Adults in Our Culture • Some Intangibles

THE DEVELOPMENTAL PROCESS

Growth, decline, change and development: all are parts of the dynamic thing we call living. All life is in a state of perpetual change. The changes that people experience over a lifetime are often described as *aging*. The rate of change is vastly more rapid at the beginning of life than it is toward the close. If you have seen a baby at the age of 1 and have been away from him until he is 3, you note dramatic changes. In contrast, changes between the ages of 50 to 52 are less noticeable.

The process of change (or aging) occurs at different rates in different individuals. Just as the age at which menstruation begins varies all the way from 10 to 16, so the time of the changes that come later in life can vary greatly. One person may be mentally alert, vigorous and active at 80, while another is aged and infirm at 60. For purposes of discussion, we may think of young adulthood as that period when the individual is establishing himself, roughly between the ages of 18 and 35; and we may think of middle life, from about 35 to 65, as the established years, when the person has found his place and is enlarging it and making it more secure. Sixty-five has become a common designation for the beginning of old age, since so many pension and retirement plans start then. This, too, is an arbitrary figure. Physiologic and mental old age may begin earlier or later. Individual differences become more marked as age progresses. Since adults pass through a variety of environments and experiences, the discussion of the periods of life is valid only in general terms.

It is important for the nurse to understand the developmental pattern of the adult so that normal changes are not confused with pathology. Some changes are familiar to all; others are not so evident. Hair gradually turns gray as age advances; reaction time changes, too. Have you ever marveled at the speed of a 17-year-old on crutches? In contrast, when you help an 80-year-old out of bed for the first time after an operation, you may think to yourself, "Why doesn't he move?" If the nurse knows what to expect from her patients on the basis of the normal characteristics for his stage of development, she can plan care more effectively, teach more realistically and avoid becoming angry and impatient at responses that should be expected.

DEVELOPMENTAL TASKS OF ADULTS IN OUR CULTURE

The baby under 2 has to learn to walk. One of the 6-year-old's tasks is to learn to read, and the adolescent is expected to establish a relationship with the opposite sex that is different from that of his childish associations. In our society one of the responsibilities of the young adult is to establish his own home and career. In middle life he has increasing community responsibility, or his responsibility may be worldwide. A job of the elderly is to lend to others the wisdom gathered through a lifetime.

Every stage of development has its own tasks— hurdles to be climbed over, things to be learned, changes to be accomplished. Developmental tasks are achieved most readily at certain ages; failure to accomplish these at one time may make their later realization difficult or impossible. The best time is the stage of life at which they normally occur. Later may be too late for a satisfactory solution.

1

It is important and appropriate for a 16-year-old to invest time and effort in the technics of dating. If he is silly and shows off too much, it is part of his learning. If he pays no attention to this social task at 16, and at 35 he is still unskilled enough to be silly and to show off, his dignity suffers both in his own eyes and in others'. What he should have learned earlier is harder to learn later. A woman who has remained dependent on her parents and has never left home or married may find adjustments in middle life to the death of her parents very difficult. A son who has never made a living, drifting from job to job and often seeking financial help from his father, may experience a rude shock when his father grows old and can no longer help him.

There is a progressive increase in the scope of developmental tasks as the individual grows from childhood to adulthood. For example, in the area of adjusting to one's own body, it is the young child's task to learn what is part of his physical self and what is not (his toy is not, but his back and toes are) and to develop skill in using his body for walking, holding a spoon, dressing, running, etc. It is the adolescent's task to make a socially satisfactory adjustment to the maturing changes that his body undergoes, and to accept and utilize well his appearance. It is the adult's task to maintain a healthful physical regimen in spite of the pressures of his life and to learn what new motor skills are needed in his work, home or recreation; and it is the task of the elder adult to adapt his living to diminished strength and agility.

Development of a satisfying sexual adjustment is one of life's tasks. It often looms large for the adolescent whose sexual drives are strong and who, before marriage, is accorded few acceptable forms of sexual expression by our society. With marriage comes the task of establishing a mutually satisfying sexual relationship with the marriage partner. Sexual adjustment is by no means a static thing—its achievement over a lifetime requires adaptability. Sexual desires of women, for example, are often affected by pregnancy. Lessening of sexual vigor with aging may affect one partner earlier in life than the other. An illness like heart disease may make it necessary to curtail marital relationships for a time. In some conditions, such as impotence due to paraplegia, sexual relations may be permanently disrupted. Patients who develop long-term illnesses, such as tuberculosis, may be separated from their families for many months, or even for years. Such lengthy separation can create problems for both husband and wife.

Although many patients do not discuss these intimate concerns with the nurse, her awareness of the diverse effects that illness can have on the patient and his family affects the atmosphere that she creates on the ward. A manner that is warm, but not prying, and that shows willingness to let patients be themselves, can help a patient to cope with his problems, whether or not he chooses to discuss them. An environment in which there is flexibility in applying rules, and encouragement of participation in diversional activities, helps patients to feel less restricted and less helpless. The nurse can create an atmosphere which at least does not make the problem worse. For example, in one day, one nurse said all of the following: "You can't stand in the hall. Patients are not allowed in the hall." "I smelled smoke in your bathroom. You must have sneaked a cigarette." "Visiting hours are OVER. Can't you see that it's 5 minutes past?" "There's to be no card playing in this room. You're too noisy when you play cards." These approaches not only are rude; they are dehumanizing. People can cope with their worries better when they are treated with respect. The restrictions imposed by hospital life are harder to bear when the nurse gives the impression that the routine is more important than the person, and that her control of the ward counts more than the patients' feelings. It would have been more helpful to allow, even to encourage, the card-playing patients to socialize, recognizing that this can alleviate tension and boredom. Imposing needless, and sometimes trivial, restrictions can increase feelings of frustration and anger, particularly in patients who have already been denied many freedoms usually taken for granted, such as freedom to come and go, to conduct business, and to live with their families. If, in the course of the card game, the patients become noisy it would be preferable to discuss this with them, helping them to recognize the need to lower their voices, or if possible, finding them a place to play away from the sicker patients. By permitting the patient activities as nearly as possible like those to which he is accustomed, strain and tension can be lessened.

If the patient initiates some discussion of sex with the nurse, she should avoid implying that he is shameful to talk of such a matter, or that he ought not have a sexual self. Instead, she can listen to him. Sometimes it is desirable to

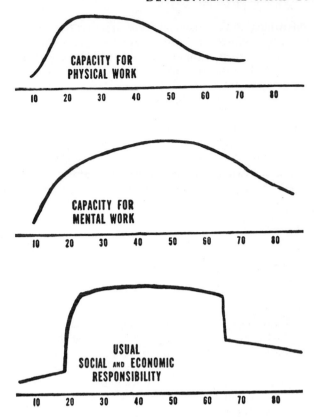

FIG. 1-1. Contrasting patterns of age relationship to capacity for physical work, intellectual work and to the usual level of social and economic responsibility. The abrupt ascent of responsibility at about age 20 and its abrupt descent at approximately 65 do not conform to actual capacities and are clearly not biologic. Curves are hypothetic and approximate. This chart does not apply necessarily to any given individual. (Stieglitz, E. J.: *The Second Forty Years*, Philadelphia, Lippincott)

suggest further discussion with the physician or clergyman.

The nurse can convey welcome to the patient's wife or husband during visiting hours and acknowledge, by her manner, his or her right to be present and to be concerned. For example, when the husband is kissing his wife good-by, the thoughtful nurse does not brusquely approach the bedside, clank down a thermometer tray and announce, "Visiting hours are over." By starting to take temperatures in another part of the ward, and allowing the couple a few moments of privacy, she conveys respect for them. This is simple courtesy. All too often the abrupt manner of the nurse and the busy routine of the hospital convey to the patient's visitor, "You are in the way.

Your expression of tenderness for the patient has no place here."

Coping with illness is part of living. Few escape it. How illness is dealt with depends on how the person has learned to handle stress, on the severity of the condition, and on the support afforded by the environment, of which the nurse may be a significant part.

Developmental tasks are in large measure culturally determined. Whereas in our culture young people are expected to become independent of their parents, in some societies young adults marry but continue to live in the parental household and to obey their parents' wishes. Although our society places great emphasis on working, making money and getting ahead, other societies place a major value on enjoying each moment of life as it is lived. After all, the future may never come, they say. In planning health care, account must be taken of cultural differences. Clinic appointments may be broken if the individual believes more in today than in tomorrow. If he feels ill on the day of his appointment, he will come; if he feels well, he may go fishing instead.

There is, and probably should be, wide variation in the degree to which adults achieve various tasks. One may be a loving husband and father but a poor provider. Another may earn a very large salary but spend little time with his family. Florence Nightingale performed a tremendous amount of work as a nurse and philanthropist during her long life after she returned from the Crimea. She is remembered for this service rather than for being a famous hostess or a devoted wife and mother. The fact that individuals achieve in such different ways is a gain for society. Discussing developmental tasks of adults does not imply that every individual should conform to a mold labeled "The Perfect Adult."

One must guard against oversimplification of the concept of developmental tasks. Adjustments must be made over and over, as each period of life, or each change in the environment, makes new demands. For example, fear of being alone which a person experienced early in life, may seem to be solved during middle life by close relationships with a growing family, only to reappear in later life when family and friends die or move away. Rather than viewing developmental tasks as achieved or not achieved, it is more accurate to recognize that people of all ages are in the process of achieving them and that the degree of success with each task may vary markedly at different periods of life.

SOME INTANGIBLES

While the more tangible accomplishments of establishing a home and earning a living are easier to observe, the search for meaning, for identity, and for lasting values involves tasks which determine the quality of the patient's life and relationships. The degree to which the patient performs these tasks influences his response to illness and other misfortunes. The effort to accomplish these tasks has different emphases at different stages of adulthood. For the youth the search for his own identity, for meaning, and for lasting values can be a new and compelling challenge. For the person in middle life it can involve re-examining his values and ideals in light of changed circumstances, such as responsibility for the care of others and to his work, and continuing his search for meaning with an understanding and humility deepened by these experiences. For the elderly person it can mean finding worthwhileness in the life he has lived, the efforts he has made, and the achievements he has earned.

Whether the individual is successfully dealing with these inner tasks is especially likely to become evident in times of stress such as occur during illness or bereavement. Some people are aided in these tasks by a strong religious faith. Illness, aging, and the loss of loved ones bring fundamental questions to the fore, such as, "What is the purpose of my life?" or "Now that I am old and cannot work, what use am I?" Patients sometimes voice these thoughts to the nurse when given an opportunity; however, many patients do not ask these questions directly, but may imply them by their attitudes and reactions. The nurse sees people under circumstances which tend to reveal inner strength, or its lack. Just as it is important to accept patients whose values and beliefs are different from one's own, it is also important to accept the patient where he is, as far as his achievement of various life tasks is concerned. The patient who has been primarily concerned with surface events may continue to focus on them during illness. The nurse should respect this and not seek to change it. However, if the patient shows that he wishes to discuss some of his concerns about the meaning of life, or of his illness, the nurse can help by listening, and showing concern. Some patients mobilize themselves after illness and misfortune; others,

seemingly no worse off, do not. The inner strength which an individual has may not be known, even to him, until it is tested by an ordeal. This inner strength is related to ability and willingness to stand the pain and anxiety of facing some of the fundamental issues of one's life, and to accept help from others when it is needed. The patients to whom you can be of most genuine and lasting service are those who can accept your help and use it to strengthen their own forces to struggle with illness or disability.

What can the nurse say to a question such as, "Why must I suffer so much pain?" or "Why did my husband have to die so young?" The nurse is not in a position to provide the answers—and especially not for another person whose values and experiences may be quite different from her own. She can, however, listen to the patient and convey concern for him as he explores these questions.

Illness is quite naturally regarded as a misfortune. For some people, though, going through illness opens up new opportunities to explore the meaning and values of life; for these patients it can be truly an opportunity for personal growth. Because the nurse cares for people during crises, such as illness and bereavement, it is often her privilege to support and help patients during these experiences.

REFERENCES AND BIBLIOGRAPHY

Coser, R. L. (ed.) : *The Family, Its Structure and Functions,* New York, St. Martin's Press, 1964.

Frankel, V. E.: *From Death Camp to Existentialism,* Boston, Beacon Press, 1959.

———: *Man's Search for Meaning,* Boston, Beacon Press, 1963.

Havighurst, R. J.: *Human Development and Education,* New York, Longmans, 1953.

Martin, H. W., and Prange, A. J.: Human adaptation, *Canad. Nurse* 58:234, March, 1962.

Murphy, G., and Kuhlen, R. G.: *Psychological Needs of Adults,* Chicago, Center for Study of Liberal Education for Adults, 1955.

Pressey, S. L., and Kuhlen, R. G.: *Psychological Development Through the Life Span,* New York, Harper, 1957.

Stieglitz, E. J.: *The Second Forty Years,* Philadelphia, Lippincott, 1952.

Strauss, A.: *Mirrors and Masks: The Search for Identity,* Glencoe, Ill., Free Press, 1959.

Tillich, P.: *The Courage to Be,* New Haven, Yale University Press, 1952.

———: *The Eternal Now,* New York, Scribner, 1963.

Thorndike, E. L.: *Adult Interests,* New York, Macmillan, 1935.

White, R. W.: *Lives in Progress,* New York, Dryden, 1952.

Williams, R. H., Tibbits, C., and Donahue, W.: *Processes of Aging,* Vols. 1 and 2, New York, Prentice-Hall, 1963.

Caring for the Young Adult

2

Physical Changes · Developmental Tasks · Implications for Nursing

The young adult has much working in his favor during illness. He is physically more resilient than the older person. Two days after an appendectomy he may be able to carry out activities which a middle-aged patient who had the same operation must postpone for a week. The young person often has an emotional resilience, too, which enables him to mobilize his energy quickly after a shock or a loss. This does not mean that he has necessarily dealt adequately with the experience inwardly. He may at a later time need to go back and re-examine the experience, and its meaning to him.

The young person's resilience is enhanced by the supports which society offers him. Our society invests heavily in the young; they are, after all, its future. Social, educational, and health facilities and opportunities are usually more abundantly provided for young people than for those in middle and later life. For example, a convalescent teenager who receives a scholarship to a nearby college has a new world opened up to him—not only an educational world but a network of contacts with other students and with teachers in a setting which emphasizes the development of his capacities. The young person is also more likely to have intact family relationships than is an elderly person. Often the young adult's ties with his parents are still strong, and in addition he may have founded a young family of his own. The situation is different, though, for a 60-year-old widow who, in addition to the challenge of recovering from illness, must learn to support herself following the death of her husband. She is less likely to receive assistance with learning new skills, and she may have fewer opportunities to make new friends, than the young person who is recovering from illness.

Because many young people have considerable support and assistance provided by others, it may be easy for the nurse to fail to notice the ways in which young patients require help. Visits from friends and family may signify that the young person has many meaningful relationships with others and that he is receiving much support. However, this is not necessarily so. The relationships may be superficial, leaving the patient very much alone. In any case personal relationships do not take the place of the professional helping role of the nurse and other members of the staff. The nurse must guard against assuming that a young person (or a person of any age) who is surrounded by cards, flowers, and candy does not need her listening ear. Perhaps he does, and the nurse should offer him this opportunity.

The patient's resilience may, ironically, be another factor which deters the nurse from recognizing his need for a supportive listener. Nevertheless, it is important to help the patient to assimilate painful experiences. Too often family and friends discourage the patient from talking about the experience. They may be eager to forget an event which is also painful for them. Because the nurse listens, the patient is helped to review what has happened and to confront some of his feelings about his illness during his stay in the hospital. Such nursing intervention may or may not suffice to help a patient deal with the experience and move on to new opportunities. Some patients require psychotherapy to enable them to cope with the experience at the time of its occurrence. Other patients may recognize the need for such assistance only later, after their physical recovery.

Young adults in our society are increasingly restless, dissatisfied with the status quo, and actively seeking participation in community affairs.

Although being fed up with the hypocrisy of some of their elders is not new to young people, there is a growing outspokenness among the young, many of whom see no point in pretending to believe the shallow contradictions with which many of them are surrounded. Although the young people who are the most openly nonconformist are in the minority, the search for involvement and for a chance to participate in righting social wrongs is widespread among youth. The search is not only for new outer experiences, but for new inner experiences as well. Some young people have turned to drugs, such as LSD, in their search for such experiences. There is much emphasis upon separateness from the older generation—the jargon of the young is not just a sprinkling of slang, but almost a vocabulary of its own. But the emphasis on separate vocabulary, styles of clothing and so forth is sometimes accompanied by feelings of alienation, and by a wish for meaningful communication with older people, and particularly with older people who have authority to effect change. Although some young people expend most of their energies demonstrating contempt for conformity and "the establishment," many are eager to use their energies to work toward alleviating social injustice.

What implications has this for nursing care of young adults? The hospital is an environment where authority and hierarchy are much in evidence, and where patients, particularly, ordinarily have little voice in making the rules. If the young person is hospitalized for more than a brief period, the rigidity of rules and authority is likely to be especially irritating to him. He may find various ways to express rebelliousness, such as by turning his radio up too loud, disregarding the doctors' orders, and so forth. To whatever extent possible, try to include the young patient in making decisions which affect him, and make a special effort to interpret hospital rules to him. Even if the rules cannot be changed, they will be less galling to the patient who understands their purpose. For instance, enforcing the rule limiting visitors to two per patient at a time makes it impossible for a young man to entertain his bowling team, but he may find his disappointment softened by realizing the impracticality of allowing each patient as many visistors as he wishes. Even if the young patient does not concede this point, he will have received the interest and concern of the nurse who, instead

of officiously quoting the rules, took time to explain them.

The opportunity provided by hospitalization for the young patient to have wider contact with adults outside the circle of home and school can be beneficial. The young person's contacts with his elders may previously have emphasized the distance between generations. The experience of illness and hospitalization brings out some very fundamental human problems, which cut across age differences and bring out the commonalities of human experience. The 20-year-old girl who is admitted to the hospital because of an impending miscarriage may find in her older roommate a source of strength and support. This young woman who may have prided herself on her separateness from older people may reach out to an older woman to share some of her intimate concerns and fears over losing her baby. Recognition of the ways that people of different ages can support one another can help the nurse avoid automatically assuming that patients of similar age should be placed together on the ward. While doing so fosters sociability of age-mates, it deprives patients of contacts with those of different ages—contacts that are already often lacking in the lives of young and old alike, in our age-stratified society.

Relationships with physicians and nurses can also bring home to the young person that the basic human questions affect people of all ages. While one's perspectives on these questions differ with age, sharing of views can lead each person to deeper understanding. The physician and nurse can also provide the young patient with experience with rational authority. Previously the patient may have viewed authority as essentially arbitrary and negative—something against which to pit himself. However, professional people, by the nature of their work, have many opportunities to emphasize the rational aspects of authority. The physician recommends bed rest, not in order to impose his will on the patient or to restrict his freedom, but because the patient's condition requires it. The nurse firmly encourages the postoperative patient to walk, not because she wants to inflict pain, but because walking will help him to recover. Emphasizing the reasons behind actions and decisions, and avoiding arbitrary use of authority, may help the young person appreciate that authority and discipline are not always negative and restrictive, but can also be positive forces enabling those with special knowledge and skill to exercise them for the benefit of others.

Idealism is one of the positive attributes of youth—idealism which can lend a glow and spark the effort and enthusiasm of older people. But inevitably the idealism of youth suffers some shocks as it comes up against reality. Being sick can increase the problem, because it brings the young person into close contact with many of the inadequacies of health care as he himself experiences them. The nurse and the doctor are not always patient and kind; the dietitian does not always remember that he prefers a hard-cooked egg to a soft-boiled one.

In contrast to some older persons who have scaled down their expectations of what life has to offer, and who accept, if not happily, at least patiently, some of their misfortunes, many young people are especially impatient when they are sick. Illness or restriction may elicit a good deal of protest. Remember that the protest can be a very positive sign that the individual is seeking, and expecting, improvement in his state. While you cannot personally provide an ideal situation for your young patient, you can serve as a sounding board as he voices some of his protest. His high expectations will present a challenge for those who provide health care. Along with some unrealistic demands, the young person often calls attention to situations which need to be and which can be changed. In so doing he may help improve the quality of his own care and that of others as well.

Many young people in our society have had few demands made on them to assist others or to share with others. In addition, their own stage of personal development requires a very necessary concern with enhancing their ability to care for themselves. Concern for and ability to care for others develop gradually as the individual achieves greater independence and mastery of himself. The experience of illness tends to make people of all ages and stages of development less able to be concerned about others. The young patient who is hospitalized may have difficulties in the necessary sharing and consideration for others required by group living.

What may seem utter willfulness in disregarding the rights of others (such as by ignoring their need for quiet) may be an inability, both because of his developmental stage and because of illness, to consider the needs of others. Rather than assuming that the patient is deliberately selfish and thoughtless, set limits firmly as to noise and so forth and stick to them. Remember that you are likely to have to remind the young person of these limits in a way which is firm, but which emphasizes the reasons for the rules.

What of the nurse's own reactions to working with young adults? For the nurse who is herself in this age group there may be a particular tendency to identify with the patient; this is especially likely to be problematic if the patient has a terminal illness, such as leukemia. Caring for a fatally ill young person is a stark reminder of the unpredictability of each person's life span. Working with young adults may make it especially difficult, also, for a young nurse to keep her professional and social roles differentiated. The nurse may find herself relating to the patient as though he or she were a chum. The older nurse may carry over to the patient some of her own conflicts with her adolescent children, and find herself responding to the patient in terms of problems she is facing with her own growing family. Sometimes the older nurse will find that she is jealous of a patient's youthful resilience and attractiveness. An older nurse may become very protective of a young patient, treating the patient perhaps as she herself would like to have been treated when she was young. For nurses of all ages the challenge in caring for young adults lies in helping the patient move forward with the developmental tasks of his age period to the extent that he is able to do so, despite illness, as well as in providing the care which is made necessary by the patient's illness.

PHYSICAL CHANGES

Following the rapid changes of puberty, physical growth ceases in the period between 18 and 20. Thereafter a slow and barely perceptible decline in many physical abilities begins. At about 20 the body and general appearance no longer change quickly. The boy who always has longed to be tall may discover that he always will be short. The girl may have to accept being flat-chested or taller than is fashionable for a woman. A young person's physical powers may or may not coincide with opportunities for their optimal use.

Visual Accommodation. The ability of the eye to adjust to near and far vision is one of the reliable physiologic indicators of age. Children can see an object clearly when it is held almost at the tip of their noses. Even before puberty this ability begins to diminish gradually, and it continues to decline during most of adult life.

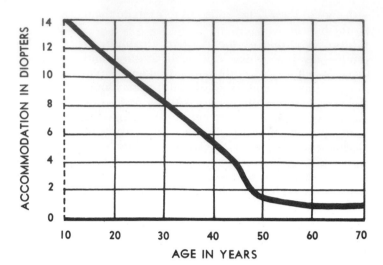

FIG. 2-1. Eye accommodation graph, showing the loss of accommodation with age. (Stearns, H. O.: *Fundamentals of Physics and Applications,* ed. 2, New York, Macmillan)

Changes in Hearing. These also occur throughout life. Loss of ability to hear high tones begins in childhood. Hearing is most acute at about the age of 14; thereafter it declines gradually. So far as this faculty is concerned, a 20-year-old is already past his prime! It has been noted that persons living in a relatively noise-free area of the Sudan had markedly less hearing loss with age than persons in highly industrialized environments. Thus, the loss of hearing that we regard as normal may be normal for us, but not for persons whose environment is different from ours. The reasons for this finding are not fully understood. It may be related to less exposure to noise over the life span, or possibly to the lower incidence of hypertension and atherosclerosis that was observed among these nonindustrialized people (Rosen).

Position Sense and Speed of Reaction. These reach their peak between the ages of 20 and 30. Some youths tend to be to sure of their fast reaction time and push they luck beyond their ability to respond. The results are disastrous enough so that insurance companies demand a higher premium for male drivers under 25. You will meet as patients some of the luckier young men and women whose accidents did not prove fatal.

DEVELOPMENTAL TASKS

A task of young adults in our culture is to work toward self-definition and self-esteem. One aspect of achieving self-definition is gradually differentiating oneself from one's parents. This process involves developing one's own values and making one's own decisions. An aspect of developing self-esteem is learning respect for one's own competence. This, in turn, forms a basis for respect for others and for their competence, as well as a basis for finding one's place as a productive member of society.

Young adults are expected gradually to become independent of their parents. This achieving of independence does not mean breaking ties with parents but gradually developing a different type of relationship with them, one in which the young person begins to accept the consequences of his own actions. Such a development does not take place suddenly; indeed, it has its beginnings when the child is encouraged to make some decisions of his own. Young people whose parents have helped them gradually to assume more independence usually find this transition period easier than those whose parents continue to exert very strict control through late adolescence.

Along with independence from his parents, the young adult is expected to learn a trade or a profession and to begin to support himself. In our technologically advanced society, becoming proficient in a profession usually entails extended schooling and prolongs the young person's economic dependence on his parents well beyond the point at which physical maturity has been reached.

Among the responsibilities of a young person are founding a home of his own, supporting it with his own money, marrying and having children. The need for extended schooling may make the achievement of some of these goals difficult. Marriage may be delayed, or the student may marry while he is still in school and will need to seek financial help from his parents. This is the time of life when, in addition to founding a home, the young person is encouraged to establish his own place in the community by taking a responsible part in community activities.

He is also expected to make decisions, stick to them and take the consequences. Society expects the adult to be able to control the display of his feelings more than a child. For instance, free expression of anger and fear are curtailed. Greater tolerance for frustration is demanded. An adult who has a temper tantrum each time things do not go his way is considered childish. Greater ability to plan for the future realistically is expected. Christmas clubs and insurance policies are examples of ways in which the adult puts off immediate satisfactions (like spending money) in order to provide for the future.

The adult is expected to face reality and to differentiate between it and fantasy. Progress in this task, as in the others, is achieved gradually throughout childhood and adolescence. Its accomplishment is of major importance in helping the young adult to sort out his own strengths and weaknesses and to set realistic goals for himself.

Each member of a family is striving to achieve his developmental tasks. At times family members are working toward similar goals; at other times the tasks which one member is trying to achieve are in conflict with those of another member of the family. Often an individual finds that there are conflicting demands made on him as he tries to achieve a variety of tasks, each of which may be important and worthwhile to him. For example, a young wife may find it difficult to remain active and interested in work outside the home because she is absorbed in the establishment of her home and family. A young husband may find that after a day filled with a variety of pressures at work, he has little energy left for tackling problems which arise in relation to his son's schooling.

IMPLICATIONS FOR NURSING

The young adult who is ill, particularly if his illness is prolonged, finds these tasks more difficult. Through understanding, all who care for him can help him to achieve to the extent possible for him.

Counsel and Encouragement. Despite illness or handicap, the young individual is part of a world that values physical attractiveness, opportunities to develop one's own capacities, a chance to work and earn and to have one's own home. Obviously, many will be prevented by illness, as well as other factors, from achieving these goals. The nurse can help the patient to develop what he has to its highest potential. For example, the young paraplegic often is impotent as a result of injury to his spinal cord. He may be confined to a wheelchair. Recognizing these severe blows to his manly pride and the limitations that they have placed on his life, the nurse will avoid the common pitfall of treating a helpless adult like a child. On the contrary, she will recognize in every way possible the need of such patients for independence and privacy. Instead of announcing, "Well, today is a nice day; you can go watch the ball game," she will encourage them to make such decisions as are open to them.

Most people have been taught through their childhood years to control the expression of strong emotion. Before surgery, the child may plainly express his fear, giving those who care for him a chance to reassure and comfort him. The young adult may be no less frightened but often shows his fear in less obvious ways. He, too, requires reassurance, but sometimes it is harder to recognize his need.

Because they are involved in achieving independence from their parents, many young people have difficulty in accepting their parents' suggestions, even when these suggestions could prove very useful to them. Adults outside the home can be especially helpful to young people by allowing them opportunities to express their ideas and to ask questions about matters that concern or interest them, and by conveying respect for the young person as an individual. Members of the health professions can offer help and suggestions that the young person might reject if his parents offered them. Counseling in matters of personal health, such as the hygiene of menstruation or care of the skin in acne, are examples of the kind of problems for which young people may seek the nurse's help. Recognizing the young person's struggle for independence, the wise nurse carefully avoids a patronizing air. She provides sound information that the young person may consider in coming to his own decisions. She is careful not to sow seeds of antagonism between the young adult and her parents, such as "Your mother says you should not bathe during menstruation? That's silly." The nurse might say instead, "Yes, many people have questioned the wisdom of bathing during menstruation. No harm from this practice has been noted, though, provided the water is not very hot or cold. Perhaps you would like to talk with your physician further about this. He will be here on Monday morning."

Pediatric units usually do not admit patients beyond the age of 13, so that the bulk of adolescents who are hospitalized are placed on adult wards. Some centers have adolescent units designed architecturally and their policies are in accord with customs of this age group, such as sociability, activity, music and food snacks. On adult wards, noncritically ill adolescents and young adults often benefit when they are assigned beds near each other, because they often have similar interests.

Respect for Privacy. The adolescent or young adult who is still developing a concept of his physical self and working through his feelings about sex often finds illness frightening. The bodily insults, such as lack of privacy, having needles forced into his skin and a thermometer pushed into his rectum, and being touched all over by a doctor or a nurse, may be difficult to accept. Illness and surgery may mean to him that his ideal picture of a beautiful body cannot be his. Surgery on or near genitals can greatly intensify the fear of castration. Embarrassment—so easily brought on—is conscious, but the underlying thoughts may be subconscious. Providing maximum protection against unnecessary exposure and fully explaining what is going to happen before a procedure is started, and why it is done, lessen some of the tension. The very fact that the nurse shows concern about these things can convey to the patient that the hospital staff is not trying to manipulate him or increase his helplessness.

Because he is not yet sure of his own strengths, the young person may worry about the impression he makes on others. The hard job of working out how much dependence he can accept without interfering with his struggle for independence can make the patient irritable. He may retort angrily when he does not mean to. A response of anger by the nurse, although understandable, compels the patient to continue his anger to save face. Youth is a period of intense testing—of oneself and one's abilities, of the endurance of one's body, of one's influence on others. Being sick and in a hospital removes the individual from the opportunity to test himself in his usual environment. It is an interruption that few welcome.

Growth has high energy requirements in addition to those for activity, so the caloric needs of youngsters who have not attained their full growth are higher than for an older person engaging in the same amount of activity. Would it not be possible to find a way to serve adolescent patients a hamburger and a milkshake instead of the usual afternoon or evening fruit juice? A patient who is led to believe that his special likes and dislikes are important and heeded may be better able to face those problems for which there is less help available. At any age, success in coping with difficult problems can increase an individual's confidence in himself, as well as his skill in dealing with similar situations in the future. The dragons of pain, fear, loneliness and anger reappear many times in the lives of most people. The young person who is helped to combat them during a personal crisis, such as illness, is girded for his future encounters.

Creating a Positive Environment. The young patient with a chronic disease or a permanent disability, is in danger of missing the challenges and the learning appropriate to his age. The nurse might search for ways in which she can change the patient's environment so that he has experiences that are more typical in our culture. Are there courses that the homebound or hospitalized adolescent can take? A party he can attend? Can transportation be provided to a church group? When parents, adolescents and nurses put their heads together and community resources are investigated, ways often can be found to provide the handicapped young person with the experiences he craves and needs.

Working with Parents. In addition to working with the young adult, the nurse has a role in working with his parents. Particularly when illness strikes, parents can be helped greatly by explanations and reassurance from the nurse. Even though they share a home, communication between family members may be inadequate. This is often the case between an adolescent and his parents.

In the tension and the conflicting demands of everyday life, many people experience twinges of regret and self-reproach for not having been, on one occasion or another, more perceptive of another's needs, or more generous in giving of their time and attention. When sudden illness occurs, such feelings sometimes surge to the fore and may be expressed as, "Is this partly my fault? Is there something I should have done to prevent it?" The wise nurse will allow the family or friends to discuss the matter but will avoid any comment which implies blame. After the sudden shock of the illness and after the patient has received initial treatment, the nurse can assist the family to recognize ways in which they can help to prevent, or detect promptly, similar problems in the future.

It is important to help the adolescent to deal with his illness, whether temporary or permanent, and to avoid unnecessary threats to his health in the future. All this requires knowledge and understanding on the part of the adolescent. He will be better able to meet his health needs in the future if he has some understanding of the reactions of his own body in health and in illness. Understanding one's own illness is never purely an intellectual undertaking; it is a combined intellectual and emotional process that includes accepting what happened and planning what to do about it.

The nurse's role often involves helping patients to recognize everyday situations that may contribute to illness, or commonplace examples of ways in which they can follow the physician's recommendations. Such assistance is never insignificant, although it may seem lacking in drama. Movies and television notwithstanding, most people learn step by step, in seemingly small ways, to deal with stress.

REFERENCES AND BIBLIOGRAPHY

BETTLEHEIM, B.: To nurse and to nurture, *Nurs. Forum* 1:60, Summer, 1962.

BRIGHT, F.: The pediatric nurse and parental anxiety, *Nurs. Forum* 4:30, 1965.

DUVALL, E. M.: *Family Development,* ed. 4, Philadelphia, Lippincott, 1970.

ERIKSON, E.: *Identity and the Life Cycle,* New York, International Universities Press, 1959.

FRIEDENBERG, E.: *The Vanishing Adolescent,* New York, Dell, 1959.

————: *Coming of Age in America,* New York, Random House, 1965.

HAMMAR, S. L., and EDDY, J. K.: *Nursing Care of the Adolescent,* New York, Springer, 1966.

KURTAGH, C.: Nursing in the life span of people, *Nurs. Forum* 7:298, 1968.

MEYER, H. L.: Predictable problems of hospitalized adolescents, *Am. J. Nurs.* 69:525, March, 1969.

NOWLIS, H.: Why students use drugs, *Am. J. Nurs.* 68:1680, August, 1968.

PRESSEY, S. L., and KUHLEN, R. G.: *Psychological Development Through the Life Span,* New York, Harper, 1957.

ROSEN, S., *et al.*: Presbycusis study of a relatively noise-free population of the Sudan, *Ann. Otol.* 71:727, 1962.

SANKOT, M., and SMITH, D.: Drug problems in Haight-Ashbury, *Am. J. Nurs.* 68:1686, August, 1968.

SMITH, D. W.: Patienthood and privacy, *Am. J. Nurs.* 69:508, March, 1969.

STEIN, M. (ed.): *Identity and Anxiety,* Glencoe, Ill., Free Press, 1960.

Caring for the Patient Who is in Middle Life

3

Physical Changes • Developmental Tasks • Implications for Nursing

INTRODUCTION

The largest proportion of the population comprises those in middle life, the long period when human beings are neither very young nor very old. Perhaps, in the natural concern for the more dependent persons at the extremes of age, too little attention has been given to the study of this group. It is they primarily who maintain the nation's homes and businesses; it is they who care for the young and the old. When illness comes to a member of this age division, other lives are particularly likely to be affected. A man of 46 who has a heart attack may be concerned not only for his own welfare but also for the welfare of his wife and children who, perhaps with his own parents, depend on him for support.

Middle life is the period when the individual's dependence is usually least acceptable, to the patient, to his close associates, and to those who care for him. For most people the middle years are more filled than any other period in life with opportunities for productivity and self-fulfillment, and with responsibilities toward others. A change from the expected independence and productivity toward dependence and curtailment of productivity constitutes a major problem for the patient and for those who care for him. We shall return to this topic later, when considering nursing implications in the care of patients during middle life. First, however, let us consider some of the physical changes which occur during middle life.

PHYSICAL CHANGES

Strength. Change occurs continuously but so gradually that it is often not noticed. Nevertheless, a particular event can bring the change suddenly into sharp focus. For example, a man of 55 is driving along the parkway and has a flat tire. Through good luck and good management it has been years since he has had a flat. He begins the job of jacking up the car. All goes well until it is time to lift the spart tire into place. It is just too heavy. He realizes with a start that he is not as strong as he used to be. This fact is emphasized painfully when a lad of 20 stops to help him. With a cheery "Stand aside, sir," the younger man easily places the tire in position. The loss of strength which seemed to make its appearance in this man's 50's had actually been going on for 2 or 3 decades but had gone relatively unnoticed until an unusual event demanded the physical prowess that he no longer possessed. However, some of the loss of strength may be attributed to disuse atrophy, suggesting that regular exercise over a lifetime contributes to well-being. The middle-aged farmer and sailor note less loss of strength than the middle-aged man who has spent most of his time at his desk.

Height and Weight. These show continuous increase until about 20. Height tends to remain constant until old age, when posture and settling of bones cause a slight decline. In contrast, weight continues to increase until about 60. Commonly there is a lessening of exercise and slowing of metabolism without a corresponding decrease in caloric intake. If an individual has reached optimum weight during young adulthood, it is undesirable for him to continue to gain weight as he grows older. However, it is often difficult for him to stay slim.

During middle life there is a gradual slowing of metabolism and reaction time, as well as a gradual decline in visual and auditory perception. During this period early signs of aging make their appearance. Sometimes these early and obvious changes are traumatic for the individual in our youth-worshiping culture. In the Orient the wisdom of old age is regarded with reverence and respect, but in America there is a tendency to deplore old age and to venerate youth. This attitude is reflected in the American preoccupation with cosmetics and youthful clothes. Bernard Shaw once said that while the 30's are the old age of youth, the 40's are the youth of old age.

Pace. During middle life the individual gradually modifies his pace. This modification by no means indicates "sitting back," for these are usually the busiest years of life. However, there is a subtle change in the tempo of living, such as walking up steps instead of racing up two at a time, and shifting participation in sports from the most strenuous and competitive to those somewhat less demanding. During active adult life many of the extremes of physical strength are not used, and their gradual loss is scarcely noticed.

Subtle but important cultural influences, as well as physical changes, cause a slow shift in activity at various ages, so that the older person often no longer seeks the more strenuous activities. Society shifts its expectations of what pursuits are considered appropriate for various age groups.

These shifts are not always consonant with desirable health practices, however. For example, in some areas of the United States little emphasis has been placed upon exercise for adults. Often it is expected that adults will merely be spectators, while exercise is left for the children.

Increasing recognition is being given to the ill effects of lack of exercise, particularly during middle and later life. Lack of regular exercise is believed to contribute to the development of atherosclerosis, one of the most prevalent and dangerous health problems of adults in this country. It also predisposes to obesity, lessened efficiency of the circulatory and respiratory systems, and decreased muscle tone and strength.

Rather than gradually slipping into a routine of too little exercise, persons in middle and later life should be encouraged to undertake regular activities that provide exercise as well as enjoyment. The type of exercise that is suitable and possible varies over the life span (for example, from football to golf) and from person to person. Brisk walking, swimming, gardening and bicycling have been suggested as activities that can be engaged in by older persons who are in good health. Social pressures exert a not wholly de-sirable influence in the kind of activities older people feel free to undertake. Emphasis on conformity and on youthful glamor in sports attire discourage some older people from activities such as swimming and bicycling. Cost must be considered, as well as availability. One physician, with a touch of humor, recommended walking to his clients; it requires, he said, no special equipment, is easily learned and readily available.

The middle-aged person who has neglected physical activity and who decides to begin a program of exercise is well advised to see his physician for a physical examination, and also to build up his exercise tolerance gradually. It is by no means unheard of for a middle-aged, sedentary person who decides to exercise in order to prevent myocardial infarction, to suffer just this occurrence during an ill-considered burst of exercise for which he has not gradually prepared himself.

Physical examinations in the middle years begin to emphasize the detection of illnesses then most common—examinations of the heart and the blood pressure, cancer detection and looking for signs of diabetes.

Menopause. Menopause usually occurs in the decade of 45 to 55. The age at which menopause appears varies considerably among different women, just as there is wide variation in the age at which puberty is reached. Whereas puberty is marked by rapid growth, maturation of reproductive organs and the development of secondary sex characteristics in response to the stimulation of sex hormones, menopause is characterized by shrinkage of reproductive organs due to the gradual reduction in sex hormones. Gradually ovulation and menstruation cease.

This period of life is often more difficult for women than for men. There is no physiologic climacteric or "change of life" among men, as there is among women, but rather a gradual decrease of sexual vigor. However, a proud new father at the age of 70 is by no means unknown. The fact that menopause usually coincides with the growing independence of children causes profound changes in women's responsibilities and activities, while men continue to be very much absorbed in their careers during middle life. Contrary to popular belief, marked diminution in sexual response does not necessarily accompany menopause. Slowing down of sexual activity is a gradual and individual matter for both men and women.

Eyesight. The point at which loss of visual accommodation, called *presbyopia,* interferes with reading, sewing and other close work usually starts between ages 40 and 50. The individual holds reading matter farther and farther from his eyes in order to see it clearly. This adjustment of position, known as the "tromboning effect," has given rise to many jokes about needing longer arms for reading. The person achieves artificial accommodation by using reading glasses for close work or by wearing lenses especially ground to provide for accommodation (bifocals, trifocals). Gradual decline in visual acuity also occurs; significant changes usually do not appear until about the age of 40. More light is needed for such activities as reading and sewing.

Many people are very sensitive about their eyesight. In their effort to disregard a decline in vision they bring great discomfort to themselves and often to others, or they may needlessly curtail their activities. Successfully holding a job may depend on the ability to see well. Help the older person to understand that change in vision is normal and that it happens to everyone. Wearing glasses is not a disgrace; in fact, they can make the wearer look distinguished. For the individual who objects to wearing conventional eyeglasses, contact lenses may provide a solution.

Hearing. Hearing gradually diminishes with age, and some persons, particularly in later middle life, find that the decrease is sufficient to interfere with their communication with others. Loss of hearing which occurs as a result of aging is called *presbycusis.*

In America loss of acuity in hearing is accepted with even poorer grace than decline in vision. Only gradually are people beginning to wear hearing aids without extreme self-consciousness. The fear that most people have of being less than perfect physically—an impossibility—makes them reluctant to call attention to a hearing defect by a visible aid. A person may attempt to conceal partial deafness if his job depends on normal hearing ability. The nurse may address an older man in her usual soft voice, only to find that he does not even look up from his newspaper. Rather than assuming that he's cranky, and ceasing further attempts at conversation, she may recall that hearing diminishes appreciably with age and repeat the greeting more loudly and distinctly. By speaking slowly and clearly, the nurse can avoid putting the patient with a hearing loss in the defensive position of asking, "What?" Face the patient while speaking so that he can note lip movement and facial expression.

DEVELOPMENTAL TASKS

In middle life the person is at the period in which society is making the greatest demands on him. He is responsible not only for himself but also for the care of his children and often of his aging parents. It is at this time that the individual acquires most of his material possessions. Usually maximum earning power is reached during this period.

Independence of Children. Often it is difficult for middle-aged parents to accept their children's growing independence. The necessary changes in attitude may be especially difficult for the mother whose entire life has been devoted to her children and her home. The fact that women are living longer and are in better health than ever before means that they are still active and vigorous when their children are grown. Keeping house for herself and her husband is usually not sufficiently challenging to women during later middle life. The menopause often coincides with these events. The woman's total reaction may be a feeling of despair and uselessness. In contrast, her husband is usually still very much involved in his work and career; therefore, he often finds it not so difficult to accept his children's growing independence. It is highly desirable for women to plan ahead for the period of perhaps 20 years when their children will be grown. Lack of planning and training often result in a woman being unable to find suitable employment, while the need for trained workers remains pressing. Seeking some opportunities for contact with her career, and for maintenance and upgrading of her skills while her children are small can help the woman in middle life to resume work outside the home, and can help her deal with the change in her role which occurs with her children's greater independence.

Dependence of the Aged. The increasing dependence of the aged also presents strains on persons in middle life, not only financially, but also socially and emotionally. Apartments and homes tend to be small in modern urban society. They were planned to accommodate only the family of parents and children. Most people in our society prefer separate dwellings for each nuclear family. Some families manage very well, however, with a 3-generation household. When families live together for economic reasons, even though they would prefer to live separately, strains and conflicts often result.

Because more people are living to very advanced age when the likelihood of physical and mental infirmity increases, their grown children become increasingly involved in care of aged parents. The needs of the parents, which become more pressing as time passes, revive the old problem of independence from parents. This time the problem is set in a new context, since now it is the child who is stronger and the parents who are weaker; the child who is richer, and the parents who are poorer.

Often the person in middle life feels squeezed by the conflicting demands of the young and the aged. Both husband and wife may have to go out to work in order to provide sufficient income for their aged parents as well as for themselves and their children. If there are very young children, the wife may understandably feel that she should not go out to work. The wife or the husband may rebel against supporting the spouse's parents, or additional problems may be created if all four parents of the couple depend on one breadwinner. With a longer life span, more and more old people live to be over 90. Their children are in the 60's and 70's, and the grandchildren (in their 30's and 40's) may have the financial responsibility for all the oldsters. It is conceivable that 12 older people could depend on one working couple. The very aged are usually in the most difficult position because ordinarily they are the least self-sufficient. When they were young there were fewer retirement plans, and many are not covered by Social Security.

If the parents become unable to care for themselves in their own homes, or are unable to afford the services of a housekeeper or home health aid, other arrangements must be considered:

- The parent shares the home of one of his children.
- One of the grown children returns to his parent's home to provide care.
- The parent resides in a home for the aged.
- The parent lives in a foster home.

Sometimes suggestions, made tactfully by the nurse, can help the family. Permitting the older person and his adult children as much privacy and freedom as possible is important. A room of his own and a place to keep treasured possessions makes the older person more comfortable. Opportunities for members of each generation to entertain their friends, though often overlooked, are also important.

If the family's decision is to provide care in a home for older persons, nurses can be of assistance in helping the family choose one where standards are high: where the menus are well planned, where there is enough well-qualified staff, where the building is safe, and where there are opportunities for rehabilitation. Care in a geriatric setting need not mean severing close family ties or a termination of responsibility and participation in the care of one's parents. One institution utilizes a group program to help grown children during the early period of their parent's residence in the home (Brudno). There are group discussions, led by the staff, and tours and observations of the activities. Grown children often feel guilty about placing their parents in an institution, even though it does not seem feasible for them to take the parent into their own homes. Their guilt often leads them to express anger and dissatisfaction toward the home and the care given. The reluctance that people often have in acknowledging the declining abilities of their parents presents problems in setting realistic rehabilitation goals. In this home the grown children were encouraged to discuss the problems they were facing in relation to their parent's care. Opportunity to express feelings of guilt and anger toward the institution and its staff was helpful. Tours of the home were arranged, and the sons and daughters were given the chance to observe and participate in the programs in such areas as the occupational and recreational therapy departments. Understanding the purposes of the various treatments, such as exercises, helped to lessen the tendency of the grown children to view the home and its staff with dissatisfaction.

Foster-home care may be provided by a couple or a widow who enjoys the company of older people and who has a large house. The advantages to the older person include living in a home environment without having responsibility for its upkeep; and the possible strain of different generations of the same family living together is prevented. The older person brings income to the family who is boarding him; in some instances the state finances the foster care. Foster homes, like institutions, can be poor or excellent. Much depends on the personalities of the people providing the care.

Observing the aging of one's parents is, for many people, a difficult experience. Changes that tend to occur with very advanced age—such as forgetfulness, loss of physical strength and diminution of vision and hearing—may be very distressing. For a few people the experience of watching their parents age is so painful, particularly if the aging process is complicated by illness or marked impairment of function, that they find ways to withdraw from it. Sometimes, for example, they avoid visiting the parent or giving assistance that seems within their ability to provide.

Certain guidelines can be helpful in such situations. Remember that people vary in their ability to cope with certain kinds of stressful situations. Blaming the son or daughter for what appears to be neglect of his parents is usually ineffective in helping him to assume more responsibility. This approach may, in fact, make the son or daughter even more likely to avoid the situation, whereas an attitude of acceptance of the grown child may help him to become better able to assist his parents.

Regardless of the attitude of the grown children, the nurse can be most helpful if she recognizes that the decision concerning the future care of the older person rests with the parent and the children, and not with her. The nurse's approach to the care of her own parents may be quite different. She should not attempt to impose her views on others, but help them to find their own solutions.

The Single Person. For a variety of reasons, many people remain single. A common attitude toward the bachelor is a mixture of sly admiration and pity, while the unmarried woman is often considered a sorrowful figure, unable to attract a husband; both are thought to be unable to accept responsibility or to adjust to marriage. However, remaining single is common enough so that it alone cannot be considered as deviant or maladjusted behavior. Creative, sometimes religious, fulfillment may be served best by remaining single; and society benefits. The single person may be lonely, as might anyone, but he or she may have a full life of varied and rich relationships. Many who remain unmarried develop a certain self-reliance that serves them well in later life because they tend to plan ahead and provide for the time when loneliness, lack of interest and too much free time are a torment to many others. Nurses, especially, need to understand that there is more than one acceptable way to live; otherwise, their disapproving attitude colors their nursing care.

Time. Some interesting changes occur in the way the person in middle life views time. Time not only seems to be shorter, but it *is* shorter. A man who feels himself to be in the wrong job and would like to enter another is aware that soon there will be no time left to make such a major change. The woman who has no children may feel that it will soon be too late to have any. The experience of seeing his parents age and his children mature is a further reminder of the "mortal span." Just as it is inevitable that his children will grow up, it is also inevitable that his parents will die in due course, probably during this period of his life. The changes in his own body also remind him that time has not stood still.

Satisfactions of Middle Age. Just as young adulthood has its satisfactions as well as its stresses, so is middle life a mixture of the two. At this period the person has a chance to reap the harvest of his early struggle to found a home and earn a living.

The process of finding one's niche in one's family and work, and of becoming aware of the particular abilities one possesses can be immensely satisfying. The person in middle life who is perceptive of his own assets, and of the ways in which he can utilize them for the good of his family, community and society, as well as for his own self-development, can harness his energies to the accomplishment of goals that to him are significant and worthwhile. He may be more able at this time of life than in his youth to differentiate what goals seem worth striving for, rather than attempting to meet a multitude of demands of society, some of which may be in conflict with one another. With a channeling and focusing of his energies may come additional time for enjoyment of the things he deems important. For one person this may be travel, for another study, gardening or volunteer work.

Middle life makes an individual increasingly aware of choices. Some of the choices he has made himself; others have been made by circumstances. If the direction of one's life is recognized as essentially consistent with one's values, middle life can be richly satisfying.

Of course, as at any period in life, all does not always go well. The person may never achieve much at home or at work. Nevertheless, it is during middle life that most people (if they are going to do so at all) bring their dreams and abilities to fulfillment. Inevitably, all the hopes are not fulfilled, and it is in late middle life that many people take stock, acknowledging, "While I have some things I've wanted, I haven't achieved others—and now I never will."

Developmental tasks of middle life may be summarized as:

- Maintaining a satisfying family life; dealing with the growing independence of children, and with the growing dependence of aged parents.
- Enhancing responsibility and contribution to work.
- Securing a home; building up financial resources.
- Enlargement of role and responsibilities in community activities.
- Coping with physical and emotional changes related to the aging process.
- Developing varied interests and relationships which can continue in later years.
- Moving toward individuation, such as by further definition of his own values, life style, and religious beliefs.

IMPLICATIONS FOR NURSING

A major problem confronting the individual who becomes ill during middle life is change of role and status, in his own eyes and in his relationships with others, from independence and productivity to dependence and curtailment of productivity. These changes create problems at other age periods, too, but their impact is particularly severe during middle life.

In what ways may the nurse assist the patient with this problem—or at least avoid adding to it? She can avoid adopting stereotyped expectations concerning the patient's response to illness, but instead be observant of his individual way of reacting. For example, there is a widespread expectation among nurses that the mother who becomes ill is more concerned about her children's welfare than her own, and that the father-provider who becomes ill is more worried about his family's welfare and support than he is about his own recovery. It seems likely that to some extent such statements reflect the expectations of nurses, rather than necessarily the reactions of patients. Some patients do respond to illness with greater concern for others than for themselves. However, a common response to illness, at any age, is increased concern for and preoccupation with one's own welfare, and diminished capacity to be concerned about the needs of others. Avoid indicating to the patient how you think he should feel. The nurse may unwittingly convey her expectations to the patient by quickly introducing a question about his children's welfare,

when the patient has voiced concern about his own condition and chances for recovery.

Just as it is important to avoid burdening the patient with stereotyped expectations of his behavior and attitudes toward others, it is also important to support the patient's remaining independence and ability to make decisions and to participate in planning his own care. Because the shift from independence toward dependence is already especially problematic for persons in middle life, it is particularly important to use nursing approaches which foster the degree of independence of which the patient is capable.

For example, a man who is recovering from myocardial infarction must rest. He must stay in bed and allow the nurse to bathe him. Frequently these patients express anger at curtailment of their activities and, particularly, at having decisions made for them. Many patients who suffer myocardial infarction are active, hard-driving people who are very much involved in their work. Suddenly, with the onset of infarction, the patient is reduced to the helpless physical dependence of an infant. If your patient expresses anger over the abrupt curtailment of his independence, one of the things you can do is consider with him the areas where he can make decisions. Although he must be bathed, he can have some part in deciding when he will have his bath. Although he must stay in bed, he can have a say about the view he prefers.

The physical decrements which accompany middle life may be especially threatening when they are compounded by illness. The woman of 37 may already be concerned about her approaching menopause. Entering the hospital to have a dilatation and curettage of the cervix, with the possibility of a hysterectomy, can greatly magnify the anxiety she is already experiencing about her reproductive capacities. As you work with patients who are about to undergo surgery, or any procedure that may alter their physiologic functions, make yourself available to listen to the patient's concerns and try to provide the patient with factual information which can help allay anxiety. Suppose the woman in the example above does require a hysterectomy, and mentions nervously to the nurse that this operation will bring on a sudden and severe menopause. The nurse can explain that removal of the uterus results in inability to bear children and absence of menstruation but not in sudden severe symptoms of menopause. The nurse can explain that the patient's ovaries continue to secrete hor-

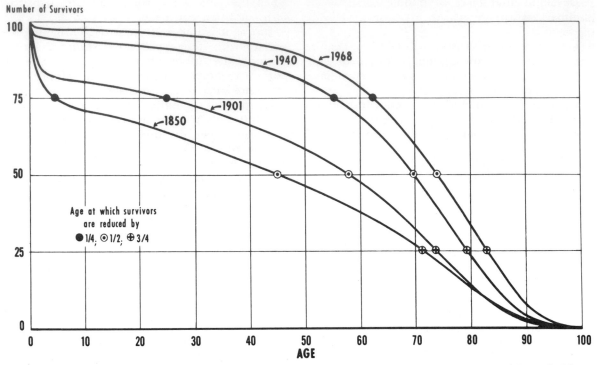

Number of Survivors

Fig. 3-2. Survivors from birth to successive ages, United States, 1850-1968. The proportion of older people in our country is increasing and is expected to continue to increase. (Metropolitan Life Insurance Co., New York, N.Y.)

mones, and that her hormonal equilibrium will not undergo sudden change.

A great variety of illnesses usually associated with emotional stress, such as asthma, peptic ulcer and colitis, are common during this time of life. Recognition of this period as one in which the individual's responsibilities and stresses are often numerous may help the nurse as she cares for patients whose illness is greatly affected by emotional strain.

The modern independent small family consisting of parents and children encounters extra problems when illness strikes. If the mother becomes ill, no grandmother or maiden aunt is there to take over the housework and the care of the children. Employing someone to do this work is often difficult and unsatisfactory even if the family can pay for it. Our emphasis on individual initiative and self-reliance has made it very difficult for the man of the house to borrow money from relatives. He is often more inclined to look to insurance or to public welfare than to his family for financial help—and to suffer eco-

nomic hardship rather than to admit that he needs money.

It is sometimes hard for those working with the hospitalized patient to recall that he is part of a family. It is so easy for nurses to sympathize only with the patient, since it is his need that they see, and to view his family only in the role of helping him. You may hear a nurse say at morning report, "And poor old Mr. Jones— his children hardly ever come to see him. It's a shame." A wave of sympathy for Mr. Jones and of disapproval of his grown children may pass through the group. The nurse who cares for Mr. Jones that morning, in response to his comments about his children, may reply, "Yes, I think it's awful that they don't visit you oftener." But the situation affecting Mr. Jones's children may be completely unknown to her. For instance, maybe Mr. Jones's son has a sick wife at home, and he has all he can do to go to work and care for his wife and children when he gets home in the evening. Or maybe the relationship between Mr. Jones and his children has never been close.

Parent-child relationships during middle and later life are an outgrowth of those developed throughout the years. Often it is useless and harmful to attempt to fix the blame for a poor relationship between parents and children on either generation, since the situation may be an outgrowth of complex emotional and social factors.

Remember that your patient's view of his family is true as he sees it. Let him express himself without your taking sides, recognizing that you do not have all the facts and that even if you did, your role is to help both the patient and his family rather than to judge or condemn. Usually the members of the patient's family are doing the best they can within the limitations of a variety of emotional, social and economic pressures.

For many people during middle life there is a quickening of interest in their own thoughts and inner experiences. No longer as concerned and absorbed in establishing a place for themselves in work, community, and family life, they begin to turn inward to greater consideration of their own values, life style, and relationships with others. Illness can spark this process by posing some profound questions concerning the meaning of life and death, as well as by providing a respite from the patients' usual activities, thus affording him time for reflection. The nurse can help the patient by listening if he wishes to discuss some of these concerns. Unfortunately, the patient's concern with the "ultimate questions" is too often looked upon as morbid preoccupation with the self, and efforts are made to distract the patient by conversation about his flowers, the weather, and so on. By recognizing that the experience of illness can bring opportunity for growth, for confronting fundamental issues of life, and for greater depth of experiences and relationships in the future, you can utilize more effectively the opportunities which you have to support the patient in his experience.

REFERENCES AND BIBLIOGRAPHY

BRUDNO, J. J.: Group programs with adult offspring of newly admitted residents in a geriatric setting, *J. Am. Geriat. Soc.* 12:385, 1964.

DONAHUE, W., et al.: (eds.): *Free Time: Challenge to Later Maturity*, Ann Arbor, University of Michigan Press, 1958.

DUVALL, E. M.: *Family Development*, ed. 4, Philadelphia, Lippincott, 1970.

FRIEDMANN, E., and HAVIGHURST, R.: *The Meaning of Work and Retirement*, Chicago, University of Chicago Press, 1954.

HAVIGHURST, R. J.: *Human Development and Education*, New York, Longmans, 1953.

KURTAGH, C.: Nursing in the life span of people, *Nurs. Forum* 7:298, 1969.

LAZARUS, R. S.: *Psychological Stress and the Coping Process*, New York, McGraw-Hill, 1966.

MURPHY, G., and KUHLEN, R.: *Psychological Needs of Adults*, Chicago, Center for Study of Liberal Education for Adults, 1955.

PRESSEY, S., and KUHLEN, R.: *Psychological Development Through the Life Span*, New York, Harper, 1957.

SKIPPER, J., and LEONARD, R. (eds.): *Social Interaction and Patient Care*, Philadelphia, Lippincott, 1965.

Caring for the Elderly Patient

4

Some Facts and Myths • Physical Changes • Intellectual
Development • Patterns of Aging • Developmental Tasks
Some Days of Later Life • Implications for Nursing

SOME FACTS AND MYTHS

As you work with medical-surgical patients, whether in general hospitals, nursing homes, or in their own homes, you will note that a disproportionate number of them are elderly. Associated with physiologic changes of aging is an increased tendency toward illness, and slowness in recovery from illness. In our society many of the aged are disadvantaged also in relation to family ties, income, housing, and opportunities to perform useful and respected work.

Although these statements are true, they do not present the whole picture. Recent efforts to highlight the plight of the aged have resulted in some exaggeratedly negative views. For example, sometimes it is assumed that a large proportion of the elderly reside in institutions. Actually, 3–5 per cent of those over 65 are institutionalized, and it is likely that this percentage could be reduced if adequate facilities for home care (such as medical and nursing care, and assistance with housekeeping) were available (Wahl).

The elderly are often portrayed as sitting on park benches, with little to do but feed the pigeons. Yes, this is true of some older people, but it does not accurately describe the majority. Interestingly, the largest proportion of the income of elderly persons comes from paid employment—much of it part-time (Wahl). This fact is all the more impressive when one considers that the labor market is becoming increasingly more resistant to employment of older persons.

Another common assumption is that the aged are increasingly abondoned by their families. A contrast with "the good old days" is often made, nostalgically idealizing the large farmhouse which sheltered not only the nuclear family but the older generation as well. While this was the case in some instances, there were other modes of responding to the issue of relationships between generations which are less widely discussed.

What about the young people who migrated across this continent, or from another land, leaving the older members of the family? In those days the leave-taking was often final. Transportation facilities frequently did not permit a return visit to those far away, nor was there telephone communication. Letters tended to become less and less frequent as family ties weakened due to prolonged separation. Sometimes the younger generation never knew what happened to their parents and other older relatives—let alone assume continued responsibility for helping them in their declining years. This, too, is part of the way things used to be. Today, despite urbanization with its smaller living quarters and the tendency for each generation of adults to reside in separate homes, families have greater opportunity to keep in touch, by visits and telephone, and many families continue to do so, despite high geographic mobility.

We are often told that the problem of aging has been with us always—but that we are just not handling it as well as did our forebears. Actually the problem is not the same as it was. In years past the person who lived longer than 65 years was a rarity. Now it is not unheard of for two generations of a family to be drawing social security: for example, one, aged 65, and his parent, aged 85. A young husband and wife may each have not only living grandparents but great-grandparents as well. The problem *is* dif-

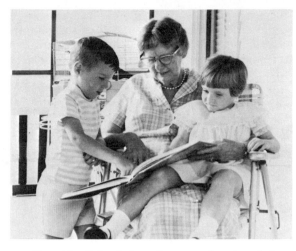

FIG. 4-1. Babysitting gives grandmother feelings of usefulness and pleasure.

ferent; it is vastly larger, and it can no longer be viewed as the sole responsibility of families, but a responsibility of society as a whole. The view that families alone are responsible for care of the aged has brought some results which are tragic for individuals and, in the long run, for society. For instance, a couple in their late 50's may be continuing to support one or two aged parents in a nursing home, at a time of life when they should be saving money for their own rapidly approaching retirement. When their retirement does come, they may be obliged to seek assistance through public welfare. Unmarried women in middle life are particularly vulnerable in this respect, as they are often expected to assume considerable responsibility for care of the aged. It is not infrequent for a woman in middle life to stop working in order to care for an aged parent. When after some years the parent dies, the woman may find that she no longer possesses the skills and confidence to seek re-employment, thus becoming, herself, a candidate for public assistance. In these examples we see the way in which the problem of care of the aged "backs up" as it were, when resources of the family are not adequate to meet the problem. Nor is the challenge only financial. It involves also the freedom of younger members of the family to marry, to seek education and satisfying work—in short, to move ahead with the multiplicity of tasks and responsibilities facing them, of which care of the aged is only one.

It is essential for nurses to view these problems broadly, over a long time span, and to recognize that the problem may significantly affect the lives of several members of a family, rather than just the aged individual alone. It is also important for nurses to recognize their role in helping families make their own decisions in these matters, rather than making decisions for them, or subtly influencing them about what course of action to take. It is essential for the nurse to distinguish between her own values, in relation to care of her own elderly relatives, and the values which others may hold. The nurse who is too quick to recommend a nursing home, and the nurse who subtly implies that placing a relative in a nursing home is tantamount to abandonment, are both imposing their own values on others; rather than helping the elderly person and his family to consider alternatives and to decide what is best for them.

What are some other myths about the aged—or views which, while once tenable, are so no longer? One is that elderly persons have so short a life expectancy that some therapeutic measures, which would be considered essential for a young person, are not worthwhile. Dentures, corrective glasses, provision of speech therapy and psychotherapy may be neglected on the assumption that the patient has very few years in which to benefit from them. But many persons aged 65 now live 20 and 25 more years! Views about care of the elderly must be re-examined in light of current life-expectancy, and also in light of values of the rights of individuals to health care, regardless of age.

Another view prevalent in our culture is that the aged are useless. But is usefulness limited to being gainfully employed? What about the values to a family, a community, or a profession, of having older members—members whose view has a different perspective and who can help those who are younger to be in touch with their own origins? What of the value to a youngster who has a close relationship with his grandfather who talks to him of family lore and of the way life used to be when he was a boy? What about the youngster who, through a grandparent who migrated to this country, is put in touch with his family's background in the "old country," and perhaps also has opportunity to learn a second language? In a fast-changing society, the aged are an important link to past events and persons who have affected our lives.

The assumption is sometimes made that later life is synonomous with incapacity. One often hears an achievement of an older person received with astonishment, "Imagine, at *his* age!" Such responses actually reveal condescension, and an expectation that the significant part of life is over, once one has passed middle age. But is it really? And even more important, does it *have* to be, or do our expectations sometimes make it so? The news that an elderly man and woman plan to marry is often greeted with a mixture of scorn and amusement, as though somehow the individuals are expected to have outlived their human need for closeness and companionship. Such views by the young are presumptuous, and can undermine the confidence and resilience of many an older person who senses that he is not expected seriously to seek new experiences, whether in work or personal relationships. The process of aging brings many doubts and uncertainties: of ability to support oneself financially, to find companionship and useful work. Attitudes of younger people, including those in the health professions, are especially important. We can convey that we see nothing odd or humorous about an older person's desire to work, or to remarry, and particularly, that we are not overcome by surprise that significant achievements can occur in later life. Instead of "Why, at your age," we can convey "Well, why not?"

We hear a great deal about the losses of aging —and it is true that the aged experience many losses—in personal relationships, income, health, agility, and opportunities to learn new things and to continue employment. However, it is necessary to view the losses not in the context of the values and goals of youth and middle life, but in the context of later life. For example, physical changes with aging are on the debit side; shortly we shall discuss these in more detail. But what does it mean to the older person that his grip is weaker than when he was 40? It means that he must live somewhat differently, and adapt to failing muscular strength. But how much of a disability is this to the older person who has gradually adapted his life style accordingly? Thus, even the stark reality of physical decline must be viewed in the perspective of the older person's life, and not just in terms of measurements of how much he has lost of his youthful vigor and physiologic efficiency.

We hear a great deal too about the older person's disengagement: his lessened concern with daily events, and increased preoccupation with his own thoughts. An increased concern with assessing one's life and accomplishments, and one's relationships with others and with work occurs for many people during middle age, and continues into later life. The older person often shows greater selectivity of involvement with certain people and with those aspects of his work which have most meaning and value for him. Whether or not this change constitutes loss depends upon one's values. In a society in which "busy-ness" and involvement with many individuals and groups is highly valued, and where little recognition is given to the importance of developing personal inner resources, these changes with age may be viewed as loss. However, if a high value is placed on development of the inner life, these changes with age are viewed as manifestations of personal maturation.

However, there is another aspect to the matter of disengagement, and that is society's disengagement from the older person. There is, if you will, a reciprocal disengagement in which society withdraws from the older person much interest and support, and the aging individual withdraws some of his involvement with society. The older person whose services have been sought because of his skill and achievements at work may no longer be consulted by his colleagues after retirement. Younger family members are busily engaged in establishing their own homes and careers, and may spend little time with older members of the family. Thus, the older individual has his tendency to disengagement greatly heightened by the disengagement of others from him, and by the lack of opportunity to become involved in significant work and new learning.

Disengagement may thus be viewed as a psychological change in the aging individual and also as an aspect of society's reaction toward the aged. The two processes together, along with physiologic changes of aging which result in decreased blood flow to the brain, sometimes result in a syndrome called senility. This word has unfortunate connotations of hopelessness; it is also frequently misused to label older people, resulting in further withdrawal of others from them, and a resultant increase in the older person's symptoms. The word "senile" is used to describe older people who are forgetful, confused, and who show feebleness and helplessness associated with advanced age. When the older person is helped to become involved with significant activities and with other people, his memory and orientation sometimes improve. Measures in the care of the elderly will be discussed later in the chapter.

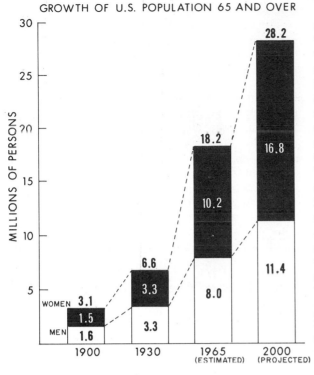

GROWTH OF U.S. POPULATION 65 AND OVER

FIG. 4-2. The United States population over 65 has grown enormously since 1900. Note the growing disproportion between number of women and number of men who survive past age 65. (*Developments in Aging 1967*, Washington, D.C., U.S. Government Printing Office)

PHYSICAL CHANGES

The elderly seek more medical care than younger people because of the higher incidence of certain health problems among older age groups. For example, the highest incidence of impaired vision and hearing occurs among older people. During later life certain prominent causes of illness and death, such as cancer, cerebrovascular accidents, and heart disease, also reach their peak. Several chronic diseases that have developed gradually often exist simultaneously in elderly people. Knowledge of normal physiologic changes which occur with aging can help the nurse plan for care of elderly patients, and can enable her to assist patients and their families to cope with the aging process.

Nutrition. There is a tendency for people to lose weight during old age, and nutritional deficiency is often a serious problem. This may be related to the lack of dentures, to boredom at eating alone or to lack of money. Chronic con-

stipation may be a problem. Diet planning for the geriatric patient should limit calories to match lessened energy output (but maintain weight unless the patient is obese), yet include well-seasoned foods, because the sense of taste dulls with age. The older person continues to need fresh fruit and vegetables, milk, eggs and meat. He should have enough fluid and roughage to encourage normal bowel function. Many older people find that a light supper (perhaps of soup or cereal, bread and fruit) is sufficient for them at the end of the day when they are tired. Their heavier meal comes, then, at mid-day. Serving unrecognizable pureed or ground foods insults the taste and the sensibilities of some elderly people, and intake increases when foods are offered in other ways, such as stews. Appetite also may increase when food is served in such a way that enables the elderly person to help himself as much as possible. It is better to have the butter soft than to spread it for the patient. The patient who cannot feed himself the entire meal may be able to eat his bread without help. Eating is a social activity and should include pleasant conversation and companionship.

Position Sense and Speed of Reaction. These show gradual decline until the age of about 70, when the decline becomes rapid. The decline of these two faculties, together with diminished vision, is frequently a cause of accidents. For example, speed of reaction and good vision are important in safe driving. Both may have diminished in the older person, but ease of transportation is especially needed in later life. It has been suggested that deterioration of the ability to make decisions and to formulate judgments involving use of short-term memory are important factors in causing automobile accidents among the aged (McFarland). For example, an older person may not comprehend quickly enough the variety of changes occurring in a traffic situation. He may fail to take account of a car emerging from a side street and fail to make a decision to stop even when his vision is adequate.

Despite problems with vision, hearing, and decision-making, older people in this country have achieved "safe driving" records which could be the envy of teen-age drivers. In light of their driving records it is apparent that many older people make realistic adaptations in their driving habits: driving only during daylight hours, avoiding heavy traffic and long fatiguing trips, and giving up their licenses when their waning abilities make this necessary. Because waiting for trains and buses is fatiguing, and since transportation is so important to the older person in maintaining his contacts with family and friends, it is important to counsel those older persons who require such guidance in measures to promote safe driving.

Diminished agility, position sense, vision, and hearing make older pedestrians prone to injury. Discourage older people from walking unaccompanied at night. If they must walk alone after dark, encourage them to use the best-lighted streets, and to be alert to the traffic.

Falls. A common cause of injury among older people, falls are related to the decline in position sense. Falls are more common among older women than men, possibly because of the difference in shoe style. When balance and agility decrease, high heels make the situation worse.

The susceptibility of older people to falls and fractures (their bones are more brittle and break more readily) should affect the planning of homes and apartments. Because of the increasing proportion of older people in the population, it is advisable to include basic safety factors in all housing and not to confine safety devices to units designed especially for older people: for example, stairs which are not too steep, which are adequately lighted and are provided with a handrail. Night lights and a sturdy handle bar near the bathtub or shower can be put up in any home.

Skin. Gradual changes in the skin and in the body's ability to adjust to heat and cold occur with age. The skin becomes drier and prone to wrinkling. In old age it may become thin, flaky and susceptible to irritation. The hair, also, becomes drier, thinner and gray. Nails, particularly toenails, often become thickened and brittle as a result of poorer circulation to the extremities.

During later middle life and old age the body gradually loses some of its ability to adjust to extremes of temperature. It is harder for an old person to keep warm in cold weather because his metabolism is slower, and he lacks physical vigor for the strenuous exercise that would help him to keep warm. In hot weather, the old person does not dissipate heat as efficiently as a younger one, because his cutaneous vessels may not dilate as much and his sweating may not function as effectively as it once did. Now there are many welcome aids for keeping older people comfortable in very hot weather and in cold weather. Contrast the comfort of heated cars with a bulky lap robe. Modern heating that provides uniform warmth in the entire house is another boon. Air

conditioning has made summers more comfortable for every one.

The nurse can help by making adjustments to keep older people more comfortable, remembering that they tolerate temperature changes poorly. If an older patient shares a room with younger people, fewer problems in regulating temperature may occur if the older patient is placed farthest from the window and is offered an extra blanket.

Teeth. Since considerable individual differences exist in the resistance of teeth to decay, some people lose their teeth as they grow old despite good dental care. Others have almost all their own teeth, and they can munch a raw apple as well as their grandchildren. The older person who needs dentures should be encouraged to obtain them, since his appearance and nutrition will benefit.

Other Physical Changes

Other important physical changes include a considerable decrease in cardiac output, from 6.5 liters per minute at age 25 to 3.8 liters per minute at age 85 (Zorzoli). Since cardiac output affects nutrition to all parts of the body, this change is of great significance. Vital capacity also diminishes markedly with age.

The aged individual has diminished ability to maintain homeostasis during stress; he has less "reserve" with which to deal with the onslaughts of exertion, infection, and fatigue. One example of the slowness of the homeostatic mechanism to adjust is illustrated by the fact that the body's ability to remove excessive glucose from the blood drops appreciably in old age (Zorzoli).

Physiologic response to exercise also changes with age. The circulatory system cannot respond as efficiently to the demands of exercise in later life; the heart and blood vessels cannot supply the increased demands of the muscles for blood as adequately as during youth. The kidneys, too, are less efficient in old age in conserving water, in situations (such as excessive sweating) where this is necessary.

INTELLECTUAL DEVELOPMENT

Teaching the Older Patient

Suppose that a 67-year-old woman has just discovered that she has congestive heart failure. The doctor has recommended rest, a low sodium diet, digitalis, and a diuretic. This woman has many new things to learn. Perhaps the most important of these will be the fact that she *can* learn. Older people themselves often have the false notion that ability to learn ceases at some point during life. Encouraging self-confidence in older people is the first big step in helping them to learn.

Unfortunately the fact that older persons perform less well on some standardized intelligence tests (older people have particular difficulty, for example, with timed tests, since they perform more slowly than young people), has led some people to the dismal conclusion that one becomes gradually less and less intelligent during middle and later life. It is more useful to consider these changes within the context of the individual's life than merely in terms of test results. We know that standardized intelligence tests are useful in predicting success of young people in school, but how useful are they, say, in predicting the success of a man in his 50's who is about to become president of his company? Many abilities, such as skill in leading others, and wisdom in decision-making, may be difficult to predict on the basis of intelligence test scores, but may more readily be predicted from past performance at work. Qualities of wisdom, tact, patience, and understanding of self and others are not readily measured by standard intelligence tests. However, these are examples of abilities in which some older persons excel. The older person also has had many experiences to which he can relate new learning.

As you begin teaching the older patient, convey to him your belief that he *can* learn. Proceed more slowly than with your younger patient, to give the older person the extra time he needs to think about and respond to new ideas. Speak slowly and distinctly to help the individual compensate not only for slowed reaction time but also for the hearing deficit so common among the elderly. If you use visual aids, such as graphs or pictures, allow the older person extra time to study them, and be sure he is wearing his glasses (if necessary) and that he has a good light. Use visual materials which are large enough to be seen easily, and which are clear and uncluttered.

Find out about the patient's past experience and relate new material to it. Because older people have accumulated a vast store of experience, helping them to draw on it aids learning. In teaching, always start with what the patient already knows, and build on that. This precept means that at first the teacher listens to the patient. Only then can she know where to start. Perhaps the patient's husband was on a sodium-restricted diet many years ago, and she recalls how she prepared his meals. Can the patient obtain her digitalis when she needs more? What problems does she have, if any, in getting to the doctor's office? Can she see the fine print on her vial of medicine? Perhaps she needs a magnifying glass to read it. How many stairs does this patient have to climb daily? Can groceries be delivered to her so that she does not have to carry them home? When can she rest during the day?

Learning is an important means of compensating for losses. Being able to master new knowledge and skill is important to self-esteem. Consider the blow which may come to the pride of a man in his late 60's who observes that the nurse is teaching his daughter how to administer his insulin injection without first evaluating whether he can learn this himself. Many times older people unnecessarily are denied the opportunity to learn new skills, thereby making it all the more difficult for them to compensate for illness and disability, and to continue their productive roles at work and in family life.

PATTERNS OF AGING

According to an old expression, as people grow older, they grow more like themselves. The old person who is cheerful and seems to be interested in everything probably has been that way for years; the person who views old age as an insuperable hardship may have found the problems of puberty and menopause insurmountable, too. Actually, preparation for later life is something that cannot be avoided. Whether planned or not, the attitudes and the abilities that individuals develop day by day will determine the kind of people they will be at 40—or 80.

Sometimes it is assumed that there is one successful pattern of aging. In our society continued active involvement in work and family affairs tends to be admired; therefore, those who adapt to aging in this way are especially likely to be considered successful. Others, however, adapt successfully by withdrawing somewhat from activities and relationships, and investing more time and energy in solitary pursuits, such as gardening, reading, and reflection.

Behavior considered maladaptive at one period in life may be an asset at another period. For example, a person who was regarded in youth as somewhat distant in his relationships may in later life seem to cope particularly well with situations in which he is alone a great deal. Conditions which for other older persons might spell intolerable loneliness may, for this person, constitute welcome relief from the pressures of maintaining close personal relationships.

DEVELOPMENTAL TASKS

Life does not cease making demands when the responsibilities of middle life have passed. In fact, some of the most difficult problems are reserved for the last part of life. Negative attitudes in our culture toward aging play no small part in aggravating the problems and decreasing the satisfactions of later life.

Society provides many educational opportunities for the young to learn to achieve the tasks set for the first half of life—tasks which are different from those of later life. For instance, during youth, emphasis is placed upon adapting to group norms, while in later life, the emphasis shifts toward development of greater individuation. Society places little emphasis on education for these significant tasks of later life. Some older people seek continued opportunities to learn and grow, through religious faith, psychotherapy, individual study and reflection, and through their relationships with significant other persons. But because some older people do not have plentiful opportunities for such enriching experiences, it is important for society to begin to develop educational programs for older people who wish help in adapting to physiologic and psychologic changes, and in dealing with the developmental tasks of later life.

Dependence. Many problems of aging revolve around dependence. People who live long enough (into their 80's and 90's) become, to some extent, dependent on others for companionship and often for financial support and physical care. Change from independence to dependence is usually gradual unless, for example, a sudden illness renders a previously self-sufficient person dependent.

Many older persons find dependence on others difficult to accept, even though they may recognize the necessity for it. Some of the elderly deny the need for any help, sometimes jeopardizing their own safety. Others readily become very dependent. Such older people tend to hang on to others, sometimes resulting in friction within the family as the demands for assurance exceed the capacities of others to meet them. Similar problems are observed in nursing homes in relationships between patients and nurses. In such instances the nurse should recognize the

patient's needs for dependence, and gradually help him to become more self-reliant. Ignoring the older person can cause him to redouble his efforts to gain the nurse's attention and support with a resultant increase of friction in the relationship. On the other hand, if the nurse shows interest and concern for the patient, the patient often begins to show interest in his progress also, initially to please the nurse, perhaps, and as a way of establishing a relationship with her, but later because he himself, with her help, has grown more self-reliant.

Employment and Income. One of the tasks of later life involves adjustment to decreased income. This is especially difficult, since in our society the degree of respect accorded a person depends to a great extent on his financial standing. Many factors are responsible for the economic plight of the aged. Compulsory retirement is an important cause. Older people who are willing and able to work, often find themselves at age 65 without any work to do and with a vastly decreased income. Physical decline plays a part, too. Sometimes the individual's working life is terminated by an illness from which he never fully recovers. The fact that more people are reaching old age means that the economic problems of this age group are multiplied many times.

That the attitudes of society have played a part in the problem is shown by the reluctance of employers to hire older workers. A popular stereotype characterizes the older worker as prone to accidents and errors, frequently absent, slow and unable to learn. There have been tendencies to emphasize the liabilities of age and to fail to recognize the assets which older workers possess. Studies have shown repeatedly that some aspects of this stereotype are not true, and that others have been magnified beyond their true proportions. It is true, certainly, that the time needed for recovery from accidents or illness tends to increase with age. On the other hand, older workers tend to be careful, accurate and dependable, although they are also likely to be slower than younger people and to have greater difficulty in adapting to change.

Attempts are being made to establish *more flexible retirement policies*. Older people who are able and willing to continue their work are being permitted to do so in some instances. Their work is re-evaluated periodically, and, when necessary, they may be transferred to less demanding types of work. However, there is little likelihood of widespread adoption of this approach, except in

Fig. 4-3. Medical expenses increase with age. (*1961 White House Conference on Aging Chart Book*, U.S. Department of Health, Education and Welfare, and the Federal Council on Aging)

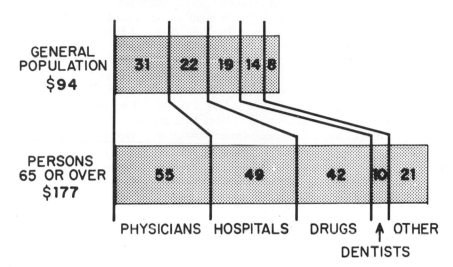

ANNUAL EXPENDITURES PER PERSON*

GENERAL POPULATION $94

PERSONS 65 OR OVER $177

PHYSICIANS   HOSPITALS   DRUGS   OTHER
                                DENTISTS

*EXCLUDING NURSING HOME CARE

fields where there is a scarcity of trained personnel, because of the need to make jobs available for younger workers.

Much has already been achieved. Social Security payments make the difference between "getting by" and destitution for many older people throughout the country. Retirement and pension plans are more numerous than they were formerly. Yet much remains to be done.

Older people particularly need money to help them to overcome or to compensate for some of the infirmities of age. Medical expenses increase with age, and the older person is in need of services to carry out tasks now physically beyond him. A newspaper article lauded an 84-year-old for the way he went to his office every day and still kept in touch with his work. Further reading disclosed that the gentleman had a chauffeur to drive him to and from work! Surely, wealthy older people are in a better position to cope with the physical decline of age than are the great majority of persons in this age group.

The enactment of federal legislation (Medicare) providing health benefits to the aged has been an important advance in helping the elderly to deal with the costs of health care. This program of federal assistance has also indirectly eased the burden for the families of some elderly people, since families often bore the entire cost of an elderly person's medical care.

Lack of money is not the only problem caused by retirement. Idleness, boredom, and loneliness often result, since work has absorbed so large a portion of most people's time and interest and has provided many contacts with other people. Because the ability to earn his way has been removed, a person may suffer from a loss of self-respect and feel that others are judging him as severely as he may be judging himself.

Time. The problem of how to spend time looms large because the individual has so much free time. During his working life the leisure after a day's work was highly prized because it was limited. Too much leisure may lead to feelings of futility and uselessness. Much has been written about the value of hobbies and interests in later life. However, older people tend not to develop new interests but to continue those they already have. There is an amazing continuity in interests throughout each individual's life. The interests developed throughout childhood and early adulthood tend to remain those of the later years. Of course, the manner in which he pursues them may change as time goes on. The young athlete no longer can run bases as he grows older, but he continues to like baseball. Following the fortunes of teams and players probably will become one of his great pleasures in later years. Sometimes the added leisure of old age helps a person to develop dormant interests and talents. Grandma Moses picked up a paintbrush at 80, but most of us are essentially consistent in what we like to do. For instance, the man recovering from cirrhosis who has never willingly read a book in his life is not likely to turn now into an enthusiastic scholar. He may be delighted to play cards with another patient. A woman with her leg in a cast has kept house all her life. She hates weaving baskets—calls it "useless"—but is happy to fold small pieces of linen.

When emphasis is placed on the development of hobbies during early and middle life, in later years they will then be available to cushion the problem of too much spare time. Older women who have been housewives encounter less of a transition in this respect than do their husbands, whose retirement from work is often abrupt. The older woman continues her accustomed housekeeping duties, while her husband may feel out of place when he is at home all day.

Hobbies, however, do not provide a wholly satisfactory solution for most people to the problems of increased leisure. Most individuals in our society have been taught the necessity for work, and that performing productive work is important in giving meaning to life. Hobbies are sometimes trivial; they may be merely measures to pass the time, rather than to use time productively. The elderly person requires opportunities for meaningful, productive work and relationships—opportunities that are often lacking in various clubs for the aged. The eager response of some older people to opportunities to serve, such as by helping disadvantaged children learn to read, underscores the need of older persons to occupy their time usefully and productively.

Loneliness. The problem of loneliness is acute for most older people. In addition to lack of contact with co-workers on the job, separations occur among families and friends. Inevitably, one spouse dies first. Grown children often live at a considerable distance. Regardless of physical distance, the emotional and social distance between generations may be hard to bridge. The very old person outlives most of his contemporaries, and difficulties in travel make it hard for him to see old friends or to make new ones. Those who have developed interests and activities that they can enjoy alone are in a better position to cope with the problems of loneliness than those who have rarely undertaken any project or diversion by themselves. Being able to tolerate and to enjoy periods of being alone is an important asset at any age, but is particularly important during later life.

The older person who has the capacity and energy to develop new relationships has an asset in dealing with loneliness. Some older persons seek situations, such as retirement villages, where they will have greater opportunities to meet people and form new friendships.

Housing is difficult for many older people from the standpoints of both money and companionship. Lack of money often forces older people to find cheaper and less desirable accommodations. Usually, the new dwelling is smaller. The reduction in living space makes it necessary for the older person to part with many treasured objects accumulated over a lifetime, objects which he knows he will not replace. Older people sustain so many losses that they tend to cling to their possessions, sometimes hoarding objects that appear to others to be of little value.

Objects with which the individual must part may remind him of past accomplishments and relationships and, therefore, be especially comforting to him. It is important that the elderly person be permitted to keep as many of his treasured possessions as possible, since they provide him with a link to his past and a comfortable feeling of "belonging here, among these things." Because being surrounded by familiar possessions is so important an environmental support, it is important to increase facilities for home care of the aged, and also to be as flexible as possible in permitting the older person to take some possessions with him if it becomes necessary for him to reside in an institution.

Efforts are being made to provide *more suitable housing* for older people at rents they can afford. Some small communities are being established for older people which combine a chance to live in apartments or small homes with such conveniences as an infirmary, shopping service and recreational facilities. Not surprisingly, the greatest need exists among those least able to pay for ideal retirement living. Some communities are establishing recreational and guidance centers for older people. Some centers serve a hot meal at noon, thus providing a place where older people who live in furnished rooms, with cooking facilities limited or nonexistent, may enjoy recreation and companionship as well as a good meal.

Retirement communities and separate, smaller "retirement neighborhoods" made up of several housing developments for older persons have, despite their advantages, the disadvantages of limiting older people's contacts with younger people, and vice versa. People of different age groups seem to need contact with each other,

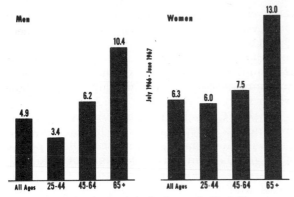

Fig. 4-4. Annual bed days of disability per person. The likelihood of disability requiring confinement to bed increases with age. (Metropolitan Life Insurance Co., New York, N.Y.)

and separate housing developments for the aged seriously limit such contacts.

In response to the increasing number of older people, many more nursing homes and homes for the aged have been established. Some of these are excellent, but others fall below adequate standards. Perhaps the most deplorable practice is that of placing indigent old people in publicly supported mental institutions simply because there is no other place for them to go, or because symptoms of mental illness were not recognized and treated promptly. Older persons possess greater insight and flexibility than is generally attributed to them, and prompt psychotherapy could benefit many older persons and prevent their hospitalization.

Many older people, despite psychiatric diagnoses, such as depression or obsessive-compulsive state, can continue to live in the community, provided the environment is sufficiently supportive. Familiar surroundings, nearness of family and opportunity to follow accustomed routines are examples of such support.

The tolerance of others for idiosyncrasies of behavior is another important factor in determining whether a patient is placed in a mental hospital. As age advances, some people become unmindful of social conventions. An elderly lady may go about in dresses down to her ankles (when this is not the fashion) and sneakers. If she is also inclined to ferret through trash left out for collection twice a week, her neighbors may decide she should be "put away." Differentiating between behavior which is eccentric, but not a hazard to oneself or others, and that which is hazardous or at least highly problematic for

others, is difficult, and decisions may be quite variable, depending on such factors as whether the individual lives in a small town or in a city, and on his socioeconomic status.

Summary

In summary, the developmental tasks of later life include:

- Increasing knowledge of oneself; further integrating the facets of one's personality to a meaningful whole.
- Developing further one's spiritual life; recognition and acceptance of life processes of growth and decline.
- Contributing one's experience and wisdom, gained through the years, to others.
- Maintaining a satisfactory home.
- Fostering close ties with family: spouse, grown children, aging siblings.
- Adjusting to retirement and (usually) to reduced income.
- Maintaining health as effectively and as long as possible; learning to live with diminished strength and vigor, and sometimes with physical disabilities.
- Maintaining ties with the community: neighbors, friends, clubs, church.
- Adjusting to loss of spouse and friends of long standing.
- Facing death.

SOME JOYS OF LATER LIFE

What about the joys of later life? For those whose lives have prepared them for it, there may be opportunities for many *activities* previously impossible because of the lack of time. In one sense older people have immense quantities of time at their disposal. In another sense they are nearing the end of their lives, and they realize the preciousness of the time left to them. Some older people with lively minds and eager curiosity take courses in subjects which have always interested them. Others rekindle interests in art, music, furniture refinishing, cooking or embroidery. It is interesting to note that a group of older people who were interviewed cited many gains during later life, stating that they were happier in many ways than they had been previously (Birren). This finding is especially interesting in view of the emphasis placed on the negative aspects of aging by some writers. Possibly the fact that most of the writing about the aged is done by persons who have not yet reached this phase of life is relevant.

Nurses and doctors tend, by the nature of their work, to have considerable contact with elderly people who are in ill health and who are not coping well with the problems of daily life. Unless this is recognized as a possible influence on one's attitudes toward aging, physicians and nurses may, without being aware of it, develop rather pessimistic views.

The longer one lives the more time one has to know oneself and to understand others better. Of course, some people just live longer and learn little in the process. The older person has been through a career, marriage, hopes that failed to come true and some ambitions that did. From this wealth of experience he may have achieved perspective that can only be envied by those younger than he.

IMPLICATIONS FOR NURSING

Attitudes. Care of the elderly evokes varied reactions. For some nurses, it can be an unpleasant reminder that they too will grow old and die. Working with elderly patients may remind the nurse of troubling aspects of her own relationship with aging parents. Sometimes the physical appearance of the aged is distasteful to nurses, since the aged do not exemplify youthful attractiveness. These reactions may lead the nurse to avoid elderly patients and possibly even to treat them with condescension.

On the other hand, the nurse may idealize the elderly person, perhaps in response to family teachings that older people are wise, and have earned a place of honor and respect. The nurse who has idealized the aged, viewing them as benevolent and kindly, and generously sharing their wisdom with the young, may also do an injustice to her elderly patients, by expecting them to exemplify her ideal of the aged. Thus nurses who have a very negative or a very positive stereotype of aging may both fail to take account of an individual patient's strengths and weaknesses.

One's views of aging can be made more realistic, perhaps, by remembering that the aged are a disadvantaged group in our society. They are disadvantaged in relation to income, employment, housing, health, and companionship—to name but some of the important ways in which most of the aged do not share equally with those who are younger. While disadvantaged people may become more patient, tolerant, and generous, in many instances the reverse is true. They may become selfish, resentful, and demanding. The latter characteristics are sometimes attributed to the aged on the basis of their age, whereas such characteristics, when observed, may actually reflect the individual's deprivations, more than his chronologic age. In addition, some people simply are more pleasant to be with than others—a fact which is true during every period of life.

Physical Care. Perhaps the older person's need to adjust to increasing physical limitations is the problem most familiar to nurses. Older people need gradually increasing amounts of help with self-care as their own ability to care for themselves diminishes. The thoughtful nurse will plan for this need, and she will help the patient's family to do so.

Many older people do not receive the kind of physical care they should. Sometimes it seems especially hard for others to carry out these measures. For instance, in the home the nurse may find that an elderly woman living with a married daughter has very poor personal hygiene. Her hair may be dirty and her clothing soiled, while the home, her daughter and the grandchildren seem to be shining with cleanliness. As the nurse begins to talk with the daughter about her mother's care, the daughter may say, "Mother doesn't seem to notice things like that any more, and I try to let her do as she wants to." Or the daughter may say that it's hard for her to remind and help her own mother with personal cleanliness.

Neglecting the physical needs of the aged is quite common in hospitals, too. It is not unusual for a nurse to say, "I can do these things for a baby. I expect him to be helpless. But with an old person—" Most people do not feel that the elderly have the appealing quality in their helplessness that infants possess. They do not seem to be cute or attractive, or perhaps no one expects them to be helpless. Nevertheless, if people live long enough (into the 80's and 90's), there comes a time when they need assistance with personal hygiene. Recognition of this necessity can help the nurse to plan for and to give this care and to teach family members to do so, too. Very old people become forgetful and unmindful of details, but it is not kind to allow them to have poor hygiene. Old people may develop severe scalp irritations, excoriated skin and pressure sores which cause discomfort and pain.

The prevention of physical discomfort is not the only reason for emphasizing the physical care of older people. It also helps them to maintain dignity and self-respect. Contrast the demeanor

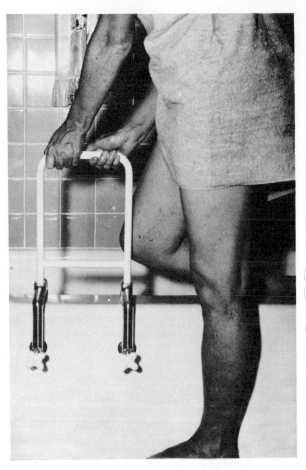

FIG. 4-5. An attachable grab bar for bathtubs helps to prevent falls. (Bollen Products, Cleveland, Ohio)

of the neglected old person with that of one whose snow-white hair is neatly coiffed, whose skin is clean and healthy and whose dress is attractive. In speaking of self-respect the following point should be made clear: the nurse should make it a rule to call each patient by name. To address an older person by his own name, rather than as "Pop" or some other patronizing nickname, helps the older person to maintain his dignity and identity. The older person should be encouraged to care for himself as much as possible as long as he is able. Many devices are available to encourage self-help.

Because circulation to the extremities is often poor, care of the feet and the toenails is important. Lessened circulation may result in injuries or infections healing poorly and even becoming gangrenous. Because the skin on the legs and the feet is usually very dry, cream or lotion should be used after bathing. Thickened, brittle nails should be trimmed carefully, a little at a time. Soften the nails first by soaking the patient's feet in warm water. Very thick nails that have been neglected may need the attention of a chiropodist. If an elderly person's feet are cold, bedsocks and extra blankets are a help. Hot-water bags and electric pads should be used cautiously because of the danger of burning. The combination of diminished sensation and lessened circulation makes this danger more acute in the aged.

Alcohol should not be used as a back lotion, since it is drying, and the skin of older people tends to be dry and scaly. Instead, cream or creamy lotion should be used. Frequent hot baths also tend to be drying. Instead of a daily tub, patients may have a partial bath on alternate days. Be very sure that all the soap is rinsed off the skin, since soap dried on the skin can be irritating. Friction from clothing and bedding should be minimized. For example, sleeves on the patient's gown should be kept down over his elbows to decrease irritation that can be caused by rubbing against the sheets.

Bath oil is helpful in overcoming dryness of the skin; particular care must be taken, however, when it is used, to avoid the patient's slipping in the tub. A rubber mat is essential so that the older person does not step on a tub made slippery by the bath oil.

A stall shower is desirable for use by the elderly, since it avoids the problem of stepping over the side of a tub, and then lowering oneself into the tub. If the patient is weak and unsteady on his feet, a chair may be placed underneath the shower, making it possible for the patient to bathe while seated. The shower provides for the most thorough rinsing of soap from the skin, thus helping to minimize skin irritations so common in the elderly. Whatever method of bathing is used, particular care must be taken to insure privacy, since many older people are especially distressed when they cannot maintain their usual standards of personal modesty.

Dentures require regular cleaning and brushing. If removed, they should be stored in an opaque covered jar. Instruct the patient not to roll them in tissues, because so concealed they can be easily thrown away or lost. If you are helping the patient to clean his dentures, put them in a small basin and take them to the sink to clean them. Avoid holding them directly over the sink—they are easily dropped and broken.

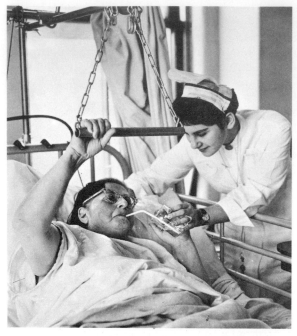

Fig. 4-6. The elderly person who has difficulty moving in bed can be helped by a trapeze. Self-help and exercise are promoted. (Free Lance Photographers Guild, Inc., New York, N.Y.)

Older women sometimes have problems with slight incontinence of urine when they are coughing or sneezing (stress incontinence) or with vaginal discharge. Late in life the vaginal mucous membrane becomes thin and subject to infection. The nurse or a family member may notice that this problem exists; the doctor should be consulted. He may recommend, among other treatments, a cleansing douche. Help the patient to keep clean through perineal care and use of disposable pads, if necessary.

Increased facial hair may be distressing to elderly women. It may be removed by careful cutting or shaving or by the use of a depilatory. Older men may need help with shaving. Tactful reminders and provision of enough clean clothing will help the patient to maintain his appearance. A predictable routine for changing clothing is helpful; for example, place clean clothes on the patient's bed, for him to wear when he has finished bathing.

Elimination may pose particular problems in the elderly. Frequency of urination is not uncommon. Many older men have hypertrophy of the prostate. Older women often have relaxation of perineal structures with less efficient emptying of the bladder. Symptoms of frequent urination should be noted carefully and reported to the doctor. Care must be taken to prevent falls when the patient gets up during the night. Leaving a urinal or a bedpan within easy reach is often helpful. Some older people have difficulty with constipation; this is likely to be especially troublesome to those who cannot get up and move around. Helping the patient to maintain adequate dietary and fluid intake and to have a regular time for evacuation may be the remedy. Sometimes enemas or mild cathartics are ordered by the doctor.

Being confined to bed has other adverse effects on older people. Older people expand their chests less fully because of loss of elasticity of structures that increase and decrease the size of the thoracic cavity. Confinement to bed accentuates this problem and often leads to development of hypostatic pneumonia. (See p. 139 for further discussion of hypostatic pneumonia.) Decubitus ulcers are common among the aged because of the lessened ability of the skin and subcutaneous tissues to tolerate pressure. Circulation tends to be lessened with age; confinement to bed often aggravates this tendency. Diminished circulation to the brain may cause disorientation. Muscle tone is readily lost by the elderly during bed rest. Extreme weakness often results and is difficult to overcome.

In view of these complications, doctors usually permit elderly patients out of bed as soon as possible. As soon as he is able, the patient should be encouraged to take a few steps with help and gradually to increase his activities. Older people, especially if they are weak from illness, have a tendency to stoop. It is important to encourage good posture at all times, whether the patient is in bed, sitting in a chair or walking about. Providing a change of scenery by helping the patient to the sitting room or the porch is a boost to morale. When you know that the patient will be allowed up shortly, ask his family to bring his clothes, particularly his shoes. Paper slippers and long sashes on bathrobes may cause falls.

Time. The older patient is slower in his movements and responses than a younger one. Attempts to make him hurry often result in confusion, irritation and accidents. It is wise to plan nursing care so that the older patient has more time for his activities. For instance, since he eats slowly, serve him his tray first and collect it last. The thoughtful nurse will prepare everything the patient needs for self-care and then let him proceed at his own pace to complete those aspects of care that he can tend to himself. Explanations of tests and treatments should be made slowly and, if necessary, repeated.

Even comparatively minor illnesses or injuries can have serious consequences for the older person, because they can tip the already precarious balance from independence to dependence. Often, the older individual unnecessarily gives up some of his usual activities, because others (and sometimes the patient himself) are too quick to assume that the patient will never be able to resume these activities.

Hospital Care. Recognizing that the older person is likely to have greater difficulty adapting to a hospital environment, the nurse can make his adaptation easier and less hazardous for him. The high beds are a potential danger, since the older person may misjudge the distance to the floor and fall as he is getting up. Hi-lo beds, which are adjustable, are ideal in permitting the ambulatory patient to get out of bed easily. If high beds are used, have a sturdy footstool in place. It is wise to leave a dim light burning in the older patient's room during the night so that he can more readily orient himself to his surroundings as he awakens, as well as avoid falling if he gets up. Some older persons need side rails at night to remind them where the edges of the bed are and to discourage attempts at getting out of bed. If these are necessary, always explain their use to the patient, so that he does not feel imprisoned in his bed. Make very certain that his call bell is handy; otherwise, he may try to climb over the side rails to go to the bathroom.

Older people usually do not require as much sleep as younger ones. Their need for less sleep may present a problem when a hospital room is shared with others. Keeping the patient awake and interested during the day often helps him to sleep better at night. If he awakens very early in the morning, encourage some quiet diversion, such as reading, so that he does not waken his roommates. Barbiturates often cause confusion and restlessness in aged patients. Whenever possible, it is preferable to encourage sleep by relying on general nursing measures than on drugs.

Even without the use of drugs, night-time confusion and disorientation are common among the elderly, and present a particular problem when an older person is moved away from his familiar surroundings, to a hospital or nursing home. These episodes of confusion, which are especially likely to occur at night, are disturbing to the patient and to others, and present a hazard to the patient's safety. Unfortunately, mismanagement of this problem is very common, leading to the patient's becoming more confused and disturbed. Initial reactions to the patient to *control* him and to lessen the noise he makes may be by such measures as scolding him and quickly closing the door of his room so that other patients are not awakened. Sometimes restraints, such as a Posey belt, are quickly applied before other measures are tried. These actions quite predictably increase the patient's agitation; he becomes more agitated and confused; at this point orders for sedation may be sought. The sedative itself sometimes exacerbates the problem. Often the use of restraints and sedatives can be avoided, and the patient can be calmed by nursing measures.*

If one of your aged patients becomes noisy and confused, go to him calmly, turn on a soft light (in addition to the night light, which should already be on), quietly explain where he is and who you are, and take hold of the patient's hand as a further measure in establishing contact with him. (Occasionally, touching the patient leads to further agitation. Note his reaction and guide your actions accordingly.) Often these episodes are precipitated when the patient awakens from a dream and has difficulty distinguishing between reality and the dream. Sometimes the episode is precipitated by the patient's awakening because he needs to void. Still half asleep, he attempts to get out of bed to go to the bathroom, notes the siderails which, especially in the dim light, can make him feel "caged in." Unfamiliar surroundings, plus the urgency of the need to void, can add to his mounting fright, and he calls out and becomes confused and agitated. The more that you can help the patient orient himself to his surroundings and to your presence, the calmer he is likely to become. After these initial measures which help the patient become calmer, ask him quietly what is troubling him. After these measures have been used, usually the patient's agitation diminishes enough so that he can realize what the difficulty is—such as that he needs the urinal, or that he had a frightening dream. If he speaks as though the dream *were* reality, such as by saying, "My son was just here," you can point out that it is the middle of the night,

---

* The following material concerning nursing intervention with the acutely confused elderly patient draws upon some material from an unpublished paper by Gertrude B. Ujhely, "The Aged Problem Patient in the General Hospital."

and that his son was not there, and ask him if perhaps it was a dream. Sometimes a glass of warm milk or a cup of tea has a calming effect, and further assists the patient to "place" himself in the real world. Usually these nursing actions will result in the patient's being ready to go back to sleep. Before you leave him, remind the patient of the location of his call bell, of the fact that you will leave his door open and the night light on, and that he should press his call bell whenever he needs you.

Measures to help the patient maintain his contact with reality are, of course, necessary at other time as well, and can serve to prevent somewhat the occurrence of episodes of acute confusion.

By talking with the patient, and finding ways to stimulate his interest and participation in activities, the nurse can help reduce his isolation and detachment. Rather than "routinely" bathing the patient, the nurse can encourage his observation and participation, by asking whether the water is comfortably warm, whether his skin feels dry, and so forth. Since most older people have diminished vision and hearing, it is particularly important to see that they have their glasses and (if used) their hearing aids, to help them become tuned in to the environment. Turning up the volume on the TV set, and obtaining books written in large print are examples of other measures which the nurse can take to help the patient maintain his sense of reality through contact with the environment.

The nurse's expectations have an important effect upon the patient. If the nurse expects her elderly patients to be disoriented and forgetful, they are more likely to be so. In contrast, the nurse who converses with her elderly patients in a way which shows she expects them to be capable of responding and remembering, is likely to foster this behavior. Much depends, of course, on the patient's capacities; it is essential to evaluate his abilities and to gear expectations realistically.

The nurse who speaks slowly and distinctly, and who presents one suggestion or request at a time, rather than a rapid barrage of instructions, is facilitating the older person's ability to respond, and showing she expects that he can do so. There is no quicker way for an older person to lose ability to care for himself than to be in a situation where he is treated as though this capacity has already been lost. The older person senses that he is no longer considered capable of managing such tasks as storing his dentures safely in the jar on his stand, or cleaning them himself; he gives over these self-care functions, which help him maintain some privacy, independence, and contact with reality. A vicious circle may ensue, in which the staff grow more impatient with the elderly person's detachment, less inclined to talk with him and encourage his participation, and he in turn turns more and more to his inner world of fantasy. Meaningful relationships are an important measure in helping the patient to maintain contact with reality; the relationship with the nurse can be significant. It is, however, difficult to bridge the gap between the generations.

The difficulty is increased if the nurse considers certain topics "taboo." For instance, some nurses believe that the aged should not talk about the past but, instead, must be engaged in conversation solely about present and future events. For many elderly persons, however, daily events are relatively insignificant compared with events in the past. Is it any wonder that a retired archeologist may sometimes prefer to reminisce about his explorations in far-off lands, rather than sticking to conversation about card parties held in the nursing home? One need of the aged involves assessing past events, achievements, and losses, and integrating these life experiences. The nurse who insists that the patient talk only of the present and future interferes with this task, in the mistaken belief that she is "keeping him from living in the past." The patient requires opportunities to talk about past, present, and future in ways that are useful to him. Sometimes nurses discourage patients from talking about death; nevertheless this is a major life experience which faces the elderly. Is it any wonder some of them wish to talk about it?

Caring for older people can be interesting and satisfying. Because they have lived so long, older people have had experiences very different from ours. The passage of time and the changes in our civilization make it unlikely that we shall ever have these experiences ourselves, but through association with older people we can share their experiences. Older people give a sense of continuity and stability amid the rapid changes of modern living. Because they are likely to adopt changes more slowly and cautiously, they can provide a balance for the impatience, the short-sightedness and the eagerness of youth. If we recognize that the older person has something valuable to contribute at home, at work and in his community, we can feel proud to have a part in helping him to maintain his health and to continue to make his unique contribution as long as possible.

REFERENCES AND BIBLIOGRAPHY

BIRREN, J. E., *et al.* (eds.): *Human Aging*, Washington, D.C., U.S. Department of Health, Education, and Welfare, 1963.

BRUDNO, J. J.: Group programs with adult offspring of newly admitted residents in a geriatric setting, *J. Am. Geriat. Soc.* 12:385, 1964.

CARNEY, R. G.: The aging skin, *Am. J. Nurs.* 63:110, June, 1963.

CLARK, M., and ANDERSON, B.: *Culture and Aging*, Springfield, Ill., Thomas, 1967.

CLEMENTS, A.: A geriatric day hospital serving a rural community, *Nurs. Times* 64:908, July, 1968.

CUMMING, E., and HENRY, W. F.: *Disengagement*, New York, Basic Books, 1961.

DAVIS, R. W.: Psychologic aspects of geriatric nursing, *Am. J. Nurs.* 68:802, April, 1968.

EISMAN, R.: Why did Joe die?, *Am. J. Nurs.* 71:501, March, 1971.

GERDES, L.: The confused or delirious patient, *Am. J. Nurs.* 68:1228, June, 1968.

HULICKA, I. M.: Fostering self-respect in aged patients, *Am. J. Nurs.* 64:84, March, 1964.

KURTAGH, C.: Nursing in the life span of people, *Nurs. Forum* 7:298, 1969.

LAMBERTSEN, E.: How can nurses function best in serving geriatric needs? *Mod. Hosp.* 111:124, July, 1968.

LARSON, L.: How to select a nursing home, *Am. J. Nurs.* 69:1034, May, 1969.

LEVINE, R. L.: Disengagement in the elderly—its causes and effects, *Nurs. Outlook* 17:28, Oct., 1969.

McFARLAND, R. A., *et al.*: On the driving of automobiles by older persons, *J. Geront.* 19:190, 1964.

MOODY, L., VIRGINIA BARON, GRACE MONK: Moving the past into the present, *Am. J. Nurs.* 70:2353, Nov. 1970.

NEUGARTEN, B. L.: Biological and psychological aspects of aging, in *Selected Readings in Aging*, St. Louis, Gerontological Society, 1968.

NEWTON, K., and ANDERSON, H.: *Geriatric Nursing*, ed. 4, St. Louis, Mosby, 1966.

RENDER, H. W.: My old age, *Nurs. Outlook* 12:31, November, 1964.

ROSEN, S., *et al.*: Presbycusis study of a relatively noise-free population in the Sudan, *Ann. Otol.* 71:727, 1962.

ROSS, E. K.: *On Death and Dying*, New York, Macmillan, 1969.

————: What is it like to be dying?, *Am. J. Nurs.* 71:54, Jan. 1971.

SCHWARTZ, D., HENLEY, B., and ZEITZ, L.: *The Elderly Ambulatory Patient*, New York, Macmillan, 1964.

SHANAS, E.: *The Health of Older People*, Cambridge, Harvard University Press, 1962.

SHANAS, E., *et al.*: *Old People in Three Industrial Societies*, New York, Atherton Press, 1968.

TAYLOR, J., and GAITZ, C.: Obstacles encountered in the rehabilitation of geriatric patients, *Nurs. Forum* 7:64, 1969.

UJHELY, G. B.: The aged problem patient in the general hospital. Paper presented at Bridgeport Hospital, Bridgeport, Conn., 1967. (Unpublished)

U.S. DEPT. HEALTH, EDUCATION, & WELFARE, and THE FEDERAL COUNCIL ON AGING: *1961 White House Conference on Aging Chart Book*, Washington, D.C., U.S. Government Printing Office.

WAHL, A.: Who are the elderly? In *Selected Readings in Aging*, St. Louis, Gerontological Society, 1968.

WEISS, A.: *Nurses, Patients, and Social Systems*, Columbia, Missouri, University of Missouri Press, 1968.

WOLFF, K.: The Elder Patient, *J. Am. Geriat. Soc.* 15:575, 1967.

YALOM, I., and TERRAZAS, F.: Group therapy for psychotic elderly patients, *Am. J. Nurs.* 68:1690, August, 1968.

ZORZOLI, A.: Biomedical factors in aging, in *Selected Readings in Aging*, St. Louis, Gerontological Society, 1968.

Nurse-Patient Relationships

5

Some Basic Concepts · Brief Nurse-Patient Relationships
Supporting the Patient During Tests and Treatments · Sustained
Nurse-Patient Relationships · Other Considerations · Guarding
Against Suicide · Patients' Complaints · The Patient Who Is
Physically Unappealing · The "Self-Care" Patient · The Patient Who
Is Unconscious · The Patient Who Refuses His Treatment · Families

As you work with adult medical-surgical patients, you may wonder how you can adapt your general knowledge about nurse-patient relationships to the particular requirements of this group of patients. Here are some guidelines:

• In most instances the medical-surgical patient has sought care for some physical condition; this condition may, of course, be aggravated by emotional stress, or even be caused by it. Usually, however, the patient's attention, and the focus of his treatment, are on his bodily ailment. Keeping in mind that the patient's attention is usually on his physical condition, and that he is not primarily concerned with seeking personal counseling will help you set the tone for your relationship with him. Your ability to give emotional support and counseling will be enhanced by recognition of the patient's view of why he is seeking treatment (to control the bleeding of his peptic ulcer, for example).

• Caring for medical-surgical patients requires a high degree of ability to consider both the physical care of the patient and his emotional reactions to illness and treatment. Often you will be able to combine these two aspects of care, particularly as you gain more experience. You will find that you can listen to the patient while you bathe him or make his bed, as well as during the times when you sit down to talk with him. Also, the way that you provide physical care constitutes an important aspect of your relationship with the patient. Is your touch rough or gentle? When you assist him out of bed, do your motions convey firmness and support, or are they gingerly and hesitant?

• Remember that others, too, may be giving the patient emotional support. Keeping this in mind will help you to maintain perspective about your relationship with the patient, so that you are less likely to conclude that supporting him emotionally is solely up to you. This is rarely the case. Particularly in the general hospital, many patients keep in touch with relatives, clergy, and friends, as well as with a personal physician. In long-term and geriatric settings the patient is likely to be more isolated from contact with other significant persons. Usually, however, you are *one* of the people to whom a patient may turn with emotional problems. If he turns to others, primarily, it is by no means necessarily an adverse reflection on the care you give. If you interpret it as such, you may interfere with the patient's relationships with others at a time when he particularly needs to maintain his ties with them.

• Frightening and painful procedures are common on medical-surgical units. Although at first you are a stranger to the patient, the stress of experiences such as undergoing surgery can lead the patient to rely on you more quickly and more fully for emotional support than would be likely if he were not faced with these experiences.

• Medical-surgical patients are often more outwardly poised than is likely to be the case among pediatric, geriatric, or psychiatric patients. One of your challenges in working with this group of patients will involve helping them maintain poise in stressful circumstances (when the patient shows that to do so is important to him), but also encouraging expression of personal feelings.

• Care of medical-surgical patients involves a good deal of physical contact. Be alert for the slight tensing of muscles which enables you to feel, rather than see, that the patient does not welcome being touched. If you notice this reaction, be especially deft and quick in your ministrations. Avoid leaning over him as you bathe him and make the bed. People vary in the amount of physical closeness they can tolerate without discomfort. If a person is up and about, he can step back when others stand too close. However, the patient confined to bed must rely on others' perceptiveness of his reactions.

• There is enormous variety among medical-surgical patients: variety of age, diagnosis, and degree of illness—to name but three variables. Some of your patients will be completely helpless; others will seem able to care for themselves. Your approaches to these groups of patients will be different.

You may be better at one mode of care than others. Working with a patient who is relatively self-sufficient may be more satisfying than working with a patient who is comparatively helpless. Or perhaps it is the other way around. The most important thing is that you know in which situation you are most comfortable. The more realistically you are aware of your own needs, the better care you will be able to give to all your patients.

Eventually, you will be able to choose the work in which your own goals and needs are met best. In the meantime you have to function in all kinds of situations. The more flexible you can be, the more service you will be able to give your patients, and the more satisfaction you will have from a job well done.

The following points will help you review some basic guidelines for nurse-patient relationships applicable in any setting:

• Be yourself. You can borrow technics from someone you admire, but do not try to imitate someone else. Sick people are perceptive, anxious and suspicious, even if they do not show it. If they feel your genuineness, they will be better able to trust you.

• Small points of care are important to the sick. Reactions to something as personal as ill-ness are not always logical and rational. The big fact of recovering may be lost in the little annoyance of being served cold coffee. But if the patient *feels* your interest in him, your concern for his welfare and comfort, he is less likely to become angry.

• Size up the situation between your patient and yourself. Do not rush in with too many busy activities at once, unless they are of vital necessity to the patient. Learn early in your career to get the feel of your patient. What is his general condition? What is he expressing? Is he in pain? Does he seem to be resigned or apprehensive? What does his attitude do to you? Can you accept it, or do you feel a need to change it? If a patient looks as if he were sinking because he has slipped down in bed, of course you will want to change this position by lifting him up. However, if he is angry or whiny, can you accept this mood and not deny him his feelings? Sometimes it helps to start the day's relationship by an objective bland phrase like "How did you sleep?"

A question like "Well, how are things going?" will give the patient an opening, and if you quietly wait or in an unbusy fashion go about your business at the bedside, he may start talking to you. Don't expect to be reassured by the patient. If he says, "Fine," but does not look as if he meant it, do not say, "Good," because again you would be cutting him off from expressing how he really feels. It often helps to repeat the patient's statement or to summarize it. This response will give him an opening to say more, if he wishes. To put your patient in the position of having to say what he thinks is expected of him is undesirable, because this might not correspond at all to his true feelings. It is all too easy to indicate to a patient what he *should* feel, and he will often parrot back what he thinks the nurse wants to hear.

Accept the statement that he feels terrible. You might reflect, "You don't feel well today?" If you try to talk him out of the way he feels, to cheer him up, he will have a new problem besides his original difficulty. He may feel guilty for not having lived up to the nurse's expectation. Learn from the beginning that if a patient is unhappy and says he is unhappy, you, personally, do not have to solve all of his problems. You may be able to help him, but your assistance will consist of helping him to help himself.

• Besides giving the expert technical care that gradually you will learn to give, there are several ways in which you can help your patient by the relationship you establish with him. One is to help him gather as many facts as possible about his situation so that he can make reasonable decisions. Another is to teach him new skills with which he can help himself either to live with or to recover from his illness. And, particularly important, you can support him as he goes through the various stages of illness and recovery.

• If the patient asks no questions and discusses none of his feelings with you, do not pry; but do not assume that he understands all, or that he has perceived nothing of what is going on around him. If it appears that he wants to know, explain treatments and tell him what to expect, so that he can use the information to orient himself to his new surroundings. But do not urge discussion on the unwilling patient.

• Such trivial reassuring clichés as "Don't worry" and "Everything will be all right" mean the same thing to a patient as "I don't want to hear about your troubles." If your patient says that he is worried or does not feel well, he has opened the door to expression of his feelings. If the nurse unperceptively pushes aside his remark by saying something like "Everything will be fine," she shuts the door, thus avoiding involvement but leaving the patient to cope with his feelings alone.

• Accept every patient as an adult who perhaps momentarily must be cared for physically as a baby. But *never talk down to a patient.* Just because a man is lying in bed instead of standing up is no reason to resort to the use of patronizing expressions, particularly the "we" which is notorious in the nursing profession. ("Now we're going to have a bath.")

• At the same time be generous with gentle ministrations. A patient needs to feel that someone cares about him.

• Never smother a patient with the kind of attention that retards his ability to do as much for himself as he can.

• When a patient is angry, let him be. He may not be angry with you, even though it is you he is scolding. Although crankiness is hard on others, it is often better for the patient than swallowing his anger and getting indigestion or worse from it. However, this depends on the patient and on the situation. Some people are more comfortable when helped to preserve their aplomb. To perceive these differences is a difficult but important part of nursing.

• Your relationships with patients will be affected not only by your concept of yourself as a nurse, but also by the patient's image of you as a nurse. When he enters the hospital, whether or not he has been hospitalized previously, he has some preconceived expectations about you. Based on stories he has heard, his reading, television and his own past experiences, he may think of nurses in a stereotyped way, considering them to be cold and heartless, or sweet and giving, ministering angels or otherwise. To a surprising extent the patient's reaction to the hospital will be governed by such notions. The newly admitted patient who expects the nurse to be gentle with him and take good care of him will behave differently from the patient who thinks of the nurse as a maid in a white uniform; both will act differently from the patient who expects the nurse to ignore him.

SOME BASIC CONCEPTS

Terms such as anger and anxiety are commonplace. Most of us have become so accustomed to these words that we sometimes use them loosely. What is the difference between fear and anxiety, for example? In the following section we shall briefly discuss the following terms: anxiety, frustration and anger, conflict, and grief.

Anxiety

Anxiety is different from fear. The person who is afraid usually can identify the cause of his fear. His knees may tremble after a narrow escape from an auto crash; trembling and a pounding heart are natural reactions to danger. In anxiety the external circumstance is identified less clearly. Often the patient feels uneasy, or he has a general feeling of impending unpleasantness or disaster but is unable to explain why he feels this way. The patient is usually not aware of the underlying cause of his anxiety, although he may be aware of situations which precipitate it. Because the patient is often unable to identify the cause of his anxiety, he frequently feels helpless and overwhelmed.

Anxiety has been defined in various ways: as an energy, and as an emotional response without a specific object; as a response to a threat to one's self respect and to the respect in which one is held by others (May). There are many facets to the concept of anxiety, of which these are but a few. Threats to survival, whether physical survival or survival as an integrated personality, elicit profound anxiety. You will observe anxiety among patients who have emphysema and coronary artery disease, for example.

The levels of anxiety vary from mild (1+) to panic level (4+). In mild anxiety the individual's ability to observe is heightened; this ability is reduced in moderate and severe anxiety, and the individual tends to focus on details. In mild anxiety the individual's ability to perceive relationships between events is enhanced; as anxiety becomes more severe, he progressively loses this ability. Ability to learn is enhanced by mild anxiety, but is impaired in moderate and severe anxiety. In panic level anxiety the individual may describe feelings of "disintegrating" or being swept away." It is important to realize that, whatever the individual's physical capacities, he is helpless while in the grip of this degree of anxiety, and requires assistance to reduce the anxiety to more manageable levels. Staying with him is one measure which is useful. Listening to him is another. He may speak of one detail, and this in distorted fashion. As the nurse listens, and as the patient becomes somewhat less anxious, he begins to "put together" in a more coherent way what he is trying to communicate, thus enabling the nurse to respond. A severely anxious person is sometimes helped by being asked to concentrate on a detail, such as counting, or by physical activity, such as walking or rocking.

We know that when a person is very anxious, he cannot see all aspects of a problem. He tends to see and to magnify only a single detail or a few details, and sometimes he makes the wrong connections. An anxious person often becomes confused and unable to follow directions or the explanation given to him about a treatment.

Avoid cutting off your patients when they begin to talk. Although verbalizing does not in itself relieve anxiety, it can be the beginning of understanding. The problem does not automatically disappear when it is understood; on the other hand, it never will be solved until it is understood. Letting a patient talk opens the way to understanding and dealing with problems. Sometimes a patient can recognize the need for further, more expert help.

The competent nurse knows when not to pursue the matter. For example, when her skills are not adequate for the amount of help the patient seems to need (in which case she assists him to find someone who is sufficiently skilled to help him), or when other factors, such as the patient's physical condition, make further discussion of anxiety-producing material unwise at that time. A patient who has just suffered myocardial infarction may, as he speaks of his recent close encounter with death, experience an increased pulse rate, restlessness, and may show signs of increasing ventricular irritability on the EKG monitor. In such circumstances the wise nurse will not encourage the patient to explore the problem further, but will suggest that the patient save further discussion until later. (After saying this, it is important for the nurse to make herself available to the patient later, when his physical condition has improved, so that "talking later" does not become a way of avoiding listening to the patient.) In the situation just described, administration of a "p.r.n." order for sedation may also be appropriate, in order to alleviate physiologic manifestations of anxiety which are particularly hazardous to a patient who has experienced recent myocardial infarction.

There are other times when it is not helpful to encourage a patient to look more closely at his problems. In these instances, instead of an approach which conveys, "Tell me more about it," measures can be used that support the patient in other ways and help him through the crisis. When a patient has a life-threatening physical need and is also terrified, attention must be given first to the physical need; psychological needs can be considered after the emergency is over. Thus, when a patient hemorrhages, all concentration must be directed first toward stopping the flow of blood. The competence with which the nurse acts will aid the patient to control, if not to understand, his fear. When a patient is in pain, the pain should be relieved, if possible, before consideration is given to how he reacts to it. Attention to physical needs is one way of communicating support to the patient. Ignoring physical needs, even such simple ones as giving fresh water or lowering the bed to a more comfortable position, is a way of telling the patient that no one cares and of increasing his anxiety. Words should not be used when action is more appropriate.

Recognize that you are a stranger to the patient. He is not likely to discuss all his thoughts with you; nor should he. Talking about some problems can help the patient to feel less alone with the other problems—often the main ones—that he does not talk about. Erroneously, it is assumed frequently that the patient is revealing his innermost thoughts, but this assumption is rarely true, particularly when the relationship between the nurse and the patient has been brief.

Some patients prefer not to discuss their emotional problems with the nurse, and the nurse should respect their wish for privacy. The nurse's need to help should be tempered by an understanding of what will bring relief to the particular patient. Some patients find it most helpful for the nurse to give support in nonverbal ways; others are benefited if they are encouraged to talk about how they feel.

Sometimes, because the patient's anxiety is so great, he bursts out with a flow of emotion-laden personal concerns even when your contact with him has been relatively brief. The patient may later worry over telling you so much about his personal life. Stay with him and listen supportively during his period of distress, but avoid questioning the patient or encouraging him at this time to go on. When the patient is calmer and has had a chance to think over what he has told you, he will be better able to assess what topics (if any) he wants to pursue. Under such circumstances the patient may seem embarrassed when he sees you later. Let him bring up the subject of his outburst if he wishes, but do not initiate the discussion. Show, by the way you care for him, that you think none the less of him because of the incident.

Dealing with Your Own Anxiety

What are some of the things you can do when you become anxious? If you can, leave the situation for a moment to collect yourself and think it through. However, there are times when you cannot leave; for instance, the patient may be bleeding. Try to concentrate on some concrete, helpful thing you can do. Hold a compress in place, or empty the emesis basin or take the patient's pulse. These actions give you time to think what to do next.

Merely learning to recognize when you are anxious often will keep you from being helpless in the grip of anxiety. When you know you are anxious—except in an emergency—stop! Think the situation through. Find help; do not race blindly ahead with what you are doing. At such times the patient gets the wrong medication, or the side rail is left down, so that he falls out of bed. Every person who deals with helpless people has the responsibility to stop work when he is unable to function. Extreme anxiety can keep one from functioning and make one a hazard. So can physical illness or excessive loss of sleep.

None of these "excuses" is accepted legally if a patient is harmed.

Knowledge and competence are an insurance against anxiety. If you do not know the proper procedure so well that it is almost automatic, you may become anxious when you find yourself fumbling. Do you know what to do if a patient has a convulsion, if he faints, if he turns blue, if he bleeds, if a fire starts? Go over the procedures so that you know them when you need them. Are you skilled in handling oxygen? When you need it in a hurry, will you be able to remember which handle does what? Can your hands manage the suction tubing so well that you can keep your eyes on the patient if he starts to choke? Do you know the locations of the fire extinguishers on the ward in which you are working now—and how to operate them?

On the other hand, do not expect too much of yourself. As you learn new things, you will have moments of insecurity. Just as the patient who is anxious concentrates on smaller and smaller details, you, too, will find that your ability to perceive the whole situation narrows with anxiety and grows with the increase of knowledge and capability. The first time you gave an enema you probably concentrated so hard on the tubing that you may not have remembered to see whether or not the patient was comfortable. As you become more at ease with the technic, you can extend what you see to include the patient. The only way not to be bound, fettered and enslaved by technical skills is to master them.

Frustration and Anger

What happens in frustration? A person sets a goal, but some barrier prevents its fulfillment. The result is frustration, which is made up of feelings of helplessness and anger. The amount of frustration one feels is dependent on how important the goal was, what similar past experiences the person has had, and how he handles feelings of helplessness and anger. If a nurse's goal is to see her patient well, she is thwarted when instead he gets sicker. If she thinks to herself that this patient's recovery is a test of her worth as a nurse, and he gets sicker in spite of everything she does, she will become more frustrated than if she had never set up this unrealistic test. A patient who fails to walk well on his new artificial leg will be frustrated, especially if his job depends on his ability to walk well. We do not always know what goals another has set for himself. Therefore, we cannot assume that the failure that does not frustrate one person will not frustrate another. One patient may be thrilled to find that he can walk around his bed; another may be dismayed to find that he will be barred from entering an athletic contest.

Frustration ends in anger. You are lucky when you are aware of anger, because then you can trace it to its origin and decide what to do. You can evaluate the goal and the barrier. Perhaps you will lower the goal (make the patient comfortable instead of trying to cure him), modify the barrier (assist in research on new methods of dealing with that disease) or attempt to circumvent the barrier by using new skills.

People can become very angry and not know it. Anger becomes subconscious when a person has to hide from himself the fact that he is angry. The anger may be too painful to face; it may interfere with the picture the person has formed of himself. Unknown anger that is still present as psychic energy is harder to handle because one does not know of its existence. Suppose the nurse's frustration at having the patient get sicker rather than better is what has made her angry; but to be aware of her anger would hurt her view of herself as a gentle person. She may be angry with the patient for not responding to her ministrations; or with herself for setting up an unattainable goal; or at the existence of incurable illness; or with the head nurse, whose assignment to this patient has led to frustration. She may take a great dislike to the patient for reasons which appear to her to originate in him. For instance, she may disagree with his outlook on life, she may blame his decline on his lack of will to live, or she may become irritated by the tone of his voice. She is trying to set up a logical reason for her anger. She is rationalizing her anger and projecting its cause from herself to the patient. Rationalization is a common mechanism which all use at times.

The trouble with feelings and reactions of which one is not aware is that they complicate and obscure the situation without offering a rational solution to the problem. Acknowledge to yourself that you are angry, when you are. Sometimes anger has a perfectly legitimate basis, and at such times the expression of it is justifiable. The more realistically you can accept anger in yourself, the better you will be able to accept it in your patients. If you can say, "I'm furious, and it's all right to feel that way," you will be more able to say, "He's furious, and it's not bad to feel that way." Then you can proceed to handle the anger-provoking situation more rationally and realistically.

Patients have many reasons for being angry. Just being sick is frustrating. To be sick and in the hospital is bad enough, but worse yet, one has to pay for it! Restriction of activity, such as that imposed by an illness or disability, is frustrating. Being unable to control the most ordinary daily routines, such as getting a hot cup of coffee, brushing one's teeth or urinating, is frustrating. The confinement to a room or a small space in a ward makes smaller and smaller details more and more important.

A patient may become angry with you. The anger from his frustration may be projected to you, so that he may disagree with your outlook on life, blame his decline on your lack of care and bristle at the tones in your voice. You are taking the brunt of the patient's unrecognized, subconscious anger at being ill, disabled or helpless. All of us prefer to be treated kindly rather than gruffly, to be liked and appreciated. It is hard not to be hurt by anger, even if we suspect that its cause is elsewhere, or that it is a cover for fear.

What can you do about such a situation? Hostility is often met with hostility. The patient is angry with you, and so you get angry with him. This reaction does not lead to any constructive end. What else can you do? You can accept the emotion, and perhaps your acceptance of it will lead the patient to accept it himself. Act as a mirror for the expression of his feelings. Let him talk. Help him to talk. If he feels angry, he has a reason for it, and it is often better for all concerned for him not to simmer silently, but to talk about what bothers him. If he is angry but does not show it outwardly, it does not mean that the anger has gone away. You can say, "Do you want to tell me about it, Mr. Johnson?" The angry patient may try to line you up on his side against a doctor or another nurse. Avoid taking sides, but do not avoid the patient's feelings. Encourage him to talk freely. Perhaps you will get to the heart of the matter.

Some of the things about which the patient expresses anger can be remedied. Try to see that he receives hot coffee if cold coffee is one of the things which make him angry. Many of the main causes of anger, however, cannot be remedied. If the patient must remain in traction for 6 weeks, and therefore misses a long-awaited trip, then there is nothing he or anyone else can do about changing the situation. In addition to giving your patient opportunities to express his anger, help him to find activities to help use up the excess energy mobilized by anger. Physical activity is especially beneficial. The patient with a lower limb in traction can still exercise his arms; these exercises can be useful not only in preparing him for crutch-walking, but also in using some pent-up energy engendered by anger, thus helping him to relax.

There may be times when you will become angry with a patient. It is nothing to be ashamed of. You are human, too. Even a superior nurse will lose her temper occasionally. When it happens, accept it in yourself and talk it over with someone else. What frustrated you? What touched off your hostility? Are your goals too high? Is there some way to get under, around, through or over the barrier? Work your way out of the trouble spots by being aware of your own feelings.

Conflict

The medical-surgical patient is often confronted with making decisions which have far-reaching consequences, and often he is expected to arrive at his decision promptly. Such situations set the stage for conflict—the patient feels torn between opposing goals. It is not uncommon for patients to have to choose "the lesser of two evils"; sometimes neither alternative is really desirable, and the question revolves around which choice has the most assets. Often the situation is complicated by the fact that no one can predict, for certain, just what the outcome of a particular treatment will be. Nevertheless, the patient must reach a decision. The nurse can act as a sounding board while the patient expresses the conflict and considers the alternatives.

When a patient is in conflict, it is important to help him get the necessary information to help him in decision making. It is also important not to try to make the decision for the patient. Realistic time pressures of course do exist; there may be only 10 minutes in which to make a decision, for example, if a patient is bleeding and requires surgery to stop the loss of blood. Avoid intensifying the time pressure beyond what is required by the situation, however.

Grief

Grief is a reaction to loss of someone or something significant to the individual. Loss of spouse, job, a body part or a capacity, are examples.

Engel has described stages through which an individual moves during normal grief. First is the stage of shock or disbelief. A woman whose husband had just died, held a straw to his lips and told him to sip the water. Her actions denied the truth of the situation, which was too hard for her to bear. The next stage involves gradual awareness of the reality of the loss. The individual experiences the pain of bereavement, anger (at oneself, at others, and at the lost person for his departure), crying, withdrawal of interest in other people and in the surroundings. Often there are feelings of emptiness, listlessness, and lack of appetite. The final stage is of restitution or recovery, when the individual renews his interest in other people and in his work, and feels a resurgence of vigor and sense of purpose in his undertakings. The duration of the grief process is variable, from a few weeks to as long as a year. Its duration and severity depend on such factors as the significance and magnitude of the loss for the individual, his capacity to deal with it, and the resources he has to sustain him during crises, such as job, family, and friends.

Think of patients you have cared for who have lost functions or body parts and see whether you note similarities to the process just described. Crying is a usual reaction following removal of a breast, for example. Unless one considers the fact that the patient has come up against a serious loss, her tears may be ascribed to babyishness, or to inability to tolerate pain. What can you do to help patients who are experiencing grief? Remember that the patient cannot be hastened through the various stages, nor can he skip over them. In fact, premature efforts to help him see the bright side, and to move ahead with rehabilitation, may only make him feel more alone and more despondent. If, instead, you can recognize the stage of grief that your patient is in, and support him as he experiences it, you will be more likely to help him move on to the next stage. For instance, a patient with partial aphasia following a stroke may be seething with frustration and anger over impairment of his ability to speak. The nurse who is sensitive to the patient's reactions will be concerned when the patient bangs down his book of speech exercises and, instead of ignoring the behavior or giving him a lecture, will take the time to listen and try to understand what the patient is attempting to communicate. Allowing him to express frustration and anger and acknowledging that he is confronted with a frustrating experience helps the patient to feel less alone, and to move on through the remaining stages of grief.

Not all patients move through grief successfully. Some become immobilized, as it were, in one stage of grief and are unable to move forward and utilize the abilities and opportunities which are open to them. It is important for the nurse to recognize when a patient seems to be reacting this way and to discuss her observation with the physician. Often such patients require the help of a psychiatrist to aid them in dealing with the problem.

Do not expect your patients to move smoothly forward through stages of grief, however. Progress is usually uneven; this in turn adds to the patient's discouragement. Sometimes, after a day of feeling his strength and interest in recovery returning, he will revert to an attitude of hopelessness. Recognize that this does not necessarily signify defeat, and help the patient to realize that the process of recovery from any significant loss is usually uneven.

Remember too that the patient grieves for what is important to him, and for those he loves, regardless of the yardstick society uses to measure the appropriateness of his reactions. Physicians and nurses often have mental yardsticks which they use to measure the appropriateness of patients' reactions, and which often blind them to what an experience means to a patient. Losses have very personal meanings to the individual who experiences them. The patient's reaction is also affected by the magnitude of other serious losses in his life, how well he has recovered from them, and his personal resources and assets. For the elderly lady who has outlived all of her relatives and close friends, the death of a beloved pet during her hospitalization may be overwhelming, while for a patient with family and friends and a challenging career the loss of a pet, although painful, may not constitute a major loss. Likewise, one patient may seem withdrawn and apathetic for months following removal of a gangrenous toe, while another patient may, a few weeks following amputation of his leg, begin learning to use his artificial limb, and start making plans to return to work.

BRIEF NURSE-PATIENT RELATIONSHIPS

As you work with medical-surgical patients you will find that your contact with some of them is limited to one 10 to 15 minute period. Your first reaction may be that 10–15 minutes do not count for anything in a relationship.

Think about it again. Have you ever had an experience in which the brief response of another person was very important to you, even though you never saw the person again? Suppose there has been a car accident. The way the policeman responds to the people who are involved is important to them at that time, and it may also affect their reactions to future situations in which they must call for help.

The patient who enters the emergency room terrified of the bleeding and pain of a scalp laceration may remember years afterward the nurse's calmness and skill, her sureness as she touched the wound, and the way she helped him gather his own strength. The nurse who can establish this kind of relationship with a patient not only helps him over the immediate crisis, but fosters his ability to respond to others who care for him later. Nurses in the operating room and recovery room are also among those whose contacts with patients are brief, but whose relationships with patients are especially important because of the patient's vulnerability during these experiences. What are some measures which help the nurse to develop a supportive relationship with a patient during a brief period? (Some of these points are also applicable to caring for patients during diagnostic and therapeutic procedures; see below.)

• Concentrate on what the patient is going through. Avoid social clichés which are not only meaningless but often offensive in such situations, because they imply denial of the stressful experience the patient is facing. At such times the patient needs to focus his energy on the situation at hand; he should not be expected to divert some of it into an effort to be sociable.

• Diverting the patient's attention toward some concrete action or observation is different from merely expecting him to socialize. The patient recognizes this difference by the context of the relationship which the nurse establishes with him. One nurse talked on and on to a patient undergoing initial treatment in the emergency room. She asked where he lived, how many children he had, what kind of work he did—all in the tone one would use when making a new acquaintance. Another nurse was helping care for a woman who had been in an automobile accident. When the nurse saw that what the physician was about to do would be painful, such as cleaning the wound or suturing, she said to the patient, "Now look at me, and squeeze my hand hard. It's going to hurt for a minute." Sometimes a patient is helped by being asked to count aloud, thus giving him something specific to concentrate on when he is anxious and in pain. The essential ingredient in all these situations is the patient's feeling of support and encouragement from the nurse.

• Establish some physical contact and eye contact with the patient. (Occasionally your patient will show that he does not welcome physical contact, in which case it should be kept to a minimum.) Gently placing your hand on the patient's shoulder may be more appropriate and more effective in some instances than verbal reassurance.

• Have your equipment handy, neat, and in good condition. You cannot concentrate on the patient if you are frantically hunting for a sterile syringe of the proper size. Also, remember that an environment which is orderly and clean can increase the patient's confidence in his care.

• Perform your technical skills with as much confidence and dexterity as possible. If some of them are new to you, practice away from the patient until you gain proficiency.

• Be alert to the patient's physiologic, as well as his emotional, reactions. Are his lips becoming cyanotic? Did his pulse rate just increase by 20 beats?

You may ask, "But how can anyone attend to so many things at once?" You will find that, with experience, you do observe many things almost automatically. You don't have to tell yourself, "Check the pulse; observe skin color." You will just *do* these things, and as you become more quickly responsive to various indices of the patient's condition, you will find that you are more alert to danger signals in the patient's physiologic and emotional state.

SUPPORTING THE PATIENT DURING TESTS AND TREATMENTS

Usually the nurse has primary responsibility for providing emotional support and observing the patient's response during various procedures, such as paracentesis, liver biopsy, or reduction of a fracture.

However routine such procedures may seem to professional staff, they usually represent stressful experiences for the patient. The points discussed in the preceding section concerning care of the patient in short-term situations, such as the emergency room and the recovery room, are also applicable to reassuring patients during various procedures which they must undergo. Additional considerations will be discussed here.

Collaborating with the Physician

The physician, nurse, and patient are typically the three persons involved during various procedures, although of course additional personnel may be required for more complex procedures such as renal dialysis. The primary focus of each of the three people is different; the interaction among them is important. The physician concentrates on the procedure, although this does not mean, of course, that he ignores the patient. Nevertheless, the main focus of his attention must be on performing the procedure. The patient's role involves getting through a painful, humiliating, frightening, or sometimes simply tedious experience with the best grace possible. The nurse functions in two roles, which may be complementary or antagonistic to each other, depending upon how she handles the situation. She supports the patient: positioning him, observing him, encouraging him. She also assists the physician by providing necessary equipment, holding test tubes, and so on. The patient's confidence is increased if nurse and physician are collaborating and genuinely appear to respect each other. One very obvious (but frequently ignored) aspect of this collaboration involves avoiding any conversation between physician and nurse during the procedure, which does not pertain to the patient's immediate care. It is not uncommon for doctors and nurses to use social conversation to ease the tension of a situation, or even to use the time to catch up on sharing information and plans about other patients' care. Do your part to avoid such conversations in front of patients. On the other hand, some procedures, particularly if the patient is already experienced with them, are not so taxing to the patient nor so demanding of staff that light conversation is out of place. Fortunately, not all procedures are performed in a solemn atmosphere. The patient may welcome the light-hearted banter which can help the time pass more quickly while he is waiting for the paracentesis to be finished. Take your cues from the patient's mood and reactions. Be sure, though, to include him in whatever light conversation seems appropriate.

The patient is usually super-sensitive to tension between the physician and nurse, since his welfare so clearly depends upon their ability to work together. Two common causes of friction between the nurse and physician involve adequacy and working order of equipment, and the preparation of the patient for the procedure. Make it a practice never to begin a procedure (especially if you have not worked with that doctor before) without requesting him to note the equipment you have prepared, and asking him whether anything additional, or different, is needed. This step will help avoid tension during the procedure which stems from requests for additional or different equipment. Particularly if the procedure proves difficult (such as a lumbar puncture, in which the spinal fluid is difficult to obtain), a minor problem with equipment may assume major proportions as physician and nurse vent their tension and frustration over the situation, thus causing the patient additional worry and strain. It is also important to mention to the physician prior to the test, what preparation the patient has had. For example, prior to proctoscopy you might say, "Mrs. Jones had the three enemas you ordered. The first two were returned with formed stool; the last one was returned clear." This will lessen the likelihood of discussing the adequacy of the patient's preparation during the procedure—such discussion held in front of the patient can seriously shake the patient's confidence.

The roles of assisting the physician and supporting the patient can be complementary ones in the hands of a skillful nurse. The way she has things ready and moves quickly and confidently to help the doctor is important in reassuring the patient, just as is her gentleness with the patient, her reminder to take a deep breath and relax, or her pronouncement of the welcome words, "We're almost finished." The more careful you have been to make certain all the equipment is ready and in working order, the less it will absorb your attention, however, and the more you will be able to concentrate on the patient. Flexibility is essential as you work with the physician. Of course, this does not mean that you insert the lumbar puncture needle, but it does mean that you are able to notice, and do, the many things which are needed to help the procedure go smoothly. Concentrate on what you see needs to be done, whether it is tilting the light, mopping perspiration from the doctor's forehead, or holding the patient's hand.

Concentrating on the Patient's Reactions

Often the nurse has a tendency to concentrate on assisting the physician, rather than combining this role with supporting the patient. What may be some reasons for this? It is frequently disquieting to observe another person's response to a painful procedure. The woman having a pelvic examination is often tense and embarrassed. Often it is less taxing for the nurse to turn her attention away from the patient, to concentrate on the slides for the Pap smear. Many nurses, perhaps, are acutely aware themselves of the distress of this procedure when they have undergone it. Sometimes, if the nurse has not personally experienced the procedure, she may exaggerate the discomfort the patient is actually experiencing, and withdraw from the patient on the basis of her erroneous perception of what he is going through. Sometimes the nurse ignores the patient because his behavior during the test does not meet her standards of stoicism. To see another person lose composure is disquieting, because the potential for similar behavior lies within all of us. The nurse is likely to be more vulnerable to experiencing anxiety as a result of these factors than is the physician, since the procedure holds his attention.

Routinization of the procedure is another problem more acute for the nurse than for the doctor. Unless the nurse concentrates on the patient's reaction, the assisting role can become quite routine, particularly if one repeatedly helps with the same tests. For example, there is little difference from one patient to another in the preparation of equipment for "routine" pelvic examination. While the physician has some variety by focusing on possible pathology (Is the cervix eroded? Are there tumors?), the preparation and cleaning up of equipment can be almost identical from one patient to another. In order to avoid falling into a highly routinized approach, it is essential for the nurse to concentrate on the patient's reaction. Each patient will respond somewhat differently and require a slightly different approach.

Another possible reason for nurses' tendency to over-emphasize assisting the physician may have to do with prestige. Society accords greatest prestige to the physician, and to the highly technical skills he performs. Therefore, the nurse may view assisting the physician as more prestigious and basically more important than supporting the patient.

Failure to provide emotional support during the stress of diagnostic tests and treatments may merely leave some patients angry and critical of this aspect of their care; others for whom emotional support is crucial are lost to treatment, or suffer serious emotional disorders precipitated by their illness and its treatment. (Of course, not all such reactions can be prevented, even by the most skillful support from the nurse and physician.) If, by your support and encouragement, you enable a patient to keep on with a series of painful procedures until he has opportunity to benefit from them, is this not just as important as performing the procedure?

SUSTAINED NURSE-PATIENT RELATIONSHIPS

Working with long-term patients provides many satisfactions; it also poses some problems. While you have the satisfaction of seeing some of your patients improve, others for various reasons will remain unchanged, or even get sicker. You will be called upon to continue working with the patient and family during extended periods often marked by exacerbations and remissions of the illness.

Maintaining a professional role with the patient presents additional challenges. Because you have known him for a long time, it may be difficult for you to differentiate between a professional role and a social role. There is also greater likelihood, because of your familiarity with family problems, of becoming a protagonist for one family member or another, rather than helping the family to assess problems and deal with them.

Long-term patients in the general hospital often get lost in the shuffle. The acutely ill surgical patient, for example, or the accident victim claim staff's time and attention in a way that an elderly man with chronic congestive heart failure may not. As you work in the general hospital, be alert to the special requirements of long-term patients. Are there activities on your ward in which they can participate, such as use of a library, playing cards and so on? Is there a place where the patient can eat his meals out of bed, with others, if he is able?

As you work with these patients, avoid reminding them that others are sicker and require more of your time. The long-term patient typically has significant problems in adapting to the restrictions imposed by his illness. Listening to these patients and their families, and helping them take stock of their situation is an important part of your role.

The care of long-term patients highlights the importance of faithfully carrying out care every day, even though there is no quick improvement. Sometimes there is no improvement at all, and one realizes that treatment is serving only to hold ground which might otherwise be lost, rather than to provide improvement. The very sameness of the care, day by day, can be discouraging to both nurse and patient. Almost anyone can perceive the drama of bringing a patient out of anaphylactic shock, but not every nurse is attuned to helping an emphysema patient do his breathing exercises daily, and to feeling joy when the patient blows out one more candle today than he did yesterday.

The relationship which the nurse has with the long-term patient is especially important since many of these patients have few ties with their families and friends. Because other significant relationships are so often lacking, what the nurse provides as a listener and as one who is concerned about the patient's welfare is especially important. Nurses can show their interest and support of patients by attending to the daily matters which help the patient toward greater freedom and mastery of his situation, aiding him to use the abilities which he has, and assisting him to keep in touch with those who are important to him. Wheeling the patient to the phone booth and helping him get the necessary change to call his family can be just as significant an aspect of nursing, particularly for this group of patients, as giving back rubs or providing adequate fluid intake.

OTHER CONSIDERATIONS

The facial expression assumed by a patient is not necessarily a good indication of what is happening inside him. Cheerfulness can be a mask behind which lurk fears and anger of a most urgent nature. The need of the quiet person to talk may be great, and it may be hard for him to express himself. The patient who pleases the staff may do so at the expense of his own health. One patient was such a good sport that he told no one about the pain until his peptic ulcer perforated.

Certain other patients by their behavior may make it hard for nurses to accept them. For instance, some grown-up patients act like uninhibited children. They demand more service than anyone could give. They cry. They are stubborn, not doing what was ordered by the physician. They do not act as persons of their age usually do. Such patients sometimes cause anxiety in the nurse, because they do not meet her expectations. However, the nurse should remember that the patient who seems to be willful and obstinate may be trying to maintain his own integrity and his will to fight. The patient who acquiesces in every demand may have given up.

There may be another reason for the nurse's difficulty in tolerating patients who do not act in a grown-up way. They may remind her of parts of herself which she has learned to control, traits which she now regards as unacceptable in her standards of good behavior. If she does not like these characteristics in herself, it is only natural that her first reaction to them in others will be one of distaste.

Some patients may lose control completely, either physically or emotionally. They may soil themselves, laugh and cry at the same time, scream or climb out of bed. These patients may arouse the nurse's long-forgotten memories, which are kept out of the forefront of awareness because they are associated with too much pain. Those who were severely punished during their toilet training sometimes feel a special revulsion toward people who are incontinent. Those who as little children had to control any show of emotion for fear of punishment may be upset by a free flow of emotions from others. Another reason a patient's uncontrolled behavior may cause anxiety in others is that it may suggest that the observer (nurse, doctor, another patient) might behave in a like manner if he were that sick or in the same circumstances.

Some adults may be ashamed of their behavior when it becomes childish; but when they are sick and forced to depend on the care of others, they do cry and complain more easily. If a patient is embarrassed by his behavior, the nurse can point out to him the temporary nature of his dependence. Nurses see people *in extremis,* with their defenses badly shaken. A matter-of-fact "This is not unusual" acceptance of the situation may help to convey to the patient recognition of the temporary nature of the circumstance and a subtle tone of support. When people are temporarily shorn of their usual poise and self-control, the nurse can help them to maintain their dignity.

It is important to assess the patient's capacity for control at a given time and also to consider some possible reasons for his behavior. While it is not only useless, but also possibly harmful, to demand that a patient show greater control than is possible for him, it is important to establish a plan of care which enables the patient to maintain the self-control which he can muster. For example, a patient with multiple sclerosis had tremors of his hands; each time he tried to take a sip of water, he spilled it on the bed, and then burst into tears of frustration. The nurse, noting the difficulty, placed the water glass, half full, on the overbed table close to the patient, and she put a flexible straw in the glass. The patient could draw the table toward him when he wanted to drink and sip the water without having to handle the glass. A patient who is incontinent at night may be able to avoid soiling himself if the urinal is left where he can reach it. This approach is not likely to be effective, though, if the patient is soiling himself in order to get attention. Sometimes the nurse's reaction to such a patient is one of further rejection, cleaning him up in the most perfunctory manner possible, and avoiding him the rest of the time. Medical-surgical patients who behave in this manner are often elderly people who are severely lacking in meaningful relationships with others. Eventually the patient regresses to a childish way of seeking attention which is distasteful to others and serves only to isolate him further. This in turn leads to more soiling. The patient and nurse become victims of a vicious circle while he suffers more humiliation, isolation, and regression and she is harassed with additional work which at first glance appears wholly unnecessary. It is the nurse who must break the circle by recognizing how her own actions are aggravating the situation and by giving more attention to the patient other than that associated with changing him.

Many of the medical-surgical patients who lack emotional control have some neurologic impairment, such as results from cerebral vascular accidents and multiple sclerosis. Others lack control primarily because of anxiety. In either instance it is important to remember that the patient has diminished capacity to perceive and respond to the subtle cues relied upon extensively in social interaction. By using a kind but direct approach you help the patient avoid missing your comment altogether, or misinterpreting its meaning.

Do tears make you uncomfortable? It may be a great compliment to your relationship that the patient feels emotionally secure enough with you to cry. A flow of tears can relieve tension. Let the patient cry. The compassion of acceptance may allow a man to cry in the nurse's presence without feeling less manly because he did. A nurse has to be able to stand the discomfort of another's tears, because the tears may help to relieve the patient's tension. As long as the nurse can recognize her own reaction to the tears of others, she can let the patient cry without feeling overly anxious herself. If the nurse disapproves of crying, then perhaps she should not cry herself; but it is not a part of good nursing care to impose one's own standards on others.

In working with patients with a variety of illnesses—many of which have no ready cure, and some of which have none—there is a great temptation for the nurse to adopt a manner which implies to the patient that there is no cause for concern. One nurse said to an elderly lady who had just learned that she had cataracts developing in both eyes, "You have nothing to worry about." Such an attitude, in effect, denies the patient any opportunity for help with the very real worries of how to get along with impaired vision (for example, if he depends on his car for his livelihood); how to deal with the possibility of blindness; how to defray the expense of surgery and how to meet the other direct and indirect effects of the operation. It has been said that the only really minor operation is the one someone else is having. Doctors and nurses sometimes have a tendency to speak of diseases as more amenable to care and cure than is actually the case, leaving the patient and family to find out the truth for themselves and to deal with their plight unaided. Dismissing the problems of patients with the statement, "Don't worry," is probably a self-protective mechanism for health personnel; they should remember that it is good practice to allow patients and families to voice their misgivings.

The nurse may find herself shying away from a patient for reasons other than personal behavior. He may speak a different language, or his customs may be so strange that the nurse feels that there is no common meeting ground for communication. Many of us have a tendency to shy away from the unfamiliar, because it usually provokes more anxiety than the familiar. We may be uncertain what to do or say. Because we do not know what to expect next, we feel uneasy. Yet there is a certain sense of adventure in exploring the unknown. What are the thoughts and the feelings of a person different from us in background or age? As the unknown unfolds, we find that we have grown, and that our own perspectives have been enriched.

Not all cultures view cleanliness in the same way. Most Europeans do not consider themselves clean without frequent cleansing of the rectal and genital regions, especially after a bowel move-

ment. There are people in other groups who do not believe in a daily bath. If a patient enters the hospital with nits clinging to the shafts of his hair and black lines under his fingernails, will his condition color your feelings about him as a person? If your answer is "Yes" (and it may well be), try to draw a distinction between a person's standards of hygiene and the person as an individual.

You may become attached to some patients. You have cared for them a long time. They like you, and you like them. They are *your* patients. You may be unwilling to relinquish them to their families or to death. Although you should not be afraid to like your patients, emotional involvement with a patient does not mean the same thing as emotional involvement with an old friend, a family member or your fiancé. Relations with patients are more temporary. You are maintaining a tacitly understood relationship based on service. Usually, you do not call your patient by his first name; you do not display your personal life to him; you are not coy. Satisfy your need to talk about the party, the picnic, your new hairdo to someone who is not the patient. You can be warm and express your interest in a different fashion. You show a patient that you like him by taking him as he is, by perceiving his needs and meeting them promptly. The tender touch at just the right moment, the word of encouragement when he is feeling low will bring satisfaction to both of you. The more you understand what comforting the patient means to you, the more free you will be to do it well.

If a man misinterprets your ministerings, idealizing your relationship into something more personal than you intend, you may occasionally have to sidestep a pass or two. One nurse who encountered the problem said firmly but kindly, "I don't want you to do that." The patient never used the behavior again with that nurse. The nurse brought the matter up in a team conference, where the question was raised of whether the patient's behavior could be due to extreme loneliness. The patient responded well when all the nurses straightforwardly voiced their objections to his "wandering hands," and, in addition, spent more time with him and encouraged him to join in ward activities.

GUARDING AGAINST SUICIDE

The depressed patient bears watching. He may be thinking of suicide. Signs of depression are: lack of enthusiasm, prolonged insomnia, listlessness, reluctance to speak, neglect of appearance, withdrawal, lack of interest in anything and feelings of worthlessness. It may be difficult to get the patient to say anything. Suicide in the nonpsychotic patient is often an attempt to escape from an overwhelming situation, which frequently is the loss of love. Hostility is often a factor, too. Anger at self, the wish to hurt those close to him who have hurt him—usually such influencing factors are unrecognized by the patient. In some instances it is possible to avert suicide if the patient thinks that one person in the world will listen to him and is concerned for him. That one person can be a nurse. The background leading to suicide is a long, complicated web of events and feelings. The nurse is expected to recognize depression and protect the patient by reporting her observations promptly to the doctor. Obvious hazards, such as a razor in the patient's stand, can be removed quietly.

If a patient threatens suicide, pay attention to him. He may mean it. Do not leave the patient alone. Communicate with the doctor. Alert the rest of the nursing staff. Chart your observations. Where pain, incurable disease, crippling disability and impending death are present—as they may be on any general hospital floor—suicide, like fire, is an ever-present possibility.

PATIENTS' COMPLAINTS

Some patients continually complain about pains and aches or the service of the hospital. These patients are often disliked, particularly by the nursing staff. Perhaps complaints about which little can be done leave the nurses feeling helpless. What is it that lies at the root of the patient's bitterness and continual complaints? Has anyone tried to find out? Is this the only way the patient can get any attention? In the course of this patient's day does he have any warm human contact? Any opportunity for a feeling of accomplishment or satisfaction? A patient, because he is a patient, is cut off from his family and friends, his work and his own fireside. His habitual sources of satisfaction are usually not available in the hospital, where his sore toe and his elevated leukocyte count may receive attention while his own self is starved for human contact. A nurse, even though she may fumble some in the trying, can delight this patient by piercing his loneliness.

The all-too-prevalent practice of calling patients who complain frequently (and some who do not) by such terms as "crocks" reveals eloquently the lack of perception and understanding in the speaker. Perhaps nurses label patients as a way of putting distance between themselves and the patients who make them anxious. The subconscious reasoning may be that a patient who is labeled as "unco-operative" is so unworthy that nurses are excused for avoiding him. A patient who does not meet the nurse's expectations, one whom she has not the knowledge and the competence to deal with, may make her anxious. By stereotyping and labeling him she in a sense dismisses him. Stereotyping can be done by a whole group, with disastrous effects on the patient. The night nurse reports to the day staff, "He's unco-operative," and sets up the climate and expectations. Once a patient is labeled as unco-operative, he probably will not disappoint anyone. He will be unco-operative.

Who are the "good" patients? Many nurses think that submissive patients are "good," and by bestowing approval on the quiet ones they force patients to hide their feelings. Often the behavior expected of patients is made evident to them subtly but very clearly. "Mrs. Glenn is a wonderful patient, Doctor. She's always smiling." Therefore, Mrs. Glenn must go on smiling, even if it kills her. Her ulcer may grow bigger, but she's smiling. If one morning she could frown or cry, maybe the nurses would not approve of her and therefore not take care of her.

Some patients do not complain because they are at the mercy of the nurse. They dare not antagonize her, or the doctor, or the orderly. A patient lying in bed, sick and in pain, depends on the hospital staff. He is in a vulnerable position, and the danger of being ignored—psychologically and physically—is a real one. A patient may be afraid to complain, no matter how miserable he feels, because he may observe that the more cranky patients are left thirsty and in wet beds. But fear of expressing one's feelings is not a stepping stone to health.

THE PATIENT WHO IS PHYSICALLY UNAPPEALING

Our culture places heavy emphasis upon cleanliness, pleasant odors, and attractive appearance. The patient who has had radical head and neck surgery for removal of cancer is badly disfigured; the patient with infected skin lesions has an unpleasant odor; patients with tuberculosis or staphylococcal infection can transmit the condition to others.

Try not to expect yourself to be impervious to unpleasant sights and odors, and do not be afraid to discuss your reaction to these problems with your instructor and with other students. Having been brought up in a society which places emphasis upon the elimination of body odor, for example, you will quite naturally be unaccustomed to, and at times distressed by, unpleasant odors. Gradually you will learn how to handle yourself in such situations, how to deal as effectively as possible with the problem (such as by lessening odor), and you will begin to accept that nursing, like all kinds of work, has some aspects which are more difficult or less pleasant than others.

As you work with patients whose physical condition is unappealing to you, try, as far as possible, to be aware of your reactions toward the patient. If you really feel slightly nauseated, or like excusing yourself on some pretext, acknowledge to yourself that this is the case. You will then be more likely to be aware of your interaction with the patient and better able to control the response you convey to him.

It is also helpful to ask someone else (such as your teacher) to observe unobtrusively as you give care to the patient, and to let you know afterward her impression of your interaction with the patient. Sometimes you will be unaware of how your facial expression or gestures come across to another person, and a candid impression from someone else can alert you to trouble spots, as well as help you become aware of your strengths. Another important barometer of your approach is the reaction of the patient. Of course, if he shows embarrassment or withdrawal, it may be entirely due to his own reaction to his situation; it may also, however, be an indicator that he perceives that you do not accept him.

Accepting the patient definitely does not mean accepting disarray of the surroundings and inattention to the patient's personal hygiene. One nurse entered the room of a patient with an infectious disease. The door was closed and when she opened it, she found 3 left-over meal trays, a bedpan which needed to be emptied, and an irritable, resentful, disheveled patient. The first step in relating to him involved concrete measures to help improve his situation, not with an air of "Oh, what a mess you are" but, "You look uncomfortable; let's see what can be done about it."

If you have questions about whether a patient's condition is infectious, ask and find out what measures you must take to protect yourself. Having made sure that your knowledge is adequate, you will find it easier to use a sure touch, rather than a gingerly one.

THE "SELF-CARE" PATIENT

A good many medical-surgical patients are described as "self-care." Some are on general wards; others are on separate units designed especially for them. These patients present no less of a challenge than the more physically helpless patients, in the establishment of the nurse-patient relationship, but the challenges are somewhat different.

Among the "self-care" patients are many who are undergoing diagnostic tests. Frequently the patient has a good deal of free time; in fact some patients describe the experience as one of interminable waiting: waiting to go to scheduled appointments, waiting for test results. Frequently the waiting is accompanied by anxiety. Until a diagnosis is made, the patient has no concrete "enemy" to grapple with. Instead, he may have many vague fears about what may be wrong and a general feeling of powerlessness.

One important aspect of care of these patients involves explaining diagnostic tests to them, and helping the patient understand the results. Both should be done in close collaboration with the physician. It is his responsibility to provide the patient with initial information about what tests are needed and why, and to interpret the test results to the patient. The nurse should talk with the physician so that she knows what explanations the patient has received. Within this framework, the nurse reviews and clarifies information with the patient.

One important thing to know is whether your patient realizes that the physician suspects a peptic ulcer, and whether he knows what a peptic ulcer is. Unless you have such background information some casual comment of yours about ulcers may be very disturbing to the patient. If you find that a patient is scheduled for some test or procedure about which he seems to know nothing, bring this to the physician's attention. Maybe the patient's preparation for the test has escaped the doctor's notice. If so, it is appropriate for you to mention it, just as you would expect a colleague to remind you if you left a siderail down. On the other hand, the patient may have been so anxious that he understood none of the doctor's explanation. This is important to notice, if it is the case, since it means that, unless it is a dire emergency, time must be spent with the patient to discover what is troubling him, before the procedure is undertaken.

Patients need opportunities, too, to review with the nurse the results of their tests, the diagnosis the doctor has made, and the treatment which he has prescribed. Often, after the physician has given the patient the information, the patient wants a chance to talk about it again—to review what was said, to clarify terms, and the like.

If the patient needs an operation it may be necessary to refer his questions to the physician. Usually the patient has forgotten, or become confused about what the doctor told him initially. Opportunity to discuss this again with the physician is helpful to the patient once the first shock of the diagnosis has diminished. If the situation is very threatening to the patient, he will require repeated opportunities to talk with the nurse and physician in order to prepare himself for treatment.

Do not encourage the patient in brooding over "What if it's ____?" If no one really knows what is wrong, it is best not to engage in a type of conversation with the patient which, under the guise of "instruction," really provides "worry data." Instead, encourage the patient to occupy himself with ward activities and, when you talk with him, encourage him to concentrate on the specific measures the physician has ordered, such as how to prepare himself for diagnostic tests.

Although this discussion has concentrated on preparing patients for diagnostic tests as an illustration of how the nurse can relate helpfully to a patient who does not require physical care, many other examples could be given. The main point is that the nurse assess the situation in which the "self-care" patient finds himself, and that she consider ways in which she can, by her relationship with him, help the patient cope with his situation.

THE PATIENT WHO IS UNCONSCIOUS

Your first thought may be that if the patient is unconscious, there can be no relationship. However, the nurse does not turn off her reactions because a patient is unconscious. Sometimes imperceptibly, the patient who appears comatose begins being aware of the nurse and she, in any case, is aware of him.

Some nurses find it very difficult to care for a patient who cannot respond in some way; others may find it a relief not to have to relate verbally to the patient. The nurse must try to avoid, on the one hand, treating the patient as though he were an object, rather than a person, and on the other hand, feeling overwhelmed by the seriousness of his condition. As you care for these patients try to think of concrete, individual nursing needs which you observe, and plan ways to meet them. Is the skin on the patient's sacrum redder? How can you position him to promote good body alignment and prevent pressure sores? Has he shown any sign of returning consciousness—the flicker of an eyelid? Concentrating on such practical and individualized observations will help you avoid being overwhelmed by the gravity of the patient's condition and also to avoid thinking of the patient as an object.

Care of an unconscious adult, particularly if he is heavy, is best undertaken by two nurses working together. The physical and emotional burdens for the nurses are made lighter when they are shared. Each can encourage the other in how best to give mouth care, prevent obstruction of catheters, and so on. However, it is essential to keep in mind that the patient may hear you, even though he cannot respond. Make it a rule never to say anything in your patient's presence which you do not want him to hear.

As you work with the patient, if there seems to be any possibility of returning consciousness, speak to him slowly and gently, saying what you are about to do. Occasionally you will observe someone shouting at an unconscious patient—or slapping his face brusquely. Such actions are never warranted and may reflect the nurse's anxiety over working with an unconscious patient.

Just as the experienced nurse seeks help when moving a heavy person, to avoid straining her back, she will also seek help with situations (whatever their nature) which are emotionally overburdening. Talk with your teachers and supervisors about your reactions to very ill patients, as an aid in helping you understand these reactions and dealing with them.

THE PATIENT WHO REFUSES HIS TREATMENT

A teacher, lawyer, or salesman is, upon admission to the hospital, expected to "take orders" unquestioningly. A host of indignities surround him. No matter how necessary these may be from the standpoint of running the hospital, they can be galling to the patient. The abrupt change from being in charge of his own affairs to acquiescing to directions of others is difficult for many patients. Anxiety over the diagnosis and its implications plays a part in patients' refusal to follow treatment. The patient may refuse treatment because he cannot acknowledge that he could be sick enough to need it. When a patient refuses treatment, he places the nurse in a difficult position. The nurse is expected to see that prescribed treatment is carried out, whether this involves taking medication, staying in bed, or keeping within a prescribed diet. Frequently the nurse assumes more responsibility than she can handle in such situations, and her frustration may then get in the way of effectively dealing with the patient who refuses treatment. What nurse has not been reminded, for example, that it is *her* responsibility to see that the patient stays in bed, sticks to his diet, or whatever. Yes, it is the nurse's responsibility, but it is not hers alone, as is often implied. It is also the patient's responsibility to follow his treatment and, except in unusual circumstances when the patient is unable to make his own decisions, it is basically a matter for the patient to decide, once he has acquired the necessary facts. It is also the physician's responsibility to see that his patient has necessary information concerning the treatment, and encouragement to follow it. Keeping these factors in mind will help you maintain perspective concerning your role and your responsibility. By concentrating on what your responsibility really is, and recognizing the limits of your authority, you will be less likely to feel overwhelmed by the situation, and more able to concentrate on what you can do to help the patient. For example, suppose you are informed during morning report that a coronary patient refuses to stay in bed, and that it is your job to see that he does. The entire responsibility for seeing that he remains in bed does not rest solely on your shoulders, nor will it be "all your fault" if he keels over during one of his trips to the bathroom. You do, however, have a responsibility to do all in your power to help the patient follow his treatment. With your responsibility cut down to more manageable size, how will you approach the patient?

Start by thinking of his situation. What may be some reasons for his not staying in bed? Did his physician explain the need for bed rest fully, and did the patient understand the explanation? Is his call bell answered promptly, or does he feel that he must choose between wetting the bed and getting up to the bathroom? Does the thought that he has had a coronary make him so **anxious** that he does everything possible to deny

his illness? These are among the possibilities. How can you find out what is troubling the patient?

If you scold him, he is likely to tune you out. So instead, try starting to give him care, and then gently asking him what makes it so difficult for him to stay in bed. Listen carefully to what he says, and avoid cutting him off. The most important reason may not be mentioned until some of the lesser ones have been expressed. Avoid giving the patient a lecture on the pathophysiology of myocardial infarction, and of the possibility of dire consequences if the order for bed rest is not followed. Most patients are already only too well aware of the seriousness of heart attacks. Emphasizing this is likely to frighten the patient further, and make him more prone to deny his condition.

As you listen to the patient, keep attuned not only to underlying fears which he may express, but also to his recounting of daily annoyances. Often these patients, in their frustration and anger at being suddenly stopped in the midst of a busy life by a serious illness, start out by listing cold coffee, no one to empty the urinal, and so on. Let the patient know that you will do what you can to remedy these problems. When the patient senses your concern about his daily frustrations and notices that you are interested in seeing what can be done about them, he may be more likely to confide other concerns to you.

Diabetics are another group of patients with whom the nurse is often asked to enforce rules concerning treatment. Here again, it is essential that you examine your role and responsibilities. Suppose, for instance, that when you are assigned to care for a diabetic patient you are told "Watch him. He sneaks food from other patients' trays." What is your role here? Can you, in light of your other patients' requirements, watch this one so closely that you are sure he does not help himself to extra food? Probably not. It is the patient's responsibility to stick to his diet, and it is your job to help him do so, by finding out what the difficulty is, and helping him to deal with it. But you cannot force him to follow a diet against his will.

One crucial consideration, when working with a patient who refuses his treatment, is acknowledgment that the patient (except under unusual circumstances which are dealt with in literature on the legal aspects of nursing) has the right to refuse his treatment. The nurse who proceeds with this realization will do so with a more realistic assessment of the patient's role and of her own. It is then the nurse's job to help the patient make the best possible decisions for his own welfare, rather than to place herself in the false position of deciding for him what he may and may not do.

FAMILIES

Nurses have specialized knowledge and skills that help patients to recover. But a loved member of the family can make many contributions to the peace of mind and the comfort of a patient that because of the closeness of the relationship is beyond even the most skilled tongue and hands. When it is appropriate, capitalize on what the family can do for the patient; do not exclude them. Help the family to encourage the patient in the hard things that he has to learn. Is he walking better? A word of praise from a loved one may mean more to the patient than the applause of the entire hospital staff. Is a patient worried about his new diet? Let his wife show him how she will fit it into their daily lives. Perhaps Mr. Cole will eat better if his wife brings some food from home. With permission of the doctor and the physical therapist, encourage the family to participate in the rehabilitation program in speech and exercises.

It may not be easy for a daughter to sit passively by while others care for her mother. The illness alone makes her uneasy, and her inactivity may make her feel even more powerless. Action is a good antidote for this kind of feeling. Instead of allowing her to feel left out, suggest that her mother might be cheered by the evening paper, or ask her to encourage fluids (if the patient needs fluids). Say something like this: "Your mother will probably take the fluids better if you give them to her."

Feelings of guilt about illness are common and often irrational. A son might think, "If I had spent more time home, Father would not have had this heart attack." A wife may think, "If I had gone on that trip with John, he wouldn't have been in this car accident." That these thoughts may be irrational does not lessen their sting. Being able to participate in the care of the patient may help the family to feel in some small measure less guilty. The nurse should provide opportunities for the family to talk about the experience, if they wish.

Visitors should be made to feel welcome. They are the patient's contact with his usual life. Show them how to cheer the patient without tiring him. Is the visitor standing at the bedside, awkwardly clutching his coat? Draw up a chair for him; show him where to hang his coat.

Several other challenges must be considered when working with patients' families, particularly in long-term illness. (Although the terms "relative" and "family" are used here, remember that what is really meant is those persons closest to the patient. For some patients this is a close friend.) It is easy for nurses to view family members only in their role of helping the patient and to disregard their other responsibilities. In an acute illness, it is common for relatives to discontinue other responsibilities temporarily in order to help the patient. If illness continues, however, the patient's family must begin to resume other obligations. As you talk with the patient's relatives, try to consider the situation which that person faces. One aspect of it, to be sure, is the patient's illness. However, do not close off other topics of conversation, if the family member wishes to introduce them. As you listen to some of his other concerns, such as the fact that one of his children has cerebral palsy, or that he belongs to a union that is now out on strike, you will gain greater appreciation of his situation and you will have less tendency to consider him solely in the role of the patient's helper.

Society sets certain standards concerning responsibility when a family member is ill. Perhaps nowhere are these standards so forcefully upheld as in health care institutions. At morning reports and team conferences one frequently hears negative comments about patients' families: the family does not take the patient home; they do not visit, and so on. This criticism is understandable, as health personnel must rely on families to fulfill their role in helping the patient. When families do not meet these expectations, not only does the patient lack the support and encouragement that he needs, but also the work of physicians and nurses is made more difficult. Remember that not all families can meet your expectations in helping the patient for a variety of reasons, many of which may remain unknown to you. As you work with the patient's family, be alert to their attitudes and to their resources for helping the patient, rather than establishing, according to your values, what the family should do. This approach will enable you to help the family use the resources they do have. What questions do they have about the patient's care? What community resources may be of help to them?

Evaluate your own intervention with family members. Do you, without meaning to, encourage a family member to withdraw from her usual relationship with the patient? Suppose you are teaching the patient's wife how to irrigate and dress his colostomy. In your emphasis on the procedure, and your zeal to help her perform it correctly, are you losing sight of the fact that you and she are beginning to talk as though she were another nurse rather than the patient's wife. The family member, particularly if he or she is well informed about medical and nursing matters, may have a tendency to substitute a highly "clinical" approach for the personal relationship with the patient if the illness poses problems affecting this relationship. For instance, although the patient's wife may spend a great deal of time at the hospital, most of it may be focused on concern for her husband's diet, his dressing, the condition of the skin around the stoma, and so on. Such an approach may be one indication of failing to deal with the implications of the husband's illness for their personal relationship. The patient is often acutely aware that his role has suddenly shifted exclusively to that of a patient in his wife's eyes. Although a relative's reluctance to learn to care for the patient is usually quickly noted, an overly "clinical" approach may not attract attention, since it fits in with the staff's expectations. If you notice that a relative is beginning to speak of the patient's care almost as though she were the "assistant nurse," perhaps you can spend some time talking with her—other than the time you have allocated to teaching her the various procedures. By showing interest in her, and in her concerns, rather than just in her ability to carry out her husband's care, you may make it possible for her to talk over some of her personal reactions with you. No matter how well informed a patient's wife may be about her husband's condition, she is still his wife, and not another nurse.

Keep in mind that illness, such as cancer or heart disease, in a family member is a powerful force in mobilizing the anxiety of relatives. They may show their anxiety in various ways: by withdrawing, by becoming too "clinical," by talking about the patient rather than to him, or even by ascribing whatever difficulties the family may be having to the patient's illness. The more you can recognize that anxiety plays a part in such reactions, the better able you will be to help the family care for the patient.

The transition from hospital to home can be a stressful experience for the patient and his family. Often it is possible for the patient to reestablish his ties with family and friends when he returns home. Sometimes it is not, and the patient must recognize that the place he had filled in the lives of others, to which he was so eager to return, no longer exists, and that he must begin all over again to develop new relationships. As you work with patients who are making the transition from hospital to home, your appreciation of these factors will help you to assist the patient's family to assess the situation realistically.

REFERENCES AND BIBLIOGRAPHY

AASTERUD, M.: Defenses against anxiety in the nurse-patient relationship, *Nurs. Forum* 1:34, 1962.

ASHBROOK, J. B.: Not by bread alone, *Am. J. Nurs.* 55:164, 1955.

BETTELHEIM, B.: To nurse and to nurture, *Nurs. Forum* 1:60, 1962.

BIRD, B.: *Talking with Patients*, Philadelphia, Lippincott, 1955.

BURSTEN, B., and DIERS, D. K.: Pseudopatient centered orientation, *Nurs. Forum* 3:38, 1964.

BROWN, E. L.: *Newer Dimensions of Patient Care. Part 1, The Use of the Physical and Social Environment of the General Hospital for Therapeutic Purposes*, New York, Russell Sage, 1961.

———: *Newer Dimensions of Patient Care. Part 2, Improving Staff Motivation and Competence in the General Hospital*, New York, Russell Sage, 1962.

———: *Newer Dimensions of Patient Care. Part 3, Patients as People*, New York, Russell Sage, 1964.

ENGEL, G. L.: Grief and grieving, *Am. J. Nurs.* 64:93, September, 1964.

FARBEROW, N. L., and PALMER, R. A.: The nurse's role in prevention of suicide, *Nurs. Forum* 3:93, 1964.

FRANCIS, G., and MUNJAS, B.: *Promoting Psychological Comfort*, Dubuque, Iowa, Wm. C. Brown, 1968.

GLASER, B. G., and STRAUSS, A.: The social loss of dying patients, *Am. J. Nurs.* 64:119, June, 1964.

GOLDSBOROUGH, J. D.: On becoming non-judgmental, *Am. J. Nurs.* 70:2340, November, 1970.

GREGG, D.: Reassurance, *Am. J. Nurs.* 55:171, 1955.

———: Anxiety—a factor in nursing care, *Am. J. Nurs.* 52:1363–1365, 1952.

HANDEL, G. (ed.): *The Psychosocial Interior of the Family*, Chicago, Aldine, 1967.

HAY, S. I., and ANDERSON, H. C.: Are nurses meeting patients' needs? *Am. J. Nurs.* 63:97, December, 1963.

HILTNER, S., and MENNINGER, K. (eds.): *Constructive Aspects of Anxiety*, New York, Abingdon, 1963.

HUNGLER, B. P.: What every patient needs, *Am. J. Nurs.* 64:112, October, 1964.

HYDE, R. W., and COGGAN, N. E.: When nurses have guilt feelings, *Am. J. Nurs.* 58:233, 1958.

INGLES, T.: Do patients feel lost in a general hospital? *Am. J. Nurs.* 60:648, 1960.

KNOWLES, L. N.: How can we reassure patients? *Am. J. Nurs.* 59:834, 1959.

LEWIS, J. A.: Reflections on self, *Am. J. Nurs.* 60:828, 1960.

McGREGOR, F. C.: *Social Science in Nursing,* New York, Russell Sage, 1960.

MAY, R.: *The Meaning of Anxiety,* New York, Ronald, 1950.

MENNINGER, K. A.: *Man Against Himself,* New York, Harcourt, 1956. (Section on Suicide.)

———: *The Vital Balance,* New York, Viking, 1963.

NEHREN, J., and GILLIAM, N. R.: Separation anxiety, *Am. J. Nurs.* 65:109, January, 1965.

ORLANDO, I. J.: *The Dynamic Nurse-Patient Relationship,* New York, Putnam, 1961.

PEPLAU, H. E.: *Interpersonal Relations in Nursing,* New York, Putnam, 1952.

PETERS, D.: The Kewanee story, *Am. J. Nurs.* 61:74, October, 1961.

QUINT, J.: *The Nurse and the Dying Patient,* New York, Macmillan, 1967.

SKIPPER, J. K., and LEONARD, R. C.: *Social Interaction and Patient Care,* Philadelphia, Lippincott, 1965.

SKIPPER, J. K., TAGLIACOZZO, D. L., and MAUKSCH, H. O.: What communication means to patients, *Am. J. Nurs.* 64:101, April, 1964.

SMITH, S.: The psychology of illness, *Nurs. Forum* 3:35, 1964.

THALER, O. F.: Grief and depression, *Nurs. Forum* 5:9, 1966.

THOMAS, M. D., BAKER, J. M., and ESTES, N. J.: Anger: A tool for developing self-awareness, *Am. J. Nurs.* 70:2586, December, 1970.

TRAVELBEE, J.: What's wrong with sympathy? *Am. J. Nurs.* 64:68, January, 1964.

———: *Interpersonal Aspects of Nursing,* Philadelphia, Davis, 1966.

UJHELY, G. B.: *The Nurse and Her Problem Patients,* New York, Springer, 1963.

———: *Determinants of the Nurse-Patient Relationship,* New York, Springer, 1968.

———: Basic consideration for nurse-patient interaction in prevention and treatment of emotional disorders, *Nurs. Clin. N. Am.* 1:179, June, 1966.

———: Grief and depression—implications for preventive and therapeutic nursing care, *Nurs. Forum* 5:23, 1966.

———: What is realistic emotional support? *Am. J. Nurs.* 68:758, April, 1968.

Fundamental Processes of Health and Illness

6

Homeostasis · Concept of Stress · Nursing and Stress · Disease Terminology · Water and Electrolyte Regulation · Intravenous Therapy · Body Defenses · Body Responses to Infection · Allergy Incidence · Substances Commonly Causing Allergy · Diagnosis Treatment · Anaphylactic Shock

Nursing, as one of the health professions, is concerned with helping people to obtain and maintain optimal health as well as with preventing disease and caring for those who are ill.

Health and illness are relative states. Constantly in flux, they depend on the satisfaction of biological, psychological, and sociological needs and the ability to make suitable adaptations to stresses affecting these needs as they arise from within or without the individual.

HOMEOSTASIS

Homeostasis is the term used to describe the state of the body when it is in a dynamic state of equilibrium. The word dynamic is used because in order to maintain this equilibrium the body of man is constantly at work to balance the components of his internal environment: endocrine secretions, water, electrolytes, proteins, vitamins and oxygen. The body must obtain the materials needed and convert or eliminate what is superfluous. Thus pathology can arise from deprivation such as vitamin deficiency, or from excess such as too many sodium ions. Endocrine disturbances can arise when one has too little of a hormone or too much. The work of scientists such as René Spitz (1954) showed that deprivation of psychological and social factors could provoke serious disease and even death though physical needs were met.

CONCEPT OF STRESS

Another derivative from the concept of homeostasis is the concept of stress. Stress, according to Engel (1953), can be "any influence, whether it arises from the internal environment or from the external environment, which interferes with the satisfaction of basic needs or which disturbs or threatens to disturb the stable equilibrium."

In Selye's theory (1956), stress is a specific physiologic condition manifested by a general adaptation syndrome. No matter whether a stressor be biologic, such as surgical trauma or bacterial toxins; psychological, such as worry, fear, rage; or sociologic, such as a new job or increased family responsibilities, the same nonspecific general adaptation syndrome results if the stressor is excessive in degree, ill-timed, or too sudden in onset.

The general adaptation syndrome consists of three stages: the alarm reaction, stage of resistance, and stage of exhaustion or death. Most stressors evoke the first two stages of response. An individual goes through these defensive stages a great many times during life. They are purposeful homeostatic reactions.

The general response to a stressor is accomplished through the coordinate efforts of the endocrine and nervous systems. Acting through the nerves, stressors produce adrenalines and acetylcholine in nerve endings; and a few nerve filaments go directly to the adrenal medulla. Also, through the endocrine system, stressors stimulate the pituitary to secrete ACTH, which then stimulates the adrenal cortex to produce predominantly anti-inflammatory corticoid substances or glucocorticoids, namely cortisone and cortisol. Glucocorticoids tend to be inhibitory and catabolic.

The adrenal is also stimulated to produce pro-inflammatory corticoids or mineralocorticoids, namely aldosterone and desoxycorticosterone. Mineralocorticoids tend to be stimulative and anabolic.

Selye found that imbalances between these two types of hormones as well as an excess of ACTH can be responsible for disease through their effect on certain "target organs." These include the thymus and lymphatic system; joints and connective tissue; blood vessels; the liver, kidney, pancreas, and gastrointestinal tract.

The adaptive hormones of the pituitary-adrenal system appear to be necessary to maintain life during the alarm reaction of the general adaptation syndrome when large tissue regions are under stress. The body then gains the time necessary for the development of specific local adaptive phenomena in the directly affected region.

During the stage of resistance the directly affected region can cope with its local task without the help of adaptive hormones.

At times, when the body uses one organ system repeatedly to cope with a threatening situation, disease can result from its disproportionate excessive development, or from its eventual breakdown due to wear and tear. Specifically, Selye uses the term "diseases of adaptation" to refer to those maladies resulting from an excessive or insufficient amount or an improper mixture of adaptive hormones. Nephritis, nephrosis, peptic ulcer, keloid formation, hypertension, arthritis are among those so classified.

Stress is obviously not an entirely negative concept. Inherent in each individual's growth and development are markedly stressful situations which, if mastered, give zest and fullness to life. In the oyster the pearl is produced in response to a stressor. One needs stress to live. At each stage of development there are stressful tasks to be learned and mastered which ready one for the next stage of development.

The person who subjects himself to the stress of physical conditioning involved in a daily two-mile run gradually increases the efficiency of his cardiovascular system. This is beneficial compared to the person who limits his exercise to changing the channels on his television set.

Trying something for the first time, whether it be a new job, a new skill, or a new role in life, is often a stressful experience. But as one perseveres and grows in ability and confidence, the apprehension diminishes and life is enriched because one made the effort to continue to learn and grow.

Biologically, the individual's mode of adaptive responses is limited by genetic endowment as well as by morphology and physiochemical structure. Psychological adaptation also depends on genetic endowment plus one's relationships to significant others, finite and the Infinite. Though individuals have greater latitude sociologically for new adaptive modes, inertia and cultural tradition often impede the development of new coping mechanisms, particularly if they condradict old values.

The body, with its marvelous capacity for coping with large variations in the assaults of various stressors sometimes reaches a point when quantitative excesses cannot be compensated for and symptoms result. Symptoms represent the evidence of damage or the defense reaction to excessive stress. Though symptoms have been categorized classically as mental or physical, each disease process involves all tissues of the body, directly or indirectly and in varying degrees.

Though symptoms may indeed reflect an organic disturbance, cellular pathology may not necessarily have initiated the symptom complex. Disease is usually the result of multiple factors. A female diabetic patient, well controlled with diet and insulin may be looked upon as being in a state of equilibrium. But the social and psychological stressors of her husband's sudden death may be sufficient to provoke acute symptomatic illness. Organic disorders are concomitants in the complex of biologic, psychologic, and social patterns of adaptation, and illness should be looked upon as a breakdown in total living. Good treatment, then, emphasizes the function of the individual in all his dimensions.

NURSING AND STRESS

How does nursing fit into this more comprehensive view of health and illness? Examining some of its dimensions, nursing care involves:

1. Preventing, modifying, reducing, or removing stressors.

Nurses can anticipate the adaptive tasks facing an individual through a knowledge of the developmental needs and tasks facing him at his particular stage in the life cycle. The prevention of illness at crisis points in life is enhanced when individuals are prepared for new adaptive tasks. Nurses can assist in the maintenance of homeostasis by participation in programs of health education. Participating in immunization programs, encouraging routine Pap smears, or speaking to members of a Golden Age Club on the prevention of falls are other ways.

In the hospital, the nurse who cares for the patient with an acute myocardial infarction monitors his electrocardiogram continuously to detect the added stressor of dangerous cardiac arrhythmias from interfering with the heart's effective function and healing.

2. Supporting the adaptive processes utilized by the patient in his attempt to establish a new state of equilibrium.

To support adaptive processes one must know the nature of such processes. Nurses study such subjects as anatomy and physiology, pathophysiology, psychology, and cultural anthropology so that they can understand patients' modes of adaptation, assess where they may need assistance, establish priorities, and intervene appropriately.

During illness, support of the patient's natural defenses and adaptive processes can be accomplished while working with the physician and other members of the health team. Management of the internal environment through such activities as the control of pain with drugs, the administration of fluids and electrolytes, or antibiotics and other medications offer specific kinds of help.

Understanding the mental mechanisms patients use to cope with threats to their integrity enables the nurse to be supportive. Just nonjudgmentally listening to the patient as he confronts his weaknesses, identifies his strengths, and attempts to reassess the direction of his life relieves the patient's autonomic nervous system of the burden of carrying this load internally. The nurse who listens supportively may help the patient to deal with an amputation although she cannot prevent the amputation. Nor can she solve the patient's problems for him. She can assist him to identify what the problems are and where she and the other available resources can be of assistance.

Management of the external environment is often necessary to promote rest, a major treatment for many illnesses. Nursing activities which promote rest include arranging for a comfortable room temperature, providing a cotton instead of a wool blanket for the allergic patient, noise control, provision for a pleasant appropriately cheerful environment, and spacing nursing activities for the benefit of the patient rather than for the convenience of hospital departments.

Using good judgment regarding the number of visitors and the length of visitation assists the patient in his attempt to regain equilibrium. The elderly lady might greatly benefit by having the rules relaxed and her daughter near at hand most of the time whereas the active businessman might need to be protected from the over-solicitude of his office associates.

3. Recognizing that applying stressors is a necessary part of the treatment process and that, in moderation, stress is necessary for life.

Patients have optimum stress tolerance levels. These need to be accurately assessed so that patients are guided to use their adaptation energy at a rate and in a direction appropriate to the capacity of their minds and bodies.

The patient in shock has very limited and only essential physical activity so that his metabolic demands are minimized.

The nurse who encourages the postoperative cholecystectomy patient to cough up secretions introduces another stressor, but minimizes its effect by splinting the incisional area. Stress is also minimized by teaching the patient to cough properly preoperatively when he is apt to be more comfortable. Letting the patient know what is expected of him, commending his often heroic efforts, and giving him pain medication as warranted after he has performed his task are ways of supporting the patient through this stressful experience. Introducing minimal stress through coughing and deep breathing exercises prevents the major stress resulting from atelectasis and hypostatic pneumonia.

Though bed rest is a treatment designed to reduce stress in many illnesses, it can be hazardous in itself. The nurse who uses good judgment in encouraging deep breathing, in turning and properly positioning her bed-rest patient prevents more stressful complications. Providing the usually very active business executive on enforced bed rest with diversional material of his preference reduces his discomfort and promotes his adaptation.

When the nurse attempts to teach a diabetic patient how to inject himself with insulin, she indeed may introduce a stressor. His normal emotional response may result in trembling, pallor, or profuse diaphoresis.

Thus, the diabetic should learn self-care after he has some control of symptoms and he is not in severe disequilibrium. The judgment that comes from knowledge and experience enables the nurse to determine how much stress is appropriate for the individual patient, when to apply it, and when to lessen or remove it.

DISEASE TERMINOLOGY

The word *acute* can be misleading to patients and their families. It does not refer necessarily to the seriousness of disease; rather it describes the rapid nature of the onset and the progress. In contrast, the term *chronic* describes the lengthy, sometimes endless persistence of a condition without much change for the better.

The seriousness of the problem is graded as *severe, moderate* or *mild*. A stage of the disease may be described as *early, late* or *terminal*. *Terminal* usually means a stage preceding death. *Terminal pulmonary insufficiency* would describe a state in which the patient is approaching death from inadequate lung function.

A disease may be described also as *primary* or *secondary*. A *primary* condition is assumed to have developed independently of any other. A subsequent disorder that develops as a result of an original illness is called *secondary*.

Morbidity means sickness. It usually is expressed as a rate in relation to population. If 39 people are ill in a population of 1,000, the morbidity rate is 39 per 1,000. *Mortality* means death. If 25 people die in a population of 1,000, the mortality rate is 25 per 1,000.

Hereditary Conditions. Heredity can be an etiologic (causal) factor. From the moment of conception the destiny of thousands of traits is decided. Some of these inherited traits can impair the function of the body, and the individual is born with hereditary disease or a tendency to develop it. Hemophilia and color blindness are disorders transmitted by the genes from parent to child. Many hereditary diseases are carried in the genes as recessive traits and are not manifested in every generation.

Congenital Defects and Diseases. Although they are often confused with hereditary conditions, congenital diseases are not necessarily the same. Although congenital disease is present at the time of birth, it is not always transmitted by the genes. It can result from some unfavorable event or unfortunate environmental condition experienced by the fetus during the period of pregnancy. For example, drugs and radiation

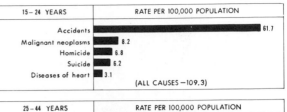

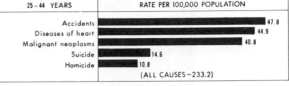

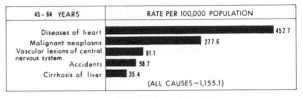

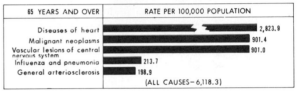

FIG. 6-1. Leading causes of death, according to age group, in the United States, 1967. (U.S. Department of Health, Education and Welfare: *The Facts of Life and Death*, Washington, D.C.)

can affect the developing fetus. The mother can transmit an infection of her own, such as syphilis, to the fetus, and at birth the child has congenital syphilis. An illness of the mother, such as German measles, may impair normal development of the fetus, and the resulting defects would be termed *congenital*.

The etiology of the congenital defect may be unknown. Until it is known, it is difficult to take steps to prevent it. The cause of congenital heart disease is obscure in most instances. The congenital irregularity may be a serious threat to life, as when a baby is born missing a vital organ; or disfiguring, as in polydactylism (more than the usual number of fingers or toes); or so slight as to escape notice completely. One woman lived for 76 years with a congenital diaphragm across her duodenum before it caused her enough trouble to have a roentgenogram taken. Any part of the body, inside or outside, can be anomalous (deviating from the usual).

Few, if any, people are born perfect. The flaw may be tiny, a mole or the deviation of a minor

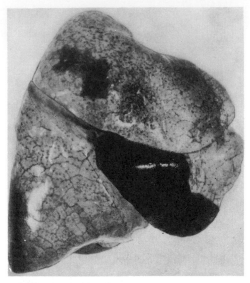

FIG. 6-2. A blood clot has prevented adequate circulation to the middle lobe of the lung, and destruction of tissue (infarct) has resulted. (Hardy, J. D.: *Pathophysiology in Surgery,* Baltimore, Williams & Wilkins)

blood vessel; or the defect may be important to appearance or health. The thought of being deformed is troublesome to most people. Through the ages such persons as dwarfs, whose anomalies were evident, have been objects of morbid curiosity, social ostracism and fear of ill omen; and the present is not entirely free of this attitude. Those with obvious major deformities have the constant reminder before them of their imperfection, their "wrongness." The experienced nurse can come across the grossly deformed person and show no surprise, shock or curiosity, but instead an acceptance of the patient as a fellow human being.

Trauma. The term *trauma,* meaning injury, applies to both physical wounds, such as those a person suffers in an automobile accident, and to psychic wounds, such as those suffered in the loss of a loved one.

Deficiency Diseases. Disorders resulting from the lack of essential dietary substances required by cells for their normal function and maintenance are deficiency diseases. Some specific deficiencies can produce clear-cut disorders; for instance, lack of vitamin C causes scurvy—historically, the disorder that affected seamen on long voyages without fresh foods. It was found that citrus fruit, commonly limes or lime juice, prevented the disease, and the world had a treatment for scurvy long before its etiology was understood.

Dietary Excesses. The body is harmed not only by the deficit of materials that it requires but also by the excess. Too many calories produce obesity, and overdoses of certain vitamin and mineral preparations can be harmful.

Hypoxia. Hypoxia (insufficient oxygen) produces dramatic effect, for all body cells require an adequate uninterrupted supply of oxygen. Mental impairment often quickly follows hypoxia and anoxia (lack of oxygen). The cells of the central nervous system are damaged by an oxygen deficiency most easily. The tissues responsible for the control of heart rhythm are readily affected by hypoxia. Insufficient oxygenation of these tissues can lead to cardiac arrhythmia and arrest.

Local areas may receive insufficient oxygen while the rest of the body is properly supplied. Such a problem results from a decrease of local blood flow (ischemia). Among the more frequent causes of ischemia is the plugging of an artery with material that either forms there, as in thrombosis, or is delivered there by the circulation (embolism). Ischemia can be produced accidentally by applying an encircling bandage or cast too tightly on a limb.

Ischemia may damage nerves irreparably. Less sensitive tissue, like muscle, also can undergo damage. If the ischemia is relieved and has not been too severe or prolonged, healing may occur in time. However, serious and long-continued ischemia can cause necrosis (death) of the involved tissues. Decomposition of the necrotic tissue begins, and gradually the area darkens to purple and eventually to black. This massive death of tissue is called *gangrene.*

When an area of tissue is deprived of blood supply long enough to become necrotic, the affected tissue is described as an area of *infarction.*

Neoplasia. This term refers to the new formation of abnormal tissue. Such growths are called *tumors.* A *benign tumor* is one usually similar to the tissue in which it originates, and it is covered by a capsule of fibrous tissue. It may have little activity except local growth, or it may carry on the processes characteristic of the tissue from which it started. Benign tumors of endocrine glands can produce the hormone of the gland. A certain benign tumor of the pancreas is capable of making insulin. Benign tumors typically stay within their capsules and do not spread to other sites.

A benign tumor may cause trouble for several reasons. In certain locations it is disfiguring. In other cases it grows to occupy too much space and crowds the normal structures so that they cannot function properly. A hormone-producing tumor may function outside of the organized body commands, secreting the hormone in excess or at inappropriate times.

Once located, benign tumors usually can be excised and will not regrow. However, while benign tumors usually are viewed as not so dangerous as cancer, they can prove to be just as deadly. A benign tumor in the brain or the spinal cord that grows in an inoperable site can be fatal.

Malignant tumors (collectively called *cancers*) grow and act in total disregard of body order. Their cells may differ considerably from those of the tissue of their origin. They tend to spread (metastasize) to other parts of the body. To track down all the metastatic "seeds" of a malignant tumor may be impossible. The malignant tumor can invade, crowd and weaken normal structures. For example, bones become fragile, and blood vessels break open. The tumor can absorb nutrients so greedily that normal tissue is malnourished in its presence. Some cancers arising from endocrine glands may secrete hormones and produce additional disorder. So great is the capacity of cancer for causing destruction, pain and ultimately death, and so difficult is the control of many of the malignant neoplasms, that cancer is one of the most dreaded of all diseases. For further discussion of cancer, see Chapter 13.

Infection. Many species of plant and animal parasites are offensive to living cells in the human being. These organisms, classified as protozoa, yeasts, molds, bacteria, rickettsiae and viruses, can harm human cells by growing within them or producing *toxins*.

Infection is invasion of the body by an organism that produces harm (called a *pathogenic organism* or *pathogen*). Each organism must live in an environment suited to its needs, and not all tissue sites appeal to it. For example, the bacillus that causes typhoid fever thrives in lymphoid tissue. The organism of tetanus cannot survive in oxygen; hence, to multiply and produce the toxins of its serious disease it needs to live deep in a wound. Viruses live inside cells and may be very selective as to which kind of cell they will inhabit. The polio virus inhabits selectively the anterior horn cells of the spinal cord.

Because we do not live in a sterile environment, we are constantly bombarded by organisms, but we are not always sick. Becoming infected depends on several factors: (1) the number of invading organisms, (2) how virulent they are, and (3) the resistance of the host.

As a rule, foreign material, dead or alive, is tolerated poorly by the tissues. Whether the organisms consume nutrients needed by the cells, invade them and disturb their structure or activity, or in some other unknown way offend the tissue, they do produce injury and death of body cells. The group of organisms finds food in the host, adapting its enzymes to the chemical compounds in the host. This is the incubation period, and during it the host is usually unaware of the organisms and may be symptomless. The organisms thrive on the food, and they multiply. The host may become a patient. (See p. 69 for a discussion of the body's response to infection.)

Idiopathic (Unknown) Etiology. Though they are being extensively studied, cancer, diabetes and rheumatoid arthritis are diseases of unknown origin. The effects of aging are apparent, but *why* these changes take place is not clear. There are many other disorders of obscure etiology. For some of them there is a satisfactory treatment. As a general rule, cure must await knowledge of cause, but this order is not always true. Recall the case of scurvy.

WATER AND ELECTROLYTE REGULATION

Normal Functioning of the Body Fluids

Approximately 75 pounds of a human body that weighs 125 pounds is made up of water. Much as appearance may belie it, approximately 60 per cent of the adult human body is water. Body water is kept within the cells (*cellular* or *intracellular*), between the cells (*interstitial*) and in the bloodstream (*intravascular*). The interstitial and intravascular spaces are called, somewhat misleadingly, the *extracellular* (outside the cells) *compartment*.

Every one of the countless number of cells that make up an inch of skin, muscle or any tissue is a tiny pond of fluid, held together by the cellular membrane. Around these skin cells is the bath of interstitial fluid. Within each cell is constant chemical activity, along with constant interchange with the interstitial fluid.

Electrolytes are in the water of both the cellular and the extracellular spaces. These electrolytes include such ions as potassium, magnesium, sodium, phosphate, sulfate, calcium, chloride, bicarbonate, protein and organic acids such as carbonic acid and the amino acids. There is a striking difference between the extracellular and the cellular fluids in terms of the concentration of the ions. The sodium, calcium, and chloride concentrations are many times higher in the extracellular fluid than in the cellular. In contrast, potassium, magnesium and phosphate concentrations are many times higher cellularly than extracellularly. These differences are responsible for electrical potentials that develop across the cell membrane and perhaps also for the degree of permeability of the membrane.

Most cell membranes are apparently completely permeable to water, and the total exchange is enormous. The net exchange of water is governed by the osmotic pressure changes in the two compartments. *Osmotic pressure* is a drawing power for water, exerted by concentrated solutions on one side of a semipermeable membrane drawing water from dilute solutions on the other side. Osmosis takes place whenever a concentration gradient exists across a semipermeable membrane. If the concentration is higher within the cell, water will be drawn through the membrane into the cell from the interstitial space until the concentration of particles in the fluid is the same on both sides of the membrane. If the concentration is higher in the interstitial space, water will be pulled from the cell. By means of osmosis the system tends to achieve a situation of uniform osmotic pressure.

Ordinarily, a healthy person consumes more water and electrolytes than the body needs. Water is in everything he eats. Water is formed also within the body during the metabolic processes. Fluid requirements vary, depending on the size of the person, his activity and conditions in the external environment that affect fluid loss, like temperature. Normal daily fluid requirements for an adult range from 1,500 to 3,000 ml.

Water and electrolytes normally leave the body by way of skin, lungs, kidneys and bowel. *Insensible fluid loss* is that which is lost through skin and lungs. Perspiring is the primary cause of insensible loss, but water is exhaled also from the lungs as vapor. Breathing on a mirror makes it cloudy with moisture. The largest amount of fluid is excreted by the kidneys, and a relatively small amount is lost in feces. The tubules of the kidneys select and return to the general circulation electrolytes needed by the body. Those ions not needed by the body are excreted in the urine. As the kidney is in contact only with the extracellular compartment, to affect the composition of intracellular water it first must make changes in extracellular water; these changes in turn will affect the composition of cellular water. The kidneys form approximately 180 liters of glomerular filtrate each day, making continuous adjustments in ion selection according to the needs of the cells. All but approximately 1 liter of the 180 liters of glomerular filtrate is reabsorbed into the blood. The remaining liter passes into the renal pelvis in the form of urine. The total daily urinary output for the average adult is usually under 2 liters, and total fluid output ranges from 1,850 to 3,600 ml. To keep the body in good condition, the amount of fluid lost each day should be balanced approximately by the amount taken in.

The normal functioning of the body depends on the maintenance of constant conditions within the body's internal environment. Body fluids carry nutrients and oxygen to the cells and remove waste products from them. Relative quantities of water and electrolytes must not be disturbed; if they are disturbed, severe symptoms, damage to tissues and even death may result.

Observations and Nursing Care

Do you see the pitting edema on the ankle of a patient with cardiac disease? The clear fluid in a blister? The sweat on the forehead of a patient

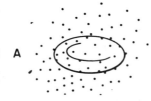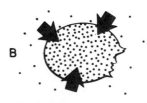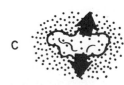

FIG. 6-3. Concentration of particles in cells in relation to surrounding fluid. (A) Isosmotic: the number of particles within the cell and in the fluid surrounding the cell are approximately equal. Water passes across the cell wall in both directions. (B) Hypo-osmotic: the number of particles in the fluid is less than the number inside the cell. Water flows into the cell until the concentration is equal on both sides of the wall, or until the cell bursts. (C) Hyperosmotic: the number of particles in the fluid is greater than the number inside the cell. The cell becomes dehydrated as the water leaves it.

in pain? The mucoid return at the bottom of a gastric suction bottle? Vomitus in the basin? Diarrheal stool in the bedpan? There are valuable electrolytes in each, as important to the patient as his blood.

Careful observation of fluid intake and output is important in the early detection of water and electrolyte imbalance. The amount of vomitus should be measured and charted, and the amount of perspiration should be noted and described as accurately as possible. Since water and electrolytes are lost through the abnormal drainage that is part of therapy, such as aspiration of secretions of the gastrointestinal tract, it is essential to measure the contents of all drainage bottles accurately. Note by measurement the amount of blood or other drainage coming from a wound or a body orifice, or, if this observation is impossible, estimate the amount as accurately as possible. Although accurate tabulations of intake and output are singularly rare in hospital practice, *this phase of nursing, on which the doctor may judge his replacement therapy, is of the greatest importance to the patient.*

Keeping an accurate intake and output record is a matter of communication among aides, nurses and doctors. Sometimes the patient can help, too, by keeping track of what he drinks and measuring his own urine in a graduate. For your patients:

1. Be sure that you know whether or not they are on Intake and Output. It is not necessary to wait for a doctor's order. Use your nursing judgment.

2. Find out how many ml. are in a cup, a glass, a bowl.

3. Be sure that the ambulatory patient has been cautioned not to discard his urine before it is measured.

4. Record intake and output at the time the patient has intake or output.

5. Check his intake and output record for completeness before leaving the floor.

6. Remember that output includes vomitus, diarrhea, drainage—any output.

Daily weight is often requested as an aid in determining loss or retention of body fluids. One liter of water weighs 2.2 pounds. Always weigh the patient at the same time of day in the same amount of clothing and on the same scale. If there is a marked change in the patient's weight, notify the doctor.

Unless contraindicated by the type of surgery, such as that on the gastrointestinal tract, it is important to encourage fluid intake during the preoperative and the early postoperative periods. Postoperative orders will indicate when and whether the patient may have fluids. If the amount is to be in any way unusual, this will be specified by the doctor—for example, "encourage fluids to 2,000 ml." or "restrict fluids to 750 ml./day." Taking fluids helps to regulate water and electrolytes and reduces the need for prolonged intravenous therapy, thereby canceling some discomforts. Patients usually tolerate fluids best when they are given frequently in small amounts. Whenever the patient's preferences for certain fluids do not conflict with the doctor's orders, giving him the fluids that he likes will increase his intake. Some postoperative patients can retain carbonated beverages, like ginger ale, better than plain water.

INTRAVENOUS THERAPY

Parenteral Replacement Therapy. Some of the solutions commonly used for parenteral replacement therapy are the following:

• Glucose in water, given in 5 per cent or 10 per cent solutions, supplies carbohydrate in a readily usable form, or is used slowly only to keep a vein open for emergency purposes.

• Isotonic solution of sodium chloride (sodium chloride 0.9% solution). Other substances, such as potassium, vitamins or antibiotics, may be added.

• Plasma expanders, such as Dextran, can be used as substitutes for whole blood and plasma to maintain the volume of circulating blood and to prevent shock. Dextran contains an unusually large sugar molecule. Because of these large particles it increases the amount of circulating fluid in the bloodstream by pulling tissue fluid into the blood vessels. The volume of circulating fluid is expanded, thus lessening shock due to too little fluid in the vascular system. The use of plasma expanders is especially applicable when adequate supplies of whole blood and plasma cannot be quickly obtained.

• Whole blood is used to supply red cells and plasma. Plasma (blood minus red blood cells) alone may be given when additional red blood cells are not needed. Because plasma can be stored for long periods, and whole blood cannot, plasma is more readily available in emergencies.

• Electrolyte solutions contain many of the electrolytes found in the cellular and extracellular spaces. These solutions are chosen for replacement therapy on the basis of the patient's needs for electrolytes and water.

• Amino acid solutions also may be given intravenously. Their use is especially important in conditions involving prolonged malnutrition. Amigen is one preparation containing amino acids for intravenous use. It should be administered slowly so as not to produce such untoward symptoms as nausea and a feeling of warmth.

• Emulsified fats are available for parenteral administration. Their use, however, is attended by a high incidence of untoward reactions.

Although the procedure for intravenous therapy can be reviewed readily in texts on the fundamentals of nursing, several points are especially important and should not be overlooked even on busy wards:

• The rate of administration is important. While the doctor usually regulates the flow initially, the maintenance of the correct rate is almost always the responsibility of the nurse. The usual rate of flow is about 60 drops per minute. The physician may request more rapid administration if the patient is severely dehydrated, or he may ask for slower administration with a microdrip set in elderly persons, those with cardiovascular disease, or for those solutions containing potent drugs.

• Find out what your patient's attitude to intravenous therapy is. He may think of it as a last measure resorted to by desperate doctors. Allowing him to express his thoughts and explaining to him that it is merely another way of eating may help to lessen his fear. If preoperatively the patient sees others getting intravenous fluids, the nurse can tell him that he also may get some fluids this way after his operation.

• Promptly after the absorption of the solution in the bottle the intravenous infusion should be discontinued, or more solution should be added as ordered. Allowing the solution to run out and the blood to clot in the needle closes the vein, with the result that the needle must be reinserted, and the patient caused needless pain.

• In some hospitals nurses are asked to add some medications to intravenous solutions when the solution is being prepared for administration. In other hospitals only the physician adds medications to intravenous solutions. Always indicate what is added by labeling the bottle clearly.

• Never administer medication by injecting it into the tubing after the intravenous infusion has been started, unless such administration has been specifically ordered, and unless the administration of intravenous medications is considered part of the nurse's function in that hospital. Injecting medication into the tubing gives the patient a more concentrated dose than does adding medication to the bottle.

• Unless there is a specific, written order to the contrary, solutions containing potassium should not run into a patient's vein at a rate faster than 40 mEq. every 8 hours for fear of too rapid rise in serum potassium and cardiac standstill. In emergencies, the maximum rate is 40 mEq. every 2 hours.

• Watch the site of injection carefully for infiltration of solution into the tissue, evidenced by swelling and blanching of the skin. This observation is always necessary and is especially important when certain substances that can cause sloughing of tissues, such as levarterenol (Levophed) are being administered.

• If a needle is used and it enters an arm vein at a joint or in the back of the hand, the arm or the hand should be supported. Use a wooden splint or a special metal holder. If the arm does not have excessive hair, fastening it loosely to the board with adhesive tape at both ends and near the needle will sometimes hold better than gauze bandage. If the patient has much hair it can be shaved off over the area to be taped. Whether gauze or tape is used, be sure that it is snug enough to hold but not so tight that it compresses the blood vessels. Venous catheters allow more flexibility and are tolerated for longer periods of time.

• The administration of intravenous infusions should not interfere with postoperative nursing care. If the arm is supported carefully in the correct position, the patient can be turned without dislodging the needle or intracath. Keep the arm well splinted and the tubing loose while turning the patient.

• Transfusion reactions may occur from administration of the wrong blood, allergic response or bacterial contamination. Watch carefully for chills, fever, dyspnea, cyanosis, and sudden sharp pain in the lumbar region. If any of these symptoms appear, stop the transfusion and seek additional direction from the physician. If it is decided that the transfusion is not responsible for the symptoms, it can be restarted. However, if the blood is at fault, permitting additional blood to enter the patient's body while you are seeking advice may cause serious and even fatal consequences. Careful checking of labels on the blood to be administered is of crucial importance.

• Be careful! Plain distilled, sterile water *never* is given intravenously. It is hypo-osmotic and will destroy the patient's red blood cells. Some head nurses keep the supply of sterile distilled water away from the supply of intravenous fluid bottles to prevent its accidental use.

BODY DEFENSES

Sources of Body Protection

The body maintains many reserves. When a blood vessel fails, often the body can replace its function with the development of other vessels to the stricken part (collateral circulation). Oxygen cannot be stockpiled, but the body does have a supply of minerals, vitamins, food and fluid beyond immediate requirements. There is a reserve capacity for many vital functions of the body. For example, there is more lung tissue than is normally required. There are two kidneys, although one could provide satisfactory renal function. There is reserve liver function, and dual organs of sight and hearing.

Hyperplasia. This extra growth of normal tissue is a mysterious body asset resulting in *hypertrophy* (enlargement). We do not always know how the body commands this extra growth, but it occurs in certain tissues in time of extra need. If one kidney is removed, the remaining kidney may enlarge, increasing the amount of available kidney function. Other examples in endocrine glands, muscles, heart and lymphatic tissue are common.

At times hyperplasia can occur when no apparent need for it exists. There may be hyperplasia in the thyroid gland, with such excess secretion that it is toxic to the body.

(With disuse some tissues and organs decrease in size and in capacity to work [*atrophy*]. In a limb confined for a long time in a cast, bone as well as muscle may show this effect. Atrophy from disuse usually reverts to normal with the return of normal demand on the involved structure. Atrophy can occur without evident reason, and it may resist reversal to normal.)

The Autonomic Nervous System. Another source of body protection is the organized provision for *adjustment* through the autonomic nervous system. If a normal person stands up, the momentary rush of blood toward the lower limbs causes immediate orders from this system to constrict the blood vessels in the lower body. Since there is no room in the constricted vessels for an undue proportion of the body blood, a fair share is ensured for distribution to other parts of the body, particularly the brain, where arterial flow is not aided by gravity.

Orders through the autonomic nervous system regulate sweating, alter the size of the pupils of the eyes, speed and slow heart beats, and direct many other adjustments in the body that are beyond voluntary control. Moment to moment,

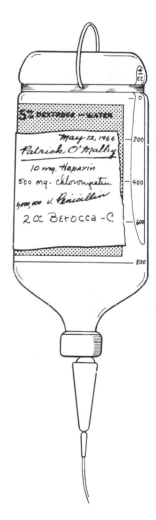

FIG. 6-4. The label on an infusion bottle should include the name of the patient, the date of preparation, and every ingredient in the bottle. The patient's label is taped on the bottle so that it does not cover the name of the solution.

whether human beings are awake or asleep, the autonomic nervous system is making adjustments in response to the ever-changing environment around and inside them.

Provisions Against Hazards. Externally, the skin shell, with its superficial layer of dead cells, is a relatively impermeable covering. As long as it remains intact, it is the major protection of the body from invasion by organisms. The outer layer of the skin prevents soaps, lotions, perfumes and other chemical irritants from coming in contact with living cells.

Openings into the body are not without protection. Hydrochloric acid in the stomach creates an environment in which bacteria do not thrive. The reflexes of blinking and sneezing guard the eyes and the respiratory tract. Secretions in these areas have antimicrobial activity. The unprescribed use of washes, gargles, douches and irrigations often do not offer as much protection as the natural material they wash away. Body openings have a rich blood supply and abundant lymphatic tissue to serve the cells of the area, if they are invaded by organisms.

The hard bony skull is protection for the delicate tissues of the brain. The rib cage is protection for the thoracic organs. A whole series of defensive barriers protects the lungs from infection by organisms of the air and the teeming bacterial population of the nose and the throat, through which every breath passes. Tears and mucus wash away particles of dust and microorganisms. Tiny cilia beat against foreign matter to hasten its exit from the body.

Major Internal Defenses. These are the highly organized reactions called forth when the body is threatened. These reactions can originate in the endocrine glands, through their chemical messengers, the *hormones.* For example, in times of sudden, urgent distress everyone has experienced the sensations of a large dose of epinephrine (Adrenalin). When the sympathetic division of the autonomic nervous system orders this hormone released from the adrenal medulla, it enters the bloodstream and produces a massive body-wide reaction. The alert state of the body produced by epinephrine has been described as preparation for "fight or flight."

A second hormonal reaction can occur when the pituitary gland orders the adrenal cortex to discharge its adrenal cortical steroid. Hydrocortisone constitutes a major part of the substance released. (A study of this material, which we have available as a drug, can be found in Chapter 28, Rodman and Smith, *Pharmacology and Drug Therapy in Nursing,* Lippincott, 1968. See also p. 187.) Blood pressure, water and electrolyte regulation, the membranes covering cells and the metabolism of glucose are only a few of the structures and the mechanisms affected. Particularly during periods of prolonged stress the hormonal activity of the adrenal cortex provides a key to the widespread reaction that defends the body. (See beginning of this chapter.) Hormones also regulate many processes to maintain a normal cellular environment. The hormones help to avoid the harm that could follow those occasions when excess fluid, sugar or salt ingestion otherwise would upset radically the normal environment of the cells.

The Inflammatory Response

A wound is a break in the continuity of tissue, caused by physical means, such as a knife or burns. How does the body handle the problem of injury or necrosis, in which some special attention is required that is not routine for the rest of the body? First, there must be some way for the injured area to signal its distress. There must be provision for the removal of dead cells, and some kind of replacement must fill in the defect left behind.

Inflammation is the body's response to damage of cells. Regardless of the cause, whether a cut, a burn, a bruise or a pinch, the reaction is similar. The signal that starts the reaction may be the release from dead or injured cells of some of their internal substances, such as histamine. These substances have a profound effect on the capillaries they contact. The capillaries dilate widely and thus bring greatly increased amounts of blood to the area. If the action takes place in the skin or in tissues close under it, the redness produced by this flushing is visible. This site is warm to touch, because it has a greater supply of blood than the tissue around it.

Not only do the capillaries dilate, but the "mesh" of their walls also is opened. Normally, capillaries are permeable to the passage of water and electrolytes, but in this situation they permit extra fluid and some protein of the plasma to escape. This extra content in the tissue spaces produces swelling. Often the swelling is sufficient to stimulate the receptors for pain. The blood vessel changes are responsible for the *cardinal symptoms of inflammation: swelling, pain, redness and heat.*

The patient is made uncomfortable by the throbbing often felt in the part. The tense tissues of the damage-area no longer cushion the impact of the heartbeat in the vessels. The jolt is transmitted by the nerves, and the patient feels the throb of each heartbeat.

Among the substances released by the injured cells is one which attracts leukocytes. They pass through the capillary walls into the damaged tissues. When there is extensive tissue damage, with consequently great release of the substance that attracts leukocytes, this material may be absorbed and circulate in the blood. It appears to stimulate the production of more white blood cells. A blood count taken at this time will demonstrate an increase in the white cells of the blood far beyond normal (leukocytosis).

Fever often accompanies inflammation. How inflammation influences the temperature-regulating center is not clear. Possibly a substance absorbed from the injured cells is the signal that stimulates this response.

These effects of inflammation might prove to be beneficial. The protein escaping into the damaged tissue tends to gel and impede movement of materials within the site. Swelling and pain encourage the individual to keep the injured part at rest, which prevents activity from dispersing the contents of the injured area. Bacteria or an offensive substance, such as a foreign chemical, could create additional harm if distributed beyond the local tissue. Fever may be beneficial by speeding the rate of chemical reactions, thus bolstering the chemical defenses.

Inflammation attracts attention. The patient feels its effects, and the doctor relies on its features to help to locate and to identify the place and the type of body injury. By watching the sequence of symptoms it is possible to decide whether the body is overcoming its problem successfully or needs help to master it.

At times it is desirable to combat inflammation by countering the vascular dilatation. For example, cold compresses may be prescribed for a sprained ankle, because there is no apparent benefit from the painful swelling, and no microorganism needs to be isolated. The removal of necrotic tissue still takes place, although at a slower pace because of the vasoconstriction induced by the cold. Sometimes the doctor prescribes cold compresses for the first 24 hours to impede swelling, and then warmth to increase blood supply and to hasten the removal of waste.

In summary, important effects of inflammation include:

- The capillaries dilate to bring more blood to the part, and in the blood more oxygen, nutrients, leukocytes and heat.
- Swelling occurs as fluid escapes from blood vessels into tissues.
- Pain is felt because these changes cause pressure on nerve endings.

Tissue Repair

As damaged tissue is being cleared of its debris, the signal for repair is given. One of two types of repair follows: replacement with tissue identical with that destroyed or replacement with scar tissue.

When there is a break in tissue, cells bordering the defect multiply and fill it. However, if the defect is large, the ability to re-establish identical cells is diminished or lost. To encourage repair with normal or near-normal structures, the sides of identical tissue are brought together. The surgeon lines up each of the surfaces of tissue he cut through at the time of operation. The sutures hold the tissues firmly in this position and allow the patient reasonable freedom of movement without worry that the wound edges will shift. Optimal healing occurs with some normal cells and a narrow line of scar cells the length of the incision. This ideal healing is called "healing by first intention."

Sometimes the edges of a traumatic wound are so far apart that they cannot be pulled together satisfactorily; sometimes the products of infection separate the tissue surfaces. The open skin is a way of escape for dead cells and other debris that must be removed from the area before regrowth can be complete. In such cases, packing may be used to keep the wound open and methods to promote drainage, such as irrigation, may be ordered. Scar tissue is allowed to fill the defect from the bottom. This is called "healing by secondary intention." In "third intention healing" a large gaping wound is filled in with granulation tissue.

The scar mass is formed by cells called *fibroblasts.* These cells locate throughout the protein gel and start to extend little fibrils or threads from the cell body. As the threads weave and intertwine, a network is formed from side to side. To nourish the working cells in this area, otherwise deprived of circulation, capillaries from normal tissue bud out and crisscross the defect.

They give a pink or bright-red appearance, and at this stage the tissue being formed is called *granulation tissue.*

Granulation tissue is delicate and very vascular. Great gentleness should be used when changing dressings to avoid damaging newly forming tissues, as well as to prevent unnecessary discomfort to the patient. Packing or gauze that adheres to the tissues should be moistened with sterile saline before removal, to avoid pulling the delicate tissues apart.

When the union of tissues is satisfactory, a signal stops further work by the fibroblasts. In the weeks to follow their fibrils tend to harden and contract. The drawing tight of the network of tough fibrils can cause deformity. The pull of a contracted scar is strong enough to tilt the head or keep an entire limb in a contorted position. This problem is one of the reasons for attempting care that allows healing with a minimum of scar formation.

The scar is as strong at 3 weeks as it ever will be, but it continues to change for a long time. With contraction, the scar squeezes out the capillaries that once richly infiltrated its network. It begins to blanch, and over months and years it becomes colorless.

Blood flow is the key to healing. Healing is poor where there is normally a poor supply of blood. The anterior portion of the lower leg is such a site, and injuries there heal slowly. Because adipose tissue has poor vascularity, it heals slowly. The surgeon knows extra care and time will be required for healing in an obese person in whom great pads of fat have been joined together within the wound. Circulation must never be impaired by carelessness. Tight garments or dressings on or above a wound should not pass without notice. When there is a leg wound, the patient must be encouraged to move from an unfavorable position, such as crossed legs. Excessive tension or pulling on wound edges can delay healing. Be alert for any signs of impaired circulation, such as swelling, coldness, absence of pulse, pallor or mottling, and report them. In applying a dressing, particularly to an extremity, make certain that it is not so tight as to impair circulation.

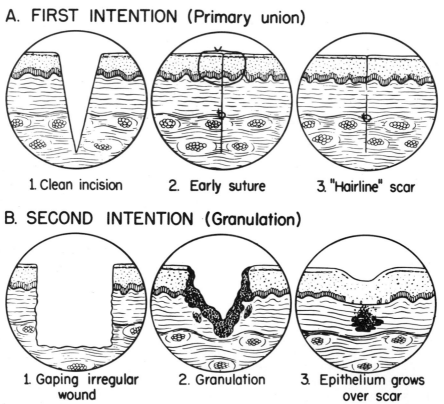

A. FIRST INTENTION (Primary union)

1. Clean incision 2. Early suture 3. "Hairline" scar

B. SECOND INTENTION (Granulation)

1. Gaping irregular wound 2. Granulation 3. Epithelium grows over scar

Fig. 6-5. First and second intention wound healing. (Rhoads, J. E., *et al.: Surgery—Principles and Practice,* ed. 4, Philadelphia, Lippincott)

BODY RESPONSES TO INFECTION
Inflammation

The inflammatory defense in infection is usually greater than that in which no pathogen is involved. The patient with an injured area of heart muscle due to a coronary occlusion will have an inflammatory response: a slight fever and a slight leukocytosis; whereas in infection the leukocytosis is usually pronounced. Infection also influences the kinds of white blood cells that will appear. In viral disease the response may

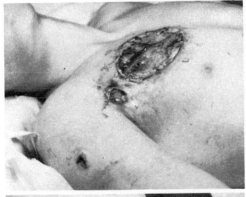

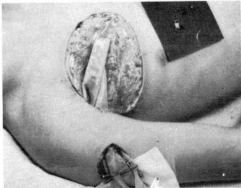

FIG. 6-6. Gunshot wound of arm and anterior thorax. The wounds were débrided, and adequate drainage was established. A graft was required to close the chest wound. Note the granulation tissue in the second picture. (Hardy, J. D.: *Pathophysiology in Surgery*, Baltimore, Williams & Wilkins)

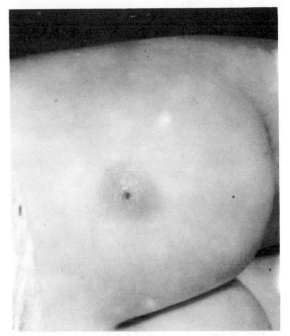

FIG. 6-8. This painful abscess followed an intramuscular injection. Note the swelling and the redness. (Medichrome—Clay-Adams, Inc., New York, N.Y.)

not be characteristic, or there may be little response. However, in many bacterial infections rapid changes occur that demonstrate how the body is handling the infection. When a doctor suspects that a patient may have an early appendicitis, he can watch the white blood cell count, taken a few hours apart. If there is a growing inflammation and infection, the white cells increase in number.

An infection that has not spread is said to be *localized*. A white, thick exudate of dead cell debris develops inside an outer shell. This material is pus, and a pocket of pus is called an *abscess*. A furuncle (boil) is an abscess of the subcutaneous layers of skin. Around its edges the fight between leukocytes and bacteria continues and adds to the pus accumulation. The pressure of the pocket of pus causes pain.

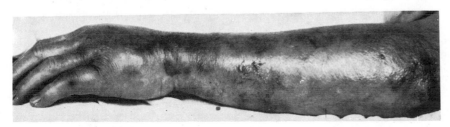

FIG. 6-7. Streptococcal infection of hand and arm. There is no localization. (Rhoads, J. E., *et al.: Surgery —Principles and Practice*, ed. 4, Philadelphia, Lippincott)

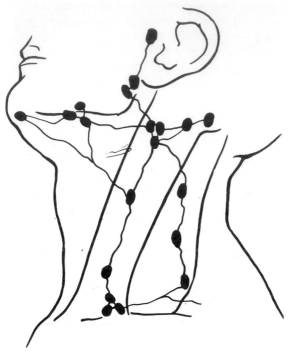

Fig. 6-9. Lymph nodes of the neck help to prevent spread of infection from a primary site in the head or neck to the rest of the body.

When the infection is conquered in the tissue surrounding the abscess, the doctor may drain the abscess safely. If a rim of a furuncle reaches the skin surface, the abscess may rupture spontaneously. A liver abscess may rupture and evacuate its contents into the abdomen. The abscess can join two surfaces with a channel between them (fistula). For example, a gonococcal infection of the vagina can invade the adjoining tissue of the overlying bladder, resulting in a fistula between vagina and bladder. Urine then would not stay in the bladder but would seep through the fistula and drain from the vagina.

Infections caused by certain organisms localize more readily than do others. The streptococcus, for example, can produce products that tend to break down the confining protein gel of the inflammatory exudate. Therefore, its ability to spread in the tissues and to invade lymphatic channels is greater than that of some other organisms. Wide tissue inflammation without pus is characteristic of its infection.

The infection caused by the staphylococccus tends to become walled off. The organisms can multiply rapidly inside the walls, but they have less chance to extend into surrounding structures.

The lymphatic system has nodes at frequent intervals. These nodes are a defense against infection, but sometimes they become infected themselves. Inflammation of the lymph glands is called *lymphadenitis*. The swelling in the lymph gland at the node produces a tender, firm lump—a signal that organisms have reached this point. If the organisms are sufficiently numerous and virulent, they may resist destructive forces in the lymph channels and pass through node after node. Eventually, the lymph glands drain into the veins, and bacteria are deposited in the bloodstream. When infective organisms circulate in the blood, the condition is called *septicemia*. Although organs such as lung, spleen and liver are rich in lymphatic tissue traps, septicemia threatens by blood-borne delivery every tissue in the body in which the organism might find living conditions suitable to its taste. Once in the blood, although defensive forces continue to wage war, the organisms may spread throughout the body to infect many tissues.

Fever is a cardinal sign of infection. It is almost always present when there is septicemia. The temperature may increase as the infection grows. A very sudden high fever is not uncommon in infection. The superficial blood vessels constrict to avoid loss of warmth from the blood. Sweating stops, and circulation is diverted to the deepest, most protected blood vessels. The patient feels cold. Muscles begin to contract in uncontrollable shivering and shaking. Heat is being produced by the activity of the chill. Suddenly the patient feels extremely hot. Sweating and vasodilation occur. Fever at this time can be dangerously high. It tends to subside gradually over a period of hours, but in some patients the new excessive temperature level remains relatively unchanged hour after hour. (See Chap. 58 for a discussion of the care of the patient with hyperthermia.)

A chill often is a signal that the body is responding to microorganisms that have entered the bloodstream. It is, therefore, an opportunity to identify the organisms. If the patient is in the hospital his doctor should be notified so he can draw blood for culturing if he wishes.

A severe chill is both uncomfortable for the patient and frightening. The chattering of his teeth and the shaking of his body—movement that he cannot control—may be so violent that the whole bed shakes with him. He can stop only after his skin is warmed. He may need several blankets over him. Bath blankets placed next to his skin will help. So will hot-water bottles and heating pads, especially at the feet. A doctor's order is needed before these are applied. External heat may help, but the chill ceases in response to the internal mechanism of the body. Antipyretic-analgesic drugs are useful for reducing temperature and making the febrile patient more comfortable.

As soon as the chill is over, some of the covers from the patient should be removed. Sudden extremes of temperature should be avoided, but too much covering will increase the patient's temperature unduly. Since a chill is a result of peripheral blood vessel constriction, it is not infrequent for a patient to have a fever of 103° and be shaking with the cold he feels. Check his T.P.R. every 15 minutes, or as ordered. A patient who has experienced a chill should have his temperature taken at least every hour until the temperature is stable. The patient may be drenched in sweat as the temperature starts to drop. To prevent too rapid cooling and to lessen discomfort, replace his gown with a dry one and change any damp bed linen.

Hospitals present a problem in infection because they have a high population of pathogens donated by patients whose infections release billions of organisms of proved virulence. These pathogens become resident organisms on the skin and the mucous membranes of hospital personnel. They also live on the hospital floors and equipment. When such numbers of available virulent organisms come in contact with many vulnerable hosts, such as the patients debilitated by other diseases or those with wounds, infection can become extremely common. Many organisms, especially staphylococci, have developed resistance to certain antibiotics. Because of these known hazards, rules have been developed to govern practices in the hospital, rules about isolation, changing dressings, housekeeping, and operating room activities. In essence, all the rules apply the principle that in a hospital the only way to avoid infection is to separate the organisms from the potential hosts.

Immunity

Two reactions to infection may occur—the basic response of inflammation and the response related to immunity.

The body reacts to any substance not normal to it. Some of the reactions are common to all people while others develop from each individual's experience. The response depends on material called *immune bodies*. They are capable of altering the nature of foreign material (*antigen*). Immune bodies can produce many kinds of alterations, but the successful outcome is the destruction of the antigen. The immune bodies that destroy organisms are called *antibodies*. The immune bodies that destroy toxins are called *antitoxins*.

Human beings are born with some immune bodies. The tissue of other animals and of other people, when present in a person's body, usually is destroyed by native immune bodies. In addition to natural immunity, the body responds to some foreign substances by producing antibodies and antitoxins to destroy them. When an antigen is introduced into the body for the first time, the lymphatic tissue begins to manufacture an immune body. Sometimes the original experience with a specific antigen is so profound that the tissue can pour out antibodies at any time for the rest of the person's life. This state is *permanent immunity*. *Temporary immunity* requires the renewed stimulus of antigen to produce antibodies.

Killed organisms or those that are alive but attenuated (lacking in virulence) are made into a vaccine, which can be injected to stimulate the body to produce antibodies against that organism. When a virulent form of the organism subsequently invades the body, the defense has already been prepared. In a similar way, modified toxins (toxoids) can be injected to stimulate the body to make antitoxin. This kind of immunity is *active immunity*.

If another individual or animal has become actively immune to an organism or a toxin, a special preparation of the serum from that person or animal can be given a threatened individual to provide some defense, even though the recipient has played no part in producing it. If the use of this serum is protective, the individual is said to be *passively immunized*. When the donated serum disappears, the individual has no immunity left. His own lymphatic cells have not been stimulated to produce antibodies.

ALLERGY

There is no general agreement on what the term *allergy* means. It is a term bearing a close relationship with immunity which is customarily regarded as indicating protection against infectious agents. However, to most of us allergy is synonymous with hay fever, asthma, hives, anaphylaxis and other illnesses or phenomena which cannot be interpreted as protective. In its most general sense, then, allergy refers to a state of *altered* immunologic reactivity whereby the body is injured in the course of its immune response against an agent "recognized" as something foreign to the body. Thus an *immunogen,* a substance capable of stimulating the host to produce an immune response, becomes an *allergen* when that immune response injures the host. The immunogen may be a bacterium, virus, pollen particle, drug (e.g. penicillin) or it might even be a normal constituent of the host such as the red blood cell in so-called autoimmune hemolytic anemia. In this last example it is assumed that through some unknown mechanism the body perceives its own red cell as foreign and mounts an immune response against it resulting in its own destruction. It would be more consistent with our definition to call this *autoallergic* hemolytic anemia.

INCIDENCE

It has been estimated that approximately 10 per cent of the population has a tendency to develop clinically significant allergies. However, sensitivity to certain substances is widespread among the population. Individual susceptibility to such substances often varies. For example, some persons develop poison ivy merely from walking past the plant without contact with the plant itself; others develop it only if the leaves rub against the skin. Almost everyone who has been host to the tubercle bacillus has a positive skin reaction to tuberculin.

Allergy can occur at any age, and in the same individual the pattern of allergic response often varies over the years. A person may show suddenly an allergic reaction to a substance with which he has had contact for years. On the other hand, allergic responses to one agent may disappear gradually even without treatment, to be replaced by sensitivity to another substance, or the person may be left entirely free of symptoms. Why these changes occur is not clear. They may be related to changes in the body's metabolism at different periods of life, to unusual physical or emotional stress or to changes in the environment (e.g., moving to a new part of the country and being exposed to different pollens or to larger doses of pollen). As in many other conditions, fatigue, emotional stress and the presence of infections contribute to development of symptoms of allergy in susceptible persons. Symptoms of allergy may appear when the patient is tired or emotionally upset, or they may be aggravated by tension and fatigue.

SUBSTANCES COMMONLY CAUSING ALLERGY

Allergens may be classified as those that are inhaled or ingested and those that come in contact with the skin. Here are some common examples:

INHALANTS	INGESTANTS	CONTACTANTS
Dust	Eggs	Wool
Feathers	Seafood	Nylon
Animal danders	Nuts	Dye (such as hair dye, shoe dye)
Pollens	Chocolate	Cosmetics

Drug allergy is common and can be caused by almost any drug. Certain drugs, such as penicillin, quinine and thiouracil, are especially likely to cause allergic reactions. An allergic response to drugs is a different phenomenon from toxicity due to overdosage; even a minute amount of a drug to which the patient is sensitive can cause symptoms. Such commonly used and relatively safe drugs as aspirin can produce severe allergic response. Sometimes in giving a new drug to an allergic patient, small doses are given initially to determine the patient's reaction, or an antihistamine is administered simultaneously. Allergic reactions to drugs may be immediate, or they may be delayed for several hours or days. A variety of common allergic responses may occur, although some drugs are noted for causing a particular type of reaction, such as the rash that follows the administration of penicillin.

If a patient says, "Is that aspirin? I'm allergic to it," take his word for it. Withhold the drug (whatever it may be) and check with the doctor. Never assume that a small dose will not matter, or that the patient is mistaken. You are the one who administers many potent drugs—often drugs that the patient has never received before. Be alert for any symptoms that may indicate allergy, and report them promptly.

When you are preparing medications, you can lessen the contact of drugs with your skin by working neatly, avoiding spilling and washing your hands afterward. Never out of curiosity taste the drugs that you are administering. These simple measures will help you to avoid allergies due to contact with drugs during your work.

DIAGNOSIS

The diagnosis of allergy may be the simplest and the most clear-cut matter, or it may tax the resources of the most astute physician and require a high degree of assistance from the patient, his family and the nurse. A patient may develop typical symptoms of allergic rhinitis only when ragweed is pollenating, leading the doctor to suspect immediately that ragweed is the offender and to perform a skin test to confirm this diagnosis. The cause-and-effect relationship may be so clear that the patient himself may affirm, "I can't eat strawberries. They give me hives." On the other hand, a patient may have repeated asthmatic attacks throughout the year without any apparent relationship to the substances that he eats or inhales. Sometimes by very careful observation and skillful interviewing the doctor may discover clues that previously had passed unnoticed. For instance, the patient or a family member may recall that each attack occurred after visiting friends who had a dog. Such a clue is followed with skin tests for sensitivity to animal dander and further observation of the relationship between allergic symptoms and contact with dogs.

The diagnosis is made more complicated by the fact that the patient may be allergic to several things, and that his tendency to develop symptoms varies with the degree of fatigue or emotional stress and with the presence of infection. Symptoms may not occur each time the patient is in contact with the allergen.

• Skin tests. Skin testing is begun by making a scratch on the skin and applying the test antigen to the scratch. This lessens the danger of a severe reaction in a highly sensitive individual. There have been reports of sudden anaphylactic reactions from intradermal injection of penicillin in persons suspected of penicillin allergy. If the scratch test is negative then tiny amounts of the suspected antigen are injected intradermally. After about 20 minutes the physician inspects the site of the injection. If the area has a wheal, surrounded by erythema, a positive reaction to the antigen has occurred. Extracts of various pollens, animal danders and so on may be administered in this way, and the patient's reaction is noted. Sometimes, even though the patient has a positive skin test, he encounters no symptoms when he is in contact with the substances; or despite a negative skin test, all the evidence seems to point to one substance as being responsible.

The Nurse's Role. The nurse can help with diagnosis by being alert to the possible relationship between the patient's symptoms, his contact

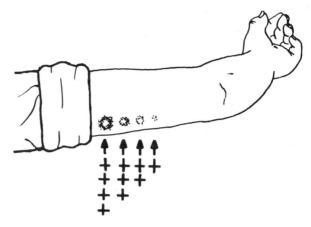

Fig. 6-10. Positive skin tests. Positive reactions are characterized by a wheal surrounded by erythema. The severity of the reaction frequently is described as ranging from 1+ to 4+.

with substances in the environment and his physical and emotional state at the time the symptoms appear or grow worse. These observations must be made unobtrusively and then reported to the doctor. Avoid constant reminders or suggestions like "Maybe it's those flowers—we'll have to get rid of them," or "I'll bet it's that fish you ate for lunch." Continued reminders of possible allergens may make the patient feel that his environment is filled with lurking danger and cause him to fear contact with things that may have nothing to do with his symptoms.

The nurse assists also with skin tests. In addition to assembling and preparing equipment for the doctor to use (syringes and needles, extracts of various antigens), the nurse often is asked to observe the patient during the interval between the injections and the reading of the test. During this period of approximately 20 minutes the patient may note the development of itchy wheals, indicating a positive skin reaction to the substance injected at that site. Assure the patient that the wheals and the itching will subside soon, just as mosquito bites do, and advise him not to scratch them.

Observe the patient very carefully for any sudden sneezing, difficulty in breathing, pallor, faintness or sweating that might indicate a severe generalized allergic reaction. If you notice any such symptoms, tell the doctor at once.

Observing the patient can be achieved without staring or even making him aware that you are watching. Just stay nearby and glance at him frequently while you are busy with other tasks.

The doses used in skin testing are so small that severe reactions are unusual. Nevertheless, they do happen occasionally. Epinephrine 1:1,000, syringes and needles for intravenous injection and tourniquets are kept unobtrusively ready whenever antigens are given, because the substances being injected are those to which the patient may be extremely sensitive. If a severe reaction occurs, the doctor may give epinephrine either subcutaneously or intravenously, and he may apply a tourniquet on the patient's arm above the point where the injection was given in order to diminish absorption of the antigen. The doctor may ask you to apply ice to the site of the injection as another way of diminishing absorption.

TREATMENT

Avoidance of the Allergen. When it is feasible, this is the surest, safest treatment. For example, avoiding strawberries is a simple matter, but avoiding eggs is more difficult, since they are so often an ingredient of other foods. While the patient cannot avoid house dust entirely, he can diminish his contact with it by:

* Avoiding dust catchers. Heavy draperies that are not easily laundered are a good example. Curtains that can be tossed into a washing machine and need no ironing are preferable, so that they can be laundered very frequently. 'Bedspreads and blankets should be easily washable.
* Using a vacuum cleaner rather than a dust mop or broom for cleaning. The dust is sucked into the machine, and less of it flies about the room during cleaning. Of course, it is preferable to have someone else do the cleaning while the patient is out of the house. Sometimes this arrangement is not possible, and the patient must learn to clean in a way that stirs up as little dust as possible.
* Dusting with a damp cloth rather than a dry one. Using a commercially treated cloth that causes dust to cling to it is often a help.
* Wearing a face mask while cleaning if the doctor recommends it.
* Obtaining an air conditioner, if the patient can afford it. Air conditioners decrease dust as well as pollens.

If the patient is allergic to feathers, he will need to eliminate all pillows and comforters filled with feathers and to substitute those filled with foam rubber or a variety of synthetic fabrics. Help the patient to learn specifically what the allergens are that he must avoid and to develop the habit of examining labels. By reading the labels he can find out just what ingredients are in commercially prepared foods and just what material is used to stuff pillows. When a person who has food allergies eats out, he should avoid mixtures, confining himself instead to plain foods of known composition.

When avoidance is not possible as, for example, when the patient is allergic to pollen, and circumstances require that he continue to live and work where the pollen is troublesome at certain seasons, he may be treated by desensitization and/or antihistamines.

Densensitization is accomplished by administering tiny doses of the antigen subcutaneously and gradually increasing the dose. In this way the patient slowly develops increased tolerance for the substance and fewer symptoms. Sometimes symptoms can be relieved completely in this way.

Desensitization is started usually before the season begins, if the patient's allergy is seasonal, and it may be continued throughout the season. If symptoms persist throughout the year, as is often the case when such substances as house dust are involved, treatment must be continued during the entire year. Injections may be given once a week or more or less frequently, depending on the patient's particular needs. Some patients find that their symptoms eventually disappear and require no further treatment, but others must continue to have the injections for many years. While many patients are helped by desensitization, it is a prolonged and usually a costly treatment. Some types of allergy cannot be treated successfully by desensitization.

The same precautions required during skin testing are necessary during desensitization. The patient is observed with special care when treatment is first begun, and whenever the dose of antigen is increased. Doses are measured in syringes so finely calibrated that $\frac{1}{10}$ or even $\frac{1}{20}$ ml. can be measured accurately. Under no circumstances should the patient leave the clinic or the doctor's office before 20 minutes have elapsed. Severe reactions are most likely to occur during this period. The patient is instructed to place ice on the site of injection, to take an antihistamine and to call his doctor, if he notes an increase in symptoms after he returns home.

Drug Therapy. The rationale for use of drugs is in their ability to interrupt the inflammatory cycle and antagonize the effects of released pharmacologic mediators.

Antihistamines are given to provide symptomatic relief. It is believed that their effectiveness is due to inhibiting the action of histamine within the body. While they give temporary relief, they do not decrease the patient's hypersensitivity, and symptoms recur when the drugs are discontinued. Antihistamines are especially useful in relieving symptoms of short duration, such as hay fever, which occurs for a few weeks in the fall, or allergic reactions to drugs. Therapy with antihistamines may be combined with desensitization in long-term management of allergy.

Overuse of antihistamines can worsen the situation in asthmatics by drying secretions and increasing the difficulty with which they are removed.

Many antihistamines cause drowsiness. Occasionally, dryness of the mouth and dizziness also are noted. Since many different preparations are available, if one preparation causes marked side-effects, the doctor usually prescribes a different one. It is important that medication used during the day not make the patient sleepy, particularly if he drives a car or performs other activities requiring alertness. A number of these preparations are available in tablets having prolonged action. Thus, instead of taking the drug every 4 hours, once every 8 to 12 hours may suffice.

Adrenergic Agents such as epinephrine and Isuprel are used principally for their relaxation of bronchiolar smooth muscle spasm. They also reduce congestion of bronchial mucosa and constrict small blood vessels in the skin.

Corticosteroids may be given to relieve the symptoms. Usually these drugs are given only during a brief period when symptoms are very severe. Therapy then is continued with other measures, such as desensitization. Prolonged administration of corticosteroids leads to side-effects, such as edema and moon face.

ANAPHYLACTIC SHOCK

Anaphylactic shock is a term used to describe a sudden, severe allergic reaction in which the patient's blood pressure falls sharply, his pulse becomes rapid and weak, he is pale, sweaty and faint, and he often loses consciousness suddenly, especially if he is in an upright position. Symptoms of shock may follow quickly such allergic manifestations as severe asthma, urticaria or diarrhea and vomiting, when the patient has received a large dose of a substance to which he is allergic or even a small dose of an allergen to which he is extremely sensitive. The exact mechanism of anaphylactic shock is not understood fully. It is believed that the sudden liberation of large amounts of histamine causes heavy loss of plasma from the bloodstream. Capillary damage permits plasma to flow out through the walls of the blood vessels, thus diminishing suddenly the volume of circulating blood. An insufficient volume of blood is returned to the heart; therefore, the heart cannot pump enough blood to maintain adequate circulation. As in any case of shock regardless of the cause, the patient may die quickly due to insufficiency of the blood supply to the vital organs, such as heart and brain.

Prompt treatment is essential to avoid irreversible shock—the condition in which the damage to the tissues from the lack of blood supply makes it impossible for the patient to respond to treatment. First aid involves that for shock in any condition. The doctor immediately gives treatment to increase the circulating blood volume, to restore the normal blood pressure and to combat hypoxia.

- It may be necessary to perform a tracheotomy if laryngeal edema interferes with breathing.
- Epinephrine may be life-saving. Small amounts are given intravenously. Its actions have been briefly discussed.
- Antihistamines are of value in emergency treatment.
- Drugs such as levarterenol (Levophed), which raise blood pressure (vasopressors), may be added to the infusion.
- Intravenous solutions such as plasma or balanced electrolyte solutions are occasionally necessary to increase circulating blood volume.
- Corticosteroids have no role in emergency treatment except to potentiate the action of vasopressors. Their anti-inflammatory properties take several hours to become effective.
- Oxygen may be given to help to compensate for the poor oxygenation of tissues that occurs when adequate circulation is not maintained.
- Corticosteroids and antihistamines may be administered to combat the allergic response.

Treatment and observation do not stop when the patient recovers from shock. Although use of intravenous solutions and vasopressors is limited usually to the treatment of sudden acute symptoms, corticosteroids and antihistamines usually are continued for several days or longer to avoid any further symptoms. The patient is observed carefully for any evidence of further allergic reactions.

SUMMARY

The homeostatic processes by which the body protects and defends itself are constantly in use, and most of the time they are impressively successful. Their activity is noticeable only when they are severely challenged. If the defenses are weakened, inhibited or destroyed, the body can be an easy victim of unfavorable influences that a normal individual could be expected to counteract without difficulty. In general, the very young, the old and the poor are an especially easy prey to complications. Malnutrition and fatigue lower body defenses. The smooth, methodical healing of a bone can be slowed by an attack of pneumonia, and vice versa. One disease almost always makes another worse, in itself a compelling reason for the avoidance of secondary complications by every known nursing measure.

When the patient's adaptive responses, time, or therapy falter, one complication can follow another. Then the struggle between health and death is on in full force, and the attention to nursing details can make all the difference to the patient.

REFERENCES AND BIBLIOGRAPHY

APPERLY, F. L.: *Patterns of Disease on a Basis of Physiologic Pathology*, Philadelphia, Lippincott, 1951.

AYRES, S., and GIANELLI, S.: *Care of the Critically Ill*, New York, Appleton-Century-Crofts, 1967.

BEESON, P. B., and McDERMOTT, W. (eds.): *Cecil-Loeb Textbook of Medicine*, ed. 12, Philadelphia, Saunders, 1967.

BERGEN, A. J.: Sensitivity reactions, *Am. J. Nurs.* 55:948–949, 1955.

CANNON, W.: *The Wisdom of the Body*, New York, Norton, 1932.

CAMMER, L.: *Outline of Psychiatry*, New York, McGraw-Hill, 1962.

DUBOS, R., *in* LIEF, H., LIEF, V., and LIEF, N.: *The Psychological Basis of Medical Practice*, New York, Harper, 1963.

ENGEL, G.: Homeostasis, behavioral adjustment and the concept of health and disease, *in* GRINKER, R. (ed.): *Mid-century Psychiatry*, Springfield, Ill., Thomas, 1953.

Facts on the Major Killing and Crippling Diseases in the United States Today, The National Health Education Committee, Inc., New York, 1966.

FOSTER, M.: *Claude Bernard*, Longmans, 1899.

GALDSTON, I. (ed.): *Beyond the Germ Theory*, New York, Health Education Council, 1954.

GUYTON, A.: *Textbook of Medical Physiology*, ed. 3, Philadelphia, Saunders, 1966.

JAMES, G., *in* TALCO, P., and REMENCHEK, A.: *Internal Medicine Based on Mechanisms of Disease*, St. Louis, Mosby, 1968.

LANDRUM, F. L.: Nursing in an allergist's office, *Am. J. Nurs.* 58:677–678, 1958.

LAZARUS, R.: *Psychological Stress and the Coping Process*, New York, McGraw-Hill, 1966.

MacBRYDE, C. M.: *Signs and Symptoms*, ed. 5, Philadelphia, Lippincott, 1970.

MARTIN, H., and PRANGE, H. J.: Human adaptation: a conceptual approach to understanding patients, *Canad. Nurse* 58:234, 1962.

METROPOLITAN LIFE INSURANCE CO.: *Statistical Bulletin*, vol. 50, January, 1969.

MILLER, H., and BARUCH, D.: *The Practice of Psychosomatic Medicine as Illustrated in Allergy*, New York, McGraw-Hill, 1956.

RODMAN, M., and SMITH, D.: *Pharmacology and Drug Therapy in Nursing*, Philadelphia, Lippincott, 1968.

SELYE, H.: *The Stress of Life*, New York, McGraw-Hill, 1956.

SPENCER, R.: Helping your asthmatic patient to breathe, *RN*. 34:36–37, April, 1971.

SPITZ, R.: Unhappy and fatal outcomes of emotional deprivation and stress in infancy, *in* GALDSTON, I. (ed.): *Beyond the Germ Theory*, New York, Health Education Council, 1954.

VODA, A. M.: Body water dynamics—A clinical application, *Am. J. Nurs.* 70:2594–2601, December, 1970.

The Interaction of Body and Mind

7

The Concept of Psychosomatic Illness • The Reality of Psychosomatic Illness • Treatment of Psychosomatic Illness • The Delirious Patient

THE CONCEPT OF PSYCHOSOMATIC ILLNESS

Psychosomatic illness is defined by Dorland's Dictionary as "having bodily symptoms of a psychic, emotional or mental origin." The first part of the word, *psycho,* refers to mind, and the second part, *soma,* to body.

Mind and body are not separate; one affects and is affected by the other. Who has not experienced some physical manifestation of emotional stress? Such experiences as a headache after a quarrel, urinary frequency or diarrhea before an important athletic contest or an examination are part of everyday life, and for most people they are of a transitory nature. The symptom disappears and is forgotten quickly after the crisis has passed. No treatment may be needed, or the patient may use simple remedies to relieve the discomfort. One person may find that a leisurely walk in the fresh air is the best cure for a headache; another may take aspirin.

Certain conditions have been considered classic examples of psychosomatic illness. Peptic ulcer, eczema, colitis and asthma are examples. Personality profiles have been developed to describe the typical characteristics of persons who develop such illnesses. Another point of view is that human beings are more complex and varied in their responses than such profiles would indicate, and that the type of illness a patient develops in relation to stress varies with many additional factors, such as heredity and environment. Much remains to be learned about the relationship between stress and physical illness.

Often physical symptoms are related to *anxiety.* When anxiety mounts, the patient may develop symptoms, or his symptoms may become more severe. Unlike the transitory fear reaction anxi-ety may persist. Physical symptoms, such as pal-pitation, tachycardia, sweating or disturbance of sleep, which may reflect anxiety, often occur over a prolonged period. The symptoms may seem mysterious and threatening, because the patient is unaware of their cause. The patient whose heart beats more rapidly and forcefully as a mani-festation of anxiety may report this symptom to his doctor, and that he feels something is wrong with his heart. Often the patient is not aware that he is anxious. He knows only that his heart keeps pounding for no apparent reason.

Almost any symptom can have its origin in emotional stress. Some patients almost invariably have the same symptom when they become anx-ious. One may have diarrhea, another asthma, and a third may develop hives or eczema. Some people develop two or several different symp-toms; often the symptoms are experienced in an alternating fashion. One man was troubled with colitis and eczema. When his eczema was severe, his colitis subsided. When his colitis was severe, his eczema subsided. The patient's physician believed that both illnesses were manifestations of anxiety.

Prolonged anger can contribute also to psycho-somatic illness. For example, one theory of the relationship between anger and hypertension postulates that unrecognized and unrelieved an-ger results in structural changes in blood vessel walls. In this state of mind the autonomic nerv-ous system is stimulated to constrict the arteri-oles, thus raising blood pressure. The heart beats faster to push the blood through the narrowed lumen of the vessels. Respiratory rate increases as blood passes more quickly through the lungs. These changes prepare the person to fight, to flee or otherwise to take action. They are reversed after action has been taken, and the emotion has been relieved. The theory states that when anger is subconscious, unrecognized and undischarged for a period of years—as it might be in a person who, having to live with an anger-producing situation, has no adequate avenues of expression for his feeling—the physiologic changes become structural and permanent. According to this theory, the arterioles lose their elasticity, and the blood pressure is elevated permanently.

Emotional stress can lessen the body's resistance to disease, and it is one of several factors that can lead to illness. For example, a patient may develop bronchitis when under intense emotional stress. Skin tests may reveal allergy to dust and feathers. However, when the patient is relaxed, he may show few or no symptoms of bronchitis, even when he is exposed to dust or feathers. Emotional strain often intensifies allergic symptoms. Stress also may play a part in causation of infectious diseases by decreasing the body's resistance.

The development of bodily symptoms is only one manifestation of anxiety. It may show up also in symptoms that are primarily mental, such as the inability to concentrate or to remember. Such symptoms, too, vary in degree. Many people occasionally experience symptoms like moodiness or depression. When such symptoms are severe or long-lasting, they interfere with the functioning of the individual in daily life and with his relationships with others.

Sometimes a person subconsciously develops an illness as a way of handling a desperate need, such as that for affection. The only real cure is to satisfy the primary desire. An example is a woman who has pain in her heart, not because of organic heart disease, but because the symptom is a way of gaining, if only temporarily, the love and the attention for which she longs. Her husband cannot leave her when she is so sick; her children are concerned. Her pain is just as severe as if it were the result of a physical cause.

THE REALITY OF PSYCHOSOMATIC ILLNESS

Is the patient with psychosomatic illness really sick, or does he merely imagine that he is sick? Many people, including the families of patients and members of the health professions, believe that the influence of emotional stress on physical illness makes the latter less real or wholly imaginary. But psychosomatic illness is real. Acknowledging the reality of the patient's illness is important; it is the first step in helping him.

The patient with psychosomatic illness often is neglected. The same staff who give excellent care to patients whose illness does not carry the stigma of the word *psychosomatic* not uncommonly ignore, scorn or ridicule the patient whose illness is believed to be related to emotional stress. Some possible reasons for the stigma may include the use of the term *psycho* as a prefix. Perhaps this conveys the idea that the patient is mentally ill, making him subject to the contempt and avoidance so often the lot of the mentally ill. Perhaps the patient is considered a weakling. One hears comments like "He could snap out of it if he wanted to." Prejudice against these patients may be due to a belief that the patient is feigning illness in an attempt to get attention or favors, or that the illness is wholly imaginary.

A patient with psychosomatic illness is confused often with a malingerer, one who deliberately shams illness in order to achieve some secondary gain, such as financial compensation or excuse from work. Pretending illness is considered an unhealthy and unsatisfactory solution to the problems of life. Often it adds to the patient's difficulties, as he makes elaborate attempts to avoid detection. Malingerers can be helped sometimes to find other ways of coping with their difficulties. The essential difference between psychosomatic illness and malingering is that the malingerer feigns symptoms. It is a conscious process. The patient is aware that he is pretending to be sick. The patient with psychosomatic illness develops symptoms as a manifestation of largely unconscious psychic conflicts. The symptoms are real.

Condemnation of the patient with psychosomatic illness can persist despite intellectual understanding of theories about the causes of psychosomatic illness. The patient can sense immediately whether those who care for him are trying help him, or whether they are belittling him. It is important to understand that:

• The patient with psychosomatic illness is really sick. He is not pretending or imagining his symptoms.

• The idea that he can "snap out of it" at will is no more true than it is of those with diseases like pneumonia, whose need for care is readily acknowledged.

The patient with psychosomatic illness is in a difficult position. Sometimes his therapy consists of being told to go home and forget it. How can he forget the pain or the nausea, or whatever symptom is nagging him? He often detects veiled contempt behind the ministration of physicians and nurses. Frequently, his symptoms are ignored by those who care for him. "Keep his mind off it" may be the ward's watchword in dealing with these patients. The patient who feels that he is about to faint, vomit, or both may be told cheerily, "Now you go watch television—or would you like to join a card game?"

Is it any wonder that these patients feel misunderstood and neglected? Because the patient does not understand how his symptoms come about, he often feels helpless. He feels sick, but no one seems to believe him. He may begin to wonder whether he is imagining the symptoms. Many of these patients long for the concreteness of an underlying physical cause. They may say, "If only the doctor would find something definite wrong!" The patient knows that a diseased appendix can be removed, and that an infection can be cured by drugs. But what can be done for symptoms that seem to have their origin in emotional stress?

TREATMENT OF PSYCHOSOMATIC ILLNESS

The first step in helping the patient is to accept and acknowledge his illness. The cause of his symptoms must be found, and measures must be taken to relieve them and to prevent their recurrence. Thorough examinations are essential. Although the physician may suspect that the illness is due to emotional rather than physical causes, he must search carefully for any evidence of physical disease. It is not unknown for a patient whose illness is considered psychosomatic to be found later to have cancer or some other disease. The thorough search for physical causes of the symptoms helps to gain the patient's confidence. He knows that his condition and welfare are being taken seriously. If no organic basis for his complaints is found, he usually will find this news easier to accept when he knows he has had a thorough examination.

Finding no physical cause for the disorder points the way to understanding the patient's condition. What is the cause? Is it emotional stress? If so, what kind? What are the problems which are upsetting the patient? Knowing that it is only "nerves" does not help the patient, because it does not help him to learn what to do about it.

Sometimes, by talking with the patient the physician can learn about the emotional difficul-ties the patient is experiencing and can help him to see the possible relationship between his symptoms and emotional stress. Until the patient himself begins to see this relationship, the relief of symptoms is transitory and random. When he begins to understand the cause-and-effect relationship, he may begin to find other ways of handling his emotional problems. Almost any example is an oversimplification, because the situations have many diverse and subtle aspects. Perhaps the patient will be helped by learning to express some of the anger he feels, as well as by beginning to modify some of the situations that make him angry.

Sometimes the patient's physician recommends the services of a psychiatrist. The two physicians may work together closely in helping the patient, one concentrating largely on the emotional causes and the other on the relief of physical symptoms. Some hospitals have separate units for the care of psychosomatic patients, where emphasis is placed on both the emotional and the physical components of the illness.

The patient's physical discomfort should not be ignored. While the emotional factors responsible for his illness are being studied, he needs to feel that others are concerned about his symptoms, and that he will be helped to be more comfortable. The patient's symptoms indicate the type of treatment that may provide relief. Sometimes sedatives or tranquilizers are prescribed to lessen the patient's anxiety, thus helping to relieve his physical symptoms. However, these drugs do not provide a substitute for the patient's understanding of the relationship between his symptoms and stress situations. Sometimes psychotherapy is carried on individually; sometimes, in groups. One of its objectives is to help the patient to become aware of the deep-rooted and often unconscious causes of his anxiety.

There is no easy cure for psychosomatic illness. Discovering the causes of the patient's illness and helping him to understand and to find more satisfactory ways to cope with his problems are challenges to all who work with the patient. Frequently, the process takes many years. Some patients are unable to accept the idea that their symptoms originate in emotional conflicts; therefore, they cannot begin to move toward identification of their emotional problems. These patients may continue to be treated symptomatically by such measures as diet and medication. At some future time it may be possible for them to recognize a relationship between their physical symptoms and their emotional conflicts.

Nursing Considerations

Nursing care of the patient with psychosomatic illness requires a great deal of tact, insight and judgment. The patient needs someone to listen to him, to be concerned about his symptoms and to respect him. Prying or attempting to force on the patient an acceptance of a relationship between his symptoms and emotional problems can make him more anxious, and such efforts may result in intensification of his physical symptoms and resistance to any later suggestion by the physician that he have psychotherapy.

Often the nurse makes certain observations that seem to show a relationship between the patient's physical symptoms and other events in his life. It is important to make these observations. Do symptoms come and go, leaving the patient free of discomfort for part of the day, or do they persist most of the day and night? What kinds of things tend to relieve the symptoms? Medication? Diversion?

It is also important to know how to act on your observations. For instance, the nurse may note that an asthmatic patient almost always has an attack after his mother visits him. Recognizing that this sequence may be an important clue in determining the cause of the patient's symptoms, the nurse should discuss this observation fully with the patient's physician. Through such collaboration the nurse can share in helping the patient, increase her understanding of his emotional needs and receive guidance from the physician in how best to proceed in relation to this aspect of the patient's care. She can listen carefully to the patient. Perhaps he will begin talking about his mother, or, equally significant, he may avoid carefully any mention of her. This information, too, can be shared with the physician and may prove to be very useful in planning the patient's treatment. The nurse's observations thus form a basis not only for her own intervention, but also for collaboration with others who care for the patient.

Observing such a relationship between the patient's symptoms and events in his life is a clue that the patient may experience considerable anxiety in relation to these aspects of his life. It would be unwise to make a blunt statement (which might or might not be true), interpreting the patient's symptoms in light of these events. For instance, it can make the problem worse to remark, "You always have asthmatic attacks after your mother comes. She must upset you."

However, as the nurse gradually develops a relationship with the patient, she can listen with greater sensitivity to his concerns, and often she can find opportunities, during this process, to assist the patient to see connections between his symptoms and his reactions to daily experiences. By being available to listen and to support the patient, the nurse can help him to make his own connections of cause and effect. In the example just cited the nurse might stay with the patient who is disturbed after his mother's visit, caring not only for physical relief of symptoms of asthma but also listening as the patient expresses emotions such as fear or anger. In this process the patient himself often begins to see a relationship between the bodily symptoms he is experiencing and the emotion which he is describing. Helping the patient to see relationships between physical symptoms and emotional experiences is an important aspect of nursing care of patients with psychosomatic illness.

Avoid stereotyping the patient as soon as you learn his diagnosis. These patients cannot be neatly separated and labeled. All patients have some anxiety. Do not decide, on meeting your patient, "Oh, I know all about what you're like." Each person is an individual. Let him show you what he is like.

The nursing of all patients, including those whose illnesses have been diagnosed as psychosomatic, includes considerations of both physical and mental comfort. For example, if an antacid has been prescribed for such an illness, administer it without any words or actions that would convey to the patient, "You really don't need this, but here it is anyway."

Use of Placebos. Sometimes the physician prescribes a placebo (a medication given not for pharmacologic effect but for the relief which may result from suggestion). A sugar pill or an injection of sterile water is sometimes used for this purpose. Administration of any drug carries with it expectation of relief, as well as tangible assurance of the doctor's and the nurse's interest in lessening the patient's discomfort. These effects are enhanced by a statement from the person administering the drug concerning the benefit that may be expected.

Some patients are more likely to be relieved by the placebo action of a drug than others. The fact that help is obtained from a plecebo does not mean necessarily that the patient has a psychosomatic illness. One man with cancer was kept comfortable for several weeks by injections of sterile saline. Later he required narcotics for control of pain. His physician's comment was, "We'll use the placebos as long as they'll help him. When they don't, we'll start using narcotics." The patient was spared temporarily some of the undesirable side-effects of narcotics, including the development of tolerance for the drug and the consequent need of larger doses to produce relief. Whether or not the patient's symptoms can be relieved by a placebo is sometimes a clue to the cause of his illness. Observe and report whether the symptoms have subsided and for how long.

Suggestibility is a highly complex phenomenon. It can be a most useful therapeutic tool, extending to hypnosis as an anesthetic. The various factors in suggestibility are not fully understood, but it has been noted that anxious patients are especially likely to have good results from placebo therapy. The physician's and nurse's demonstration of interest in the patient's treatment and progress is believed to enhance the success of placebo therapy.

Placebos, like any medication, are ordered by the physician for a definite purpose—either to relieve certain symptoms or to aid in diagnosing their cause. Never should the decision to use a placebo be made independently by the nurse. There is nothing wrong or dishonest about the legitimate use of placebos. Make sure that you understand the reason for their use and what kind of preparation is to be used. (For instance, the patient would become suspicious if one nurse used a pink placebo tablet and another nurse a white one.) The doctor will indicate whether the placebo is to be given orally or parenterally.

Let the Patient Talk. It may be the nurse to whom the patient turns to talk over the physician's findings that his illness is due primarily to emotional rather than physical causes. Frequently, the patient initiates the conversation after he has undergone a series of tests and examinations. He may find it upsetting that he has no physical disorder curable by such measures as drugs, diet or even surgery. He needs time to think this fact through, as well as help and support. If psychotherapy has been recommended, this thought, too, may be very disturbing. Let the patient talk about his thoughts on the subject. Convey to him that he is not odd because he has physical symptoms as a result of emotional stress. Many people reflect emotional stress in physical symptoms. If he is doing so to the extent that he is often uncomfortable, it is merely an indication that he needs treatment.

People are under more stress than most of us realize. Our culture emphasizes presenting a brave, smiling face. Even close friends and members of the same family are often unaware of the degree of stress other members are experiencing. Psychosomatic illness is understandably very common.

Because the effects of emotional stress on physical symptoms are being studied in relation to such a wide variety of diseases, this aspect of study will be found throughout this book. The concept that mind and body continually interact and affect each other is one which is applicable to the care of all patients in any setting.

THE DELIRIOUS PATIENT

Delirium is a state of disorientation and confusion caused by interference with the metabolic processes of the neurons of the brain. The condition is usually temporary and reversible. Delirium usually subsides when its cause has been removed.

The delirious patient is disoriented as to time and place and may have illusions and hallucinations. An *illusion* is an inaccurate interpretation of stimuli within the environment. The patient may think that his sister is calling him, when actually the nurse is calling him. *Hallucinations* are subjective sensory experiences that occur without stimulation from the environment. The patient may hear a voice calling him, when no one is calling him.

The delirious patient is restless and confused. He has defects in memory and judgment. He often behaves impulsively and acts on incorrect interpretations of his environment. For instance, he may believe that a window is a door and attempt to escape through it. Often delirium develops suddenly; it can subside equally quickly. A patient may seem well oriented at bedtime but be delirious an hour later. Symptoms are usually worse at night. Often the patient becomes quite anxious, because he senses that his ability to cope with his environment has lessened.

Nursing care of the delirious patient involves protecting him and others from harm and helping him (as far as possible) to minimize the disorientation and confusion. The basic cause (drug intoxication, fever, alcoholism) is treated medically. In the meantime the following nursing measures can help to lessen the patient's confusion and to protect him from harm:

• Keep sensory stimuli to a minimum. The room should be quiet. Avoid unnecessary conversation. Chatter, especially if it concerns abstract subjects, is likely to confuse the patient further. Be concrete and repetitive in your conversation. For example, repeating, "You're in the hospital, and I am your nurse," can help the patient to orient himself to his environment. Keep explanations brief and simple, such as "Here is your soup" or "I'm going to wash your back." Try not to reflect the patient's restlessness and agitation. Feelings can be contagious. Speaking quietly and slowly may help to lessen the patient's apprehension.

• Keep the patient's room softly lighted during the night. Soft light will help to prevent the increased disorientation that usually occurs when the patient is left in a darkened room, and it will contribute to his safety by enabling others to observe him.

• Protect the patient from harm. If he tries to act on his illusions, he may fall out of the window, thinking it a stairway and an escape route from the danger that he perceives around him. Most hospitals require a doctor's order before restraints can be used. If your delirious patient has such an order, be sure that the restraints in no way impair circulation, and that they give the patient as much movement as is compatible with safety. Many people, delirious or not, react to physical restraint with anger; the delirious patient may be made more excited by them. Remove the restraints whenever there is adequate supervision so that the patient can move about. If he has been pulling against them, his skin may be reddened—or worse, broken—where he was restrained. Help him to sit up as much as possible, if he is permitted to sit up.

• The delirious patient usually is incapable of feeding himself. Feed him slowly and allow him to assist, if he is able. Encourage fluid intake, unless the doctor has left orders to limit fluids.

• Side rails can help to keep the patient in bed. Try to help the patient to understand their purpose, so that he is prevented, if possible, from considering the rails a confining cage from which he must escape. A patient who is physically strong enough can climb over side rails.

• Having someone remain with the patient, assuring him that he is being cared for, can help greatly to lessen his agitation and to prevent him from hurting himself. Sometimes a family member can stay with the patient, if shortage of staff makes it impossible for nursing personnel to do so.

• Keep objects with which the patient could harm himself away from him. For instance, a paper drinking straw should be used instead of a glass one and a paper cup instead of a water glass. Cigarettes and matches should not be left within reach.

• Remember that the patient cannot control his behavior. Scolding him is both inappropriate and ineffective.

Delirious patients require a great deal of nursing care. Their unpredictable behavior often interferes with the goals of those caring for them. For instance, the patient may spill a glass of water on the bed just after you have changed it. Do not show impatience or anger to the patient, although it is important to recognize that you are annoyed, if you are. As far as possible, modify the environment and the plan of care to help to prevent incidents that can upset the patient and those around him. For instance, it is better to hold the glass for the delirious patient than to allow him to hold it himself.

REFERENCES AND BIBLIOGRAPHY

BARUCH, D.: *One Little Boy,* New York, Dell, 1952.

CLEGHORN, R. A.: Psychosomatic principles, *J. Canad. Med. Assoc.* 92:441, 1965.

COHEN, S., and KLEIN, H. R.: The delirious patient, *Am. J. Nurs.* 58:685, 1958.

Dorland's Illustrated Medical Dictionary, ed. 24, Philadelphia, Saunders, 1965.

DUNBAR, F.: *Mind and Body: Psychosomatic Medicine,* New York, Random, 1947.

———: *Emotions and Bodily Changes,* ed. 4, New York, Columbia University Press, 1954.

EVERSON, T. C., and COLE, W. H.: *Spontaneous Regression of Cancer,* Philadelphia, Saunders, 1966.

FORRERR, G. R.: The therapeutic use of placebo, *Mich. Med.* 63:558, 1964.

FRANK, I., and POWELL, M.: *Psychosomatic Ailments in Childhood and Adolescence,* Springfield, Ill., Thomas, 1967.

GARNER, H. H.: *Psychosomatic Management of the Patient with Malignancy,* Springfield, Ill., Thomas, 1966.

GOODWIN, D. W.: Psychiatry and the mysterious medical complaint, *JAMA* 209:1884, Sept. 22, 1969.

JORES, A., and FREYBERGER, H. (eds.): *Advances in Psychosomatic Medicine: Symposium of the Fourth European Conference on Psychosomatic Research,* New York, Basic Books, 1961.

KISSEN, D. M., and LESHAN, L. L. (eds.): *Psychosomatic Aspects of Neoplastic Disease,* Philadelphia, Lippincott, 1964.

KOLB, L. C.: *Noyes' Modern Clinical Psychiatry*, ed. 7, Philadelphia, Saunders, 1968.

LAZARUS, R. S.: *Psychological Stress and the Coping Process*, New York, McGraw-Hill, 1966.

MENNINGER, K. A.: *Man Against Himself*, New York, Harcourt, 1956.

————: *The Vital Balance*, New York, Viking, 1963.

NODINE, J. H., and MOYER, J. H.: *Psychosomatic Medicine*, Philadelphia, Lea, 1962.

PEPLAU, H. E.: *Interpersonal Relations in Nursing*, New York, Putnam, 1952.

PRICK, J. J., and VAN DE LOO, K. J.: *The Psychosomatic Approach to Primary Chronic Rheumatoid Arthritis*, Philadelphia, Davis, 1964.

SELYE, H.: *The Stress of Life*, New York, McGraw-Hill, 1956.

————: The stress of life: New focal point for understanding accidents, *Nurs. Forum* 4:29, 1965.

————: The stress syndrome, *Am. J. Nurs.* 65:97, March, 1965.

SHAPIRO, A. K.: Etiological factors in placebo effect, *JAMA* 187:712, March 7, 1964.

SHOCHET, B. R., et al.: A medical-psychiatric study of patients with rheumatoid arthritis, *Psychosomatics* 10:271, Sept.-Oct., 1969.

UMPHRESS, A., et al.: Adolescent enuresis, *Arch. Gen. Psychiat.* 22:237, March, 1970.

WAHL, C. W. (ed.): *New Dimensions in Psychosomatic Medicine*, Boston, Little, Brown, 1964.

WARSON, S. R., et al.: The role of intentionality in recovery: Operational concepts, *Psychosomatics* 10:225, July-Aug., 1969.

WENAR, C., et al.: *Origins of Psychosomatic and Emotional Disturbances*, New York, Hoeber, 1962.

WITTHOWER, E. D., et al.: A global survey of psychosomatic medicine, *Int. J. Psychiat.* 7:499, Jan., 1969.

WOLF, S., and WOLFF, H. G.: *Human Gastric Function: An Experimental Study of a Man and His Stomach*, London, Oxford, 1943.

WOLF, S., et al.: *Life Stress and Essential Hypertension*, Baltimore, Williams & Wilkins, 1955.

The Patient in Pain

8

Pain · Observations · Nursing Care · Intractable Pain
Surgery to Relieve Pain

PAIN

"Physical pain is not a simple affair of an impulse traveling at a fixed rate along a nerve. It is the resultant of a conflict between a stimulus and the whole individual" (Leriche).

Pain is a disagreeable sensation elicited by a potentially harmful stimulus. Its purpose is mainly protective. It is the symptom that most often prompts the seeking of medical help. The destruction that can occur in the absence of pain demonstrates its value. Some cancers are painless until they have become well entrenched and have spread to adjacent areas. A patient whose legs are without sensation owing to a spinal injury will not feel the pain of an overheated hot-water bottle, and severe burns may result.

Sources. Pain occurs whenever tissues are being injured. Pain receptors may be stimulated by chemical, thermal, electrical, or mechanical agents. (Even minor stimuli, such as a too tight cast or taut drainage tubes, stimulate pain receptors.) Pain arising from cutaneous receptors is called *superficial* or *surface* pain. That arising from deeper structures, such as muscles and joints, is referred to as *deep* pain, while pain arising from the viscera is referred to as *visceral*.

Surface pain stimulates the sympathetic nervous system into a series of reflex actions. Adrenalin is poured into the system; blood pressure, pulse and respiratory rates rise; and blood is drained from the brain, the skin and the gastrointestinal tract and flows into the muscles. This is the "alarm" reaction which, physiologically speaking, readies the patient for action to fight against or flee from the cause of the pain. On the other hand, deep pain is more likely to cause failure of the defense reaction. The patient feels weak and nauseated, and he may vomit or faint. He may be very tense or restless. Hypotension, bradycardia, pallor and sweating occur. These

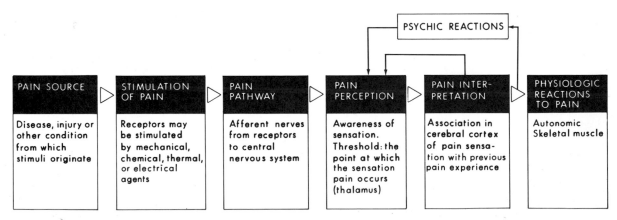

Fig. 8-1. The pain experience. (Adapted from Newton, M. E., *et al.: A Study of Nurse Action in Relief of Pain*, Columbus, Ohio, Ohio State University Research Foundation, 1964, *in Am. J. Nurs.* 66:1096, May, 1966; reprinted with permission from the American Journal of Nursing)

signs and symptoms are frequently observed in patients with such conditions as acute myocardial infarction or perforations of abdominal viscera.

Severe pain may cause shock and even death. Continued pain can result in added damage to the body organs because of the prolongation of such physiologic reactions.

The psychic reaction to pain is far more subtle than reflex reactions. Following comparable degrees of pain stimuli, the reactions of individuals vary tremendously. The way an individual responds to pain depends on many factors. His physiologic and psychological state and his adaptive resources, his cultural background and beliefs, his previous pain experience, the location of the pain and the response of the people around him all influence his reaction.

Distractions make a vast difference. A small wound received while playing basketball or doing housework scarcely may be noticed. The same amount of pain caused, let us say, by a needle being injected into a vein, seems to be much more severe, because the patient concentrates all his attention on the procedure. During the injection physiologic and psychological attention are focused on one set of impulses. Nurses sometimes find that a patient experiences pain more acutely at night and during early morning hours, when his mind and body are unoccupied by the activities of the day.

Pre-existing anxiety lowers the threshold for pain perception, increases pain sensation and intensifies the pain reaction. The intense sensation of pain further increases anxiety, thus setting up a vicious cycle.

OBSERVATIONS

The patient in pain who does not complain shows discomfort by other means. He may curl up in bed or assume an abnormal posture, such as kneeling, or toss about. His pulse is often elevated, and he may perspire. Observe the facial expression of your patients; those in pain will look tense, with taut muscles, clenched teeth, fixed eyes and a drawn expression. Some express pain covertly through such mechanisms as focus on detail, demandingness or argumentativeness. Interaction with the patient as well as observation and examination are essential for an accurate assessment of the patient's condition.

When observing and reporting (to the doctor, to the nurse who follows you or on the chart), do not state simply that the patient has pain. Also look for, and report, its:

- Nature (sharp, dull, burning, aching, knife-like, squeezing, deep, pulsating, gnawing, pressing)
- Intensity (mild, moderate, severe)
- Location (left lower abdomen, inner aspect of right upper midthigh, entire left chest)
- Onset (occurred suddenly, slowly, slowly building up to present intensity, similar to pain that the patient had at home, first occurrence)
- Duration (intermittent, returning at 5- to 6-minute intervals and lasting about 30 seconds; persistent since 3:30 A.M.; brief, lasting 15 minutes)
- Spread (radiates down left arm, extends from groin to knee)
- Relation to circumstance (before or after eating, as the patient turns to the right side, when the patient moves his foot)
- Control (apparently relieved by elevation of the limb; patient reports that pain stops when he lies still; sleeping 25 minutes after medication)

Because of the subjective nature of pain, it is best to report only what you actually see, and what the patient does or says. For example, on one chart the nurse wrote: "Patient was observed rocking on his knees in bed. He complained of severe colicky pain in his entire lower abdomen. The patient said the pain started suddenly about 10 minutes ago. Pulse 132, respiration 40. Profuse diaphoresis. While nurse was calling the doctor, patient vomited 120 cc. of undigested food."

Note that the nurse did not say, "The patient had pain," but rather, "He complained of . . . pain." The nurse also charted what she did about the symptom. In this case she called the doctor.

Sometimes pain is relieved or intensified by a change in the course of the disease. The severe pain of acute appendicitis suddenly vanishes when the appendix ruptures. The sudden absence of pain is both a dangerous symptom and an important observation to make. On the other hand, an increasing amount of pain under a cast after the fracture has been reduced means that something is wrong. Report changes in pain to the doctor.

NURSING CARE

Whatever the patient's response to pain, there are no rights or wrongs about it. A person who complains loudly may antagonize a nurse who admires stoicism more. On the other hand, a patient who silently suffers may neglect to call attention to a serious condition; therefore, he may fail to get medical attention. Beware of judging how severe pain *should* be, and how much the patient *should* show his suffering.

Sometimes, when pain is severe, such as in acute myocardial infarction, a patient may be hesitant to accept narcotics for some psychosocial reason. Recognizing his stoicism, the nurse explains the rationale for the ordered medication and plans with him to discuss his reaction at a later time when pain relief has been obtained. The patient who absolutely refuses narcotics should not have them forced upon him. The matter should be promptly discussed with his physician.

The patient in pain is preoccupied and unable to respond to people and events in the same way as he does when he is not in pain. Small talk not only does not distract him but is an added burden. Pain makes noise especially bothersome and tires the patient. The nurse can help visitors to understand the patient's need for quiet and his inability to respond to them in his usual manner, while assuring them that all possible is being done to help the patient to become more comfortable.

Planning. The planning of care is important. Because movement usually increases pain, the patient often tries to remain as still as he can. However, measures to prevent complications frequently require movement. For example, postoperative deep breathing, turning from side to side and ambulation may increase the immediate discomfort of the patient. Explain why these measures are necessary. Talk to the patient before surgery so that he knows what to expect. If the patient is forewarned to expect pain, he may be helped to understand it as necessary and transitory, and this knowledge may help him to relax and feel less worried and tense. Frequently, painful dressings can be timed so that they are undertaken after the patient has had an analgesic. Organize the patient's day so that periods of necessary activity are followed by rest periods.

Movement. Some patients are able to find ways to move that hurt them the least. The patient in pain should be consulted before he is moved. One may wish to roll over unaided, while another can tell you where to place your hands.

Other patients in pain, however, need not be burdened with the additional decision-making involved in movement. Rather, they need the gentle but firm, sure motion of a nurse or a team who explains first what is about to happen. Asking the patient when and where it hurts as he is moved and positioned can give the kind of information needed to retain the approach or try a different method.

Splinting a painful part often helps. This can be accomplished with an abdominal binder, manual support of a limb or holding the operative site when coughing after chest surgery. Supporting the joints helps to move a painful limb in one piece and is far more comfortable than allowing a part to lag. A limb may be moved on a pillow, or the whole body on a turning sheet. Move slowly and steadily, stopping when the patient requests it. Jerky and swift motions increase pain.

Nursing Measures. Sometimes pain can be lessened to a tolerable level by the presence of a nurse who takes care of small but important details. The patient who is alone in a room can be comforted by a nurse who expresses a word of encouragement or sympathy, massages tenseness from an aching shoulder, rests a sore muscle by supporting it with a pillow, elevates an edematous hand, gives a refreshing mouthwash, cools bed-weary feet with an alcohol sponge or tightens a rumpled sheet. In some instances heat, cold, ultrasonic therapy, oxygen, or physical therapy technics may be more effective than drugs in relieving mild or moderate pain.

Drug Therapy. Analgesics should not be used to replace nursing care and never to quiet a patient because the nurse is weary of his complaints. When they are ordered, use them as necessary to keep the patient comfortable.

Three important points to remember in drug administration are:

1. Pain is relieved more readily before it becomes too severe. Often an analgesic should be given before the pain has developed completely.

2. A drug can mask symptoms that the doctor may need to observe to establish a diagnosis. Give analgesics only for the pain for which they are ordered, not for another pain. For instance, if the patient has an order for aspirin for headache, do not give aspirin to him for a pain in his calf.

3. If the patient with acute pain does not obtain relief from the drug within the time of

its predicted effective action notify the physician. Do not insist that the patient wait until the next ordered dose without other measures for his comfort.

The very act of giving medication is proof to the patient that someone cares that he is uncomfortable, and that there are measures available to help him. The action of a drug can be reinforced by a patient's faith in it. In administering a drug for pain the nurse should inform the patient of the expected effect, because the power of suggestion will be valuable in itself.

Give the patient the necessary care and attentions that will help him to rest before he receives the medication. After the medication for pain has been administered, keep him from being disturbed. If he is awakened from the sleep that follows the administration of morphine, he may be unable to recapture relaxation. Pain is wearying, and rest is hard to come by. Do not allow the patient to be awakened to have his temperature taken (unless specifically ordered at this time), for routine housekeeping chores or for a social call on the telephone.

Report in detail the effects of relief measures. It is important to note whether or not the rectal tube helped the patient to expel gas that was causing distention. Relief of pain often brings better physiologic functioning (for example, pain can decrease renal efficiency), and these changes should be noticed. Accurate reporting may help the doctor to adjust the drug dosage. Perhaps he will wish to decrease the amount given, or to increase the dose, if the pain is unrelieved.

When analgesic ointments are ordered, restrict their application to the specific area, because the larger the surface (especially when denuded) to which they are applied, the more systemic absorption there will be. Various types of systemic relief-giving drugs also are available. Many of them affect the patient's "alarm" reaction more than his perception of pain, but in any event they do bring comfort.

INTRACTABLE PAIN

Intractable pain is pain that is not managed easily. The term usually is applied to chronic pain. Acute pain is different from chronic pain in some important ways. When a man crushes his finger in a car door, he is aware of the emergency nature of the situation and expects that the pain will end in the foreseeable future. There is no such time limit to the severe pain

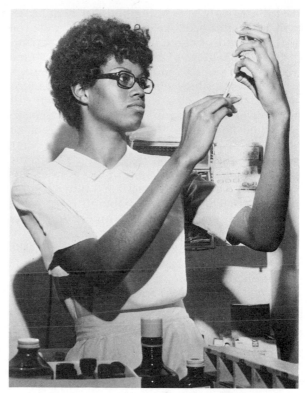

FIG. 8-2. Having reviewed her patient's need with the instructor and nursing team leader, a nursing student promptly prepares medication for pain.

associated with such conditions as disseminated cancer and advanced chronic pancreatitis. Patients with these conditions often have days so filled with intense pain that all other thoughts are excluded from consciousness. Pain demands an almost exclusive concentration on itself, and almost every other consideration becomes secondary or nonexistent.

Some patients with chronic pain say that it seems senseless to them, and that this is its most difficult aspect. Renal colic calls attention to a pathologic condition and serves as a warning, but the repetitious pain of arthritis seems to them to have no purpose. Meaningless suffering is damaging to the integration of personality. So the patient with chronic pain makes endless efforts to control his reaction to it and to maintain a sense of himself.

Nurses may be able to help such patients to build defenses against pain. It is necessary for the nurse to think first about her own reaction. If severe pain so frightens her that she avoids the patient, cannot listen to what he has to say, and thinks only of sedating him, her helpfulness will be diminished. Religious counselors can be a great comfort to both the nurse and the patient.

Help the patient to maintain his dignity. One way to do this is by minimizing his helplessness as much as possible. Provide him with as much decision-making and activity as the situation will warrant. Find something for the bed patient to do, when he is able, that truly interests him, so that he does not spend relatively pain-free time just lying there, waiting for the pain to become more severe. The patient will be groping for both an answer to the question "Why?" and a way to behave that is acceptable to him in the very difficult circumstance of pain in the present and the promise of pain in the future.

If it is not time for his medication and the patient is in pain, staying with him and giving attention to comfort measures often is effective in lessening his distress and helping him to wait until medication can be given safely.

When the patient is dying slowly and in pain, the doctors may be able to regulate the dosage of narcotics so that increasing tolerance does not rise so rapidly that the drug is no longer effective. Addiction is unlikely when a narcotic is given for only a few days; it becomes more likely as the drug is given for longer periods. The nurse and the doctor work together to try to keep the patient comfortable without giving the narcotic so frequently that its effectiveness is lost, and the patient is left with no help for his pain.

The patient in continuous, severe pain may be contemplating suicide. If he has intractable pain due to some incurable disease, he may worry about becoming a burden to his family, and he may dread the future, fearing that the time will come when narcotics will relieve his suffering no longer. Details of the nursing care of patients with long-term pain are discussed in the chapters on cancer, arthritis and peripheral vascular diseases.

SURGERY TO RELIEVE PAIN

Sometimes intractable pain can be eliminated by cutting the nerves that transmit it. There is usually a price to pay in disability, numbness or less control over a function, but relief from pain is usually worth it to the patient. Surgery to relieve pain may be performed when the patient has distress in a localized area from cancer. Pain that is widespread throughout the body cannot be eliminated by neurosurgery. More rarely, surgery may be performed for continuing pain

following herpes zoster, frequent gastric crises in tabes dorsalis, continuing painful phantom limb following an amputation and neuralgia after peripheral nerve injury.

A *chordotomy* is an interruption of the pain-conducting pathways in the spinal cord. After the operation there will be loss of temperature sensation (attended, therefore, by a danger of burning the skin) and of pain on the affected side, but no loss of tactile sensation. In addition, there may be some weakness of the limb on the side opposite the operation. If a bilateral chordotomy is performed, the patient's legs may be so weak that he is unable to walk. Difficulty in bladder control is to be expected. Because this operation is most often done for patients with uncontrolled cancer, the relief of severe pain for the remaining days of the life of the patient is usually more important than mobility or bladder continence. When several roots are severed, the patient has a loss of position sense.

A *rhizotomy* is division of a sensory root just as it enters the spinal cord, an operation that may be used for patients with cancer of the lungs. It may cause loss of position sense and numbness below the level of the incision. A *tractotomy* is division of the pathways in the brain stem, eliminating the senses of pain and temperature, but leaving the sense of touch and other sensations undisturbed. A *neurectomy* is an interruption of peripheral or cranial nerves by cutting the nerve fibers (rather than the roots). Movement and position sense are affected.

Both chordotomy and rhizotomy involve a laminectomy, and the postoperative care of the patient is similar to that of a patient operated on for a herniated disk or a tumor of the spinal cord. (See p. 247.) Because there usually is diminished sensation below the level of the incision, extra care must be taken to prevent decubitus ulcers. An alternating air-pressure mattress may be used. Back care should be given several times a day, and the patient should be repositioned at least every 2 hours. Muscular weakness and a loss of position sense may make the patient lie more quietly in bed than he should. Be sure to use a footboard and to prevent outward rotation of the feet and the legs. Exercises should be done several times a day. When the patient gets out of bed, he may need a walker or a cane.

If bladder and bowel sensations are diminished, the patient will need to be taught to regulate these functions. For example, he will feel no longer the usual signs of needing to defecate. He may be able also to learn to void regularly. Tidal drainage may be used initially to help to re-establish bladder tone.

Sometimes a second chordotomy is necessary, especially if the patient had general anesthesia during the first chordotomy and could not describe his sensations during the operation. For this reason observing and charting the exact location of any postoperative pain is important.

Percutaneous chordotomy involves the insertion through the skin of a spinal needle into a cervical interspace. An electrode is then directed into the cord to destroy by coagulation the sensory fibers in the lateral spinothalamic tract. These fibers transmit pain as well as temperature sensation. Since it is a relatively innocuous procedure which is well tolerated by patients, it can be performed on those too debilitated to withstand laminectomy. Postoperative care involves appropriate neurologic observations and supportive care.

The experience of pain with its concomitant suffering has elements of fear, anxiety, loneliness, and the unknown. One can never comprehend the extent of another's suffering. But it is in the effort to comprehend it that much relief of the patient's pain and the loneliness that accompanies it can be found. The way the nurse gives a medication, and the other relief measures she uses, can be as helpful to the person in chronic pain as the medication itself.

It is not an easy task of nursing to stand by helpless in the face of another's pain. But it is unrealistic to assume that technically competent, compassionate, collaborative nursing care can eliminate all suffering. The nurse who assists the patient to best bear his unrelieved pain in his own way makes a significant contribution toward the alleviation of suffering.

REFERENCES AND BIBLIOGRAPHY

BUTTENDJICK, F. J. J.: *Pain: Its Modes and Functions,* University of Chicago Press, 1962.

BLAYLOCK, J.: The psychological and cultural influences on the reaction to pain: a review of the literature, *Nurs. Forum* 7:262, 1968.

CARTER, B.: Comparison of individual pain reactions to injections of distilled water and normal saline, *ANA Reg. Clin. Conf.,* p. 219, 1967.

CHAMBERS, W., and PRICE, G.: Influence of the nurse upon effects of analgesics administered, *Nurs. Res.* 16:228, Summer, 1967.

CLEMENCE, SR. MADELEINE: Existentialism: a philosophy of commitment, *Am. J. Nurs.* 66:500, March, 1966.

DAVIS, L., and PENDLETON, S.: Nurses' inferences of suffering, *Nurs. Res.* 18:100, March-April, 1969.

FENSTERMACHER, J., and ZELLWEGER, G.: Patients can relieve postoperative pain by using electronic injection devices, *Hosp. Topics* 47:104, March, 1969.

FINNESON, B.: *Diagnosis and Management of Pain Syndromes,* ed. 2, Philadelphia, Saunders, 1969.

FRANCIS, G., and MUNJAS, B.: *Promoting Psychological Comfort,* Dubuque, Wm. C. Brown, 1968.

GUYTON, A.: *Textbook of Medical Physiology,* ed. 3, Philadelphia, Saunders, 1966.

HARDY, J. D., WOLFF, H. G., and GOODELL, H.: *Pain Sensations and Reactions,* Baltimore, Williams & Wilkins, 1952.

HANKEN, A.: Pain and systems analysis, *Nurs. Res.* 15:139, Spring, 1966.

KEATS, A., and LANE, M.: The symptomatic therapy of pain, *Disease-A-Month,* June, 1963.

LERICHE, R.: Surgery of pain, in STRAUSS, M. (ed.): *Familiar Medical Quotations,* Boston, Little, Brown, 1968.

LeSHAN, L.: The world of the patient in severe pain of long duration, *J. Chronic Dis.* 17:119, 1964.

MacBRYDE, C. M.: *Signs and Symptoms,* ed. 5, Philadelphia, Lippincott, 1970.

McBRIDE, M.: Pain and effective nursing practice, *ANA Clin. Sessions,* p. 75, 1966.

———: Nursing approach, pain, and relief: an exploratory experiment, *Nurs. Res.* 16:337, Fall, 1967.

McCAFFERY, M., and MOSS, F.: Nursing intervention for bodily pain, *Am. J. Nurs.* 67:1224, June, 1967.

MOSS, F.: The effect of a nursing intervention on pain relief, *ANA Reg. Clin. Conf.,* p. 247, 1967.

MOSS, F., and MEYER, B.: The effects of nursing interaction upon pain relief in patients, *Nurs. Res.* 15:303, Fall, 1966.

MULLEN, J. F., and VON SCHOICK, M. R.: Intractable pain, *Am. J. Nurs.* 58:228, 1958.

NOEL, L.: Suffering in man's world, *Cath. Nurse* 16:36, December, 1967.

Pain. Basic concepts and assessment, Part 1. *Am. J. Nurs.* 66:1085, May, 1966. Rationale for intervention, Part 2. *Am. J. Nurs.* 66:1345, June, 1966. Programmed Instructions.

Pain, *Ther. Notes* 75:30, Fall, 1968.

Reduction of postoperative pain by encouragement and instruction of patients: a study of doctor-patient rapport, *New Eng. J. Med.* 270:825, 1964.

RODMAN, M., and SMITH, D.: *Pharmacology and Drug Therapy in Nursing,* Philadelphia, Lippincott, 1968.

SEEMAN, B.: *Man Against Pain: 3,000 Years of Effort to Understand and Relieve Physical Suffering,* Philadelphia, Chilton, 1962.

Symposium: Common pain problems, *Med. Clin. N. Am.* 42:1465, 1958.

THERRIEN, B., and SALMON, J.: Percutaneous chordotomy for relief of intractable pain, *Am. J. Nurs.* 68:2594, December, 1968.

WANG, R. I. H.: Control of pain, *Am. J. Med. Sci.* 246:590, 1963.

WHITE, J. C., and SWEET, W. H.: *Pain, Its Mechanisms and Neurosurgical Control,* Springfield, Ill., Thomas, 1955.

ZBOROWSKI, M.: Cultural components in responses to pain, *J. Social Issues* 8:16, 1952.

———: *People in Pain,* San Francisco, Jossey-Bass, 1969.

Dependence on and Abuse of Alcohol and Drugs and Tobacco

9

Incidence and Economics · Treatment · Alcoholism · Drug Abuse and Dependence · Habituation to Smoking

Repeated consumption of some drugs leads to dependence—a complex interaction between physical craving and psychological longing. Most habit-forming drugs are harmful when taken in excess over long periods of time. They can compel enslavement that overrules the better judgment of the user, and they may ruin his health.

In 1957 the World Health Organization Expert Committee on Addiction-Producing Drugs defined drug addiction and drug habituation in this way:

DRUG ADDICTION

Drug addiction is a state of periodic or chronic intoxication produced by the repeated consumption of a drug (natural or synthetic). Its characteristics include:

1. An overpowering desire or need (compulsion) to continue taking the drug and to obtain it by any means;

2. A tendency to increase the dose;

3. A psychic (psychological) and generally a physical dependence on the effects of the drug;

4. Detrimental effect on the individual and on society.

DRUG HABITUATION

Drug habituation (habit) is a condition resulting from the repeated consumption of a drug. Its characteristics include:

1. A desire (but not a compulsion) to continue taking the drug for the sense of improved well-being which it engenders;

2. Little or no tendency to increase the dose;

3. Some degree of psychic dependence on the effect of the drug, but absence of physical dependence and hence of an abstinence syndrome;

4. Detrimental effect, if any, primarily on the individual.

When the topic of drug dependence is discussed, one tends to think first of narcotics. Alcohol frequently is not regarded as a drug but as a beverage. However, alcohol has potent pharmacologic effects, and dependence on alcohol is common. Dependence on smoking is in still a different category. Recent emphasis on the harmful effects of smoking has led many smokers to try to stop the habit. Many have found the process difficult; some have found it impossible. The report of the Advisory Committee to the Surgeon General of the United States Public Health Service states that "habituation" is the correct term to apply to cigarette smoking.

The Need. Understanding the urgency of the need is difficult for the nonaddict. The person addicted to narcotics is a victim of his own need; everything in life becomes secondary to it. The patient believes that he must have the drug to continue to live through the next hour.

To their own amazement, smokers in countries where both food and cigarettes were scarce after World War II found themselves forgetting long-established manners and morals, not for bread and meat, but for a cigarette. A respectable middle-class man to his own horror searched the streets for smokable butts. Another known for his honesty bought cigarettes on the black market. The need defies usual social sense. Outlawing smoking in Russia in 1634 did not prevent it, even though a penalty for persistent use of tobacco was death. A farmer's helper smokes in a corner of the barn and jeopardizes the winter supply of hay. A nurse refuses a job if there is no place for her to smoke. The comfort of others and sometimes their safety are ignored in the face of the need. Those so attached to cigarettes and narcotics require daily consumption. The need for alcohol is equally compelling but different in that drinking every day may be less necessary.

Onset of Dependence. In varying degrees, according to the agent and the individual dependence on alcohol and drugs includes a strong need to continue taking the agent, ambivalence toward it, and withdrawal symptoms. Drug dependence takes time to develop. There is no clear-cut point at which the person who drinks changes from a social drinker to an alcoholic who can no longer control his drinking but is controlled by it. There is no warning that heroin will become more important than family or job. By the time the person realizes that he is dependent, he has changed. He has lost control over the habit before he knows that he has. It may take 10 years for alcoholism to develop fully, and several more years before it is identified as a problem by the patient. However, addiction to narcotics may occur in a few weeks.

Ambivalence Toward Habit. At first the intake of the agent has a pleasant effect. Heroin and alcohol can reduce tensions, perhaps making an unbearable world less difficult, perhaps creating an aura of self-liking instead of self-loathing. Later, a craving for the agent is noticed at odd moments—on a bus, in a theater, during reading. Finally, the dependence is fully established.

Now the intake of the drug is accompanied by anxiety as well as pleasure.

A drink is downed or a narcotic is hastily injected rather to relieve a state of tension than to seek a pleasurable sensation. The factor of diminishing pleasure seems to operate more fully in some persons than in others. For some who stop taking the drug, the loss of pleasure is intense, and sometimes it is compounded by the inability to find a satisfactory substitute.

Tolerance. When tolerance develops, the dose that was previously effective no longer gives relief, and an increased dose is necessary to obtain the original effect. As the dependence progresses, the alcoholic can indulge in heavy drinking without getting drunk, and the drug addict requires higher and higher doses. Tolerance buildup is a major problem in drug dependence. However, although tolerance to these substances can increase, it is limited, and can be exceeded. When tolerance is exceeded, poisoning results. For instance, although the alcoholic may be able to consume several drinks and show no ill effects from it, downing a bottle of whiskey in an hour or two can render him stuporous. Over a period of time, such excessive intake of alcohol can lead to profound and serious physical effects, such as delerium tremens (DT's) and cirrhosis of the liver.

Withdrawal Symptoms. A strong psychological and physiologic dependence on the substance is established. When the drug is no longer taken, the patient suffers psychological and physical symptoms.

INCIDENCE AND ECONOMICS

Dependence on alcohol and drugs is increasing. Of particular concern is the rising incidence of drug abuse among young people.

Drug dependence is a major health problem. Alcoholism is responsible for loss of time from work and for inefficiency at work. It is unusual for the drug addict to be able to work in a regular job. Also, the care of both types of patients in general and mental hospitals and penal institutions is costly to the community.

Drug dependence is as expensive to the individual as to society. Most alcoholics are between 35 and 55—years when responsibility to home and job are heavy, and the tasks of building a career and a home assume particular importance. The person addicted to a narcotic is placed in an impossible financial position. He can obtain the narcotic only by illegal means; he depends on the pushers who sell it. He has no recourse if the price is exorbitant, if he does not have the money, or if the drug he buys is diluted. Many addicts soon find themselves without funds, and their stealing is related directly to their need for the drug.

When addiction to alcohol occurs, the need becomes insatiable. Alcoholic beverages are expensive. Besides, excessive drinking often leads to intemperate spending. A person who is sensible about money when he is sober may, when he is inebriated, invite everyone he sees to dinner or treat his companions to shopping sprees. These excesses, plus loss of time from work, often wreck the budget.

TREATMENT

Treatment comprises two phases. Initially, it is aimed at overcoming the physical symptoms caused by withdrawal of the drug and giving psychological aid to help overcome the acute sense of loss that the patient suffers. After physiologic adjustments have been made so that physical craving has diminished, the psychological craving remains and requires continued, long-term consideration. Treatment and nursing care that ignore the long-term rehabilitative aspects of a therapeutic program are doomed to fail. Unless the patient solves some of the underlying emotional and social problems which led to addiction, there is great likelihood that he will relapse after the first phase of treatment.

Overcoming physical dependence on drugs is sometimes the beginning, but it is never the end of the patient's struggle to overcome his drug dependence. He may be offered individual or group psychotherapy, a "buddy" system (such as that used in A.A.).

Facilities for treatment of the drug addict are not as widespread as those for the alcoholic, but are increasing as more attention is being paid to these health problems. Sometimes community resources exist, but the patient is unaware of them. Helping patients to find facilities as well as helping communities to develop them are a part of creative nursing that can make the difference between health and disease.

ALCOHOLISM*

Many efforts have been made to differentiate excessive drinking and alcoholism, but there are no wholly-agreed-on criteria that differentiate the heavy drinker from the alcoholic. One definition states that an alcoholic is any individual who relies on alcohol to meet the ordinary demands of living even after alcohol has brought him difficulty in family and job relationships (Bier).

Etiology

Some believe that the reaction of the body of the alcoholic to alcohol is different from that of the body of the person who is not an alcoholic even though he drinks, and sometimes heavily. In other words, there may be a physiologic as well as a psychological basis for alcoholism. Although there is no agreement on this point among authorities on alcoholism, this view has assisted some individuals to acknowledge their dependence on alcohol and to seek treatment. In our society conditions which are physiologically, rather than psychologically based, are the

* Some material dealing with the physiologic and pharmacologic aspects of alcohol consumption has been adapted from: Rodman, Morton J., and Smith, Dorothy W.: *Pharmacology and Drug Therapy in Nursing*, Philadelphia, Lippincott, 1968, with permission of the authors and publisher.

more acceptable. The disadvantage of this view is that by encouraging the patient to focus on physiologic causes for his drinking, he may be discouraged from learning about factors within his emotional life which may contribute to his excessive intake of alcohol.

Personal problems often lead to excessive drinking. Drinking is one way to relieve anxiety and to escape from problems that seem insurmountable. A psychoanalytic view of causation states that alcoholics are fixated at the oral stage of development, and that they use alcohol as a way of returning to feelings of warmth and security experienced during infancy. Some authorities state that alcoholics often have a sense of never having been loved enough, and that they react to this feeling with rage and frustration. Alcohol is commonly used as a means of allowing the individual to express hostility. Frequently, the rage and the frustration are turned inward on the alcoholic himself. Self-destructive tendencies are common. Often alcoholics feel such hopelessness that they see little point in taking ordinary measures to protect themselves against illness, exposure and accidents. The high incidence of pneumonia and tuberculosis among alcoholics is related closely to personal neglect. Suicide is a particular problem among alcoholics. It has been stated that low self-esteem and conflicts over dependence are important factors in the causation of alcoholism.

Incidence

Alcoholism is most prevalent during middle life. Only a small percentage of alcoholics live in the skid-row sections of our cities; they come from all occupational and social groups, and they are scattered throughout the community from the rich to the poor, from executives to laborers.

Despite the manifold problems associated with alcoholism, many alcoholics have an amazing ability to maintain themselves in the community. Despite desperately heavy drinking, many alcoholics manage to continue to work and, sometimes, to conceal their disability from all but their families and closest friends. Often the condition continues with varying degrees of severity for a large part of the individual's life.

Women as well as men become alcoholics. However, because women typically confine their drinking to their own homes, sometimes the mistaken assumption is formed that alcoholism is largely a man's disease. Women alcoholics are less well accepted by society than men alcoholics.

Although the effects of women's drinking are less noted in public places, the effect of a woman alcoholic on her family is devastating.

Because many alcoholics try to hide their condition, it is especially important to show sensitivity when dealing with the alcoholic whose condition brings him to health-care facilities. Illness and accidents associated with drinking are occasions when alcoholism comes to the attention of nurses and physicians, and are opportunities for the patient to acknowledge his problem and to seek help. Unfortunately, the alcoholic is often rebuffed by health professionals, and the opportunity to assist the patient to acknowledge and deal with his drinking is lost.

Physiology

Alcohol is absorbed directly from the stomach and small intestine into the blood stream, without digestion. The rate of absorption of alcohol is slowed by the presence of food in the stomach. However, when alcohol is taken on an empty stomach, its effects are felt quickly, and reach a peak in about 20 minutes.

Alcohol acts directly on the central nervous system. It is a depressant with sedative-hypnotic, analgesic, and even anesthetic properties. The highest intellectual functions, such as judgment, are the first to be impaired, and the vital physiologic functions such as breathing, which are under control of the brain stem, are the last to be affected. Thus, the inebriated individual may lose his life due to an error in judgment while driving, although the same level of alcohol intoxication would not jeopardize his vital physiologic functions such as respiration.

Alcohol is not a stimulant, although many persons regard it as such because an inebriated person may feel or act stimulated due to lessening of inhibitions.

The effects of alcohol on the central nervous system are related to the levels of alcohol in the blood and brain tissue. When alcohol enters the capillaries it diffuses into all body tissues. The tissues which have the best blood supply have a particularly rapid accumulation of alcohol. For example, the level of alcohol concentration in the brain quickly comes into balance with that of the blood. Later, alcohol is taken up by tissues with lesser blood supply, thus drawing some alcohol away from the brain. However, the most important factor in reducing brain levels of alcohol is oxidation of alcohol by the patient's body.

Between 90-95 per cent of alcohol is metabolized to carbon dioxide and water. Most of the rest of the alcohol is excreted unchanged in the breath and urine. The first steps in metabolic breakdown of alcohol occur in the liver. Later, metabolism of alcohol occurs in all cells of the body, where the acetate derived from alcohol is fed into the cellular system for obtaining energy from food (Krebs cycle).

Energy is produced in the process of oxidation of alcohol to carbon dioxide and water, and in this sense alcohol is a food. Alcohol produces 7 calories for every gram oxidized. However, alcohol does not contain essential nutrients such as vitamins and amino acids. Therefore, although the individual who uses alcohol as a significant source of calories may maintain or even gain weight, he frequently suffers malnutrition because he relies substantially on alcohol, rather than on nutritive foods for his caloric intake. The prevalence of malnutrition among alcoholics is believed to be a factor in causing cirrhosis of the liver. However, there is also evidence that prolonged excessive consumption of alcohol has, in itself, adverse effects upon the liver and leads to fibrosis and to fatty infiltration which gradually impair the functioning of the liver.

Alcohol affects other parts of the body besides the central nervous system and the liver. Alcohol can irritate the mucosa of the mouth, the throat, and the stomach leading to hoarseness and gastritis. Moderate intake of alcohol has little effect upon the heart; in fact the sedative and analgesic effects of alcohol may help relieve the pain of coronary insufficiency. Prolonged excessive alcohol intake, however, can lead to myocardial damage.

Korsakoff's psychosis is a condition resulting from prolonged toxic effects of alcohol on the brain. The individual shows memory loss, particularly for recent events. The prognosis for recovery is poor. Peripheral neuropathy is common among alcoholics. Damage to motor and sensory nerve fibers leads to numbness, tingling, and weakness of the extremities. The nerve damage is not due to the direct action of alcohol but is believed to be caused by multiple vitamin deficiencies resulting from the alcoholic's inadequate diet.

Symptoms

Drinking patterns vary widely. Some alcoholics maintain themselves most of the time in a state of intoxication that dulls their reactions to personal problems, interferes with judgment and human relationships, but permits them to perform some routine tasks. Other alcoholics alternate periods of sobriety with drinking sprees, when they continue drinking until they are unconscious. The alcoholic may stick to one drinking pattern, or he may vary the pattern at different periods of his life; no one pattern invariably characterizes his behavior. However, the person developing alcoholism often feels the need to drink regularly during the day, and often he drinks furtively and alone. Others who are developing the condition drink heavily in the evening but abstain during the workday. Later the individual usually finds that he must drink also during working hours.

Usually the alcoholic does not talk about his drinking, although he may say that he is not feeling well. The patient often becomes terrified of his condition, but he is afraid to admit to others (or even to himself) that anything is wrong.

Hangovers increase in severity; nausea, vomiting, weakness and headache are the typical symptoms. The patient misses work more and more frequently, and he has blackouts (amnesia). He sneaks drinks and gulps them as fast as he can.

The patient's disease has serious repercussions in the rest of his life. His employer notices increased absence from work and lessened efficiency when the patient is at work. (Most of Monday may be spent at the water cooler or in the rest room while the alcoholic tries to pull himself together.)

The alcoholic is so horror-stricken by the havoc his disease has brought that he drinks to dull the pain. He rationalizes to keep his guilt down to a more manageable size. He tells himself that he drank today only because his supervisor had accused him wrongly; anybody would take a drink with that kind of provocation. Or his children were so noisy and disrespectful. Or it was so cold out that he could not face waiting for the bus in that weather without something to warm him. As the reasons he gives himself for drinking come one at a time, it is difficult for him to see that they deny truth by their variety and number. A very common reaction of the alcoholic is to blame others, particularly his spouse and employer, for his condition.

He tells himself that he can stop drinking any time he wants to. This statement is true. He can and does stop drinking—sometimes for months. He stops long enough to convince himself that he can stop; but he goes back to it, sure that he has it under control. His ability to have lapses in his drinking proves to him that he is not dependent on the stuff. Unfortunately, the "proof" is not true; he *is* dependent on it.

Often the alcoholic becomes so overwhelmed with guilt over the effects of his drinking on his family, as well as on himself, that he drinks increasingly, thus establishing a vicious circle.

About 4 per cent of alcoholics with an 8- to 10-year history of heavy drinking have brief episodes of mental disorder called *delirium tremens* or the DT's. The onset of delirium tremens is sudden, although before it an alcoholic is often restless, anxious and sleepless. DT's are especially likely to occur when the patient cannot maintain his usual high alcohol intake. Gastrointestinal disturbance, hospitalization, or imprisonment are examples of circumstances which may precipitate delirium tremens because the patient is temporarily unable to drink alcoholic beverages. Characteristics of DT's are tremors that may shake the whole body and hallucinations. The patient sees—and less frequently hears—things that are not there. Most commonly he sees fast-moving animals of grotesque shapes and colors. Some patients see small people running over the floor or climbing on the chair. Restless, violent, unceasing activity that may take the form of running from the animals accompanies DT's. The activity is so great that it may lead to death from heart failure or exhaustion, especially if the patient is malnourished.

The patient experiencing DT's is in the throes of extreme anxiety. He knows who he is, but he may misidentify other people or identify objects incorrectly. He may understand that he is having hallucinations, but this realization does not make the animals go away. He perspires, and therefore dehydration and electrolyte imbalance are further increased. Respiration, pulse, blood pressure and often temperature are elevated. If DT's come when the body has an added strain, such as pneumonia, the body's resistance to alcohol poisoning is decreased.

Effects on the Family

The alcoholic's wife may suffer from lack of money and attention as the need for drink takes up more and more of her husband's thought, time and earnings. There may be many nights when he does not come home at all. Often his wife feels ashamed—ashamed before others who notice her husband's condition—and sometimes guilty, too, concluding that he may have turned to alcohol because she has failed him in some way. She tries to shame him into stopping, but he is so ashamed already that he only drinks more. She gets rid of the liquor, and he buys more. She asks the liquor storekeeper not to sell him any, and he goes to another store. She hides the family supply, but he hides his private stock even more cleverly. There seems to be no answer. She threatens to leave him, and sometimes she does.

In some instances the wife's personality seems to foster the patient's alcoholism in various and subtle ways of which she may not even be aware. For example, she may seek as a marriage partner someone whom she can dominate and hold in low esteem. (Although it is generally believed that the basis for alcoholism is developed largely during childhood, it is recognized also that relationships during adult life can help or hinder the individual in his personality development and his ability to cope with problems.) In many instances the patient's wife is able to help her husband overcome the condition. However, the strains on the marital relationship are severe, and divorce is common.

Often the effect on children in the home is disastrous. Relationships between their parents are strained, and the alcoholic parent's reactions to his children are unpredictable. He may be kind and affectionate when sober, but harsh and violent when drinking. In such a situation it is difficult for children to obtain the consistent affection and security they need, and to develop trust in the alcoholic parent. The expectancy of future alcoholism among these children is high.

Because alcoholism is socially so unacceptable, the family usually makes every effort to conceal the problem from others. They are thus cut off from the kind of help and support they might receive if the condition were more acceptable.

Problems in family relationships often are compounded by the way in which alcohol affects the patient's behavior. For example, gross neglect of the usual standards of dress and of personal cleanliness during intoxication tends to lower the esteem of others and himself, as do his angry outbursts.

Perhaps the most difficult aspect of all for the family is the fact that the patient cannot be treated successfully until *he* seeks treatment. The family may find many community resources for treatment, but they are useless to the patient unless he himself decides to use them. One of the commonest errors of the family is to attempt to arrange for treatment when the patient does not accept it. Success in treatment of alcoholism rests on the patient's desire for help, not on his family's wish (or desperate need) that he be helped.

Often the patient does not seek help until he has hit bottom—perhaps he has lost his job and alienated his family. Experiences like waking up in a jail or a hospital with no recollection of how he got there sometimes shock the patient so much that he becomes able to admit the need for help and begins to seek it.

Treatment

The patient brought to the hospital in acute poisoning is highly agitated, and he may have or soon develop DT's. His blustering, noisy behavior may be part of his defense against feelings of utter helplessness and fear. The nurse must protect the patient from injury. If he perceives that he is being chased by animals, he may run, and an open window may look like a welcome escape from his pursuers. Physical restraints are avoided whenever possible, because they often aggravate the condition by making the patient feel fettered and more helpless. maximum protection with a minimum of direct physical restraint. Closing and locking the window and placing side rails on the bed are examples of measures that can help to protect the patient. The presence of a nurse or a nursing assistant who is calm, firm and watchful helps to protect the patient from injuring himself, as well as lessening his extreme agitation.

Drug therapy for acute alcohol poisoning includes:

• Vitamins, especially the vitamin B group. Alcoholics usually suffer from vitamin deficiency; vitamin B deficiency may be so severe that the patient develops pellagra.

• Paraldehyde often is used as sedation during periods of acute agitation.

• Tranquilizers are widely used to lessen the patient's restlessness and agitation. Some, such as chlorpromazine (Thorazine), also help to relieve nausea and vomiting. Meprobamate (Miltown, Equanil) is another tranquilizer commonly administered.

Phenothiazine-type tranquilizers must be administered cautiously, however, because they potentiate the depressant and hypotensive effects of alcohol. Tranquilizers are also used to control withdrawal symptoms such as nervousness and tremulousness, when the patient is being helped to abstain from alcohol. Continued use of these drugs presents hazards, however, as alcoholics are likely to become dependent on tranquilizers and sedatives, such as phenobarbital. Medical supervision of drug therapy is particularly essential for alcoholics, who so readily transfer their dependence on alcohol to other agents.

Intravenous fluids and electrolytes may be given until anorexia, nausea and vomiting are controlled sufficiently to permit the adequate intake of oral fluids. Encouragement of a nutritious diet is essential as soon as the patient can tolerate it.

After the acute phase has passed, the patient requires long-term treatment. Disulfiram (Antabuse) is a drug sometimes used an an adjunct to other kinds of therapy for chronic alcoholism. The drug causes no apparent effects when given alone, but the ingestion of even small amounts of alcohol by a patient taking Antabuse causes flushing of the face, nausea, vomiting, diarrhea, rapid pulse, fall in blood pressure, palpitation and sometimes collapse. The patient must consent to the use of Antabuse and be fully aware of the symptoms he will experience if he takes a drink. The use of this drug is not without danger. The patient may be unable to resist the temptation to drink, and then he will become seriously ill.

Antabuse is given orally. Usually the patient takes 500 mg. a day for the first few weeks, and then he is placed on a daily maintenance dose of 125 to 500 mg. daily. The rationale underlying the use of Antabuse is that it will deter the alcoholic from drinking because he knows the alcohol will make him very ill.

Citrated calcium carbimide (Temposil; CCC) is another drug which is used to deter the alcoholic from drinking. CCC takes effect more rapidly than Antabuse, but its action is of relatively short duration. CCC is reported to produce a lower incidence of side effects, such as gastric distress, headache, and drowsiness, than Antabuse.

The alcoholic is particularly perceptive of the attitudes of others toward him. Because of unfortunate past experience, he often expects to be treated with scorn and condescension, and he may be ready to defend himself in a demanding, restless manner. Such behavior may be a cover for feelings of helplessness, anxiety and self-loathing. By your kindness, patience and tact you can show him that you consider him a worthwhile individual. By your actions as much as by your words you can convey to him that you regard him as a sick person who needs treatment, that your relationship to him is based on helping him toward recovery, and that you believe recovery is possible. Try not to lecture the patient about anything, even Alcoholics Anonymous. Instead, emphasize acceptance of him as he is and give him opportunities to talk about his situation and his feelings. Let the patient say what he wishes, but avoid prying. Avoid giving advice. It is not likely that you can give him advice that he has not heard already many times.

Another important aspect of caring for the alcoholic involves setting limits. This has nothing to do with punishment or feeling superior to the patient. It means simply that the nurse must keep the patient's demands within limits that she can reasonably fulfill. This rule holds for any patient, not just alcoholics. However, the alcoholic patient may present a particular challenge in this aspect of nursing. For instance, if you are the first person who has seemed to accept him, he may want you to spend more time with him than you can. It is helpful to state how much time you can spend with the patient. Often such a statement helps to avoid misunderstanding later.

Rehabilitation

Some hospitals have carefully planned programs of follow-up care for their alcoholic patients. The patients may come back to the hospital one evening a week for group discussions shared with other alcoholics. The hospital dietitian may lead a discussion on planning an adequate diet, and a member of Alcoholics Anonymous may talk with the group about the work of that organization. Others who may be invited to participate in this type of discussion are physicians, clergymen, nurses and social workers.

Psychotherapy may help the patient to gain greater insight into the emotional problems that have led him to dependence on alcohol. Psychotherapy may be carried out individually or in groups.

Alcoholics Anonymous is an organization composed of and run by alcoholics who by helping each other find that they themselves have been helped. The organization has been notably successful. Often it has helped people who have failed to be helped by other means.

The philosophy of A.A. is disarmingly simple. It is expressed in a prayer its members use, "God grant me the serenity to accept the things I cannot change, courage to change the things I can, and the wisdom to know the difference."

DRUG ABUSE AND DEPENDENCE

Drug abuse and dependence are problems of vastly increasing importance, particularly among young people. Misuse of drugs is a matter of serious concern, especially in such settings as university campuses where a significant proportion of students have had personal experience with one or more drugs such as marihuana and LSD. Because of the magnitude of this health problem, the reader is urged to study widely in the growing literature on this subject. The remainder of this chapter will be devoted to a very brief discussion of some principal forms of drug abuse and dependence. Suggestions for further reading will be found in the bibliography.

Some Characteristics of Drug Users and Abusers

The question of use of drugs is highly charged emotionally, making it especially necessary for nurses and other health professionals to be aware of their own emotional reactions to drug use, and to try to avoid having their personal views interfere with ability to work with patients who have this problem.

Although we shall try to indicate here some of the personality traits believed characteristic of people who abuse drugs, it is becoming increasingly clear that many different kinds of people use drugs for many different reasons, and that it is not useful to deal with this group of people according to a stereotyped concept of "the drug addict." It is essential to consider the differences among drugs (there is considerable difference between occasionally smoking marihuana and becoming addicted to heroin) as well as among drug users, in relation to personality, motivation in using drugs, and patterns of drug use. With this qualification, we shall now briefly consider some characteristics of drug users and abusers.

Low self-esteem is believed to be a significant characteristic of persons who misuse and become dependent on drugs. The drug experience temporarily conveys a feeling of competence, power, and excitement which increases the individual's sense of worth while he is experiencing the effect of the drug. Drug abuse is also a way of withdrawing from problems, and of making problems seem insignificant, and therefore not worth the effort needed to solve them. Persons who use drugs often do so as a form of protest and an expression of anger against others: parents, school administrators, and employers. Their purpose in using drugs may have much to do with shocking, humiliating, and punishing persons in authority.

On the more positive side, some individuals seek drug experience as a way of expanding their consciousness, and of helping them gain insight into the nature of being. Disenchanted with the emphasis upon competitiveness and materialism, some people turn to drugs in their search for meaning and values. Such "mind-expanding" drugs as LSD, by altering the person's perception, are reputed to assist him to achieve insight which may help him experience life more fully. Use of drugs such as LSD carries significant hazards, however, a point which will be discussed subsequently in relation to particular drugs.

Although drug use occurs among young and old alike, it is of particular significance among young people of high school and college age. Among these groups, especially, drug experience is often sought as a way of temporarily relieving loneliness. In contrast with the solitary habits of many drug abusers in the past, young people today often use drugs in groups, seeking through drugs to develop a greater feeling of relatedness to others. Other motives mentioned above, such as rebellion against authority and disenchantment with values emphasizing competition and materialism, are also especially prominent among young people.

Although it used to be assumed that drug abuse was primarily a problem of persons who are economically, socially, and educationally disadvantaged, it has become clear in recent years that the problem exists, and is sometimes especially common, among the "haves" socially, economically, and educationally. Despite such obvious advantages, these young people are sometimes seriously lacking in parental love and concern, and in opportunities for meaningful and satisfying participation with adults.

Relevance to Nursing

As the role of the nurse expands toward greater involvement with the community (rather than being confined largely to hospitals), problems such as drug abuse assume increasing significance in nursing practice. Not many years ago many nurses' involvement with drug dependence and abuse was confined largely to such problems as care of terminally ill patients with cancer, who became addicted to narcotics as a consequence of therapy with these potent pain-relieving drugs. As nurses become more active in care of teen-agers and young adults in school health services, in community mental health centers, and, as public health nurses, in caring for families in their homes, the problem of drug abuse and dependence is brought increasingly to the attention of nurses. The young nurse, particularly, may experience a feeling of interest in and loyalty to the youth-culture which encourages use of drugs, while at the same time, an identification with and loyalty to a profession which seeks to limit use of potent and hazardous drugs without medical advice, and whose members, regardless of age, tend to be viewed as authorities on matters affecting health.

The nurse-student has a particular professional stake in this matter, because, while some forms of drug abuse may be viewed almost as an adolescent prank among many young people, the consequences of being known as a drug abuser can be very serious for members of the health professions, such as nurses, physicians, and pharmacists, whose work requires a high degree of responsibility in adherence to laws concerning use of drugs. Their work also provides easy access to certain types of drugs commonly used in therapy, such as sedatives, amphetamines, and opiates. Thus, the nurse-student is faced with the problem not only of delineating her own values in relation to drug use, but also considering the implications of her values and her behavior, in relation to drugs, upon her future career.

One important attribute of the nurse who works constructively with drug users is approachability. Whatever her personal beliefs in terms of her own conduct, it is important to convey to young people concern, interest, and a willingness to talk frankly with them about the problems of drug use.

One of the tragedies of the current situation is that young people tend to turn to each other, furtively, for information, rather than ask nurses and physicians who could help them to gain more reliable and accurate information. An attitude of silent avoidance on the part of health professionals is not useful. Students already are involved with the problem. Silence does not serve to keep young people from knowing about and using drugs, but it does keep them from gaining accurate information, and from obtaining the emotional support in thinking through the problem which a concerned adult can give.

Drugs*

Some of the more common drugs which are taken without medical advice, and which are often misused, are briefly described below.

Amphetamines. Amphetamine (Benzedrine), dextroamphetamine (Dexedrine), and methamphetamine (Methedrine) are commonly used drugs of this type. Amphetamines are central nervous system stimulants. They increase the individual's sense of alertness and wakefulness, and they also alter mood. They are sometimes called mood-elevating drugs because they help depressed patients to feel more energetic and optimistic. This group of drugs is sometimes prescribed for mildly depressed patients, for treating patients who have taken overdoses of sedatives, and, in conjunction with low calorie diets, to lessen appetite when the patient must lose weight. However, we shall limit our discussion to the misuse of amphetamines.

Ampehetamines are widely misused, particularly among young people, who use them to keep awake while studying for examinations or during long drives. The person who takes amphetamines for this purpose masks his fatigue and his need for rest, and can continue to work, study, drive, or whatever, beyond his usual period of endurance. Misuse of amphetamines varies from brief and relatively infrequent use of moderate amounts of these drugs in order to postpone fatigue, to drug-abuse by "speed freaks" who take massive doses, seeking extended periods of euphoria and wakefulness until they "crash" in a toxic psychosis.

After using amphetamines to produce an unnatural wakefulness and alertness, the individual often experiences a "let-down" characterized by physical and mental exhaustion. If the individual goes to bed and permits himself the rest he urgently needs, he may experience no serious physiologic disturbance from brief use of the drug. If, however, he takes more of the drug,

---

* Some material dealing with the physiologic and pharmacologic aspects of drug abuse and dependence has been adapted from Rodman, Morton J., and Smith, Dorothy W.: *Pharmacology and Drug Therapy in Nursing*, Philadelphia, Lippincott, 1968, with permission of the authors and publisher.

either in an attempt to continue working, or because he enjoys feeling "high" or euphoric, the individual exposes himself to serious sequelae, among which are mental and physical collapse from exhaustion, marked nervousness and tremulousness, weight loss, and, in some instances, psychosis. A further serious effect of misuse of amphetamines is development of dependence on the feeling of euphoria, which can lead the individual on more and more "speed sprees" regardless of their harmful consequences.

LSD (lysergic acid diethylamide) is a drug which produces mental states said to be similar to those observed in some psychoses. For this reason LSD is often called a psychotomimetic drug (a drug which mimics psychosis). The drug causes visual hallucinations and illusions, as well as mood changes. The results are highly variable and individual, from one person to another, and in the same person, when the drug is taken under varying circumstances. The current clinical status of LSD is that of a research drug, administered under carefully controlled conditions, to aid in understanding and treating alcoholism and other conditions characterized by emotional disturbance. However, it is also widely used without medical supervision to induce states of altered consciousness. (These states are referred to as "trips.")

The weight of evidence to date indicates that self-medication with LSD constitutes a serious form of drug abuse, even though the drug is not addictive in the sense that narcotics are. Among the reasons for this belief are:

• LSD, has precipitated prolonged psychotic reactions and suicide attempts. It is not without risk even when administered by a psychiatrist after careful study of the patient, and under circumstances which provide continuous observation of the patient and measures to safeguard him from harming himself during the period of altered consciousness.

• Persons who are experiencing an LSD "trip" can seriously hurt or kill themselves, because they may believe themselves invulnerable to hazards, such as falling from heights, or being struck by cars.

• A sense of extreme terror sometimes occurs as a result of using LSD. This result is variable and unpredictable, and is referred to as a "bad trip." Because the individual is in a state of panic, he requires the calming presence of another person and prompt treatment with a phenothiazine-type tranquilizer. Prompt administration of the latter can quickly reduce the patient's terror and help him reorient himself to his surroundings.

• Administration of LSD to experimental animals during pregnancy has reportedly resulted in the birth of litters with malformations and brain defects. Although the long-range genetic effects of LSD in humans are still not fully understood, current knowledge gives considerable basis for alarm over its possible effects upon unborn children.

Advocates of self-administration of LSD emphasize its "consciousness-expanding" properties and its use in providing extraordinary experiences. These persons stress the greater perceptiveness, and the emotional growth and insight which they attribute to LSD. These are goals which others seek through psychotherapy and through religious experience. The question which must be raised is whether the seeking of quick results in expanded consciousness through use of LSD can be justified, in view of the serious hazards in use of this drug. In light of current evidence concerning its hazards the drug is still restricted to research use with psychiatric patients.

The nurse can make an important contribution by helping young people appreciate the hazards and the variability in effects of LSD, and by helping them to consider other safer ways of expanding their consciousness and insight. The nurse who takes seriously a young person's search for meaning, insight, and heightened awareness is in a better position to guide the youth to seek these experiences in safer ways than the nurse who scorns the young person for searching for new dimensions of experience which have, by various means, been sought throughout the ages of human existence.

Marihuana is derived from the cannabis plant, and is popularly referred to as "pot." The drug is usually inhaled by smoking although it is occasionally taken orally. Considerable controversy exists concerning the harmfulness of marihuana. It is generally believed to be one of the least harmful substances falling into the category of frequently abused drugs. It has not been shown to produce lasting physical or mental damage, and its use does not lead to physical dependence and tolerance. The effects of smoking marihuana are variously described by users as subtly pleasurable changes in mood, perception, and consciousness, a feeling of bodily lightness, and sometimes hallucinations. While the use of marihuana does not necessarily lead to experimentation with other more harmful substances such as LSD and narcotics, numerous studies have shown that the likelihood of using these more harmful drugs is markedly higher in the group of marihuana users than it is among non-users (Louria, D., *The Drug Scene*). That use of marihuana may be one aspect of initiation into the drug culture seems indisputable, and constitutes an important danger to youth. There is some discussion that the illegal status of use of marihuana may foster its popularity among young people as a way of expressing rebellion against authority. Its use is illegal in the United States.

Marihuana has until recently been used most widely among persons who are poor and underprivileged, in order to relieve the starkness and harshness of daily existence. Its use in the U.S. has, until recently, been most widespread in the urban ghettoes.

The present widespread use of marihuana among young people of all social and economic classes probably has much to do with rebellion against authority and middle-class values, as well as heightened interest in introspection and altered states of consciousness. Use of this drug, particularly, has become a symbol of the new movement among young people. It seems to arouse intense emotional reactions among young people and their elders which often obscure the facts concerning this drug's physiologic and psychologic effects.

Barbiturates, Nonbarbiturate Sedative-Hypnotics, and Minor Tranquilizers. These drugs are commonly referred to, among drug abusers, as "downs," leading to sedation and somnolence. The barbiturates and minor tranquilizers are dangerous when misused by persons who seek to control their nervousness by self-medication with these agents. Particularly dangerous is the use of amphetamines and barbiturates in combination, and combinations of alcohol with barbiturates or with other sedatives, hypnotics, and minor tranquilizers such as Miltown and Librium. Because alcohol potentiates the depressant and hypotensive effects of these sedative drugs, this combination can be especially hazardous, leading even to coma and death.

Because of the frequency with which sedatives and minor tranquilizers are prescribed to help control anxiety, many persons who misuse these

drugs have been introduced to them through a physician's prescription. However, when other measures to deal with anxiety are not promptly also undertaken, the individual sometimes finds himself relying on the drug for this effect after the supply permitted by the physician has run out. Then the individual begins to purchase the medication illegally, or to obtain it through a friend whose physician prescribes it freely. An important nursing measure which can help prevent dependence on sedatives involves assisting the patient to consider what other measures he can begin to use to reduce anxiety. For example, a public health nurse who knows that her patient has just received a prescription for barbiturates or for a tranquilizer can talk to the patient about other measures he can begin to use in addition to the drug, in order to reduce anxiety. Too often the patient sees the medication as the solution rather than as a temporary aid until other measures are found. For one patient this may mean dealing with a disturbing situation at home or at work. For another it may mean finding some relaxing activities unrelated to his work, such as swimming or dancing, which can help him relax and prepare him for a good night's sleep.

Use of barbiturates and similar sedatives, hypnotics and tranquilizers can lead to serious physical dependence and to withdrawal symptoms when the drugs are abruptly discontinued. Withdrawal symptoms are characterized by nervousness, extreme restlessness, and insomnia. Prolonged insomnia and agitation sometimes lead to hallucinations or to a full-blown psychosis. Muscular tremors and even convulsions may also occur. Withdrawal of barbiturates in persons dependent on them must be undertaken gradually, under close medical supervision. Physical dependence on minor tranquilizers can also occur. This is manifested by an abstinence syndrome when the tranquilizer is abruptly withdrawn. Its signs and symptoms are similar to those for withdrawal of barbiturate: nervousness, tremors, hallucinations, delirium, and convulsions.

Potent Narcotic Analgesics. Misuse of narcotics is one way of temporarily relieving anxiety and escaping from personal problems. As is often the case with alcohol, heroin and related drugs are used to relieve emotional pain and then their continued use adds to the individual's pain, anxiety, and emotional disturbance. Sometimes misuse of narcotics is related to hostility in a conscious or unconscious effort to hurt oneself or others.

Even though the production and the distribution of heroin (diacetylmorphine) is prohibited in the United States, it is the most commonly used narcotic, the one especially favored by the younger addicts. It gives an intense euphoria without nausea and vomiting. It is a potent analgesic, and tolerance is developed rapidly. Opium and morphine (an alkaloid of opium), preferred by older addicts, also lead to euphoria. When morphine is taken intravenously (or by the "mainline," as addicts say), the person feels an acutely pleasurable sensation in his abdomen. Before the letdown, which follows in 4 or 5 hours, there is an increase in phantasy attended by a decrease in anxiety. Pain, hunger and sexual urges are forgotten. Morphine contracts smooth muscle, and tolerance is not developed to this action of the drug, as it is to other effects. Most morphine addicts remain constipated as long as they take the drug.

The consistent administration of a powerful analgesic, such as morphine, can allow pain from another disease to go unrecognized and therefore untreated. Whenever an addict requires treatment for any disease, it is essential that doctors and nurses know that he is an addict. Addicts usually require larger doses of premedication and anesthesia for surgery. Because he is engaged in an illegal activity, an addict often will hide the fact that he is addicted, yet this information is important to the anesthesiologist. The observation of constricted pupils, which may mean that the patient is addicted to morphine, would be a most valuable observation to make. Because the addict's technic may not be sterile, he may develop complications like local infections or hepatitis from the use of unsterile syringes and needles.

Withdrawal Sickness

Withdrawal sickness, a self-limiting but extremely uncomfortable illness, occurs when addicts do not take the narcotic to which they are addicted. The symptoms of withdrawal from narcotics begin to become severe about 24 hours after the last dose, and they reach their peak in 36 to 72 hours, after which they taper off. The patient feels sick and apprehensive. Soon his eyes tear, and his nose becomes congested. Withdrawal from morphine causes repeated yawning. The patient perspires and feels hot and cold flashes. "Goose bumps" are raised on his skin.

He feels anxious and restless. Temperature, blood pressure and pulse are elevated. Vomiting, diarrhea, anorexia, headache, muscular aching and twitching and severe abdominal cramps follow. Coma and collapse are possible. The patient is most comfortable lying on his side in a flexed position, and he will naturally assume this position. Keep a blanket over him, even on hot days. Because cigarettes are distasteful to him, he will refrain from smoking while withdrawal symptoms persist.

It is important to differentiate between *physical* withdrawal and psychological dependence. Physical withdrawal symptoms are of a few days' duration, but psychological dependence, and the craving for the euphoria produced by the drug, can last for years even when the patient is prevented from obtaining the drug during that prolonged period. This emphasizes the need to focus on helping the addict deal with his psychological craving which can, after several months in a hospital, lead him to seek narcotics upon his release.

Treatment

People addicted to heroin and other opiates are often weaned away from these drugs with the aid of methadone. This drug is itself addicting, but its use seems justified in some circumstances. Its main advantage when used as an adjunct to the gradual withdrawal of opiates is that it keeps the patient comfortable without itself producing a euphoric "high." Eventually, when dosage of the opiate has been gradually reduced and finally eliminated, the doctor must also withdraw the methadone that he has been administering. Fortunately, this is usually accomplished with only relatively mild discomfort, as physical dependence on this drug is not as powerful as dependence upon heroin.

Recently methadone has been used in still another way to aid in the long-term rehabilitation of narcotic addicts. In this so-called "methadone maintenance" therapy, methadone is not withdrawn, but it is instead administered indefinitely much as insulin is administered to diabetics. It is claimed that patients taking methadone are unable to experience the characteristic euphoria produced by heroin. Similarly, patients taking methadone in doses that reduce or eliminate the craving for heroin are able to carry on activities requiring mental alertness and motor coordination. Thus, it is claimed that former heroin addicts can hold jobs, go to school, and in other ways also perform the activities expected of them.

As a result of recent reports of successful rehabilitation programs based upon the adjunctive use of methadone, clinics are now being set up in some large cities where addicts are treated with a combination of methadone, counseling, and assistance with finding and keeping jobs and homes.

When methadone is used to aid in withdrawal of opiates, symptoms of lassitude, nausea, vomiting, dizziness, sweating, anorexia and insomnia still may occur and last for weeks, but the most acute symptoms of withdrawal illness are largely avoided. Barbiturates may be given for sleep, but there is danger of further addiction with this prescription. Prolonged baths are given for sedation, aspirin for pain and intravenous fluids for dehydration.

Withdrawal is complete in about 4 days for adolescents and 10 days for adults. Then the hardest part of the treatment starts, an attack on the underlying cause of the addiction. Psychotherapy is an important aspect of treatment. Treatment involves not only breaking the pattern of addiction to a narcotic but, even more difficult, treatment of the underlying personality disorder and dealing with the complex web of social problems that accompany the addiction.

Prevention

Addiction to drugs of a person with severe, long-term pain is a tragedy. Use of narcotics to relieve the pain of such conditions as arthritis and peripheral vascular disease usually is avoided for this reason. Some patients, such as those who require relief from severe pain due to terminal cancer, cannot obtain relief by any other therapy. If addiction to narcotics occurs in such instances, it is viewed as an unavoidable complication during treatment of an acutely painful terminal illness. In most hospitals narcotics must be reordered by the physician at frequent intervals (such as every 48 hours), thus bringing to the attention of the physician the question of whether the patient should continue to receive the drug. If you observe that a patient seems to be relying on narcotics, consult the physician. Above all, never use narcotics ordered by the physician for the relief of pain merely to quiet a patient who is making difficult demands on the staff. Instead, consider the reason for the patient's behavior, and in consultation with the physician develop a plan for dealing with the patient's discomfort.

Any person who regularly receives narcotics for whatever reason can become addicted. Addiction is *not* limited, as is commonly supposed, to those who are socially and educationally disadvantaged.

Doctors, nurses and pharmacists have a special responsibility in prevention and early detection of drug addiction, because they are the ones who handle narcotics as part of their work. Destroying disposable syringes and needles before discarding them to prevent their possible use later by addicts is an example of something nurses can do to help to combat the problem. Keeping the medicine closet locked is another. Those whose work involves handling narcotics are especially vulnerable to addiction. Honest recognition of this possibility has helped many a professional person to avoid the pitfall of taking unprescribed drugs with the idea that it will be all right "just this once."

HABITUATION TO SMOKING

Any discussion of habituation and dependence syndromes would be incomplete without some attention to the problem of habituated tobacco smokers. It has become increasingly apparent that the undesirable effects of smoking constitute a real health hazard to the large segment of the population who are heavy smokers. Consequently, the problem of tobacco habituation is a rightful concern for all those engaged in the health field.

Lung Cancer

The risk of developing lung cancer increases with the number of cigarettes smoked per day and decreases when smoking is discontinued. Pipe and cigar smokers, who usually do not inhale, develop cancer of the lung more frequently than non-smokers, but less frequently than cigarette smokers. Pipe smokers are especially prone to cancer of the mouth. (Smoking and Health, U.S.A., 1964)

Physical Effects of Tobacco

Besides cancer of the lung, cigarette smoking is important in the morbidity and mortality from bronchitis and emphysema. It causes breathlessness, decreased pulmonary function and, as every heavy smoker knows, a chronic productive cough. Smoking can cause paralysis of the cilia; this prevents the clearing away of foreign particles, such as those found in tobacco smoke, which are then deposited on the epithelium. In addition, pathology seen in chronic bronchitis can be caused by smoking. Smoking has not been as clearly identified as a cause of emphysema, but the rupture of alveolar septa and the fibrosis caused by smoking seem to be related to this disease. And, it is known that the death rate from emphysema, like that from bronchitis, is higher in the smoker than in the non-smoker. In a group of smokers who coughed, were dyspneic or had a history of asthma, 70 per cent of those who stopped smoking showed improvement of symptoms, whereas among those who continued to smoke, only 1 per cent improved (Smoking and Health, U.S.A., 1964). The symptoms of bronchitis and emphysema tend to be progressive, especially in smokers, and may result in respiratory crippling to the extent that the patient is unable to work or even to walk because he cannot breathe adequately.

Effects of Withdrawal. When a habituated smoker stops smoking, he may experience such physical signs and symptoms as ankle edema, gastrointestinal instability, profuse diaphoresis, sleep disturbances, slowing of the pulse and lowering of blood pressure (Knapp *et al.*). Chest pain, anorexia and hunger also have been reported. In addition, it is not uncommon to have impaired concentration and memory, a rise of anxiety, distorted time perception, restlessness and great irritability. The craving is so urgent that it leads to some remarkable mental gymnastics, in the course of which some compelling and subtle arguments are put forward in the person's mind

as to why he should have a cigarette now, that he often takes one in spite of his resolve not to do so. This process is hard to believe unless one experiences it. Although the craving may disappear after a few days or months of distress, no one can hold out this hope to patients, because the acute discomfort may recur for years.

Decreasing the number of cigarettes smoked a day may be the most satisfactory solution for some people. Many, however, soon find themselves smoking the same number of cigarettes as before. The longing is kept alive.

Some people report that they feel wonderful after giving up smoking; there is no morning cough, food tastes better, they have more energy, and there is the thrill of accomplishing a difficult task. Others find the depression, irritability and craving not worth the compensations.

Some Ways of Assisting the Patient. The attitudes of those in contact with the person who is attempting to become an exsmoker are of prime importance. Although the nurse may be in a position to inform the patient about the dangers of smoking, fear technics and preaching are known to fail. Authoritatively telling people to stop smoking because cigarettes are harmful may be like daring them to continue. Such an approach may instill fear but not change the habit, an undesirable psychological situation. The decision and the action must lie with the patient, with the nurse supporting him. Otherwise, the patient may feel that the nurse is trying

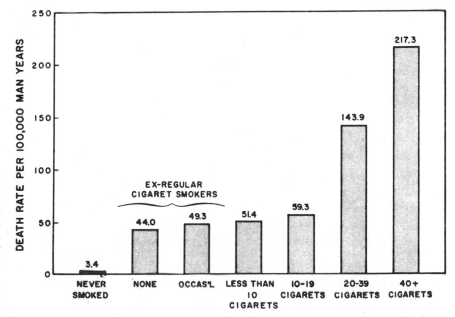

FIG. 9-1. Death rates: lung cancer (confirmed diagnosis). Age standardized death rates from verified cases of bronchogenic carcinoma (exclusive of adenocarcinoma), by number of cigarettes smoked daily. (American Cancer Society: *Cigarette Smoking and Cancer,* New York, The Society)

to manipulate him and reject her message. Backsliding is to be expected. The nurse should respond to these lapses by helping the patient realize that he is not outstandingly weak-willed because he failed in his resolve this time, but that each time he stops it can become easier to do so.

Irritability seems to be one of the most consistent symptoms observed during abstinence. Unless it is recognized as a symptom, it can create tensions between people, which, among other disadvantages, leads to resuming smoking. Helping someone to stop smoking can be exacting for spouse, friend or nurse. Responding to irritability with irritability is not therapeutic for the patient. Responses that do not imply disapproval, impatience or manipulation are desirable, but difficult.

The nurse should be familiar with the following considerations about stopping smoking, because some of them may be useful to her patients:

• Delaying tactics, such as delaying the first smoke by an hour a day. Within 15 or so days the time for smoking will not be until long after the time for retiring. A variation of this, for those whose need for the first cigarette of the day is most compelling, is not to smoke at a certain time or place, or while doing something specific, such as between 2 and 5 P.M., or while watching television, or while in the bedroom, and then to increase the nonsmoking times and areas. The point here is to encourage the patient to try for something that is possible for him and then to build on success.

• Most people need help in fighting the arguments that they put to themselves for taking a cigarette when the craving comes over them. Making a list of private reasons for not smoking and referring to it at those times may help. Being forearmed is often useful, especially if the patient has prethought ways to redirect himself, like a quick walk, a substitute thought, a treat he can anticipate. Allowing the mind to rest on the thought of a cigarette usually leads to reaching for one. Perhaps the most helpful measure is to have a person to talk to who will listen sympathetically. A nurse could be such a person. So could another patient who also is trying to stop, or who has stopped. Being able to talk to someone who understands how overwhelming the need is when the craving strikes, night or day, seems to help.

• Advance planning and creating a psychological buildup for the day when smoking will be decreased or stopped seems more effective than deciding to stop on the spur of the moment. The time should be carefully chosen. Some people find that vacation is a good time, when they are in a strange place without the precedent of having smoked there and without the usual pressures of work and home. Illness may be another good time to break away from smoking, especially when one has a disease that makes smoking distasteful. On the other hand, some hospitalized patients need cigarettes more than ever, because they are tense and worried. The campaign to stop must be planned so that it is most suitable to the person it is to serve.

• Many find that making the promise to stop provisional and private (or shared with only 1 or 2 trusted people) encourages abstinence, because the pressure of having to keep face is avoided. Others find that telling everyone they know that they are stopping helps them to do so, because they are ashamed not to.

• For the first hard days of nonsmoking there are measures that may decrease the severity of the physical symptoms. Some physicians prescribe a regimen of sedation to overcome restlessness and insomnia, and mild stimulants to replace the arousal effects of cigarette smoke. Patients should be warned not to take these drugs without a prescription. Lobeline is a substance that simulates the action of nicotine. Opinions of its effectiveness are divided. Some researchers find it helpful for people who are motivated to stop smoking. Others find it no more useful than inert tablets.

• Some patients are helped by hypnosis. This therapy should be under the direction of a physician. It is not a cure, but, like tranquilizers, it may be part of a total treatment program.

• Some mechanical aids are: using a dummy cigarette (such as an unfilled cigarette holder); biting on a clove or chewing on root ginger (a cigarette tastes terrible afterwards); following a pre-established day-by-day regimen for abstinence (such as that presented in *The Cigarette Habit* by Arthur King); letting the cigarette burn unsmoked (this may diminish some of the loneliness, but it is difficult not to draw on it); not smoking to the very end of the cigarette (the unburnt part acts as a filter); switching to brands enjoyed less than the favorite one; changing to pipes or cigars.

• Efforts to interrupt the cues (such as finishing a meal) which stimulate the desire for a cigarette are helpful to some people. Shapiro and Tursky of Harvard Medical School have developed a program using a "beeper" paging device to assist people to stop smoking. The "beeper" gives a signal from the user's pocket or purse, in response to which the individual lights a cigarette. The "beep" signals are not in pattern with the individual's usual cues, however; thus, smoking at the signal is a way of interrupting the individual's usual smoking pattern. The signals gradually become less and less frequent, and the individual whose smoking pattern has been interrupted, gradually cuts down on his use of cigarettes and sometimes eliminates their use altogether.

• Groups which are formed to help their members stop smoking are useful. Sometimes a physician is the group leader; in other instances, a physician and nurse serve as co-leaders for the group. The opportunity to discuss personal problems concerning smoking, combined with group support as well as group pressure to stop, can help with the lonely and discouraging task of overcoming the craving for a smoke.

• Chewing gum and eating, especially candy, sometimes are substituted. Then a gain in weight can become a problem. It is often most helpful to encourage the patient not to fight battles on too many fronts at once. After the need for cigarettes has been lessened, the patient can lose the weight he gained.

• Perhaps the most effective approach is a multidirectional one in which drugs are used to help quell the physical symptoms, and group and individual interviews are held to encourage insight into the needs met by smoking and the reasons for the great difficulty in stopping.

These suggestions apply to patients who have made the decision either to stop smoking or to decrease the number of cigarettes consumed. It may be that the cigarettes serve certain needs so well for some people that they do not want to change their use of them in spite of the health hazards. In any case, it is the patient's decision to make and not the nurse's. The nurse's function is to help the patient to understand the facts he needs to make a decision, and to help him to stop or to diminish his smoking if he wishes such help.

If the person is not under the care of a doctor, the nurse should advise him to consult one. With all patients the nurse's approach should be supportive. She should be especially careful not to push the person who reacts to stopping smoking with increased anxiety. Instead, encourage the patient to seek further help, and assist him to do so, if he wishes, by providing him with names of resources where individual and group counseling are available. In this way he can receive expert assistance with personal problems which may be affecting not only his problem with smoking, but other aspects of his life as well.

Prevention

Because it is so difficult to stop smoking, it is logical to pay attention to its prevention. Studies indicate that reaching high-school students is probably too late to begin the educational process; teaching 5th and 6th graders may be more effective. This finding places a special responsibility on school nurses to provide children with information about the health hazards associated with smoking, so that fewer children will become smokers.

Other measures that may lessen the health dangers of smoking include:

• Making cigarettes less easily available. Some cafeterias, especially those serving young people, have removed their cigarette vending machines.

• Changing what is smoked from tobacco to some other substance, such as papaya leaf. Palatability, acceptance, finding a nonharmful substance, and enjoyment replacement are a few of the problems here.

• Effective filtration. What is to be filtered out of the hundreds of components of smoke is a problem. One hundred per cent filtration would result in smoking hot air.

• Restriction of smoking in public places.

• Increased taxation on tobacco products.

• Restriction of advertising of cigarettes.

• Labeling packages for tar and nicotine contents, and placing a warning on each pack of cigarettes.

REFERENCES AND BIBLIOGRAPHY

American Cancer Society: *Cigarette Smoking and Cancer,* New York, The Society, 1963.

The Anti-Smoking Clinic, *Lancet,* 2:353, August, 1963.

Aspects of the cigarette problem: III. Nicotine addiction, *Canad. Med. Asoc. J.* 88:1120, June, 1963.

Auerbach, O., Stout, A. P., Hammond, E. C., and Garfinkel, L.: Changes in bronchial epithelium in relation to cigarette smoking and in relation to lung cancer, *New Eng. J. Med.* 265:253, 1961.

Barrett, K. A.: High school students' smoking habits, *Canad. J. Public Health* 53:500, 1962.

BARTER, J. T., and REITE, M.: Crime and LSD: the insanity plea, *Am. J. Psychiat.* 126:531, October, 1969.

BIER, W. C. (ed.): *Problems in Addiction,* New York, Fordham University, 1962.

BLANE, H. T.: *The Personality of the Alcoholic,* New York, Harper, 1968.

BLUM, E., and BLUM, R.: *Alcoholism,* San Francisco, Jossey-Bass, 1967.

BRADEN, W.: *The Private Sea, LSD and the Search for God,* New York, Bantam, 1968.

BURTON, G.: An alcoholic in the family, *Nurs. Outlook* 12: 34–37, May, 1964.

CAMERON, D. C.: Narcotic drug addiction, *Am. J. Psychiat.* 119:793, February, 1963.

CATANZARO, R. S.: *Alcoholism: The Total Treatment Approach,* Springfield, Ill., Thomas, 1968.

CHAFETZ, M. E., and DEMORE, H. W.: *Alcoholism and Society,* New York, Oxford University Press, 1962.

CHEVALIER, R. B., BOWERS, J. A., BONDURANT, S., and ROSS, J. C.: Circulatory and ventilatory effects of exercise in smokers and nonsmokers, *J. Appl. Physiol.* 18:357, 1963.

Consumers Union Report on Smoking and the Public Interest, Mt. Vernon (N.Y.), Consumers Union, 1963.

DOLE, V. P., *et al.:* Methadone treatment of randomly selected criminal addicts, *New Eng. J. Med.* 280:1372, June, 1969.

DOLL, W. R., JONES, F. A., and PYGOTT, F.: Effect of Smoking on production and maintenance of gastric duodenal ulcer, *Lancet* 1:657, 1958.

FOX, R. (ed.): *Alcoholism,* New York, Springer, 1967.

FERNEAU, E. W., and MORTON, E. L.: Attitudes of nursing personnel regarding alcoholism and alcoholics, *Nurs. Res.* 18:446, Sept.-Oct. 1969.

FRIEDMAN, S. H.: I choose not to smoke, *Nurs. Outlook* 12: 40–42, March, 1964.

GELPERIN, A., and GELPERIN, E.: The inebriate in the emergency room, *Am. J. Nurs.* 70:1494, July, 1970.

GILLESPIE, C.: Nurses help combat alcoholism, *Am. J. Nurs.* 69:1938, September, 1969.

GRINSPOON, L.: Marihuana, *Sci. Am.* 221:17, December, 1969.

HAGUE, SR. BETSY: In San Francisco's tenderloin, *Am. J. Nurs.* 69:2180, October, 1969.

HAMMOND, E. C., and HORN, D.: Smoking and death rates, report on 44 months of follow-up of 187,783 men: II. Death rates by cause, *JAMA* 166:1294, March 15, 1958.

HAMMOND, E. C., and PEREY, C.: Ex-smokers, *New York J. Med.* 58:2956, 1958.

HORN, D.: Behavioral aspects of cigarette smoking, *J. Chronic Dis.* 16:383, 1963.

HORN, D., COURTS, F. A., TAYLOR, R. M., and SOLOMEN, E. S.: Cigarette smoking among high school students, *Am. J. Public Health* 49:1497, 1959.

JAMES, G.: A stop-smoking program, *Am. J. Nurs.* 64:122–125, June, 1964.

KING, A.: *The Cigarette Habit: A Scientific Cure,* Kingswood, England, World's Work, Ltd., 1959.

KING, S. H.: *Youth in Rebellion, Drug Dependence,* Washington, D.C., National Institute of Mental Health, July, 1969.

KNAPP, P. H., BLISS, C. M., and WELLS, H.: Addictive aspects in heavy cigarette smoking, *Am. J. Psychiat.* 119:966, 1963.

KRAMER, J. C., *et al.:* Amphetamine abuse, *JAMA* 201:305, 1967.

LARSON, P. S., HAAG, H. B., and SILVETTE, H.: *Tobacco, Experimental and Clinical Studies,* Baltimore, Williams & Wilkins, 1961.

LINGEMAN, R.: *Drugs from A to Z,* New York, McGraw-Hill, 1969.

LOURIA, D. B.: *The Drug Scene,* New York, McGraw-Hill, 1968.

————: Lysergic acid diethylamide, *New Eng. J. Med.* 278: 435, February, 1968.

LUCIA, S. (ed.): *Alcohol and Civilization,* New York, McGraw-Hill, 1963.

McFARLAND, J. W.: Lifeline for ex-smokers, *Nurs. Outlook* 12:50–52, July, 1964.

OSTROW, S.: Drug addiction—The medico-legal conflict, *Am. J. Nurs.* 63:67, July, 1963.

PARLEY, K.: Supporting the patient on LSD day, *Am. J. Nurs.* 64:80, February, 1964.

PATTISON, E. M., *et al.:* Evaluation of alcoholism treatment: A comparison of three facilities, *Arch. Gen. Psychiat.* 20:478, 1969.

PEARSON, B. A., KROMBERG, C. J., and PROCTOR, J. B.: Methadone maintenance in heroin addiction, *Am. J. Nurs.* 70:2571, December, 1970.

PODOLOSKY, E.: *Management of Addictions,* New York, Philosophical Library, 1955.

POPLAR, J. F.: Characteristics of nurse addicts, *Am. J. Nurs.* 69:117, January, 1969.

Report of Committee on Alcoholism and Drug Dependence: Dependence on LSD and other hallucinogenic drugs, *JAMA* 202:47, October, 1967.

Report of Committee on Alcoholism and Drug Dependence: Dependence on cannabis (marihuana), *JAMA* 201:368, August, 1967.

RHODE, M.: Drug addiction—The addict as an inpatient, *Am. J. Nurs.* 63:61, July, 1963.

RODMAN, M. J.: Drug abuse and its medical management, *RN* 30:47, August, 1967.

————: Drug therapy today: Drugs used against addiction, *RN* 33:71, October, 1970.

RODMAN, M. J., and SMITH, D. W.: *Pharmacology and Drug Therapy in Nursing,* Philadelphia, Lippincott, 1968.

RUSSAW, E.: Nursing in a narcotic-detoxification unit, *Am. J. Nurs.* 70:1720, August, 1970.

SIMON, W., and LUMRY, G.: Alcoholism and drug addiction among physicians, *Drug Dependence,* Washington, D.C., National Institute of Mental Health, July, 1969.

Smoking and Health: a Report of the Royal College of Physicians of London on Smoking in Relation to Cancer of the Lung and Other Diseases, London, Pitman, 1962.

Smoking and Health, Report of the Advisory Committee to the Surgeon General of the Public Health Service, Public Health Service Publication No. 1103, U.S. Department Health, Education, and Welfare, Public Health Service, Washington, D.C., U.S. Government Printing Office, 1964.

SORENSEN, K., and FAGAN, R. J.: The hospitalized skid row alcoholic, *Nurs. Forum* 2:88–112, 1963.

STRACHAN, J.: *Alcoholism,* Vancouver, Mitchell Press, 1968.

WORLD HEALTH ORGANIZATION: *WHO Expert Committee on Addiction-Producing Drugs, 13th Report,* Technical Report Series No. 273, 1964.

YOLLES, S. F.: The drug scene, *Nurs. Outlook* 18:24, July, 1970.

Care of the Dying Patient

10

Care of the dying patient is a topic which has been long neglected among all health professionals. However, it is now receiving more attention, and the reader is referred to the Bibliography for references on this important subject. Space allows only a very brief discussion here.

There are many indications that death has become a taboo subject in our society, much as sex was a taboo topic in the Victorian era. Euphemisms are widely used in place of the word "death," and great effort and expense are often employed to prepare and to show the body of the deceased in a way which makes it appear that death has not occurred at all.

Many people have little contact with death occurring naturally in the home. Frequently death occurs among awesome equipment and busy physicians and nurses dedicated to saving lives, to whom the death of a patient may signify to them their failure as healers. Seldom, in the hospital environment, is death viewed and discussed as a natural and universal experience. The role of health workers in supporting the patient and his loved ones during this experience is often de-emphasized in the stress on details of therapy which, though necessary and important, do not in themselves convey human caring. Nurses, because of the nature of their work, have opportunity to be involved with patients and families at the time of death—an opportunity which can enable them to help others during one of life's crucial experiences, as well as to grow personally in their understanding and acceptance of death as a part of life.

Attitudes of falseness and denial interfere with provision of supportive care for the patient and family. The patient whose illness is terminal is often dealt with by evasion and a false and superficial cheerfulness which he is usually quick to detect. Family members who realize that death of a loved one is near frequently have little opportunity to discuss their feelings with nurses and physicians. Avoidance of the dying patient and his family is common, and serves to protect staff from confronting their own anxieties about death, and their own feelings when one of their patients has a terminal illness.

Although death can occur in any clinical setting, its most frequent occurrence is on medical-surgical units and, of course, in geriatric services. In years past most people died at home; death in the hospital was primarily the lot of persons who were destitute or without family to care for them.

In this chapter we shall consider the nurse's role in care of the dying patient, and some ways in which the nurse can help the patient and family during this significant experience. We shall consider the nurse's role primarily in relation to:

- herself
- the patient
- other patients on the ward
- the patient's family

Because it is less usual in our society for neighbors and friends to gather round when death occurs—providing lodging and food for visitors, and companionship and support for the family, many persons have their first experience with death in a highly charged emotional situation where the death is of a close relative. Patients and their families, as well as health workers, tend to come to this experience relatively unprepared by experience with death as they grow up in their own neighborhoods and communities.

A primary concern, then, is for the nurse to consider her own views about death, and to recognize that many of her patients and their families come to this experience quite unprepared to deal with it. The person whose only experience with death has been a visit to a funeral parlor, where someone has explained, "See, he is not dead; he is sleeping" is not well prepared for the reality of the change which occurs with the cessation of breathing and sudden stillness, as the patient crosses the threshold between life and death.

The development of one's philosophy and religious beliefs concerning death, and of one's ability to accept the reality of death is a lifelong task to be dealt with again and again as life makes new demands and presents new challenges. The individual who thought he understood his views on death may find that he has really hardly begun this process when confronted by the sudden death of his young wife. And, as he grows old and the time of his own death draws near, he is again challenged to deal with death. For the nurse, as for all people, considering death is a process of personal growth which can occur over a lifetime. Persons in the health professions are among those who have opportunity, by care of patients and their families at the time of death, to enhance their own personal growth in the process. The nurse's ability to help patients and their families at the time of death is based upon her own understanding and inner growth. It is through her own understanding, her own humility, and her own recognition and acceptance of death as part of life that the nurse ministers to dying patients and to their families. Emphasis is upon recognition of what this experience means to the patient and to those close to him, helping them to express their thoughts and feelings, and supporting them as they pass through the various stages of the experience, such as stages of denial, and anger—and (it is hoped)—finally, acceptance.

One consideration is especially important in work with dying patients. Often the nurse avoids talking with the patients in any but a very superficial way, out of uncertainty about how she will respond when the patient asks "The Question." Tension over this increases when the nurse (usually unrealistically) views herself as the only one to whom the patient can turn for help in dealing with his illness. Often the patient gradually recognizes clues in the behavior of others toward him that indicate that his illness is terminal. Thus the view of the patient as thoroughly unaware and seeking a disclosure from the nurse is often incorrect, and it greatly interferes with the nurse's relationship with the dying patient. When patients are given the opportunity, they often bring up awareness of their own approaching death by a remark about plans for providing for their children—leaving gifts for their families, and so on. Such comments, when they reflect the patient's realistic assessment of his situation,

should be accepted rather than refuted by such replies as, "You shouldn't talk like that." Sometimes no verbal reply is necessary, as the feeling of acceptance of what has been said is expressed nonverbally in the way that the nurse conveys caring.

Three important aspects of nursing care of dying patients are: (1) supporting the patient as he begins to consider his approaching death; (2) fostering communication with the patient so that he does not face this experience in increasing isolation from others; and (3) talking with family members and with others who care for the patient, such as the physician and clergyman, concerning observations about the patient and plans for his care.

The patient requires thoughtful attention to his physical comfort: to position change, sips of fluids, if he is able to tolerate them, a quiet restful environment. Primarily, he needs consideration as a human being, in all the varied ways that this can be demonstrated through thoughtful care. He requires particularly to be protected from routine, impersonal care typified by large numbers of health workers arriving to carry out, impersonally, the taking of his temperature, the provision of a water pitcher, or a check on the liter flow of oxygen being administered to him.

It is important to spend time with the dying patient which is over and beyond that required for physical care and treatments. The patient may bring up his concerns during his bath and treatments, too, of course. However, because of the tendency for dying patients to become isolated from others, it is particularly important to provide additional time, regularly, with them, when the primary objective is listening to them and suporting them as they come close to the time of their death.

It is important to be sensitive to the patient's spiritual concerns and to help him obtain the religious counseling and rites which he wishes. If the patient is too ill to express his wishes, the family should be consulted concerning spiritual care.

The patient can grow and mature as a person when he approaches death. The patient's philosophical and religious views may mature; he may develop a broader view of his life as part of the cosmos, and his death as a natural event in the ebb and flow of life. He may experience a tenderness and closeness toward family and friends which he has not felt before. On the other hand, the patient may become progressively disengaged from others as death approaches. If so, his family, particularly, will need help in understanding this change. Often the patient has a particular need for familiar and treasured possessions. It is especially important to keep the possessions the patient shows he values near him. Pictures of loved ones and articles which are gifts from people he cares for may be especially precious to the patient at this time.

Frequently the dying patient is placed apart from other patients. If there is no private room, he may be wheeled into a treatment room, or even into the hallway. Although such measures are often undertaken in the belief that the patient and his roommate will be more comfortable, this is not necessarily the result. It is preferable to talk with the other patients in the room about their reaction to having the dying patient with them, and also to talk with the dying patient himself, about moving him, if he is still aware of his surroundings and able to respond, rather than to move the patient suddenly and without explanation or discussion. Such sudden transfers of the dying patient can arouse anxiety both in the person who is moved and in the other patients. Sometimes after death has occurred, all doors to patients' rooms are closed, without any explanation, as the stretcher on which the deceased person is being wheeled to the morgue passes down the corridor. Patients' questions about what has occurred are often met evasively.

The important question for the nurse to consider is: "Do these approaches make the dying patient and other patients on the ward more comfortable and less anxious?" Responses are highly individual, and no one approach, therefore, is suitable in all situations. If a dying patient's roommate is disturbed because of the patient's condition, or because of the frequent presence of visitors, then it is best for him not to share a room with the dying patient. If, on the other hand, a close relationship has been developing between these two patients, both patients may prefer to continue to share a room. Considerable support and comfort may be offered to the dying person by his roommate who, in turn, may grow in the process of offering such support. Removing the dying person from view and evasively answering questions about his condition do not necessarily relieve anxiety when a dying patient is on the ward. In fact, these approaches may heighten anxiety. When patients are quite certain what has happened, and ask the whereabouts of the patient when they see his bed

is empty, it is preferable to say calmly that the patient has died, and to make oneself available to patients who want to discuss the fact that death occurred on the ward.

Families of dying patients particularly need the support that a nurse can give. Often their own process of grieving begins when they learn that the patient's illness is terminal. Some family members begin to withdraw emotionally from the patient at this time because they find the experience too painful. Others draw closer, realizing the shortness of the time left with the loved one. The family's feelings do not conform necessarily to others' idealized views of what these feelings should be. For instance, the family may feel anger that the patient is about to leave them. The more the family member can express his feeling to an understanding listener, the better, because it helps the family member to recognize the emotion, and to consider whether it is one which would be beneficial to share with his dying relative. He can thus avoid burdening the patient and he can free himself to relate as constructively as possible to the dying patient. However, the possible harm from direct expression of feelings between relatives and the dying person is often overestimated. Family members may be so cautioned against showing any but cheerful feelings that they assume an air of false cheerfulness when visiting the patient. The patient senses the "mask" and feels isolated from the persons to whom he turns for closeness. When the family member finally can no longer keep up the pretense, but shows grief, both the relative and the patient often experience relief at the honest communication between them. Of course this does not mean that it is helpful for family to burden the patient again and again with their grief, or with their refusal to let him go when death is near. However, one big problem among family members of dying patients in our culture seems to lie in the inability to communicate frankly with the dying person—to express feelings and accept his expression of feelings. The regret at tenderness unexpressed, and thereafter unable to be expressed, is among the most poignant problems of grieving relatives. The nurse who can accept direct, straightforward communication from families can help them be more direct with the patient, thereby assisting them to have this enriching experience.

Perhaps nowhere is the stereotyped expectation of what the family *should* do, and how they *should* react, so strong as it is toward relatives of dying patients. The family may have their opportunity to experience this significant event in their lives impaired by the expectations of others about how they should react. Notice how the patient's relatives respond, and what they seem to want and need.

One patient's husband may want to stay with his dying wife most of the day, sitting quietly with her. To argue with this man that he should "get more rest" may be useless and irritating both to him and the nurse. Instead, it would be more helpful to provide him with an easy chair, encourage him to visit the coffee shop for nourishment, and help him to feel comfortable and accepted as he does what he shows he wants to do: remain with his wife. On the other hand, for the husband who shows that short visits are best for him, or may be all that is possible for him in light of responsibilities to others and to his work, it is important to help the husband and wife to have these short visits free of other interruptions: make a special effort not to schedule treatments during the husband's visit and avoid conveying to him any attitude of "It's about time you came," or "Where have you been?" Some family members will openly express their grief—and it is helpful if they can do so to the nurse, in a private room or office, away from the patient. Others seem to need a "stiff upper lip" in order to cope with the experience. In either case it is important to respect the way the relative is dealing with the situation.

It is important for family to have some room near the ward where they can go and have privacy to talk with other relatives, to cry, and to rest. Facilities are extremely limited in this regard, and often family members are seen standing for long periods in the corridor (while one or two relatives remain with the patient). Use every effort to find a place where the family can have some privacy, and can be seated comfortably. Make frequent visits to them if they show they wish this contact. Just sitting with the family for a short time and expressing concern for their comfort and welfare, and listening to some of their concerns, can bring comfort. The family frequently worry about how much the patient is suffering. It is helpful to explain that, as life ebbs, so usually does awareness of pain and discomfort. Thus, as the patient's death draws near, he may seem "detached," very often he slips into unconsciousness. It is then that the family's suffering is likely to be acute, although the patient's suffering is lessened.

Helping the family to express their emotions and, as much as possible, to understand what is occurring can help them bear their grief after the patient's death, and to recover from it. The nurse has many opportunities gently to assist the family to deal with the reality of death. For instance, if the patient's wife keeps calling to her husband who has just died, and trying to rouse him, the nurse can gently lead her away to a private room and stay with her. Often, after some brief agitation and denial, the relative will burst into tears, with the support of the nurse and her comforting presence.

When death has occurred, it is usual for the relatives to leave the hospital at once. However, some may wish to remain for a time with the body of the deceased, and it is important to provide them a period of privacy before postmortem care is given. Particularly if only one relative is present at the time of death, it is important to offer to stay with the relative for a time, before he leaves the hospital. If the relative seems very distraught, it is wise to telephone another family member to come and be with him, or to call the hospital chaplain.

REFERENCES AND BIBLIOGRAPHY

ASSELL, R.: An existential approach to death, *Nurs. Forum* 8:102, 1969.

BLEWETT, L. J.: To die at home, *Am. J. Nurs.* 70:2602, December, 1970.

BRAUER, P.: Should the patient be told the truth? *in* SKIPPER, J., and LEONARD, R. (eds.): *Social Interaction and Patient Care*, Philadelphia, Lippincott, 1965.

EISMAN, R.: Why did Joe die? *Am. J. Nurs.* 71:501, March, 1971.

ENGEL, G. L.: Grief and grieving, *Am. J. Nurs.* 64:93, September, 1964.

FEIFEL, H.: *The Meaning of Death*, New York, McGraw-Hill, 1959.

GLASER, B. G., and STRAUSS, A. L.: *Awareness of Dying*, Chicago, Aldine Press, 1965.

————: The social loss of dying patients, *Am. J. Nurs.* 64:119, June, 1964.

HINTON, J. M.: *Dying*, Baltimore, Penguin, 1967.

HOFFMAN, E.: Don't give up on me! *Am. J. Nurs.* 71:60, January, 1971.

KASTENBAUM, R., and AISENBERG, R.: *The Psychology of Death*, New York, Springer, in press.

PEARSON, L. (ed.): *Death and Dying*, Cleveland, The Press of Case Western Reserve University, 1969.

QUINT, J. C.: *The Nurse and the Dying Patient*, New York, Macmillan, 1967.

QUINT, J. C., STRAUSS, A. L., and GLASER, B. G.: Improving nursing care of the dying, *Nurs. Forum* 6:369, 1967.

ROSS, E. K.: *On Death and Dying*, New York, Macmillan, 1969.

————: What is it like to be dying? *Am. J. Nurs.* 71:54, January, 1971.

Nursing in Emergencies

11

Safety in the Hospital • General Principles of First Aid
First Aid in Various Emergencies • Emergency Nursing in
the Hospital

SAFETY IN THE HOSPITAL

Many factors contribute to making hospitals less safe than most industrial plants. There are weak and disabled people, oxygen, an unusual concentration of pathogenic organisms, radiation, and waxed floors with people hurrying over them. When the staff is aware of these dangers, accident rates fall. More accidents are caused by unsafe acts than by unsafe conditions (Kesner).

The following is a safety checklist for nurses. How many of these items were you aware of during your last week in the hospital?

Safety Checklist for Nurses

1. Did you wash your hands before going on and off duty?
2. Did you wash your hands between patients?
3. Do you know where the emergency tray is? Is it complete?
4. Is the suction machine ready for immediate use?
5. Is emergency oxygen ready for immediate use?
6. Did you attach your patient's call bell within easy reach?
7. If your patient was ambulatory, did he know about the call bell in the bathroom?
8. If your patient took a tub bath or shower, was there a nonskid mat in the tub or on the floor of the shower stall to prevent slipping? Are there grab rails?
9. Did you read all medication labels carefully?
10. Was the overbed table clear before you put a tray with hot soup, tea or coffee on it?
11. Were any wet spots on the floor not immediately wiped up?
12. Did any objects fall on the floor that were not immediately picked up?
13. Did you use good body mechanics when lifting patients?
14. Were side rails secured when it was necessary?
15. Do you know where the fire extinguishers are?
16. Do you know how to operate them?

The following points of safety are equally important:

• In one study 29 per cent of all accidents to nurses comprised lacerations, bruises and burns (Carner) A dustpan and broom should be used to remove glass slivers from the floor. Protect your hands with gauze when breaking ampules. Wrap broken glass in paper toweling before discarding it, to prevent cutting anyone who may handle the trash.

• For precautions against radiation injury, see Chapter 14.

• Use a footstool when you are helping a patient out of bed if the bed cannot be lowered. If the patient is elderly or tends to become disoriented, especially at night, put side rails on, for he may try to get up alone, forgetting how high the bed is. When you are working evenings and nights, check all your patients frequently. An elderly patient may be sleeping soundly one moment, and the next he may be climbing over the side rails in the dark to get to the bathroom. Leave a Hi-lo bed in low position when the patient is allowed up or has a tendency to get up. Be sure the night lights are on. When the patient is in bed, be sure that the casters on the bed and the bedside stand are locked, so that the bed and the stand do not separate if the patient reaches for something. When you are moving a patient to or from a stretcher, hold it securely against the bed, so that the patient does not slide down between it and the bed.

• Protect patients from falls. Porters should wash and wax one side of a hallway or ward at a time, always leaving a dry path. Nonskid wax should be used. Handrails in the halls are helpful. Patients in wheelchairs should be taught to use the brake. Stairs should be well lit and have nonskid abrasive strips. Watch out for long electrical cords.

• Use "Busy" signs instead of locks on hospital bathrooms. A patient in trouble (faint, in pain, etc.) in the bathroom should not be locked inside. Call bells should be in easy reach.

• Stretchers are narrower than beds, and the patients on them may not be well oriented. They should be strapped on, and they should be covered by a blanket to prevent chilling from the drafts of the hallways. Arms and legs should be under the blanket, so that they do not get caught in the elevator door or squashed between the stretcher and the bed.

• Use equipment correctly. If you are not familiar with some piece of equipment, read the manufacturer's instruction booklet. Ask your instructor, the head nurse or the doctor for a demonstration. Trying to muddle through with an unfamiliar piece of equipment can be dangerous. For instance, if the nurse does not know how to use a Hoyer lift correctly, the patient may fall. If the nurse does not know what not to touch on the Bird respirator, the pressure applied to the lungs may be too great.

• Take the temperature of the water before filling hot-water bottles. Test for leaks, and be sure that the cap is on tight. Warn patients not to touch heating lamps or the nozzle of an inhalator.

• Do not put metal beds against metal radiators, because if the light socket is defective and the patient touches the light switch, he may receive a fatal electrical shock. Immediately report all defective electrical equipment. All electrical equipment should be checked regularly and be properly grounded, preferably through the use of a 3-prong plug. The "cheater" adaptor, a device used to make a 3-prong plug fit into a 2-blade socket, is of no use as an effective ground unless the little pigtail ground wire is connected to the outlet face plate.

Fire

What would you do if a fire broke out on the floor on which you are working? Time is vital; the right things done in the first few minutes are worth more than hours of work later. Which would you do first: close the windows, call the telephone operator, get the fire extinguisher, or remove the closest patient? Here is a suggested order of action:

1. Remove the patients nearest to the fire.
2. Call the operator, report the location of the fire. (If there is a firebox, set the alarm.)
3. Have someone else close the doors and the windows, and turn off the gas, the electrical, the oxygen and the ventilating equipment.
4. Remove the helpless patients from the area.
5. Try to put out the fire, using the fire extinguishers, or wet blankets or linen.
6. Remove wheelchair patients from the area.
7. Remove ambulatory patients from the area.
8. Remove staff from the area.

Of course, if the fire is still a small one, such as a sheet just starting to smolder, douse it with water and put the fire out before doing anything else. If an oxygen tent is burning, turn off the oxygen and lift the canopy up before doing anything else. (Oxygen, you will remember, does not itself burn, but it supports combustion.) A special fire extinguisher is necessary for electrical fires.

Detection, containment (of smoke, heat and flame) and extinguishment are the main principles of fire control. Closing doors and windows helps to contain smoke as well as flames—an important point because of the damaging effects of inhaled smoke. Most deaths in fires come from smoke inhalation.

Smoking in the hospital must be limited to those areas where it is permitted. This applies to everyone—patients, staff and visitors. An aide who smokes in the linen room is inviting disaster. So is the visitor smoking in a hallway through which oxygen tanks are passing. Patients who smoke in bed are a major cause of fires in hospitals. If the patient is allowed to smoke, be sure that he has an adequate ash tray. Furtive smoking is hazardous; the patient quickly crushes a lit cigarette in a wastepaper basket or a bedside paper bag full of tissues. Be sure that patients are attended if they smoke after they have had

Demerol, morphine or other sedation. Do not be punitive about this—have someone stay with the patient if he wants a cigarette.

Decorations, such as those for Christmas, may be a fire hazard. They should be without electrical attachment, and they should be fireproof. Trash that collects also may be a fire hazard, and it should be removed. Be careful in the use of all appliances that give off heat, such as hot-water bottles, steam inhalators, and heat lamps. Know the location and the operation of the fire extinguisher on each floor on which you work, and the type of fire each extinguisher is designed to put out. Oxygen tanks should not be covered, because the drape might conceal a leak. Because ether is highly inflammable, never use it near flame; for example, do not clean the adhesive marks off a patient's skin while he is smoking. A patient who has been anesthetized with ether exhales combustible fumes for a considerable time postoperatively. Do not light a match near him.

The operating room has its own special hazards. Many anesthetics are combustible: for example, cyclopropane, ether and ethyl chloride. Never put a tank of explosive gas by the radiator. To avoid igniting the combustible gases, clothing made of silk, rayon, wool, nylon and plastic never is worn in the operating room, because a spark from the static electricity that these materials generate could ignite one of the gases. All operating rooms have protective rules. Be sure that you are familiar with the ones for your hospital before entering.

Reports

Reporting accidents in writing is standard procedure in hospitals. The purpose of this is not to fix the blame on individuals but to identify the causes and to prevent repetition of the accidents. Some hospitals establish safety committees to study the reports and to provide safer working conditions.

GENERAL PRINCIPLES OF FIRST AID

First aid is not the amateur practice of medicine; it consists of measures that keep the patient alive and prevent further damage until definitive medical treatment can be initiated.

The right kind of first aid depends on the situation; and your judgment in an emergency should be adjusted to the particular circumstances.

Some important general principles of first aid, which you will adapt to particular situations, are the following:

- If there is a sucking wound of the chest, cover it and keep it sealed at once, even if sterile materials are not available. Seconds can make the difference between life and death.
- Stop the injured person's bleeding.
- Establish an airway and adequate respiration.
- Give first aid for shock.
- Get medical help as rapidly as possible.
- Whenever it is possible, get a doctor to the patient, or the patient to a doctor, as rapidly as is consistent with safety. Many police departments have emergency squads. If you cannot immediately contact a doctor, call the police and describe the nature of the problem.
- Do not move the patient unless he is further endangered by staying put (for instance, if he is on a cliff, in danger of falling, or if he is on a railroad track that may be used). A minor injury can become a major one when the patient is moved incorrectly. The rule is to keep the patient lying flat until he is seen by a doctor, or until a plan to move him has been evolved on the basis of the nature and the extent of his injuries. If the patient *must* be moved immediately, handle him as little and as gently as possible, and keep his body as straight as possible. Do not jackknife him. Handle any injured parts as little as possible. Get enough help—for the patient's sake and your own. Sometimes, in the excitement of the moment, people forget others are around, and they try single-handedly to move a heavy person.
- Search for injuries systematically. Carry out this search after stopping the patient's bleeding and establishing respiration, but before you do anything else. Start at the head and work down to the toes. A wound may be tiny, hidden by clothing and very dangerous. There might be a small puncture wound in the chest that penetrates to the pleura. An abdominal wound or hidden bleeding also could be present.
- Prevent chilling. Almost all emergency conditions entail some degree of shock, and so chilling should be avoided. Do not make the patient too warm. Excessive heat can increase shock.
- Consider each injury as maximum. If you see blood, think of hemorrhage. If you suspect a sprain, splint it as you would a fracture. If the patient feels faint, treat him as if he were in

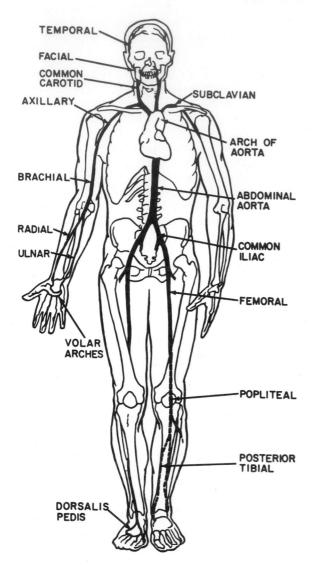

TEMPORAL
FACIAL
COMMON
CAROTID
AXILLARY
SUBCLAVIAN
ARCH OF
AORTA
BRACHIAL
ABDOMINAL
AORTA
RADIAL
ULNAR
COMMON
ILIAC
FEMORAL
VOLAR
ARCHES
POPLITEAL
POSTERIOR
TIBIAL
DORSALIS
PEDIS

Fig. 11-1. Arteries that may be palpated (except the aorta and the common iliac) and compressed. The dotted line on the left leg indicates that the arteries travel along the back of the leg.

shock. Nothing is lost by caution, and an injury actually may be more serious than it looks.

• Think of the underlying anatomy and physiology. For example, if the patient has a hole in his chest that sucks in air with every breath, it is a sign that the wound extends to his pleural cavity. When his rib cage expands, he is pulling air into the pleural space through the wound. The immediate first aid measure is to close that wound to prevent further collapse of the lung. Use a pressure dressing or, if one is not available, the palm of your hand.

• Do not give the patient anything to drink or to eat until the full extent of his injuries has been diagnosed by a physician. Never give an unconscious person anything to drink, and never give an injured person alcohol. Among the disadvantages of giving alcohol to the injured is that alcohol acts as a vasodilator, so that heat loss from the body is increased, thus increasing shock; and vasodilation increases bleeding.

• Stay with the patient until a doctor arrives, unless there are a large number of casualties, and you must leave one to attend another.

• Prevent further injury by transporting the patient flat and carefully, and by taking command, so that untrained persons do not harm the patient. Do not add to the problems by, for example, using material to cover wounds that may stick to them.

• Report accurately. If you can stay with the patient until the doctor sees him, tell the doctor, concisely and accurately, what happened, what injuries you suspect, and what first aid was given. Otherwise, write the report and attach it to the patient.

• Communicate calmness. Every emergency is psychologically traumatic. The very suddenness of becoming a casualty is shocking. Give the patient a sense of security by your manner. Even if you do not feel calm, demonstrate calmness. Fear and confusion in others can be minimized by your manner of competence. Do not tell the patient or bystander what you think the diagnosis is. Convey to them that you have the situation under control.

• Apply to psychological emergencies the same principles as you would for any emergency nursing: prevent further injury and seek medical care. Anyone who has attempted suicide requires medical attention. Anyone who is acutely confused, disoriented or disturbed needs help. Stay with the patient. If he has erroneous impressions of reality, do not argue about them. If possible, do not touch the patient, but talk to him and allow him to talk to you.

FIRST AID IN VARIOUS EMERGENCIES

Hemorrhage

Look for bleeding, and stop it quickly. Most people can tolerate the loss of a pint of blood, but losing a quart or more leads to shock. A patient can hemorrhage to death in less than one minute from a large artery that is severed, but most bleeding can be stopped by pressure and elevation. To control bleeding:

• Apply direct continuous pressure on the wound, which usually will stop the hemorrhage. If you do not have a sterile bandage to place over the wound, use a clean handkerchief or a piece of cloth. Lacking these, use your bare hand.

• Apply pressure on a major artery leading to the wound. Press the artery against the bone.

• Elevate the part.

• The American Medical Association advises that a tourniquet should be applied *only* for an amputated, mangled or crushed extremity. Tighten it only enough to stop the bleeding. Be sure to write a note stating that a tourniquet has been applied. The tourniquet should be loosened every 20 minutes to allow blood to flow to the part. Since a tourniquet may mean the loss of the part distal to it because of reflex arterial spasm, apply one *only* when all other measures have failed to stop the hemorrhage, and only when the arm or leg already is missing, crushed or mangled.

Cessation of Respiration

This condition may be due to drowning, electric shock, carbon monoxide or other gaseous poisoning, or to disease. Treatment must be begun at once.

• Mouth-to-mouth breathing is the most effective method of resuscitation (see figure on p. 654). Properly performed, it can maintain in good physiologic condition a patient who is not breathing for himself. Speed in initiating the procedure is important.

• Clear the airway. An obstruction in the mouth, the trachea or the bronchi will prevent ventilation of the lungs. Wipe the inside of the patient's mouth with a handkerchief. If it is necessary, turn him on his side and sharply slap his back. This procedure may dislodge an obstruction in a bronchus.

• Make sure the tongue does not obstruct the airway.

• Hold the patient's nose, so that the air you blow into his mouth does not escape.

• Take a breath, and blow into the patient's mouth until you see the chest rise. Listen for the rush of expired air while you take your next breath. Watch for relaxation of the chest wall.

• Reinflate the patient's lungs as soon as his

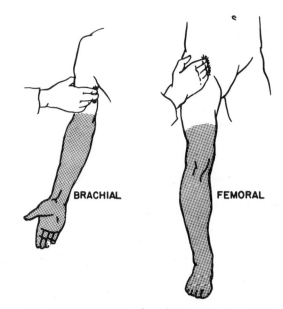

Fig. 11-2. ·Methods of occluding the brachial and femoral arteries to control bleeding from injuries in the shaded areas. Pressure is applied to artery and bone behind it.

expiration is complete. Repeat about 12 times a minute.

If some air is being blown into the stomach, you can expel it by gentle pressure just below the diaphragm. Be careful not to take such large breaths that you become dizzy, because artificial respiration may be necessary for hours. Make your breaths just deep enough to inflate the patient's lungs. There will be enough oxygen in such breaths for both of you. Continue until the patient breathes for himself or is declared dead by a physician. When the patient does start to breathe for himself, watch him continuously for at least an hour.

Many people recoil from this close physical contact, and more so if the patient is old or looks dirty. If you wish to place a thin cloth between your mouth and the patient's, do so. It will not impede ventilation. If a double-ended plastic airway (Resuscitube) is available, it can increase the efficiency of artificial respiration considerably.

Shock

Keep the patient lying flat with his feet 8 to 12 inches higher than his head (unless there is dyspnea in this position). If there is a head injury, keep the patient flat. Do not allow him to exert himself at all. He should be as still and as quiet as possible. Keep him warm, and yet not hot. Excessive heat induces vasodilation, which can increase shock. Do not use hot-water bottles, and do not induce sweating, because valuable electrolytes and water are lost in perspiration. Do not give anything by mouth to an unconscious patient, or to one with a head injury or an abdominal wound, or to any patient who will receive medical attention within 2 hours. If a long interval is anticipated, and the patient is not vomiting, start him on sips of water. If sips of water are tolerated, give an electrolyte solution made up of 1 teaspoon table salt and ½ teaspoon bicarbonate of soda (baking soda) to a quart of water.

Electric Shock

When a person is in contact with a live conductor of electricity, be careful that you do not become a part of the circuit yourself while you are attempting to rescue him. Avoid standing on a wet surface during the rescue. Use a dry, nonconducting object—for instance, loose clothing or a piece of wood—to push or to pull the person away from the conductor. Do not touch his skin directly; otherwise, you yourself may have to be rescued.

A severe electric shock results in cardiac arrest

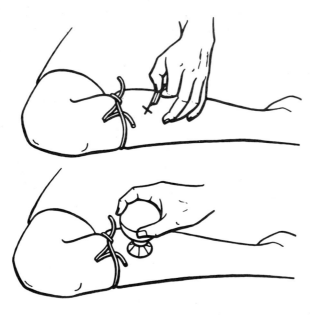

Fig. 11-3. First aid for a poisonous snakebite. A tourniquet is applied proximal to the wound, a crisscross cut is made into it, and suctioning is instituted. A suction cup such as this one is included in snakebite kits.

from ventricular fibrillation. The only definitive treatment for this is electric defibrillation. If a defibrillator is not immediately available, the patient must be given mouth-to-mouth respiration and closed chest cardiac compression while being transported to the nearest treatment facility.

Wounds

Unless you have a sterile bandage, most wounds should be uncovered and left exposed to the air until they are treated surgically. Cut clothing away so that threads do not fall into the wound, but expose the patient as little as possible. Do not allow anyone to wash the wound or to put any antiseptic, or anything else, into it. If the patient has to be transported, and you have a sterile bandage available, dress the wound until it can be seen by a physician. Evisceration of intestine through an abdominal wound should not be pushed back inside the abdominal cavity. Cover the wound with a wet gauze or handkerchief (sterile, if it is available, or as clean as possible).

If there are several casualties, the patient with a penetrating abdominal wound receives first priority in removal to a hospital. When the doctor arrives at the scene, direct his attention to this patient first. If the patient with an open wound will not be seen by a doctor for many hours, you may flush the wound with sterile water and cover it with a dry sterile dressing.

Snakebite

If a patient has two small puncture wounds close together, assume that the snake is poisonous. If you are in doubt, give first aid as if it were poisonous, and try to identify the snake (or at least be able to describe it). Note the snake's size, color, design, and the shape of its head.

Even an apparently dead snake can bite, and most have enough poison to harm a second victim, so be careful in handling or examining the snake.

Persons bitten by snakes native to the United States usually recover, but the bite may be fatal, depending on the size and the type of snake and on the amount of venom that has been injected into the patient. Ten to 35 per cent of snakebites are fatal. In all likelihood the person who is bitten will be extremely apprehensive.

First aid is directed toward removing as much of the venom as possible and preventing the spread of the venom throughout the patient's body. Apply a tourniquet above the wound. This tourniquet should be tight enough to occlude venous and lymphatic circulation, *but it should not be so tight that there is no pulse.* Speed is important; the quicker the tourniquet is applied, the less venom will be circulated throughout the patient's body. Every 10 or 15 minutes move the tourniquet up just above the progressively swelling area. With a razor blade or other clean, sharp instrument, make a crisscross incision into the wound. The incision should go through the skin but not the underlying muscle. Suction the wound by syringe or suction cup, if it is available; otherwise, by mouth. Venom is not toxic when it is ingested (but spit out what you suction by mouth), and therefore this technic is not dangerous unless you have a cut on your lips or mouth. Continue suctioning until nothing more can be extracted from the wound. Transport the patient to a doctor.

Contrary to popular opinion, whisky is not "snakebite medicine." Antivenom is the only specific medication. Because it is made from horse serum, many people are allergic to it. The doctor also will give antitetanus injections.

Snakebite kits include a tourniquet, suction cup, razor blade, antivenom powder, iodine, a vial of sterile water, and instructions. Take one along when you go camping in snake country. Also, wear high boots when you walk in areas inhabited by snakes.

Animal Bites

Bites from any warm-blooded animal must be regarded as potential rabies threats and must be reported at once to a local health officer who will specify the treatment to be used. As a first-aid measure, thorough washing with either tincture of green soap or benzalkonium chloride solution (1:100 or 1:1,000) *but not both* is helpful. There should be a predetermined policy at each emergency room for handling animal bites.

Poisoning

Food poisoning can be caused when food is contaminated with such organisms as *Staphylococcus aureus, Clostridium botulinum,* and *Clostridium perfringens.* The toxins produced by the organisms cause the illness. In infection transmitted by food, the food serves as a vehicle that transfers pathogenic organisms (such as *Salmonella*) from a contaminated source to the victim.

Food poisoning may be of nonmicrobial origin, for example in cases of contamination by insecticides. Naturally toxic plants, such as certain strains of mushrooms, some berries, and some wild plants, may be ingested through accident or ignorance.

Clostridium botulinum produces a neurotoxin that may cause nausea and vomiting, headache, lassitude, double vision, muscular incoordination and inability to talk, swallow or breathe. This organism, an anaerobe, is found most often in foods that have been improperly canned at home.

Botulinus toxin is destroyed by heat just below the boiling point; therefore, food which has been boiled in the previous few hours is considered safe. However, the *spores* of botulinus are not killed by boiling, even for hours. Therefore, food which is boiled and then kept in closed containers for several days can be lethal. Botulism can also be acquired from improperly cured sausage and fish. Ordinarily, this bacterium doesn't grow in a highly acid medium, so most fruit preserves are quite safe. Any can which is swollen or seems to contain gas should be discarded unopened. Foods suspected of being contaminated should not be tasted. There have been some deaths from a single taste. Smoking, salting, marinating and drying food do not necessarily kill the spores of *Cl. botulinum.*

Botulism is treated with antitoxin, a positive-pressure respirator and intravenous therapy. Early treatment is important; the mortality rate is about 65 per cent. Death often is due to respiratory failure.

Staphylococci grow in food, especially creamed food that has not been sufficiently refrigerated. Symptoms may include weakness, diarrhea, nausea, vomiting and abdominal cramps that develop a few hours after ingesting the contaminated food and last for a day or two. Death is rare. Food poisoning may not be recognized until the food is absorbed, and the patient has symptoms, usually diarrhea and vomiting. Keep the patient quiet, and obtain medical help as quickly as possible. Parenteral fluids and sedation may be given. To prevent food poisoning, nurses should teach the importance of cleanliness in food preparation, and of prompt and adequate cooking and refrigeration. For example, in preparation for a picnic, the arrangements must include refrigeration. Sometimes food such as potato salad is prepared in large quantity and left out of the refrigerator for hours before it is consumed because of lack of room on the shelves. This is a dangerous practice.

Drug poisoning in adults results sometimes from suicide attempts and sometimes from the theory that if one pill is good, several must be better. Drug poisoning may or may not be recognized promptly. First try to discover what the patient ingested. Look for the container or, if the patient is conscious, ask him. Read the label, and follow its antidotal instructions, if any. Look for burns on the mouth that suggest a corrosive acid or alkali. If the container is not found immediately, try to dilute the poison by giving the patient (if he is conscious) as much milk or water as you can. Rapid action is important.

Induce vomiting unless the poison is ammonia, or a strong acid or alkali (which burn tissue on contact), or any petroleum product, such as gasoline, lighter fluid or kerosene. Vomiting is not induced in these instances because of the danger of aspiration. Vomiting should not be induced if the patient is already comatose or convulsing. If the patient complains of severe pain or a burning sensation in his mouth and throat, do not induce vomiting.

Smell the breath for fumes. If you see no burns and smell no fumes, induce vomiting by putting your finger down the patient's throat or by making him drink copious amounts of water to which you have added several tablespoonfuls of bicarbonate of soda. Turn the patient's head to one side while he is vomiting; take every precaution to avoid aspiration. After he has vomited, give more antidote (if it is known), or (if it is not known) 4 egg whites in a glass of milk, or 2 teaspoonfuls of flour or any other starch in a glass of water or milk. Do not give alcohol.

Call the doctor or arrange for the patient's transport to a hospital. If the container is found, it should be saved. If not, save a specimen of the patient's vomitus. If the patient urinates, try to obtain a specimen for the doctor. The observation of vital signs and the prevention of chilling are important first aid measures.

If the poison has been absorbed, the first aid is suggested by the symptoms. For instance, if the patient is not breathing, administer artificial respiration. If he is convulsing, prevent the aspiration of saliva and keep him warm and free from further harm. If he has taken an overdose of barbiturates, try to keep him aroused; however, avoid any exertion that may tire him unnecessarily. You may give him black coffee while he is conscious. He should be transported to the hospital as rapidly as possible. Estimate the amount of urine, if any. The patient who develops kidney shutdown may be placed on dialysis (Chap. 56). If the drug poisoning is due to a suicide attempt, it is not usually helpful to discuss this with the patient, nor to try to reassure him by saying, "Everything will be all right." Let him know that you are interested in caring for him, and that you are taking adequate steps for his safety. After the patient is in the hospital, he needs to be attended constantly, for he may attempt suicide again.

Poisoning by Gas. When gas poisoning is suspected, remove the patient from the area of the fumes. If he is overcome at home, immediately throw open the window and remove the patient from the room. If he is not breathing, start mouth-to-mouth resuscitation. There is no other first aid measure that you can take. The patient should be hospitalized as rapidly as possible. The ambulance or an emergency squad may have resuscitating and oxygen equipment.

Exposure to Temperature Extremes

Heatstroke (Sunstroke). In this disorder, the body's normal responses to increasing temperature are not functioning. The patient feels dizzy, weak and nauseated, and he may have a headache, but there is no perspiration. The skin is red, hot and dry to the touch. There may be convulsions or collapse. Without treatment the patient probably will die.

The immediate first aid measure is to cool the patient. Remove him from the sun, and sponge him. If he is conscious, he may have cool drinks. If ice is available, it can be put in packs and placed on forehead, axillae and around the body and the legs. Cold water can be poured on the patient, or he can be fanned or put into a cool tub. Take his temperature frequently, and continue cooling him until his fever is down to about 101°F. Sustained high fever will result in brain damage. These patients need hospitalization even if they respond to first aid measures. The patient may have a lifelong problem with heat regulation after an episode of heatstroke, possibly necessitating a move to a cooler climate or the regulation of his life so that he is not exposed to heat for long periods of time.

Heat Exhaustion. This disorder is characterized by circulatory disturbances brought about by an excessive loss of salt and water by prolonged sweating. The patient feels dizzy and faint, and he may have headache, muscle cramps and nausea. In contrast with heatstroke, the skin is pale and damp. Uncorrected, the condition leads to collapse, but it usually is possible to rouse the patient.

Heat exhaustion is treated as if it were shock, except that it is necessary to cool the patient. Give water with a teaspoon of table salt in each glass. To relieve muscle cramps, apply firm pressure against the muscle with the flat of your hand. Heat exhaustion often can be prevented by taking adequate salt and water during a time of excessive exposure to heat and by observing such commonsense precautions as avoiding strenuous exertion and wearing suitable clothing.

At times, patients may have a combination of heatstroke and heat exhaustion, and the physical signs may not be as distinct as descriptions suggest.

Overexposure to Cold. Warm the patient as quickly as possible. Gradual warming is not necessary.

Frostbite. Severe cold causes injury to tissues; frostbite is a degree of cold injury. There is extreme vasoconstriction, thrombosis, as well as direct injury to the walls of the blood vessels and the cells. Exudate escapes from the damaged vessel walls, resulting in edema. There is ischemia of the tissues, and the skin blanches. The frostbitten part becomes numb and stiff. As it warms, it turns a bright pink and blisters.

Experience in World War II and the Korean War showed that the previously common practice of slowly warming a frostbitten part causes more tissue damage than rapid warming.* Bathe the affected part in comfortably warm water for 10 minutes. Be sure the temperature of the water is comfortable for the patient. Let him test it; water that may feel warm to normal skin may feel hot to frostbitten skin. After bathing, blot the skin dry, and apply a dry sterile dressing, using sterile gauze to separate skin surfaces. Elevate the part. Do not rub the part with snow or anything else, and do not apply cold water or allow cold air to touch it. Hot-water bottles and heat lamps should not be used. If legs or feet are involved, the patient should not walk. Frostbitten fingers or hands can be wrapped in warm covering, such as wool, or placed in the patient's axillae while he is being transported.

When the patient arrives at a treatment center,

---

* *Bureau of Medicine and Surgery Syllabus of Lesson Plans for Teaching First Aid,* NAVMED P-5056, Under the Authority of the Secretary of the Navy, Washington, D.C., 1957.

therapy includes rest with the part elevated. Débridement and grafting may be necessary. Because deep circulation is less affected than is superficial circulation, this surgical treatment usually is effective.

The degree of injury varies in severity. In mild cases, recovery is complete. In severe cases, amputation may be necessary. Patients who have been severely frostbitten may, for years afterward, experience numbness and tingling when the affected part is exposed to cold. Patients are advised to protect the affected part in the future from injury or exposure to cold.

Prevention of frostbite includes:

- Avoiding skin contact with the CO_2 in fire extinguishers
- Avoiding constricting clothing, such as shoes and socks that are too tight, or the use of circular garters in cold weather—these further impair blood supply to the part
- Keeping the entire body as warm and dry as possible when in extreme cold
- Teaching persons likely to be affected, such as soldiers, to exercise legs, feet, arms and fingers if they are in a situation likely to cause frostbite
- Teaching persons vulnerable to frostbite to observe each other's skin for the development of yellow-white patches (on the ear lobe for example) and to heed such sensations as pricking or pain, which may herald frostbite

First Aid in Minor Emergencies

Fainting. A momentary deficiency in cerebral oxygenation causes fainting. It can be distinguished from other forms of unconsciousness by its temporary nature. Usually, the patient regains consciousness as soon as he has attained a horizontal position.

If a person feels faint, he should lie down flat, without a pillow. Loosen tight clothing around the neck and the waist. Prevent falling when possible, since the injury sustained by the fall may be far more serious than the faint. If the patient cannot lie down, he should sit down and put his head between his knees. He should be seen by a doctor to determine the cause of the fainting.

Sunburn. A first-degree burn may be soothed by cool compresses. Handle the person gently to avoid further trauma to his skin. Blisters should be dressed with sterile gauze. They should not be punctured. If the burn is extensive, seek medical aid.

Bites and Stings. *Ticks.* Kill the tick with a few drops of turpentine, or touch it with a hot needle to make it release its hold. Then, using tweezers, remove it very gently from the skin. Do not crush the tick since this could transmit to the patient virulent pathogenic microorganisms which some ticks carry. Do not use excessive force in trying to remove a tick. Scrub the area with soap and water.

Bees, Wasps, Hornets. Remove the stinger with a sterile needle or tweezers (only honey bees shed their stinger). Apply an icebag and baking soda (one tablespoon per quart of water) to reduce the swelling and the itching. If the person is allergic to the sting of that insect, the sting may be fatal. Any symptoms of allergy after a sting demand immediate medical attention.

Poisonous Spiders, Tarantulas and Scorpions. Death of a healthy adult from spider bite or scorpion sting is rare, but the symptoms can be extremely painful. Deaths have occurred in children and in adults in a weakened condition. The best known toxic spider is the black widow which secretes a neurotoxin. This spider is a shiny black color with a red to orange hourglass on its ventral surface. A less well-known spider is at least as dangerous. The brown recluse spider originally was reported in Missouri but seems to have spread throughout the continental United States. It is somewhat smaller than the black widow, and ranges from light tan to dark brown in color. It has a banjo-shaped spot on its *dorsal* surface. The brown recluse is a shy animal and is usually hidden from view. It bites when it feels trapped. Unfortunately, it sometimes lives in old clothing or shoes kept in a garage or basement. When a person tries to put these garments on, the spider, presumably in self-defense, bites. The initial bite is seldom painful and often is unnoticed. The toxin, however, contains an extremely potent digestive enzyme, and after a few hours, it destroys a large amount of tissue, leaving an open wound which may not heal for many months. Secondary infections can ensue. For this reason, a report of a spider bite must be taken seriously, even if there is no pain, and no initial evidence of toxicity. If possible, the spider should be identified. If this cannot be done, any person bitten by a spider of unknown species should be referred to a physician for immediate observation and definitive management. A spider bite should not be incised by a first-aid worker (as is done with snakebites). The incision is likely to do little good, if any, and may cause a serious infection. For temporary relief, cold applications to the bitten area are helpful, but freezing of tissues must be avoided. There are specific medical treatments for black widow spider bites, including the intravenous injection of calcium gluconate and the use of an antivenom. Thus far, there is no antivenom available for brown recluse spider venom, but one may be developed. The part should be kept lower than the rest of the body for several hours.

The tarantula, a giant spider of fearsome appearance, has venom of such low toxicity that it poses no danger to human beings. Unfortunately, the appearance of the spider, and its use in several movies and television programs as a symbol of great danger may produce undesirable psychologic effects in someone who has been bitten. The victim, who may have seen even the valorous James Bond cringe before a tarantula, is not likely to accept the nurse's reassurance that he is in no danger. Accordingly, in such situations, the use of some harmless procedure to relieve the patient's concern or terror is advisable. A paste made of bicarbonate of soda and water placed over the bite can be reassuring. The patient is in much greater danger from his own fear than he is from the bite. The nurse, aware of this, should show concern and attention to the bite and its treatment but avoid communicating her own fear, which she may have, to the patient.

Scorpion stings are often painful, but the scorpions found in the United States can rarely produce lasting harm to an adult. Cold applications are helpful until the patient is seen by a physician.

Hiccups (Singultus). Hiccups are caused by recurrent spasms of the diaphragm. They can usually be cured by breathing into a paper bag, accumulating carbon dioxide (but *not* a plastic bag). Sometimes, drinking water while holding the nostrils closed will stop the attack. If hiccups persist more than 30 minutes after these maneuvers have been tried, a doctor should see the patient.

EMERGENCY NURSING IN THE HOSPITAL

Some large hospitals have emergency wards in which patients stay during the first hours or days of an acute disorder. For example, an emergency ward in a large hospital might have the following patients in one evening:

A woman in cardiac failure
A woman recovering from diabetic coma

A woman being prepared for the operating room for treatment of multiple injuries sustained in an automobile accident

A man from the same accident, in coma from head injuries

A man with severe burns

A fireman with smoke poisoning

A man in coma due to an overdose of barbiturates

When the emergency is over, the patients are transferred to regular hospital wards, where their treatment is continued. Hospitals without emergency wards use the regular wards or the intensive care unit to treat the patients having acute difficulty.

Of course, any illness can become severe enough to require emergency care, and all nurses should be prepared at all times to give it.

For example, a man recovering from a herniorrhaphy may have a myocardial infarction; a woman who seemed to be doing very well on a Sippy diet may suddenly hemorrhage from her peptic ulcer; a patient who seemed to be moody when he was admitted may try to jump out the window.

Below are some principles of emergency nursing in the hospital. They apply to any nursing situation—on the ward, in the clinic, in the emergency ward itself.

• Recognize an emergency. Know enough about each patient under your care to recognize when his illness becomes serious. Know the diagnosis of each patient for whom you are responsible, and learn what the danger signs are. For example, if you have a diabetic patient, you must know not only what the general symptoms of insulin shock are, but what symptoms usually precede insulin shock in this particular patient. Does he become irritable? Drowsy? Dizzy? An important part of good emergency nursing involves recognizing impending disaster and knowing when to call the doctor.

• Apply first aid. The nurse may be the first person to see a patient in an emergency. Whether the patient is hospitalized or comes into the nurse's care from the street, the principles of first aid apply. Do first things first. Have the patient lie down; establish his respirations; stop his bleeding; call the doctor.

• Adjust your pace to the rapidly changing situation. The nurse must move fast to aid respiration, stop the bleeding, and call the doctor. Her report to the doctor must be as accurate as it is prompt. She must move quickly enough to take care of what needs to be done, and yet not in such a manner as to add confusion to the scene.

• Since the nurse is often the first one to greet the terrified patient and his family, she must not, in her haste, neglect the kind word of encouragement. And because her contact with the patient may be brief, she must relate to him quickly, perceive his feelings and respond to them. The right word at the right moment, the touch on the arm, the chair offered, the assurance that the doctor is on his way, the deft application of a dry sterile dressing—all can help to make the patient and his family feel secure in the knowledge that he will be cared for at the time when he desperately needs help.

• Support the patient in every way possible. Call for the priest, minister, or rabbi if the patient so wishes. If the patient seems apologetic for what he now considers a foolish accident, an offhand remark by the nurse that he was wise to come for treatment, or that the accident is a common one, may help him to feel less embarrassed. Providing dramatic treatment and concentrated care often helps to allay anxiety. On the other hand, the extent of the patient's injuries should realistically be explained by the doctor, so that the patient will not imagine that his injuries are more or less serious than they actually are. The patient should be allowed to discuss what happened and his reactions to it; ignoring the patient does not help him to assimilate the traumatic experience. The nurse should be especially observant for symptoms which seem in excess of the injury, or for denial of the injury, and report these observations to the doctor. They can signal extreme anxiety.

• Remember the legal implications of the situation. The patient's valuables should be collected carefully and sent home with a relative or deposited in the hospital safe. Handle all clothing with care, even if it is bloody or dirty. A patient who sees the nurse handle his clothing as if it were repugnant to her considers himself rejected. If the clothing must be cut, cut along a seam, when it is possible, so that it can be repaired.

The nurse may work with the police to help to establish the identity of an unaccompanied, helpless person. For example, if the patient is unable to sign a consent for surgery, his family must be located.

• Be alert to your function in relation to others on the health team. An acute emergency demands smoothness, with each member of the team contributing his share of efficiency. The nurse should anticipate the information that the doctor will want. For instance, if the patient is bleeding or in shock, she should take his pulse, respirations and blood pressure, so that the doctor will have this information already available when he arrives.

• Be sure that supplies are ready for use. Such emergency equipment as oxygen, cardiac pacemaker, etc., are of no value unless they are available when needed. It is every nurse's responsibility to know where the emergency supplies and the equipment are, and how to use them. Are the sterile goods outdated? Is there oxygen in the oxygen tank? Are the appropriate medications on the emergency drug cart? Are all the necessary parts of all the emergency equipment in good working order?

• Be clear and complete in regard to follow-up care. Because patients and their families tend to be anxious, instructions are easily confused or forgotten. Did the doctor say to take the pill every 4 hours for 2 days, or every 2 hours for 4 days? *Write instructions down.*

Emergency nursing requires judgment, timing, alertness and knowledge. There is no substitute for knowing the basic principles of physiology, sterile technic and first aid so well that when the pressure is on, you can function without hesitation. Do not expect to manage your first emergencies as well as you will the later ones. Review mentally the emergencies that you encounter, and learn from each of them.

REFERENCES AND BIBLIOGRAPHY

AHLES, SR. M. A.: Disaster nursing . . . death to ideals? *Cath. Nurse* 10:50, June, 1962.

AMERICAN MEDICAL ASSOCIATION: *First Aid Manual,* Chicago, The Association, 1962.

AMERICAN RED CROSS: *Disaster Handbook for Physicians and Nurses,* rev., Washington, D.C., 1966.

ARENA, J.: The treatment of poisoning, *Ciba Clin. Symp.* 18:3, January, February, March, 1966.

BOETTCHER, E. N.: Evacuation: Outmoded as fire plan mainstay? *Hospitals* 39:68, 1965.

BRAUNSTEIN, P. W., *et al.:* Preliminary findings of the effect of automotive safety design on injury patterns, *Surg. Gynec. Obstet.* 105:257, September, 1957.

BRAVERMAN, S., and JENKS, N.: California quake, *Am. J. Nurs.* 71:708, April, 1971.

CARNER, D. C.: Safety saves nurse, *Am. J. Nurs.* 52:1477, 1952.

COLE, W. H., and PUESTOW, C. B.: *First Aid: Diagnosis and Management,* ed. 6, New York, Appleton-Century-Crofts, 1965.

COSTELLO, D., and ELLEMAN, V. B. (eds.): I, Emergency nursing; II, Disaster nursing, *Nurs. Clin. N. Am.* 2 (complete volume), June, 1967.

COWAN, L.: Emergency! *Am. J. Nurs.* 64:123, April, 1964.

Disaster Fatigue, Washington, D.C., American Psychiatric Association Committee on Civil Defense, 1956.

DOLMAN, C. E.: Botulism, *Am. J. Nurs.* 64:119, September, 1964.

Electric currents that stray and shock, *Medical World News* pp. 30–31, August 23, 1968.

FEERICK, J. P.: Fire! What do you do first? *Am. J. Nurs.* 70:2578, December, 1970.

FRAZIER, C. A.: Those deadly insects, *RN* 34:49, April, 1971.

GARB, S., and ENG, E.: *Disaster Handbook,* ed. 2, New York, Springer, 1969.

HADDON, W., *et al.: Accident Research,* New York, Harper, 1964.

HERSHEY, N.: The nurse who works alone, *Am. J. Nurs.* 62:91, December, 1962.

———: When the nurse is injured, *Am. J. Nurs.* 67:1458, July, 1967.

HILDRETH, E. A.: Penalty for unconsciousness (editorial), *Ann. Intern. Med.* 61:794, 1964.

HORNIBROOK, J. W.: Snake bites, *Am. J. Nurs.* 56:754, 1956.

KESNER, B. J.: Accident control for nursing personnel, *Am. J. Nurs.* 51:565, 1951.

MAHONEY, R.: *Emergency and Disaster Nursing,* ed. 2, New York, Macmillan, 1969.

MAMMEN, H. W.: The need for employee health services in hospitals, *Arch. Environ. Health* 9:750, 1964.

METROPOLITAN LIFE INSURANCE CO.: *Statistical Bulletin,* vol. 50, January, 1969.

MONEY, R. A.: The medical aspects of road safety and traffic accidents, *Med. J. Aust.* 48:655, 1961.

PERRY, J F., and McCLELLAN, J.: Autopsy findings in 127 patients following fatal traffic accidents, *Surg. Gynec. Obstet.* 119:586, 1964.

Psychological first aid in disasters, *Am. J. Nurs.* 55:437, 1955.

RIDGWAY, J. M.: The nurse in disaster medical and health programs, *Nurs. Outlook* 5:41, 1957.

SHAW, B. L.: Emergency care for near-drowning victims, *RN* 33:49, July, 1970.

The *new* E. R. nursing—is it for you? *RN* 33:37, November, 1970.

WALLER, J. A., and MITCHELL, H. W.: Is "accident proneness" a useful concept for medical practice? *Med. Times* 93:36, 1965.

WINDSOR, R. B.: Factors in automobile accidents, *Wisconsin Med. J.* 60:288, 1961.

The Surgical Patient

12

The Preoperative Phase • Immediate Preoperative Preparation
Preoperative Apprehension • Preoperative Explanations
The Patient's Family • Preoperative Medication • Physical
Preparation and Hospital Procedures • The Postoperative
Phase • Post-anesthesia Recovery • Possible Postoperative
Complications • Early Ambulation • Visitors

THE PREOPERATIVE PHASE

Initially, the patient sees his doctor in the office or at the clinic, or the patient is seen by a surgeon called in consultation after the patient is hospitalized. When surgery is decided upon, the surgical suite at the hospital is notified in advance so that an operating room will be available. The patient's admission to the hospital sets the preoperative phase into motion.

In the hospital admitting office, the patient's preadmission medical history form is used to minimize delay in preparing hospital records. The face sheet of the patient's chart carries significant information that is used by all team members throughout the hospital stay.

It is very important that the admitting record be accurate especially in specifying the site of operation. This is particularly true if the designation "right" or "left" is used because this record is the basis for all future considerations for the patient in the hospital.

An identification bracelet is applied to the patient's wrist to assure safe administration of medications and treatments and to prevent misidentification of the patient in the operating room.

Permission for Operation. The operative permit is part of the admitting record, granting permission for such treatments and procedures as the doctor prescribes. The patient is asked to sign the consent form showing that he agrees to have the surgery performed and stating ex-

ceptions if he has any to make. The consent, or operative permit, implies that the patient understands the nature of the treatment. The patient usually is asked to sign a consent for diagnostic procedures such as cystoscopy and bronchoscopy as well as for major surgery. If the patient has more than one such procedure or operation during his hospital stay, he signs a permit for each of them separately. The signed consent protects the patient, the hospital and the doctor. The patient is protected from having surgery to which he has not consented, and the hospital and the doctor are protected against claims that unauthorized surgery has been performed.

For the consent to be valid, the person giving it must understand what he is doing. The consent is signed while the patient is alert. Do not allow the patient to sign a permit after he has received preanesthetic medication. A patient who is intoxicated, mentally incompetent or otherwise incapable of understanding, cannot sign his own consent; a relative or guardian must sign for him. A child who is too young to understand the procedure or its consequences may not legally consent to have an operation. One of his parents or his legal guardian must sign the permission for him. It is customary to require the signature of a parent if the patient is under 21 years of age. To save the patient's life, it may be necessary in emergencies to obtain verbal consent by telephone from a responsible

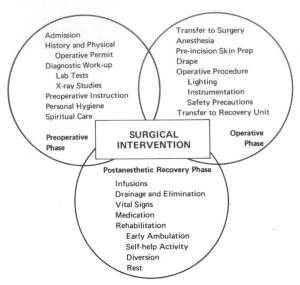

Preoperative Phase
- Admission
- History and Physical
- Operative Permit
- Diagnostic Work-up
- Lab Tests
- X-ray Studies
- Preoperative Instruction
- Personal Hygiene
- Spiritual Care

Operative Phase
- Transfer to Surgery
- Anesthesia
- Pre-incision Skin Prep
- Drape
- Operative Procedure
- Lighting
- Instrumentation
- Safety Precautions
- Transfer to Recovery Unit

SURGICAL INTERVENTION

Postanesthetic Recovery Phase
- Infusions
- Drainage and Elimination
- Vital Signs
- Medication
- Rehabilitation
- Early Ambulation
- Self-help Activity
- Diversion
- Rest

FIG. 12-1. The phases of care of the surgical patient. The preoperative phase, the operative phase, and the postanesthetic recovery phase are interrelated and interdependent.

relative.* Two surgeons, in consultation duly recorded on the patient's record, may proceed with surgery in an extreme emergency if the patient is unconscious and where there is no one to give consent.

Any person who has the ability to understand the consequences of his own actions may refuse consent for surgery or any other treatment. The doctor explains the reasons and recommends treatment, but the patient may refuse.

Admission to the Nursing Unit. When the patient is admitted to the nursing unit, he is welcomed by someone on the nursing team, preferably by the team leader, who introduces him to the team members assigned to care for him. The nursing interview content along with the medical plan is then worked into an initial program of care and communicated to the oncoming nursing team.

Initial instructions to the patient will depend on how much and what kind of information the doctor has given to him and his family. Baudry and Weiner have given some general principles of what they call "family management" that can assist the nurse to relate effectively with the persons involved in this admission phase. In addition to this, the doctor usually has an initial

working plan, sometimes called standing orders, that are individualized for each patient. The nurse explains to the patient that the doctor has been notified of his admission and will leave orders to be carried out. The nursing team leader or the nurse who has been assigned to the patient, carries out the important initial procedures and gives appropriate information to the patient while he, in his turn, has the opportunity to give information that the nurse can incorporate into the plan of nursing care. Such matters as the degree of self-help ability, any physical handicaps, personal preferences or strong dislikes that the patient has may be noted to be used by the nursing team in planning for nursing care based on understanding of the patient.

Accurate recordings of the patient's vital signs, blood pressure, weight and physical appearance are made so that there is a basis for comparison throughout the phases of the patient's care. Such diagnostic tests as the electrocardiogram (EKG or ECG) and the additional laboratory studies of the blood, urine, or of body organs by means of x-rays or isotopes will be explained when and as they pertain to the patient. Whenever possible, in the measure of his ability to understand, the patient is encouraged to participate in his own care or, at the very least, to have the information which helps him feel more secure, and which enables him to cooperate intelligently with the doctor, the nurse and the technologists in carrying out their work.

Personal Hygiene. The majority of patients who enter the hospital for surgery are able to care for their own personal needs, but they need instruction and encouragement while they prepare for the experience of an operation. The nurse provides assistance with personal hygiene if the patient requires it.

The patient should bathe thoroughly either the evening before or the morning of surgery. If surgery is scheduled very early in the morning, it is best to have the patient bathe the evening before. If surgery is scheduled late in the morning, the patient should be allowed to sleep later than usual. There will still be time to complete his care, and he will be spared many anxious hours of waiting. Most patients are up and about before surgery and can take a tub bath or shower using hexachlorophene for thoroughly cleansing the skin. For those patients who are able to use them, these facilities are preferable to a sponge bath from a small bath basin. Not

---

* For further information concerning consent for surgery and other treatments, see Lesnik, M. J., and Anderson, B. E.: *Nursing Practice and the Law,* ed. 2, with revisions, Philadelphia, Lippincott, 1962.

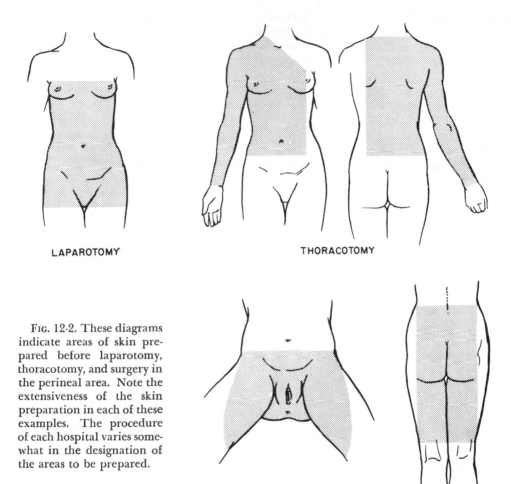

LAPAROTOMY

THORACOTOMY

FIG. 12-2. These diagrams indicate areas of skin prepared before laparotomy, thoracotomy, and surgery in the perineal area. Note the extensiveness of the skin preparation in each of these examples. The procedure of each hospital varies somewhat in the designation of the areas to be prepared.

PERINEAL

only is the patient's bath facilitated, but he is spared being made dependent on others before this is necessary. Most patients can assume responsibility for their own cleanliness; however, some will need assistance or encouragement because their habits of personal hygiene are poor.

Most patients who are up and about at home before surgery shampoo their hair before coming to the hospital, because they will be unable to do so for a time after surgery. If the patient has been hospitalized for some time preoperatively, he may, if he is able and the doctor gives permission, have a shampoo at the hospital.

IMMEDIATE PREOPERATIVE PREPARATION

The immediate preoperative preparation of the patient takes place on the nursing unit. A nursing assistant from the operating room presents a written "call slip" on the unit to obtain permission to take the patient, with his chart, to

surgery. At this time, the nurse on the unit and the nursing assistant from surgery use a preoperative checklist to be sure that each detail required for safe patient care has been carried out. This same checklist is the guide the nurse uses to organize the assignment of caring for the patient in the preoperative phase. The preoperative checklist differs somewhat depending upon the policies of particular hospitals. It consists of a list of observations to be made and tasks to be carried out just prior to surgery. Typical items include making sure the operative consent has been signed, and that the patient has voided. When these details have been carried out with careful attention and due consideration for the patient and his family, both unit nurse and the assistant from surgery help the patient onto the stretcher for safe transportation to the surgical suite.

The patient who consents to have surgery, particularly when this involves taking a general anesthetic, renders himself completely dependent on the knowledge, the skill, and the integrity of those who care for him. In accepting this trust, members of the surgical team have an obligation to make the patient's welfare their first consideration during the period when they are ministering to him. The handling of the patient should be as gentle as possible; every effort should be made to prevent injury. The patient should not be left alone until he has recovered from the anesthetic. The most meticulous attention is given to preventing infection and other complications, such as hypostatic pneumonia. It is the conscientious attention to each detail and the teamwork and concern of all who care for the patient that translate knowledge of modern technics into a miracle of healing.

PREOPERATIVE APPREHENSION

What fears may the surgical patient have? Consider the woman who is to have surgery of the breast. Fear of the diagnosis probably looms large. Today most women recognize that a lump in the breast may be cancerous, and they know that the diagnosis will be determined during surgery and the subsequent examination of tissue. She may fear mutilation: amputation of the breast would alter her appearance irrevocably. (Even though a prosthesis may be worn that keeps others from realizing she has had surgery, the patient will experience a change in body image.) She may be very much concerned about her husband's reaction to her changed appearance. The possibility of cancer—and of major surgery—may arouse fears of pain and death. The thought of being unconscious and unable to know or in any way control what is happening to her is disquieting. Fear of unrelieved pain after surgery is often a source of apprehension.

Patients who are extremely frightened respond poorly to surgery; they seem to be particularly prone to complications like cardiac arrest and irreversible shock. Unless the operation is an emergency, many surgeons defer surgery if the patient is very frightened. If the patient has been extremely fearful before surgery, he may show unusual behavior afterward, perhaps not recognizing changes in his body that have resulted from surgery, or withdrawing from others and seeming very depressed. Be alert for symptoms of unusual emotional reaction during the preoperative period and report them carefully. Baudry

and Weiner point out that the task of preoperative instruction is a dual one, giving information and correcting misconceptions. Throughout preoperative instruction, the nurse recognizes mechanisms of defense as part of a process that does not necessarily imply pathology or illness in the personality.

In one study patients who had had the opportunity to explore with the assistance of the nurse the meaning of surgery to them and to ask questions concerning the surgical experience were compared with a control group who had received only routine care limited largely to the physical aspects of preparation for surgery. A far lower incidence of postoperative vomiting occurred in the first group than in the second (Dumas and Leonard). The nurse's skilled attention to the patient's emotional needs can lessen the likelihood of postoperative vomiting, with its discomforts and dangers. It is also undoubtedly true that preoperative patients who are helped to understand and to cope emotionally with the surgical experience are spared much anxiety, the effects of which can influence recovery—even after the patient has gone home. Vomiting is obvious. Many of the other effects of preoperative anxiety are more subtle, and all too often they are ignored in practice. Modern nursing practice is becoming better informed of the meaning of behavior and significant cues to which the health team can respond. If the nurse recognizes anxiety and knows how to respond she also learns to seek the assistance of other persons skilled in the helping art. The nurse discusses with the doctor the patient's behavior patterns which the observations of an alert staff bring to the nursing care conferences. The preoperative phase is a crucial time to assist the patient to begin his journey to recovery or to work at his postoperative limitations of rehabilitation. For some situations, a psychiatric consultant or a clinical specialist in psychiatric nursing works with the nursing unit team during the pre- and postoperative phases (Kolouch).

Preparation for elective surgery (surgery to improve the patient's health, not emergency surgery) begins well before the day of operation. A careful, clear explanation by the surgeon of the reason for the surgery and of the results to be expected is necessary. It is important for the nurse to talk with the doctor, so that she knows what his plan of care is for the patient. When the team knows what information the doctor has given, nurses are in a better position to help the patient to understand any points that are not clear, or to help the patient in overcoming any misconceptions he or his family may have.

After the doctor has discussed the surgery with the patient, the nurse explains the plan for preoperative and postoperative nursing care and ways in which the patient can participate in helping himself to recover. For example, the nurse explains the purpose of the deep breathing exercises. Turning and range of motion exercises are prescribed. She might say, as she demonstrates the deep breathing exercises, "After your surgery, we want you to take deep breaths, like this, so you can get rid of sputum or mucus so that your lungs can expand fully." Then she lets the patient practice the exercises and praises his successful efforts.

PREOPERATIVE EXPLANATIONS

Before surgery the patient usually is alert and free of pain. During the immediate postoperative period he is drowsy from medication and anesthesia, and often he has pain. Pain and sleepiness interfere with learning. Apply this understanding by teaching your patients during the preoperative period. Repetition and review will be necessary postoperatively, but your patient then will be better able to participate, because he knows what to expect. Remember that the patient probably is anxious, and that anxiety may interfere with learning. For this reason, the nurse learns to recognize defenses, such as denial or forgetting, and plans her explanations in accord with the patient's readiness and ability to receive instructions. Planned use of simple, factual explanations that are adjusted to the patient's ability and need are an essential part of the nursing care plan. A patient who is helped to understand what he can do to help himself is prepared to cooperate with the health team.

The patient who enters the hospital for emergency surgery must be prepared as quickly as possible. There is not a great deal of time for reassurance and explanation. However, even in this situation the nurse's manner can convey to the patient and the family a sense of calmness and a feeling that the patient is in good hands. Even though explanations must be brief, they should be given if the patient is aware enough to understand them. As soon as emergency measures have been carried out, it is especially important to spend time talking with the family, helping them to understand what has happened. When the patient recovers sufficiently, extra thought

and attention should be given to helping him to understand the illness or the accident that has overtaken him.

Religious faith is a source of strength and courage for many patients. Opportunities for contact with the clergyman of a patient and for the sacraments of his church are especially important during a crisis like an impending operation. Every effort should be made to help the patient to maintain ties with his church, either through the services of the patient's own clergyman or through the hospital chaplain.

THE PATIENT'S FAMILY

Family members need to understand what measures are necessary to prepare the patient for surgery, so that they can participate intelligently in his care and provide him with further explanation and encouragement. Sometimes the patient can accept the necessity for surgery better if it is explained further to him by a relative whom he loves and trusts. Many family members want to be near the patient and to help in any possible way to prepare him for surgery. Their presence helps the patient to feel less alone and assures him of his family's concern and interest.

The nurse who believes that family members have a right to be with the patient, and that their presence can be helpful, will reveal this attitude in her manner toward the family. On the other hand, if she believes that the family is in the way or likely to upset the patient, she will behave in a way that is conducive to this very occurrence.

PREOPERATIVE MEDICATION

Barbiturates, such as phenobarbital and sodium pentobarbital, often are given the evening before surgery to help the patient to sleep. Sometimes tranquilizers, like meprobamate, are given for 1 or 2 days before surgery to help the patient to remain calm. About an hour before surgery a narcotic, such as morphine or Demerol, usually is administered to relieve apprehension. (Because morphine depresses respirations, some doctors prefer to use Demerol preoperatively.) If a general anesthetic is to be given, atropine often is administered with the narcotic to lessen respiratory secretions, thus decreasing the likelihood of respiratory complications resulting from aspiration of secretions. If your patient receives atropine, mention to him that it will make his mouth feel dry. To make sure that the maximum effect is obtained, the nurse will plan the work so that there is no delay in giving a preoperative medication. The optimum time for the medication is 30 to 45 minutes before surgery.

Most patients who enter the hospital for surgery are unaccustomed to taking sedatives and narcotics. Elderly people particularly may become restless and confused after the administration of barbiturates. Often another type of sedative, such as chloral hydrate, is ordered for them. Explain to the patient that the preoperative injection will make him very sleepy. Ask him to stay in bed, once the drug has been administered, and to call the nurse if he needs anything. Impress on him the importance of not smoking after the injection has been given; he is likely to fall asleep, drop the cigarette on his bed, and suffer severe or fatal burns. If the patient feels he must smoke one last cigarette just before surgery, have someone stay with him while he is smoking. When the patient is left alone, side rails are put up into position and the call button is left where the patient can reach it. Instruct him to stay in bed and advise him that the medication will be in effect about 20 minutes after it is given.

On the day of surgery the patient's care should be planned in such a way that he need not be disturbed after the narcotic has been given, so that the medication can exert its beneficial effect. The patient need not be left entirely alone, if someone's quiet presence would make him feel more secure. While the patient is resting in bed or in the operating room suite, he should not be approached with social chitchat that serves to keep him alert and awake. If the patient has been carefully prepared before the narcotic is given and is not disturbed afterward, he will go to sleep after the narcotic has been administered. Although often he may awaken when he is taken to the operating room, the medication dulls his awareness of the experience and makes it easier for him to relax and to take the anesthetic.

The best nurse-patient relationship can be marred if the nurse seems confused and disorganized in carrying out physical aspects of preoperative care, or if her lack of knowledge and technical skill jeopardizes safe preoperative preparation. Because it is especially important to appear calm and well organized, even during a first experience in preparing patients for surgery, make a list of important points and carry it in your pocket the first few times you get patients ready for the operating room. It will free you from excessive concern over forgetting important details, and enable you to concentrate more on the patient's reactions and special needs.

PHYSICAL PREPARATION AND HOSPITAL PROCEDURES

Preoperative preparation may extend over a period of several weeks, and it may include many tests, x-ray studies and laboratory procedures, as well as education of the patient and the family. The nurse plays an important part in explaining the necessity for preoperative tests and in carrying out the preparation for them. For instance, she may have the patient fast until blood specimens have been drawn, or she may give enemas prior to x-ray studies of the gastrointestinal tract.

Preoperative patients have their medical histories taken and a complete physical examination performed. In addition, certain laboratory tests, such as urinalysis, complete blood count and hemoglobin determination, are usual. These procedures are carried out to discover any pre-existing disease that might alter the patient's response to surgery or his recovery from it. For instance, urinalysis may suggest the presence of diabetes mellitus or chronic nephritis. In many hospitals a routine chest roentgenogram is taken to make certain that the patient has no unsuspected pulmonary disease, such as tuberculosis. If unsuspected disease is discovered, the operation may be delayed while measures to treat or to control the condition are instituted.

Often surgery must be undertaken despite the presence of other illnesses. The patient with multiple sclerosis may require surgery for a broken leg, or a patient with heart disease may have to have his appendix removed. These long-term illnesses affect plans for medical and nursing care. The surgeon often consults the patient's medical doctor concerning the management of the co-existing disease. For instance, the patient with heart disease may require daily doses of digitalis, as well as a low sodium diet. The patient with multiple sclerosis may need considerably more assistance with the activities of daily living than would most surgical patients. A diabetic patient needs special treatment before, during and after surgery. These needs have to be considered in planning nursing care.

Immediate Preoperative Care

Immediate preparation for surgery starts usually the afternoon before the patient is to have his operation.

Skin Preparation. The purpose of skin preparation is to make the skin as free of microorganisms as possible, thus decreasing the possibility during surgery of the entrance of bacteria into the wound from the skin surface.

Most hospitals have manuals describing specifically the areas of the skin to be prepared for certain types of surgery and the procedure to be used. Figure 12-2 shows areas of the body customarily prepared for common types of surgery. Before commencing any skin preparation, look up the procedure and the area to be prepared in the hospital manual. If you are in doubt, consult the doctor. It is very important to have the skin preparation meticulously complete before surgery, because last-minute additional preparation, along with the tension generated among the staff by the necessity for this procedure, is very upsetting to the patient and may shake his confidence in those caring for him.

Although the procedure for skin preparation varies in different hospitals, cleanliness of the skin and the removal of hair from its surface without injury to or irritation of the skin in the process are fundamental. The skin cannot be made completely sterile, but the number of microorganisms on it can be reduced substantially. Hair is shaved because microorganisms readily cling to it. Long hair, as on the head, the male chest, and the pubic-perineal area, is shaved when surgery is to be performed in that region. This is necessary in order to prevent the presence of hair in the wound, which acts as a foreign body to prevent healing. Plain soap and water are sometimes used for cleansing the skin. Solutions effective in decreasing the number of microorganisms on the skin are now very widely used. Because of the controversy concerning its use, preparations containing hexachlorophene (pHisoHex) are used only with caution today. Alcohol removes hexachlorophene from the skin, and therefore it should be used as a rinse when cleansing is done with hexachlorophene. Rinse with plain water and dry the skin. The umbilicus should be cleaned carefully with cotton swabs dipped in the soap or antiseptic solution.

Shaving is made easier if long hair, such as that in the axilla and the pubic region, is first trimmed with scissors. In shaving, use a sharp, new blade for each patient, and be sure that the razor is sterilized before it is used for another patient. Hold the skin taut and be very careful not to cut the patient; even a small cut can cause

infection later in the operative area. Shaving the pubic hair can be very embarrassing for the patient. Before starting the procedure explain briefly what you are going to do and why it is being done. (Of course, this advice holds true for all preparations.) Drape the patient and screen him to prevent unnecessary exposure. In most hospitals a male nurse or nursing assistant takes care of the skin preparation for male patients. Preparation for orthopedic surgery must be especially careful, because infections of bone are very difficult to cure.

Elimination. Before certain types of surgery it is particularly important that the bladder be empty. For example, distention of the bladder makes lower abdominal surgery more difficult and increases the possibility that the bladder may be traumatized during the operation. For this reason some surgeons ask that the patient be catheterized, and that a catheter be left in place just before surgery on the lower abdomen. If the patient is not to be catheterized, make certain that he voids just before surgery. Even in operations far removed from the region of the bladder, such as surgery of the nose, the patient will be more comfortable and at ease if he has voided just before going to the operating room. Too often the patient is given the bedpan or the urinal hastily, with little attention to position or to privacy, when the stretcher arrives to take him to the operating room. Under these circumstances many patients become tense, are unable to void, or void in insufficient quantity. Plan the patient's care in such a way that there is time for the important details of positioning and privacy, without obvious haste or impatience.

Enemas are ordered often (but by no means always) before surgery. The reasons for their use are apparent—for example, when the patient has surgery of his gastrointestinal tract, and the tract must be as free of feces as possible. The act of straining to have a bowel movement is painful after any abdominal operation. If fecal matter is left in the bowel preoperatively, it may become hard and even impacted before the patient is able to bear down painlessly enough to evacuate.

Sometimes, enemas are ordered for patients whose surgery involves distant organs. For instance, enemas often are ordered before eye surgery, so that the patient will be spared the strain and the exertion of moving his bowels in the immediate postoperative period; this exertion might cause hemorrhage in the operative area.

General anesthesia produces muscular relaxation; having the bowel empty prevents the possibility of involuntary bowel movement during or immediately after the operation. The patient's comfort and peace of mind are enhanced if he has moved his bowels before going to the operating room. Small-quantity commercially prepared enemas are being used with increasing frequency for preoperative preparation. Most patients find them more comfortable and less tiring than the large-quantity enemas, and they are usually quite effective.

Read the doctor's preoperative orders carefully. Each patient's needs are different; each doctor has his own individual preferences concerning preoperative preparation. One patient may be given an enema the evening before surgery. Another patient's doctor may order a Dulcolax suppository and no enema. When thorough preoperative cleansing of the bowel is essential, doctors often order "enemas till clear." This expression means that the enema is to be repeated until no more fecal matter is expelled with the solution.

Food and Fluids. The doctor will leave specific directions concerning the length of time during which food and fluids are to be omitted preoperatively. Usually, midnight preceding surgery is specified as the time for terminating food and fluids. Before this time the patient should be encouraged to eat and drink in order to maintain fluid and electrolyte regulation and to provide nutrients necessary for wound healing. Protein and ascorbic acid (vitamin C) are especially important in promoting wound healing. Except in emergencies, a patient whose nutrition is poor usually has surgery deferred until deficiencies of food, fluids or electrolytes can be corrected. Parenteral administration may be necessary if the patient is unable to take a sufficient amount of oral fluids.

Care of Valuables. Attention is given to the care of valuables on admission. Sometimes, despite these measures, the nurse finds that the patient has valuable jewelry or documents with him on the morning of the operation. It is the policy in most hospitals that valuables be placed in the hospital safe before the patient goes to surgery. Always chart what has been done with valuables (such as depositing them in the safe). You may not be working when the patient asks for them, but if you have written the information

on the patient's chart, another nurse can locate them readily.

Nails and Hair. Details of personal grooming, such as trimming the nails and shaving, should be completed before surgery. Women are asked to remove bobby pins, because these might cause injury if the patient is restless during or immediately after surgery. Long hair should be braided to keep it neat and out of the way. The ends of the braids may be secured with elastic bands. Regardless of the length of a woman's hair, help her to arrange it so that it will be away from her face and mouth.

Attire. The patient is given a clean hospital gown. If she asks permission to wear her own gown or pajamas, explain that sometimes patients perspire a good deal and need to have their gowns changed while they are in the operating or recovery rooms. Her own clothing is harder to remove, and it might be put with the hospital laundry. For added warmth, patients in some hospitals are provided with long, white cotton stockings to wear to the operating room.

Prostheses. In most hospitals the patient is asked to remove dentures, so that they will not become dislodged and cause respiratory obstruction during the administration of anesthesia. However, some anesthetists prefer that well-fitting dentures be left in to preserve the contours of the face. Acquaint yourself with the policy at your hospital. If dentures are to be removed, tactfully ask the patient if he has any. If he does, give him an opaque denture jar; then, unless he needs help, leave him alone for a few minutes while he removes and cleans them and places them in the jar. In most hospitals the denture jar is left in the patient's bedside stand until he returns to the ward. Other prostheses, such as eyes or limbs, must be removed before surgery.

Mouth Care. All patients should have thorough mouth care before surgery; a clean mouth makes them more comfortable and prevents the aspiration of particles of food that may be left in the mouth. Needless to say, chewing gum is not permitted, since it, too, could be aspirated!

Makeup and Jewelry. Because the color of face, lips and nailbeds is watched carefully for cyanosis during surgery by the anesthetist, patients are asked to remove their makeup. Jewelry should be removed for safekeeping; a valuable ring might slip off the finger of an unconscious patient and be lost. If the patient is reluctant to remove her wedding band, it may be tied to

FIG. 12-3. This patient is on his way to the operating room. The stretcher is held tightly against the bed. The drawsheet is being used to help him slide onto the stretcher.

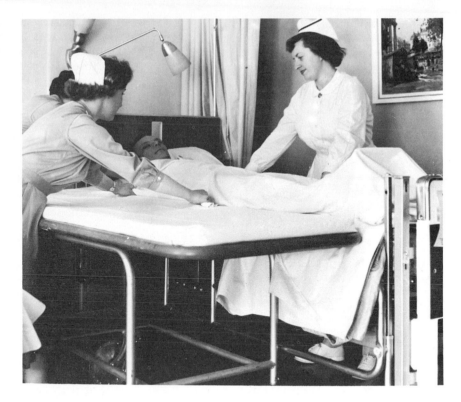

her wrist with a piece of gauze. Just slip the gauze under the ring; then loop the gauze around the finger and the wrist. Be careful not to tie it tightly enough to impair circulation.

Transportation of the Patient to the Operating Room

When it is time for the patient to go to the operating room, he is placed on a stretcher and covered with cotton blankets. All necessary information should be recorded on the chart before the patient leaves the ward: medications, T.P.R., voiding, disposition of valuables and dentures, and pertinent observations concerning the patient's condition. The chart and x-ray films are taken to the operating room with the patient. The blood pressure is taken and recorded by the nurse before the patient goes to the operating room; it is helpful to have a record of the patient's preoperative blood pressure so that it can be compared with blood pressure readings during surgery. The blood pressure should be taken before narcotics are administered, since they may lower the blood pressure. Always check the patient's identification bracelet and bed tag before taking him to the operating room to be sure the right patient is being taken for surgery.

Checklist for Preoperative Care

Here are a few hints on organizing preoperative care. Some hospitals put a checklist or reminder sheet on the front of the chart of each preoperative patient. In any case, you can make your own checklist this way.

A. General goals for the whole preoperative period
   1. Emotional support
   2. Instruction
   3. Spiritual needs; visit from clergyman
   4. Planning with family; teaching family

B. The afternoon before surgery
   1. Check preoperative orders carefully; note orders for enemas, catheterization, medications, and any other procedures that are to be carried out preoperatively
   2. Have patient sign consent
   3. Prepare skin of operative area
   4. Safeguard valuables
   5. Give sedative, if ordered, to promote sleep
   6. Withhold food and fluids as ordered (usually after midnight)
   7. Make certain that all specimens requested have been collected (urine, blood)

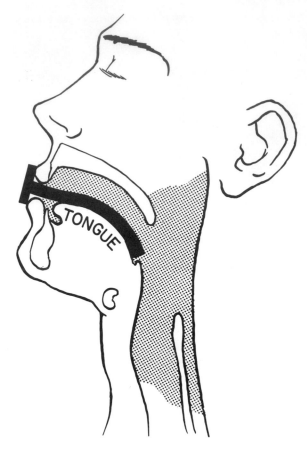

FIG. 12-4. A pharyngeal airway in place. Note how the airway prevents the tongue of the unconscious patient from blocking the air passages. As long as the airway is unobstructed and in place, there is a free route for air between the pharynx and the outside.

C. The morning of surgery
1. Take and record, T.P.R., B.P.
2. Assist the patient with personal hygiene as necessary
3. Help the patient to dress for the operating room
4. Remove prostheses (including dentures, if it is hospital policy that they be removed)
5. Administer preoperative narcotic, as ordered
6. Have patient void
7. Leave patient resting in bed, with call bell handy
8. Make certain that all charting is complete

These measures cannot and should not be carried out always in this order. *The needs of each individual patient are more important than any routine.* Recognition of this difference was shown by a wise surgeon whose patient had said that she did not want to see her pastor before surgery. Just before going to the operating room, the patient became agitated and asked to see her clergyman. The operation was scheduled for 8 A.M., and it was then 7:45 A.M. When the nurse called the surgeon to say that the patient wanted to see her pastor, the surgeon's reply was, "Of course, I'll wait. Call me when she's ready."

THE POSTOPERATIVE PHASE

Postoperative nursing care involves intensive nursing designed to:

- Prevent and detect complications
- Protect the patient from injury during his period of helplessness
- Relieve discomfort
- Help the patient to regain independence

Factors in the case such as age of patient, nutritional status, or disease conditions requiring more intensive therapy will affect the duration of the postoperative period. The kind of surgical intervention will have a bearing on how long the patient will require continuous surveillance beyond the immediate postanesthetic period.

During the immediate postoperative period, the patient is in the recovery room or in an intensive care unit. These are rooms specially designed for the care of the patient while he requires close observation and prompt care in the event of a sudden complication. Patients who go to the intensive care unit are sent there because the doctor anticipates a more prolonged stay (over 24 hours) while patients in the recovery room usually stay just long enough to recover from the anesthetic. The intensive care unit may be equipped with electronic monitoring equipment which is used to carry on the continuous and/or intermittent monitoring of vital signs begun in surgery.

POST-ANESTHESIA RECOVERY

The recovery room (P.A.R. or R.R.) is usually a very large room with accommodations for a group of patients to be under the continual surveillance of highly skilled personnel. Patients are in cubicles which can be curtained off for privacy during nursing procedures or examinations, in consideration of the patient's need for privacy, as well as thoughtfulness for other patients who are nearby. Equipment at each bedside and at the nursing station is available for immediate application in case of need. Recordings of vital signs are made at frequent intervals and the progress of the patient's recovery from the anesthetic is charted on the patient's bedside record.

As a general rule, the endotracheal tube is removed by the anesthesiologist before the patient leaves the surgical suite. A complication which can arise during this critical time is laryngospasm. The natural respiratory response to noxious gases is a forced expiratory grunt as the thoracic and abdominal muscles tense into a protective shield. The same reflex can be stimulated by action on nervous structures of the body, notably, the rectal or perineal muscles, the periosteum, and a pulling action on abdominal viscera. Too light a plane of anesthesia allows this protective reflex to narrow the laryngeal space, resulting in high-pitched inspiratory stridor. This condition requires that the patient be assisted with respiration manually, along with being supplied a slightly higher oxygen content than ordinary air. An oropharyngeal airway is inserted to prevent the tongue from obstructing the air passage during this phase of the patient's recovery from anesthesia. This airway is left in position until the patient begins to regain consciousness, giving evidence of the return of the swallowing and cough reflexes. Even then, the patient is so positioned that vomitus or secretions will not be aspirated into the tracheobronchial passages. If necessary, suction is used to promptly remove vomitus and secretions so that the patient will not aspirate them.

When the patient is fully reacted and there is no evidence of complications, he is prepared to return to the nursing unit. The length of time varies, but an average duration of the postanesthetic period is about one and one-half to two hours. If the surgery is of such a nature that intensive nursing care is required, the patient may be sent to the intensive care unit. In this unit, similar measures are taken as in the recovery room to foresee and prevent critical complications.

The chief responsibilities of the nurse during the immediate postoperative recovery period are (1) to assure a patent airway, (2) to help maintain adequate circulation, (3) to prevent and/or treat shock, and (4) to attend to proper positioning and the function of drains, tubes and intravenous infusions.

Positioning the patient is an important measure in preventing interference with circulation; normal body alignment should be maintained.

Precautions are taken to prevent displacement of the infusion needle because maintenance of the infusion is important to adequate circulatory function. If the patient is in one position for any prolonged period, measures are taken to prevent pressure over bony prominences and delicate tissues like the ear. A skin surface that rests against another is protected to prevent excoriation. A patient with a cast is observed closely to detect interference with circulation either because of swelling or a malposition. Change in the color of the skin (cyanosis or blanching) with either hyperemia or loss of heat would necessitate careful checking and, if necessary, splitting or trimming of the cast. The doctor should be notified early at the onset of these symptoms or in the event that the patient's complaints of persistent pain are not relieved by nursing measures.

Nursing care and observation are important after spinal anesthesia, although the fact that the patient does not lose consciousness simplifies some aspects of postoperative care. Even though the patient is conscious, it is important to remember that he usually has had medications that may make him dizzy and confused. When you leave the patient, make sure that the side rails are in place and that the call bell is handy. Later, when you observe that he is sufficiently alert, you may lower the side rails.

At first the patient's lower extremities will feel numb and heavy. Even though an explanation of this feeling was made before surgery, it is important for the nurse to repeat the explanation that numbness is usual and will subside in a short time. Many patients become apprehensive because of this symptom, and fear that the anesthesia has resulted in paralysis of their legs.

The patient usually is kept flat in bed for 6 to 12 hours after the surgery. Unless the doctor has ordered otherwise, he may be turned from side to side. As the anesthesia wears off, he will begin to have sensation in the anesthetized parts. Often he describes this as "pins and needles." He also will begin to experience pain in the operated area; analgesics usually are ordered to relieve the pain. Those patients who develop headache may have to remain flat for a longer period. There has been so much discussion about "spinal headache" that patients sometimes think it an inevitable sequel to spinal anesthesia. Remember not to contribute to this impression by the power of suggestion. A statement like "I'll keep your bed flat so you can doze" is preferable to "I'll keep the bed flat so you won't get a headache."

Postsurgical shock due to blood loss, fluid shifts and neurogenic factors, is usually mild and amenable to therapy. Intravenous fluids are regulated to prevent overhydration but are specified in amount and rate of flow to treat dehydration. The kind and specific amount of intake for fluids and blood depends on the patient's requirements and the kind of surgery performed. The rate of flow is carefully determined at the start and checked frequently to keep it flowing at the number of drops per minute ordered by the physician. Medication for pain relief or sedation is ordered by the surgeon. The recovery room nurse exercises judgment in administering the first postoperative medication. Judgments in this matter are based on knowledge of the drugs used for anesthesia and their effect on the action of drugs used for pain relief. The physician is guided by these considerations when ordering analgesics for postoperative patients. For example, it is known that smaller doses of narcotic are indicated when fentanyl (Innovar) is given for the anesthetic. The pattern of the vital signs gives the nurse a clue to the degree of shock and the value of judiciously administered sedation for control of the autonomic nervous system, which regulates many of the reflex mechanisms involved in shock.

The number and kind of drains and tubes vary with the surgical intervention. Specific details of the use of drains in surgery are discussed in relation to those procedures that require them. What is essential is that the nurse determines the adequacy of drainage so that when drains are not functioning properly, measures may be instituted to correct the malfunction. In order to prevent further complications and delayed healing, indwelling drains must be kept in proper position and in working order. Catheters and tubes must be checked to prevent kinking or clogging that interferes with adequate drainage of urine or bile. Calm, patient and, if necessary, repeated explanations will be required to help the patient understand these drains and tubes. This is much more difficult to do in the postoperative period if adequate explanation has not been included in the preoperative instruction, according to the patient's level of understanding.

Intravenous fluids are usually administered throughout the operation and into the recovery phase until the patient's blood pressure is stabilized. This is a routine precaution that is desirable in the event of sudden reaction which might precipitate shock. Maintenance of adequate circulation is essential for prompt treatment of vascular collapse even in a mild form. If the surgical procedure is a major one, fluids are needed to maintain nutritional status until the patient is able to resume oral nourishment.

POSSIBLE POSTOPERATIVE COMPLICATIONS

The first 24 hours after the surgery require alert attention to the prevention of possible occurrence of 4 important complications of the immediate postoperative period: hemorrhage, shock, hypoxia, and vomiting. The patient may have been moved from the recovery room so that each member of the nursing team must be alert to the signs of change that result from or point to these complications.

Hemorrhage

Hemorrhage can be either external or internal. If it is internal, it is noted, not by visible bleeding, but by pallor, fall in blood pressure, rapid pulse, restlessness and dehydration. Dressings must be inspected regularly for any sign of bleeding. Also the bedding and the dressing under the patient is inspected, because blood may run under the patient's body and be more evident under him than on his dressing. (See Chap. 51 for a discussion of hematogenic shock.) In such an eventuality it may be necessary for the patient to be taken back to the operating room for ligation of bleeding vessels. Frequently, transfusions are ordered to replace the blood lost.

When reporting bleeding, always note the color of the blood. Bright red blood signifies fresh bleeding. Dark, brownish blood indicates that the bleeding is not fresh. When the patient first is transferred to your care, find out whether drains have been inserted, and what type of drainage is expected. If you know that a drain is in place, you will not be surprised when brownish-red drainage appears on a dressing. Dressings that become soiled may be reinforced, but they never should be changed except at the direction of the surgeon. If drainage is to be expected, always explain to the patient that the drainage is a normal consequence of the surgery and does not indicate any complications.

The color and the amount of any drainage should be reported accurately on the patient's chart.

Shock

The loss of fluids and electrolytes, trauma (both physical and psychological), anesthetics and preoperative medications may all play a part in precipitating shock. The symptoms include pallor, fall in blood pressure, rapid, weak pulse and cold, moist skin. Narcotics never should be administered to patients in shock or to a patient in whom shock seems imminent, unless the patient's condition has been evaluated by the doctor, and he expressly orders that the medication be given. Narcotics given to a patient in shock may not be absorbed, due to the decreased volume of the circulating blood. As the patient recovers from shock, and the circulation improves, several doses of the narcotic may be absorbed at once, resulting in an overdose. Narcotics may precipitate shock in patients in whom this complication is imminent.

Patients in shock are placed with their heads lower than their feet. Patients who have had brain surgery or spinal anesthesia should be kept flat; for these patients the foot of the bed should not be elevated. (The spinal anesthetic might travel upward and paralyze the diaphragm; placing the head lower than the rest of the body following brain surgery may increase cerebral edema.)

The treatment of shock includes the administration of whole blood, other parenteral fluids, such as plasma expanders, and drugs that help to raise blood pressure. Medications usually are administered intravenously to patients who are in shock.

Hypoxia

Hypoxia may complicate postoperative recovery. Sometimes anesthetics and preoperative medications depress respirations, thus interfering with oxygenation of the blood. Because mucus may block tracheal or bronchial passages and interfere with breathing, the amount of oxygen entering the lungs may be lowered. Oxygen and suction equipment always should be ready for emergency use, and the patient should be watched carefully for cyanosis and dyspnea. Remember that if breathing is obstructed (for example, by the tongue falling backward), the first thing to do is to relieve the obstruction (in this instance by bringing the tongue forward).

Other factors such as residual effect or overdose of drugs, pain, poor positioning causing pressure or an obstructed airway also predispose to hypoxia. Restlessness, tracheal tug, jerky and grunting respiratory efforts, perspiration, bounding pulse and rising blood pressure all arouse suspicion of embarrassed respiration.

When indicated, positive pressure ventilation is applied by the use of a mechanical respirator. Any one of several types may be used. Many hospitals have the advantage of inhalation therapy services. Personnel in these services are specially trained to take care of the equipment and to assist with this important aspect of care.

Pain

Because a certain amount of pain is expected after surgery, the doctor will leave orders for analgesics, so that the patient will be as comfortable as possible. The most severe pain occurs during the first 48 hours. Pain arouses varying degrees of anxiety in different people. Some take it in stride; others greatly fear it, and their tenseness and fear increase the pain.

It is the responsibility of the nurse to evaluate the need of the patient for the narcotic. Usually the medication, such as morphine or meperidine hydrochloride (Demerol) can be repeated at 4-hour intervals, if necessary. In no aspect of nursing is sound judgment more vital than in the administration of narcotics to postoperative patients. What at first appears a simple procedure (he has pain; you give the drug) is really a complex one.

Here are some factors that must be considered before administering the narcotic:

• Narcotics are not without side-effects. For example, morphine may depress respiration or lead to constipation. Demerol often makes patients dizzy.

• Consider the timing of narcotics in relation to getting the patient out of bed. It is sometimes unwise to get a patient up shortly after he has had a narcotic, because he is more likely to feel dizzy and faint after receiving such medication. However, the timing of narcotics in relation to ambulation is a matter requiring astute judgment. Some patients require medication for the relief of pain before they can tolerate the additional discomfort entailed in getting up. In such instances it usually is wise to allow the patient to rest in bed for about an hour after administering the medicine to permit some relaxation, and then, when assisting him out of bed, perhaps to have the assistance of a second person in case the patient should become faint or dizzy.

• If narcotics are continued for prolonged periods, the danger of addiction arises. However, their use during the first 2 or 3 postoperative days does not cause addiction.

• Have nursing measures been tried to relieve the pain? Narcotics never should be administered as a substitute for nursing care. Sometimes helping the patient to turn, rubbing his back, and letting him express some of his worries about his condition are all that is required. Many a nurse who has left her patient to check on a narcotic order, after carrying out these measures, has returned to find him asleep.

• If the narcotic is required, it will have greater effect when the patient first has been made as comfortable as possible. A comfortable patient can rest undisturbed and receive the full benefit of the medication without being disturbed for ward routines.

• Never give a narcotic to a patient whose blood pressure is low and unstable without first consulting the physician. If shock is imminent, administration of a narcotic can precipitate it.

• Usually it is advisable to wait until the patient has reacted fully from anesthesia before giving a narcotic. While he may mumble about pain, he often is not fully aware of it until he opens his eyes and knows where he is. The patient's condition and recovery from anesthesia can be evaluated more accurately if the medication is withheld until he has reacted.

• The purpose of the medication is to relieve pain, not to render the patient stuporous. Oversedation makes it impossible for the patient to practice such preventive measures as deep breathing and coughing.

• Morphine depresses respirations. Withhold it and consult the doctor if the patient's respirations are less than 12 per minute.

• Narcotics and sedatives should be given with special caution to older people, because they have a tendency to become restless and disoriented as a result of the medication.

• When giving medicine for the relief of pain, take advantage of its psychological as well as its physiologic effect. All medicines convey some psychological meaning, along with their physiologic action. For example, do not rush in and give an intramuscular injection of Demerol, saying only, "Turn over." The patient may be receiving penicillin or Prostigmin also as part of his therapy, and he may think that nothing has been done to relieve his pain. You might say, "I'm going to give you some medicine to lessen the pain. In a few minutes you'll find it will be much less severe. Maybe you can doze off for a while."

• Give the medication promptly when it is required. Minutes seem like hours to patients who are in severe pain.

• Determine whether the pain is incisional pain, for which the narcotic is ordered, or whether it stems from another source. It is not enough to know that the patient has pain. Find out where the pain is. If he had abdominal surgery and the pain is in his chest, do not give the narcotic. Call the doctor instead, so that he can discover the cause of the pain.

• Most patients do not require narcotics after the 2nd or the 3rd postoperative day. If the patient continues to complain of pain and ask for medication, tell the doctor. Perhaps a complication like wound infection is developing. Or perhaps the patient is beginning to rely on the drug to relieve worry and anxiety rather than pain. This tendency should be noted early, because it can lead to addiction.

Exercises in the early postoperative period also can increase the patient's pain. Assisting the postoperative patient to carry out measures to forestall complications and discomforts requires a great deal of tact, patience and skill. It is all very well to say that the patient must turn, cough and take deep breaths. Persuading him to do these things when they cause him considerable apprehension and pain is not so easy.

Vomiting

Vomiting is especially likely to occur after the administration of ether. In current practice other agents usually are used to commence anesthesia, even though ether may be added later. Some patients receive no ether at all but have a spinal anesthetic or some other type of anesthetic. Postoperative nausea and vomiting are not as severe now as they used to be, when more patients received ether.

If vomiting is severe or prolonged, oral feedings are discontinued temporarily, and the patient is fed intravenously. Gastric intubation and suction may be necessary. However, this procedure is not usual. Most patients can begin to take food and fluids a few hours after surgery, unless it has involved the gastrointestinal tract. The nurse's own attitude is important. Never suggest to the patient that he will vomit after surgery. The skillful nurse keeps an emesis basin nearby but not prominently displayed during the postoperative period.

Oral Fluids and Diet

Regardless of how much intravenous fluid the patient is receiving, nothing soothes his parched, dry mouth and throat like cool liquids that he can swallow. Patients usually ask for water almost as soon as they begin to complain of pain in the incision. Several important points must be considered, though, before giving the patient fluids by mouth:

- Check to make sure that the doctor's order indicates that fluids may be given postoperatively. Sometimes the order reads, "Food and fluid as tolerated." At other times it may say, "Nothing by mouth."

If the patient is not allowed oral fluids, rinsing his mouth and placing a cool, wet cloth or some ice chips against his lips will help to relieve the feeling of dryness.

- Make certain that the patient has recovered sufficiently from anesthesia to be able to swallow. Ask him to try swallowing without drinking anything. If he can, give him a small sip of water.
- Give only a few sips at a time. It will taste so good that the patient may gulp it, unless you instruct him to take only a few sips. Gulping the water will make him more likely to vomit it. Give fluids through a straw rather than directly from the glass, so that the patient does not have to sit up.

If the patient vomits, assure him matter-of-factly that he will be able to retain fluids later. Offer him mouthwash to help to get rid of the taste of anesthetics and of vomitus, and make sure that he is kept dry and clean. Try not to make him feel that the vomiting was a great calamity, or that it is likely to continue for a long time.

However, emphasis on neatness and cleanliness should not obscure other essentials. For instance, if an unconscious or partly conscious patient starts to vomit, and an emesis basin is not handy (perhaps someone just went to empty it), do not leave the patient to look for a basin. Stay with him and turn his head to the side. Soiled bedding is more easily managed and less harmful than aspirated vomitus!

Urinary Retention

Patients who have had abdominal surgery, particularly if it has been in the lower abdominal and pelvic regions, often have difficulty voiding after surgery. Operative trauma in the region near the bladder may decrease temporarily the patient's sensation of needing to void. The fear of pain also causes tenseness and difficulty in voiding. The discomfort and the lack of privacy associated with using the bedpan may play a

part. Position is very important. Many women cannot void lying down, but they can void if allowed to sit up. Men often have difficulty voiding when recumbent, but they can void normally if permitted to use the urinal while standing at the bedside.

Catheterization in the postoperative period formerly was used quite widely. Because the procedure entails the risk of bladder infection, it should be avoided when simple nursing measures, plus a little patience, can result in adequate voiding.

Record the time and the amount of each voiding for 1 or 2 days after surgery (the length of time that this part of the record should be kept depends on how quickly normal function is resumed). No order is necessary for this record, and usually none will be given. The doctor will expect you to know the patient's intake and output and to record them. Follow any specific orders the doctor may leave concerning the measuring of intake and output.

If the patient is unable to void, 8 to 12 hours is the usual time that is allowed postoperatively before catheterization is considered. Overdistention of the bladder must be avoided. Not only does it make the patient restless and uncomfortable, but it can lead to infection of the urinary tract. There are several indications that the patient needs to void:

- Restlessness
- Distention of the area just above the pubis. Palpation of this areas causes discomfort and makes the patient feel that he has to void.
- Large intake of oral or parenteral fluid, with no unusual loss of fluid, such as that from prolonged vomiting or profuse sweating

Distention

Abdominal distention results from the accumulation of gas (flatus) in the intestines. It is caused by a failure of the intestines to propel gas through the intestinal tract by peristalsis, and it is aggravated by the tendency of some patients to swallow large quantities of air, especially when they are frightened or in pain. The handling of the intestines during surgery may cause postoperative distention, because the trauma of handling temporarily inhibits normal peristalsis. Contributing factors are immobility following surgery and interruption of the diet necessitated by surgery.

Sometimes, if the symptoms are mild, they can be relieved by nursing measures. If the patient is permitted out of bed, help him to walk about and to go to the toilet. Sometimes the walking, plus some privacy in the bathroom, will help him to expel the gas. Encourage him to eat as normally as possible within the limits specified by the doctor's orders.

Taking only fluids, particularly if these are always iced, often aggravates the problem. For instance, when the patient eats breakfast on the morning after surgery, suggest that he take a few bites of toast and cereal in addition to the liquids. Hot liquids, like tea and coffee, sometimes help to relieve distention.

If the patient's discomfort is severe, or if it is not relieved promptly by nursing measures, the doctor should be notified. Usually he orders one or several of the following measures:

• Insertion of a rectal tube to dilate the anal sphincter and to release the gas that may have accumulated in the rectum. Insert the tube as though you were going to give an enema. Protect the bedding, in case some fecal matter should be expelled with the flatus, by covering the end of the tube with an absorbent disposable pad. The best results are achieved by leaving the rectal tube in place for about 20 minutes, removing and cleaning it, and then inserting it an hour or so later. The constant presence of the tube both day and night makes the patient uncomfortable and messy, and using it continuously can render it ineffective.

• Application of heat to the abdomen. A hot-water bottle or an electric heating pad usually is used. Be careful not to burn the patient. If available, use a pad that makes accurate regulation of the temperature possible. A device that permits the nurse to set the temperature and to maintain it constantly is preferable to devices that provide uneven amounts of heat.

• Use of neostigmine (Prostigmin) intramuscularly to stimulate peristalsis, thus helping the patient to expel gas. The usual dose is 1 ml. of a 1:1,000 or a 1:2,000 solution. Some doctors routinely order Prostigmin postoperatively to prevent distention.

A very serious condition called *paralytic ileus* sometimes occurs. The patient has paralysis of the intestines and thus absence of peristalsis.

Acute gastric dilatation, a condition in which do not pass normally through the gastrointestinal tract, is another complication similar to that of paralytic ileus. The patient frequently may regurgitate small amounts of liquid, his abdomen appears distended, and, as the condition progresses, he may develop symptoms of shock. Acute gastric dilatation is treated by passing a Levin tube to the patient's stomach, applying suction, and removing the gas and fluid. Some surgeons use suction of the gastrointestinal tract routinely to prevent paralytic ileus and acute gastric dilatation.

Pneumonia and Atelectasis

Pneumonia may result from failure to expand the lungs sufficiently, accumulation of fluid in the lungs, which is favored by lying quietly in one position, and by failure to cough up mucus. Patients with chronic respiratory diseases, such as bronchitis, and elderly patients whose breathing has become more shallow are especially susceptible to postoperative pulmonary complications. Pneumonia of this type is sometimes called *hypostatic* or *postoperative pneumonia*. It occurs because the condition of the patient's lungs favors infection (any fluid which stagnates in the body tends to become a culture medium for bacteria) rather than because the patient has been exposed to virulent organisms, such as those that often cause pneumonia in healthy people. Because conditions in the patient's own respiratory system offer so little resistance to infection, it may be set up by organisms normally harbored in his mouth and throat, organisms that usually are not harmful.

The symptoms of pneumonia include fever, cough, expectoration of purulent or blood-streaked sputum, dyspnea and malaise. The treatment involves the use of antibiotics, such as penicillin. If a mucous plug should obstruct a bronchial passageway, causing the part of the lung served by that portion of the bronchial tree to fail to expand normally, this condition is called *atelectasis*. (Since unconsciousness and immobility are important predisposing factors, these complications can develop also in nonsurgical patients.)

The nurse should help the postoperative patient to maintain conditions in his respiratory tract that help to avoid pneumonia and atelectasis. Specifically, she can

• Suction mucus from his nose and mouth while the patient is unconscious.

• Have the patient rid his respiratory tract of mucus by taking deep breaths, coughing and expectorating mucus.

• Help him to change his position frequently.

Thrombophlebitis

When patients lie still for long periods without moving their legs, particularly if there is pressure on their legs from a tight strap or a pillow roll under the knee, venous circulation may be impaired. Blood may flow sluggishly through the veins (venous stasis). This condition predisposes a patient to the development of inflammation, with consequent formation of clots within the veins, a condition called *thrombophlebitis*. There is another condition in which clots form, but in which inflammation is minimal or absent. This is called *phlebothrombosis*. These conditions occur most frequently in the legs. Inflammation helps the clots to adhere to the walls of the veins; therefore, thrombophlebitis is considered to be less dangerous than phlebothrombosis.

Clots that do not stick to the wall of the vein but travel in the blood stream are called *emboli*. By lodging in a distant blood vessel they may obstruct circulation to a vital organ, such as a lung, and cause severe symptoms and even death. For example, a patient with pulmonary embolism may have dyspnea, cough and cyanosis.

The nurse may help to prevent thrombophlebitis by avoiding prolonged pressure on the patient's legs which might impair circulation, and by encouraging him to exercise his legs. Although it is usually necessary to place a restraining strap across the patient's legs during surgery, the use of such straps during the recovery period is not a good practice and, except in unusual situations, is even unnecessary. If the patient is placed in a bed equipped with side rails rather than on a narrow stretcher during his recovery from anesthesia, he can move about without danger of falling. Moreover, on regaining consciousness he will be spared the uncomfortable feeling of finding that his movements are restrained. Often the patient's arm must be restrained because of infusions. To restrain his legs as well will cause him to feel shackled and will increase his restless attempts to free himself.

In contrast with previous nursing practice, pressure on the legs resulting from the placing of pillows under the knees and elevating the knee gatch, and having the patient "dangle" (sit on the edge of his bed, with his legs hanging down over the side) now are avoided. Formerly, these measures were used to relieve strain on the incision and to make the patient more comfortable. But in addition to causing pressure and possibly

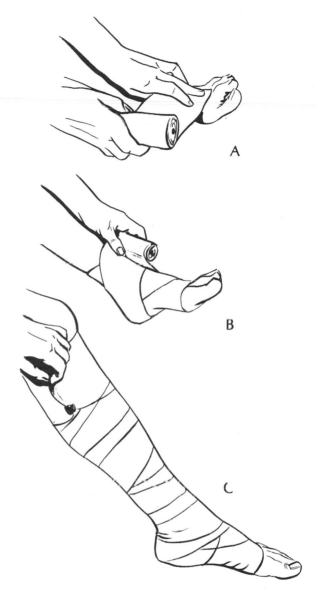

Fig. 12-5. Steps in applying an elastic bandage. (A) Use 4-inch bandages, starting as close to toes as possible to assure maximal venous return. (B) Anchor bandage around ankle, completely covering heel. (C) Overlap one-half to two-thirds of bandage. Continue wrapping to knee or thigh. Use additional bandages as needed. Secure with fasteners.

interfering with circulation, these practices discouraged movement and exercise of the legs. Providing support for the veins by wrapping both legs with Ace bandages from the ankle to the midthigh also is considered helpful in preventing thrombophlebitis.

Exercises. Unless the physician leaves orders to the contrary, postoperative patients should begin to move their legs as soon as consciousness returns. These exercises are not complicated, can be taught readily by the nurse during the preoperative period and then reviewed with the patient postoperatively. Instruct the patient to move his toes and his feet, alternately flexing and extending them. Then have him flex and extend his legs by bending his knees and then straightening his legs. These exercises should be repeated regularly. It is much more effective to advise the patient, "Exercise each leg the way I have shown you 10 times every hour," than to say, "Move your legs as much as you can." Remind the patient to exercise each time that you check vital signs. If he is still sleepy from anesthesia, he cannot be expected to remember to do exercises.

Wound Infection

The postoperative patient must be observed carefully for symptoms of wound infection. The first symptom may be increasing pain in the incision. (In normal recovery pain in the incision decreases.) Other symptoms of wound infection include localized heat, redness, swelling and purulent exudate. Systemic symptoms of infection include fever, chills, headache, and anorexia.

If a patient develops wound infection, every precaution must be taken to prevent the spread of the infection to others. The rational use of medical aseptic technic is essential in preventing the spread of infection.

The treatment of wound infections involves local and parenteral use of antibiotics, measures to drain pus, if any, and maintenance of the patient's resistance through rest and nutritious diet. Local applications of heat, such as hot compresses, sometimes are ordered to bring more blood to the part to help fight infection.

Wound Disruption

Dehiscence means the separation of wound edges without the protrusion of organs. *Evisceration* means the separation of wound edges with the protrusion of organs. These complications are most likely to occur between the 6th and the 8th postoperative days, when the sutures hold the wound less firmly, and the wound itself may not yet be strong enough to hold the edges together. Predisposing factors include those that interfere with normal healing, such as malnutrition (particularly insufficient protein and vitamin C), defective suturing, or unusual strain on the wound from severe coughing, sneezing, retching or hiccups.

The patient may say that he has a sensation of something "giving way." Pinkish drainage may appear suddenly on the dressing. If you suspect that wound disruption has occurred, place the patient at complete rest in a position that puts the least strain on the operative area. If evisceration has occurred, place sterile dressings moistened with sterile normal saline over the protruding organs. Report the symptoms immediately. Emotional support and reassurance are as necessary as in any other emergency. You might say, "Just lie there very quietly. I'm going to ask Dr. Jones to check your dressing. I'll be right back."

EARLY AMBULATION

The term *early ambulation* is used widely to describe one aspect of postoperative treatment. *Ambulation* means walking. The patient is helped to walk about early in his postoperative period.

Help the patient to a sitting position at the side of the bed. If dizziness is more than momentary, help him to lie down again. Stand right at the bedside so that he will not fear tumbling to the floor. The nonadjustable hospital bed is much farther from the floor than the usual bed. If the height of the bed can be adjusted, place it in the lowest position possible. If this type of bed is not available, use a footstool. While you support the patient firmly with one hand under his axilla and the other on his forearm, let him step to the floor and take 1 or 2 steps to the chair. He may be surprised to find that he can accomplish the walk within hours of having been on the operating table without having all his stitches pop open.

The exercise and the erect posture help the patient to breathe more deeply, and the change of position helps to prevent congestion of the lungs with fluid. Walking stimulates circulation in the lower extremities, thus lessening the problem of venous stasis. Erect posture and exercise also help to overcome problems of urinary retention, constipation and distention. Early ambulation helps patients to regain their appetites, and greater activity during the day helps them to sleep better at night. Several important points are:

• Early ambulation is a therapeutic measure. Its primary purpose is to prevent complications.

• Although early ambulation helps the patient to become self-sufficient more quickly, he continues to need attention and psychological support from the nurse in ways that do not interfere with his being up and about.

She is still very much needed—to give skin care, backrubs, advice, attention to diet, and to help him to carry out gradually more of his own care and to plan periods of rest and activity.

• Ambulation means walking, not sitting. Frequently the treatment is misunderstood to mean just getting out of bed, and the patient is assisted to a chair in the morning, where he sits until evening! Prolonged sitting, by putting pressure on the legs, may predispose a patient to thrombophlebitis. The patient should sit for short periods, take frequent short walks, and alternate these with resting in bed.

• Walking soon after surgery often causes the patient pain and apprehension. He needs a great deal of explanation about the purpose of the treatment, so that he does not consider it merely a lack of attention or concern for his comfort.

• Special equipment, like catheters and infusion bottles, need not restrict the patient to bed. However, their management does require some ingenuity, so that the treatment may be continued safely and effectively while the patient is out of bed.

• Having plenty of assistance will add greatly to the patient's confidence, as well as ensure his safety. Don't hesitate to ask a male nursing assistant or another nurse to help you, particularly if it is the patient's first time out of bed, or if the patient is aged.

Early ambulation helps the patient to feel less helpless, and it tells him that he is recovering quickly and satisfactorily from his operation. One of the dangers of early ambulation is this same confidence. Because patients look more self-sufficient, they themselves may be misled to walking down a hospital hall that is too long, returning to work too soon, resuming their full routine or going on a camping trip before they have recuperated sufficiently.

VISITORS

The patient's relatives usually feel less worried when they are kept informed of the patient's condition, given opportunities to express their interest and concern, and allowed to participate, when possible, in the patient's care.

Seeing the patient, if only for a few moments, often does a great deal to assure a relative that the patient really is all right—that he actually has come through the operation. Careful explanation of what to expect (for example, that the patient is drowsy or confused, or that he is receiving intravenous fluids) is essential in lessening apprehension. A brief visit from a relative just after surgery often assures the patient that his family is there, and that they are concerned about him.

Although visitors usually are not permitted in the recovery room, it is important to keep family members informed of the patient's condition and of the time when he returns to his own room. Some hospitals provide a visitors' lounge adjacent to the area of the operating room and the recovery room. Opportunities for contact with the staff are fostered by such an arrangement because of its convenience to all concerned. If the surgeons and the nurses know that the family are nearby, they can more easily stop to speak to them. The provision of such areas for the family conveys concern for them as well as for the patient. Such an arrangement is in marked contrast with the still prevalent practice of providing no particular place for the families of patients to wait during the surgery and recovery period. Especially in multiple-bed rooms the presence of the family over an extended period can be disturbing to the other patients.

It is sometimes possible and desirable to allow a responsible member of the family to sit quietly beside the patient during the early postoperative period. Having a member of the family near is especially helpful if the patient is aged or extremely apprehensive, or if he is unable to speak English.

REFERENCES AND BIBLIOGRAPHY

ADLER, R. H., and BRODIE, S. L.: Postoperative rebreathing aid, *Am. J. Nurs.* 68:1287, June, 1968.

ALDRICH, C. K.: *An Introduction to Dynamic Psychiatry,* Chap. 9, The later years, p. 204, New York, McGraw-Hill, 1966.

ALEXANDER, E. L.: *Care of the Patient in Surgery, Including Techniques,* ed. 4, St. Louis, Mosby, 1967.

AYRES, S. M., and GIANNELLI, S., JR.: *Care of the Critically Ill,* New York, Appleton-Century-Crofts, 1967.

BENDIXEN, H., *et al.: Respiratory Care,* St. Louis, Mosby, 1965.

BERNZWEIS, J. D.: *Nurse's Liability for Malpractice: A Programmed Course,* New York, McGraw-Hill, 1969.

BORDICKS, K. J.: *Nursing Care of Patients Having Chest Surgery,* New York, Macmillan, 1962.

BRUNNER, L. S., *et al.: Textbook of Medical-Surgical Nursing,* ed. 2, Philadelphia, Lippincott, 1970.

BURGESS, M. G.: Nursing care plan for the postoperative patient in the recovery room and intensive care unit, *Nurs. Clin. N. Am.* 3:499–502, September, 1968.

CARNES, M. A.: Postanesthetic complications, *Nurs. Forum* 4:46–55, 1965.

CLEMONS, B.: The OR nurse in the patient-care circuit, *Am. J. Nurs.* 68:2141, October, 1968.

DUMAS, R. G., and LEONARD, R. C.: The effect of nursing and the incidence of vomiting, *Nurs. Res.* 12:12, Winter, 1963.

DURRANT, C. W.: Postanesthetic suggestion, *J. Am. Ass. Nurs. Anesth.* 36:35–42, February, 1968.

GIBBON, J. H. (ed.): *Surgery of the Chest*, Philadelphia, Saunders, 1962.

GREGG, D. E.: Anxiety—a factor in nursing care, *Am. J. Nurs.* 52:1363–1365, 1952.

HEALY, K.: Does preoperative instruction make a difference? *Am. J. Nurs.* 68:62–67, January, 1968.

HOELLER, SR. MARY LOUISE: Visible file improves O.R. schedule, *Hosp. Prog.* 15:84, 1959.

————: *The Operating Room Technician*, ed. 2, St. Louis, Mosby, 1968.

INGALL, J. R.: That much discussed preoperative visit, *AORN* 5:44–46, February, 1967.

JARVIS, D.: Following open heart surgery, *Am. J. Nurs.* 70:2591, 1970.

JOHNSON, J. E.: The influence of purposeful nurse-patient interaction on the patient's postoperative course, *ANA Reg. Clin. Conf.* 2:16–22, 1965.

LESNIK, J. J., and ANDERSON, B. E.: *Nursing Practice and the Law*, ed. 2, rev., Philadelphia, Lippincott, 1962.

LYNCH, J. D.: Anxiety and anxiety reduction in surgical patients, *AORN* 6:58–60, July, 1967.

McCARTHY, R. T.: Vomiting, *Nurs. Forum* 3:49, 1964.

MONTEIRO, L. A.: Tape recorded conversations: a method to increase patient teaching, *Nurs. Res.* 14:335–40, Fall, 1965.

O'BRIEN, M. J.: The reaction of coronary patients to the sacrament of the sick, *Cath. Nurse* 16:36–43, June, 1968.

PAYNE, J. P.: Modern concepts of anesthesia, *Nurs. Mirror* 121:242–44, November, 1965.

RODMAN, M., and SMITH, D. W.: *Pharmacology and Drug Therapy in Nursing*, Philadelphia, Lippincott, 1968.

SARNER, H.: *The Nurse and the Law*, Philadelphia, Saunders, 1968.

SUTTON, A. L.: *Bedside Nursing Techniques in Medicine and Surgery*, ed. 2, Philadelphia, Saunders, 1969.

TITCHENER, J. L., and LEVINE, M.: *Surgery as a Human Experience*, New York, Oxford University Press, 1960.

TODD, J. C.: Wound infection: Etiology, prevention and management, *Surg. Clin. N. Am.* 48:787, August, 1968.

VILJOEN, J. F.: Postoperative-respiratory adequacy affected by drugs, positioning, *Hosp. Top.* 46:95–6, May, 1968.

WIEDENBACH, E.: *Clinical Nursing: A Helping Art*, New York, Springer, 1964.

ZEPERNICK, R. G.: New trends in anesthesia, *Nurs. Forum* 4:41–45, 1965.

Care of the Patient with Cancer

13

Pathology and Epidemiology · Etiology · Symptoms
Diagnosis of Cancer · Treatment · Prevention and Control
The Patient's Reaction to Diagnosis · Nursing the Patient
with Cancer

PATHOLOGY AND EPIDEMIOLOGY

For reasons that continue to confound scientists, certain body cells sometimes undergo changes in their structure and appearance; they begin to multiply and give rise to a colony of cancer cells. They may arise in any part of the body, at any time, and from any cell that can proliferate. They multiply rapidly, invading and destroying surrounding normal tissues by pressure and competing with normal cells for nutrients and oxygen. Cancer cells, though changed in appearance, usually retain enough resemblance to the tissues from which they arose to be recognized, if found, in any other part of the body. For example, if a tumor from the neck shows malignant cells arising from breast tissues, it is recognized as having spread from the breast. Sometimes the secondary tumor is found even before the primary tumor has been discovered.

Although all forms of malignant growth may be referred to as cancer, more specific terms are used to describe the particular types of cells that have undergone malignant transformation. The suffix "oma" refers to new growth or tumor. Two of the more common terms are:

Carcinoma—a malignant tumor arising from epithelial tissues.
Sarcoma—a malignant tumor arising from connective tissues.

Malignant tumors may arise from any or all three embryonal tissues. When a tumor contains all three embryonal components it is referred to as a teratoma.

The embryonal tissues are as follows:

Ectoderm—outer layer of the embryo—which produces the skin and nervous system.
Mesoderm—middle layer of the embryo—which produces the bones, cartilage, muscle, fat, blood and all other connective tissues.
Endoderm—inner layer of the embryo—which produces the linings of the gastrointestinal tract, respiratory system, spleen, liver etc.

It is customary to name tumors after the types of tissues from which the tumors arise. Over the past century at least 100 different cancers have been identified. This number can be increased if finer morphologic details are elaborated. Sometimes the cell disorganization is so complete that no recognizable cell structure remains. This is referred to as anaplasia. Some examples of the names of tumors, related to the types of tissue from which they arise, are:

Tissue	Malignant Tumor
Epithelial	Squamous cell carcinoma
	Malignant melanoma
	Adenocarcinoma
Connective	Liposarcoma
	Osteogenic sarcoma

Malignant tumors differ from benign tumors in several ways. Benign tumors are usually encapsulated while malignant tumors tend to infiltrate surrounding tissues and even metastasize. Breast cancer for example shows a special predilection for metastasizing to the lungs or bone. Cancer is known to spread to the lymph

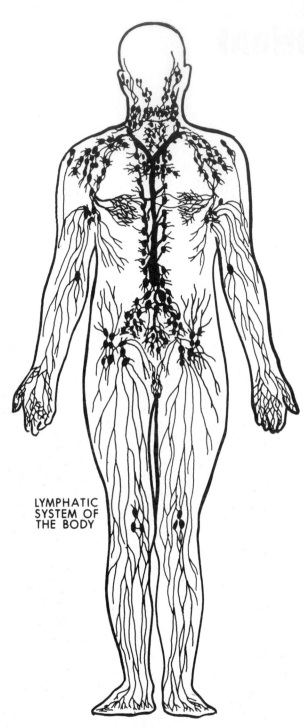

LYMPHATIC
SYSTEM OF
THE BODY

FIG. 13-1. One route by which malignant cells can spread to other areas of the body is the lymphatic system. Cancer cells can also be carried by the blood.

nodes that drain the tumor area. For this reason a lymph node dissection is often performed in addition to wide excision of the tumor (Fig. 13-1).

Cancer can spread by:

- Direct extension to adjacent tissues
- Extension from lymph vessels into the tissues which lie alongside lymphatic vessels
- Being carried in the stream of lymph or blood, often to distant sites (embolism)
- Diffusion within a body cavity

The area in which malignant cells first arise is called the primary site. The regions of the body to which cancer cells are spread are termed secondary or metastatic sites. The metastasis phenomenon is one of the most discouraging characteristics of cancer. Even one malignant cell can start a metastatic lesion in a distant part of the body. Today, however, these metastases are treated aggressively with one of the three modalities of therapy or a combination of two or all three; as a result, we now have more long-term survivors. The importance of good follow-up care with an interval history and physical examination must be emphasized to the patient and his family.

Benign tumors remain at the original site of their development. They may grow larger, but their rate of growth is slower than that of malignant tumors. Benign tumors usually do not cause death unless their location impairs the function of a vital organ, for example: thymoma, meningioma. On the other hand malignant tumors grow rapidly and unless they are removed completely before metastases have occurred they are likely to spread widely so that palliative therapy may be the only form of treatment available and death will occur sooner than necessary.

The term cancer is associated often with a solid tumor, e.g., a breast tumor. There are other conditions which do not involve solid tumor formation. For instance, in leukemia malignant cells aggregate and produce infiltrates (sometimes referred to as soft tumors). These infiltrates may concentrate anywhere in the body and produce such symptoms as pain, seizure and bleeding. Leukemia is characterized by the maturation arrest of a certain type of white or red blood cell (erythroleukemia) at the blast or stem cell level. The disease process is not completely reversible even with the ever increasing newer chemotherapeutic drugs. Although today the patients live longer and are more comfor-

Fig. 13-2. Cancer incidence by site and sex. (The American Cancer Society)

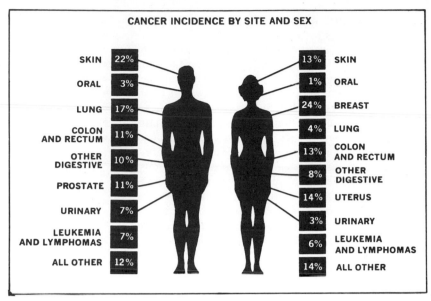

CANCER INCIDENCE BY SITE AND SEX

SKIN 22%	13% SKIN
ORAL 3%	1% ORAL
LUNG 17%	24% BREAST
COLON AND RECTUM 11%	4% LUNG
OTHER DIGESTIVE 10%	13% COLON AND RECTUM
PROSTATE 11%	8% OTHER DIGESTIVE
URINARY 7%	14% UTERUS
LEUKEMIA AND LYMPHOMAS 7%	3% URINARY
ALL OTHER 12%	6% LEUKEMIA AND LYMPHOMAS
	14% ALL OTHER

TABLE 13-1. CHARACTERISTICS OF TUMORS

BENIGN	MALIGNANT
1. Grow slowly.	1. Grow rapidly.
2. Often encapsulated.	2. Rarely encapsulated.
3. Do not infiltrate surrounding tissues.	3. Infiltrate surrounding tissues.
4. Remain localized.	4. Metastasize via lymphatic or blood vessels.
5. Usually no recurrence after surgical extirpation.	5. May recur after surgical extirpation.
6. Cells well differentiated in resembling those of parent tissues.	6. Cells are not well differentiated and may be anaplastic.
7. Produce minimal tissue destruction.	7. Produce extensive tissue destruction generally.
8. Do not cause death as a rule except when the size and position impair a vital function.	8. May cause death unless treated aggressively and early.
9. Do not produce cachexia.	9. Produce typical cachexia.

table, the disease is progressive and fatal.

Cancer can occur at any age. However, it is more common after the age of 40. Youth, however is no guarantee against cancer. Cancer is now the second leading cause of death in children, second only to trauma.

ETIOLOGY

So far the cause of cancer has eluded definite determination. Much stress is being placed on early detection but not enough stress is being placed upon the prevention of cancer which in some instances is preventable.

Cancer is considered as a large category of diseases all of which are concerned with the spread of malignant cells. There is question about whether one cause or a combination of causes is responsible for the development of cancer. Much investigation concerning the inci-

dence of cancer and its relation to possible causative factors is being carried out.

Environmental and social factors strongly influence the incidence of some types of cancers. Cancer of the cervix is more frequent in the lower socioeconomic group. The incidence of lung and stomach cancer in men in the lower socioeconomic group is higher than among those in the highest income group. Skin cancers are the most common of all cancers and are often induced by prolonged exposure to sunlight. Fortunately, such cancers are easy to detect and are highly curable. Physical agents such as X-rays and gamma radiations are well established causes of squamous cell and bone sarcomas. Cutting oils and other chemicals have been known to produce skin cancers in industrial workers. The inhalation of cigarette smoke over a period of many years has been implicated as a major cause of lung, pharyngeal, oral, and laryngeal cancers.

Some factors are thought to predispose to cancer. Leukoplakia of the mouth or genitals, for instance, may remain benign or undergo malignant change, and should be removed when feasible. Extensive research is being conducted in an effort to determine whether cancer in humans can be caused by viruses. No virus has yet been identified with the causation of human cancer, although viruses have caused cancer in animals. Parasites have been implicated in the development of cancer of the colon, bladder and liver in Near Eastern countries where schistosomiasis is endemic. Some researchers believe that the development of cancer is related to emotional factors. Numerous studies indicate that symptoms of cancer often appear after an individual has experienced significant personal loss (Kissen and LeShan).

It is considered likely that cancer occurs only when a certain combination of factors favors its development. These factors may include heredity, hormonal state and exposure to carcinogens. In addition to efforts to find the causes of cancer, attempts are being made to understand factors that affect host resistance in the hope that susceptibility to the development of cancer can be decreased.

SYMPTOMS

Cancer is an insidious disease that tends to develop slowly and with few or no early symptoms. Every effort must be made to discover it in its earliest stage, for early discovery facilitates complete extirpation and a good prognosis. It is now believed that cancer may develop even more slowly than was originally believed. Cancer cells may exist in the body (in situ) for many years without causing symptoms. According to one theory, if host resistance is good, these cells will not multiply and cause disease, but if conditions are favorable to malignant growth, the cells will multiply and cause symptoms. Two examples of this are the malignant cells present in the sputum of mine workers long before there is evidence of lung cancer and the malignant cells present in the cervix long before there is evidence of cancer. A routine "Pap" smear will disclose the presence of preclinical cancer.

Everyone should be familiar with the 7 warning signals of cancer listed by the American Cancer Society.

- A sore that does not heal
- A lump or thickening in the breast or elsewhere
- Unusual bleeding or discharge
- Any change in a wart or mole
- Persistent indigestion or difficulty in swallowing
- Persistent hoarseness or cough
- Any change in normal bowel habits.

If the disease progresses untreated, pain, weakness, weight loss and anemia are characteristic. However these symptoms frequently do not appear until late in the disease. Delay in seeking medical attention is still common. We need to direct our attention to early diagnosis and treatment and to place emphasis on the prevention and avoidance of cancer. We must teach people that cancer can arise from self neglect. Cachexia is generally characteristic during the terminal stages of cancer.

Other symptoms relate to the disturbed function of the part of the body that is affected. Intestinal cancer may cause partial or complete obstruction, cancer of the larynx typically causes hoarseness. These symptoms are discussed more fully in later chapters dealing with specific organs involved.

DIAGNOSIS OF CANCER

The diagnosis of cancer begins with the recognition that cancer may assume many forms and guises. Sometimes the symptoms are so typical that the patient proclaims the diagnosis himself. At other times the doctor's suspicion is aroused by an apparently minor condition that does not respond to therapy.

A complete regular physical examination is the first weapon in the struggle to discover cancer in its early stages. Every physician's office, clinic, and industrial clinic should be a cancer detection center. With effective team work the doctor, nurse, laboratory technicians, and others, can make the cancer detection examination a simple, routine, and sometimes, a life-saving procedure.

A pelvic examination should be a part of every woman's physical examination. In situ cancers can be discovered early with the proper application of the "Pap" smears. Sputum examinations should be performed on all patients with a history of cough. Cytologic tests are performed to detect cancer cells that have been shed from malignant tissue. These tests are useful because in the normal scaling or "exfoliation" of

Fig. 13-3. Appearance typical of cachectic patient.

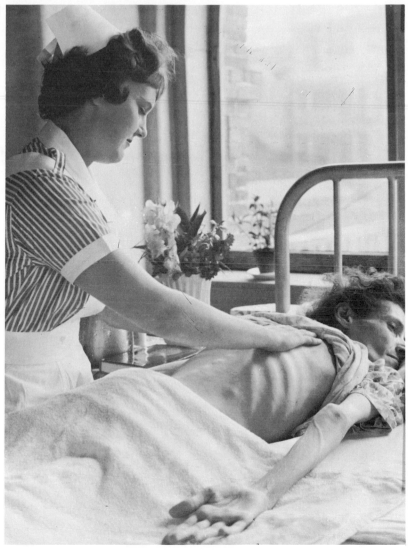

epithelial cells, malignant cells may also be present in the secretions after they have been shed from a malignant lesion. Cytologic tests are now widely used, especially among groups where the risk of developing cancer is high. The patient at this time usually shows no symptoms of illness, thus it is possible to diagnose the disease in an earlier stage. Cytologic tests are called "Pap" or Papanicolaou tests in recognition of the doctor who developed this important technic.

TREATMENT

Complete destruction or removal of malignant tissue is the only cure for cancer. There are three forms of therapy available for the patient with cancer: surgery, radiation therapy and chemotherapy.

Surgical treatment involves wide excision of the tumor and the node-bearing areas to which the disease might have spread. The need to remove all of the malignant tissue sometimes necessitates radical or disfiguring surgery or surgery that results in the alteration of body function, such as an opening of the colon on the abdomen (colostomy), or removal of the larynx (laryngectomy). In later chapters specific types of operations will be discussed in relation to the part of the body affected.

Radiation therapy is used to destroy cancer tissue. Some forms of cancer are destroyed readily by radiation. The location of the tumor and its radiosensitivity help determine the usefulness of this form of treatment. Radiation therapy is given to cure, palliate or control the spread of

TABLE 13-2. ANTINEOPLASTIC AGENTS*

GENERIC OR OFFICIAL NAME	SYNONYM OR PROPRIETARY NAME	USUAL DOSAGE RANGE
Alkylating Agents		
Busulfan U.S.P.	Myleran	1 to 6 mg. orally
Chlorambucil U.S.P.	Leukeran	2 to 12 mg. orally
Cyclophosphamide N.F.	Cytoxan	100 mg. orally maintenance
Mechlorethamine U.S.P.	Mustargen; Nitrogen mustard	200 to 600 mcg./Kg. I.V.
Melphalan	Alkeran; 1-Phenylalanine mustard	6 mg. orally; then regulated in accordance with weekly blood counts
Pipobroman	Vercyte	1 mg./Kg. per day orally initially; 0.1 to 0.2 mg. per day maintenance
Thiotepa U.S.P.	Thio-TEPA; TESPA, etc.	Up to 200 mcg./Kg. parenterally
Triethylenemelamine N.F.	TEM	2.5 mg. daily for 2 or 3 days; then 0.5 to 5 mg. weekly
Uracil mustard	—	1 mg. daily orally maintenance
Antimetabolites		
Cytarabine Cytosar	—	0.5 to 4 mg./Kg. per day, depending upon the patient's response and the method of administration which may be by rapid I.V. or slow I.V. infusion, or subcutaneously
Fluorouracil	—	7.5 to 15 mg./Kg. by intravenous infusion, up to a maximum daily dose of 1 Gm.
Mercaptopurine	Purinethol	2.5 mg./Kg. orally
Methotrexate	Amethopterin	Children 2.5 to 5.0 mg./Kg. orally or parenterally. Adults 5 to 30 mg./Kg. orally or parenterally
Thioguanine	—	2 to 3 mg./Kg. orally per day
Alkaloids and Antibiotics		
Dactinomycin	Actinomycin D; Cosmegen	Adults 0.5 mg. I.V. daily for up to 5 days. Children 15 mcg./Kg. daily for 5 days
Mithramycin	Mithracin	25 to 30 mcg./Kg. per day I.V.
Vinblastine sulfate	Velban	0.1 mg./Kg. increased up to 0.5 mg./Kg. I.V. no oftener than once every 7 days
Vincristine sulfate	Oncovin	2 mg./sq. meter of body surface per week intravenously
Radioactive Isotopes		
Radio-gold Solution Au[198]	Aurocoloid; Aureotope	35 to 150 millicuries parenterally
Sodium Iodide I[131] Capsules and Solution U.S.P.	Theriodide; Oriodide; Radiocaps; Tracervial	Oral or I.V., the equivalent of 1 to 100 millicuries for therapy, or 1 to 100 microcuries for diagnosis
Sodium Phosphate P[32] Solution U.S.P.	—	Oral or I.V., the equivalent of 1 to 5 millicuries for therapy, or 250 microcuries to 1 millicurie for diagnosis
Miscellaneous		
Hydroxyurea	Hydrea	*Intermittent therapy:* 80 mg./Kg. orally as a single dose every third day. *Continuous therapy:* 20 to 30 mg. orally as a single dose daily
Procarbazine HCl	Matulane	50 mg. to 300 mg. per day orally
Quinacrine HCl U.S.P.	Atabrine	200 to 1,000 mg. daily by intracavitary (intrapleural or intraperitoneal instillation)
Urethan	Ethyl carbamate	3 to 6 Gm. orally daily

* Modified from Rodman, M. J., and Smith, D. W.: *Pharmacology and Drug Therapy in Nursing,* Philadelphia, Lippincott, 1968.

cancers. Some destruction of normal tissues around the tumor also occurs. This is inevitable if the tumor is to be completely treated by radiation.

It is known that increased oxygenation of poorly oxygenated malignant cells increases their susceptibility to radiation therapy. For this reason, some patients with cancer are being treated with a combination of radiation therapy and hyperbaric oxygen therapy. Hyperbaric oxygen therapy provides oxygen in an atmosphere at increased atmospheric pressure, resulting in an increased amount of oxygen being dissolved in body tissues and body fluids. This treatment is administered in a special pressure chamber which resembles an iron lung, and accommodates the patient. There are several different types of hyperbaric oxygen chambers. The principle of treatment, however, remains the same.

Chemotherapy. With the exception of many cures for choriocarcinoma with methotrexate and actinomycin D, no drugs have been discovered so far that can cure cancer (Shimkin). Some drugs can slow down the progress of the disease and provide relief. Patients with leukemia and lymphoma are living longer and more comfortably thanks to some of the newer chemotherapeutic drugs and better medical management. Chemotherapeutic drugs are toxic to normal cells, or they disturb the body's hormone balance. Much research is being done to discover drugs that destroy malignant cells without harming normal cells.

Several types of drugs are used: Alkylating agents, such as nitrogen mustard, are injurious to cells, particularly to the rapidly proliferating cancer cells. It is believed that this action results from reaction of the alkylating agent with the nucleic acids in the cells. Antimetabolites of which folic acid antagonists are examples, interfere with cell growth and metabolism. Methotrexate and 6-mercaptopurine are examples of folic acid antagonists.

Both of these groups are potentially dangerous. Depression of the bone marrow, oral ulceration, nausea, vomiting, and diarrhea are some of the toxic effects encountered. The usefulness of these drugs lies in the greater susceptibility of malignant cells to their effects and their ability to exercise some control over the malignant process.

Vincristine and vinblastine are derived from a species of the periwinkle plant. The mechanism of their action is to produce mitotic arrest

and thus prevent new cancer cells from forming. Side effects from this group of drugs are bone marrow depression areflexia, and muscular weakness.

Dosage of antineoplastic drugs is carefully adapted to the patient's particular form of disease and his response to the drug. Bone marrow depression resulting in decreased numbers of blood cells such as leukocytes is watched for by periodic blood counts. If the depression is marked, the chemotherapist may wish to modify the dosage or temporarily discontinue the drug, until the bone marrow recovers. Many chemotherapeutic drugs are not effective until toxic levels have been reached. The dosage of the drug is in large part determined by the patient's weight in kilograms. It is important therefore to weigh the patient at the same time each day, for example before breakfast, using the same scale and wearing the same attire.

The nurse's role in care of the patient receiving chemotherapy for cancer involves observation for toxic effects of the drugs, using nursing measures to lessen discomfort caused by drug therapy, explaining (within the framework already established by the physician) the purpose of the drugs and how the patient may participate to receive the best results possible, and supporting the patient emotionally during this treatment. For example, the patient receiving fluorouracil may experience diarrhea as a result of taking this chemotherapeutic agent. The nurse's role involves noting and reporting the symptoms, and using measures to promote cleanliness, relieve anal irritation, and provide ready access to bathroom or bedpan, as well as helping the patient to recognize that this unpleasant side-effect is but a part of the drug's effects; that its use also involves helping him combat the illness. During such explanations it is essential to use terminology which has been agreed upon by all members of the health team, so that there is a coordinated approach to the patient. Sometimes the patient is told some of the truth, but not the whole truth. He may be told that the drug is being used to arrest his disease, but he may not be told that this effect of the drug probably will be only temporary (if this is the case). Such decisions must be based on the individual patient's situation and needs.

Hormones. Certain hormones slow the growth of malignant cells by providing a less favorable environment for their growth. For example, men with disseminated prostatic cancer may have symptomatic improvement when the effects of male hormones are counteracted. This counteraction is achieved by the administration of estrogens to the male patient or by removal of the testes (bilateral orchiectomy).

Adrenal steroid hormones (ACTH and cortisone) are used in the palliation of cancer. By a mechanism not fully understood, they inhibit proliferation of malignant cells temporarily, providing symptomatic relief.

Supportive Therapy. Transfusions of whole blood, platelets, fluids, electrolytes, drugs for the relief of pain, high protein and high vitamin diet are all important in the supportive therapy for the patient with cancer.

PREVENTION AND CONTROL

Educating the Public. Public education has accomplished a great deal to encourage the awareness of warning signals and the willingness to seek diagnosis and treatment. Today more women are aware of the need to seek early treatment for breast tumor or abnormal vaginal bleeding. Some people have become so fearful of cancer that every symptom, however minor or transient, causes near panic. Such reactions do not indicate less need for public education. On the contrary, this points to the extreme fear that people have of cancer and the need for continued education in the ways by which cancer can be controlled and cured. These reactions emphasize the importance of teaching in a manner that does not provoke needless alarm. People who are very frightened may react with apathy. Patients who refuse to go to doctors or clinics are not necessarily uninterested or even uninformed. Their fear of cancer may be so great that they are unable to face examination and the possible discovery that they have cancer.

Besides teaching the 7 warning signals of cancer and advising early diagnosis and treatment, nurses can encourage people to avoid practices believed to favor the development of cancer. Nurses can help people to correct misconceptions about cancer. Some people still believe cancer to be contagious even though no evidence to support this belief has been found. Another misconception involves cancer odor. With the use of power sprays and radiation therapy for ulcerating wounds one rarely encounters the odor that used to be prevalent in cancer wards many years ago. Today's cancer hospital looks and smells no different from the general hospitals in the community. Much is being done also to maintain the nutrition of the patient with incurable cancer so that the patient does not develop the severe cachexia that used to distinguish the patient with cancer from other patients. Patients with cancer are no longer segregated or consigned to some back ward of the general hospital as they once were. This change has come about slowly as a result of public education and improved therapy.

THE PATIENT'S REACTION TO THE DIAGNOSIS

Illness other than cancer can cause death and disability. Most patients with heat disease know their diagnosis, and heart disease outranks cancer as a cause of death in our country. Why, then, does the question of knowing the true diagnosis loom so large in the care of the cancer patient? Most people associate cancer with a lingering, painful death. This accounts for some of the widespread discussion over the advisability of telling cancer patients their diagnosis. Early diagnosis and modern treatment have altered this grim picture substantially. Today many patients with cancer can be cured. Others have had their lives extended and made more comfortable by advances in therapy. The new advances in therapy are changing the old attitudes towards the disease. The problem of "telling or not telling" reflects not only the nature of the disease, but individual attitudes toward it.

Probably there is no one best way of answering the question, "should the patient be told?" Much depends upon the patient's personality and his ability to cope with stress. Most will agree that the patient whose inner resources enable him to cope with the diagnosis should be told, and that the patient who is likely to react with panic or depression should not. Determining beforehand how the patient is likely to respond is the problem. Sometimes several people who know the patient well discuss the problem and decide. For example, the patient's doctor, pastor and family can discuss the pros and cons of whether the patient should be told. Sometimes the doctor informs the family fully and leaves up to them the decision concerning what to tell the patient. In other situations the doctor assumes entire responsibility for deciding what and how much to tell the patient. Often the decision is left to the patient himself, in the sense that he is given the information he specifically requests.

How does this affect the nurse? She may or may not have a part in making the decision.

If she is asked, she must suggest what she believes is best for that particular patient, whether or not this decision is what she would want done for her in like circumstances. Often nurses do not participate in making the decision. In such instances, they must accept the decision of others and be guided by it. Inconsistency and conflict among those who care for the patient are extremely upsetting to him. If he is told he has arthritis, everyone should know this decision and be guided accordingly. It is always a good idea to have this information in the nursing care plan so that all staff members will be aware of just what the patient was told.

The approach used initially may need to be modified later on. The depression of one patient on being told that he had cancer became so great that he could neither sleep nor eat. After a conference with the staff and the family, the patient was told that further tests had shown he did not have cancer. Eagerly accepting this explanation, he became calmer and more optimistic. Another patient who was told merely that he had a tumor seemed to be satisfied at first, but later began asking everyone whether he had cancer. After his doctor frankly discussed the diagnosis with him, the patient became more composed and showed more confidence in the staff. It is important not only to know what decision has been made and to work within the limits of that decision, but also to observe and report the patient's reaction to it so that the plan can be changed as necessary.

NURSING THE PATIENT WITH CANCER

The nursing needs of the patient with cancer are varied and complex. They depend on his and his family's reaction to the diagnosis of cancer, the location and consequent impairment of body functions that may result from the disease or its treatment, the stage of the disease and the prognosis. The quality of the care the patient receives depends not only on the scientific advances in drug therapy, surgery, radiotherapy, and on the availability of equipment, but also on the attitudes towards cancer of those who take care of him. To know how she feels about the disease is important to a nurse as the first step in working with the patient. Most patients with cancer are extremely sensitive. They can detect any insecurity and distaste on the part of the nurse as she performs her duties. If her attitude is calm, able and understanding, the patient's confidence in her will help in his rehabilitation.

In similar vein, the nurse's attitude and care of the patient also affect the patient's view of the staff generally, and his responsiveness to therapy. Each staff member's actions and attitudes are important and affect the patient's response to others on the health team.

A matter of particular concern involves communication among those who care for the patient. Evasion and subterfuge are common, lessening the patient's confidence in those who care for him. Two guidelines can help the nurse in communicating with the patient, and with colleagues.

• Do not avoid the patient's questions and concerns. Let him express them without being interrupted, or having the subject changed. When you have heard a patient's question, decide whether it is one which you can, and should answer. Remember that because a patient asks a question, it does not follow that you must answer it. But you can help him to find the answer, or refer him to the appropriate person with whom to discuss it. For instance explanation of the diagnosis and plan of therapy is the responsibility of the physician.

• Be clear about what others, particularly the physician, have explained to the patient. Ideally such matters should be discussed regularly among all staff. But since in many instances regular staff conferences are not yet established, it is essential to take the initiative in establishing such communication. It is unwise to work with any patient without knowing the framework of explanation given to him by the physician. However, with the cancer patient it is especially necessary that communication be kept open among all who care for the patient. Sensitivity and judgment are required concerning what to tell the patient, in order to promote his comfort and well-being.

Helping the patient maintain dignity and equanimity is important. Perhaps in no other disease is there such a threat to "wholeness" as exists in cancer. The disease itself and the treatment are often destructive of tissue, and sometimes disfiguring. Some patients who know they have cancer state that they fear the pain or disfigurement or any other specific aspect of the illness not so much as they fear possible overall loss of self control and dignity during the final stages of the illness. The nurse must not lose sight of this important concern of her patients. The process of physical care is often demanding: tubes to keep patent, skin care, and many other tasks which can tax the resources of the nursing staff. Every effort should be directed towards helping the patient maintain his self-respect. Care in draping him during treatments, strict attention to cleanliness, allowing him to participate in planning his care as long as he is able to do so are all measures to help him maintain his dignity. It is essential for the nurse to assist the patient and his family to recognize that a diagnosis of cancer is not synonymous with death, to help them avail themselves of available treatment, and to establish a regimen which encourages as full a return to usual activities as possible. The patient who is physically able to continue working is encouraged to do so, as well as to continue his usual home life and recreation. Family members can assist the patient as they themselves are helped by professional staff to realize that the patient is likely to benefit (as will those in close association with him) if he is encouraged to live as full a life as possible. Patients who have cancer and who nevertheless continue most of their usual activities have many realistic concerns. The nurse can help by listening, clarifying, and assisting the patient and family to find their own solutions.

More patients are being cured of cancer, and these patients, too, require assistance of health professionals. Usually it is not certain, at the outset, whether or not the patient has been cured. A patient with cervical cancer may undergo hysterectomy. The physician explains to the patient that he believes all malignant tissue has been removed. Nevertheless, it is of the utmost importance that the patient return regularly to the clinic or to the physician's office, for periodic examinations, so that any new evidence of the disease can be promptly detected and treated. Many patients, however, having been through the ordeal of facing the diagnosis of cancer and having surgery or radiation, or both, want nothing so much as to forget the experience. A visit to the clinic or physician not only reminds them of the experience, but brings with it suspense and dread concerning what may be found at follow-up examinations. Nurses, especially nurses in public health and industrial settings, can help by encouraging and supporting the patient, by showing understanding and acceptance of the patient's feelings, and also by stressing the necessity for, and the advantages to the patient of follow-up care. As the years go by, and no new evidence of cancer is found, the patient usually relaxes more, as each favorable report brings greater feeling of security that he is, in fact, cured.

If the patient's disease becomes widespread, certain nursing considerations become especially important. The patient may conjure up dreaded fantasies of agonizing pain and mutilation. Too often his opening and sometimes fumbling comments and questions to express these concerns are met by avoidance or by an overly jolly approach which denies the seriousness of his situation. It is important to consider what the patient says, to patiently assist him in expressing his fears, and to discuss them with him. In so doing, some of the vague, enormous, and very threatening fears can be lessened and become more manageable. For instance, the patient who has opportunity to express the fear that the pain may later become unbearable can consider, with the nurse and doctor, what is available to relieve his pain, and also important, can receive reassurance from them that they will not desert him—that they will be there, and help him remain as comfortable as possible. It has been observed repeatedly that patients who receive emotional support from staff and who are in an atmosphere which fosters dignity, self care to the extent possible, recreation and companionship, experience less pain. Other fears, which patients often voice, and which also can become less paralyzing to the patient once he can speak of them, are fears of death, of separation from loved ones, loss of control, and mutilation.

During the spread stage of cancer it is especially important to observe the patient for complications. Bleeding or even serious hemorrhage may occur if a blood vessel is eroded by malignant tissue. Infection, manifested by such symptoms as fever and chills may occur since the tissues undergoing malignant change are vulnerable to infection. Pathologic fractures may result if the patient has metastases to bone. In addition, complications may occur as a result of physical inactivity: thrombophlebitis is an example. Vigilant nursing care is required to prevent complications when possible, and to detect their occurrence promptly.

For the patient who is not cured, it is important to realize that the illness involves many stages, physically and emotionally, and to plan care appropriate to each stage. Upon first learning of the disease the patient usually experiences shock and disbelief, followed often by anger, and, when his personal resources and the help he receives enable him to do so, a stage of acceptance. In the patient who is not told of his diagnosis and who does not find out about it in some way, there may be growing distrust of therapy and staff, resentment, and withdrawal. Or the patient may seem to manage quite well and to maintain hope for his recovery. Physically, there may be a prolonged period when the patient is able to maintain his accustomed activities, followed by decline as the disease overpowers the patient's resistance and the benefits which therapy can provide.

It is important to assist the patient during each of these stages, not rushing him prematurely toward a phase which has not yet arrived, nor failing to recognize when a change in the patient's situation requires a change in his care. For the patient whose resistance has been overcome by the disease it is necessary to consider care required by the dying patient and by his family.

REFERENCES AND BIBLIOGRAPHY

AMERICAN CANCER SOCIETY: *A Cancer Source Book for Nurses*, New York, American Cancer Society, 1968.

———: *Cancer, a Manual for Practitioners*, ed. 4, Boston, American Cancer Society, 1968.

———: *Cancer Management*, Philadelphia, Lippincott, 1968.

———: *1970 Cancer Facts and Figures*, New York, American Cancer Society, 1970.

BARCKLEY, V.: A visiting nurse specializes in cancer nursing, *Am. J. Nurs.* 70:1680, August, 1970.

BOUCHARD, R.: *Nursing Care of the Cancer Patient*, St. Louis, Mosby, 1967.

CRAYTOR, J. K.: Talking with persons who have cancer, *Am. J. Nurs.* 69:744, April, 1969.

CRAYTOR, J. K., and FASS, M. L.: *The Nurse and the Cancer Patient*, Philadelphia, Lippincott, 1970.

DAVIS, M.: Cancer dwells here, *Nurs. Forum* 6:379, 1967.

DONALDSON, S., and FLETCHER, W.: The treatment of cancer by isolation perfusion, *Am. J. Nurs.* 64:81, August, 1964.

ENGEL, G. L.: Grief and grieving, *Am. J. Nurs.* 64:93, September, 1964.

EVANS, R. B., et al.: Some psychological characteristics of men with cancer, *Cancer* 17:307, 1964.

EVERSON, T. C., and COLE, W. H.: *Spontaneous Regression of Cancer*, Philadelphia, Saunders, 1966.

FEIFEL, H. (ed.): *The Meaning of Death*, New York, McGraw-Hill, 1959.

FOX, J. E.: Reflections on cancer nursing, *Am. J. Nurs.* 66:1317, June, 1966.

FRANCIS, G. M.: Cancer: the emotional component, *Am. J. Nurs.* 69:1677, August, 1969.

GARNER, H. H.: *Psychosomatic Management of the Patient with Malignancy*, Springfield, Ill., Thomas, 1966.

GRANT, R.: Nursing the cancer patient, *Nurs. Forum* 4:57, 1965.

GRIMES, ORVILLE: Neuromuscular syndromes in patients with lung cancer, *Am. J. Nurs.* 71:752, April, 1971.

GUTHRIE, D.: *A History of Medicine*, Philadelphia, Lippincott, 1946.

KISSEN, D. M., and LESHAN, L. L. (eds.): *Psychosomatic Aspects of Neoplastic Disease*, Philadelphia, Lippincott, 1964.

KLAGSBRUN, S. C.: Cancer, emotions, and nurses, *Am. J. Psychiat.* 126:1237, March, 1970.

———: Communications in the treatment of cancer, *Am. J. Nurs.* 71:944, May, 1971.

LESHAN, L. L., and GASSMAN, M. L.: Some observations on psychotherapy with patients suffering from neoplastic disease, *Am. J. Psychotherap.* 12:723, 1958.

MEDICAL NEWS: Cancer respects neither regions nor persons, *JAMA* 189:38, July, 1964.

METTLER, C. C.: *History of Medicine*, Philadelphia, Blackiston, 1947.

NEELON, V. J.: Hyperbaric oxygenation, *Am. J. Nurs.* 64:cer, Philadelphia, Saunders, 1965.

NEELON, V. J.: Hyperbaric oxygenation, *Am. J. Nurs.* 64:73, October, 1964.

NOWAK, P. A.: Nursing care in isolation perfusion, *Am. J. Nurs.* 64:85, August, 1964.

PAYNE, E., and KRANT, M. J.: The psychosocial aspects of advanced cancer, *JAMA* 210:1238, 1969.

PUBLIC HEALTH SERVICE: *Survival Experience of Patients with Malignant Neoplasms*, Washington, D.C., U.S. Government Printing Office, 1960.

———: *The Facts of Life and Death*, Washington, D.C., U.S. Government Printing Office, 1963.

ROSENFELD, L., and CALLAWAY, J.: Snuff dippers' cancer, *Am. J. Surg.* 106:840 844, 1963.

SHIMKIN, M. B.: *Science and Cancer*, Washington, D.C., U.S. Department of Health, Education and Welfare, 1969.

STANDARD, S., and NATHAN, H. (eds.): *Should the Patient Know the Truth?* New York, Springer, 1955.

WYNDER, E. L., ONDERDONK, J., and MANTEL, R.: An epidemiological investigation of cancer of the bladder, *Cancer* 16:1388–1407, 1963.

WOLF, E. S.: Where hope comes first, *Nurs. Outlook* 12:52, April, 1964.

WOLF, I. S.: Should the patient know the truth? *Am. J. Nurs.* 55:546–548, 1955.

WOLSTENHOLME, G., and O'CONNOR, M. (eds.): *Carcinogenesis*, Boston, Little, Brown, 1959.

Nursing Management in Radiotherapy   14

Clinical Application of Radiotherapy • Radiation Protection
Radioisotopes • Nursing Care of Patients Receiving Radium or
Cobalt • Radioactive Iodine • Radioactive Gold • Radioactive
Phosphorus • Cobalt Therapy

The term "radiotherapy" refers to the therapeutic application of ionizing radiation from x-ray machines or radioactive materials. Radiotherapy deals mainly, but not exclusively, with the treatment of cancer. The aim of radiotherapy is an orderly destruction of malignant, rapidly dividing cells, while leaving the rest of the body well or able to recover and capable of eliminating the killed cancer cells. This destruction is accomplished by x-rays or radioactive materials. When the malignancy is far advanced, radiotherapy is used palliatively to cause a remission of symptoms so that the patient will be more comfortable. Radioactive isotopes are used both for diagnostic and therapeutic procedures.* Radiotherapy is used to heal lytic lesions in the bones. As the lytic lesions heal, pain diminishes. Radiotherapy is both palliative and therapeutic in late-stage malignancy.

That radiation is invisible and inaudible makes it seem menacing and difficult for some patients to understand. Diagnostic tests and treatments often involve the use of large machines that are, for the patient, strange to behold. Because radiotherapy is used for the treatment of cancer more often than for any other condition, and because most patients know this, radiotherapy itself suggests a serious condition. The nurse whose practice is based on understanding of the physical laws that govern radiation will be able to protect herself from possible damage that can be produced by radiation. Her skill in applying the principles underlying nursing care

* The diagnostic uses of radiation are discussed in the various clinical chapters where appropriate.

is necessary for the safe and effective use of radiotherapy.

An adequate knowledge of radiation is necessary not only for the safety and protection of personnel, but also for countering the superstition, misconception and fear brought about by the atom bomb. A more realistic attitude concerning clinical uses of radiation is necessary if we are to be truly successful in the management of patients receiving radiotherapy. Uncertainty or confusion on the part of hospital personnel will only increase the patient's fears and damage his morale.

Radiation deserves the same respect given to other modalities of therapy for cancer. Radiotherapy is one of three accepted forms of treatment for cancer and allied diseases. Surgery attempts mechanical removal of the cancer. Chemotherapy attempts to kill cancer cells by means of chemical agents. Radiotherapy attempts to kill cancer cells with physical agents (ionizing radiation). These methods are used singly or in combination. The choice is left to the judgment of the physician. It must always be remembered that it is the patient rather than the cancer which is being treated. All available means must be used to support the patient while he is receiving radiotherapy for his disease.

CLINICAL APPLICATION OF RADIOTHERAPY

Radiotherapy is an exacting science. Its administration is as meticulous and often as tedious as that of surgery or chemotherapy. The application can be as extensive as that of an operative procedure. Major and minor procedures are often performed concomitantly for the express purpose of treatment with radioisotopes, e.g., a thoracotomy with an implant of either radon or iodine seeds into an unresectable lung tumor. Radiotherapy is not an easy way out in the management of cancer. Like surgery, it can result in painful and unpleasant complications.

The patient's basic needs for information must be met. Silence or vague answers can be more disturbing to him than the truth. It is well to use the exact terms the therapist has used to explain the effects of treatment ("melting" or "shrinking" of the tumor). This should be noted on the nursing care plan. Lay terminology is best understood by most patients. Technical terms may add to the patient's fears. Most patients tolerate therapy and bear some discomfort if they are given simple explanations. Discussion of the side-effects of therapy should be minimized until they are imminent or actually occur.

When preparing the patient for radiation therapy and assisting him during the period of therapy, it is important not only to explain the treatment to him, but also to listen to his views, doubts and concerns about the treatment.

Sensitivity of Tissues to Radiation. Rapidly dividing cells are more sensitive to radiation than those which divide slowly. This generalization was made by Bergonie and Tribondeau (1906) who stated that "cells are sensitive to radiation in proportion to their proliferative activity."

The following is an outline of cells arranged according to their sensitivity to radiation, with the most sensitive cells listed first:

1. Lymphocytes
2. Erythroblasts
3. Myeloblasts
4. Epithelial cells
   a. Basal cells of testes
   b. Basal cells of intestinal crypts
   c. Basal cells of the ovaries
   d. Basal cells of the skin
   e. Basal cells of secretory glands
   f. Alveolar cells of the lungs and bile ducts
5. Endothelial cells
6. Connective tissue cells
7. Tubular cells of the kidneys
8. Bone cells
9. Nerve cells
10. Brain cells
11. Muscle cells

This summary is now called the law of Bergonie and Tribondeau (Behrens *et al.*).

Radiosensitivity does not imply curability of cancer. The lymph nodes in Hodgkin's disease or in the leukemias are quite radiosensitive, and radiotherapy is the treatment of choice, but the disease itself is a progressive one. Great strides have been made in the treatment of the lymphomas with the newer supervoltage machines and mantle technics employed, so that the malignancy is held in check for longer periods of time. On the other hand, a basal cell cancer, usually of the face, is quite radiosensitive and the cure rate by radiotherapy is usually very good.

Individual Reactions. Individual differences may alter the patient's response to therapy. Infection or ischemia may decrease the radiosensitivity, and poor response is evident more often among the cachectic than in well nourished patients. On entering tissues, radiation produces ionization of atoms with chemical alteration of tissue proteins. Ionization is facilitated by the large amounts of water and oxygen present in the tissues. The maintenance of good hydration of the patient receiving radiation therapy is an important nursing responsibility. When the oxygen carrying ability of the blood is impaired as a result of anemia, there is a reduced response to radiation therapy. It is important therefore to maintain the patient's hemoglobin at near normal levels. Hypoxic cells within a tumor are protected to some extent from radiation destruction. Based on this concept, clinical trials have been undertaken in administering radiation therapy while the patient breathes in oxygen under increased barometric pressure. This involves the use of the hyperbaric chamber. Hyperbaric radiation therapy is still in the clinical trial stage and more experience is needed to make definite statements about its value.

Nursing Care in External Beam Therapy. Most patients know that they are receiving x-ray therapy for cancer. The physician discusses the diagnosis with the patient and his family. In some instances a young or frightened patient is not told that he has cancer and a term such as "cyst," "ulcer" or "inflammation" is used to describe the disease. It is important that all members of the health team be aware of this. The nurse is perhaps of greatest help when she listens and allows the patient to express his feelings. By her quiet acceptance of his emotional state, she can help him accept therapy and come to terms with his illness. Many social and psy-

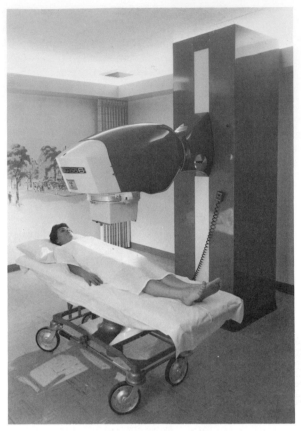

Fig. 14-1. A vertical teletherapy unit. The radioactive source is Cobalt[60]. (Atomic Energy of Canada, Ottawa, Canada)

chological problems can be resolved once the diagnosis and its implications are openly or tacitly accepted. If the patient's disease is curable, this fact should be stressed to the patient and his family. The discomforts of therapy can be tolerated better, knowing that a cure is imminent. For the patient with incurable disease, the palliation achieved may permit normal or near normal activities for a long period of time. If radiation reactions should become severe, the therapist may halt treatments to give the body a chance to recover. The reason for this should be explained to the patient and his family to avoid misunderstandings, feelings of discouragement and setback. It should be explained that deviations from the original plan of therapy are not unusual. Normal activities are encouraged as much as possible. Rest periods should be provided after therapy as some patients tire easily.

Radiation Reactions. A systemic effect known as radiation sickness is sometimes experienced by patients undergoing radiotherapy. The amount of radiation sickness depends upon the site, dose, and volume treated; for example, a patient undergoing therapy for a small basal cell cancer of the face will not be expected to experience radiation sickness. Patients who have larger areas of the body treated may experience radiation sickness. The symptoms may include weakness, nausea, vomiting, diaphoresis and sometimes chills. The symptoms are handled prophylactically and symptomatically.

To avoid nausea and vomiting, the nurse and dietician should plan the patient's meals to be served so that food is avoided at least one hour before and after therapy. Some therapists may decide to order an antiemetic to be given one half hour before therapy. Rushing the patient should also be avoided, and diagnostic tests should not be scheduled immediately before or following therapy. Emphasis upon emotional support and a program including necessary rest and pleasant diversion often obviate the problem of nausea.

With better radiation technics and patient management, many side-effects have been reduced or nearly eliminated. It is unwise to burden the patient by telling him of side-effects which may or may not occur. However, the patient should be advised to report any discomforts he experiences to the staff. When the patient reports symptoms, such as itching or burning, it is essential to take his statements seriously and to see that the appropriate member of the health team receives the information about the patient's symptoms. The patient should know that the skin in the treated area may become reddened, and that this is a normal reaction to therapy. The term "burn" should never be used as it may connote overtreatment or carelessness. The patient is instructed to keep the radiated skin clean and dry, and to avoid unprescribed ointments or creams. The radiated skin should be protected against extremes of heat or cold. Heat pads, ultraviolet light, diathermy, whirlpool, sauna or steam baths, and direct sunlight must be avoided. Careful bathing is advised and soap and friction over the treated skin must be avoided. Loose clothing is advised to avoid irritation. Intense itching, especially in patients with Hodgkin's disease, is sometimes experienced. A steroid type cream or aerosol spray is sometimes prescribed for relief. Corn starch may be used over radiated areas where two skin surfaces are in contact, e.g., axillary and groin areas, and areas under the breasts, provided there is no breakdown of the skin. When therapy is completed, talcum or zinc stearate powder may afford some relief from itching. If the scalp is being irradiated, shampoos, tinting and permanent waving should be avoided. Upon completion of therapy, the therapist may recommend a mild baby shampoo. Partial temporary hair loss is seen. This epilation is temporary, regrowth occurring in from 4 to 6 months, and the patient should be reassured that this condition is temporary. A wig is recommended to restore appearance and morale.

Patients receiving radiotherapy may develop varying degrees of bone marrow depression. The need for periodic blood counts and occasional small blood, packed cells or platelet transfusions to tide over the patient until his therapy course is completed must be explained to the patient. The lowered leukocyte count makes the patient easy prey to infection. Visitors and hospital personnel with colds or other infections should not be in close contact with radiotherapy patients. If the leukopenia is severe, the therapist may temporarily halt treatments and perhaps put the patient on reverse isolation precautions.

Fluids and Diet. Most patients tolerate a well balanced diet. Because large amounts of tumor are being lysed during therapy, it is important to maintain effective kidney function to avoid uric acid crystalluria and possible kidney shutdown. Good hydration and maintenance of dilute urine are measures used to prevent this rare complication. The patient should take up to 3000 ml. of fluid daily. If the fluid intake is inadequate, the therapist may wish to order a supplementary intravenous infusion to make up the deficit. Accurate intake and output records are essential. Most patients who are able like to do this themselves once they have been taught. Unless the patient has been on a special diet for some medical reason, a regular diet is usually recommended. Allopurinol is sometimes prescribed when the uric acid level in the blood is high.

Prophylactic Management. Radiation sickness is often influenced by the emotional state of the patient. He should be reassured that side-effects are not frequently encountered today. Care of the patient should emphasize support, explanation, and a program of rest and diversion in pleasant surroundings. It is possible for most patients to remain at home among familiar surroundings, and to continue accustomed activities.

Follow-up Care. The patient is encouraged to live as normal a life as possible. The help of the patient's family is often enlisted toward that end. When the family is offered the opportunity to express their own misgivings and questions to the staff, they are better able to offer assistance and support to the patient. The patient is referred to the social worker for assistance with such matters as housing, transportation and family problems. In some instances homemaker or housekeeping services may also be necessary.

It is important for the nurse in all clinical settings to be alert to the need for continuity of care and to initiate referral to other nurses when necessary. For example, if the patient is treated initially in the hospital and subsequently as an outpatient, referral to a public health nurse may be indicated. Side-effects from therapy can occur after the course of treatment has terminated. The therapist will therefore prepare the patient for this possibility and stress the importance of returning to the clinic if he experiences any discomfort, so that medication and treatment can be prescribed if necessary.

RADIATION PROTECTION

All persons involved in the care of patients receiving radioisotopes must recognize the necessity for limitations to radiation exposure. The degree of possible hazard depends upon the type and amount of radioactive material used for treatment.

Generally, no special precautions are required when patients receive small amounts of radioactive material for diagnostic studies (less than 200 microcuries). If any precautions are necessary, they are specified by the radiologist. There is usually no hazard to personnel or visitors. Patients receiving moderate or large amounts (200 microcuries to over 5 millicuries) may present a hazard unless simple precautions written by the radiation safety officer are carried out.

The safety principles of time, distance and shielding (where applicable) should always be borne in mind.

Time. This refers to the length of exposure. The less time spent in the vicinity of a radioactive substance the less the radiation received. Nurses should plan carefully so that less time will actually be spent at the bedside. The nurse must learn to work quickly and efficiently. Careful psychological preparation helps the patient to accept the limited amount of nursing time.

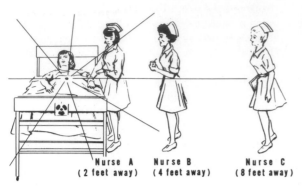

FIG. 14-2. Examples of distance. Nurse B (4 feet away) receives approximately 25 per cent of the radiation received by Nurse A (2 feet away), and nurse C (8 feet away) receives approximately 25 per cent of the radiation received by Nurse B.

Distance. This refers to the distance from the radioactive source. The patient's bed assignment and degree of isolation are determined by the radiation safety officer after monitoring the patient. The inverse square law applies to radiation exposure. The rate of exposure varies inversely as the square of the distance from the source (patient). A nurse standing four feet away from the source of radiation receives 25 per cent as much radiation as she would if she were standing two feet away from the source (patient). (See Fig. 14-2.)

Shielding. This refers to the use of any type of material to attenuate radiation. The material usually used is lead, but other materials have the capability of shielding. Examples include the concrete walls usually found in radiation therapy and diagnostic radiology departments. Lead lined gloves, leaded aprons and drapes are also examples of shielding.

Since radiation produces no immediate symptoms, one can receive radiation injury without being aware of it. The National Committee on Radiation Protection publishes guides for radiation safety for all hospitals, clinics and laboratories engaged in the handling of x-rays and radioactive materials. Many of the early radiation pioneers were not afforded the benefits of radiation safety rules and regulations, and many received radiation damage as a result of prolonged and unnecessary exposures. The effects of long and short exposures must be taken into account. The latent period between the exposure and the accumulated biologic effect is often long. Today, great care is taken to protect occupation-

ally exposed workers from radiation injury which can accumulate over the years.

However, absolute protection for all personnel is not possible and those who work in this field must deal with the small risk involved. Radiation risks are very small. We have come a long way in reducing radiation exposure to the barest minimum. However, all women who are pregnant (whether staff or visitors) should avoid any exposure to radiotherapy.

RADIOISOTOPES

In certain instances it may be more advantageous to use radioactive sources within the tumor itself (interstitial), as opposed to using a distant source (external beam therapy). This method has the advantage of delivering the highest dose within the tumor, with a rapid fall off of dose in the surrounding tissues. Radioisotopes also may be administered orally or intravenously for systemic effect, and into body cavities for local effect. Radioisotopes also may be applied topically for local lesions using various kinds of applicators.

NURSING CARE OF PATIENTS RECEIVING RADIUM OR COBALT

The highly radioactive qualities of radium make it dangerous to handle because of its destructive effects on normal tissues. Therefore, extreme caution must be exercised in the use, storage and transportation of radium and cobalt. Since its discovery, radium has been used extensively for practically every form of cancer. Today, its advantages and disadvantages are better understood. Radium continues to have a definite place in the treatment of cancer in specially selected sites such as the cervix, uterus, tongue, nasopharynx, and other sites which may lend themselves to the use of applicators. In many European countries radium is used more extensively than in the United States.

Physical and psychological preparation of the patient are important. As with all radiotherapy procedures, the radiation therapist is responsible for explaining the procedure and for obtaining the patient's consent. The nurse reinforces the physician's explanations and supports the patient as he goes through the preparation and the treatment. The need for enforced bed rest when indicated, as well as limited activity and temporary isolation must be explained to the patient and his family. Careful attention to these details will help the patient and his family accept and cope with the temporary enforced isolation. Necessary nursing care should be given without rushing the patient. The radiation safety officer will specify safety precautions such as the time and distance required for safe visiting. A narrow strip of adhesive is used on the floor of the patient's room in some centers to designate safe distance for visiting. A wristlet reading "RADIATION PRECAUTIONS" is placed on the patient's wrist. This must remain until removed by the radiation safety officer. This precaution is applied to all patients treated with internal sources of radiation. The bed, door and patient's chart are also appropriately identified with radiation tags and adhere type labels. The radiation principles of time, distance and shielding (when applicable) are observed. Film badges must be worn by all personnel involved in direct care of the patient, and rotation of nursing assignment, if recommended, is carried out.

Be alert to the number and types of applicators used to hold the radioactive source, the time the applicator(s) was inserted, and the time the applicator(s) is to be removed. The applicator(s) must be checked periodically to avoid displacement or loss. The removal of the applicator(s) must be done at the specified time, and the therapist should be notified at least one half hour in advance. If an applicator should fall out, it should be picked up carefully, using long handled tongs, and placed in the lead container (pig) which is usually kept in the patient's bathroom. This is a rare occurrence, but occasionally does happen with cervical or intraoral applicators. With cervical or uterine applicators, the Foley catheter is removed just prior to removal of the applicator. The radiation therapist will remove the applicator. The nurse, wearing disposable gloves and using long handled tongs and brush, will wash the applicator in a basin of soapy water before returning the applicator to the container. The container is then placed on a cart and removed to the radium room by the radiation therapist. The applicator is handled carefully and never opened. Body excretions, vaginal tampons, Foley catheter, and urine are not radioactive and do not require special handling. The patient should be checked for bleeding and should remain in bed for one hour after removal of the applicator. A plain water douche is usually ordered and the patient may be transferred to a multi-bed room. Radiation precautions are no longer necessary.

NURSING CARE OF PATIENTS RECEIVING RADIOACTIVE IODINE

Radioactive iodine (^{131}I) is used for the treatment of thyroid cancer, thyroid metatases, and some types of hyperthyroidism. For therapy, radioactive iodine is administered orally in liquid form. This isotope is usually contraindicated in pregnancy, children, and most people below the age of 40. The therapeutic dose is from 1 to 100 millicuries. It is a clear, colorless, tasteless preparation administered in a half glass of water. The patient will need to fast, because food delays the absorption of the isotope. The precautions set forth by the radiation safety officer must be strictly observed. In some clinics visitors are not permitted for 40 to 72 hours, or the period of greatest radioactivity. In some institutions visitors may visit for a brief period (10 min.) provided they sit near the entrance of the room. The radiation safety precautions of time and distance are thus observed. Contamination from perspiration, vomitus, or diarrhea will present the greatest hazard within the first 24 hours. Unnecessary or sustained contact must be avoided and only essential nursing care is performed. If close contact becomes necessary an isolation gown and disposable gloves should be worn. Urine is collected carefully by the patient and put into gallon jugs which are contained in a lead lined box kept in the patient's bathroom. Linen which is wet is placed in a plastic laundry bag in a linen hamper also kept in the patient's bathroom. These items are safely disposed of according to the directions of the radiation safety officer after monitoring. In case of accident, e.g., spillage of urine, suspend all activity while the radiation safety officer is notified for instruction and supervision of proper decontamination. With large doses some patients may complain of neck soreness or difficulty in swallowing. A rare severe reaction may threaten tracheal obstruction or compression of the larger blood vessels if the gland is retrosternal. A rare severe general collapse related to acute endocrine imbalance (thyroid crisis, storm) may also occur. Severe reactions of this type are generally treated with steroids. Following completion of therapy, the room is thoroughly cleaned, then monitored before new occupancy (Benna and Rawson).

NURSING CARE OF PATIENTS RECEIVING RADIOACTIVE GOLD

Radiogold (^{198}Au) is used to retard the accumulation of malignant effusions in body cavities.

Also, this isotope is sometimes injected interstitially (liquid form) directly into an unresectable tumor, or interstitially in stainless steel seeds as a permanent implant. Small amounts of this isotope are eliminated in the urine, while most of it remains in the injected area. Contamination may easily be seen by the appearance of a pink or red stain on the dressing, gown or bedding.

With intracavitary use, radiogold produces irradiation of the lining of the cavity. It will reduce or suspend tumor activity and will deliver a lethal dose to tumor cells. The radiation therapist will use and remove his own equipment, usually sterile disposable paracentesis or thoracentesis sets. When the isotope is used in body cavities, the position of the patient must be rotated every 15 minutes for at least two hours. This will assure equal distribution of the isotope throughout the cavity. Sometimes the polyethylene tubes used for administering the isotopes are clamped and left in place to facilitate further treatment at a later date.

NURSING CARE OF PATIENTS RECEIVING RADIOACTIVE PHOSPHORUS

This isotope (^{32}P) concentrates in the nuclei of cells where it forms an important constituent of their chemical structure, nucleic acid. The nuclei of rapidly proliferating cells tend to have more nuclear material than normal cells, so they concentrate the radiophosphorus. Temporary isolation is not necessary because the patient's own body serves as an effective shield. Contamination can easily be seen by the appearance of a blue stain on the dressing, gown or bed linen. Contaminated items must be handled carefully wearing disposable gloves and using waterproof containers. Contaminated items are removed for proper disposition by radiation safety personnel after monitoring. Radiophosphorus may be administered orally or intravenously for the treatment of chronic leukemia or polycythemia vera. The isotope tends to deposit in bones and in the cells of the reticuloendothelial system. Some of the isotope is excreted in the urine and stool in the first few days. The patient should flush the toilet three times and should wash his hands thoroughly. As with radiogold and all radioisotopes the patient's chart should contain the appropriate labels. The patient's bed should have a radiation tag as a reminder that a possible hazard can exist if there is contamination. The patient should also wear a wristlet reading "RADIOACTIVE PRECAUTIONS." The radi-

ation safety officer should always be consulted for problems.

NURSING CARE OF PATIENTS RECEIVING COBALT THERAPY

This isotope (^{60}Co) is never used as a permanent implant. Cobalt-60 has many applications in the treatment of tumors. The nursing considerations are the same as for radium and radon when the isotope is used in applicator form. No contamination problems occur because the isotope is in a sealed container. The patient will need to be isolated while the radioactive source is in place. He is assigned to a single room and maximum precautions are observed.

Cobalt teletherapy is external beam therapy. The isotope is used as a distant source for treatment. This form of therapy is generally used to treat deep-seated tumors. There is no hazard except in the treatment room when the shutter on the installation is open during actual treatment. The patient does not become a radioactive source.

REFERENCES AND BIBLIOGRAPHY

BARNETT, M.: The nature of radiation and its effect on man, *Nurs. Clin. N. Am.* 2:11, March, 1966.

BEHRENS, C. F., KING, E. R., and CARPENDER, J. W. J.: *Atomic Medicine*, p. 135, Baltimore, Williams & Wilkins, 1969.

BOEKER, E.: Radiation safety, *Am. J. Nurs.* 65:111, April, 1965.

————: Radiation uses and hazards, *Nurs. Clin. N. Am.* 2:32, March, 1967.

BOUCHARD, R.: *Nursing Care of the Cancer Patient,* St. Louis, Mosby, 1967.

CRAYTOR, J. K., and FASS, M. L.: *The Nurse and the Cancer Patient,* Philadelphia, Lippincott, 1970.

HILKEMEYER, R.: Nursing care in radium therapy, *Nurs. Clin. N. Am.* 2:83, March, 1967.

ISLER, C.: Radiation therapy-2: The nurse and the patient, *RN* 34:48, March, 1971.

KAUTZ, H. D., STOREY, R. H., and ZIMMERMANN, A. J.: Radioactive drugs, *Am. J. Nurs.* 64:124, January, 1964.

LIEBEN, J.: The effects of radiation, *Nurs. Outlook* 10:336, 1962.

MILLER, A.: The nurse on the radiological team, *Am. J. Nurs.* 64:128, July, 1964.

NEALON, T. F., JR. (ed.): *Management of the Patient with Cancer,* p. 784, Philadelphia, Saunders, 1965.

OVERMAN, R. T.: *Basic Concepts of Nuclear Chemistry,* New York, Reinhold, 1963.

PROSNITZ, L. R.: Radiation therapy-1: Treatment for malignant disease, *RN* 34:42, March, 1971.

PUCK, T. T.: Radiation and the human cell, *Sci. Am.* 202: 142–153, April, 1960.

RUMMERFIELD, P. S., and RUMMERFIELD, M. J.: What you should know about radiation hazards, *Am. J. Nurs.* 70:780, April, 1970.

ZAINO, H.: Eliminating the hazards from radiation, *Am. J. Nurs.* 62:60, April, 1962.

The Patient with a Fracture

15

Types of Fractures · The Pathology of Fracture and the Physiology of Bone Repair · Incidence · Symptoms · First Aid · Hospital Treatment of Fractures · Care of the Patient in a Cast · Traction Care of the Patient in Traction · Crutch Walking · Other Fractures Dislocation and Sprains

TYPES OF FRACTURES

A fracture is a break in the continuity of a bone. A simple classification of fractures follows:

- *Open* (compound)—the bone breaks through the skin. Because there is an open wound, the danger of infection is increased greatly.
- *Closed* (simple)—any fracture that is not open is a closed fracture.
- *Displaced*—the bone ends are separated.
- *Greenstick*—the bone bends and splits, but it does not break clear through. This kind of fracture occurs primarily in children.
- *Complete*—the fracture line goes all the way through the bone.
- *Comminuted*—bone is broken in several places.
- *Impacted*—one portion of the bone is driven into another.
- *Complicated*—a fracture with injury to the surrounding tissues, such as blood vessels, nerves, joints or internal organs.
- *Pathologic* (spontaneous)—the bone breaks without sufficient trauma to crack a normal bone. This kind of fracture occurs in such conditions as osteoporosis (porous bones), cancer, certain instances of malnutrition, Cushing's syndrome, and as a complication of cortisone and ACTH therapy.

THE PATHOLOGY OF FRACTURE AND THE PHYSIOLOGY OF BONE REPAIR

For 10 to 40 minutes after the fracture the muscles surrounding the bone are flaccid. Then they go into spasm, and when they do, they cause increased deformity and additional interference with the vascular and the lymphatic circulations. Traction at this later stage is accomplished only with difficulty. The application and the maintenance of traction immediately after a fracture avoids the later complication of spastic muscles.

When there are bone fragments as a result of fracture, the local periosteum and surrounding blood vessels are torn. The tissue surrounding the fracture shows an aseptic inflammation (unless the skin is broken), with swelling due to hemorrhage, inflammatory exudate and edema. The blood in the area clots, and fibrin network forms between the bone ends. This changes into granulation tissue. The osteoblasts, proliferating in the clot, increase the secretion of an enzyme that restores the alkaline pH, and the result is the deposition of calcium in the callus and the formation of true bone. At the stage of the consolidation of the clot (6 to 10 days after the injury) the healing mass is called a *callus*. The callus holds the ends of the bone together, but it cannot endure strain.

Interference with the removal of the debris will interfere with the healing process. Nonunion of the fracture may result—a permanent break in the continuity of the bone. Nursing measures that promote adequate circulation in the affected part foster deposition of calcium and healing of the bone. This is one reason that elevation of the affected limb, which helps to reduce edema, is so important. Because early mobilization of the patient encourages favorable nitrogen balance and counters sluggish circulation, many patients with a fractured hip are treated with pin fixation instead of traction.

Consolidation of bone takes about half as long in a 6-year-old as in a 60-year-old; but, interestingly enough, once a person becomes an adult, age does not affect healing. Nor does generalized disease, including the atrophy of bone, influence the time it takes for a fracture to heal, although the older or debilitated patient is in greater danger of not surviving the injury because of complications. Bone repair is a highly local process. About a year of healing must take place before bone regains its former structural strength, becoming well consolidated, remolded and possessing fat and marrow cells.

INCIDENCE

Most accidents occur in the home and on the highways. Slippery, wet tubs, scatter rugs, highly polished floors, roller skates on a dark stairway, and activities involving a precarious balance, such as standing on a rickety chair to hang a curtain—all can be hazardous. The incidence of fractures is greater among persons who have predisposing conditions, such as osteoporosis and cancer which affects bone. Poor coordination, diminished vision and hearing, the frequency of dizziness and faintness, and general feebleness make falls and resultant fractures a common problem among the aged. Other high-risk groups include patients with diseases affecting locomotion, such as arthritis, Parkinson's disease, and multiple sclerosis. The fact that bone breakage in older persons is more frequent across the neck of the femur is attributed partially to atrophy of bone. Up to the age of about 45, men suffer more fractures than women. After that age the frequency is higher in women.

SYMPTOMS

- *Pain*—one of the most consistent symptoms of a broken bone is pain. It may be severe, and it is increased by attempts to move the part and by pressure over the fracture.
- *Loss of function*—skeletal muscular function is dependent on an intact bone.
- *Deformity*—a break may cause an extremity to bend backwards or to assume another unusual shape.
- *False motion*—unnatural motion occurs at the site of the fracture.

- *Edema*—swelling usually is greatest directly over the fracture.
- *Spasm*—muscles near fractures involuntarily contract. Spasm, which accounts for some of the pain, may result in the shortening of a limb when a long bone is involved.

If the sharp bone fragments tear through sufficient surrounding soft tissue, there will be bleeding and black and blue discoloration of the area. If a nerve is damaged, there may be paralysis.

FIRST AID

Bleeding. If the nurse is present at the accident, she first should notice any bleeding and take measures to stop it and to combat shock. The average amount of blood lost to the general circulation in a closed fracture of the femur is 800 to 1,200 ml., and, of course, there may be a great deal more bleeding in an open fracture.

Evaluation. It is safe to assume that a fracture has occurred if the limb is misshapen, if the patient states that he has heard the bone snap, or if there is a loss of function. Overcaution is never misplaced. It is better to splint a sprain than not to splint a fracture.

"Splint them where they lie" is the motto. The ragged edge of a broken bone can do great damage to the soft tissues around it. Fragments of bone can cut through periosteum, fascia, muscle, nerves, blood-vessel walls and even skin. The protrusion of a fragment of bone through skin is very dangerous, since dirt or perhaps bits of clothing may be introduced into an otherwise clean wound. Frantic efforts to remove the patient to a hospital in all haste are perilous. Pulling a patient to the side of the road and lifting him into a car without supporting the fracture can create an open fracture from a closed one. It is far better to stop hemorrhage, treat shock and immobilize the fracture before the patient is moved at all from the place where he fell.

Getting the Right Kind of Help From Others. The patient with a possible fracture needs protection against well-meaning but ignorant passersby who try to sit him up or to move him immediately. Such interference usually can be stopped by the self-assured presence of the nurse who identifies herself. Although she may feel neither calm nor self-assured, others will listen if she can convince them that she knows what she is doing. Immediately taking the patient's pulse gives her valuable information about his condition. Also, this professional gesture often will convince even a stubborn lay bystander that one more competent than he has taken charge. Taking the patient's pulse has the added advantage of giving the nurse a full minute to collect her thoughts and to plan what to do next. If the patient is lying in a busy street, let the cars go around him until the ambulance comes. Cover him and keep the crowd away. Perhaps one bystander can take the responsibility of keeping people back, and another can call for the police or an ambulance, and a third can direct traffic to protect the patient and those ministering to him from being struck by oncoming cars.

Splinting. Before the patient is moved, his limb must be splinted. To splint an arm or a leg, use padded wood, a folded telephone book, or anything that is stiff. If nothing else is available, a broken leg can be splinted to the intact leg. If possible, the splint should be applied so that it includes the joints above and below the fracture site. For example, if the tibia is broken, include both the ankle and the knee in the splint. Be sure to pad the appliance, so that the soft tissues are protected uniformly. Remember that the arm and the leg bones are especially close to the skin, and that extreme gentleness is needed in handling a fractured limb to prevent a simple fracture from tearing the skin and becoming a compound fracture. Tie the splint in place securely but not so tightly that circulation is impaired. For further details see first aid manuals, such as that published by the American Red Cross.

Traction. As the ends of broken bones in the arms and the legs tend to override, traction should be applied before splinting, except in open fractures. Traction holds the broken edges of the bone still, thus preventing further damage to soft tissues and reducing pain and shock. Traction is accomplished by steady pulling of an intact part that is distal to the fracture, such as the wrist, the head or the ankle. Be sure that the pull is steady. A jerky movement can cause more damage to muscles, nerves and blood vessels. The amount of traction should be just enough to support the extremity in such a way that motion of the fracture area is minimized. Traction is not necessary in every fracture, but it should be applied to fractures that are unstable or those that cannot be externally splinted.

Open Fracture. In first-aid treatment of an open fracture, cover the open wound with a sterile dressing. If none is available, at least keep dirt away from the wound. The inside fold of

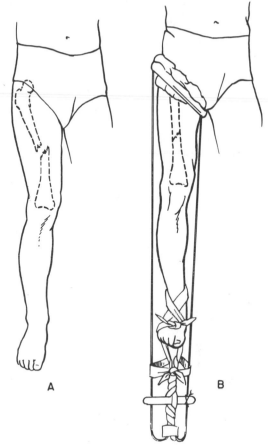

FIG. 15-1. Application of a Thomas splint to a fractured femur. (A) Diagram of a fractured femur, showing the bone fragments pulled out of alignment by muscle spasm. (B) Application of Thomas splint at the scene of the accident. Traction maintains the alignment of the bone fragments and prevents their injuring nearby tissues.

a clean handkerchief may be placed over the wound. If the bone disappears into the wound, surely carrying some dirt back with it, write a note that the bone has broken through the skin, and pin the note to the clothing of the patient. When he gets to the hospital, the doctors then will know that deep, thorough cleansing will be necessary. Do not apply traction if the bone protrudes through the open wound; you should immobilize the area by splinting. Try to prevent the contaminated end of the bone from slipping into the wound.

Infection is a prime concern in an open fracture. For this reason early débridement of the wound in the operating room is considered essential. Excision of necrotic and severely traumatized tissue, plus careful cleansing and flushing out of the wound, helps to remove the contaminated foreign materials, thus decreasing the likelihood of infection. Osteomyelitis can be a catastrophic complication of open fractures. In compound fractures the incidence of delayed union and nonunion tends to be increased, especially if infection occurs.

Although authorities are not in complete agreement, the prevailing current opinion is that the emergency use of tourniquets and antiseptics is dangerous. A tourniquet may control venous flow while the patient bleeds to death from an artery; or if the tourniquet occludes the artery, the resulting ischemia may cause gangrene, nerve compression or further soft-tissue damage. Elevate the injured part and use direct pressure over the bleeding instead of a tourniquet. Compress pressure points. Use a tourniquet only if bleeding cannot be stopped by these other methods. After a tourniquet has been applied, it should remain in place until the patient is seen by the doctor, although it should be loosened every 20 minutes to allow blood to flow to the part. Antiseptics may traumatize the tissue further, without truly disinfecting the wound. Do not use them. The doctor will order a cleansing procedure once the patient is in his care.

Patients with fractured ribs should be transported in a sitting position.

Fractures of the Spine. See Chapter 20 for first-aid measures.

HOSPITAL TREATMENT OF FRACTURES

When the patient arrives at the hospital, traction is maintained if it has been started earlier. If the patient arrives with a splint, do not remove it. X-ray films are taken before any treatment is given. If the fracture was not splinted outside the hospital, a splint is applied to immobilize the part while the patient goes to the x-ray department and waits for the x-ray films to be developed and read. The patient should travel in a wheelchair or on a stretcher. Keep the injured part elevated to minimize edema. The doctor usually orders medication for pain. Immobilization of the part also helps to reduce pain.

In removing clothing, help the patient to keep the injured part as motionless as possible. For example, to remove a jacket when the left arm is broken, have the patient remove his arm from the right sleeve first, freeing the jacket, so that it can be slipped off his left arm without moving

that arm. On occasion it may be necessary to cut clothing away. When it is possible, cut along the seam, making sure that no threads fall into any open wound.

When a patient is admitted to the hospital with multiple injuries, the doctor decides which problems are to be given prior attention. Bleeding and shock will be first on the list. The nurse and the doctor work as a team, the nurse supplying the doctor with materials as he needs them, such as intravenous setup, fluids and bandages. She observes the patient, checking on vital signs, color, urinary output, etc., and she helps to make him as comfortable as possible by such measures as providing an emesis basin, covering him with a blanket, and promptly giving him the medications ordered.

The aim of treatment is to help the body of the patient to re-establish functional continuity of the bone. One aspect of treatment does pose a dilemma: the fragments will not heal unless they are immobilized absolutely; at the same time, it is necessary to treat the limb in such a fashion that circulation is maintained and muscles will not atrophy. Early, active use of nearby muscle groups is one of the most effective ways to encourage adequate circulation. The solution to this problem is active use of the injured part without disturbance of the injured bone.

Types of Reduction

The method of treatment selected by the doctor for a fracture depends on many factors: the first aid given, the location and the severity of the break, the age and the overall physical condition of the patient. First, the doctor *reduces the fracture* (replaces the parts in their normal position) by manipulation of the fragments. He takes the broken limb in his hand and, by gentle manipulation, redirects it to its normal position. This kind of reduction is a *closed reduction.* Then he immobilizes the part by bandage, cast, traction or internal fixation.

In an *open reduction,* which is performed in the operating room, the bone is exposed and realigned under the direct vision of the orthopedist. The operation usually is performed under general or spinal anesthesia. A cast is applied, and roentgenograms are taken while the patient is still anesthetized so that any needed correction can be made without giving him more anesthesia. This method is used most frequently for dealing with soft tissue, such as nerves or blood vessels, caught between the ends of the broken pieces of bone; for wide separation of the fragments; for comminuted fractures; for fractures of the patella and other joints; for open fractures when débridement of the wound is necessary; and for internal fixation of fractures.

Skin Preparation for Open Reduction. Because osteomyelitis (infection of bone) is extraordinarily difficult to cure and may result in the patient's being permanently crippled, careful attention is paid to the preparation of the skin before any orthopedic surgery. In an emergency, shaving and cleaning the skin may be done in the operating room. When there is time, preparation begins usually the day before the surgery. The skin is shaved and scrubbed with pHisoHex, and an antiseptic is applied. The area then may be wrapped in a sterile covering, which is removed the next day, when scrubbing with pHisoHex and application of an antiseptic are repeated. A new sterile covering may be put on and left in place until the operation. In some hospitals the scrubbed area is left open.

Cast Application

Other fractures, such as those of long bones in which there is no impaction, are immobilized by casts. Casts hold the bone in place while it heals, and often they permit early ambulation even when a leg is broken. The patient may be given a narcotic before the cast is applied, or general anesthesia may be used. Sometimes a local block is performed, such as infiltrating the brachial plexus with procaine when reduction of a fracture of the arm is to be undertaken.

The doctor positions the patient as he wishes the parts to be immobilized. An assistant holds the arm or leg exactly in place. Casts that include joints usually are applied with the joints flexed to lessen stiffness later. A break in the lumbodorsal spine is corrected by allowing the patient to assume a position of hyperextension and immobilizing him in that position in a cast.

During the application of the cast the nurse stays in the fracture room, handing the doctor what he needs, perhaps giving manual support to the patient's arm or leg while the doctor's hands are busy, and giving verbal support to the patient. The doctor may be concentrating too hard to talk to the patient. A quietly spoken word from the nurse reminds the patient that he is not forgotten.

After the fragments of bone have been manipulated into place, and the cast has been applied, a second x-ray film is taken, so that the doctors

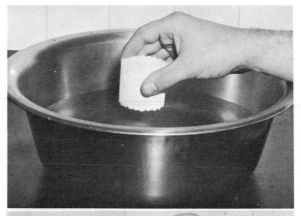

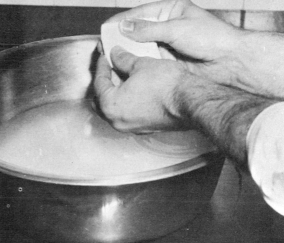

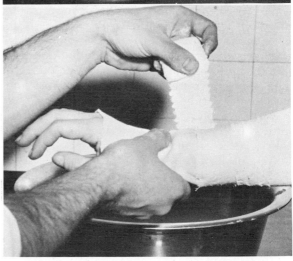

FIG. 15-2. Applying a cast. (*Top*) The roll is soaked in an upright position. (*Center*) The water is pressed out evenly and gently. (*Bottom*) The part is supported in the proper position during the bandaging.

can see that the alignment is proper. Whenever a cast is removed or applied, an x-ray picture is taken.

Drying and Finishing the Cast

Although plaster of Paris becomes hard in only a few minutes, it takes 24 to 48 hours for a cast to dry completely. During this time it needs protection. A nurse's thumbprint on the cast can leave an indentation that may cause a pressure sore on the patient's skin. Support the cast with the palm of the hand rather than the fingertips. The damp cast may feel cold, and on a winter day a warm blanket over the rest of the patient may be appreciated. If it is a hot day—on a hot day the inside of a cast feels like an oven—or if the patient is very anxious, a cool bath or the use of fans for good ventilation may help. However, no draft ever should be allowed to fall directly on a patient in a wet cast.

The cast itself must be left uncovered so that water can evaporate from it. Many doctors prefer natural evaporation, but some ask the nurse to use cast dryers to speed the drying. Never use intense heat. Not only is there danger of burning the patient, but the heat will dry the outside of the cast and leave the inside wet, so that later, perhaps, it becomes moldy. Intense heat can crack the plaster.

The damp cast never should be placed on a hard bed, where it automatically will flatten over bony prominences, later causing damage to the soft tissue between the cast and the bone. Instead, place the cast on a pillow or a series of pillows, covered with oiled silk, rubber or plastic to protect the pillow from the dampness of the cast. The pillow prevents flattening of the cast and elevates the part.

A spica (body cast) is supported on pillows until it is dry along its entire length. After several hours, turn the patient as directed by the doctor to allow the undersurface of the cast to dry. Handle the damp cast with a flat hand, keeping your fingertips away to avoid indenting it. Never lift a spica cast by the foot or the ankle; rather, slip your hand under the buttocks of the patient.

After 48 hours, when the cast is thoroughly dry, it can lie on a hard surface. Although casts are durable, like bones, they do break. A particularly active patient may need to be told of this possibility.

Edges. After a cast is dry, the nurse can finish the edges. The roughened edges of plaster crum-

ble, and cast crumbs can find their way up under the cast and cause decubitus ulcers wherever they settle. If the cast is lined with a stockinette, pull it over the edge and tape it to the cast. Some doctors secure the stockinette over the edge of the cast with plaster. If there is no stockinette, the nurse can line the edge with adhesive tape.

Spica casts need special attention to the finishing of the area near the buttocks. If there is not enough room for defecation, tell the doctor, so that he can enlarge the space. To protect the cast from getting wet and soiled, the nurse can fit some waterproof material—oilskin or plastic—around the edge and tape it to the cast. She may prefer to shellac or varnish the section of the cast that is in danger of becoming wet. A consistently damp cast will become moldy and very malodorous.

Whenever the patient is turned, inspect the buttocks, and brush away any cast crumbs that may have accumulated. You will note that the buttocks are creased where the cast has pressed against the skin; these creases are lines of potential skin breakdown. The physician should be consulted concerning any local medication that may be applied. Sometimes he recommends rubbing the involved areas with skin cream or oil, or painting them with tincture of benzoin.

CARE OF THE PATIENT IN A CAST

Elevation of Limb

While the patient wearing a cast is in his bed, the injured limb should be kept elevated to help prevent edema. A pillow or an intravenous pole can be used. Tie one end of roller gauze to the cast and the other end to the top of the pole. Inspect the skin near the edge of the cast frequently to observe whether excessive pressure is exerted there by this position. If the limb is elevated by being tied to an I.V. pole, explain the purpose of the position to the family, who may become upset by the appearance of the setup.

Observing the Patient

The nurse uses four of her senses in observing the patient with a cast:

• **Sight.** The nurse uses her trained eyes to look at all edges of the cast—top and bottom—for any place where the edge cuts into the skin. Although this possibility is more likely to occur during the first 24 hours, it can happen at any time. In cases of pressure against the skin where no edema causes pressure, the doctor may split

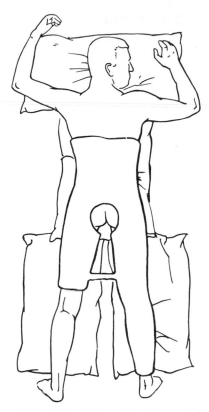

FIG. 15-3. The wet spica cast is supported on pillows until it dries. When the patient lies on his abdomen, his feet are positioned over the edges of the pillows, which are so placed that they support the patient in good body alignment.

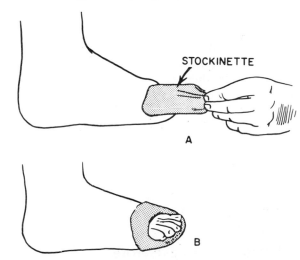

STOCKINETTE

A

B

FIG. 15-4. The edges of this cast are made smooth by pulling out the stockinette (A) and fastening it to the outside of the cast (B).

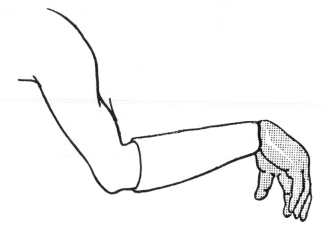

FIG. 15-5. Wristdrop caused by compression of the radial artery by a cast that is too tight. The hand is swollen and cyanotic.

the position or loosely pad the area with cotton. If the cast cuts because there is edema of the part, the doctor must be notified at once. If edema causes pressures, the doctor may split the entire cast and stockinette to release the pressure. Trimming the cast usually does no good, since the edema moves along to the trimmed edge.

Color is another useful index of pressure. The skin showing at the ends of the cast should be the same color as that of the rest of the body; it should not be white or cyanotic. Be sure that you see 5 fingers or 5 toes. The little toe has a tendency to get lost and to be compressed inside a cast that covers most of the lower leg. Teach the patient to move his fingers or his toes at the end of a cast periodically. Look to see that they move freely. One of the benefits of motion is that it helps to reduce edema in a nearby area.

The *blanching sign* is a useful color index. The nail of the great toe or of the thumb is compressed briefly and then released. The blood should rush back into it as quickly as it does into your own thumb. This test is a handy one, because you have always a standard of comparison with you—your own reaction.

• **Touch.** Make sure that the fingers and the toes at the end of a cast are as warm as the fingers and the toes on the other side of the body. If they are not, notify the doctor at once—day or night. Compression of blood vessels and nerves by a cast can cause irreparable damage. The diminished supply of oxygen and food to the tissues may cause their death. Volkmann's contracture apparently results from pressure, perhaps on the radial artery. The etiology is not entirely clear, but compression of vital structures in the arm plays a large role. The hand is swollen and blue, and the radial pulse is diminished or absent. This permanent, ugly crippling is prevented easily by a nurse and a doctor who are alert. When the nurse notices swelling and blue nails, she calls the doctor immediately, who cuts the cast and lets blood flow back into the part. Volkmann's contracture is a most serious complication of a fracture of the arm. There is no adequate treatment of the condition, but it can be prevented.

• **Smell.** Every day, as long as the patient is in her care, the nurse puts her nose right up to the edges of the cast. Because the patient can develop anesthesia in a pressure sore, sometimes the only indication that tissues inside the cast are undergoing necrosis is the odor emitted. Needless to say, the sooner a skin infection is discovered, the better for the patient.

• **Hearing.** Listen. Many a leg has been denuded of skin and muscle because nobody listened to the patient. Although some pain at the fracture line is expected the first few days, continued pain means that something is wrong.

Listen. Pay attention when the patient complains of numbness or tingling. The compression of a nerve or a blood vessel can lead to permanent damage and crippling.

Using a Cast Window. A window cut in a cast over the area of discomfort will permit visualization of that area of the skin.

Some doctors have a window cut over the radial pulse in an arm cast for the express purpose of feeling the pulse. The purpose is not to check on the patient's general condition so much as to check the circulation of the affected arm. Observe the window for edema that may puff the flesh through the opening.

If a cast is put on a patient after an open reduction, and there is bleeding from the wound, it may take longer for the blood to seep through the plaster than it would to pass through an ordinary bandage. If the nurse sees a red spot, she should encircle it with a pencil, note the time, and call the doctor. If the red spot enlarges beyond her penciled boundaries, she knows that the bleeding is continuing.

The patient may return from the operating room with a drain inserted inside the cast. In 24 hours the drain may be removed through a window.

Maneuvering the Patient

Most patients in casts become amazingly adept at locomotion in a very short time, but in the beginning, turning in a spica cast is frightening. Perhaps the worst aspect is that the patient feels and is helpless. He is encased in plaster, unable to help himself if he falls—a possibility that seldom escapes the attention of patients.

The first day or two, while the cast is still damp, and the patient is unsure of himself, two people should help him to turn, one standing at each side of the bed. Since the damp cast should not be placed directly on the bed, the covered pillows are laid in position to receive the cast while the patient is at one side.

To turn a patient in a body cast, have the patient move to one side of the bed. You stand on the other side of the bed. If you are turning him alone, be sure that he does not move so far to the opposite side of the bed that he falls out. The affected leg is the one that swings up and over. Before turning, the patient should put his arm on the unaffected side over his head, to get it out of the way. Remove the head pillows. With one hand on the patient's shoulder and the other on his hip, using good body mechanics so that you do not hurt your own back, turn the patient toward you. Do not pull on the abduction bar to turn the patient. It is more fragile than it looks. If the patient was lying on his back, he is now prone. Do not leave him with his toes digging into the bed. You can have the patient move down so that his toes hang free over the edge of the mattress, or you can elevate the cast, making sure that support all along its length leaves his toes hanging free over the end of the pillow. Each time after turning the patient, look at the exposed skin along the cast edges to see whether the new position is exerting excessive pressure.

To place a patient in a spica cast on a bedpan, pad the space just behind the pan, and elevate the head of the bed slightly to keep the fluid from running up the patient's back. Support the legs with pillows to avoid strain on the cast. Sometimes the head of the bed is elevated on blocks. The nurse cleans the patient after he has used the bedpan, if he cannot reach far enough to clean himself.

Small Objects; Itching; Exercise

The very old patient or the very young patient may push any kind of object into his cast. Coins, knitting needles, spoons, etc., may disappear inside. The pain of pressure may pass off in a few days as the wound becomes anesthetized. But a hot spot may develop on the cast over the trouble-area, and perhaps a stain will appear.

Itching, especially during hot weather, can torment the patient. Corset stays—of all things—can help. Wrap one in cotton and dip it in alcohol. Then, ever so gently, slip it down the cast to rub the itchy spot. Or a long piece of turkish towel threaded through the cast at the back can be pulled back and forth to scratch an itchy back. An applicator dipped in alcohol can be used to clean the fingers and the toes.

The patient should exercise the unaffected parts of his body. Dr. Watson-Jones sets his younger convalescent patients in body casts to running foot races and playing volley ball. No sluggish circulation, no time to brood and feel sorry for oneself when the team is losing! Although this much activity would not be possible in all conditions that demand a body cast, patients should engage in as much interesting exercise as is permitted them.

Psychological Problems

Anger and Resentment. The physical discomfort of a cast, especially a body cast, can cause serious psychological problems. A full body spica can reduce a grown man to the helplessness of a baby. He cannot go to the faucet to get a drink of water; he cannot go to the bathroom by himself. The prevention of the elementary impulse of motion is one of the most unendurable of constraints. Although most patients are grateful for the care they receive, it is natural, normal and healthy for them to resent the restrictions imposed by the cast. Many orthopedic patients who are in a state of sustained anger are not necessarily aware of why they feel that way. The nurse who can understand that her patient, for reasons beyond the control of both, may be deeply resentful has mastered an important part of orthopedic nursing. The anger is not directed purposely at the nurse, but she may be the only person around on whom the patient can vent his feelings. Usually, what he says is not meant personally.

The nurse helps the patient to dispel some of his anger by not becoming upset herself when her orthopedic patient shows anger, by encouraging as much self-sufficiency and motion (good antidotes to helplessness) as are allowed, and by listening to her patient without becoming defensive. Activities should be encouraged which allow the patient an outlet for some of the energy mobilized by anger. The stated purpose of exercise sessions conducted by a physical therapist for bed-bound orthopedic patients may be improved circulation and prevention of contractures. However, such sessions are useful, too, in dissipating energy aroused by anger. If such activities are not already scheduled on the ward, think of ways that you can initiate them. Group singing is another useful measure. It, too, can serve more than one purpose. Besides providing release of pent-up energy, it fosters deep-breathing, and helps to prevent hypostatic pneumonia.

Encouraging Self-Help. Arrange the implements for the care of the patient so that he can do as much for himself as possible. Even in a spica cast, a patient can wash the upper parts of his body. Put his food tray on a table or a stand at the same level as that of his mattress so that he can feed himself. If he cannot pour his coffee or cut his meat, perform these services for him before he asks you. A wooden prop may be used to support the patient on his side while he eats, or he may eat while lying prone. Put a shoe bag at the head of his bed to hold toilet articles. An electric razor and portable mirror will make it possible for most male patients to shave themselves. Keep the patient's water pitcher, reading material and urinal within easy reach, so that he can help himself without needing to ask for aid. Whatever helps the patient to feel adequate instead of helpless benefits him psychologically. To engage the assistance of some patients in ward tasks, such as folding pillowcases or writing headings on charts, is not only helpful to the nurse, but also is therapeutic for the patient. The nurse's expression of gratitude can do a great deal to restore the patient's self-esteem. Remember, too, that exercise with a purpose is a better morale builder than exercise for its own sake, which can be a bore. Exercise which the patient can undertake with others, and projects he can do in a group are helpful in providing companionship as well as exercise. Patients who are in private rooms require particular thought, since they lack opportunity for group activities available to ward patients. Sometimes patients in private rooms can be moved to the ward for exercise sessions or group singing.

Explanations. The doctor may show the patient his x-ray films, which are not only interesting to him, but also enable him actually to visualize the fracture. Explaining what to expect, the length of time that he probably will spend in the cast, what he will be able to do, and what limitations he will have, helps the patient to know what to expect, and, therefore, it lessens his fear of the unknown. For example, if a man knows about how long his cast will be on, and about how much limitation of motion he will have, he can make plans for returning to his job. If he has no idea about the outcome of his treatment, he may worry unnecessarily about a permanent loss of income or other things that may never happen. To be crippled is a fearful thought. Most people are afraid of the possibility, and a fracture can create deep-seated anxiety.

Later Care

If the patient is kept in the hospital only overnight or not at all, he and his family must be taught to care for his cast. Because the patient is likely to be excited from his accident, it takes a skillful teacher to reach him so that he fully understands and remembers the important points. If the hospital does not have a printed form of instructions for patients with plaster casts, the nurse should write out just what he should do: elevate the part; watch for coldness, numbness, blueness, swelling; return to the doctor the next day; do not allow the cast to get wet, etc.

Following is an example of a printed instruction sheet that gives directions for home care:

INSTRUCTIONS FOR HOME CARE—
PATIENTS WITH PLASTER CASTS

1. Go to bed as soon as you get home. Stay in bed for the next 24 hours. You may get up to go to the bathroom.

2. While you are in bed, keep the injured arm or the leg elevated on a pillow. (Protect the pillow with plastic material as long as the cast is damp.)

The hand or the foot should be the highest part of the body.

3. Whenever you get out of bed, keep the injured arm in a sling. If your leg is injured, and you sit for longer than 15 minutes, elevate your leg on a chair or a stool.

4. Move your fingers (arm cast) or toes (leg cast) for several minutes every half-hour.

5. If the cast feels tight, exercise the fingers or the toes and elevate the limb. If the tightness is not relieved, come to the hospital (emergency entrance). Immediately (day or night) report to the hospital if you notice any of the following:

Numbness of fingers or toes
Swelling of fingers or toes
Blueness of fingers or toes

Severe pain in the limb
A crack or break in your cast (if noticed at night, wait until morning to report to the hospital)

6. Return to the clinic for cast check at 8 A.M. on _____.

7. Return to the clinic for an x-ray picture at 8 A.M. on _____.

The usual sequence for a fractured arm or a fractured leg is: x-ray examination, reduction; cast application; x-ray film; the patient stays in the hospital overnight and returns to the clinic the next day for a cast check; 5 days later another x-ray film is taken; the cast may be changed; x-ray film; remove the cast after 6 to 8 weeks; x-ray film.

When the patient with an arm fracture gets out of bed, the arm that has been elevated on a pole or a pillow still has to be kept raised. Use a sling to support it. It is important to remember that the sling supports the entire arm. Include the wrist. If the wrist is allowed to drop over the edge of the sling, the fingers can become edematous, circulation can be impaired, and the nerves can be compressed. A permanent deformity could result. Make sure that the knot does not rest exactly at the back of the neck, or it will hit the cervical vertebra with each step that the patient takes.

To prevent edema of the fingers, adjust the sling so that the fingers are higher than the elbow. Never allow the sling to become so loose that the arm hangs down lower than the waist. Advise the patient to exercise the shoulder that bears the weight of the sling and the cast. If the elbow is outside the cast, it, too, should be exercised.

Removal of Cast. Casts are removed by a mechanical cast cutter. Although cast cutters are noisy and frightening, the patient should be assured that the machine will not cut him.

When the cast is removed, continued support to the limb is necessary. An Ace bandage may be put on a leg; the arm may be kept in a sling. The elastic bandage may be kept on for 5 to 6 weeks, or perhaps for several months.

The patient will have pains, aches and stiffness, and the limb will feel surprisingly light without the cast. The skin will look mottled, and it may be covered with a yellow crust composed of exudate, oil and dead skin. It may take a few days to remove this crust, but there is no hurry. Olive oil and warm baths will soften it.

Fig. 15-6. (A) The arm is positioned with the fingers higher than the elbow. (B) The knot is kept to one side of the neck, and the entire arm is enclosed in the sling. (C) The flap is pinned snugly around the elbow.

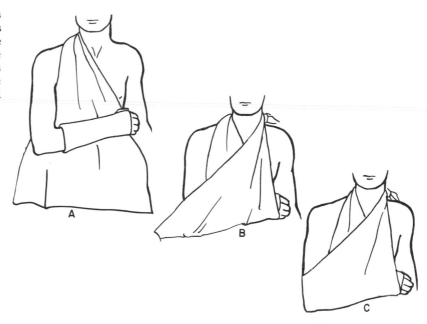

Exercise. The patient's muscles will be weak, and his circulation will be sluggish. Graded active exercise, directed by the doctor or the physical therapist, should help the extremity to regain its normal strength and motion. Resistive exercises that are beyond the patient's capacity result in increased hyperemia, fibrosis and further limitation of motion. Exercises should be active, not passive, and progressively graded so that muscles and joints are coaxed rather than forced into full range and strength of motion.

Bivalve Cast. If a cast is put on an extremity before edema has developed fully, compression of the tissues will result, because there will be no room for expansion inside a cast. To avoid this possibility, the doctor may apply the cast and, as soon as it is dry, split it along both sides. The cast sides then are refitted on the patient's limb and bandaged in place. This kind of cast is called a bivalve cast. It may be used also for a patient who is being weaned from a cast, when a very sharp x-ray film is needed, or in the treatment of such conditions as arthritis, in which the method is a convenient one for splinting the part intermittently. A bivalve cast should be removed daily, unless the doctor orders otherwise. Note any pressure areas on the skin. While the patient is out of the cast, his skin can be washed, rubbed, oiled or powdered, and the exercises ordered by the doctor can be given. Be careful not to pinch the skin when you reapply the cast.

TRACTION

Traction is used both as a temporary measure to disengage the fragments and a continuous measure to maintain the alignment of the bones. Suspension traction (using weights and pulleys) is commonly used in oblique and comminuted fractures of long bones, especially those of the legs, on which the muscle pull is strong. The pull of the traction is just enough to correct the overriding of the fragments caused by muscle spasm and to place the fragments in the position in which they should heal. Eight to 10 pounds of pull is the usual weight for the leg of an adult. Traction must be continuous and, obviously, not jerky.

Traction can be applied by means of adhesive or moleskin tape attached to the skin, or it can be applied directly to the skeletal system (skeletal traction) by inserting a pin or a wire through the end of a bone. A Steinmann pin or a Kirshner wire is threaded through the bone in leg fractures. Crutchfield or Vince tongs are attached to the skull, when traction is used in the treatment of fractured cervical vertebrae.

Explanations. The array of bars, ropes and pulleys may frighten the patient at first. Most fracture patients come to the hospital on an emergency basis, and they are in traction before they have fully gathered their senses. They have not had time to recover from the shock of their experience. At first, simple and direct ex-

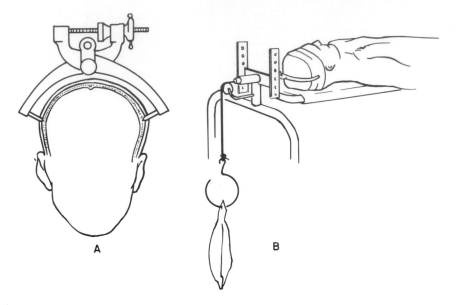

Fig. 15-7. Crutchfield tongs. (A) The prongs are inserted into the skull and securely clamped in place. Note that there is ample bone between the tongs and the brain. (B) The patient is on a Stryker or a Foster frame, which allows turning of the patient while constant traction is maintained.

planations should be given to the patient. Most important of all, he should be assured that his needs will be taken care of. Be sure that his call bell is within reach, that he knows how to use it, and that his light is answered quickly. Concerned nursing care soon will minimize his feeling that he is helplessly anchored in one place with no one to hand him a needed urinal or a blanket.

It is important for the nurse and the doctor to correct later any misconceptions that the patient may have as to the purpose of the equipment, the approximate length of time that he will be in it, the pains and the aches to be expected and the probable outcome. If these matters are not discussed with the patient, he will make up his own answers to his questions, and these may be completely wrong. It is also important to remember that severe anxiety can result in perceptual distortion. This can be a particular problem when a patient is placed in traction after the stress of an accident. The patient may, for instance, call the nurse during the first night of his hospitalization, and, in an agitated way, ask why he is "caged." Some patients, in their anxiety and confusion, perceive the traction apparatus as a cage, or in other ways experience distorted perception of their surroundings. If this occurs, turn on a light (in addition to the small night light), stay with the patient, and calmly and slowly explain to him that he is in the hospital, the purpose of the bars and ropes, and that you are close by and will come if he presses his call bell. The patient may not remember what happened, or how he got to the hospital. Help him gradually to piece together what occurred, to the extent that you have the information. If the patient has family and friends who visit him, they too can help him understand what happened. The patient's anxiety, confusion, and problems with recalling the events that brought him to the hospital are often overlooked on a busy ward in the concern to institute treatment of the physical injury. Help with the emotional impact of the event is also important, however, and can lessen anxiety and confusion and enable the patient to begin to help himself toward recovery.

Placing the Patient in Traction. The mattress on the traction bed should be firm and level. If it is not, get another. A patient in traction should never lie on a lumpy or a soft mattress. A bed board may be used under the mattress.

The doctor places the patient in traction, and the nurse helps him. If skin traction is applied, shave the limb carefully. Careless shaving removes epithelium and invites infection under the tape. Some doctors prefer that the limb remain unshaved. To toughen the skin, tincture of benzoin is swabbed on the area that will receive the adhesive. The doctor applies the tape, sets up the pulleys and weights, and positions the part in traction.

Russell traction permits the patient relative freedom to move about in bed. The knee should be bent, not kept straight. The traction cord passes first through the overhead pulley, attaches to the Balkan frame, then goes to the foot of the bed, then back to the pulley on the spreader at the patient's foot, then to the second pulley at the foot of the bed, and finally to the weights. The resulting pull on the leg is in a forward, upward direction. To keep the patient from slipping down in the bed, the foot of the bed may be elevated to provide a countertraction force. Gravity then will help to pull the patient's body toward the head of the bed.

Buck's extension is a simpler traction. It may be used to align bone fragments temporarily while the patient awaits internal fixation. Foam-rubber strips, moleskin tape and then an elastic bandage are applied to the skin of the leg; traction is accomplished with a single pulley.

CARE OF THE PATIENT IN TRACTION

After the patient is put in traction, firm pillows sometimes are placed under the leg. Some physicians disapprove of the use of pillows, because there is danger that pressure on the back of the knee may cause thrombosis. Other doctors approve of using pillows for extra support. When they are used, pillows support the thigh and the calf along their entire length. The covering on the pillows should be slippery (powdered oiled silk works well) to decrease friction, which impedes traction (the bandage will be between the limb and the silk). The patient's heel always is beyond the edge of the pillow. A Thomas splint may be used on the leg. When it is, and the traction is of the balanced suspension type (the entire leg moves up when the patient raises his hips), no pillows are used.

Observations

Check frequently to see that the patient's hand or foot is warm and of normal color—that is, it should not be white or blue, and it should match its opposite member in color. Sensation should be normal when the foot or the hand is touched. There should be no numbness or tingling.

See to it that all the ropes are in their grooves. During movement a rope can jump its track. When it does, it no longer moves. A frayed cord should be replaced before it breaks, and the weights fall to the floor. Manual traction is applied to the extremity while the cord is being changed.

Make sure that the patient's footpiece does not touch the pulleys at the foot of the bed. There is no traction when it touches the pulleys.

If suspension traction is working properly, the patient's leg will rise when he lifts his hips. If his leg does not rise, check to make sure that the traction rope is in the grooves of the pulley, and that the weights are hanging free. If the leg still does not rise, inform the doctor. He may wish to adjust the traction.

The affected leg should be straight, not twisted inward or outward.

Check the knots for tightness. Are the knots tied securely, and are their ends taped together?

The weights should swing free. A visitor or cleaning man inadvertently might have pushed a chair against them, or they may have caught on the bed.

Do the pulleys squeak when the patient moves? Not only can this annoy the patient, but free movement of the cord may be impeded. Apply a drop or two of oil to the pulley.

Make sure that the angle between the bed and the hip is approximately 20°.

The tape on the skin must not bunch or wrinkle. If it does, it can irritate and denude the skin. In Russell traction, be sure that the skin under the popliteal space, where the pull of the hammock is exerted, is protected with sponge or foam rubber. Inspect it daily for irritation.

Check to see that the patient's elbows are not becoming sore from rubbing the sheet. Long-sleeved gowns may help to protect them. After the patient's bath, apply lanolin, followed by tincture of benzoin. Teach the patient to use the overhead trapeze to lift himself in bed; he should not push up with his elbows.

Use pillows behind the bedpan to raise the patient and to prevent excreta from running down his back. Never, for any reason, remove weights without a doctor's order.

When your patient is resting, make sure that he is in a good position. Watch the patient to see that he does not slump down, so that his chin digs into his chest, now concave. Be sure that the extremity in traction is in good alignment. It should not rotate externally. A leg or an arm in traction should not be covered with a blanket, which would hamper the movement of the cord. A baby blanket or a towel so placed over the foot that it does not touch the cords may cover the foot to keep it warm. A fracture (split) blanket can be used to keep the rest of the patient warm.

Bathing and Back Care

The nurse should encourage a patient who is in traction to bathe as much of himself as he can by reaching without twisting his body out of line with the traction. The activity is both good exercise and a point in self-reliance. However, do not allow the patient to roll on his side without the doctor's permission, as this position may twist his leg out of position. To wash his buttocks and to put him on a bedpan, have the patient lift himself straight up off the bed, using the overhead trapeze. To prevent decubiti, be sure to wash and powder his buttocks well and to keep the drawsheet free of wrinkles. It is better to give back care while the patient lifts himself off the bed by using the trapeze than to have the patient turn on his side. (However, there are some instances in which the patient is allowed to turn slightly to one side. Check with the doctor.) The nurse and the patient synchronize their movements. While he pulls himself up on the trapeze, she washes his back or his buttocks. When he gets tired, he should say so. While he rests, the nurse changes the water, or she does something else for a moment. Then he lifts himself up again, and she completes the back care. Be sure to bend down and to look at the back and the buttocks. You will not be able to feel the redness of an area affected by too prolonged pressure.

Deep Breathing

Guard against hypostatic pneumonia, which is a frequent secondary cause of death in the older patient who breaks his hip and is put in traction. This dread complication is a danger for any patient who remains long in one position. Engage the patient in periodic deep-breathing exercises every 3 to 4 hours by such activities as blowing bubbles into a glass of water with a straw or blowing up balloons.

Motion

The patient's doctor will order the amount of motion allowed the patient. If you are not sure, confer with him. Patients are allowed more movement in balanced suspension traction, because the limb moves in good alignment when the patient raises his hips. Lying on the side or sitting up usually breaks the line of traction and is not allowed. The patient must carry out consistently as much motion as he is allowed. The unaffected leg must exercise up and down and engage also in knee flexing. It should go through its full range of motion. Keep in mind that as little as 2 weeks of bed rest is enough to bring on contractures of important muscle groups.

Prevent Footdrop

Footdrop is a paralytic deformity that results in an inability to hold the foot in normal position. The foot in traction should be in a natural walking position. A small splintlike footboard is used with traction. The other foot must not be allowed to grow weak from disuse. It must be exercised, and when it is at rest, it should not be pushed down with covers. A footboard not only will keep the covers off the patient's toes but also will help to prevent him from slipping down in bed. Walking is a precious ability; as patients cannot walk if they develop footdrop, every effort should be made to prevent this deformity. The most dangerous position for the unaffected leg—and this statement applies to all bed patients—is outward rotation. Although it may feel comfortable for the patient in bed, it leads easily to contractures of the strong abductor muscle groups. Teach all your bed patients to "toe in" while they are resting on their backs. If necessary, use sandbags for support, although they are a poor substitute for muscular control. Be careful that the patient does not become confined in one position for many hours.

Removal From Traction

When a patient is removed from traction, first soak the adhesive tape with ether or acetone. Then use a swab moistened with ether or acetone to help loosen the tape from the skin. Wash the leg and oil it. Find out from the physician how much movement of the affected part the patient is allowed, and make certain that the patient understands what movement is permitted. If the limb has been in traction for a considerable time, it will at first feel stiff, and there may also be some atrophy of muscles, making the limb look thinner than the other. Explain to the patient that the feeling of stiffness will disappear as he becomes able to exercise, and that the muscles will gradually grow firm and strong again as he uses his leg.

Internal Fixation. Because the patients usually are elderly, prolonged traction, which requires prolonged, debilitating bed rest, is avoided when possible. Early mobilization is desirable and possible with the use of the Jewett, the Neufeld, and the Austin Moore pins, the Smith-Petersen nail and the Thornton plate, the Pugh and the Ken nails, the Massie nail and plate, screws, and bands. Other types of devices for internal fixation of fractured hip include the

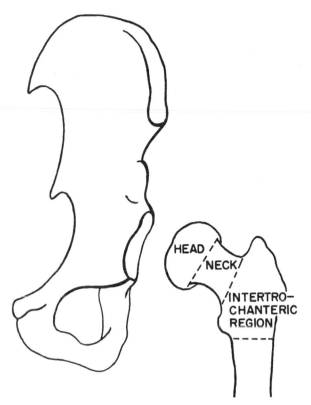

FIG. 15-8. Areas in which hip fractures are most common.

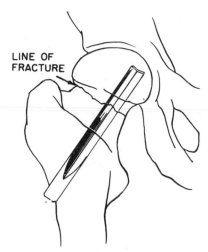

FIG. 15-9. A Smith-Petersen nail through the fractured neck of a femur.

Modny apparatus, Dyarele pins, and modification of these. These appliances are made of non-electrolytic metals, such as Vitallium and stainless steel. The bone heals around the metallic device, which in the meantime holds the bone together. Thus the bone is united immediately, and patients can be mobilized much earlier than they can be with treatment by traction. Plates, bands, screws and pins are removed only after the bone has healed, and only if they become loose or otherwise troublesome to the patient.

Another device to produce internal fixation is the intramedullary rod, which is inserted in long bones. It may be used when, for example, the patient has had a pathologic fracture. Such a patient is likely to suffer additional pathologic fractures. The patient usually is placed in traction after this procedure and may bear weight in about 3 weeks.

Bone Grafts. Sometimes cancellous bone (the reticular tissue of bone) is packed around the fracture line to stimulate bone growth. Heterogenous bone (bone from another species), homogenous bone (bone from the same species but another person), or autogenous bone (bone from the body of the patient) may be used. Autogenous bone, which may be taken from the tibia or the iliac bone, seems to be accepted best by the body. The grafted bone eventually is replaced by the growth of new bone.

Complications. Blood vessels run close to the neck of the femur. When the bone fragments produced by the fracture divide these vessels, the neck and the head of the femur suffer a loss of blood supply, which may cause avascular necrosis (called also aseptic necrosis). Dead bone looks like live bone on an x-ray film. Dead bone will unite with the live part of the femur and may even support the weight of the patient for some months following an internal fixation, but then it collapses. The incidence of nonunion is also attributed to divided arterial blood supply. Aseptic necrosis and secondary arthritic changes in the joint may occur.

Postoperative Nursing Care

Because these patients usually are elderly and have suffered two major physical insults (the trauma of the fracture and the surgery), alert, supportive nursing care and careful judgment are especially important to the life and the comfort of the patient. Hemorrhage is an immediate postoperative concern. So is postoperative pain, which may be severe. Narcotics should be administered judiciously and with consideration of the dangers of disorientation and depression of respiration. The postoperative exercises of deep

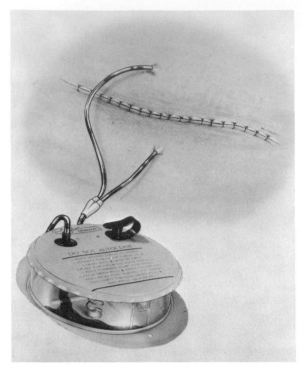

Fig. 15-10. The Snyder hemovac. This is one type of low pressure suction device which is used to drain blood and other exudates from wounds, thus facilitating healing. (Zimmer Company, Warsaw, Ind.)

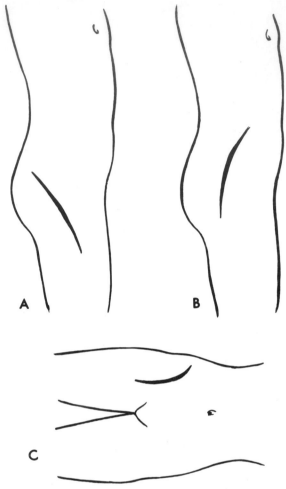

Fig. 15-11. Lines of incisions. (A) Posterior approach. (B) and (C), anterior approaches.

breathing and moving the unaffected extremities are often even more of a trial for the older patient, who might not have been agile when well. Yet the complications resulting from not participating in these exercises are life-threatening.

When there is a surgical wound in which a large skin flap covers a dead space, the patient may come from the operating room with a drain that may be connected to a low suction drainage device, such as the Hemovac; the drain may be left in place for 1 or 2 days to prevent the collection of fluid in the space (Fig. 15-10).

When a bone is nailed, there is no need for a cast. Postoperatively, the doctor will order to which side the patient may be turned. If it is toward the affected leg, the bed provides a comfortable splint and reduces the pain of movement. Place a pillow lengthwise between his legs before turning him. Turn the patient all at once, keeping the fractured leg in a straight line with the trunk. If the patient may be turned to his unaffected side, use one pillow lengthwise under his upper leg and another behind his back.

Depending on the condition of the patient, possibly on the day after the operation, exercises prescribed by the doctor are started by the physical therapist. The role of the nurse is to encourage the patient, to make the exercises as pleasant as possible, and to see that they are done at least 4 times a day. Again, the nurse reminds the patient to avoid external rotation while he is in bed by "toeing in."

After pinning for internal fixation some patients are placed in traction for 1 or 2 days to help to relieve muscle spasm. Then they are helped out of bed, sometimes to ambulate without weight-bearing on the affected leg and sometimes just to use a wheelchair. Weight-bearing on the operative side is avoided until evidence of healing is seen on x-ray film.

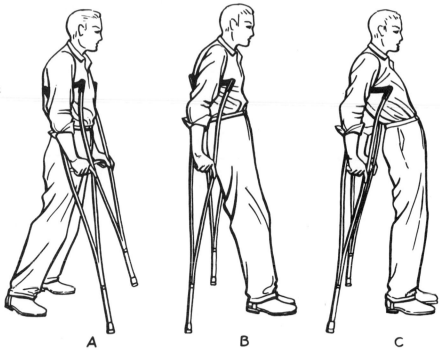

FIG. 15-12. A man with paraplegia using the swing-through gait. (A) He puts the crutches well in front of him. (B) The swing through. (C) The position in which he lands. He next puts the crutches in position (A).

When there is necrosis of the femur after a pinning, the patient will have pain and muscle spasm, and he will limp. Early recognition is important, because further weight-bearing will cause crumbling of the bone. Depending on the age, the condition and the degree of disability of the patient, reoperation for the insertion of a prosthesis may be considered.

After the insertion of a prosthesis, the position of the patient is determined by the line of the incision in the capsule. The objective is to prevent strain on the incision that would result in pushing the prosthesis through it. When the surgical approach has been posterior, the patient is kept relatively flat in bed, with the operative leg somewhat abducted and in external rotation (here is an exception to the rule). When the incision is anterior, the leg is kept in internal rotation, and the patient may sit up. He is helped out of bed on the first postoperative day and is encouraged to walk with weight-bearing as soon as the soft tissues have healed. X-ray films are taken about every 3 months the first year.

CRUTCH WALKING

The physical therapist measures the patient for crutches. It is important that they be the proper height, so that as the patient learns to walk he can hold himself erect and experience as little strain as possible. A principle of any rehabilitative measure is that it should produce the most natural situation possible. Crutches that fit properly allow the patient to walk more naturally than do ill-fitting ones.

The patient has time to think about crutch walking. It can become a goal. Warn him that progress will be slow, but mark each hard-won advance with the praise that it certainly deserves.

In preparation for walking with the aid of crutches, the patient may be taught the following exercises to strengthen his arm and his shoulder muscles: to lie on his abdomen and do push-ups, to lift sandbags up while he is lying on his back, and to sit up with both palms on the mattress and to push up until his buttocks clear the bed. Sawed-off crutches may be given to him for practicing straight elbow push-ups. At this stage he learns not to hunch his shoulders and not to lean on his crutches. In crutch walking the weight is carried on the hands, not the axillae. Branches of the brachial plexus run through the axilla; the patient who leans on his crutches may damage these nerves, so that paralysis of his arm results. This condition, known as *crutch palsy,* has been known to develop after only 4 hours of leaning on crutches without the use of handgrips.

For a day or two the patient stands before he walks. Parallel bars may be used before he tries his crutches. Standing gives him the feel of being upright with crutches. He is taught the tripod position, with the crutches ahead of him and to the side. He leans forward slightly from the ankles—not from the neck, the waist or the hips. A mirror helps the patient to obtain and to maintain good position. The patient with a pinned hip does not touch his affected leg to the floor. Shoes should fit well and have nonslip soles and heels. Women should not wear high heels. The patient is taught by diagram and demonstration before he actually tries his crutches.

Ordinarily, the physical therapist teaches crutch walking. (If there is no physical therapist, the teaching then is carried out by the nurse.) The nurse should work with the physical therapist and know what he has taught the patient. When the patient practices crutch walking in his room, on the ward or in the hall, the nurse should tell the patient what accords with the teaching of the physical therapist.

It is a tragedy if the patient falls down in the early stage of ambulation. He may be hurt, and a fall deals a severe blow to his self-confidence. Therefore, take all possible precautions. Inspect the crutch tips for wear, and teach the patient to do likewise. If the rubber shows signs of wear, discard the tip and use a new one. When the patient first starts to walk, one person stands behind him, and one stands in front. Physical therapy workers often stand behind the patient and hold him by his belt. Watch that the way is clear for the patient, and teach him to do the same. There must not be a wet or oily spot on the floor, no dropped piece of gauze, no footstool or anything else on which he can slip or trip. After looking down to see that the way is clear, he then can walk with head erect and eyes up.

OTHER FRACTURES

Fracture of the Spine. The patient with a fracture of the spine usually is placed in a position of hyperextension, a position that best reestablishes the normal position of the spinal column and exerts least pressure on the spinal cord. Continuous hyperextension may be accomplished by a cast or by immobilizing the body with head traction and sandbags over a gatch bed. Traction may be accomplished by making small burr holes in the skull into the outer layers of the parietal bones on each side and inserting tongs, such as Crutchfield tongs, which then are connected with a pulley and weights. Sandbags may be placed at the shoulders to help to keep the patient down in bed, or the head of the bed may be raised for countertraction. The patient may turn from side to side only if a doctor gives an order. The patient must be turned without bending his spine. If the patient may be turned, a Stryker or a Foster frame (Chap. 20) facilitates care. When head traction is used, place the head of the patient at the foot of the bed.

If, as rarely may be the case, the patient is not allowed to turn, his body may be held still by sandbags at his sides, or a drawsheet may be placed over his abdomen. As the patient may have to lie still in the same position for as long as 6 weeks, the care of the skin is of the utmost importance. Back care is given by compressing the mattress with one hand and slipping the other hand under the back of the patient. All of the back cannot be washed and rubbed at one time, but no area should be neglected. Beware of the development of decubiti at the back of the head. The patient is not allowed to have a pillow, but a thin piece of foam rubber under his head may help to prevent a pressure sore. Because the traction relieves pain, patients often are more comfortable in tongs than they appear to be. However, the family may need to be assured that the tongs grip only the bones of the head, and that there is no danger of puncturing the brain of the patient. Watch for signs of infection around the burr holes.

Sometimes traction is accomplished by leather or webbed straps on the head and under the chin. These can cause considerable skin irritation. Thin strips of foam rubber between the skin and the leather may help. Traction may be released momentarily for skin care only if the head is supported in the same position with the other hand, and only if the physician allows it. Use alcohol and powder. A doctor's order is required for release from traction long enough for a barber to shave a male patient. Be especially careful that there is no jerk when traction is reapplied.

Patients in the position of hyperextension may have difficulty swallowing. Feed the patient slowly. Have a suction machine nearby in case he needs it. The position is a tiresome one. There is little for the patient to look at, and his body grows weary from lying so still. A radio, a mirror and visits from family and friends may help his morale. Prism glasses enable him to read.

Massages of the parts of his body on which he lies, and range-of-motion exercises for his limbs help to maintain muscle tone. Patients who are in casts and traction are particularly susceptible to hypostatic pneumonia. Deep-breathing exercises, blowing into a bottle of water through a straw or singing should be carried out 5 or 6 times a day. If a patient has a fracture of a cervical vertebra, he may graduate to a neck brace. Since he cannot look down with this brace on, he has to be careful when he walks that he does not trip.

Fracture of the Mandible. Fractures of the mandible are treated frequently with wires that splint the lower jaw to the upper jaw. The nurse should be familiar with the wire loops that can be unhooked, and she should keep a pair of scissors strapped to the head of the bed for use in case the patient vomits. Because the patient cannot chew, the diet is liquid or, at best, semi-liquid, and he may be fed through a straw. The patient's mouth should be cleansed thoroughly after each meal and every 2 hours. Retract the cheeks with a tongue depressor, and use a flashlight to see into the mouth. These fractures usually are compound. Complications include primary hemorrhage, asphyxia and infection, which may lead to osteomyelitis.

Fracture of the Clavicle. A fractured clavicle may be immobilized by a figure-of-8 bandage. When a fractured clavicle is immobilized with plaster, the cast usually is placed over padding applied in a figure-of-8 design. Felt is placed in the axilla to protect the axillary vessels and nerves. Initially, the patient may be uncomfortable. Pressure against the axilla can be relieved by abducting the arm or resting the elbows on the arms of a chair or a table. Encourage the patient to use his arms as naturally as possible. Motion will help to prevent "frozen shoulder."

Fractured Ribs. Broken ribs are uncomfortable, since they must move when a person breathes. Often they are strapped for support, and usually they heal without trouble. They are treated with adhesive strapping, which crosses the midline to the unaffected side, front and back, and is applied as the patient exhales. Shave the skin first to facilitate the removal of the tape. Pad the nipple area.

DISLOCATIONS AND SPRAINS

Dislocations occur when the articular surfaces of a joint are no longer in contact. In adults they are caused by trauma or, less frequently, by disease of the joint. The symptoms are pain, malposition, leading to an abnormal axis of the dependent bone, and loss of the function of the joint. Treatment consists of manipulation of the joint until the parts are again in normal position, followed by immobilization by Ace bandage, cast or splint for several weeks to allow the joint capsule and surrounding ligaments to heal.

Manipulation never should be attempted by anyone except a physician, who usually makes an x-ray examination first and may anesthetize the patient for the procedure. Amateur attempts at reduction may injure further the capsule of the joint and surrounding structures, and sometimes cause fractures or hemorrhage.

If the patient must be transported to the doctor, the affected joint should be splinted. After the reduction of the dislocation the nurse watches for compression resulting from tight bandages or a tight cast.

Sprains are injuries to the ligaments surrounding a joint. They are accompanied by pain, swelling and loss of motion. They may become ecchymotic because of the rupture of the nearby blood vessels. An x-ray film may be taken to differentiate a sprain from a fracture. Treatment consists of elevation of the part and application of an elastic bandage. Buccal Varidase may be used early to minimize swelling. An injection of hydrocortisone and lidocaine at the point of maximum tenderness helps to relieve pain. There is a tendency now to treat sprains by having the patient continue to use the affected part after providing support with elastic bandage. An ankle, for example, may be strapped, and then the patient is allowed to walk.

REFERENCES AND BIBLIOGRAPHY

BLAKE, F.: Immobilized youth—a rationale for supportive nursing intervention, *Am. J. Nurs.* 69:2364, November, 1969.

COMPERE, E. L., BANKS, S. W., and COMPERE, C. L.: *Pictorial Handbook of Fracture Treatment,* ed. 5, Chicago, Year Book, 1963.

DAVIS, L.: *Christopher's Textbook of Surgery,* ed. 9, Philadelphia, Saunders, 1968.

FRANCIS, SR. M.: Nursing the patient with internal hip fixation, *Am. J. Nurs.* 64:111, May, 1964.

FRANCIS, G., and MUNJAS, B.: *Promoting Psychological Comfort,* Dubuque, Wm. C. Brown, 1968.

GARTLAND, J. J.: *Fundamentals of Orthopaedics,* Philadelphia, Saunders, 1965.

GOULD, M. L.: Nursing care of the patient with a fractured hip, *Am. J. Nurs.* 58:1561, 1958.

HARVEY, J. P.: Treatment of common fractures, *GP* 29:122, 1964.

HOWORTH, B.: *Injuries of the Spine*, Baltimore, Williams & Wilkins, 1963.

KNOCKE, L.: Crutch walking, *Am. J. Nurs.* 61:70, October, 1961.

LARSON, C., and GOULD, M.: *Calderwood's Orthopedic Nursing*, ed. 6, St. Louis, Mosby, 1965.

LIFE REPORT: Brave man fights on, a pictorial account of rehabilitation of Roy Campanella, fracture of cervical vertebra, *Life* 45(3):82, July, 1958.

LINDSEY, D.: Effective emergency splinting, *Am. J. Nurs.* 56:1120, 1956.

MERCER, W., and DRATHIE, R.: *Orthopaedic Surgery*, Baltimore, Williams & Wilkins, 1964.

MOORE, M., JR.: Ambulation following fractures of the lower extremity, *Am. J. Nurs.* 53:174, 1953.

NAYLOR, A.: *Fractures and Orthopedic Surgery for Nurses and Physiotherapists*, ed. 5, Baltimore, Williams & Wilkins, 1964.

NEUFELD, A. J.: Surgical treatment of hip injuries, *Am. J. Nurs.* 65:80, March, 1965.

POWELL, R.: *Orthopedic Nursing*, ed. 5, Baltimore, Williams & Wilkins, 1966.

ROBINSON, M., and VAN VOLKENBURGH, S. T.: Intermaxillary fixation: immediate postoperative care, *Am. J. Nurs.* 63:71, January, 1963.

SCHMEISSER, G.: *A Clinical Manual of Orthopedic Traction Technique*, Philadelphia, Saunders, 1963.

STAMM, T. T.: *A Guide to Orthopaedics*, ed. 2, Philadelphia, Davis, 1964.

TAYLOR, J., and GAITZ, C.: Obstacles encountered in rehabilitation of geriatric patients, *Nurs. Forum* 8:64, 1969.

TUREK, S. L.: *Orthopaedics*, ed. 2, Philadelphia, Lippincott, 1967.

VIEK, P., and MANCUSO, C.: *Guide to Hospital Orthopaedic Practice*, Philadelphia, Davis, 1963.

The Patient with Disease of Bones and Joints

16

Arthritis · Rheumatoid Arthritis · Ankylosing Spondylitis
(Rheumatoid Spondylitis) · Degenerative Joint Disease
(Osteoarthritis) · Gout · Bone Tumors · Osteomyelitis

ARTHRITIS

Arthritis means inflammation of a joint. The disease has been known throughout human history. Evidence of arthritis has been found in Egyptian mummies, and clear descriptions of the disease go back almost as far as the written word.

Arthritis has many forms. The term is applied usually to diseases in which a major symptom involves joints. The etiology and the relationships of the various arthritic disease entities are subject to various interpretations. It has been suggested that rheumatoid arthritis is a collagen disease. Considerable medical attention has been focused on attempts to understand the pathology, the cause and the interrelationships of the collagen diseases, including rheumatic fever, systemic lupus erythematosus, periarteritis nodosa and rheumatoid arthritis. Because there is as yet no agreement concerning the cause of rheumatoid arthritis, the way in which the condition is classified varies widely in the literature. We shall include a discussion of different types of arthritis in this chapter. Other diseases to which it may be related are discussed in other chapters.

At the present time in the United States rheumatic diseases rank first among the causes of disability. Between 15 and 16 million people suffer from some form of rheumatic disease. Some 300,000 are disabled.

Types of Arthritis

A partial classification of the complex disease entities usually included in the term *arthritis* is:

- Polyarthritis of unknown etiology (example, rheumatoid arthritis)
- Degenerative joint disease (example, osteoarthritis)
- Infectious arthritis
- Traumatic arthritis
- Arthritis associated with biochemical or endocrine abnormalities (example, gout)
- Tumor
- Allergy and drug reaction

Infectious arthritis is caused by a specific microorganism. For example, in untreated tuberculosis, the tubercle bacillus may proceed to invade the joints. Staphylococci or streptococci may infect a joint, as may many other microorganisms. Usually only one joint is involved, and that joint shows infection by the usual signs: warmth, redness, pain and swelling. Joints normally are sterile, and the products of bacterial growth are harmful to the lining of the joint. In an effort to dilute these harmful products, fluid is poured into the joint cavity. This fluid accounts for some of the pain and much of the swelling. After the infectious organism has been identified (a culture may be taken from aspiration of the fluid in the joint), the arthritis is treated with a drug to which that organism is

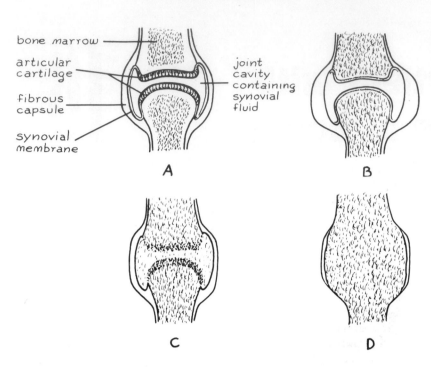

bone marrow

articular cartilage

fibrous capsule

synovial membrane

joint cavity containing synovial fluid

A

B

C

D

FIG. 16-1. Pathologic changes in rheumatoid arthritis. (A) Normal ball-and-socket joint. (B) Same joint, showing progression of pannus formation, destruction of cartilage and acute inflammation. (C) Inflammation subsided; fibrous ankylosis. (D) Bony ankylosis; the joint is immobile.

sensitive. In the case of bacterial infection, the antibiotics are administered systemically, and sometimes they are injected directly into the joint as well. Happily, the use of modern drugs has made infectious arthritis uncommon.

Arthritis due to direct trauma may be caused by a sudden twist, a direct blow to the joint or a multitude of small insults. In this category fall such disorders as arthritis of the feet of ballet dancers.

In adults the two major causes of disability due to arthritis are rheumatoid arthritis and degenerative joint disease.

RHEUMATOID ARTHRITIS

Rheumatoid arthritis is an inflammatory disease of connective tissue, characterized by chronicity, remissions and exacerbations. Constitutional symptoms and joint changes, which may become permanent deformities, are part of the disease.

Incidence

Rheumatoid arthritis is found throughout the world. In the United States, 4 million people are estimated to have this form of arthritis; half of them are under the age of 45. This crippling disease strikes during the most productive years of adulthood. Eighty per cent of the cases start between the ages of 25 and 50 (Primer on the

Rheumatic Diseases). Three times as many women as men are affected (Kellgren).

Pathology

Rheumatoid arthritis is a systemic disorder; its nature' is not fully understood, and its etiology is as yet unknown. However, the local effect in the joint can be described. Some of this effect is due to the disease itself and some to the body's reactions against it. For example, the replacement of damaged tissue by fibrosis is a defense mechanism of the body. However, scars due to fibrosis can lead to crippling contractures.

Synovitis, inflammation of the synovial membrane surrounding a joint, the earliest pathological change, causes congestion and edema. Pathophysiologic changes follow, leading to the formation of a tissue which adheres to the opposite joint surface, inhibiting motion. This is the stage of *fibrous ankylosis* (abnormal immobility of a joint).

When the restricting band of tissue becomes calcified, as it may, the stage of *osseous ankylosis* has arrived, and the joint no longer exists. This process from nonspecific synovitis to complete ossification of the joint may take years, and it may proceed at different rates in different joints in the same patient.

About 15 per cent of the patients develop subcutaneous nodules (Hollander). These appear

FIG. 16-2. Appearance typical of arthritic hands. The joints become sore, swollen and deformed. (Medichrome—Clay-Adams, Inc., New York, N.Y.)

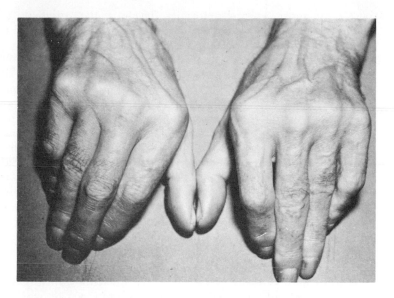

over pressure points, such as the elbow or the base of the spine. Though usually painless, they may be quite painful, especially if continuous pressure is put on them, as in a chair-bound patient who has nodules at the base of his spine.

Muscles become weak and atrophy, partially from disuse. Because of connective-tissue changes and neurovascular changes, the extremities often have a smooth, glossy appearance, and they may be cold and clammy.

Etiology

The causative factors of rheumatoid arthritis have not yet been discovered. It is probable that one or more factors trigger the onset of arthritis (Hollander). Although many types of organisms have been implicated as etiological agents in rheumatoid arthritis over the past 50 years, none has withstood the test of close scrutiny. In spite of this, there is a strong feeling that a viable agent (probably virus-like) will be found as research technics improve. The organism itself may be the cause of the abnormal autoimmune reaction which causes the body to produce antibodies against its own tissues. These autoantibodies are of both diagnostic and pathologic significance. Faulty adaptation to physical stress as an etiological factor is applied more often to degenerative joint disease; the theory of faulty adaptation to psychic stress remains unproved. Some observers have remarked that arthritis patients have dependent personalities, but the analysis was made after the disease had started, after pain and disability had taken their toll.

Children of arthritic parents have a greater tendency to develop the disease than those whose ancestors have no such history. Heredity may be a factor, but the evidence pointing to this theory could be explained also by environmental factors. Perhaps a latent virus infection was passed from the mother to the child.

Although the causes of rheumatoid arthritis have not been found, some previously suspected theories have been ruled out. This disease is not caused by faulty diet, lack of vitamins, overdose of vitamins or cold and damp weather.

Symptoms

In 75 to 80 per cent of the patients the onset is insidious. Over a period of time patients notice that a joint or two is stiff when they wake up in the morning. There are twinges of momentary discomfort in a finger or two. Slowly some joints, usually the fingers, become moderately sore, red and swollen. Over a period of weeks other joints become involved. Swelling and pain come and go. In the meantime the patients find that they tire easily. They lose weight, and they may develop a fever and a feeling of malaise. Tolerance for any kind of stress is lessened. Even temperature changes are tolerated poorly. Although the diet may be adequate in iron, patients characteristically have a persistent anemia because of the effect of this chronic disease on the blood-forming organs.

As the disease progresses, the muscle-wasting around affected joints accentuates the appearance of swelling. The proximal finger joints swell the most, and as deformity develops, the fingers point toward the lateral aspect of the hand. Extremities become cold, moist and mauve-colored. Patients in this stage of the disease have considerable pain even at rest and especially on motion.

Arthritis is a capricious disease. The symptoms may vanish suddenly for reasons apparent to neither the doctor nor the patient. Inflammation leaves the joints that were sore and red; the patient is not stiff, he has no fever, and his pain is gone. However, the symptoms almost invariably return after the patient has had a symptom-free period. Inflammation causes more joint damage, and then there is another remission. The pattern of remissions and exacerbations continues over the years.

Without treatment—and sometimes with it—the joint may be destroyed totally. As the synovial space is replaced with bony growth, motion is lost. When the joint becomes immobile, the pain of the inflammation is lessened, but there still is discomfort because of contractures and immobility. One of the aims of treatment is to decrease the inflammation of the joint before it has become one bone.

Treatment

Although the cause of rheumatoid arthritis is still a mystery, and the disease cannot be cured, much can be done to lessen its damage. Early treatment before the onset of fibrous or bony ankylosis gives the best results. Treatment is designed to make the patient more comfortable, to prevent or to correct deformities, and to maintain or to restore function of the affected parts of the musculoskeletal system.

Optimal health conditions should be maintained, since supporting the resistance of the body to the inflammation is one of the few truly therapeutic steps that medicine has to offer. Rest, both systemic and local, is balanced carefully with exercise. Even during an acute phase of the illness some movement of the affected parts usually is prescribed in order to help to lessen the possibility of bony ankylosis, muscle wasting, osteoporosis and the debilitating effects of prolonged rest. Deep breathing and prescribed exercises, graded to the condition of the patient, strengthen general body tone and keep specific muscle groups from atrophy. The patient should be encouraged to eat an optimum diet, even though he may have little appetite. Unless there are other medical complications such as

diabetes or hypertension, this diet need not be modified from that of a normal individual.

Drug Therapy

Drug therapy in rheumatoid arthritis is not curative, but it helps the patient to feel less pain, and in some instances it depresses the inflammatory process (antiphlogistic action). Because of the long-term nature of this disease, the relief of pain by the use of narcotics is avoided.

The Salicylates. Aspirin (acetylsalicylic acid) is the major drug in the group. In early rheumatoid arthritis it seems to have an antiphlogistic action as well as to afford the patient specific relief of joint pain. In chronic rheumatoid arthritis the relief appears less dramatic, but it still is present, and probably it is more related to the general analgesic properties of the drug than to any specific action (Beckman). The manner in which this common drug works still is not fully understood.

The usual dose in rheumatoid arthritis is 2 to 4 (0.3 Gm.) tablets 2 to 6 times a day. Some doctors give the drug until the serum level of salicylates reaches 25 mg. per cent (Primer on the Rheumatic Diseases) to 35 mg. per cent (Beckman).

Large doses of aspirin, which may help the inflammatory process to subside, also may give rise to the side-effects of salicylism: nausea, vomiting, tinnitus, deafness, drowsiness, hyperpnea, slow pulse and peripheral vasodilation.

A serious problem is that aspirin may erode the mucosa of the stomach, leading to multiple small spots of bleeding. Patients on high doses of aspirin should be instructed to watch their stools for evidence of gastrointestinal bleeding (black, tarry stool). Rarely, there may be interference with kidney function or blood clotting.

Hyperpnea, rare in adults, may lead to alkalosis through an excessive loss of carbon dioxide. These effects are reversible by stopping the medication. Some individuals may have an allergy to aspirin, which commonly manifests itself as a skin rash. Dehydration should be prevented since it can lead to serious salicylate toxicity (particularly in children), during hot summer months.

Milk and crackers taken before the drug may help to prevent gastric distress. Buffered or enteric-coated aspirin sometimes are ordered. If the patient experiences distress that seems to be related to his aspirin intake, the doctor should be notified. Some patients decrease the dose or omit the tablets entirely without consulting the doctor, and yet control of the symptoms depends on a high, sustained blood level of the drug. If the patient is experiencing toxic side-effects, the physician should know.

Phenylbutazone (Butazolidin). This drug has been found to be effective as an analgesic and antiphlogistic in about 50 per cent of the patients with rheumatoid arthritis (Hollander). If phenylbutazone is not effective within 1 to 2 weeks, it is discontinued. It is given by mouth in doses of 100 to 400 mg. a day. Side-effects include nausea, abdominal pain, skin rash, visual disturbances, dizziness, lethargy, fever, anemia and edema from sodium retention, especially in patients with cardiac problems. Serious toxic reactions may occur, such as the reactivation of a peptic ulcer with gastric bleeding, agranulocytosis, leukopenia, thrombocytopenic purpura, exfoliative dermatitis, psychosis, hypertension and toxic hepatitis. Many patients receiving this drug have adverse effects. Patients maintained on phenylbutazone need periodic blood counts.

Oxyphenbutazone (Tandearil) is a related compound with much the same effects and dosage.

Indomethacin (Indocin) in the dosage of 25 mg. t.i.d. or q.i.d. is used with good effect in some patients.

Antimalarials (Atabrine, Chloroquine, Plaquenil). These drugs show an affinity for connective tissue, and so they are used sometimes to help to control the inflammation of arthritis. They usually require some time to show their effects (3 to 6 weeks). Atabrine is used rarely, because it turns the skin yellow. Toxic effects may include anemia, such eye symptoms as blurred vision, halo around lights, and difficulty in adjusting to glare, and gastrointestinal symptoms. Deposits of Chloroquine in the eye may cause retinal damage. The gastric distress usually is alleviated by taking the medication with food. The usual dosage of Chloroquine is 250 mg. a day.

Soluble Gold Salts (gold sodium thiosulfate, gold thioglucose). The results of therapy with gold seem less dramatic than the effects of therapy with corticosteroids (below). There may be 2 or 3 months between the start of gold therapy and the therapeutic results of decrease in inflammation and pain. The time lapse may be very discouraging to the patient. Therapy with gold is not always effective. Although approximately one third of the patients will show

a reaction, most of these reactions are mild skin rashes that may or may not have anything to do with the gold. The patient is observed carefully with blood counts and urinalysis, as well as questions regarding skin manifestations, in order to detect early the more severe toxic effects. Among the serious reactions are jaundice, blood dyscrasias, hepatitis, hematuria, toxic nephritis, and severe gastrointestinal upsets. In a small number of patients the arthritic process may flare up. When there is a severe toxic reaction, it is necessary to discontinue the drug, and this action usually brings on a sharp exacerbation of the disease. The usual dosage is 50 mg. of the salt weekly to a total of 1.0 gm.; and then the dose is changed over gradually to a maintenance dose of 50 mg. a month for a prolonged period. The drug is given intramuscularly.

Steroids. These hormones do not cure arthritis, but they do give the patient prompt relief from pain and stiffness. Both physical and mental well-being are improved. However, the long-term use of a steroid may cause side-effects that result in a greater disability than that which would have come if no steroid at all had been used. Close supervision by the physician of the dosage is imperative for safety.

Corticosteroids. These drugs are synthetic reproductions of the adrenal cortical hormone, hydrocortisone. Among the functions of hydrocortisone are the regulation of carbohydrate metabolism and ionic balance and the ability to stand stress.

Hydrocortisone (Cortisol) is administered orally. The dosage used commonly is 10 mg. q.i.d.

Prednisone (Meticorten, Deltra, Deltasone) and prednisolone (Delta-Cortef, Meticortelone, Hydeltra, Sterane) are given orally: Most patients respond to doses of 3 mg. to 5 mg. a day (Hollander).

Corticotropin (ACTH, Acthar). This drug is derived from the pituitary gland and acts to stimulate the adrenal cortex. It is given to patients to stimulate their own production of hydrocortisone. When ACTH is given to a patient, his natural anterior pituitary gland production is reduced, and his adrenal cortices hypertrophy as they are stimulated to do increased work.

Because ACTH is destroyed in the gastrointestinal tract, it is given intramuscularly or intravenously rather than orally. A usual dose is 10 U. o.d. I.M. of corticotropin gel.

Side-effects of both the corticosteroids and ACTH are frequent, as patients usually are kept on these drugs for long periods of time. The lower the dose, the less is the chance of developing serious side-effects.

One of the most dangerous effects, the suppression of inflammation, is what makes the arthritic patient feel better; but this advantage carries with it a penalty. Inflammation is a body defense that serves the dual purpose of fighting infections and, by pain and swelling, calling attention to the troubled part of the body. A patient on steroids loses along with the pain of inflammation much of his ability to fight infection. Symptoms are suppressed, and because they can go unnoticed, they can go untreated. An arthritic patient on high dosage of steroids may have an infected tooth or appendicitis and never know it because the symptoms are masked. The unchallenged infection can proceed to septicemia or a burst appendix, as the steroids depress the symptoms of inflammation without curing the infection. One of the most important points in the nursing care of the patient on steroid therapy is observation for the slightest sign of trouble anywhere in the body. The smallest rise in temperature or the slightest discomfort in a new area is reported immediately to the doctor.

Another common side-effect is weight gain due both to an accumulation of fat and to a redistribution of ions in the fluid compartments of the body. Sodium is retained, and potassium is lost. The patient frequently becomes edematous; he acquires a moonface and perhaps a buffalo hump. These changes are not usually considered an indication to discontinue the drug. A low sodium diet may be ordered. Because of the possibility of developing edema, the patient's weight is observed carefully both in the hospital and at home. Instruct the patient to keep a record of his weight, weighing himself at intervals recommended by his doctor.

Steroids can give rise to peptic ulcers. Pay attention to complaints of gastric distress, and report them promptly to the doctor. Acne may appear in a patient who believed that he was far enough beyond adolescence never again to be troubled with it. There also may be increased pigmentation of skin, hirsutism (hairiness), amenorrhea (cessation of menstruation), osteoporosis, weakness and mental depression. The blood becomes more coagulable, increasing the danger of thrombi and emboli. The patient may bruise easily. In one study (Rothermich) of 160 patients on long-term steroid therapy, 67 had an increase in appetite with weight gain, 65 developed cosmetic problems, 62 had edema, 24 had dyspepsia, and 11 developed psychiatric disturbances. Other adverse effects included fracture due to osteoporosis, easy bruising and gastrointestinal bleeding.

The patient usually is concerned about such side-effects as moonface, as well as other possible effects which without altering his appearance may have serious effects on his health. He is helped by the knowledge that side-effects subside once the drug is discontinued.

Supplements. Since therapy with corticosteroids results in a negative nitrogen balance in the body, supplementary gonadal hormones, because of their anticatabolic action, also are prescribed by some physicians, especially for elderly and postmenopausal patients. Unexpected vaginal bleeding should be reported to the doctor, and the female patient should have regular pelvic examinations.

Since the various preparations of cortisone depress natural adrenal cortical activity, and ACTH depresses natural anterior pituitary activity, the sudden withdrawal of the drugs causes severe symptoms. When cortisone is discontinued abruptly, the patient has headache, nausea, retching, severe anorexia, weight loss, malaise, aches and pains, restlessness, insomnia and fatigue. To allow the body to resume its own production of hormones, both cortisone and ACTH are tapered off slowly; each day a little less is given.

After a course of steroid therapy patients seem to do well with their own hormones able to function adequately, unless there is an unusual stress of the body. For example, if a patient has been on steroid therapy during the past year and requires surgery, hydrocortisone or one of the other steroids is readministered, since without these supplements he may suffer from an acute deficiency of steroids because of the failure of his adrenal glands to respond adequately to the stress of surgery.

Other Aspects of Treatment and Nursing Care

During an early acute phase of rheumatoid arthritis the patient feels both ill and frightened. If he is febrile, he may be kept in bed, and no effort is spared to reduce his pain. A cradle or a footboard keeps the bedcovers from pressing tender feet into abnormal positions, such as outward rotation.

A patient at the early stage of rheumatoid arthritis—or any chronic disease, for that matter—needs accurate information about the probable course of the disease, so that he can plan for the future. As rheumatoid arthritis progresses slowly in about 80 per cent of the cases, the immediate way of life of a patient need not change drastically. If he understands the disease process, there are things he can do at the very early stages that will be helpful in preventing present fatigue and later deformity.

He will need to learn about the pathology of the joint changes, so that he will understand why he must both exercise and rest, and that the disease has spontaneous remissions. He should be told what does *not* cure arthritis, so that he can avoid spending money on worthless "cures."

Exercise. The use of exercise in rheumatoid arthritis has three objectives: (1) to preserve or to increase the function of the joint by preventing ankylosis, (2) to maintain muscle tone and to improve strength, and (3) to improve the ways of moving so that coordination is promoted. Disuse of a joint leads to stiffness, which leads to more disuse. The patient with deformities tends to avoid the use of deformed joints or to move in ways that increase the deformities.

Relative amounts of rest and exercise are planned carefully for each individual patient. Reparative processes are favored by rest, but prolonged immobilization may lead to ankylosis. Some exercises may be done while the patient is lying down; thus he avoids the extra work of overcoming the pull of gravity. The joint needs protection against overuse, wobbling and partial dislocations. If it is possible, after heat and perhaps light massage, each joint should be exercised several times a day.

Only gentle stretching is permissible. Excessive activity to the point of pain or fatigue, vigorous exercise of an inflamed part, or movement that increases joint instability and abnormal deviation and dislocation can cause further damage. Active exercise is more therapeutic for the muscles than passive movement.

Many hospitals and public health agencies have physical therapists who will be responsible for teaching the patient his exercises, applying heat, massage and perhaps whirlpool baths or contrast baths to limbs. The nurse keeps herself up-to-date with the patient's current exercises and helps him to do his exercises at the prescribed times. Where there is no physical thera-pist, the nurse has the responsibility for teaching the exercises. Some rules for exercises are:

1. The number and the duration of the rest and the exercise periods change as the patient's condition changes. These are determined by the doctor and governed by how the patient feels. The exact nature of the exercises is prescribed by the doctor.

2. Exercises can seem a tiresome chore, and they may be uncomfortable. Discomfort during or immediately after an exercise should be expected. However, exercise that causes excessive pain should be decreased.

3. Affected joints should go through their prescribed exercises several times a day.

4. Several short periods (of 5 to 10 minutes) are better than fewer, longer ones (of 20 to 30 minutes).

5. As the tolerance of the patient improves, the number of exercise periods can be increased from a starting number of about two a day, and the number of times each exercise is repeated during a period can be increased, starting with about two times.

If the patient is very uncomfortable, he may benefit from taking his dose of aspirin a half-hour before exercising. However, there is danger that a joint still affected with active disease but less painful because of aspirin or corticosteroids may be exercised beyond its capacity to sustain exercise without damage. Many patients find that the application of heat before exercising makes them more comfortable. Each exercise period can start with deep breathing.

Rest. The arthritic joint, to maintain motion, needs rest as well as exercise. Because joints limited in motion tend to take the form of flexion, which leads to contractures, rest should be in the position of greatest possible extension without actual pain. Therefore, the frequent, necessary rest periods are not as comfortable for the patient as they might be if the line of least resistance were followed. The proper position for rest is flat on the back on a well-supported bed. A small pillow or folded towels can be placed under the head, under the elbow to extend the arm, and under the wrist to extend it. The hands should be turned with the palms upward. A small pillow under the ankles straightens the knees. A pillow under the knees would be more comfortable, but it would cause flexion rather than extension. Sandbags placed against the outside of the feet keep them from rolling outward and straining the knees. Use rolled blankets instead of sandbags in the home—or in the hospital, for that matter—unless you are sure that there will be someone available and knowledgeable enough to move them and to help the patient to change his position often. Because this rather uncomfortable position does help to postpone the deforming effects of arthritis, it should be maintained intermittently for about 10 of the 24 hours in a day. The patient should lie flat and prone some of the time.

Heat. Heat is more of a comfort than a curative measure. Because it improves circulation and relieves muscle spasm and pain, it allows the part better rest and easier exercise. Heat can be applied dry or wet. Dry heat sometimes is applied by a heating pad (on low—watch out for burns), a paraffin bath, an infrared bulb, a hot-water bag or an appliance such as the Aquamatic pad which maintains a constant degree of heat. The ordinary heating pad is not as effective as other measures. Infrared heat penetrates deeper than the level of the skin. Even superficial heat affects deeper-level blood vessels by reflex action. Diathermy and ultrasonic therapy do not seem to have a special advantage in rheumatoid arthritis (Beeson and McDermott). Many arthritic patients prefer wet heat, claiming that it penetrates better. Wet heat can be applied in the form of baths, either local or tub. Patients who have advanced disease may find getting in and out of a tub too much of a struggle; in such cases, towels dipped in water at 116° F., wrung out and applied are effective. Heat in any form should be applied for 20 to 30 minutes. The application of pure lanolin or other lotions may help to counter the drying effects of this treatment.

There has been an increasing interest on the part of physicians and physical therapists in the use of cold rather than heat for relief of pain and spasm. There are strong advocates for both modalities. Patients frequently find much greater relief with one modality over the other.

Massage improves the flow of both blood and lymph, but it is not used on a joint that is actively inflamed, as it may aggravate the disease.

Equipment. Various mechanical aids have been devised to help the disabled in the performance of day-to-day tasks. Rare is the arthritic for whom a mechanism cannot be fashioned that helps him to feed himself, to comb his own hair, to select his own programs on the television set, and to cope with more complex and specialized problems. Some mechanical aids are currently on the market; others can be custom-built, very often of improvised materials, if a little ingenuity is employed. A device should be lightweight and as simple as possible. If the patient finds it inconvenient or does not like it for any reason, he will not use it.

Not every action of the arthritic should be governed by a gadget. Indeed, his life will be simpler if he has to take care of only a few appliances; but if a device can give a patient the independence of necessary self-help, by all means encourage him to use it.

Important things should come first. If playing gin rummy is a source of great pleasure to Mr. Jones, then finding a way for him to hold his cards is given priority. If Mrs. Stewart loves to read, she will probably follow her instructions to rest more faithfully if she has a pair of prism glasses. If Mrs. Bishop's self-esteem is damaged because she no longer can iron for her family, find a way for her to iron without hurting herself. Extensive information on self-help devices can be obtained by writing to The Arthritis Foundation.

Braces, bivalved casts or splints to joints that are painful and in spasm help to prevent dislocations and deformity and to keep the rest of the joints mobile (Rotstein). Splints have three basic functions: (1) immobilization for local rest during an active phase of the disease; (2) remedial, used to correct deformities, such as a long brace with a turnbuckle across the back of the knee to help place that joint in extension; and (3) supportive, to help overcome weakness. If poor posture is imposing an abnormal strain on weight-bearing joints, the patient may be fitted with a corset that improves posture. The splint or brace must fit well, be neither constricting nor loose, be lightweight, and it must maintain the joint in a good functional position. Observe for friction on the skin. Adequate padding and good skin care protect the skin. Check for rough edges that might tear the skin of the patient. Once a week the leather parts should be saddle-soaped, and the metal joints should be oiled.

The bed should be flat and firm with only one small pillow. A bed board that fits should be placed under the mattress and firmly attached, so that when the patient moves near the edge, he is not in danger of tipping the bed board over. The height of the bed should be level with that of the wheelchair, if the patient moves back and forth between the two.

Surgery. The use of surgery to overcome or prevent deformity is becoming an increasingly important aspect of early treatment. Previously surgery was resorted to only late in the disease after extensive damage had been wrought. Synovectomy (removal of the diseased lining) performed early is being extensively investigated as a means of preventing destructive changes in affected joints, particularly those of the hands, feet and knees. When muscle spasm is causing progressive deformity, tendons may be transplanted to change the direction of pull to a corrected one. An artificial angling of the bone through surgical fracture (osteotomy) may improve the utility of a deformed limb. Arthroplasty, the fashioning of a new joint with artificial material (such as a vitallium cup), may be resorted to. When all hope of salvaging a joint is gone, but it is still painful and troublesome to the patient, an arthrodesis (fusion of the joint surfaces) may be performed, eliminating the joint but relieving the pain.

It is especially important that postoperative exercises be applied when and as prescribed by the surgeon. For example, following synovectomy and arthroplasty of the fingers there may be lateral instability, and exercises requiring wide spreading of the fingers with abduction and adduction motions must be avoided (Flatt).

Living With Arthritis

The 80 per cent of patients whose rheumatoid arthritis creeps up slowly do not have to change their way of life right away, but when they first hear the diagnosis, this is their fear. Eventually life does change, though. Friends may be lost, and work may be interrupted. Many patients with rheumatoid arthritis force themselves to do more than they can comfortably, because they fear being a bother to others more than they fear joint damage.

However devoted the family may be, the progressive helplessness of the arthritic is a 24-hour burden that invariably leads to tensions. Arthritis can make other existing problems worse. Children, especially, who begin by resenting the disease, slowly and without realizing it often end by resenting the diseased.

Some arthritic patients have deformities that are far advanced, and the nurse finds them seemingly beyond rehabilitation. Sometimes the disease is overpowering; treatment was not begun in time, or it was inadequate. Perhaps the methods of treatment that are known today were not available when the illness started.

Whatever the condition of the patient, the nurse should concentrate on making the most of his remaining capabilities. The best way to begin is to look for little things that hold promise of improving the situation. For example:

What activity has the patient not yet tried that seems likely to succeed? Can you devise a way for him to do it? Dusting? Doing dishes? Cooking? Remember it is the patient's goals that are important. The nurse's job is to help the patient to reach his own objective.

The patient is not the only one to be considered. How do the other members of the family feel? Talk with them without prying. Remember, they cannot talk it out with the patient as they can with you. They may be unable to say in front of the patient how guilty they feel (if they do) at not doing more, and how angry, impatient and resentful they become at times.

What other people could be of help? Look around. Maybe a volunteer of some medical or social group could take the patient for a ride occasionally. Are there women in the church who could wheel the patient out in the air once a week? Talk to the doctor and the social worker. Remember that one person's interest can spark the interest and the enthusiasm of others. It is easier to tackle a hard problem with someone else than to face it alone. Sometimes the nurse is the catalyst; sometimes it is the doctor or the social worker or a family member.

ANKYLOSING SPONDYLITIS (RHEUMATOID SPONDYLITIS)

Ankylosing spondylitis is a chronic inflammatory disease of the joints of the spinal column that is characterized by progressive stiffening and pain. It was formerly believed that this disease was a manifestation of rheumatoid arthritis, hence the name rheumatoid spondylitis. It is now generally felt, however, that while related, the two diseases are distinct entities. The condition has many other names, one of the most common being Marie Strumpell's disease.

Incidence. A disease mainly afflicting young men, its onset is almost always before 50. It is seen in men 10 times more frequently than in women.

Pathology. The synovitis of the spinal joints starts usually in the sacroiliac region and moves upward. Ossification gradually occurs, eventually fusing the spinal column into a rigid unit.

Symptoms. In 85 per cent of the patients the onset is gradual, starting with aches and pains and frequent remissions. There is limitation of chest expansion, subjecting the patient to the possibility of pulmonary complications. As the spine stiffens, the normal lumbar curve is lost, and there may be kyphosis (humpback curvature) of the thoracic spine. As the neck and the head become immobilized, the patient must rotate from the hips to see from side to side.

Although the overall health of the patient may remain robust, he has considerable joint pain and muscle spasm.

Treatment. Salicylates relieve the pain. Moist heat relieves muscle spasm. Phenylbutazone, indomethacin and corticosteroids may be given. Properly graded exercises are planned to keep the spine mobile and especially to preserve chest expansion. Exercises are important to maintain the spine in a position of function, even though ankylosis occurs frequently.

DEGENERATIVE JOINT DISEASE (OSTEOARTHRITIS)

This type of arthritis is a disease of the joints that is characterized by a slow and a steady progression of destructive changes. Unlike rheumatoid arthritis, degenerative joint disease has no remissions and no systemic symptoms, such as malaise and fever.

Incidence and Etiology

This is a wear-and-tear disease that may start as early as the middle 30's, but it is mainly an affliction of later middle life and old age. Repeated trauma may lead to degenerative changes. Obese people, whose joints must bear heavy weight, are more likely to develop early symptoms than lean people. It has been suggested that osteoarthritis is more common in people who use muscular effort as a way of coping with anxiety and aggression. Men and women are affected equally.

Pathology

Osteoarthritis is a reflection of generalized aging. The cartilage that covers the bone edge becomes thin and ragged, and then it no longer springs back into shape after normal use. Finally, the bone end is bare.

The synovial membrane, which at first is normal, becomes thickened. The fibrous tissue around the joint ossifies. These changes, which occur slowly, give the patient pain and limited motion of the joint. Ankylosis does not occur.

Symptoms

Degenerative joint disease starts slowly with morning stiffness, especially in damp weather or after a period of heavy activity. General health is not affected. Slowly the involved joints, which may be any in the body, are uncomfortable, and finally they are painful when they are exercised. The joints most commonly affected are hips, knees and spine. There is little or no swelling, and no regional loss of muscle bulk. The discomfort yields to rest, aspirin and warmth, only to reappear with activity. Over the years there is limitation of motion.

Treatment

Proper local rest of the affected joints is more important than total body rest. Short periods of moderate exercise are helpful. Exercises never should be a strain to the patient. Normally repeated 5 to 6 times a day, they should be regulated by the feeling of the joint. Postural defects that add to the strain on a joint theoretically should be corrected; but since posture is the result of the habit of a lifetime, it probably will not be changed after middle age. Heat to the part is a comfort to the patient. If massage is used, it must be done gently to avoid further damage. Obese patients should lose weight. Anything that helps to relieve strain on the sore joints helps the patient. Support may be given with strapping, belts, braces, canes or crutches. In some instances the patient may gain relief while he is in traction.

Aspirin affords relief from pain. Narcotics are to be avoided. Corticosteroids may be injected into areas of inflammation during an acute stage. Daily traction and swimming may be prescribed.

Because both osteoarthritis and rheumatoid arthritis are called "arthritis," and patients may know that rheumatoid arthritis causes deformity, those with osteoarthritis may worry that their disease also will result in deformity. But this disease does not have the crippling effect of rheumatoid arthritis, and this worry of patients with osteoarthritis can be relieved.

GOUT

Gout is a metabolic disease, a familial arthritis that may attack any joint, but often it settles in the big toe, the ankle, the knee or the instep. There are periodic acute episodes of swelling and pain, which can be excruciating, with eventual limitations of motion. Ninety to 95 per cent of the patients are men, and the disease is rare in women before the menopause (Committee of the American Rheumatism Association).

Pathology

The basic disorder in gout seems to be an inability to metabolize purines, which are products of the digestion of certain proteins. This inability results in an accumulation of uric acid in the blood stream. Deposits of sodium urate crystals (tophi) occur in the margins of the joints, in the cartilage of the ear, in the kidneys, on the skin and, rarely, in the heart and other organs. Fibrous or bony ankylosis of the joint may develop.

Symptoms

An attack of gout begins usually with sudden, agonizing pain. The skin turns red, and the part swells. The attack lasts 3 days to several weeks and then disappears, to return in a month or perhaps a year later. The joint recovers completely after the early attacks.

During an attack the pain usually is so severe that the weight of the bedclothes or even the touch of a passing draft is intolerable. Movement of the joint is out of the question. Spontaneously, in about 2 weeks—or sooner with treatment swelling, redness and pain are gone, and the joint appears to be as good as ever. However, after years of attacks the permanent damage to the joint becomes evident. With recurrent attacks the involvement of the joints becomes migratory and polyarthritic.

The tophi that form in joints can eventually result in a chronic inflammatory reaction that causes structural damage and deformity. Sodium urate deposits in the kidney can endanger the life of the patient. The occurrence and the size of tophi are not necessarily related to the frequency of acute episodes.

Attacks become more and more frequent over the years. An attack may be triggered by surgery, trauma, infection elsewhere in the body, allergy, alcohol, nitrogenous or fatty foods, a weight-reducing diet, emotional upset, and such drugs as liver extract, vitamin B, antibiotics, ergotamine tartrate, a mercurial diuretic or environmental changes.

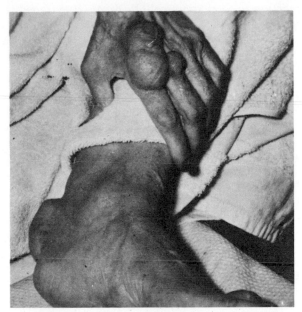

FIG. 16-3. Gouty tophi. (Vakil, R. J., and Golwalla, A.: *Clinical Diagnosis,* Bombay, Asia Pub. House)

Treatment

Although gout cannot be cured in the sense of removing the basic metabolic difficulty of constant or recurrent hyperuricemia, the attacks usually can be controlled to the point that they no longer occur. The regimen must be individualized for each patient and changed from time to time in response to the changes in the course of the disease. Understanding the nature of gout, self-discipline and conscientiously maintained contact with his physician are all necessary for success.

The aim of treatment is to decrease the amount of sodium urate in the extracellular fluid, so that the chalky deposits do not form, and to dissolve the tophi that have precipitated. This is attempted in two major ways: (1) by decreasing the amount of purine ingested, and (2) by using uricosuric drugs, which promote the renal excretion of urates by inhibiting tubular reabsorption of urates. The excess uric acid in the body of a patient with gout is derived from a process of internal biosynthesis; consequently, except for severe tophaceous gout, there is less emphasis on strict diet restriction than on the uricosuric drugs. The majority of patients are not placed on a rigid diet, although they are instructed not to take high-purine foods. The reaction to food and alcoholic drinks is extremely individual.

The prescribed diet is adequate in proteins—with concentration on low-purine proteins—low in fat and rich in carbohydrates. Large fluid intake and no alcohol usually are recommended. High-purine foods, to be avoided, include liver, kidneys, brains, anchovies, sardines, herring, smelts, bacon, goose, haddock, mackerel, mutton, salmon, turkey and veal, yeast, beer, meat broth, and leguminous vegetables, such as beans.

Low-purine or purine-free foods, usually allowed, include chocolate, coffee, tea, fruit juices, fruits, breads, caviar, cereal and spaghetti, eggs, gelatine, milk, nuts, pies (except mincemeat), sugar, and other than leguminous vegetables.

When she is instructing a patient with gout about his diet, the nurse avoids any implication that he is "bad" if he goes off his diet, although she points out that the nature of the chemical disorders will cause pain if he takes food that markedly increases the urates in his body.

During an attack a bed cradle is placed over the affected joint to protect it from bedclothes, breezes and bumps. This is one bed that never should be jarred. A sign "Don't Bump the Bed" may remind auxiliary personnel and visitors to be careful. Either warm or cold compresses may be ordered and applied very gently. Elevation of the joint may make the patient more comfortable. Only after the pain and the redness have disappeared is the joint to be exercised. Then early ambulation is a necessity to ensure good joint function.

Drugs. Because of the urgent nature of the pain, narcotics may be justified. However, they are rarely used, because more specific drugs are known.

Colchicine is a blessing to the patient with gout. Although this drug has been known to mankind for many centuries, in spite of intensive research and many theories nobody knows to this day how it works. It relieves the symptoms of an acute attack, even though, strangely enough, it is not analgesic or antiphlogistic in any other type of joint pain. Nor does it affect uric acid metabolism. If it is given promptly enough, colchicine gives relief within 12 to 24 hours. It is given by mouth in tablets of 0.5 to 0.6 mg. every hour until either the joint symptoms are relieved or nausea, vomiting or diarrhea appear, but no more than 16 tablets of colchicine should be given within a 24-hour period. More than this number of tablets may produce severe toxic gas-trointestinal reactions with shock or acute renal failure, leading even to death. Intravenous therapy may be used, but intramuscular and subcutaneous injections never are used, because colchicine is very irritating to tissues. A positive response to colchicine can be considered a diagnostic test for gout, since this is the only rheumatic disease that responds to this agent.

Patients with gout should always have colchicine tablets handy. The earlier the pills are taken in an attack, the quicker the attack will be over. If the drug is not taken early, more of it may be needed for relief, which then may not be accomplished before nausea, vomiting or diarrhea start. Regular, small amounts may be prescribed to prevent attacks.

Phenylbutazone (Butazolidin), used for stubborn attacks, is given in the dose of 100 mg. to 200 mg. by mouth q.i.d. for 2 to 3 days. When the patient takes this drug, watch for edema, nausea, epigastric pain, vertigo, stomatitis and a rash. Toxic reactions can be serious. Phenylbutazone is considered by many physicians to be the drug of choice in treating the acute attack of this disease. Usually it needs to be taken for such a short period of time that toxic effects do not appear. This drug is uricosuric. Indomethacin is also effective.

Probenecid (Benemid) also increases the excretion of uric acid. It is given in doses of 0.5 to 2.0 Gm. daily. A newer uricosuric agent is Anturane. Constipation, nausea, anorexia and rash are toxic reactions. When patients are treated with one of these drugs, encourage the intake of fluids, at least 3,000 ml. a day, to prevent kidney stones. Salicylates interfere with the action of Probenecid, and so the patient should be instructed not to take the two drugs together. Allopurinol (Zyloprin), a recent advance in treatment, inhibits the enzymes leading to the formation of uric acid. This leads to more effective renal excretion and diminution of body stores. It is of particular value where kidney disease is present.

Other treatment of advanced gout includes hemodialysis when there is renal involvement, and surgery to remove large tophaceous masses. Surgery may be employed also in an attempt to correct crippling deformities that may result when treatment is delayed, and to fuse unstable joints to increase their function.

BONE TUMORS

There are two kinds of bone tumors: (1) primary, those that originate in bone, and (2) secondary, those that are metastatic, starting somewhere else in the body and traveling to bone. The older the patient, the more likely the bone tumor is to be malignant. Many tumors never invade bone, but uncontrolled cancer of the breast, the prostate, the kidney, the lungs and the thyroid do have a tendency to settle in bone as a secondary site of involvement.

Pain and swelling are the principal symptoms of a bone tumor. Biopsy of marrow tissue may be taken to establish the type of tumor. Treatment may consist of excision of a primary tumor (if it is caught before it spreads) and roentgen therapy, which all too often is unsuccessful. Sometimes the affected section of bone is removed, and the defect is filled with bone graft chips. In other instances there is amputation of an entire part of the body, and the surgery may be extensive. For example, in a hemipelvectomy, half of the pelvic bone with its entire adjacent limb is removed. Chemotherapy temporarily may suppress the progress of malignancy. The aim of the palliative treatment is to help the patient to remain as comfortable as possible. The ingenuity of the nurse is called on to keep the patient from suffering unnecessarily.

OSTEOMYELITIS

Osteomyelitis, infection of bone, can result from a compound fracture in which the bone, usually protected, is exposed to the bacteria of the outside world, or a nearby infection can erode into bone. However, the infection is more often blood-borne, starting at a parent focus of infection somewhere else in the body, perhaps a boil or a squeezed pimple. Staphylococcus is the most common offending organism, and streptococcus is the second. Penetrating wounds that extend to bone are a good breeding ground for anaerobic bacteria. Streptococcal infections start with more violent symptoms than those caused by staphylococcus, but they have less tendency to become chronic.

No matter what the organism, the onset of the illness usually is stormy, and the danger of chronicity is ever present. The patient has a fever and feels severe pain, perhaps a headache or nausea. His leukocyte count is increased. There is local swelling.

The pain of osteomyelitis is caused by pressure due to pus formation and also to the destruction of bone. The infection spreads within the shaft of the bone, and the resultant pus gathers beneath the periosteum, stripping it. The infection

within the bone itself causes necrosis. Dead bone, called *sequestrum*, becomes detached and must be removed. The periosteum begins the formation of new bone, called *involucrum*. Thus a chronic process of bone destruction and regeneration may occur.

Treatment. The doctor has three weapons to combat osteomyelitis: (1) the patient's own defenses, aided by rest and good nutrition; (2) antibiotics; and (3) surgical drainage of the pus that forms. In the early stage of treatment the antibiotic may be given by continuous drip infusion. Some doctors make a series of drill holes in the bone to evacuate pus and to relieve the pressure. Antibiotics are put directly into the wound, and a catheter may be left in place for periodic irrigation or continuous drip of antibiotic solution. The wound is kept open for drainage, and the extremity positioned so that the mouth of the wound is down, utilizing the help of gravity in draining the pus. Sometimes a closed irrigation and drainage system is used, with a low pressure pump providing intermittent suction that allows the wound to fill periodically. The affected part may be immobilized with plaster, such as a half cast.

Nursing Care. The nurse caring for a patient with osteomyelitis must be especially mindful of the patient's pain. Movement causes great distress to the patient; yet he cannot lie continuously in one position. When she turns the patient, the nurse's hands are extremely smooth, careful and unhurried. The limb is well supported over its entire length, perhaps splinted with a pillow, and never allowed to lag behind. A firm pillow supports it, and sandbags hold it still. Immobilization of the part, which is a comfort to the patient while slightest movement is agony, can be accomplished by a cast, a brace, or the judicious placement of sandbags. The nurse takes extra care to see that the patient's bed is placed where it is least likely to be jarred. She avoids bumping into it, and she warns visitors, cleaning maids and others to be careful.

Whenever it is possible, give the patient the foods that he enjoys. He needs a nutritious diet. The doctor may order a high caloric diet. Fluids are encouraged.

The nurse, aware that the infection can spread to other bones, is quick to tell the doctor of any swelling, redness or pain elsewhere over a bone. She knows also that pathologic fractures (fractures that occur without severe trauma) may occur. These are singularly difficult to recognize, because the pain of osteomyelitis is so great that the pain of the fracture is masked.

Complications. The diseased bone may lengthen as bone growth is stimulated, or it may shorten because of the destruction of the epiphysial plate. Another complication of osteomyelitis may be the result of negligence on the part of the nurse. If dressings become too routine over a period of months, she may become careless with her aseptic technic, and fresh organisms may be introduced into the wound.

Perhaps the most discouraging complication of all is the tendency of osteomyelitis to become chronic. The sinus from the bone to the outside may drain for years. The inactivity of the part, the muscle spasm and the despair of the patient take their toll. The patient with chronic osteomyelitis frequently is wasted, weak and burdened with a deformed extremity. Sometimes amputation is necessary. Fortunately, antibiotic therapy has lessened the incidence of chronicity and heightened the chances of recovery.

REFERENCES AND BIBLIOGRAPHY

THE ARTHRITIS FOUNDATION: *Arthritis and Related Disorders,* New York, (n.d.).
———: *Home Care in Arthritis,* New York, 1966.
———: *Arthritis Quackery Today,* New York, (n.d.).
———: *Primer on the Rheumatic Diseases,* New York, 1964.
BECKMAN, H.: *Pharmacology—the Nature, Action and Use of Drugs,* ed. 2, Philadelphia, Saunders, 1961.

BEESON, P. B., and McDERMOTT, W. (eds.): *Cecil-Loeb Textbook of Medicine,* ed. 12, Philadelphia, Saunders, 1967.
BROOKE, J. W.: *Arthritis and You,* New York, Harper, 1960.
COMMITTEE OF THE AMERICAN RHEUMATISM ASSOCIATION: Primer on the rheumatic diseases, Part III, *JAMA* 190(6): 509-530, 1964.
DRAIN, C. B.: The athletic knee injury, *Am. J. Nurs.* 71: 536, March, 1971.
FLATT, A. E.: *The Care of the Rheumatoid Hand,* St. Louis, Mosby, 1963.
FROHMAN, I. P.: The adrenocorticosteroids, *Am. J. Nurs.* 64:120, November, 1964.
GARTLAND, J. J.: *Fundamentals of Orthopaedics,* Philadelphia, Saunders, 1965.
HERMANN, I. F., and SMITH, R. T.: Gout and gouty arthritis, *Am. J. Nurs.* 64:111, December, 1964.
HOLLANDER, J. L.: *Arthritis and Allied Conditions,* Philadelphia, Lea, 1966.
LAMONT-HAVERS, R. W.: Personal communication.
———: Arthritis quackery, *Am. J. Nurs.* 63:92, March, 1963.
LOWMAN, E., and KLINGER, J.: *Aids to Independent Living,* New York, McGraw-Hill, 1969.
MAGGINNISS, O.: Rheumatoid arthritis—my tutor, *Am. J. Nurs.* 68:1699, August, 1968.
MIALE, J. E., and PLOTZ, C. M.: Nursing care of patients with rheumatoid arthritis during therapy with cortisone, *Am. J. Nurs.* 53:290, 1953.
OSTROW, E. K.: *The Effects of Arthritis on the Life Adjustment of a Group of Arthritis Clinic Patients,* New York, Arthritis and Rheumatism Foundation, (n.d.).
REYNOLDS, F., and BARSAM, P.: *Adult Health: Services for the Chronically Ill and Aged,* New York, Macmillan, 1967.
ROTSTEIN, J.: *Simple Splinting,* Philadelphia, Saunders, 1965.
TALBOTT, J. H., and RICKETTS, A.: Gout and gouty arthritis, *Am. J. Nurs.* 59:1405, 1959.

The Patient with an Amputation

17

Indications • Management • Training with Prosthesis

Usually, the loss of a limb is psychologically damaging. The patient may fear that an amputation will make him less acceptable to others; loss of any part of one's body can lessen one's self-esteem, and it affects the patient's image of himself. He can be expected to experience grief over his loss and, depending on his adjustment, work through the various stages of the grieving process. The nurse helps by assessing the stage of grief the patient is in and providing appropriate support.

Not only does the loss of a limb mean that the person may consider himself to be no longer whole, but also it may create some difficult practical problems. According to his situation, the patient will face the possibility of loss of locomotion, lifelong invalidism, a change in homemaking practices and perhaps the loss of a job.

Even if the mechanics of rehabilitation can be accomplished perfectly, the loss of a limb may cause such anxiety and grief that the patient is unable to use a prosthesis. A young healthy person who loses a leg in an automobile accident, often is able to make the necessary physical adjustments, so that after only a relatively short time he can continue a full, active and productive life. On the other hand, the young college athlete or cheerleader who has an amputation due to cancer of the bone has overwhelming adjustments to make. Yet these people need rehabilitation also. Persons who undergo amputation for metastatic disease survive for an average of 3.5 years and occasionally for 5 to 10 years (Dietz). The young war amputee has his own problems to cope with and these will be different from the young patient with bone cancer. The military casualty who has multiple amputations faces the developmental tasks of the young adult, such as mobility, courtship, marriage and choice of lifetime occupation, with considerable physical and psychological handicap (Speers). The entire response to amputation is highly individual, but is affected by such factors as age, reasons for amputation, prognosis regarding underlying condition, and the patient's emotional state and developmental level.

The older person requiring an amputation has a greater likelihood than the younger person of having widespread concomitant disease that may be disabling in itself. There may be generalized weakness, poor vision or the aftermath of a cerebral vascular accident. Changing lifelong habits requires stamina, courage, patience, help and a certain degree of health. Yet some elderly patients, especially those who are supported emotionally by loved ones, do very well in adjusting to great changes in their lives.

The doctor may decide that it is better for the family to learn of an impending amputation before the patient does, so that they will have time to adjust to the idea and can help the patient when he learns about it.

If the amputation is necessitated by trauma, and the patient is brought to the operating room directly from the ambulance or the emergency room, the psychological adjustment is even more difficult. That morning the patient rose from sleep with an intact body. He thought, perhaps, that a usual day lay ahead of him. That night he is minus a leg. An amputation is irrevocable, carrying a deep sense of loss, even for the patient who has had severe pain in the leg. The patient who awakens from anesthesia to find a limb amputated needs people around him who can help to cushion the emotional impact by their acceptance of his feelings and their faith in his ability eventually to cope with the problems.

INDICATIONS

The causes of amputation are: (1) accidental extensive violence to extremities, (2) death of tissues from peripheral vascular insufficiency or from peripheral vasospastic diseases such as Buerger's disease and Raynaud's disease, (3) malignant tumors, (4) longstanding infections of bone and other tissue which leave no chance of restoration of function, (5) thermal injuries, both heat and cold, (6) a useless deformed limb which is objectionable to the patient, (7) other conditions which may endanger the life of the patient, such as vascular accidents, snake bites and gas bacillus infections and (8) congenital absence.

MANAGEMENT

The successful management of amputees requires cooperative teamwork among doctors, nurses, therapists and prosthetists. Although amputation involves loss of a significant body part with all this entails for the patient, it can also be viewed as reconstructive surgery. A functioning organ is left, the amputation stump, capable of using one of the modern designs of prostheses from which the patient can gain the greatest degree of functional performance.

Medical treatment for control of diabetes, nutrition, peripheral circulation, systemic infections and tissue metabolism can save some limbs. It is important for the nurse to give accurate dosages of insulin and other medications on time and to dress open lesions meticulously to help bring threatening disorders under control and to save the limbs. Surgical procedures such as bypassing obstructed vessels, endarterectomy, and sympathectomy, may be performed in an attempt to save the limb.

Preoperative Phase

When amputation is inevitable, the physician discusses with the family and ultimately with the patient, the extent of physical disability, the psychological, esthetic, social and vocational implications, as well as the realistic possibilities for prosthetic restoration. He promptly attempts to reduce anxieties and misunderstandings because radical surgery constitutes a severe threat to most people. Nevertheless, the patient is still faced with a crisis. However, this approach establishes the groundwork for assisting the patient to accept and to adjust to the realities of the situation. Not all amputees can benefit from a prosthesis and the surgeon is careful not to make casual promises to soothe a patient prior to surgery.

Patients vary in their reaction to the impending loss of a limb. These reactions are based upon such variables as age, the educational, intellectual, economic and emotional status of the individual, what the loss of the part means to him, and how he has dealt with previous losses. In general, a gradual state of depression and a degree of hopelessness are most common. Those with diabetes, for example, may be angry because in spite of the extra care they gave their legs and their dietary deprivation, they lose their limb, after all.

If the operation is not an emergency, there is time to prepare the patient for some of the things he will be required to do after amputation. A good diet, including plenty of fluids, helps the patient to withstand the shock of the operation. If the patient's condition permits it and if the doctor or head nurse approves, prepare him for postoperative exercises by starting them preoperatively. Have the patient do pushups while he is lying prone. In anticipation of crutch walking, have him push down on the bed with his hands while he is in the sitting position. Have the patient practice until he can lift his buttocks off the bed. Put the three unaffected limbs through the normal range of motion. If the patient is old, ill or weak, be careful not to tire him. An exercise done two or three times a day is better than one done ten times all at once. Have a Balkan frame and trapeze put on the bed.

The nurse can help the patient and family by accepting their reaction of shock and grief at the news and by letting the patient and his family talk about their feelings. Before the operation, help them to learn how others have managed with one arm or one leg, how the patient can help himself (by diet and exercises), and what to expect during the postoperative period. She can resist the temptation to make preoperative promises that cannot come true when attempting to aid the patient to accept the thought of an amputation. Although it has been stated frequently that nurses should encourage patients by showing enthusiasm and optimism themselves, this does not necessarily result in the patient sharing this attitude. Sometimes, in fact, it results in the patient perceiving the subtle message that he is expected to smile bravely and undertake his rehabilitation exercises with enthusiasm. This he may do as a facade to smooth relationships with the staff. He meets their need for an eager, smiling patient, rather than his own needs. Although it is important for the nurse to feel and show confidence in the patient's ability, a forced cheeriness may not be the best way to do this. It is usually preferable to listen while the patient discusses his concerns, realizing that he is likely to express grief and anger. If it is possible, have an amputee who has coped successfully with his handicap visit the patient.

Many of the serious psychological problems at the thought of amputation are lessened by recently improved surgical procedures, making it possible for amputees to ambulate almost immediately after surgery. Despite immediate post-surgical fitting and early amputation, the patient cannot be hurried through his stages of grieving and each needs support to proceed at his own pace to fully integrate the experience.

Most physicians assure a patient who will lose one limb and has three remaining normally functional limbs that he will derive practical function from the use of a prosthesis. This applies to almost all lower extremity amputees and most upper extremity amputees, regardless of age. The great majority of amputations in the lower extremity are performed on patients over the age of 60. Unfortunately, it is in this older age group that co-existing debilitating and degenerative diseases exist, many of which are disabling in themselves. The nurse must be careful not to become over-enthusiastic about how much function will be regained after the amputation, since in the older age group the quality of performance with prostheses falls far short of the normal, both for upper and lower extremity amputations. Some patients are unable to accept the amputation. Many of these, unfortunately, do not receive the help which is sufficient for their emotional requirements. One task of the nurse is to continually support those patients who initially cannot accept it. At a later time they may begin to progress toward acceptance, especially if they have family and friends as well as nurses and doctors who don't give up on them.

Phantom Limb. The surgeon also informs the patient of the phenomenon of phantom limb sensation (not phantom limb pain). This is the patient's sensation of the presence of the amputated limb. It is a normal, frequently occurring physiologic response following amputation surgery. If the phantom is painful, however, it can be an extremely serious problem with regard to the emotional status of the patient and his ability to use a prosthesis. The phantom should be explained to the patient as a normal phenomenon so that he will not be disturbed by his awareness of the amputated part. After a patient learns to use a prosthesis for practical purposes, although he still is aware of the phantom, he usually learns to ignore its presence. The patient may merely feel that the foot or the hand is still there. Let him tell you about the sensation. He may be embarrassed, or he may fear that he is losing his mind or fear that you will think that of him. The experience of phantom limb as a usual occurrence after amputation consists of somesthetic and kinesthetic sensations which feel as real as those in the opposite limb or as in the phantom limb before amputation. Amputation phantoms can persist for months or decades, or can come and go.

Aldrich suggests that the incidence of painful phantom limb is less likely if the patient's physician helps him to express his feelings about the amputation, both pre- and postoperatively. The nurse, by her supportive listening presence, helps the patient to accept and deal with the loss. The reactions of patients who lose limbs resemble reactions of grief at the loss of a friend or relative. The patient's failure to communicate or even to recognize his reactions may result in later emotional problems. For example, the doctor may say, "The operation is safe and necessary," but the patient may hear, "You will feel better after it." When during the postoperative period the patient does not feel better, he feels deceived and angry at the surgeon.

The amount of grief is thought to be proportional to the symbolic significance of the part and the resultant degree of disability and deformity. It is recommended that the physician in his preoperative explanation emphasize the necessity for the amputation without criticizing the patient for his reservations and recognize the anger the patient may feel about the threat to his body integrity. This helps clear the way for the expression of grief as well as the patient's concern about the disposition of the amputated part. The patient usually wants the separated part of himself treated with respect, which includes decent burial of the part. The nurse discusses with the physician what was told to the patient and the patient's response, and gives the patient the opportunity to further express his thoughts and feelings.

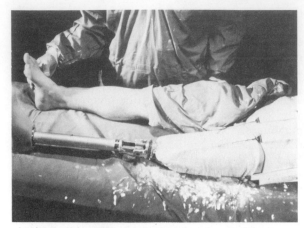

FIG. 17-1. Above-knee rigid dressing and immediate fitting in the operating room. (Institute of Rehabilitation Medicine, New York University Medical Center, New York, N.Y.)

Surgical Phase

Amputation can be performed at any level in the lower extremity. There are preferred levels of choice above and below the knee to facilitate fitting with available prostheses. A stump too long or too short creates fitting problems and discomfort. Over 90 per cent of amputations in the lower extremity are at the standard above- or below-knee levels. The ideal level above the knee is in the middle third of the thigh, the longest preferred stump being to within four inches of the knee. The standard below-knee level of choice is in the middle third of the leg, but not lower than the musculocutaneous junction of the calf muscles. Hemipelvectomy and hip disarticulations are relatively infrequent and are performed almost exclusively for malignant tumors. Knee disarticulations, disarticulation at the ankle joint (Syme's amputation) and partial foot amputations are occasionally performed but are rare.

When the surgeon decides that amputation is inevitable, the first decision he makes is the level of amputation. Although he has a number of tests available, including arteriography, the final decision can be made only by observing the vascularity of the tissues on the operating table. In the upper extremity the principle followed is to save all possible length and tissue with the exception of partial hand amputations. An amputation through any part of the hand that does not leave functioning elements is obstructive to the use of a prosthesis. In such cases, amputation is generally by disarticulation through the wrist

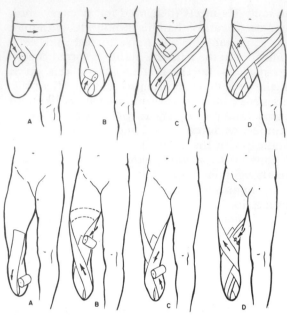

FIG. 17-2. In bandaging a stump of the upper leg, the bandage is anchored at the waist. Apply the bandage while the patient is standing on his unaffected leg. A crisscross (rather than a circular) pattern is followed around the leg, starting at the stump end. Each loop overlaps the previous one by at least half its width. The same principles apply to bandaging a stump of the lower leg. Note that anchoring is accomplished without a circular turn around the leg.

or just proximal to the wrist. In the lower extremity, unless there is unequivocal evidence that the knee cannot be saved, an attempt is made to amputate below the knee. Amputation above the knee is considerably disabling. Since function is achieved in relationship to agility, older people do not do as well with an amputation above the knee, although the majority of them can be fitted with a prosthesis.

With modern technics and the use of a rigid plaster dressing (cast) applied at the time of surgery, a good many of the borderline cases which in the past were considered to be candidates for above-knee amputation, particularly in diabetics with gangrene of the toes, can survive with below-knee amputations in greater proportion than was previously recognized.

If the rigid dressing is not used at the time of surgery, the amputation stump must be shaped and conditioned by bandaging with elastic bandages or the use of elastic stump shrinking socks or both (Fig. 17-2). With the use of the rigid dressing and immediate or early ambulation, the entire preprosthetic management period is altered since the most efficient way of conditioning, shrinking, and shaping the amputation stump is by using it. Even when immediate ambulation is not anticipated, the use of the cast considerably lessens the former lengthy period of stump conditioning for prosthesis fitting.

Other Amputations. Hemipelvectomy, interscapulothoracic amputation and translumbar amputation (hemicorporectomy) are radical procedures used in specialized centers when the patient has a bone or soft tissue malignancy. The nursing care is complex depending upon the patient's disturbance in self-image, loss of function, and involvement of other organ systems. Special prostheses are required for some return of function. In one report a 49-year-old male underwent total amputation of the lower body at the level of L4-L5 for cancer of the bladder and intractable pain. Four and one-half years later he was ambulating and driving a car with the use of a full lower body prosthesis. The patient with hemipelvectomy may have a sitting prosthesis initially (Hampton).

Postoperative Phase

When the patient is returned to the unit and the immediate postoperative reaction is past, the nurse plays an important role in making observations with regard to the status of the amputation stump. Some oozing will take place and stain the rigid plaster dressing. If the stain is marked with a pencil and observed periodically, one can determine whether or not excessive bleeding is taking place, and if so, the doctor should be notified immediately. When the rigid dressing is not applied, the same principle is used in observing the compressive dressing with the Ace bandages.

There is the possibility of hemorrhage in an amputation stump when a rigid dressing is not applied, and the nurse observes carefully the degree of bleeding. Have a tourniquet in view, tied to the bed in the event that massive bleeding is evident. With the use of the rigid dressing, however, hemorrhage is not possible.

Most of the amputations that are done on an elective basis are completely closed without the use of a drain. It is not necessary to drain a stump which is encased in a rigid dressing since it cannot bleed and cannot swell. If there is any possibility of infection, the rigid dressing is not applied and a closed amputation is not performed.

Open amputations (guillotine operation) are often performed in the presence of infection. These are left open and the skin placed in traction so that a secondary closure may be accomplished at a later date. In these cases close observation by the nurse is necessary to observe the degree of oozing from the amputation stump. Be alert for the odor which is characteristic of infection. A doctor should be notified with regard to both bleeding and the development of an odor from the amputation stump.

The traction must be continuous. The surgeon may arrange the traction so that the patient can turn over in bed and even get up in a wheelchair with a specially designed traction board without interrupting the pull of the weights. If the patient is incontinent, secure waterproof material around the outside of the bandage to prevent soiling of the wound.

If the wound is infected, reoperation or perhaps amputation at a higher level may be performed after clearing the infection and getting the patient in good condition. Sometimes the stump is allowed to heal without revision (reamputation). Sometimes revision is done. For instance, a guillotine operation may be revised later to provide a stump suitable for the prosthesis.

When a flap operation (closed amputation) has been performed and a rigid plaster dressing is not used, the surgeon often does not insert a drain if the wound is clean. The patient returns to the ward with a pressure dressing and perhaps a splint. The splint may be applied to prevent contractures at the knee or the elbow. The splint should be padded well to prevent skin irritation and the breakdown that may be caused by the pull of muscle spasm against the splint.

Bed positioning of the patient is important. With the rigid dressing there is no danger of the development of flexion contractures of the stump. When the rigid dressing is not used, bed positioning to prevent contractures is quite important. The patient can be made comfortable by placing a pillow under the thigh or under the knee if he has a great deal of pain. No harm is done in the first day or two in this position. The amputated limb, however, should be kept in extension alignment with the body thereafter at all times. The nurse may assist in the prevention of contractures by:

• Assisting and teaching the patient in rolling from side to side and in the face lying position in order to create extension for the amputation stump. Know what the doctor and physical therapist permit. Because the patient may experience a great deal of pain in the immediate postoperative period, a good time for placing him prone is about a half-hour after he has received medication for pain. Then he will be more comfortable and better able to move.

While he is lying on his abdomen, the patient may be instructed to adduct the stump so that it presses against his other leg. Be sure that his toes extend over the end of the mattress and are not pressed down into the mattress. When the patient lies on his unaffected side, he may be taught to flex gently and to extend his stump. When a patient with a BK amputation (below the knee) is in the supine position, and a pillow has been placed momentarily under his knee on the operative side, he can flex gently and extend his knee. Teach him to pull himself up in bed by using his arms and the overhead trapeze rather than to push with his heel, which may become sore.

• Being sure that the patient is lying on a firm mattress. A sagging mattress can cause a flexion contracture.

• Elevating the foot of the bed on blocks, if this is permitted, instead of using a pillow. Do not raise the foot gatch. Raising the foot gatch would have the same effect as using a pillow.

• Working with the physiotherapist so that a program of exercises to prevent contractures is implemented for the patient who progresses to the point where he is up in a wheelchair most of the day. For example, to prevent hip flexion contracture, the patient can be taught to suspend his stump over the edge of the bed and go through the full range of joint motion before he gets up and when he returns to bed. Attention is paid to the remaining limb as well as to the stump. Good muscle tone is maintained by range-of-motion exercises, with the patient doing the work. Footdrop is avoided by ankle exercises and the use of a footboard.

Amputation is major surgery and a great strain even for the young and the robust. Be careful that the patient, especially the older one who may be in poorer physical condition, does not overstrain himself and become fatigued.

Temporary Prosthesis. When immediate fitting of a temporary prosthesis is performed in the operating room, it is intended to get the patient up as soon as possible. Thus, the patient with a rigid dressing may be allowed to sit on the edge of the bed and dangle his unaffected leg on the day of surgery. If he has the stamina the next day or the second postoperative day, he may be permitted to stand and regain his sense of balance. Touching down on the floor with the improvised prosthesis and weightbearing of about 10 per cent of body weight is permitted.

The patient then progresses to walk with crutches or in parallel bars or with the use of a walkerette, one, two or three days after the amputation with a high degree of safety if the rigid dressing is properly applied. He is not permitted to put full weight on the amputation stump until six weeks after amputation. The reason is that the skin may heal in two weeks, but the deep tissues take at least six weeks for maturity of the scars to withstand the forces of full weightbearing. If a walking pylon ("peg leg") has been applied, he will then be ambulating under the supervision of the physical therapist. The nurse works with the physical therapist by providing for the patient bed positioning, exercises, supervision of his standing and weight transfer and balance in his room, in addition to the activities in which the patient participates in the physical therapy department. Keep in touch with the physical therapist, so that you know what exercises to continue on the ward.

Whenever the patient returns from the physical therapy department, the nurse should question him with regard to shortness of breath, the presence of pain, his response to exertion, the condition of the phantom and encourage the patient to continue his program so that he may make progress. Two or three weeks after amputation, he progresses to the point where the cast is removed for taking out the skin sutures.

After removal of the sutures, the patient is fitted with a temporary prosthesis with which he walks until his stump is in condition to tolerate a permanent prosthesis (Fig. 17-3). Under these conditions it is possible for the patient to leave the hospital ambulatory on two legs about a month after surgery if the scar is healed and all other conditions are satisfactory.

In some centers, upon removal of the initial cast socket as a rigid dressing, the patient is fitted with a removable plastic socket (Fig. 17-3). Under these conditions, the amputation stump

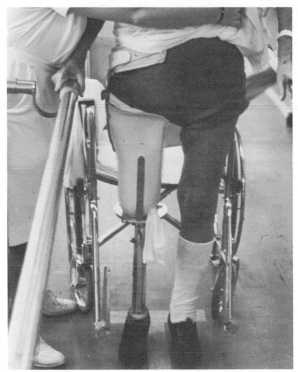

Fig. 17-3. Temporary, removable above-knee socket and walking pylon. (Institute of Rehabilitation Medicine, New York University Medical Center, New York, N.Y.)

will have a tendency to swell and the nurse may be required to bandage this amputation stump or apply an elastic stump shrinking sock so that the patient may sleep in it. This prevents excessive swelling so that the limb will fit in the morning when he is ready to use it. The amputation stump will have a tendency to swell for about three weeks. This is why in most centers where immediate or early ambulation is carried out, the initial cast is left on for about 21 days, so that a removable prosthesis can be applied rather than the reapplication of another plaster socket.

The whole process of postoperative management has changed in recent years since it is known that even if a standard amputation is performed and the stump heals in a reasonable length of time, the patient can be fitted with a prosthesis three or four weeks after amputation. If he is using a walking pylon, the concept of doing exercises and strengthening muscles is less important since the patient is active during the postoperative period, rather than passive, and the activities in which he is engaged are precisely the ones which he needs to keep his muscles

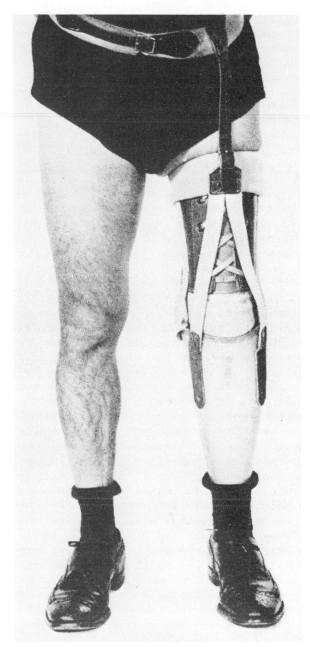

Fig. 17-4. Conventional below-knee wood socket with knee joints and laced thigh corset. (Institute of Rehabilitation Medicine, New York University Medical Center, New York, N.Y.)

strong and functioning without additional exercise.

Upper Extremity. A similar approach is used in amputations in the upper extremity. The surgical objective here is to create a gently tapering stump with muscular padding over the end. The upper extremity amputation stump moves within the socket more and is subject to more variations in friction than the lower extremity stump. For this reason the myoplastic closure and loose approximation of the skin flaps is essential. Tight skin across a subcutaneous cut bone end is the primary cause of the pain in an upper extremity amputation at any level.

Most patients with upper extremity amputations can be measured for a prosthesis shortly after the surgical scar has healed. It is necessary to maintain a full range of motion in the remaining joints and build up strength in the muscles by the time the prosthesis is finally delivered. This is accomplished by passive exercises and encouraging the patient to perform active exercises within his tolerance. The application of a rigid dressing can simplify the postoperative care of the upper extremity amputee, but it is only seldom used. The reason is that most upper extremity amputations are performed following extensive trauma or infection and the greatest length is being preserved. In emergency circumstances, the application of a rigid dressing adds to the risk since frequent inspection of the part is necessary. The dressing of an upper extremity stump usually consists of a thin strip of nonadherent material such as Telfa, silk or petrolatum gauze, covered with fluffy gauze and kept in place with a gently compressive bandage. This bandage is not designed for shrinkage, but simply for external support to hold the dressing on and to some extent control post-traumatic and surgical edema.

During the healing period the patient may become ambulatory and is made aware of the importance of good posture. In amputations above the elbow and higher, there is a tendency for the trunk to tilt away from the side of the amputation and for the head to tilt toward it. Eventual foreshortening of the shoulder girdle results in scoliosis. This is of greater importance, of course, in growing children. For this reason, deep breathing, bilateral adduction and abduction exercises for the scapulae, and shoulder shrugging should be practiced several times daily. The nurse gives the patient support and supervision as necessary and is guided by the physical therapist.

Only when there is no longer the possibility of infection and the scar is well on the way to healing is shrinking bandaging done. The elastic bandage is applied in the same manner as for lower extremity stumps. Compression proximally is achieved by spirals and doubling back the bandage to avoid circular constriction. Upper extremity stumps do not need massive shrinkage over a long period as do those of the lower extremity. They will not be subjected to the great forces of body weight support even while using a prosthesis, and usually stabilize in about six months.

A person who loses his dominant hand has the choice of learning to do everything (write, light a match, count change, eat, etc.) with his other hand or of learning to use a prosthesis. There are many things a one-handed person cannot do for himself. For example, he cannot wash his hand. Since the loss of a hand is a devastating disability, one that makes a difference to the patient almost every minute of the day, early restoration of the sense of purposeful use is important and can be accomplished by placing a temporary cuff over the stump and fitting it with a clip or clamp which can hold a pencil, piece of chalk or a spoon. The patient can then have the satisfaction of practicing writing on paper or a blackboard and attempting to feed himself as training procedures.

The upper extremity phantom is more active and liable to be more painful than the phantom of the lower extremity. The more violent the injury or the more painful the condition for which the amputation was performed, the more troublesome will the phantom tend to be. Many patients feel that the absent hand is bleeding, or is in a cramped position. A common complaint is that the thumb is dug into the palm of the hand. Exercising the muscles of the stump as if the limb were still there should be part of the daily routine. For example, have the patient close his eyes and move the stump as if he were putting the limb through full range of motion. Bilateral opening and closing of the hands, movements of the individual fingers and shaking of the wrists are part of the phantom exercise routine. The nurse can play a very important part of this preprosthetic training program in association with the occupational therapist. With persistence and support, the painful phantom is eliminated by purposeful use of a functional prosthesis, whether the upper or the lower extremity is involved.

Complications that may occur late in the postoperative course include chronic osteomyelitis (following persistent infection) and, rarely, a burning pain (causalgia), the etiology of which is not known. Pain may also be caused by a stump neuroma, which is formed when the cut ends of nerves become entangled in the healing scar. A neuroma may be treated with injections of procaine, or reamputation may be necessary.

Caring for the Stump. The type of surgery performed influences the length of time for stump conditioning, shrinking, and shaping. However, there are some general principles to be observed.

To help the stump shrink and shape properly for the wearing of a prosthesis, two or three elastic bandages may be sewn together and applied to the stump. Learn from the doctor how he wishes the bandage to be applied. The stump usually is bandaged first with an over-and-under motion and then with a spiral motion (Fig. 17-2). Be sure that all parts of the wrapped limb are equally compressed. If the proximal part of the stump is compressed more tightly than the rest of the limb, edema will result in the end of the stump (bulbous edema). In applying a bandage to an above-knee amputation, continue the spirals as high as possible to avoid a roll of flesh above the bandage. Change the bandage at least twice during the day and before the patient retires for the night, inspecting the underlying skin. In the summer especially, when the patient perspires profusely, wash the stump each time that the bandage is changed, and apply talc. If the skin is dry, use a little petrolatum or cold cream.

If the patient will have to bandage his stump at home, teach him, and perhaps a member of his family, how to apply the bandage and how to care for the stump. Teach the patient who soon will return home to wash the bandages between wearings, to rinse them well and to lay them flat to dry, since hanging tends to decrease the elasticity. When the bandages are dry, they should be rolled without stretching. If the patient uses a leather shrinker, teach him to use it with the same precautions that he would use with elastic bandages, giving special attention to cleanliness, frequent changes, prevention of tightness on the top and skin irritation. It is safer to use safety pins instead of clasps to secure the end of the bandage.

The nurse should check to make sure that the patient is applying the elastic bandage or any other device for shrinkage with even pressure from the tip of the stump on up the limb. The patient and the nurse should look for shrinkage without pockets of flabbiness. The patient should

return to his physician if the stump becomes uneven.

Successful ambulation depends on maintaining both the stump and the prosthesis in good condition. The patient should learn to protect both. Trauma to the stump may necessitate a return to the wheelchair or even to surgery, and repair of the prosthesis is an added expense. The stump is protected also by good daily care. It should be inspected for skin irritation, bathed, aired and powdered twice a day. Stump socks should be washed every day. When they tear or stretch, they should be discarded; the roughness of a darn or the crease of a stretched sock may cause a decubitus ulcer.

TRAINING WITH PROSTHESIS

A prosthesis is not designed to replace the lost part and its functions or its appearance. Therefore the function achieved should not be compared to the normal, but is to be evaluated against the patient's best potential. The amputee's potential depends upon such variables as his age, type of amputation, condition of the amputation stump, physical status, condition of the remaining leg, concurrent debilitating illness, visual motor coordination, motivation, acceptance, cooperation and insight. Patients vary greatly in their capability of deriving function and in their learning capacity with their prosthesis; the period allotted for their training varies and is affected by such factors as the speed with which the patient learns and his potential for rehabilitation.

For some a prosthesis signifies tragedy; to them it is a constant reminder of inadequacy. For others a prosthesis is an expensive, sometimes troublesome piece of machinery that nevertheless enables them to walk. Al Capp, the cartoonist, who lost a leg at the age of 9, said:

. . . I had learned how to live without resentment or embarrassment in a world in which I was different from everyone else. The secret, I found, was to be indifferent to that difference. . . . As you sway through life on a wooden leg, an odd and blessed thing happens. The rest of the world becomes accustomed, and then forgets that you have one, just as it becomes accustomed to, and then forgets the color of your eyes or whether you wear a vest. And you become accustomed to the limitations of one-legged life, such as not being able to pole-vault or drive a shift car, or being limited to half as much athlete's foot as other people have (Capp).

A prosthesis is expensive. If mental depression prevents its use, it is of equal importance to relieve the depression as well as concentrate on ambulation. For some, alleviation of despair is a more important consideration than the mode of getting from one place to another.

The purpose of a lower extremity prosthesis is to provide weight support and comfort as well as the capacity to ambulate with safety, with or without mechanical aids. The process is begun by teaching the patient to apply the prosthesis properly without assistance. His training starts with standing and weight shifting to get the feel of weight support and balance, between parallel bars. He is then taught heel and toe balance and rocking and hip hiking to get the prosthesis off the ground. Early steps begin by advancing the prosthesis first and bringing up the other leg to the standing position. With practice, alternate steps and increasing weight bearing are progressively accomplished. Initially crutches, the walkerette or canes are used until the patient has sufficient confidence and stability to discard them. It takes about two weeks of daily training to determine what any individual patient's best function will be. Daily practice for about two months thereafter usually permits the patient to achieve a satisfactory level of function. Learning to walk correctly takes time and practice. The patient may learn this skill in a doctor's office, a rehabilitation center or a hospital clinic.

Any discomfort caused by the prosthesis itself should be corrected as soon as possible. The nurse is in a position to discuss the progress with the patient and to examine the stump. Any observations relating to fit, comfort or general physical stress should be reported to the physician, the physical therapist, or the prosthetist.

Upper extremity amputees are trained by occupational therapists and assisted by the nurse. The training consists of teaching the patient to apply and operate the prosthesis. He is taught procedures to bend and lock the elbow and proper use of the harness. He is given very small increasingly difficult operations to perform with the terminal device, whether it is the hook or the hand. All of the operations of the elbow and terminal devices are controlled by the shoulder on the amputated side.

One of the most important advances is the concept of the teamwork approach in the rehabilitation of the amputee. The nurse has more personal contact with the amputee than any other member of the team. In this role she is in a position to encourage and to help him become motivated, and to keep his wounds clean, and gain his confidence and participation.

Rehabilitation is not an all-or-nothing proposition. It does mean assessing strengths and liabilities and helping the patient to make the most of what he has. It is equally vital that the doctor, the nurse, the physical therapist, the family, and the patient be realistic about what is expected. Help the patient to set goals that are possible for him. A 71-year-old man with generalized arteriosclerosis and diabetes may never be able to walk without a cane for extra support. That he can ambulate at all is an important consideration.

The nurse can help the patient to realize that he has assets as well as problems. When people are discouraged, they sometimes fail to see that they have strengths with which to work. The nurse who can help her patient to see both sides of the ledger will be better able to help him to become self-directing. She herself must not give in to hopelessness, nor must she expect her efforts to yield spectacular results. Effective action— even, at times, unexpected success—will lie somewhere between these extremes.

REFERENCES AND BIBLIOGRAPHY

Bosanko, L. A.: Immediate postoperative prosthesis, *Am. J. Nurs.* 71:280, February, 1971.

Brady, E.: Grief and Amputation, *ANA Clinical Sessions*, p. 297, New York, Appleton-Century-Crofts, 1968.

Committee on Prosthetic-Orthotic Education: *Amputees, Amputations and Artificial Limbs. An Annotated Bibliography*, Washington, D.C., National Research Council, 1969.

———: *Review of Visual Aids for Prosthetics and Orthotics*, Washington, D.C., National Research Council, 1969.

Hull, P., and Thomas, E.: Nursing regimen for the care of the amputee with contracture, *ANA Clinical Sessions*, p. 103, New York, Appleton-Century-Crofts, 1968.

Hodkinson, M. A.: Some clinical problems of geriatric nursing, *Nurs. Clin. N. Am.* 3:675, December, 1968.

Kirkpatrick, S.: Battle casualty: amputee, *Am. J. Nurs.* 68: 998, May, 1968.

Larson, C., and Gould, M.: *Calderwood's Orthopedic Nursing*, ed. 6, St. Louis, Mosby, 1965.

Russek, A.: Immediate postsurgical fitting of the lower extremity amputee, *Med. Clin. N. Am.* 53:665, May, 1969.

Sarmiento, A.: Recent trends in lower extremity amputation, *Nurs. Clin. N. Am.* 2:399, September, 1967.

Sternbach, R.: *Pain—A Psychophysiological Analysis*, p. 117, New York, Academic Press, 1968.

Zilm, G.: Hyperbaric oxygen units—high pressure nursing, *Canad. Nurse* 65:37, February, 1969.

The Patient with Neurologic Disturbance

18

Levels of Consciousness · Nursing Care of the Comatose Patient
Encephalitis · Parkinson's Disease · Epilepsy · Multiple Sclerosis
Headache · Trigeminal Neuralgia

Neurologic nursing challenges observational powers and bedside skills. The patients are often extremely ill, and they demonstrate physical signs (such as tremors or weakness) and personality derangements that require detailed observation, thoughts for the safety of the patient, and highly skilled hands to make the patient more comfortable. Neurologic lesions that change physical function or the ability to think and to communicate are especially distressing to both the patient and his family. The patient who cannot think clearly, or who must learn to feed himself again, or who is in deep coma for weeks requires both psychological understanding and such thorough attention to nursing details that visitors leave the bedside with the comforting thought that the patient is receiving the best possible care. The nurse should be alert for early opportunities to help the patient to become self-sufficient. Throughout the hospital stay of the patient the nurse makes the detailed observations that may be of diagnostic importance, such as where the convulsion started, the slight drag to the left leg, the transient nystagmus.

Neurologic Examination

The nurse may be asked to assist with a neurologic examination. Her role then is no different from that of assisting the physician with any other physical examination (she prepares the equipment and keeps the patient comfortably positioned and draped during the examination). However, understanding some of the special tests for neurologic diseases and their results will help the nurse to understand the condition of the patient better, so that she can plan his care more

intelligently. For instance, if the doctor discovers that the patient has no sensation in his right foot, the nurse can take special precautions to avoid burning the foot, and she can inspect the skin of the foot daily to detect the beginning of any pressure areas that the patient cannot feel.

During the neurologic examination the doctor will note carefully any disturbances in motor function, since these often reflect damage to the nervous system. He will note tremor, incoordination, imbalance. He will test reflexes, such as the knee jerk, and the reaction of the pupils to light. Muscles of the neck and the face, as well as those involved in locomotion, will be tested. For instance, some patients have drooping of an eyelid (ptosis) or difficulty in moving the tongue.

Disturbances of sensory function also are important. The doctor will note whether the patient can perceive pain (such as a pin prick) or sensations of heat and cold (often tested by placing a test tube filled with hot or cold water next to the skin of the patient). Abnormalities of sensation may be described, such as paresthesia (abnormal sensations, like burning, or the prickly sensations that patients often call "pins and needles") or hyperesthesia (intensified or exaggerated sensation).

Vision, hearing, taste and smell may be disturbed by neurologic disease, and examinations of these senses are an important part of the neurologic examination. Taste and smell are ascertained by asking the patient to identify the odor and the taste of common substances like peppermint.

In addition to the equipment used in a general physical examination, extra equipment is needed

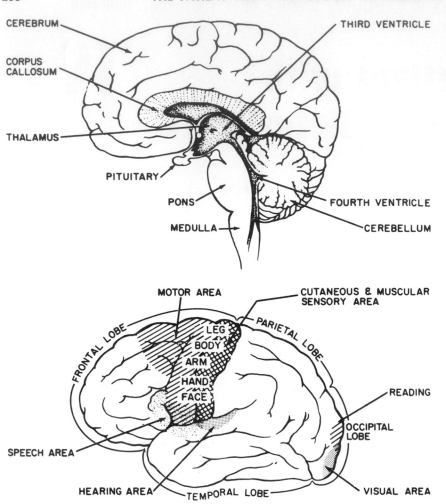

Fig. 18-1. (*Top*) A diagram of the major structures of the brain. (*Bottom*) Diagrammatic representation of approximate areas of the brain that control various functions.

for the neurologic examination: substances for testing taste and smell, pins for testing sensation, test tubes of hot and cold water, a tuning fork to test vibratory sense, and a dynamometer to measure strength of grip.

Neurologic disturbances can cause alteration of consciousness and of intellectual and emotional functioning. In a neurologic examination do not be surprised if you hear the doctor ask the patient who the President of the United States is or similar questions that most people can answer. The purpose of the questions is to ascertain the orientation of the patient to his environment. The state of consciousness can vary from normal to deep coma.

Emotional lability (fluctuations in mood) is a common symptom among patients with neurologic disease. They may burst into tears for no apparent reason, and shortly afterward they seem to be euphoric.

Special Tests

Most hospitals require that a patient sign a statement of consent for any of the following tests. Hospital procedures and equipment vary. Check the hospital procedure book before assisting with any of these tests. You will want to be sure that the desired equipment has been prepared, and that the patient has an idea of what to expect.

Lumbar Puncture

Cerebrospinal fluid surrounds the brain and the spinal cord. By acting as a cushion it protects them and helps to maintain a relatively constant intracranial pressure.

Lumbar puncture is performed to obtain specimens of cerebrospinal fluids for examination, to inject medication (for example, in spinal anesthesia), to measure the pressure of the cerebrospinal fluid, to withdraw the fluid for the relief of pressure, and to inject dye or air before taking roentgenograms of the brain and the spinal canal.

Normally, cerebrospinal fluid is crystal clear and colorless. It contains small amounts of protein, sugar, and, occasionally, a few lymphocytes. The normal pressure is 80 to 200 mm. of water; compressing the jugular veins increases the pressure of cerebrospinal fluid, if the circulation of the fluid is unobstructed (Queckenstedt's sign).

Changes in cerebrospinal fluid occur in many neurologic disorders. For example, meningitis (inflammation of the membranes that surround the brain and the spinal cord) causes a marked increase in the number of leukocytes in the cerebrospinal fluid, making it appear to be cloudy or even purulent. Often in a cerebral hemorrhage blood will be present in the spinal fluid, causing it to contain many red blood cells and to appear reddish. When a spinal-cord tumor completely obstructs the flow of the fluid, no rise in pressure will occur during the Queckenstedt test. A partially obstructing tumor causes an unsatisfactory rise or a fall. Fluid pressure is increased when intracranial pressure is increased, whether the cause be an abscess, a blood clot, a tumor, or any lesion that takes up space.

Bacteriologic tests on specimens of spinal fluid may reveal the presence of pathogenic organisms, such as the tubercle bacillus. Serologic tests for syphilis may be performed on spinal fluid.

Glucose will be decreased in bacterial meningitis. Protein usually is elevated when there is a spinal cord tumor or a brain abscess. Special analysis of the cerebrospinal fluid proteins (electrophoresis, immunophoresis) are frequently helpful in multiple sclerosis and other diseases.

To perform a lumbar puncture a hollow needle is inserted by the doctor into the subarachnoid space of the spinal canal below the level of the spinal cord. (The cord extends to the region of the 1st and the 2nd lumbar vertebrae; the needle usually is inserted between the 3rd and the 4th lumbar vertebrae.)

Here are some important points to remember when you are assisting with a lumbar puncture:

• Find out where the test is to be carried out and what position the doctor wishes the patient to assume. The test may be performed at the bedside or in the treatment room. Usually, the doctor wants the patient to lie on his side, with his knees drawn up to his chest and his head drawn down to his knees. The arching of the back separates the vertebrae, so that the needle

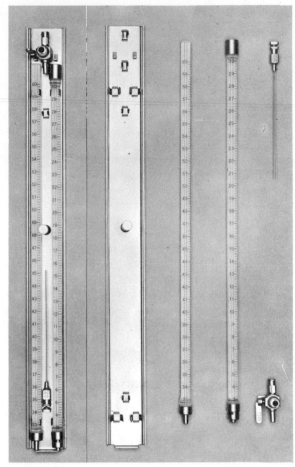

Fig. 18-2. Manometer set for measuring the pressure of cerebrospinal fluid. Both halves of the tube are fitted together, and the tube then is attached to the spinal needle. (Becton, Dickinson and Company, Rutherford, N.J.)

may be inserted more easily. Sometimes the test is performed with the patient sitting up on the treatment table.

• Make sure that the patient understands the test, and that he has signed the consent. The doctor explains the necessity for the test in the light of the condition of the patient, but it is possible that the patient will have additional questions just before the test is performed. Before the test is begun, show the patient how to assume the desired position. Emphasize the importance of lying still during the test. (Movement while the needle is in place may cause injury.) Sometimes patients experience a shooting pain in one leg. Explain to the patient that he may experience some pain during the procedure, and that the pain does not indicate nerve damage. Knowing this possibility will help him to avoid sudden movement.

• Check the procedure manual, and assemble the necessary equipment. Before the test is begun, confer briefly with the doctor to make sure that you have the needed equipment. (For instance, find out what size gloves he wears, so that you can have them ready.) An atmosphere of haste and confusion can be very upsetting to the patient. Careful preparation of equipment also will avoid your having to leave the patient to procure additional supplies.

If you are the only nurse present, your responsibility is twofold:

1. To help the patient to assume and to maintain the desired position, to reassure him by your presence and attention to his comfort, and to observe his reaction to the test.

The nurse sometimes must remind the patient to hold still during the procedure. If it is hard for him to maintain the acute flexion of his back, the nurse should stand on the side of the treatment table that is opposite to the doctor and, being careful not to contaminate the sterile field, put one arm around the patient's neck and the other around his knees, thus supporting him in the desired position until the test is over. Try not to become so intrigued with watching the procedure that you forget the patient.

2. To assist the doctor. Once the equipment has been assembled, and the patient positioned and draped with a bath blanket over his hips and legs, the nurse handles the unsterile equipment needed during the procedure. After the doctor has put on sterile gloves, he touches only sterile equipment. For instance, the doctor may pick up a sterile syringe and needle for use in injecting a local anesthetic, such as procaine. The nurse will help him by holding the vial of procaine (the outside of which is unsterile), while the doctor withdraws the drug. After the doctor has allowed cerebrospinal fluid to drip into test tubes, he will hand them to you to be labeled and sent to the laboratory. Stand the tubes upright in a container, such as an ordinary drinking glass, until the procedure has been completed. Check with the doctor to make sure that you know just what tests are to be performed on the specimens, so that laboratory slips can be made out correctly.

Occasionally, two nurses are present to assist with the procedure. Then one nurse assists the doctor while the other observes and helps the patient.

Headache occurs sometimes after lumbar puncture. Its exact cause is unknown, but it is thought to be associated with the loss of the cerebrospinal fluid. Many doctors ask their patients to stay flat in bed for several hours after the procedure, because they believe that this position minimizes the likelihood of headache.

Pneumoencephalography

A pneumoencephalogram enables the doctor to visualize lesions of the brain by the use of roentgenograms. In this diagnostic procedure a lumbar puncture is performed with the patient sitting upright, cerebrospinal fluid is withdrawn, and filtered air is injected into the subarachnoid space through the spinal needle. The air rises in the spinal canal and fills the ventricles of the brain so that their size, shape and position can be seen; then x-ray films are taken. If there is a brain lesion nearby that occupies space, such as a tumor, the contour of a ventricle may be distorted. Since the brain is held within the inflexible skull, abnormalities that take up space cannot cause herniation outward (except into the upper cervical spine via the foramen magnum) but cause distortion of the surrounding tissue inside the cranial vault.

The preparation of the patient for pneumoencephalography is similar to that of a preoperative patient. The patient must give written permission for the procedure. An enema may be ordered the evening before the procedure. A sedative usually is ordered the night before, and often it is repeated the morning of the procedure. Ordinarily, an injection of atropine and Demerol or other premedication is administered one-half to one hour before the pneumoencephalogram is begun.

Other aspects of preoperative care that are applicable to patients being prepared for pneumoencephalography include:

• Attention to personal cleanliness
• Removal of hairpins and dentures
• Noting and recording vital signs on the patient's chart
• Omission of food and fluids for 6 hours befor the procedure

Patients usually experience a severe headache after pneumoencephalography. Some also have nausea, vomiting and fever, and they may have shock, convulsions, respiratory distress, or symptoms of increased intracranial pressure (see Ch. 58). The patient may hear a splashing noise when he turns his head. This reaction is due to the presence of air in the ventricles. The symptoms gradually subside over a period of about two days, as the air is absorbed gradually, and cerebrospinal fluid is produced to replace that which was removed during the test.

After a pneumoencephalogram has been taken, the patient is placed flat in bed, at complete rest. The movement of his head tends to increase the severity of the symptoms. An ice cap to the head, codeine and aspirin may be ordered. The patient should be fed, bathed, and given assistance when he turns. Fluids are encouraged in order to increase production of cerebrospinal fluid. Level of consciousness, state of pupils, pulse, respiration and blood pressure are observed and recorded frequently, on the basis of the doctor's order. Usually, these observations are taken every 15 minutes or every half-hour at first. On the 2nd or the 3rd day after the test, the patient usually is assisted to get up. He should sit up first and then slowly assume a standing position. If he experiences headache, he may be placed on bed rest for another day.

A serious complication in patients with brain tumors is a shift of the tumor, caused by the injection of air. In its new position the tumor may encroach on brain centers vital to the patient's life. Emergency surgery to remove the tumor may be necessary. Tumor shift may be evidenced by a change in vital signs, level of consciousness or the development of such neurologic symptoms as paralysis, altered sensation in a part, or a dilated, poorly reactive or nonreactive pupil on one side. What symptoms appear will depend on which area of the brain the tumor presses. The physician should be notified immediately if any new neurologic symptoms appear, or if there is intensification of preexisting symptoms.

Ventriculography

The procedure for ventriculography is similar to that for pneumoencephalography, except that the air is injected into the ventricles of the brain through burr holes made in the skull. Ventriculography is used when pneumoencephalography is not possible. For example, obstruction of the spinal canal may make it necessary to secure a ventriculogram rather than a pneumoencephalogram. Since the air injected during a lumbar puncture could not rise to the ventricles if the

spinal canal were blocked, the air is injected into the ventricles. Ventricular puncture is the procedure preferred by many neurosurgeons when increased intracranial pressure is known or suspected, because lumbar puncture may permit shifts of brain tissue downward through the foramen magnum from loss of fluid below.

Hair that covers the area where the burr holes are to be made must be shaved before the ventriculography is performed. Other preparation is similar to that for pneumoencephalography. Ventriculography is performed in the operating room under local or general anesthesia.

The care of the patient after ventriculography is similar to that of a patient after pneumoencephalography. However, the patient is less likely to suffer from a headache, because during ventriculography there is less chance the air will enter the subarachnoid space. Keep sterile brain cannulas in a sterile test tube taped to the head of the bed. If there is a sudden increase in pressure after the ventricular puncture, the doctor may need to do an immediate tap.

Cerebral Angiography

In cerebral angiography a radiopaque substance is injected into one or more of four arteries: left and right carotid arteries and left and right brachial arteries. X-ray films then are taken of the blood vessels of the brain. This test can reveal abnormalities of intracranial lesions, such as aneurysms or the displacement of blood vessels by a tumor. Usually, one vessel is injected at a time; sometimes bilateral carotid angiography is done at one sitting, followed in one or two days by brachial angiography.

After angiography, ice usually is applied to the sites of the injections to lessen edema and to help to prevent oozing of blood. Edema around the sites of the carotid injections may cause pressure on the trachea and so cause respiratory difficulty. An ice collar is applied to the neck.

Although most patients experience few complications after having an angiogram, there may be serious sequelae, including fibrillation, hemiparesis, aphasia and respiratory distress due to edema or a hematoma near the trachea. Patients should be watched for signs of muscle weakness on the side of the body opposite to the injection; these would appear if trauma to the brain had occurred during the test. Note any weakness of the extremities or of facial muscles. Blood pressure, pulse and respirations are taken frequently. After brachial artery angiography the pulse in both arms should be taken. If it is not palpable in the arm on which the test was performed, the doctor should be notified. Because of the possibility of respiratory difficulty, a tracheostomy set should be kept handy. The patient may have difficulty in swallowing. Ice chips may be offered first, and then sips of water until the patient can be graduated to his usual diet.

Myelography

A lumbar puncture is performed in myelography, and a radiopaque substance is injected through the spinal needle into the spinal canal. X-ray films then are taken to demonstrate abnormalities of the spinal canal, such as tumors or a ruptured intervertebral disk. When the roentgenograms have been taken, the dye is removed via the spinal needle to prevent irritation of the meninges by the dye. Movement of the spinal needle is necessary in order to remove the dye. This manipulation of the needle sometimes causes pain, due to the contact of the needle with the nerve roots. If the patient is told just before this procedure that some pain commonly is felt, and that it does not indicate any untoward response to the procedure, it will be easier for him to tolerate the discomfort. Afterward the patient rests flat in bed for a few hours. He should be watched for signs of meningeal irritation (stiffness of the neck and pain when an attempt is made to bend the head forward).

Electroencephalography

The electroencephalogram is a record of the electrical impulses generated by the brain. Electrodes are placed on the patient's scalp, and the graph is recorded by a machine called an *electroencephalograph*. Usually, the patient is taken to a separate room, where a technician carries out the test. The procedure is not painful, and it does not cause after-effects. The patient is instructed to sit comfortably in a chair, or to lie on a bed or a stretcher, and to relax while the machine makes the recording. The test is run for varying lengths of time (½ to 2 hours). It is important to explain the test to the patient before it is begun, so that he will not fear that the wires and the machine will give him a shock. The patient follows his usual activities after the test. No special care or observation is necessary. If the doctor approves, a shampoo may be given after the test to remove the conducting jelly from the patient's hair. If a shampoo is contraindicated, the patient's hair can be gently and

briskly rubbed with a towel and combed until the jelly is removed.

Brain Scanning

Because certain brain lesions have a tendency to accumulate radioactive substances more readily than healthy tissue, a radioactive isotope, such as radio-iodinated serum albumin (RISA), radioactive mercury or technetium may be given intravenously. Two to three hours later a scanner is passed over the head in search for isotopic concentration.

When mercury is used, the doctor usually orders a mercurial diuretic, such as Mercuhydrin, to be given on the morning of the test. The kidney tends to take up large amounts of mercury. Giving a mercurial diuretic first saturates the renal cells and allows a larger and more concentrated amount of the radioactive mercury to circulate and to reach the tissues to be scanned.

LEVELS OF CONSCIOUSNESS

The following classification of *levels of consciousness* applies to altered consciousness from any cause, including increased intracranial pressure, cerebral vascular accident; edema; effect of a drug, such as alcohol; anesthesia; fever; and disorders of brain physiology that may be brought about by such deviations as hypoxia and hypoglycemia.

Alert Wakefulness. The patient responds immediately, fully, and appropriately to visual, auditory, and other stimulation.

Somnolence or Lethargy. This is a state of drowsiness in which responses to stimulation are delayed or incomplete and in which increased stimulation, usually by verbal or manipulative means, is necessary to get the patient to respond. He may be delirious and restless, or quiet, falling asleep again when left alone. Although he can answer questions, he may be confused.

Stupor. The patient can be aroused only by vigorous and continuing stimulation, usually by manipulation or perhaps by strong auditory or visual stimuli. Such stimulation may arouse him enough to answer simple questions with one or two words or his response may be only restless motor activity or purposeful behavior directed to avoiding further stimulation.

Semicoma. The patient is unresponsive except to superficial, relatively mild painful stimuli to which he makes some purposeful avoiding motor response. Spontaneous motion is uncommon, but the patient may groan or mutter.

Coma. He is unresponsive to all but very painful stimuli to which he may make fragmentary, delayed reflex withdrawal or, in deeper stages, may lose all responsiveness. There is no spontaneous movement and respirations may be irregular.

NURSING CARE OF THE COMATOSE PATIENT

Maintaining Air Passages. Unconscious patients need continuous protection against asphyxiation. Both by positioning and suctioning, the nurse keeps the air passages free. Patients in coma must be observed by someone competent to suction when it is necessary. Aspiration of mucus may lead to pneumonia. The nurse suctions the patient as frequently as necessary, being careful not to traumatize the tissues. If the tip of the catheter is pushed roughly against the tissues of the nose or the throat, or if suctioning pressure is applied directly to a tissue, the injured membrane may become edematous, it may bleed, or it may produce even more mucus. Apply suction only when you are withdrawing the catheter and never when you are inserting it. Oxygen by nasal catheter or tent may be ordered.

Mouth Care, Feeding and Diet. Give mouth care as often as it is needed. The comatose patient's mouth is often wide open, as he breathes through it. His mouth becomes dry, saliva sticks to his teeth, and his lips crack unless mouth care is repeated frequently.

When you first try the patient on oral fluids at the return of consciousness and on the doctor's order, allow only a small amount in the patient's mouth at one time and have the suction machine ready. Even though he is conscious, his swallowing reflex may not have returned, and he may choke or aspirate the fluid.

The patient who is unable to suck through a straw may be fed with a spoon or with a rubber-tipped Asepto syringe. Replace dentures as soon as it is safe to do so, because the patient will feel more comfortable and be better able to eat. The patient's teeth should be brushed or cleaned with an applicator after he eats.

While the patient is unconscious, fluids are given parenterally and by Levin-tube feedings. Avoid giving the patient too much at one time, because overloading the stomach may cause vomiting. The danger in vomiting is aspiration. Some patients cannot tolerate more than 200 ml.

at a time and will need to be fed more frequently than those who can take more.

Whatever is the patient's capacity, he should ingest an adequate diet in liquid form. Protein, carbohydrate, fat and caloric needs can be met through tube feedings. If the patient's skin seems dry, his mouth cracked, and he shows other signs of dehydration, ask the doctor if you may increase his fluid intake. Water or fruit juice may be given between his scheduled feedings.

Watch for changes in vital signs and levels of consciousness. Look at the pupils. Are they equal in size, and do they accommodate to light? Note skin color and muscle tone. Increasing spasticity may indicate increasing cerebral involvement. Changes in pulse, respiration or blood pressure may precede or accompany a new pathologic process. Rigidity of the neck may indicate involvement of the meninges. Daily descriptions of the patient's response to his environment should be made in the nurse's notes.

Eye Care. If the patient's eye is held open, ask the doctor if you may irrigate it with sterile saline. A drop of sterile mineral oil or colloid suspension ("artificial tears") can be applied to protect the cornea from drying, and a patch can be put on to keep the eye closed. If the doctor orders a patch, change it daily, looking at the eye for such signs of irritation as redness and excessive dryness.

Incontinence. The patient may be incontinent of urine. An indwelling catheter may be used. If one is not, keep your patient dry and clean.

Bowel Movements. Note the frequency of bowel movements. Impactions are not infrequent. Diarrhea may occur around an impaction without relieving it. An enema every two to three days may be ordered for the unconscious patient. Hold the buttocks together for retention of the enema solution. After all the fluid has run in, turn the patient onto a bedpan. Sometimes it is necessary to siphon the fluid back. If no stool is returned, the enema will have to be repeated.

Positioning the comatose or partially unconscious patient is of the greatest importance. When there is paralysis, such as after a cerebral vascular accident, the devitalized tissues of a paralyzed side easily break down to decubitus ulcers. The patient cannot prevent his arms from being crushed by his own body. No matter how busy the ward is, the patient must be turned every two hours. He will lie absolutely still in any position in which you put him, and, therefore, be sure that the position does him no harm while he is in it.

Never allow the comatose patient to lie on his back. Aspiration is too much of a risk in this position. Whatever position is used, take special care to avoid pressure in areas where peripheral nerves may be easily injured, namely the elbows and lateral aspect of the knees.

Turning, Skin Care, Cleanliness. Turning a heavy comatose patient or a partially comatose patient may require two people. If you have a member of the family to help you, be sure that he uses good body mechanics (using the thigh instead of the back muscles, bending at the knees, etc.). Be sure that the limbs are well supported while the patient is being turned. A leg that is allowed to flop over may pull the ball of the hip joint right out of its socket. If the patient is heavy, it is helpful to use the drawsheet to help to turn him.

Each time that he is turned, briefly rub the bony prominences on which he has been lying. The skin of the shoulder and the hip on that side may be red and show the marks of each wrinkle in the sheet. Use lanolin, cold cream, lotion or powder (alcohol is too drying). Brief rubbing of reddened areas is a good assignment for a family member who is visiting the patient and eager to do something to help. Explaining the importance of preventing skin breakdown will help the visitor to feel that he is making a real contribution to the care of the patient, as he is, and less like a spectator standing helplessly by while strangers care for the one he loves.

Exercise. As the patient is turned, his breathing pattern alters. He may be stimulated to take a deeper breath and to fill resting alveoli with air. His circulatory pattern also alters. More blood can enter the skin areas that were partially deprived of circulation when they were pinched between the bone and the bed. As the patient is turned, you can exercise briefly the arm and the leg that have been lying motionless under him for the previous two hours. Because footdrop will cripple the patient, so that he will not be able to walk when he recovers from coma, pay attention to the position of the feet every time that the patient's position is changed.

Dependency. *The unconscious patient is totally dependent.* If his tongue falls to the back of his mouth, he is powerless to move and to prevent asphyxiation. He has lost both position sense and the ability to catch himself, if he starts to fall out of bed. He may be cold, but he cannot cover himself or protect himself from a draft. He needs protection. Put bed rails on every time that the patient is alone. If you alone are changing his position, turn him toward you and not away from you.

Because the patient does not respond, it cannot be assumed that he does not hear, think and feel. He may be aware of those who are with him, even though he cannot indicate that he is. Keep his environment peaceful and quiet. Say nothing in his presence that you do not wish him to hear. Tell him what you are about to do, even though there is no indication that he understands you. Some patients with neurologic disorders begin first to make contact with the outside world in response to talk directed to them when they appear to be entirely unresponsive.

Helping the Family. The care of the decerebrated patient is a difficult experience for the physician, the nurse and the patient's family. A person who was well now lies abed, unable to speak, to feed himself or to think. When there is no chance for cure, the hopelessness of the situation can be very difficult for the family.

It is the responsibility of the physician to explain to the family the extent of the damage and to encourage them to seek a less expensive means of care than that in the general hospital. It is the responsibility of the nurse to give the best possible care to the patient. The nurse may be able to help the family to accept the fact that no amount of medical or nursing therapy can restore the patient to his original mental and physical state. Dealing with such a difficult task requires time and much support of the family, who must go through a process of grief before they can accept the situation.

SOME COMMON NEUROLOGIC DISORDERS

MENINGITIS

The meninges are three layers of membranes that lie between the bones of the skull and the brain tissue. The *dura mater,* the outermost layer, lines the skull; the *arachnoid,* the middle layer, is separated from the pia mater by the subarachnoid space, which is filled with cerebrospinal fluid; the *pia mater,* the covering on the brain, is a highly vascular membrane. Meningitis means inflammation of the meninges.

Etiology. Bacteria, viruses and fungi can infect the meninges. The most common organisms causing meningitis are pneumococcus, hemolytic streptococcus, staphylococcus, tubercle bacillus, meningococcus and influenza bacillus. The meninges can become inflamed by direct extension from the infected paranasal sinuses, the mastoid process, the middle ear, or an unsterile lumbar puncture or an unsterile craniotomy. Infection also can be carried to the meninges in the bloodstream. Children are more prone to meningitis than adults.

Symptoms. The onset of this serious illness is usually sudden, with headache, high fever, pain and stiffness in the neck, nausea, vomiting and prostration, diplopia and photophobia. The patient may be stuporous or in a coma and have a generalized convulsion. There may be herpes or a hemorrhagic skin eruption.

Treatment and Nursing Care

When the patient has been admitted to the hospital, a lumbar puncture is done to establish the diagnosis and to identify the organism, so that measures can be taken to kill it. A blood culture also may be taken.

Intravenous fluid therapy and antibiotics are started immediately. Antibiotics are given intramuscularly and perhaps directly into the spinal column (intrathecally). Isoniazid, streptomycin, and PAS are sometimes given to treat tuberculous meningitis. Drug therapy for tuberculous and bacterial meningitis may be continued after the acute phase of the illness is over to prevent the recurrence of the infection of the meninges. Corticosteroid therapy may be used for the dangerously ill patient. After the meningitis episode is over, the physician may search for the primary focus of infection and take steps to eradicate it. For example, a patient might require a mastoidectomy.

During the early stage of meningitis the patient is very sick. He needs side rails, careful watch of his temperature and cooling measures if his temperature goes too high, attention to hydration and nutrition, observation of his color, his alertness and his muscle tone. The patient may be fed by tube. Constipation and urinary retention are not uncommon.

Most adults with bacterial meningitis will recover without sequelae, thanks to antibiotics. When complications occur, they are usually serious. The infection may be overwhelming, and the patient may die. Neurologic complications, such as damage to cranial nerves, and especially visual and auditory deterioration, may take place.

ENCEPHALITIS

Encephalitis is an infectious disease of the central nervous system characterized by pathologic changes in both the white and the gray matter of the cord and the brain.

Etiology. Encephalitis can be caused by bacteria, fungi or viruses. Bacterial infection of the brain is frequently referred to as *cerebritis*. Poisoning by drugs, chemicals like lead or arsenic, or carbon monoxide may clinically closely resemble encephalitis but are referred to by the term *encephalopathy*.

The disease can occur after any viral infection elsewhere in the body, such as measles, smallpox or rabies, or after vaccination. In endemic or epidemic forms it is caused by a filtrable virus. Some of these viruses have been identified, such as the St. Louis virus, the Western equine virus and the Eastern equine virus. Some viruses are transmitted by ticks; others, by mosquitoes.

Pathology. There is severe, diffuse inflammation of the brain, with intense lymphocytic infiltration, especially around the blood vessels of the brain. In patients who die, and in some who do not, there is extensive nerve-cell destruction.

Symptoms. The onset of viral encephalitis is usually sudden. The patients are admitted to the hospital with fever, severe headache, stiff neck, vomiting and drowsiness. Lethargy is a prominent symptom. There may be coma or delirium. The patient may have tremors, convulsions; rarely, spastic or flaccid paralysis; usually irritability, incoordination and muscular weakness; sometimes, incontinence, spasm of the muscles of the jaw (trismus), or eye symptoms, such as sensitivity to light (photophobia), involuntary eye movements (nystagmus), double vision (diplopia), irregular pupils, crossed eyes (strabismus) or blurred vision. In the equine types, lysis of the symptoms occurs six to ten days after the onset.

Treatment and Nursing Care

As there is no known specific antiviral measure in existence as yet, treatment is symptomatic. Sponges or hypothermia treatment may be ordered to reduce fever, which may be as high as 107° F. The room should be dimly lighted, quiet and free from excitement. The patient may be placed in an oxygen tent to provide a better supply of oxygen. Intravenous therapy is started. Accurate intake and output records are important. Because the patient may be coma-

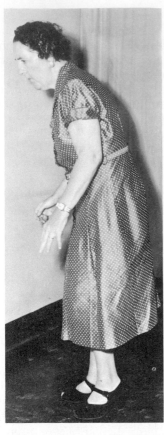

Fig. 18-3. Typical posture of a person who has Parkinson's disease. Note the tense stance, the small step and the forward bend of the patient's body. (Dr. Lewis J. Doshay, New York, N.Y.)

tose for as long as ten days, a nasogastric tube may be inserted and nourishment given through it. Suctioning to prevent choking or aspiration of secretions, and mouth care are important. A Foley catheter may be inserted to keep track of the patient's output and to keep the bed dry. Hot wet packs may be ordered three or four times a day for muscle spasm. The nurse observes the frequency and the adequacy of bowel movements, and reports constipation or diarrhea to the physician. The patient is kept clean and turned frequently. A patient who becomes confused and restless may need a harness restraint, which in most hospitals is applied only on written order of the doctor. As is true with any delirious or comatose patient, side rails should be kept in place. Observe and report the patient's eye symptoms, tremors, mental alertness, and any changes in these symptoms. Patients with extreme respiratory difficulty may require mechanical assistance with respiration.

PARKINSON'S DISEASE (PARALYSIS AGITANS, SHAKING PALSY)

Parkinson's disease is a slowly progressive disease of the central nervous system characterized by stiffness, slowed movements, and rhythmic, fine tremors of resting muscles.

Incidence. It has been estimated that approximately 1.5 million people in the United States have Parkinson's disease. Each year one person in every 1,000 over the age of 50 is newly affected. White people are afflicted more frequently than nonwhite, although the disease can be found all over the world. It is more common among men than women. It begins usually in the 5th or 6th decade of life. Rarely does it afflict more than one member of a family.

Pathology. Parkinson's disease affects primarily the basal ganglia and their connections. The main pathway of the basal ganglia is the extrapyramidal tract comprising the system of motor nerves responsible for automatic movements like blinking, walking, eating, posture, muscle tone, and the movements of facial expression. In Parkinson's disease there is a loss of the large ganglion cells of the corpus striatum. The ability to think is not affected.

Etiology. The cause of the classic syndrome of Parkinson's disease is unknown, and as yet even the nature of the pathologic changes in the nervous system is not entirely clear.

Symptoms. In 1817 an English general practitioner wrote a paper called "An Essay on the Shaking Palsy" that is so accurate in its description, so perceptive in its observations, and so thorough in its details that little since has been added to the description of its symptoms. Here are portions of the description that Dr. James Parkinson gave of the disease since named for him:

So slight and nearly imperceptible are the first inroads of this malady, and so extremely slow is its progress, that it rarely happens that the patient can form any recollection of the precise period of its commencement.

As the debility· increases and the influence of the will over the muscles fades away, the tremulous agitation becomes more vehement. It now seldom leaves him for a moment, but even when exhausted nature seizes a small portion of sleep, the motion becomes so violent as not only to shake the bedhangings, but even the floor and sashes of the room. The chin is now almost immovably bent down upon the sternum. The slop with which he is attempted to be fed, with the saliva, are continually trickling from the mouth. The power of articulation is lost. The urine and faeces are passed involuntarily; and at the last, constant sleepiness, with slight delirium, and other marks of extreme exhaustion, announce the wished-for release [Parkinson].

Although today the death rate of patients with Parkinson's disease is half again as high as that for those in the same age group without Parkinson's disease, the pitiful last stages, as described in Dr. Parkinson's paper, are seldom seen. Modern treatment often prevents this extreme.

The symptoms progress so slowly that there may be a lapse of years between the time of the patient's first observation that something is wrong and the time of the diagnosis. The symptoms may start on only one side of the body, and later they may become bilateral. The spread to the other side may occur quickly, or it may be delayed for as long as 15 years.

• The rhythmic alternating tremor is rather coarse. It occurs in the resting muscle, decreasing during activity and disappearing in sleep, except in the last stages of the disease.

• Rigidity is more widespread through the muscles of the body than is the tremor. There is a slight but continuous flexion of all limbs. Reflexes and the power of contraction are not affected, but speed of movement is.

The gait of patients with Parkinson's disease is composed of "part shuffle and part loss of balance" (Button). The patient slides his feet along with small steps in an attempt to catch up with himself before he falls down. If a patient starts to fall forward and is unable to save himself, he tries to get to a wall. A victim of Parkinson's disease falls like a dead weight. Some patients have attacks of spasm that glue both feet to the floor. It takes courage to walk under these circumstances, but staying in bed leads only to atrophy of body and perhaps also of personality.

The loss of associated movements reduces the patient's facial expression. He blinks infrequently. He fails to twist a corner of his mouth into a quick smile or to show an appropriate frown or to give any of the thousands of expressions with which human beings communicate with each other.

In late stages of the disease, when jaw, tongue and larynx are affected, the speech becomes slurred, and food is chewed inadequately and swallowed with difficulty. Rigidity that is not controlled by drug therapy and physiotherapy, or surgery, can lead to contractures.

• There is increased salivation sometimes accompanied by drooling.

• In a small percentage of patients, the eyes roll upward or downward and stay there against the patient's will (*oculogyric crises*) perhaps for several hours or even a few days. Pain may occur.

The spasm of the ocular muscles may be regular —e.g., occurring once a week—but there may be ten years between attacks. This peculiar, frustrating symptom is not found in any other disease known to mankind.

Patients with idiopathic Parkinson's disease have no disorder of sensation nor any clouding of the mind. However, anxiety can cause an exacerbation of the symptoms, and anorexia, excessive sweating, insomnia, agitation and depression may plague the patient.

Patients with symptoms similar to those of Parkinson's disease that have been caused by encephalitis or arteriosclerosis (parkinsonism) may be lethargic and have additional ocular symptoms, such as double vision (*diplopia*) and a fluttering spasm of the eyelids (*blepharospasm*).

Prognosis. Parkinson's disease progresses slowly. A patient may have the disease 20 years or more. Because of their disability, patients are susceptible to respiratory disease, which may prove lethal. The battle to minimize the symptoms by treatment goes on constantly.

Treatment and Nursing Care

Drug therapy is aimed at the control of the troublesome symptoms.

Drugs in the *belladonna group* quiet the tremor and relax the rigid muscles. Toxic reactions to be aware of are excessive excitement, restlessness and glaucoma. Watch for changes in pulse rate and blood pressure, for dizziness and for mental confusion. Dryness of the mouth and blurred vision may occur. Atropine dries the skin, impairs bladder function and may cause heat collapse by preventing perspiration.

In the belladonna group are atropine, Rabellon (containing hyoscyamine, atropine and scopolamine), and Prydon Spansules (sustained-action capsules with the same ingredients as Rabellon). Synthetic preparations are Artane (trihexphenidyl), Pagitane (cycrimine), Kemadrin (procyclidine) and Phenoxene (chlorphenoxamine).

Antihistamines decrease rigidity, with a resultant improvement in spontaneous movement, gait and speech. They do not affect the tremors. Benadryl (diphenhydramine) and Thephorin (phenindamine) may be given. The maximum effect is expected in about ten days. Watch for dryness of the mouth, gastrointestinal disturbances, drowsiness and dizziness. Dryness of the mouth may result in loosened dentures. Drinking citrus fruit juices or touching the tongue to a lemon may help.

Perhaps the greatest advance in medical treatment of any neurologic disease in recent years has been the discovery of the effectiveness of L-DOPA (levo-dihydroxyphenylalanine) in alleviating most of the symptoms in this disease. Tremor, rigidity, slowness of movement and walking, dysphagia, and drooling are all frequently dramatically improved. Although L-DOPA is a drug with many side effects, it is anticipated that it will largely replace other drugs as well as surgical therapy. L-DOPA is still under study.

Surgical Therapy. Most surgical therapy attempts to destroy a small area in the basal ganglia; when successful, this seems to give patients symptomatic relief. This type of surgery is called *stereotactic* because the surgeon is guided to the desired location in the brain by elaborate mechanical devices.

Thus far, surgery has been most successful in young patients with symptoms on only one side. A decrease in tremor is the hoped-for result. Some patients also have some lessening of rigidity. Because of the risk of hemorrhage and other complications, the older patient with bilateral symptoms is operated on more rarely. This type of neurosurgery is relatively new, and evaluation of long-term results will have to await further study.

The effectiveness of L-DOPA may in the future limit the necessity of recourse to surgery.

Postoperative Care. Postoperatively, some patients suffer a transient hemiparesis, visual field impairment, and speech impediment. Hemiplegia may prevent a patient from swallowing without choking. If he has difficulty in feeding himself and swallowing, give him foods that he can eat, and help him with his meals. If the patient has aphasia, the principles of care discussed in Chap. 19 can be applied. Protect his cornea with a drop of sterile mineral oil, if he is not blinking. Range-of-motion exercises are indicated—passive on the hemiplegic side and active elsewhere. The patient also may have weakness, decreased mentation and a headache for a day or two after the operation, during the time in which the brain is edematous.

After surgery the nurse watches for mental confusion. Side rails are kept up on the bed, and the patient's dressing is protected, so that he does not disturb it. His temperature needs to be taken at frequent intervals, as the temperature-control center in his brain may be affected temporarily. If surgery was successful in controlling his tremor and rigidity, he will need help in re-learning how to use his newly found abilities. His bowels may need retraining, and he will need to practice walking and swinging his arms, feeding and dressing himself.

Neurosurgery for Parkinson's disease is always an elective operation.

Physical Therapy. Although it cannot halt progression of the disease, physical therapy can result in the patient's maintaining greater ability for self-care than would otherwise be possible. Physical therapy is not indicated for tremor, but it is of great value in rigidity. Here, as always, early and consistent treatment will be of more use to a patient than starting physical therapy after he is doubled and twisted with contractures.

The Long-Term View. The patient should be helped by his family, friends or the nurses only when he really cannot perform a motion by himself. It is important that stress and anxiety and fatigue, all of which make the symptoms worse, be kept to a minimum, and in achieving this aim the family can help. When the patient is not present, the nurse might find an opportunity to discuss with the family his needs for serenity and peace of mind.

Parkinson's disease is discouraging for patient, family and nurse. It is a long-term affliction without remission in its symptomatology. The drooling disgusts the patient, the blank face and the slowed movements make social interchange difficult, and the rigidity is fearful and frustrating. There are large areas in which treatment facilities are scarce or nonexistent.

Yet—and the nurse can point out some of these things to a discouraged patient—present-day drug therapy does control many of the symptoms in many of the patients, and research on new drugs is going on all the time. Who knows what improvements tomorrow will bring in chemotherapy or surgery? In due time research workers may find drugs that will work even better than those available now.

EPILEPSY

Epilepsy was described by Hippocrates as long ago as 400 B.C., but modern study and treatment of the disorder began only about a century ago. Attitudes toward epilepsy have delayed both study and treatment. Until recent times epileptics were considered to be possessed by good or evil spirits. Fear of the disease was the rule, and not study of it. However, superstitions about epilepsy cannot be relegated to the Dark Ages.

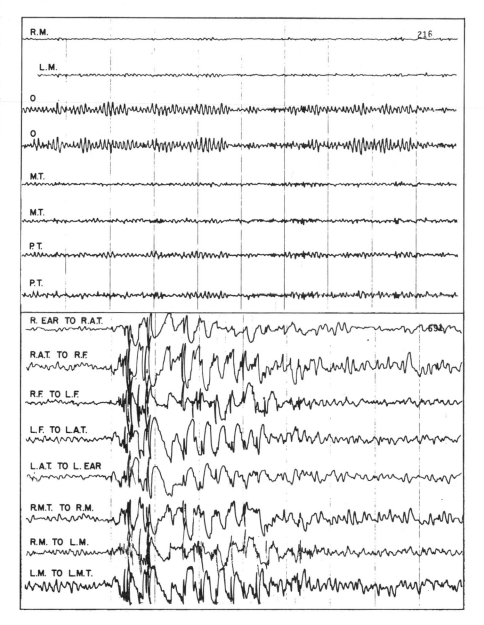

Fig. 18-4. Contrast of a normal electroencephalogram with that of an epileptic patient during a grand mal seizure. Note the sharp, spiky waves recorded during the seizure. (Dr. Julius Korein, New York, N.Y.)

Evidence abounds that even today epilepsy is held in special awe and dread. It is viewed quite differently from diabetes or heart disease. Although most people recognize that those with diabetes must receive treatment to be able to maintain usual activities, this disease is usually accepted for what it is, a long-term disorder for which most patients can compensate effectively by following their treatment. Epileptics, too, have a long-term disability, one that can be controlled in most instances by careful treatment, but another attitude tends to prevail. Epilepsy still is mentioned sometimes in hushed whispers, as if it were a disgrace. It is not discussed frankly as a disorder that affects some otherwise healthy, capable people.

Definition. Epilepsy means a tendency to have recurrent seizures. A common lay term for seizure is "fit." The seizures are not accompanied always by convulsive movements, but they do involve a temporary interruption of consciousness.

Cause. About four-fifths of all cases of epilepsy are termed *idiopathic* (of unknown cause). The remaining cases are called *symptomatic* *epilepsy* (the seizures are symptoms of some lesion in the brain). For example, injuries or tumors of the brain may cause symptomatic epilepsy.

It has been shown that epileptics frequently have abnormal electroencephalograms. Figure 18-4 contrasts a normal electroencephalogram with that of an epileptic. Note that the normal tracing has a regular, smooth pattern, whereas that of the epileptic looks jagged and irregular, with many abnormal discharges.

Although the underlying cause of idiopathic epilepsy is unknown, there is a definite hereditary predisposition to the disorder. Parents of epileptics often have abnormal electroencephalograms, although they may not have seizures. In one study it was found that only 6 per cent of the parents of epileptics had normal electroencephalograms (Sakel). Epilepsy is found more commonly among relatives of epileptics than among the general population. This incidence does not mean that every epileptic parent will have epileptic children, but that the children of an epileptic have greater chances of having epilepsy than do the children of nonepileptic parents. When both parents have epilepsy, the likelihood of the children's having epilepsy is further increased.

Incidence. An estimated 1,000,000 to 1,750,000 people in the United States have epilepsy. Usually, the seizures of idiopathic epilepsy appear during childhood and youth. When epilepsy appears late in life, it is often symptomatic of some trauma or disease of the brain. For example, arteriosclerosis may cause a lesion in the brain, which in turn causes seizures.

Types of Seizures

The interruption of consciousness characteristic of epilepsy may or may not be accompanied by convulsive movements. The seizure reflects a sudden unruly pattern of brain waves, possibly triggered by chemical changes within the patient's body. An electroencephalogram taken during a seizure shows an extremely irregular pattern. This disturbance in the brain is reflected in several ways. An epileptic may always have the same type of seizure, or he may experience a variety of types.

Many patients experience an aura or warning symptoms during the very early phases of the attack. This aura may take the form of seeing a bright flash of light, hearing a strange sound, or smelling a distinctive odor. The warning aura may occur long enough before the loss of consciousness to give the patient time to protect himself. He can lie down, thus preventing a fall, or he can get away quickly from objects that could harm him during unconsciousness, such as a hot stove. Unfortunately, only about half the patients have auras. Those who do not, have less opportunity to protect themselves.

Grand Mal (The Big Sickness). In this type of seizure the patient suddenly utters a cry and falls to the ground, unconscious. At first his whole body is rigid in tonic spasm of the muscles. ("Tonic" refers to tension or contraction of muscles.) Laryngospasm and spasm of the chest muscles cause a temporary obstruction of breathing. The patient's color, initially very pale due to the constriction of the superficial blood vessels, becomes bluish-purple during the moments when breathing is interrupted. Breathing resumes with deep, often irregular respirations. After a moment or two the clonic phase of the convulsion begins. ("Clonic" refers to alternate contraction and relaxation of muscles.) Jerky movements resulting from the alternate contraction and relaxation of muscles pervade his entire body. Frothy saliva appears on the patient's lips, a condition often described as "foaming at the mouth." During his uncontrolled movements he may bite his tongue. If he does, the frothy saliva will appear to be pinkish. When the convulsion is over, the patient's body and his clothing are moist from perspiration. Patients sometimes void involuntarily during the convulsion.

The patient usually has no recollection of the attack. He often experiences headache and exhaustion afterward, and frequently he sleeps for several hours. He may experience a "twilight state" after the seizure, a period in which he is not aware of his actions. During the twilight state he is not himself. He cannot be held accountable for his actions, since he is not aware of them; nor will he remember them later. The twilight state, if it occurs, is likely to go unnoticed if his behavior seems to be reasonable and is not conspicuous.

Status Epilepticus. Status epilepticus occurs when epileptic seizures follow one another so closely that the patient does not regain consciousness. If the repeated seizures are not stopped by treatment, the patient will die from brain damage. Fortunately, because of improved therapy, status epilepticus is much less common now than formerly.

Petit Mal (The Little Sickness). This type of epileptic seizure is characterized by brief interruptions of consciousness, sometimes accompanied by twitching of the head, the eyes, or the hands. The patient may pause suddenly in his conversation and then continue where he left off. He does not fall. Sometimes the seizures are so brief that they go unnoticed. Petit mal seizures are more common among children than among adults.

Psychomotor Attacks. Sakel defines psychomotor attacks as "circumscribed and transient disturbances of mental or emotional functions." These attacks include a wide variety of clinical phenomena: automatic, purposeless movements that may seem voluntary, like hands fumbling at opening shirt buttons, licking, smacking, chewing, or swallowing movements around the mouth; perceptual distortions like hallucinations or illusions; emotional experiences like sudden intense fear or elation; memory distortions like feeling of familiarity of a place or event never actually before experienced (déjàvu). Some patients have only psychomotor attacks; in others these attacks occur sometimes instead of grand mal seizures.

The term *epileptic equivalent* is used to refer to seizure manifestations usually not looked upon as seizures, such as paroxysmal recurrent abdominal pain or vomiting, pallor and sweating, and palpitations, among others.

During psychomotor attacks the patient may show stereotyped behavior that is inappropriate for the situation. Attempts to make him stop what he is doing are unsuccessful, because he is not aware of his actions; nor will he remember them afterward.

Jacksonian Seizure. Jacksonian seizures are a manifestation of symptomatic epilepsy. The seizure originates in a lesion in the brain, such as a scar or a tumor. Convulsive movements usually start in one part, and often they spread to involve the entire side of the body to which the part belongs. For instance, the seizure may start in the left hand and spread to the entire left side of the body. The brain lesion is on the side of the brain opposite to the side of the body having the convulsion.

Diagnosis

Epilepsy may be the easiest or the most difficult disorder to diagnose, depending on the symptoms. Recurring grand mal seizures present a very typical picture. Irregular tracings on the electroencephalogram confirm the diagnosis. The history of the onset of the patient's illness, his family history and a careful neurologic examination help the doctor to differentiate between idiopathic epilepsy and symptomatic epilepsy.

The occurrence of a single convulsion never is conclusive evidence that a person has epilepsy. Convulsions may be caused by a variety of disorders, such as severe infections with high fever.

Care of a Patient During a Convulsion

Convulsions may be caused by a variety of conditions other than those produced by epilepsy. For instance, drugs like Metrazol can cause convulsions. Children are more susceptible to convulsions than are adults, and it is not uncommon for them to experience convulsions during a high fever.

Witnessing a convulsion, especially for the first time, can be an upsetting experience, whether one is a nurse or a layman. Knowing what to do and what to observe will enable those with the patient to protect him from injury and to contribute information about the seizure that may be very important in helping the doctor to make a diagnosis. The same points that the nurse herself learns can serve as a guide for teaching the patient's family, friends or business associates. No one can predict just when or where a seizure will occur. Regardless of where it occurs, or who observes and assists the patient, the same principles are applicable. Learning what to do and, equally important, what not to do, before the situation arises will help to prevent injury to the patient and panic among the observers.

The first and perhaps the most important rule is: *stay with the patient.* There are several reasons for staying with the patient:

• Most convulsions last only several minutes. (What seems like an hour to a terrified onlooker is usually about three minutes by the clock.)

• If you leave the patient to seek help, the attack often is over before you return. The patient may injure himself, because no one is there to protect him.

• Unless you stay with the patient, you will be unable to observe and to report the necessary information concerning the seizure.

Place a padded tongue depressor between the patient's back teeth to prevent him from biting his tongue. Insert the depressor quickly, before the patient's teeth become tightly clenched. Do not try to force the teeth apart to insert the tongue blade, because you might loosen or even break his teeth. If the seizure is already in progress when you arrive, it may be impossible to insert the mouth gag safely. Never place your fingers in the patient's mouth. (You probably will be bitten.) If a padded tongue depressor is not available, substitute something like a clean folded handkerchief. Fold it several times, so that it will form a thick, soft cushion. Avoid using hard or sharp objects that might cause further injury. For instance, a table knife would not make a good mouth gag, but a folded table napkin would. If you know that a hospitalized patient is likely to have a convulsion, keep a padded tongue depressor at his bedside.

Of course, the safest environment for the patient who is having a convulsion is his own bed, particularly if it is equipped with padded side rails to prevent him from falling. Usually, the convulsion starts so abruptly that if the patient is up and about, there is not time to help him into bed. Have him lie down—on the floor, if necessary—to prevent him from falling. Place a pillow or any soft object, such as a folded coat, under his head, and turn him on his side to allow saliva to run out of his mouth rather than to be aspirated. If he has fallen already when you arrive, do not try to move him until the convulsion is over, unless he has fallen on or near something dangerous, such as a hot stove or a radiator.

Do not try to restrain the patient's movements. It is impossible to stop the convulsion in this way, and both you and the patient are likely to be injured, if you try to hold him down.

Loosen any tight clothing, especially if it is around the patient's neck (ties, scarves, collars).

Protect the patient from being a spectacle. His problem is great enough without the added embarrassment of recovering to find himself surrounded by gaping spectators. Often one person can concentrate on observing and protecting the patient, while another screens the patient or—if screening is not possible—discourages onlookers.

Observe, report and record the following information:

- Where the convulsion started. (In Jacksonian seizures the part of the body first affected often gives the doctor a clue about the location of the lesion.)
- The parts of the body involved. (It may be just one extremity, one side of the body or the entire body.)
- Position and movements of the eyes
- Whether the patient lost consciousness during the seizure
- Skin color; diaphoresis

- Respirations (character and rate)
- The type of muscle response (clonic, tonic)
- Whether he was incontinent of urine or feces
- How long the convulsion lasted. (Time the length of the seizure with your watch; most people greatly overestimate the duration of a convulsion.)
- Any injury that occurred during the convulsion, such as a bitten tongue
- The symptoms of the patient after the attack (for example, somnolence, headache, orientation to surroundings)

Treatment

There is no known cure for idiopathic epilepsy. Treatment often can reduce the number and the severity of the attacks, and in some patients it actually can prevent the occurrence of attacks. Symptomatic epilepsy sometimes can be cured, or the number and the severity of seizures can be lessened, by surgical removal of the brain lesion that causes the attacks. Regular exercise has been found to be beneficial in diminishing the number and the severity of attacks. Counseling is an important part of therapy; it helps the patient and his family to understand the nature of the disorder, and it aids them in planning for as normal a life as is possible.

Anticonvulsants make the patient less susceptible to seizures. Just how these drugs work is not fully understood, but it is known that they increase the resistance of the patient to seizures. Some patients remain completely free of seizures as long as they take the medication, whereas other patients experience a marked reduction in the frequency and the severity of the seizures.

Phenobarbital is effective as an anticonvulsant, but it has the disadvantage of causing drowsiness when it is given in large enough doses to control seizures. The average daily dose is 0.1 to 0.2 Gm. *Mephobarbital* (Mebaral), similar to phenobarbital, is given in doses of 0.3 to 0.6 Gm.

Diphenylhydantoin sodium (Dilantin Sodium), a very effective anticonvulsant, does not have the hypnotic action of phenobarbital. This makes it a very useful drug for the control of seizures, because patients can take a sufficiently large dose to control seizures without becoming drowsy. It is especially useful in controlling grand mal attacks. Although the dose needed to control attacks varies widely, many adults are given 0.1 Gm. 3 times daily. If their attacks are not controlled, the doctor may increase the dose to a total of 0.4 to 0.6 Gm. daily. The toxic effects of Dilantin include muscular incoordination and tremor, nausea and vomiting, and skin rash. Weight loss, fatigue, hirsutism and psychosis occur occasionally. Dilantin usually is given orally, but preparations for parenteral use also are available.

Trimethadione (Tridione) is used particularly in control of petit mal seizures. The usual beginning adult dose is 0.3 Gm. 3 times daily. The amount may need to be increased to control seizures. Tridione is a dangerous drug, and patients treated with it should be especially careful to report to the doctor regularly for check-ups. It can cause severe aplastic anemia, and most doctors recommend frequent examinations of the blood while the patient is taking the medication. Other toxic effects include photophobia, skin rash, and nausea and vomiting. *Paramethadione* (Paradione) is similar to Tridione in its action, dosage and toxic effects.

Ethosuximide (Zarontin) is another effective drug in petit mal and is probably safer than Tridione. Starting dosages in children may begin at 0.25 Gm. once daily. Gastric distress from the drug may be avoided by giving it with meals.

Phenacemide (Phenurone) is used in the treatment of petit mal, grand mal and psychomotor seizures. The adult dose is 1.5 to 3.0 Gm. daily. Because it is highly toxic, Phenurone usually is reserved for patients who do not obtain relief from other drugs. Toxic effects include liver damage, blood disturbances and personality disorders. Careful medical supervision is very important for patients taking Phenurone.

Methyl phenylethylhydantoin (Mesantoin) is similar in action to Dilantin. It is used primarily for the control of grand mal and psychomotor seizures. The dose is similar to that of Dilantin, 0.1 Gm. 3 or 4 times a day. The toxic effects include drowsiness, fatigue, skin rash, and, occasionally, aplastic anemia.

Diazepam (Valium), usually used as a tranquilizer, has been found to be very effective when given intravenously in the control of status epilepticus. The dose is individualized on the basis of patient's age and general condition. The doctor may request pulse and blood pressure be monitored closely during administration. The drug is generally less effective when given orally in long-term therapy, but may be used in combination with other drugs.

A number of other anticonvulsants have been developed for the control of epilepsy. They include phensuximide (Milontin), methsuximide (Celontin), and primidone (Mysoline). Acetazolamide (Diamox) is used primarily as a diuretic. However, it is sometimes used in conjunction with anticonvulsants in order to control and prevent seizures.

Patients need instruction concerning these drugs. They must understand that the drug is not a cure, but that it controls symptoms when it is taken regularly. When some patients have been symptom-free for a time, they decide to discontinue the medication, or they grow careless about taking it regularly. Most of these patients require medication for years. Since most of the anticonvulsants can cause severe toxic symptoms, patients should remain under close medical supervision while they are taking them.

Relapse. Patients who have had successful control of their seizures by drugs sometimes experience a sudden reappearance of seizures. The four most frequent causes of such recurrences are:

- Irregularity in taking prescribed medication
- Use of alcohol
- Increase in age and body weight (particularly of children), which requires adjustment in drug dosage
- Severe emotional strain
- Febrile illnesses

Patients with epilepsy are advised to abstain from all alcoholic beverages. Some patients, unable to follow this suggestion, are advised to use alcohol as sparingly as possible. As far as possible, the patient should be helped to lessen sources of emotional strain. In light of society's attitudes toward the illness, this poses a difficult problem.

Social, Emotional and Economic Implications of Epilepsy

Many epileptics suffer more acutely from the stigma attached to epilepsy than from the symptoms themselves. Every life situation is tinged with the dread of an attack and the fear of what others will think. The family of the patient often is ashamed that a close relative has epilepsy. Because of the familial predisposition to epilepsy, family members often feel that the disorder of a relative is a reflection on them, and they make every effort to conceal it. The epileptic child may be denied admission to public school; or, if he is admitted, he may find that he is the object of curiosity, pity or distrust.

Later the questions of marriage and childbearing may arise. The individual may be helped in making these decisions by personal counseling based on consideration of his particular condition.

Finding and keeping a job present tremendous problems for the person with epilepsy. Many people have the impression that epileptics are necessarily of subnormal intelligence. Although some persons with epilepsy experience alteration in their mental functioning, many of these patients are nevertheless coping satisfactorily with work, and with home and community responsibilities. The proportion of epileptics who have severe impairment of intellectual functioning, due to brain damage, and who are therefore unable to function adequately in work and other community situations is very small. Some people with epilepsy have unusual intellectual gifts, but all too often they lack the opportunity for advanced education and work commensurate with their talents.

Other misconceptions are that epileptics are unreliable, frequently absent, and a hazard to themselves and others. Epilepsy should not cause absenteeism or impair the quality of work, if the seizures are well controlled by medication. Persons with epilepsy who have frequent, severe seizures can be employed only in controlled situations, such as those afforded by sheltered workshops. It has been estimated that this group comprises only 15 per cent of persons with epilepsy.

Emotional strain often is a factor in precipitating seizures. Satisfying home and family life and suitable work are just as important to persons with epilepsy as to anyone else.

Here are some points to keep in mind concerning rehabilitation of people with epilepsy:

• The patient must recognize the importance of taking his medication and visiting his doctor regularly. The control of the seizures is the foundation on which the rehabilitation program is built. The sudden withdrawal of medication can cause a seizure.

• People who associate closely with the patient in his everyday activities must understand the condition of the patient and know what to do if an attack occurs. They need help in overcoming their own fears and misconceptions about epilepsy.

• The condition and the capabilities of each patient must be evaluated individually, so that educational and vocational plans can offer him opportunities to contribute to society without jeopardizing his own safety or that of others.

• Some types of activity are unsuitable for any person who is subject to seizures. Society has a

right and an obligation to protect its members; it cannot permit an epileptic to pursue activities that could become dangerous if they were interrupted by his loss of consciousness (for instance, piloting a plane). Such sensible restrictions do not constitute discrimination.

Public attitudes have forced the epileptic to conceal his disability. Concealment has resulted in lack of help for many who could benefit from it. How can the epileptic receive help if he is afraid to admit that he needs help? A big job still has to be done in educating people about epilepsy. We who are nurses are in a strategic position to make a valuable contribution to this need.

MULTIPLE SCLEROSIS

Multiple sclerosis is a disease of the nervous system that may lead to paraplegia. Both similarities and differences will be found in this discussion of multiple sclerosis if it is compared with the section on paraplegia. The similarities will be mentioned briefly; concepts that are relevant to the care and the rehabilitation of any patient with severe physical disability will not be repeated. Multiple sclerosis is a disease that usually causes gradual paralysis and gradual disturbance of important body functions, such as vision, speech, walking and mentation.

Regardless of the cause, if the patient's legs are paralyzed, and he is confined to a wheelchair, physical, social and emotional problems will be similar to those discussed under paraplegia. If his hands tremble when he uses them (as they often do), he may benefit from self-help devices similar to those used for quadriplegic patients. A glass equipped with a holder that slips over the patient's hand is an example of a device that can help both types of patients.

Rehabilitation, long-term illness and all the related problems are relevant there, too, but with this difference: because the disease is progressive, the symptoms of the patient keep changing. For example, plans for physical and vocational rehabilitation must be adapted constantly to the changing abilities and the requirements of the patient.

Emotional problems related to helplessness, dependence and inability to move about are common among multiple sclerosis patients whose disease is far advanced. In contrast to the patients whose disability results from trauma to the cord, the patient with multiple sclerosis usually undergoes a period of gradually increasing symptoms, in which he, his family and his physician wonder what is wrong with him. When the diagnosis is first established, its implications often are not clear to him; as he experiences the progressive symptoms and learns more about the disease, he begins gradually to recognize the seriousness of the illness.

Pathology. Many nerves are covered by a phospholipid, called *myelin,* the purpose of which is to increase the diameter of the neurones and to speed the conduction of nerve impulses.

Multiple sclerosis is a demyelinating disease: there are patchy areas of destruction of the myelin sheath throughout the central nervous system. This patchy destruction of the myelin sheath causes dysfunction of the nervous system. Where the myelin has been destroyed, hardened areas of scar tissue are formed. At first the lesions are temporary; later they are permanent. Symptoms often subside during early phases of the illness, and the patient may seem to be perfectly healthy for several months or even years. But with each reappearance the symptoms tend to be more severe and to last longer. These periods of growing better and then growing worse again are called remissions (getting better) and exacerbations (getting worse). They form a characteristic pattern.

Incidence. Multiple sclerosis is a disease of youth and early middle life. The highest incidence occurs between the ages of 20 and 40. Men and women are affected about equally. The disease is more common in north temperate zones than it is in warm climates; it is more common in the northern parts of the United States and in Europe than in the southern regions.

Cause. The cause of multiple sclerosis is unknown. Some theories implicate allergy, infection and emotional stress.

Symptoms. Usually, symptoms appear gradually, and early symptoms vary greatly from patient to patient. There may be a slight weakness or dragging of an extremity, which soon passes, a transitory blurring of vision or double vision. Often these seemingly minor symptoms are dismissed as a result of fatigue or strain. Later, when the doctor questions the patient, he may recall these episodes. Just as the symptoms themselves vary, their intensity and duration differ among different people. Some patients begin having severe, long-lasting symptoms early in the course of the disease, whereas others may experience only occasional and mild symptoms for several years after the onset of the illness.

Here is a list of some common symptoms of multiple sclerosis:

- Blurred vision
- Diplopia (double vision)
- Nystagmus (involuntary movement of the eyeball)
- Blindness
- Weakness, clumsiness, numbness and tingling of an arm or leg; ataxia (motor incoordination)
- Paralysis, usually of lower extremities (paraplegia)
- Disturbance of bowel function and of bladder function—incontinence or retention
- Intention tremor (the hand trembles when the patient uses it)
- Emotional lability
- Slurred, hesitant speech

Treatment

There is no cure for multiple sclerosis; nor is there any single treatment that reliably relieves symptoms. The problem of treatment is complicated by the uneven and unpredictable course of the disease. A new remedy may be tried, and coincidentally the patient may have a remission of symptoms. The remedy may have had nothing to do with relieving the symptoms. The difficulty in evaluating therapy is obvious.

Research is being carried on in many parts of the country to try to determine the cause and to develop specific therapy for multiple sclerosis. Organizations like the National Multiple Sclerosis Society are active in programs of education and research. In an attempt to find a way of curing the disease or of slowing its course and relieving symptoms, various drugs and diets are being tried. Nurses are called on to administer a variety of drugs and diets. Recognizing that these are experimental will help to avoid the confusion that results from seeing one treatment-regimen in progress in one hospital and a quite different type of therapy in use in another hospital.

However, all agree that the patient should be helped to maintain the best possible general health, so that he may withstand his illness better. Infections, such as colds or influenza, and emotional upsets may precipitate exacerbations of the disease.

Here are some important measures that the patient can observe to maintain his general health:

• Get plenty of rest. Do no continue an activity to the point of fatigue. Stop and rest; then resume activity.

• Avoid infections. (For instance, try to stay away from people who have colds.)

• Eat a nourishing diet, with plenty of meat, milk, eggs and fresh fruits and vegetables. Eat regularly.

• As far as possible, avoid situations that you know are upsetting.

• Keep on doing things that are enjoyable, but find ways to make them less strenuous, so that they do not produce fatigue. Does the patient like to walk in the country? Then he should drive along country roads to a pretty spot and take a short walk.

Management of the Disease; Prognosis

People can live a long time with multiple sclerosis. Living for 20 years after the diagnosis has been established is not unusual. Of course, these patients are subject to the same kinds of accidents and illnesses as are other people. We might ask: Are people with long-term illness particularly prone to accidents and other illnesses? The driver with double vision as a result of multiple sclerosis may be more likely to have an accident; the pedestrian with slow and awkward gait may be less able to get out of the way of taxicabs. Nor does multiple sclerosis make people immune to other diseases. The patient may die from heart disease or a stroke rather than from multiple sclerosis.

However, let us assume that accidents and other diseases do not intervene. Usually the patient with multiple sclerosis gradually develops more severe symptoms and shorter remissions. Weakness of a limb may progress gradually to paraplegia. Incontinence of urine may develop, and slight visual disturbances may progress to total blindness. The activity of the patient gradually is modified as these changes occur—for example, from walking to wheelchair to bed.

Although many patients experience gradual worsening of their symptoms, this is not invariably the case. Some patients have the disease in mild form, and do not experience increasing severity of their symptoms. Some people who have had the disease for 15 years are able to continue their usual activities. The prognosis is decidedly variable.

Nothing is to be gained by insisting on bed rest before the symptoms of the patient require it. If he has influenza, bed rest is an important aid to recovery. But if he has multiple sclerosis, confining him to bed before it is absolutely necessary not only fails to halt the disease, but also leads to depression, boredom and such physical complications as decubitus ulcers. Help him to maintain normal activity as long as he can.

Emotional Responses. Mood swings (emotional lability) are common among patients with multiple sclerosis. The patient may feel on top of the world one minute, and shortly later declare that life is not worth living. Two possible explanations have been given for this state. The patient may experience fluctuations of mood because of damage done to his nervous system or because of his deep anxiety about his illness and prognosis. Both may contribute to alternating euphoria and depression.

Complications. Some patients show symptoms of impaired intellectual functioning late in the course of the illness. For instance, loss of memory, difficulty in concentrating, and impaired judgment may occur. As the disease progresses, the patient is subject to many complications. With the knowledge that paralysis and incontinence often occur, it is not difficult to foresee the complications to which the patient is especially vulnerable:

• Pneumonia. It is not unusual for pneumonia to be the immediate cause of death. The patient is very susceptible to infection because of his limited activity, shallow breathing and general debility. Keep people with respiratory infections away from the patient. Encourage him to breathe deeply and to cough up mucus. Help him to change his position frequently.

• Decubitus ulcers. Incontinence and immobility, along with general body wasting (cachexia), make him an easy prey to decubiti. An indwelling catheter (to prevent soiling), changes of position and massage help to keep the skin in good condition.

• Deformities. These often occur because of weakness and paralysis. Put joints through full range of motion daily. Pay careful attention to position and body alignment.

HEADACHE

Headache is one of the commonest ailments of mankind. Few people go through life without experiencing it. Headache is a symptom and not a disease in itself. It may be caused by emotional tension, concussion, sinusitis or brain tumor—to name only a few possible causes.

Rational therapy of headache starts with understanding and, if possible, removing the cause. Treatment may involve such measures as prescription of glasses, drainage of an infected sinus, or psychotherapy. People who have occasional headaches resulting from fatigue or emotional stress often find that rest and analgesics, such as aspirin, help to relieve the symptom.

Migraine

Migraine is a particular type of headache believed to be due to initial constriction and subsequent dilation of cerebral arteries. The underlying cause of the condition is not fully understood, but it has been noted that emotional stress plays an important part in precipitating attacks. There is also a marked familial tendency toward the disease.

The attack usually begins with feelings of malaise, irritability and fatigue. Pallor and puffiness of the face may occur. Just before the headache begins, some patients experience visual disturbances, such as seeing spots before their eyes (scotomata). The headache usually starts on one side, but it may involve the entire head before the attack is over. Patients describe the headache as "throbbing" or "bursting." The headache is severe, and it often is accompanied by nausea and vomiting. The patient may be incapacitated for one day or even several days. Often light increases the anguish. Many patients feel so miserable that they can only lie in bed in a darkened room until the attack subsides.

TRIGEMINAL NEURALGIA (TIC DOULOUREUX)

The 5th (trigeminal) cranial nerve has three major branches: mandibular, maxillary and ophthalmic. It is a major sensory and motor nerve, important to mastication, facial movement and sensation. For reasons not fully understood, it occasionally becomes exquisitely painful, particularly in people over 50 years of age.

Symptoms. The pain comes in paroxysms, each lasting about 2 to 15 seconds, and they are so painful that patients have been driven to suicide. During a spasm the face may twitch, tears come to the eyes, and the hand rises to the face, without touching it. The patient has learned that a certain facial expression helps to shorten the bout, and he maintains the grimace as long as the pain lasts. After the paroxysm he is left with a dull afterglow, a tongue that feels furry, and the fear of the next attack.

Certain trigger spots cause an attack when they receive the slightest stimulus: the vibration of music, a passing breeze, or a change of temperature. Patients are understandably reluctant to wash that side of the face, and men remain unshaven. The forehead over the eyebrow is a common trigger spot when the ophthalmic branch of the nerve is affected. If the trigger zone is in the angle of the mouth, the patient gulps a mouthful of food, has a paroxysm, and pauses while he gathers courage for the next swallow.

Treatment. For some patients, inhaling trichloroethylene on a handkerchief gives temporary relief. Bartine may be given. However, surgery is the only satisfactory solution. There are three usual approaches:

• Alcohol is injected into the gasserian ganglion in the dura mater or into the branches of the nerve. This injection paralyzes the nerve, causing loss of sensation, movement and pain. The effect wears off in about 6 months, and then the nerve can be injected again, or it can be cut. With each injection the effect lasts a shorter time because of the scarring from the previous treatments.

• The dura is stripped off the ganglion. There is no loss of sensation in the face, but there may be a crawling sensation or other paresthesias.

• Partial section of the root of the ganglion is the standard operation. The effect is the same as that from the injection of alcohol into the ganglion, but it is permanent. A creeping, crawling, burning or tingling sensation may be present, but it tends to decrease in time. When the ophthalmic branch is cut, the corneal reflex is lost. Because the patient no longer blinks normally, there is danger that he will develop a corneal ulcer.

Preoperative Nursing Care

Temperature extremes stimulate the trigger zone; therefore, food and fluids should be tepid. The patient should be given food that is easy to swallow; perhaps he can take only semiliquids. The patient is in danger of becoming dehydrated and starved. After he eats, he may not be able to rinse his mouth. He may be able to use an applicator, but the nurse should not attempt to give him mouth care if this will stimulate pain. Have him talk as little as possible, since facial movement can start the pain. Avoid causing a breeze near his face, and ventilate the room in

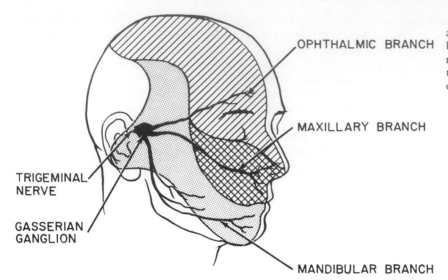

OPHTHALMIC BRANCH

MAXILLARY BRANCH

TRIGEMINAL NERVE

GASSERIAN GANGLION

MANDIBULAR BRANCH

Fig. 18-5. Diagram of the areas innervated by the three branches of the trigeminal nerve. These are the areas that become painful in tic douloureux.

such a way that no draft will hit him. Put a sign on his bed that it is not to be jarred, and avoid touching his face in any way. Hair brushing on that side may have to wait until after surgery. The patient may be exhausted from fighting the pain and need assistance with bathing, dressing and other personal hygiene.

Preoperatively, the hair is shaved to a point about 4 inches above the ear. Surgery is performed under local or general anesthesia, with the patient in a sitting position.

Postoperative Nursing Care

The elderly patient may have vasomotor changes from the sitting position in which the operation was performed. Vital signs are taken as ordered until they are stable. The head of the bed is elevated 12 inches or more to avoid a change from the position at operation. Because the dura mater was entered, watch the dressing for the yellow stain of cerebrospinal fluid leakage. The patient may have a headache from the loss of cerebrospinal fluid during surgery. Look for any change in the responsiveness of the patient that may indicate hemorrhage or a clot in the brain. Often these patients are elderly, and they may have a pre-existing cardiovascular problem.

If the ophthalmic branch was severed, the eye on the operative side will be bandaged for one or two days. When the dressing is removed, eye irrigations with sterile saline may be ordered.

Eating becomes a new problem. The patient may bite his tongue and drool without realizing it, food gets caught in his mouth, and his jaw deviates toward the operative side. Until he becomes used to the altered sensation, he may have difficulty swallowing. Since the patient may be elderly, and aspiration of fluid or food may lead to a fatal pneumonia, postoperatively he should be supervised when he first begins to swallow. See that he takes small sips, and encourage him to concentrate on what he is doing.

After he has eaten, check the inside of the mouth for particles of food that may remain and set up a site of infection. The best way to teach the patient to rinse his mouth and to brush his teeth after eating is to have him do this after each meal in the hospital. He should make regular visits to his dentist, because he will not feel the warning pain of a cavity. A pocket mirror placed at the dinner table so that the patient can observe his operative side will help him to eat in a neater way, and it may make him feel less shy about eating with others.

The majority of the patients develop a painless herpetic rash over the distribution of the nerve. Usually, it subsides in about a week. The doctor may order local application of tincture of benzoin or camphorated oil.

The side-effects of numbness and the loss of muscle power are annoying, and they require adjustment. This can be aided by the nurse's understanding of the daily living problems posed by the symptoms.

REFERENCES AND BIBLIOGRAPHY

Anderson, E. M., and Irving, J.: Uninterrupted care for long term patients, *Public Health Rep.* 80:271, 1965.

Beland, I.: *Clinical Nursing*, ed. 2, New York, Macmillan, 1970.

BURNSIDE, I. M.: Clocks and calendars, *Am. J. Nurs.* 70:117, January, 1970.

BUTTON, J. C.: *Hope and Help in Parkinson's Disease,* New York, Vantage, 1953.

BUTTS, C., and CANNEY, V.: The unresponsive patient, *Am. J. Nurs.* 67:1886, September, 1967.

CARINI, E., and OWENS, G.: *Neurological and Neurosurgical Nursing,* ed. 5, St. Louis, Mosby, 1970.

CARROLL, B.: Fingers to toes, *Am. J. Nurs.* 71:550, March, 1971.

COTZIAS, G. C., *et al.*: Modification of parkinsonism–chronic treatment with l-dopa, *New Eng. J. Med.* 280:337, February, 1969.

FANGMAN, A., and O'MALLEY, W.: L-dopa and the patient with Parkinson's disease, *Am. J. Nurs.* 69:1455, July, 1969.

GARDNER, E.: *Fundamentals of Neurology,* ed. 5, Philadelphia, Saunders, 1968.

GARDNER, M. A.: Responsiveness as a measure of consciousness, *Am. J. Nurs.* 68:1034, May, 1968.

GERDES, L.: The confused or delirious patient, *Am. J. Nurs.* 68:1228, June, 1968.

LUESSENHOP, A. J.: Care of the unconscious patient, *Nurs. Forum* 4:6, 1965.

McGINITY, P. J., and STOTSKY, B.: The patient in the nursing home, *Nurs. Forum* 6:238, 1967.

MERRITT, H. H.: *Textbook of Neurology,* ed. 4, Philadelphia, Lea, 1967.

OLSON, E. V., *et al.*: The hazards of immobility, *Am. J. Nurs.* 67:779, April, 1967.

PARKINSON, J.: *An Essay on the Shaking Palsy,* London, Whittingham & Rowland, 1817.

PLUM, F.: Axioms on coma, *Hosp. Med.* 4:20, May, 1968.

PLUMMER, E.: M-S patient, *Am. J. Nurs.* 68:2161, October, 1968.

SAKEL, M.: *Epilepsy,* New York, Philosophical Library, 1958.

The Patient with Cerebral Vascular Disease

19

Cerebral Vascular Disease • Cerebral Vascular Accident

CEREBRAL VASCULAR DISEASE

Cerebral vascular disease constitutes a major health problem, especially among older people. It ranks third as a cause of death among persons over 45, and it is a leading cause of disability among older people (Reaves).

The term "senility" sometimes is used to describe the decrements of physical and mental functioning that occur among the aged. In previous years it was widely believed that this process was an inevitable accompaniment to

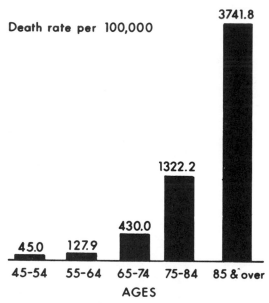

Death rate per 100,000

3741.8

1322.2

430.0

127.9

45.0

45-54   55-64   65-74   75-84   85 & over

AGES

Fig. 19-1. Death rates from cerebral vascular diseases, total of persons by age, United States, 1965. (Metropolitan Life Insurance Company, New York, N.Y.)

growing old, and that it was a normal manifestation of the aging process. For instance, many people believed that loss of memory and confusion were, like wrinkling of the skin, inescapable in older people. Currently, there is an increasing tendency to consider such changes as manifestations of pathologic processes of the cerebral blood vessels that are more frequent among the elderly, rather than to view them as normal or inevitable processes. Some persons in their 50's show symptoms of severe cerebral vascular disease, whereas others in their 80's do not. The underlying reason for the pathologic changes in blood vessels is not fully understood at this time.

Pathophysiology. The pathophysiologic basis for cerebral vascular disease involves the lessened ability of the arteries to carry blood to the brain cells. The cerebral nerve cells are extremely sensitive to lack of oxygen, which is carried to them by the blood. Complete ischemia leads in a few minutes to destruction of the cells that have been deprived of oxygen. These changes are irreversible; cerebral nerve cells that have been destroyed do not regenerate.

Atherosclerosis and Arteriosclerosis. The pathologic processes which impair the ability of the blood vessels to nourish the brain are primarily atherosclerosis and arteriosclerosis. In atherosclerosis fatty plaques (atheromas) gradually are deposited in the intima of the artery, causing its lumen to become narrowed and in some instances occluded. This process roughens the normally smooth lining of the artery, making it more prone to the development of clots that adhere to the atherosclerotic plaques. Such

FIG. 19-2. (A) A thrombus forms in a vessel. (B) The force of the flowing blood over the clot helps to break off a piece from it. (C) The embolus is loose in the bloodstream and can travel to any tissue fed by connecting blood vessels. (D) The embolus is pushed into a small terminal vessel, completely occluding it and causing anoxia of the tissue served by the occluded vessel.

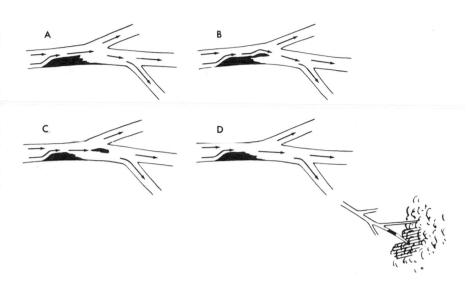

clots may form gradually and increase in size until they occlude a vessel (cerebral thrombosis), or they may travel in the bloodstream and become lodged in a narrowed portion of the blood vessel, cutting off the flow of blood (cerebral embolism).

In *arteriosclerosis* there is loss of elasticity of the artery and thickening of the intima of the artery. The combined effects of arteriosclerosis and atherosclerosis lead to a reduction of the artery's ability to transport blood. When the blood supply is completely cut off to an area of the brain, the normal tissues are destroyed and replaced by scar tissue. This region of the brain is referred to as an *area of infarction*. The episode itself in which an area of the brain undergoes infarction is called a *cerebral vascular accident*. Such an episode usually occurs suddenly, with the prompt development of symptoms of brain damage. The lay term for the condition is *stroke*.

Symptoms. The severity of the patient's symptoms depends on the extent of brain damage and its location. Damage to the brain in the area concerned with vision will result in visual impairment; damage in the area involved in speech will result in speech impairment. The following symptoms are typical of organic brain disease:

- Impaired memory, especially of recent events
- Impaired attention and concentration
- Impaired abstract thinking
- Circumstantiality. (For example, the patient introduces topics into his conversation that seem unrelated to the main point.)

- Lability of affect. (For example, the patient suddenly cries without apparent reason.)
- Perseveration. (For example, the patient may be asked to close his eyes. He does so. Then he is asked to raise his arms. Instead he again closes his eyes.)

Association with Hypertension. Cerebral arterial disease is often, but not necessarily, associated with hypertension. Although the drop in blood pressure may be to levels found in normotensive persons, it constitutes a significant fall in blood pressure in persons with hypertension.

Cerebral Hemorrhage. When this hemorrhage occurs, there is interference with the supply of blood to an area of the brain, together with pressure on the brain substance from the pool of blood that has collected. Both factors damage the brain cells. Cerebral hemorrhage is more likely to be associated with effort and activity than is cerebral thrombosis. Rupture of cerebral aneurysms is another significant cause of brain hemorrhage.

Cerebral thrombosis and embolism are more common causes of cerebral vascular accident than hemorrhage. Cerebral thrombosis is particularly likely to have its onset after unusual fatigue, or during sleep, when the patient's blood pressure is lowered. Cerebral emboli are sometimes a complication of cardiac arrhythmia, or of rheumatic endocarditis, conditions in which clots frequently form in the heart. They can enter the general circulation and become lodged in a cerebral artery, occluding it. These patients tend to suffer cerebral vascular accidents relatively early in life, for example, in their 30's or 40's.

Transient symptoms of cerebral ischemia may occur in patients who have cerebral vascular disease. Such episodes are often the first warning that the cerebral circulation is impaired, and they warrant prompt medical attention in the hope of preventing or postponing widespread brain damage. Although these patients may never experience a major cerebral vascular accident, they may, as the years go by, gradually exhibit considerable decrement of cerebral function. Symptoms of transient ischemia may include temporary weakness or paralysis of an arm, brief loss of consciousness, temporary loss or impairment of vision or speech. Unless the significance of such symptoms is recognized, the fact that they may subside completely can lead the patient and his family to believe that no medical investigation is necessary.

Special Problems of Patients with Cerebral Vascular Disease

Cerebral vascular disease is typically a condition of later life; consequently, its incidence is rising sharply because of the increased number of older persons in the population. Many advances have been made in the care and the treatment of these patients. The importance given to rehabilitation after cerebral vascular accidents and the possibility of surgical treatment have made it possible for some of these patients to live fuller lives now than in previous years. A tendency exists, however, to ignore the needs of patients who, because of the extent of their disease or the unavailability of effective treatment, continue to have marked impairment of physical and mental functioning.

The number of such patients is growing rapidly. Many of them are in nursing homes; many continue to live in their own homes. Whether they live alone, share a home with others, or live in homes for the aged, the problems involved in their care are difficult. An increasing share of nurses' time is spent caring for these patients. This is especially true of nurses employed in nursing homes and public health agencies. Efforts to care for these patients are often hampered because of the general apathy of many groups, both lay and professional, an apathy which may stem from feelings of hopelessness. Nevertheless, there are ways in which nurses can help patients and their families to deal with the problem of organic brain disease.

Nurses who work successfully with these patients are able and willing to appraise the patient's condition for what it is. If it is unlikely that 98-year-old Mrs. Winters will be gainfully employed, or that she ever will be able to care for herself again, what *is* possible? Instead of a bed bath, would it be possible to lift her into the tub? A tub bath would afford her the opportunity for stimulation of circulation, which might minimize the likelihood of decubiti, as well as provide her with relaxation and a feeling of personal freshness. Instead of dozing all day in her chair and spending restless nights, could she, by having someone to talk with and an interesting view to watch, be helped to remain awake part of the day and to sleep better at night? Why not take her to the porch on pleasant days? Is there a half-forgotten skill, such as knitting, which she could use if she were provided with the materials and simple directions?

Recognition of the Complexity of Behavior. Patients who have cerebral vascular disease are usually very much aware of the changes occurring in their abilities, unless their disease has progressed to the point that this awareness has been lost or blunted. For example, the patient's family may be talking and laughing together about an incident that occurred yesterday. The patient is painfully aware that he should know what the joke is about, but he doesn't. Observing that he is not laughing, his wife may say reproachfully, "Why, that happened only yesterday, Arthur. Don't you remember?" Nurses, too, can point up to the patient his lack of memory or his confusion by comments like "But it was only this morning that I asked you not to drink anything until the test was over. Now the test is ruined." Such small humiliations are commonplace in the lives of those with cerebral vascular disease. In a sense they are being scolded for being ill. (Yet few people scold a person for having a fever.) The patient's symptoms by their very nature are likely to prove to be irritating to others. The impatience shown by others can increase the patient's feeling of being unwanted and a burden.

In caring for such a patient the nurse should make every effort not to demand of him abilities that he lacks. As she works with the family, she can help them to do likewise. For example, the patient's wife may tactfully mention to her husband, as the group begins to laugh and she detects a puzzled look on his face, the event that is the cause of the laughter. Such measures help the patient to feel more at ease in his relationships with others.

It is important to remember, however, that motivation for behavior is complex, and that it grows not only from conscious thought processes but also from unconscious ones. If the patient's wife has been angry with her husband for many years, she may find ways to humiliate him, even though she is consciously aware of the kind or thoughtful thing to say in a given situation. Nurses also respond to patients in ways that are not wholly congruent with an intellectual grasp of their patients' needs. Recognition of the complexity of these factors does not lessen the need for their thoughtful consideration, but it does imply that one should not expect all problems to be solved by an intellectual approach.

Changes and Orientation. The realization of these patients that they suffer some confusion and memory loss tends to intensify their feelings of insecurity and fearfulness. Since changes in environment or being alone in the dark may accentuate their fears and increase their confusion, it is important to keep the patient's environment as unchanged as possible. For example, transfer from one room to another or contact with an entirely strange staff should be avoided when possible. Keeping a light on in the patient's room at night helps him to avoid the increased confusion that can result if he is left in a darkened room. Careful and, if necessary, repeated orientation to the location of the bathroom or his own room may help a patient who has been newly admitted to a nursing home.

Dependence and Independence. Because of their infirmities, aged persons with cerebral vascular disease tend to be dependent, emotionally and physically, on those who care for them. This tendency must be recognized and dealt with; otherwise, it readily engenders situations in which the patient clamors for more of the nurse's attention, while she insists that he is too demanding. For example, when a patient is newly admitted to a nursing home, it is important to recognize that his efforts to gain the attention of the nurse are necessary to him to help him feel more secure and to assure him that those responsible for him care about him. By accepting and dealing with the patient's efforts to gain her attention, the nurse can help him gradually to feel safer. She can then slowly help him to increase

his independence. For instance, she may help him to bathe and dress, if he states that he is unable to do this unaided. As she helps him, she can evaluate what aspects of self-care he seems capable of performing. As he begins to feel more at home in his new surroundings, she may encourage him to undertake aspects of care of which he seems capable, while stressing that she is available to help him if he requires her help. In the same way the nurse can help the patient to undertake recreational activities.

Families

You will learn that the families of patients with cerebral vascular disease are particularly in need of the nurse's help. To a greater extent than many other disabilities, brain damage severely taxes interpersonal relationships. Sometimes these difficulties are avoided rather than faced. Many families fail to visit a member with cerebral vascular disease if he is in a nursing home; or if he lives at home, they find ways to exclude him from most of their activities. Too frequently, such reactions by the family are censured by physicians and nurses; instead, the family needs help in dealing with the problem.

An important point for the nurse to remember in dealing with the family is that usually they are doing the best that they can in the situation. Reproaching them not only fails to help but may result in their showing even more rejection of the sick relative. Allowing them opportunities to discuss, if they wish, some of the problems they are experiencing and showing them ways that can help to provide more satisfactory care for the patient often enable the family to be more understanding and to accept the illness better. The nurse and the physician can help the family to acquire information that is valuable in making decisions concerning long-term care. However, the making of such decisions —for example, whether to care for the patient at home or in a nursing home—should follow an appraisal by the family of their own resources and the needs of the patient.

Evaluation of Orientation. A difficult problem for families and nurses is the fluctuation in the patient's mental status. Some patients with cerebral vascular disease are well oriented at some periods and grossly confused at others. Those who care for the patient must become accustomed to evaluating the patient's state of orientation and adapting their approach accordingly. If the patient typically is well oriented in the morning, select the morning hours to talk over plans with him or to provide instruction or encouragement with a hobby. In evaluating the patient's orientation, it is important to distinguish between the ability to make stereotyped responses like "Hello, how are you?" and the ability to think abstractly. Many patients with brain damage are able to continue to respond in stereotyped phrases, but have impaired ability to think through current problems. Because a patient can smile brightly and say, "Good morning," it sometimes is assumed that he is more capable intellectually than he is. In such instances nurses and family members often expect him to do things that actually are beyond his ability.

Another problem involves the patient's ability to perceive emotionally the significance of events. He may, for example, say without emotion, "My son was killed last week." Those who do not understand that he is ill may reproach him for being heartless, whereas actually the disease process has blunted his perception of the significance of events. (Remember that patients with cerebral vascular disease do not necessarily have all these symptoms. As is important in dealing with any patient, carefully evaluate which symptoms apply to your patient.)

CEREBRAL VASCULAR ACCIDENT

Symptoms

The onset of a cerebral vascular accident is sudden. Whatever the patient's activity, he may fall into a shocklike state. Coma as a symptom of cerebral vascular disease is especially common after hemorrhage. It comes on suddenly, and it may be deep or light.

Immediately after a severe cerebral hemorrhage the patient is unconscious, his face often is brick red, and his breathing is stertorous and difficult. On the paralyzed side his cheek blows out with each respiration. His pulse usually is slow but full and bounding. Initially, blood pressure is likely to be elevated. The patient may proceed into deeper and deeper coma until he dies. He may remain comatose for days or even weeks, and then he may recover. However, the longer the coma is, the poorer becomes the prognosis. Pneumonia is the most common cause of death during prolonged coma.

When the accident is due to cerebral embolism, there are neurologic symptoms, usually without loss of consciousness, although the state of consciousness may be altered.

Sometimes cerebral vascular accidents occur without warning. In other instances the patient suffers from such symptoms as dizzy spells, headache, unusual fatigue, or disturbances of speech or vision. Usually, the significance of such premonitory symptoms is recognized only retrospectively, when the physician questions the patient or his family about his health just before the cerebral vascular accident.

If the patient survives a major cerebral vascular accident, his symptoms will depend on the extent and the severity, as well as the location, of the resulting brain damage. Some areas of his brain may have suffered from hypoxia and then recover as the supply of oxygen and other essential elements carried by the blood improves; other areas have died from anoxia. During the early stage it is not possible to tell whether the symptoms will be permanent or temporary. Improvement in neurologic symptoms can occur for at least six months after the accident—a point of encouragement for the patient, and a reason for the nurse's doing everything possible to prevent deformities and to help the patient to maintain and to improve his contact with others and his orientation to his surroundings.

Hemiplegia. The most common neurologic sequela is hemiplegia. A hemorrhage or clot in the right side of the brain causes the patient to have a left hemiplegia, because there is a crossover of nerves in the pyramidal tract as they lead from the brain down the spinal cord. A right-handed person is left-brain dominant, and a left-handed person may be right-brain dominant.

The speech center of a right-handed person also is located in the left side of the brain, and the speech center of a left-handed person is on the right side of the brain. It is not uncommon for the hemorrhage or clot responsible for the patient's hemiplegia to cause aphasia by cutting off the blood supply to the patient's cerebral speech center. A right-handed person developing a right hemiplegia might have aphasia, since the speech center is in the left hemisphere.

Other symptoms of cerebral vascular accident include confusion, emotional lability, and hemianopsia. The last term refers to a condition in which the patient can see only half of his normal visual field. He cannot see, with either eye, what is going on to the right or to the left of him as he looks straight ahead. This is due to damage to the visual area of the cerebral cortex or its connections to the brain stem (optic radiations). This symptom like other symptoms resulting from cerebral vascular accident may subside completely, or partially, or not at all.

Aphasia. The loss of the usual ability to use or to understand spoken and written language is called *aphasia*. Although aphasia may exist without intellectual impairment, in aphasia resulting from cerebral vascular accident there usually is evidence of some intellectual impairment in all but the mildest forms of aphasia.

Until aphasia is seen, it is a very difficult syndrome to believe. A patient with aphasia may know what a pencil is, if he is shown one. If it is handed to him, he will write with it; but he cannot think of the word "pencil." He says, "Rag—sweater—miniature—wife." He cannot think of the correct name. The patient may be able to conceive the symbol, but he cannot express the word "pencil." This type of aphasia is *expressive aphasia*.

SOME TYPES OF APHASIA

Receptive
  Auditory aphasia (symptom: difficulty in understanding the spoken word)
  Alexia (symptom: difficulty in reading)
Expressive
  Motor (symptom: difficulty in speaking)
  Agraphia (symptom: difficulty in writing)

Any type of vascular disorder or tumor can cause aphasia if it involves the speech center in the brain. The patient may, to his horror, find that he has lost not only his speech, but, if he also has an auditory aphasia, that the words people speak to him are as garbled as an unfamiliar foreign language. On the other hand, the patient frequently does not realize that what he is saying is not what he thinks he says. He then is mystified, and sometimes he becomes angry, at the seemingly strange behavior of others, who say, "What?" when he believes that he has asked a perfectly logical and intelligible question.

Diagnosis

In an attempt to identify the cause of the cerebral vascular accident and thus to select those patients whom surgery may help, a lumbar puncture may be performed. A stroke caused by hemorrhage will show blood in the cerebrospinal fluid, whereas a stroke from a thrombosis will not.

Cerebral angiography may be done. An electroencephalogram or a pneumoencephalogram may be made.

Medical Treatment

Anticoagulant therapy of cerebral thrombosis and emboli may be used in selected patients in the hope that it will discourage further formation of thrombi at the place of their origin and, therefore, prevent pieces of clot from breaking off and becoming emboli. Anticoagulants are always contraindicated in hemorrhage.

Heparin. This drug prolongs the clotting time of blood. The dosage of heparin is calculated to keep the patient's clotting time at an increased level.

Heparin is more rapid in action than Dicumarol (see below), and its action is over sooner when it is stopped. About 80 per cent of heparin is gone one hour after administration, and about two hours after administration clotting time has returned to normal.

Heparin is given intramuscularly or intravenously. To initiate therapy, about 300 mg. are given in the first 24 hours.

Watch patients on this drug for a drop in blood pressure, racing pulse and other signs of massive hemorrhage. To counteract this effect of heparin, a transfusion of fresh whole blood may be given. If a rapid reversal of heparin effects is required, protamine sulfate, usually 50 mg. intravenously, may be administered slowly. The coagulation time is expected to return to normal limits within 5 minutes.

When heparin therapy has been used and is discontinued, it is very important that the patient be ambulatory to prevent new clot formation. If the patient cannot be out of bed, exercises of all limbs should be repeated at frequent intervals during the day.

Dicumarol. This drug decreases the coagulability of blood. Its efficacy is determined by prothrombin time. It acts more slowly than heparin, requiring 48 to 72 hours to be effective. Unlike heparin, it is given by mouth. Therapy frequently is initiated with 300 mg. the first day and 200 mg. the second day; after that the dosage is related to the patient's prothrombin time, which is tested every day before the first dose of Dicumarol. Once a Dicumarol level has been established, the heparin is discontinued.

Because of the possibility of hemorrhage, Dicumarol is a dangerous drug and never should be used if there are no reliable laboratory facilities. Vitamin K is the antidote. Fresh whole blood also may be used. Stored whole blood is less useful, because its prothrombin content is less than it is in fresh blood.

Coumadin. This drug is similar to Dicumarol. One of its advantages is that it can be given either by mouth or intravenously. Its average maintenance dose is 10 mg. a day.

Surgical Treatment

Surgical treatment of cerebrovascular disease is relatively recent. Extensive research on new surgical approaches is being carried out, and progress is rapid and encouraging. The nurse will need to supplement her understanding of this expanding field by reading current articles in periodicals, attending meetings and talking with surgeons, so that nursing care may be based on the latest available knowledge.

Cerebral Insufficiency Due to Extracranial Vessel Occlusion

The four major arteries supplying the brain are the two vertebral and the two internal carotid ateries. In about 30 per cent of the patients with cerebral ischemia, an atheroma of one of these vessels obstructs the flow of blood to the brain. The sections of blood vessel proximal and distal to the atheroma often are relatively normal.

Sometimes atheromas occur in more than one vessel, or the vessels in the neck may be normal, and the infarction results from atherosclerosis involving only the small vessels in the brain itself.

Treatment and Nursing Care. Following diagnosis, based on the history, the neurologic examination and studies of the vessels by angiography, the surgeon removes the offending atheroma, perhaps with a patch graft of the vessel, or he may bypass the obstruction with a shunt. The patient comes to the recovery room with a dressing on his neck.

Postoperative nursing care includes observations for a change in neurologic symptoms from the patient's preoperative status. Important symptoms for which to watch include headache, increased confusion, return or loss of ability to move an extremity, facial asymmetry and aphasia.

Aneurysms of the Blood Vessels of the Brain

Aneurysms are formed by the outpouching of blood vessel walls, which may occur in cranial vessels (see Chap. 32).

Because aneurysms develop slowly, they may become very large before they give rise to symp-

toms. Sooner or later they will show themselves through either nerve compression or hemorrhage. Local symptoms of pressure will depend on the location of the aneurysm in the brain. Aneurysms may leak, and then they give rise to signs of increased intracranial pressure and to edema from tissues irritated by extravasated blood. The blood vessels go into spasm as a protection against further bleeding. This causes ischemia of brain tissue. The patient will have a severe headache. It is important to note where the pain started. As the meninges become irritated and edematous, the headache will become generalized. Then the patient will have a stiff neck and blood in his spinal fluid, and he may become comatose. Diffuse intracerebral vasospasm, which elevates the pressure in both the systemic arterial system and the spinal fluid, may cause death. Therefore, increasing blood pressure should be reported to the physician immediately.

Bleeding from a ruptured aneurysm is an ever-present danger. If the patient survives one episode of leakage, he may have others. The bleeding patient should lie very still and do nothing to increase his blood pressure. He should not sit up, cough or strain in any way. Ruptured intracranial aneurysm is the prime cause of subarachnoid hemorrhage.

The presence and the location of an aneurysm is identified by cerebral angiography. As the danger of further hemorrhage from the weakened aneurysmal sac is great, particularly in the first weeks after the initial hemorrhage, often surgical repair is necessary. The operation is not without hazard, because manipulation of the small cerebral vessels may result in increased vasospasm or thrombosis and cerebral infarction. Usually, the risks of surgery are less than the dangers of recurrent hemorrhage.

Postoperative Nursing Care. The patient is observed for increased intracranial pressure, which may mean intracerebral hemorrhage, and for neurologic symptoms on the side of his body opposite the site of the surgery. The nurse talks to the patient, observing for language difficulties that may indicate the beginning of aphasia; she frequently tests the movement and the strength of the muscles on the opposite side of the body; and she notes facial and pupillary symmetry.

Arterial Clamp. As an alternative to direct repair of the aneurysmal sac when collateral circulation is believed to be adequate, a Crutchfield or a Selverstone clamp may be applied to a carotid artery. The purpose is to obstruct the blood flow to the vessel on which there is an aneurysm, thus reduce the pressure in the sac and so prevent rupture. Sometimes the clamp is tightened all at once, or the doctor may prefer to screw it down gradually over several days in the hope that collateral circulation will have a chance to develop. In either case, when the clamp finally occludes the artery, the patient should be observed frequently, perhaps as often as every 15 minutes, for aphasia or hemiparesis, which may result if the circulation to the brain is inadequate. If this occurs, the clamp must be opened promptly to prevent permanent brain damage. The doctor may instruct the nurse in this procedure, as she is usually the first to discover signs of ischemia, and speed is important. If some time has passed before signs of cerebral ischemia are discovered, removal of the clamp may be done more safely on the exposed vessel in the operating room, because a clot may have formed proximal to the clamp and be embolized to the brain when the clamp is unscrewed. The patient is not really out of danger until after the clamp has been tightened for 48 hours or more. When occlusion is complete, the doctor may snap the screwdriver off the clamp and leave the clamp permanently in the neck, or he may prefer to remove the clamp and ligate the artery.

General Points in the Nursing Care of Patients with Cerebral Vascular Accidents

Objectives in the treatment and the nursing

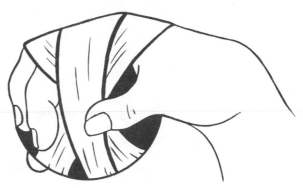

FIG. 19-3. A ball placed in the spastic hand may help to prevent contractures and keep the hand more in a position of function. It may be necessary to bandage the ball lightly in place. If this is done, inspect the hand frequently to make sure that the fingers have not curled up between the gauze and the ball, causing the gauze to cut into the skin or to impede the circulation.

care of the patient with a cerebral vascular accident include maintenance of body functions and prevention of complications, such as pneumonia, decubitus ulcers and contractures. These considerations are applicable to any unconscious patient.

When a patient first has a cerebral vascular accident, he should be turned to his side, so that his tongue does not occlude his airway, and so that he does not drown in the frothy saliva over which he has no control. Do not move him,

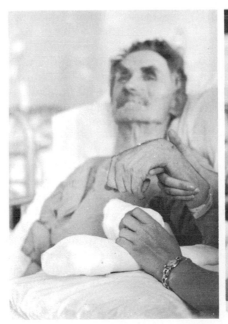
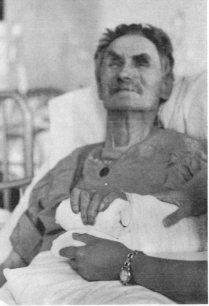

FIG. 19-4. One way to position a spastic, paralyzed hand. The bandage should be removed and the hand exercised periodically. Note finger positioning.

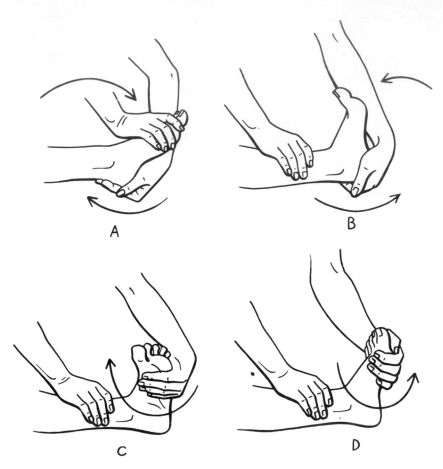

Fig. 19-5. Range-of-motion exercises for the affected foot in hemiplegia. The motions should be conducted slowly and smoothly, with a momentary pause when spasticity causes resistance. As soon as the patient has movement, these exercises should be done actively rather than passively. In the beginning of the regaining of function, the patient may start the exercises, and the nurse completes the movements. As the patient gains strength, he should do them himself entirely.

except perhaps away from any obvious hazard, such as a radiator, until the doctor has seen him. Moving him may cause further mobilization of clots or more bleeding.

Family Visits

Ordinarily, the patient is placed on the critical list, and the family can visit at periods other than scheduled visiting hours. The family make the decision on how long to stay in light of the patient's condition and their own reactions to the experience. Some family members wish to be present as much as possible. One consideration is that, if the condition of the patient changes markedly, or if he dies, they will be with him at the critical time. A family member should be helped to be as comfortable as possible. Provide a comfortable chair, and be sure he knows the location of the coffee shop, the telephone and the visitors' bathroom. Above all, convey to him that he should not hesitate to call the nurse whenever he believes her presence is needed. Some family members do not undertake a prolonged vigil at the bedside, perhaps because of responsibilities for children or their need to get away from the stressful environment to regain their composure. If they decide not to stay, assure them that you will call if there is a significant change in the patient's condition. In either case try to be perceptive of the family's reaction to the experience, and avoid implying that there is one correct way for them to behave in relation to length and frequency of visits.

The Return of Consciousness

As the patient recovers from coma, the head of the bed may be elevated further. Now, although the patient may be allowed on his back, his affected arm still should be supported on a pillow. A roll of gauze or a rubber ball placed in his hand may help to prevent the clawlike contracture deformity that so frequently follows a cerebral vascular accident. If the patient has any movement at all in his hand, encourage him to squeeze the ball periodically for exercise. As the patient sits up more, special attention is paid to

FIG. 19-6. Exercises of the affected hand and the affected arm that the hemiplegic patient should learn to do himself. (A), (B) and (C): The affected arm is grasped at the wrist by the unaffected hand and is raised over the head. (D) and (E): The unaffected hand is slipped into the spastic hand, and slowly in turn each finger is extended.

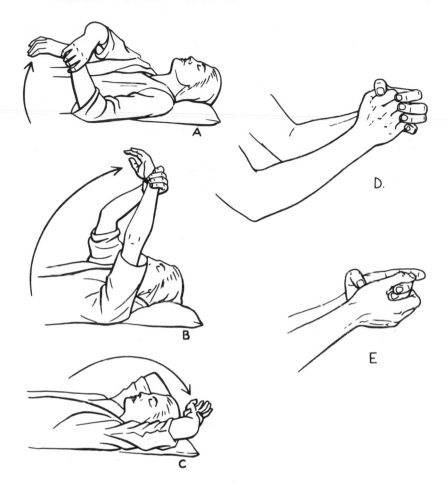

the skin of the buttocks, in an attempt to prevent skin breakdown. Change of position and frequent massage continue to be necessary. The patient's feet should press against a footboard. Beware of footdrop and outward rotation. The physician may ask that a light splint be used on an extremity, if contractures seem to be forming.

With Continued Improvement

As the patient who has had a cerebral vascular accident improves, he may be able to eat and drink, although some of what he takes will run out of the paralyzed side of his mouth. He may not be able to swallow well. His embarrassment, when he feels that he is drooling like a baby, can be minimized by turning him on his unaffected side during meals and putting only small amounts of food in the side of his mouth that has the best control. This method of feeding also will help to minimize the possibility of aspirating the food.

As the patient recovers from a cerebral vascular accident, teach him not to strain while mov-

ing his bowels. Straining may result in embolism or hemorrhage. Tell the doctor there is difficulty. A laxative or an enema may be ordered.

Anticipation of Needs. As the patient recovers, he becomes aware of new limitations, and the discovery is frightening. Perhaps one reason that most people fear paralysis is that they have no assurance their needs will be met. A patient's throat is parched, and he cannot ask for a drink. He lies on his arm until it is painfully cramped, and he is powerless to move or to complain. A patient wishes to tell his wife not to cry, but he cannot speak.

Do the little extra things that will make your patient more comfortable. Put a piece of ice in his drink, adjust the pillows, elevate or lower the bed to his exact satisfaction, and rub an aching shoulder as you change his position. If his mouth is dry, and he is allowed extra fluids, bring him a glass of orange juice or an eggnog. Anticipate what he needs before he has to try to ask you. If he has diarrhea, he will be fatigued, and fresh-

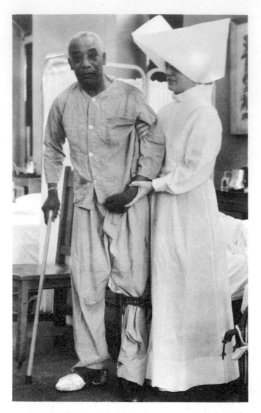

FIG. 19-7. Because this patient is helping to support himself with a cane, the nurse assists him on the affected side. She does not lead the patient; rather, he sets the pace. Note how she supports the affected arm and wrist. Her firm touch is a source of confidence to the patient.

through range-of-motion exercises several times a day—actively on the unaffected side and passively on the affected side. Teach the patient to massage and to stretch the fingers of his affected hand with his unaffected hand several times daily. Work toward having the patient passively exercise his affected arm with his good arm, for thus both arms are exercised at once. As soon as there is the slightest evidence of movement of either the affected arm or the affected leg, rejoice with the patient, and capitalize on it. This change may be the beginning of the return of function. Be careful, though, that the patient does not become tired. He is still weak. Early use of exercise not only serves to prevent contractures and wasting of unused muscles but also implies to the patient that he is not going to be a hopeless cripple.

If you are the one who is responsible for the early ambulation of the newly paralyzed patient, have someone else—preferably a strong person—assist you the first time that you help the patient out of bed. This arrangement will make both you and the patient feel more secure. Remember that the patient who has lived for a while with his hemiplegia has found ways of moving that are effective for him, but the newly paralyzed patient does not know what he can do and what he cannot.

Let the patient sit at the edge of his bed for a minute, to become accustomed to the upright position. If dizziness is prolonged, help him to lie down again, and consult the doctor. Tell the patient just what the sequence of movement will be, so that you will both be moving in the same direction. If the patient is not faint or dizzy, put his robe on while he is sitting up. Put the sleeve on his affected arm first (it would be much more difficult for him to maneuver his affected arm into the second sleeve). Later, in the same manner, the patient learns to get dressed. Stand at the patient's unaffected side and support him from that side. It might seem logical to help him from his affected side, but this arrangement is not as effective. Support the side that helps the patient to steady himself. While you hold him firmly, let the patient step onto the footstool and then to the floor with his unaffected foot. The one or two steps to a chair are probably enough for the first day. When you are helping the patient to go back to bed, tell him to step up on the footstool with his unaffected foot. The other is still too weak to lift his entire body. Many hospitals have beds that are adjustable in height.

ening the bed and providing quiet will help him to rest. If he vomits, his mouth will have a sour taste, and mouth care should be given without his asking for it. If his appetite is jaded, give him frequent snacks, attractively presented.

Exercise and Ambulation. Many doctors have their patients walk shortly after consciousness returns. Whether your patient's doctor orders bed rest or ambulation, keep your patient in enough motion to maintain muscle tone and function, but not so active that he tires. If a physical therapist is available, he is the resource person who will plan, in cooperation with the doctor, exercises for the patient. Confer with him, so that you can follow his treatment while you care for the patient.

If there is no physical therapist available, consult the doctor about the specific exercises allowed the patient. Perhaps he will be permitted to go

If this type of bed is being used, place the bed in the lowest position and help the patient to place both feet on the floor. This type of bed makes the use of a footstool unnecessary; the procedure is easier for the patient and the nurse, and it is safer.

Slowly, the patient may graduate under the guidance of the physical therapist to parallel bars, a walker, a crutch and a cane, and then to no aid. Make the goal of each day's activity one that is attainable, even if it is only one more step. Walking is a primitive activity, something that the patient doubtless has taken for granted for years. To lose it is disheartening. To the patient every small success in regaining mobility is a point of great encouragement for the future; every failure may be a sign that the future is hopeless.

Care of an Affected Arm. If the patient's arm on the affected side is completely paralyzed, consult the physical therapist concerning positioning of the arm when the patient is up. Usually, a sling is recommended to keep a completely paralyzed arm from dangling while the patient is out of bed. If a sling is used, teach the patient to remove his arm from it at intervals and to provide passive range-of-motion exercises for the paralyzed arm with his unaffected arm. It is usually recommended that the arm be left out of the sling if there is any function in the arm, no matter how feeble. Any hint of movement should be persistently nurtured.

Rehabilitation

An early start at rehabilitation is one of the best ways to prevent depression. The patient should never be given the impression that there is no use in training his muscles up to their full capacity. It is also important for the patient eventually to take a realistic account of what he can do, and what he cannot, so that he can plan his life; however, no one knows at the beginning how much function can be recaptured. Some patients recover completely. Every step forward is nurtured, encouraged and enlarged. After about six to eight months the patient's limitations, if any, will be more clear.

Family attitudes are of the utmost importance. If they become upset in his presence, his newly labile emotions (based on the recent brain damage) will make him easily subject to depression. Then it will be more difficult to help him to recover from his depression and to work toward further function. A stable emotional environment is essential for the patient who is recovering from a cerebral vascular accident. His bouts of sudden, uncontrolled weeping should not be infectious to those around him.

The family can help the patient with his retraining program if they are instructed in the necessary steps by the physician and the nurse, and if *their* emotional needs for support and help are recognized and dealt with by the professional staff, relatives, friends and clergy. Family members may understand what will catch the patient's attention. One patient may like stamp collecting; another, gathering recipes.

If the family is large and live near each other, and if they typically come to one another's aid in crises, the care of the patient can be shared in terms of both its emotional impact and its daily time-consuming activities, such as helping the aphasic patient read aloud. But in many instances such family assistance is not available, especially when the patients are elderly. When the patient does not have family members available and willing to help him, supplementary arrangements, such as the services of a visiting homemaker or a church worker, must be sought.

Long-Term Treatment. Patients with hypertension sometimes are given drugs to help to lower their blood pressure. Such drugs are avoided at the time an infarction occurs, and they are used cautiously at other times because of the possibility that a marked fall in blood pressure may precipitate cerebral infarction or increase the area of infarction. If the patient is overweight, he is advised to reduce. If he smokes, he is advised to stop, or if this is impossible, to decrease his smoking. Sometimes such drugs as phenindione, which depresses blood cholesterol levels, are ordered in the hope of preventing additional atheromas. The long-range effect of such drugs in combating atherosclerosis has not been fully evaluated. Moderate exercise that does not lead to fatigue is recommended. Excessive use of alcohol is contraindicated.

For some patients only a part-time job is advisable, due either to problems of general fatigue or to residual disability. Other patients continue to work full-time, but they curtail social and family activities to gain necessary additional rest.

Some patients find it impossible to accept the physician's recommendations. Older persons with cerebral vascular disease frequently have lost some of the adaptability that would make it possible to follow suggestions for changes in their way of living. Sometimes they reject a treatment regimen simply because it is not acceptable to them, although they recognize it may be ideal for most patients. Unfortunately, sometimes the patient's inability to follow a regimen suggested by his physician is viewed as sheer stubbornness rather than as the result of years of gradually developing a way of life that the patient cannot suddenly relinquish—possibly, too, because of problems in adaptability due to brain damage. Most patients manage best when they have opportunity to consider the suggestions made to them without feeling undue pressure from others to change themselves or their way of living. Patients who have habitually overeaten, for example, ordinarily do not suddenly eat sparingly. The patient who has made work the center of his existence, and the means of helping to fill needs not met in other areas of his life, will not be likely to agree to give up his work until his condition forces him to do so. Although nurses and physicians of necessity place health needs first in advising patients, the patient himself may decide that he would rather live in his accustomed way, however unwise it may seem in relation to his health, in order to fulfill other needs which for him may take precedence—such as the need to be self-supporting. In such instances the physician and the nurse help the patient to carry out those aspects of treatment which he can accept.

Speech Rehabilitation. Just as in retraining for arm movement and walking, speech rehabilitation is most effective when it is begun early. Ideally, the patient's speech problem is evaluated carefully and promptly by a speech therapist, and a program is developed in which the nurse can collaborate with the speech therapist. However, it frequently happens that the patient does not have the services of a speech therapist, or that his illness persists for a considerable period before these services are obtained. Although the nurse is not in a position to carry out the detailed evaluation of the type of aphasia from which the patient suffers, or to set up a program of therapy, there are ways that she can help the patient in the interim before speech therapy is started or in the absence of a speech therapist. In either instance the nurse should consult with the physician. For instance, the physician who has assessed the patient's neurologic status can help the nurse to understand the type of aphasia from which the patient suffers, whether the patient's intellectual functioning has been affected, and to what extent.

Here are some suggestions concerning ways that the nurse can help the patient with aphasia:

• Because the patient has problems of association (between word and subject, between word and concept), talk to him and expect response from him. Do not tire him; on the other hand, do not work in silence, guessing at what he wants and accepting only nonverbal communications, such as hand signals. "Do you want a blanket, Mr. Jones? Here is a blanket. *You* say: 'Blanket.'" Continuously, strengthen associations.

• Even if you are hurried, you must seem calm and unhurried to the patient. He is so frightened by his loss of speech, and he feels so inadequate in not being able to talk as he could a few days ago, that any impatience or haste on your part will inhibit him even further. Wait quietly and pleasantly while he struggles with a word. Praise him, if it comes out, but do not show impatience if he is unsuccessful.

• Never be tempted to treat him like a child, even though the tasks he must relearn are those that children learn. He is not a child, and he does not think like one.

• Capitalize on what speech he has. If he can say his dog's name, but not his own, build sentences that he can copy, using the dog's name and ask him questions that he can answer with the dog's name. Be sure to point out his successes to him.

• Do not shout. He's not deaf.

• Set attainable goals. One sound may be worked on for weeks before it is mastered.

• Involve the family as much as possible in the early stages of rehabilitation. They may catch an attitude of hope from you, and you can show them how to help with retraining.

• Minimize distraction while you are helping the patient with his speech. Since he has difficulty concentrating due to his illness, working with him in an area where others are talking loudly, or where a radio is playing, adds unnecessarily to his difficulty and quickly leads to fatigue and frustration.

• Be aware of your own reactions to the speech difficulty. Work with these patients can be taxing and frustrating for the nurse. If you work with the patient to a degree that exceeds your ability to tolerate the effort and stress, you will show impatience and frustration, which in turn can lead the patient to become discouraged or resentful. In general, both patient and nurse function best when speech practice periods are brief and interspersed with other activities.

Because social isolation is such a common response to this disability, help both the patient and his family to feel that, his physical condition permitting, there is no reason for him to live without friends, parties and outings. Group speech therapy often is the first contact that a patient has with others, but it should not be the only contact.

Care of the patient with a stroke is a tremendous nursing challenge. The nurse's knowledge, dedication, and willingness to persevere can be crucial in determining whether the patient can resume his accustomed responsibilities.

REFERENCES AND BIBLIOGRAPHY

BEESON, P. B., and McDERMOTT, W.: *Cecil-Loeb Textbook of Medicine*, ed. 13, Philadelphia, Saunders, 1971.

BELAND, I.: *Clinical Nursing*, ed. 2, New York, Macmillan, 1970.

BROWN, T., and POSKANZER, D.: Treatment of strokes, *New Eng. J. Med.* 281:594, September, 1969.

BUCK, McK.: Adjustments during recovery from stroke, *Am. J. Nurs.* 64:92, October, 1964.

BURT, M.: Perceptual deficits in hemiplegia, *Am. J. Nurs.* 70:1026, May, 1970.

CARINI, E., and OWENS, G.: *Neurological and Neurosurgical Nursing*, ed. 5, St. Louis, Mosby, 1970.

DE WEESE, J., *et al.*: Surgical treatment for occlusive disease of the carotid artery, *Ann. Surg.* 168:85, 1968.

FOX, MADELINE: Talking with patients who can't answer, *Am. J. Nurs.* 71:1146, June, 1971.

GARDNER, E.: *Fundamentals of Neurology*, ed. 5, Philadelphia, Saunders, 1968.

GARDNER, M. A.: Responsiveness as a measure of consciousness, *Am. J. Nurs.* 68:1034, May, 1968.

GREY, HOWARD A.: The aphasic patient, *RN* 33:46, July, 1970.

HODGINS, E.: *Episode*, New York, Atheneum, 1964.

LARGE, H., *et al.*: In the first stroke intensive care unit, *Am. J. Nurs.* 69:76, January, 1969.

McGINITY, P. J., and STOTSKY, B.: The patient in the nursing home, *Nurs. Forum* 6:238, 1967.

MERRITT, H. H.: *Textbook of Neurology*, ed. 4, Philadelphia, Lea, 1967.

MOSER, D.: An understanding approach to the aphasic patient, *Am. J. Nurs.* 61:52, 1961.

OLSON, E. V., *et al.*: The hazards of immobility, *Am. J. Nurs.* 67:779, April, 1967.

OSGOOD, C. S., and MIRON, M. S.: *Approaches to the Study of Aphasia*, Urbana, Ill., University of Illinois, 1963.

RAMEY, I.: The stroke patient is interesting, *Nurs. Forum* 6:273, 1967.

SMITH, G. W.: *Care of the Patient with a Stroke*, New York, Springer, 1967.

TOOLE, J. F., and PATEL, A. N.: *Cerebrovascular Disorders*, New York, McGraw-Hill, 1967.

ULLMAN, M.: Disorders of body image after stroke, *Am. J. Nurs.* 64:92, October, 1964.

WOLANIN, M. O.: They called the patient repulsive, *Am. J. Nurs.* 64:72, June, 1964.

The Patient with Spinal Cord Impairment 20

Areas of Function of the Spinal Cord • Causes of Cord and Spinal
Nerve Root Compression • Paraplegia

AREAS OF FUNCTION OF THE SPINAL CORD

The two main functions of the spinal cord are (1) to provide centers for reflex action and (2) to provide a pathway for impulses to and from the brain. The *sensory fibers* enter the *posterior* portion of the cord; the nerve fibers that transmit *motor* impulses run outward to the peripheral nerves from the *anterior* portion of the cord.

A lesion on the posterior horn cells of the cord can result in hypesthesia (diminished sensation) and anesthesia (no sensation). A lesion on the anterior horn cells can result in paresis (muscular weakness), paralysis and spasticity. Disturbance of motor and/or sensory function occurs below the level of the injury (i.e., its location in the spinal column).

Hence, the degree of injury, and its location, determine the extent of the disability. If the injury is high in the cervical region, respiratory failure and death follow paralysis of the diaphragm. Midcervical injuries result in breathing only by diaphragmatic movement, since the muscles of the upper thorax are paralyzed. Thoracic vertebrae seldom are injured, because they are protected by the rib cage. The 5th and the 6th cervical vertebrae and the 1st and the 5th lumbar vertebrae are especially vulnerable to injury; therefore, injury to the cord at these levels is frequent.

The severity of the injury to the cord also determines how much function will be lost. When the cord is completely severed, function is lost permanently below the level of the injury. If the damage to the cord is partial, some function may be maintained or at times regained.

CAUSES OF CORD AND SPINAL NERVE ROOT COMPRESSION

The lesion that presses on the spinal cord can lie inside or outside the canal. It may be *extradural, subdural* or *intramedullary* (within the cord substance). Whatever the lesion, it is the pressure on the cord that causes the symptoms. Symptoms may begin on one side and become bilateral as the disease progresses.

The pressure may be caused by:

Trauma. Violence to the back may fracture and collapse one or more vertebrae. A bone fragment pressing into the cord can intefere with the movement of the nerve impulses. Even if there is no fracture, momentary compression of the cord can lead to edema, which will compress further the cord within its bony housing. In this instance, symptoms may disappear gradually as the edema subsides. Trauma may lead to bleeding within the cord; because the blood has no place in which to drain, its mass forms a hematoma that occupies space and squeezes the nerve roots. An injury to the cord, such as a gunshot, may sever nerve fibers. When this kind of injury happens, and the complete severance of the cord results, the patient is completely and permanently paralyzed and loses sensation below the site of the injury to the cord. Because the tracts of the nerves are cut, there is no effective regeneration, and attempts to suture the pieces together have not been successful. Vertebral fracture may be caused by osteoporosis or tuberculosis of the spine.

Herniated Intervertebral Disk. Disks of cartilage act as cushions between the bones of the spine. Their spongy center (nucleus pulposus) is

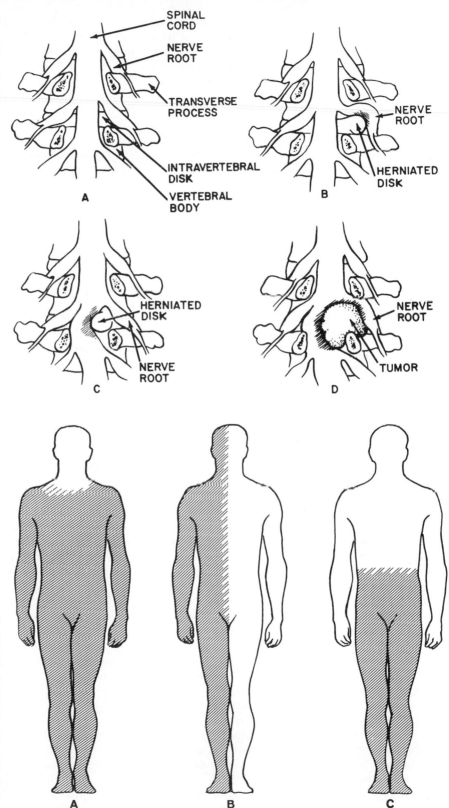

FIG. 20-1. (A) Diagram of the normal spinal column. (B) Herniated disk pressing on a spinal nerve root. (C) Herniated disk pressing on the spinal cord. (D) Tumor compressing both the spinal cord and a spinal nerve.

SPINAL CORD

NERVE ROOT

TRANSVERSE PROCESS

INTRAVERTEBRAL DISK

VERTEBRAL BODY

A

NERVE ROOT

HERNIATED DISK

B

HERNIATED DISK

NERVE ROOT

C

NERVE ROOT

TUMOR

D

FIG. 20-2. These diagrams illustrate three common types of disability: (A) quadriplegia, (B) hemiplegia, and (C) paraplegia. The shaded areas indicate the parts of the body that are affected. The location and the extent of the paralysis depend on the location and the severity of the injury. The diagrams are over-simplified. A patient may have some remaining function in an affected part.

A

B

C

encased in a fibrous coat. When stress, age or disease weakens an area in the coat or in a ligament attachment to the vertebra, and the nucleus pulposus becomes thickened and hardened, the disk herniates, causing pressure on the nerves. The most common site of the protrusion is one of the three lower lumbar disks. Because the cord ends at the level of the first or the second lumbar vertebra (L 1, 2), herniated lumbar disks compress spinal nerve roots rather than the cord itself. Pain along the distribution of the sciatic nerve is a common symptom. Anything (straining, coughing, lifting a heavy object) that causes increased pressure within the spinal cord intensifies the pain. Pain is more severe when the nerves are stretched, such as when the patient, while lying flat on his back, tries to lift his leg up without bending his knee. Also, there may be weakness and changes in sensation. The symptoms tend to be recurrent rather than steady, at least in the beginning of the disease.

Tumors. These may be primary or, more commonly, metastatic. They usually produce symptoms that become steadily worse as the lesion grows. Pain, spasm, paralysis, sensory changes and incontinence appear as compression builds up.

Cervical Spondylosis. In this disease the hypertrophic osteoarthritic ridging of cervical vertebrae can cause cord compression.

Treatment and Nursing Care

Conservative Therapy

Bed Rest. The patient with a herniated intervertebral disk is often treated first with conservative measures. For perhaps several weeks he is put to rest on a firm mattress, supported by a bed board. A horsehair rather than a foam rubber mattress should be used, because the latter is too soft. Occasionally, the patient is placed on a Stryker frame, so that he may be turned without danger of twisting. A patient with rupture of a cervical disk may have a sandbag at either side of his head to help him to maintain his head in the midline position. Pain is relieved by drugs, heat, massage and rest. Since part of the pain is due to muscle spasm, warmth to the back and muscle relaxants often are prescribed. Heat applied to the affected limb may also be a comfort to the patient, but be careful that the skin does not become burned, since there may be numbness and other sensory changes in that limb. Early in the course of the illness, the physical therapist may come to the bedside to save the patient the

strain of getting on and off the stretcher. Heat, massage and stretching exercises under water may be included in his program.

Traction by Buck's extension or a pelvic girdle for a lumbar herniated disk, and a cervical halter or tongs implanted into the skull for a cervical herniated disk, may be used to decrease muscle spasm, which may be severe. Traction also increases the distance between adjacent vertebrae. It may be continuous or intermittent, with 5 to 30 pounds of weight. The traction keeps the patient in bed in good alignment, and some patients find that it relieves their pain. Sometimes this treatment is so effective that the patient is symptom-free for a period of months or years. Some patients return to the hospital for several weeks in traction once or twice a year, when their symptoms recur.

The patient's situation suggests his nursing needs: for example, in Buck's extension, special attention to the skin of his legs; relief of pain and boredom; range-of-motion exercises in unaffected limbs.

Lying relatively still in bed with 6 or 10 pounds of weight pulling on each leg can be uncomfortable and boring, especially if the patient is no longer in pain. The physician usually regulates the time intervals in which the patient on intermittent traction is allowed out of traction. Occasionally he is permitted bathroom privileges. Some patients remove the weights during the periods when traction is prescribed. In other instances, the physician allows the patient to remove the traction at his own discretion. In either case, the patient must be assisted with reapplying the traction.

When reapplying traction, support the weights and lower them gently so that the patient does not receive a jolt. A pillow may be placed under the legs in such a way that the heels do not rub against the sheets. In pelvic traction, thick abdominal pads are placed over the iliac crest. While the nurse gives skin care she observes for symptoms of increasing compression on the cord (when the herniation is above L 1–2) or the root. Is the affected leg weaker? Does the patient say that he has less sensation in that leg, or has more pain?

When out of traction and moving in bed the patient should roll from side to side without twisting the spine. However, if his symptoms are not severe it is difficult for him to remember to move in this way. Sudden movement that strains or twists the spine should be avoided. When the patient first gets out of bed, bending over to put his slippers on or to pick up something, twisting his body, such as turning to step over the edge of a bathtub, and quick motions should be avoided. He may need to wear a lumbosacral corset.

Surgery

If conservative therapy fails to relieve symptoms of a ruptured intervertebral disk, surgery is considered. For spinal cord tumors, surgery is the treatment of choice. In a *laminectomy* operation, the posterior arch of a vertebra is removed to expose the spinal cord. Then the neurosurgeon can remove whatever lesion is causing blockage: a herniated disk, a tumor, a clot or a broken bone fragment.

Sometimes a piece of bone is taken from another area, such as the iliac crest, and grafted onto the vertebrae. This is called *spinal fusion*. The area commonly fused is from the involved vertebra to the sacrum. The fusion stabilizes the spine weakened by degenerative joint changes, such as osteoarthritis, and further weakened by the laminectomy. Fusion results in a firm union; mobility is lost, and the patient has to become accustomed to a permanent area of stiffness. When a portion of the lumbar spine is fused, the patient usually becomes unaware of stiffness after a short time because motion increases in the joints above the fusion. There usually is more limitation of motion when the area of fusion is in the cervical spine. Spinal fusion also may be done for such orthopedic conditions as fractures and dislocations of the spine and Pott's disease (tuberculosis of the spine).

Preoperative Care. Before surgery the care of the patient is similar to that of a patient being treated conservatively. When the patient has spinal compression, whatever the cause may be, make specific observations of function and sensation. Note, and chart, what activity and which position increases pain, and any gain or loss in motion or sensation since your last observation.

The patient is instructed in and encouraged to practice such exercises as deep breathing and "log rolling" turning in bed before the operation so that he has an experienced pattern to follow afterward.

Laminectomy—Postoperative Care. After a laminectomy the patient should deep-breathe at frequent intervals, but, unlike other postoperative patients, he should cough only when he needs to, since coughing increases pressure within the spinal canal. Watch for signs of compression due to edema or hemorrhage at the operative site. Compression of the cord will cause changes of motility or sensation from that point downward. Inspect the dressing for leakage of spinal fluid as well as for hemorrhage.

Incisional pain usually can be relieved by narcotics. Surgery for a herniated disk will abolish the pain that was due to stretching the nerve, but a few patients will continue to have backache, especially after standing for long periods. When there has been irritation of the nerve by pressure exerted by the herniated disk or by surgery, the pain may last for some time postoperatively. Heat and massage, when prescribed by the physician, will make the patient more comfortable. They should be used also, whenever possible, in lieu of narcotics when the patient has long-standing back pain (such as in cancer of the spine), because the problem of addiction may arise.

One of the most important principles of care after a lumbar laminectomy is to have the patient rest his back as much as possible. Twisting, turning and jerking the back are not conducive to healing. The first postoperative order concerning the position of the patient usually specifies that he not be turned for the first 8 hours, that his position be supported with sandbags and that he is to be kept flat for 12 hours. It is usually the surgeon's wish that the patient not help himself turn in bed for the first two days postoperatively. He usually is turned "log fashion." Before he is turned, the patient's bed is flattened, and he makes himself stiff as a log, with his arms at his side. Then the nurse rolls him over all at once, without bending his spine. A turning sheet is helpful, especially early in the postoperative period. Get help if the patient is heavy. Usually patients feel safer when they are allowed to participate in the turning process. At first a patient may be limited to listening to the nurse explain just how the turning will be carried out, to be as comfortable and safe as possible. Later, he will be taught to turn himself, log fashion. It is essential to avoid any abruptness in the turnings, either in manner or the movement of the patient. Most patients greatly fear that they will be moved in such a way that the results of the operation will be compromised, or that they will suffer much pain. Therefore, one proceeds slowly, with the patient's full knowledge, and his participation insofar as possible, in order to lessen anxiety by helping him have more control. Support the patient's position in good alignment with pillows. Look at his spine in the new position. If it is not straight, use small propping pillows until it is. The neurosurgeon usually allows the patient to have a pillow under his head. The patient may be placed in a bivalve cast, made preoperatively.

The patient should not lift his hips to get on a bedpan, because this motion will bend his spine. Rather, he should roll onto the bedpan. Support his back with pillows while he is on it. Tell him to call for help rather than to reach for something on his bedside stand that is just beyond his fingertips. Better still, try to anticipate what the patient will need, and put it close enough to him so that he can reach it without stretching.

The patient with a lumbar laminectomy often is kept in bed for ten days to two weeks. When he gets up, there will be less strain on his back if he walks in shoes rather than slippers.

Of course, women should not wear shoes with high heels. Only a shoe with a moderate heel that gives good support to the foot is desirable. A brace or corset occasionally is prescribed and should be applied while the patient is still lying in bed. Have him wear a thin cotton shirt under the brace, no part of which should contact the skin, and be sure that there are no wrinkles to leave marks in the skin. If the doctor does not want a shirt to be worn under the brace, be sure that there is smooth padding where the brace touches the skin.

To help the patient into a brace, have him lie on his side. Center the stays on his back, and have him roll onto the garment. While he is still lying down, after the support has been snugly fastened in place, assist the patient across the bed, so that when he sits up, his feet will be over the edge. Help him to sit up, without straining or twisting his back. In such a support, patients have to keep a straight back. Also, encourage them to maintain good posture with their muscles. The stronger the back muscles become, the more support they can give to the operative site, and the less the patient will need the external support of the brace.

Exercises in some form will be prescribed. Such calisthenics as lifting the arms and the legs off the floor simultaneously from a prone position are boring. Because swimming is equally effective in strengthening the muscles and is enjoyable to many people, it may be recommended by the doctor. Release from the uncomfortable brace is the motivation to continue whatever exercise is prescribed by the doctor.

After a lumbar laminectomy patients are more comfortable and better supported when they sit in a straight chair rather than an easy chair.

Teach patients not to bend over from the waist; instead, they should lower the body by bending the knees while they keep the spine straight.

Laminectomy With Spinal Fusion—Postoperative Care. A patient who has had a spinal fusion usually is kept on postoperative bed rest longer than the patient who has had a simple laminectomy. Even greater care must be taken that the fusion patient does not twist his back while the bones unite.

Occasionally, this patient is placed in a spica cast, from his knees to his chest. The cast may be applied several days after surgery. This interval is provided to permit visualization of the operative site to detect bleeding or drainage. During the time between surgery and the application of the cast the patient may be encouraged to move his arms, but extreme care is taken that his spine is straight at all times. The cast may be left on six to eight weeks. When it is removed it is replaced by a brace, which may be worn initially 24 hours a day.

A patient who has had a spinal fusion may have two wounds: the wound in the spinal column and the wound in the donor site (although sometimes the bone for the graft is taken from a bone bank). If bone was taken from the patient's leg, he wears an elastic bandage on that leg as long as there is swelling, possibly for several weeks. Be sure that he knows how to apply the bandage himself before he leaves the hospital.

Cervical Spine. A patient with injury or surgery of the cervical spine may not be turned at all without special equipment, such as Crutchfield tongs (see Chap. 15), a brace or halter, a Foster or Stryker frame. Two sandbags may be placed along his head or his neck to keep his cervical spine straight. If the patient is in an ordinary bed, with or without traction, be sure that he is allowed to be turned before you do so. In an ordinary bed he needs two people to help to turn him, one at the head and one at the hip. When the patient lies on his side, put a small pillow under his neck to keep his spine straight. Watch for respiratory distress. Edema of the cervical cord or the spinal nerves may temporarily paralyze the respiratory muscles. When this occurs, the patient is placed in a respirator until the edema subsides. Have a tracheostomy set and

Fig. 20-3. (*Top*) This patient was paralyzed from the waist down after an automobile accident. The Stryker frame has several advantages in his care. He can be turned easily, and his feet can be positioned readily to prevent deformity. (They extend over the mattress when he is in prone position. When he lies supine, a footboard is used to support his feet.) The tray underneath the frame is useful for holding personal belongings. The armboard, padded by a pillow, is removable. Because the frame rolls easily, the patient can be taken to the sun porch or the TV room. Because the patient is incontinent, a Foley catheter has been inserted and is connected to tubing that drains into the disposable bag (lower right corner of picture).

(*Bottom*) These two nursing students are getting ready to turn the patient from prone to supine position. The frame on which the patient will lie has been placed over him and secured with bolts, nuts and straps. After the frame has been turned, the patient will be lying on his back on the frame, which is shown over his body. The other frame then will be removed.

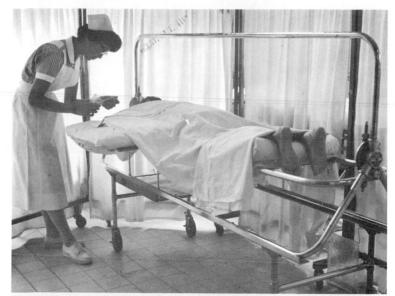

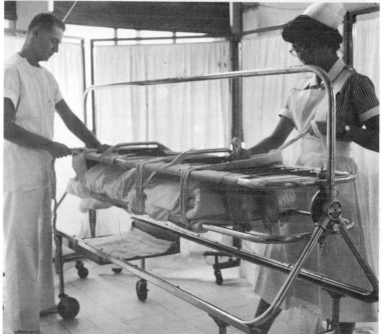

a respirator ready for use. After injury or surgery of a cervical disk, traction may be applied with a head halter. Sometimes, the patient can remove the head halter when he sleeps, and sometimes he is ordered to use it continuously. When he improves after surgery, he may wear a rigid collar to decrease neck motion.

Thoracic Spine. When surgery has been performed on the thoracic spine, a figure-of-eight dressing may be applied postoperatively. Because the dressing may constrict the axillary vessels, check the radial pulses every hour. The patient is cautioned not to stretch his arms until healing is well advanced.

Resumption of Activities; Lifting. When spinal fusion has been performed, the resumption of activities is gradual for six months to a year, after which the patient usually can resume full activity. After a laminectomy without spinal fusion the patient is allowed gradually to do light work, but usually he should do no lifting for a year, and he may never be able to lift heavy objects. The light objects he does lift should be held close to his body to avoid back strain.

PARAPLEGIA

The word *paraplegia* usually calls to mind a picture of a war-wounded veteran in a wheelchair. This picture is only partly true, for civilians become paraplegics, too. Paraplegia is paralysis of both lower extremities. (In much of this discussion the term *paraplegia* will be used broadly to include both paraplegics and *quadriplegics,* patients who have paralysis of all four limbs.) The cause may be battle injuries or any one of a variety of diseases, such as multiple sclerosis and polio, or civilian injuries, such as those sustained in automobile or diving accidents. Paraplegia is caused by injury to the spinal cord. When the injury comes from disease, such as multiple sclerosis, the paralysis is likely to develop gradually. The paralysis caused by fracture or dislocation of vertebrae during an accident or a war injury usually occurs suddenly.

Early Treatment and Nursing Care

First Aid. Suppose that someone has been hurt in an automobile accident, and an injury to the spine is suspected. The patient should be placed without flexing his back or neck, onto a firm, flat surface, such as a door that has been removed from its hinges. Do not move him until help is available, and a firm, flat support on which he can be carried has been obtained. Never permit bystanders to pick up a patient hastily, thus flexing his spine, and to toss him into the back seat of an automobile. Such careless moving may damage the cord further. Proper first aid may mean the difference between his being able to walk and having to spend the rest of his life in a wheelchair. Treatment for shock or hemorrhage may also be required as first-aid measures.

After the patient has been admitted to the hospital, the doctor will determine the extent of the injury by physical and x-ray examinations. If the vertebrae are so injured that they are squeezing or crushing the cord, measures may be taken to relieve the pressure of the bones on the cord.

Positioning. During the period immediately after spinal cord injury the patient is seriously ill and requires a great deal of care and observation. When nerve impulses to the skin are interrupted, the skin's normal response to injury is diminished. The paralyzed patient cannot engage in the almost constant movement that is normal, even during sleep, and that protects the skin from pressure sores. Decubitus ulcers form easily in these patients, become infected easily and heal very slowly. Unless his position is changed frequently by the nurse, decubitus ulcers will result. Eventually, the patient is taught to inspect his own skin. The Stryker or the Foster frame and the CircOlectric bed make it easier to turn helpless patients.

Complications. Deformities readily develop unless special precautions are taken. Footdrop is a frequent complication because of paralysis of the lower extremities. A footboard must be used from the very beginning of the patient's illness to prevent footdrop.

Because the patient is unable to move about, his breathing is shallow, and he fails to cough up respiratory secretions. Therefore, he is predisposed to the development of respiratory complications, such as pneumonia. Changing position frequently and encouraging the patient to breathe deeply and to cough up respiratory secretions are important in preventing respiratory complications.

Observations. The areas affected by paralysis must be observed carefully. Does the patient have sensation in those parts? Can he feel that water during his bath is warm or cold? Can he feel the pressure of the nurse's hand? Can he move the part? At first the paralysis is flaccid (limp). Later it becomes spastic. Severe reflex spasms that the patient cannot control are frequent. The muscle movement is spasm and not the return of voluntary function. Physical activity helps to decrease spasm. Passive exercises and changes of position, when they are used regularly, also reduce spasms.

Many patients have pain in the affected area, even though sensation in the usual sense has been lost. The pain is associated with scar formation or irritation around a nerve root. In most patients the pain decreases gradually with recovery from the initial injury.

At first the patient will not perspire below the point of injury. Later, he may perspire profusely and require frequent bathing.

Site of Injections. When possible, intramuscular injections should be given above the level of the paralysis. Because capillary circulation is sluggish below the injury, the medicine will be less well absorbed, and injury to the tissues, due to the injection, is more likely to occur.

Fig. 20-4. The CircOlectric bed permits vertical rather than lateral turning of the patient. The power for turning the bed is provided by electricity. The student is showing the patient the switch that controls the movement of his bed.

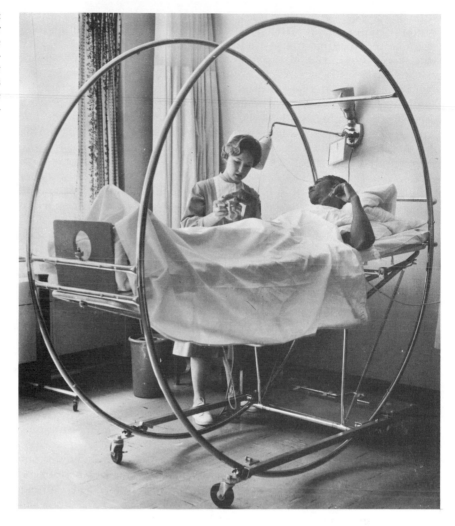

Elimination. Cord compression can interfere with the patient's control over the bladder and the bowel. There may be incontinence or retention of feces, and fecal impactions are frequent. At first there usually is retention of urine; later the patient voids involuntarily. Even when the patient is incontinent there often is some retention of urine. A retention catheter is used in the bladder. If the bedding of the patient becomes wet, the likelihood of decubitus ulcers increases. Enemas may be given daily or every other day to evacuate the bowel and to lessen the problems of fecal impaction or incontinence.

Fluids and Food. The fluid intake and the nutrition of the patient must be maintained. High-fluid intake helps to lessen the possibility of urinary-tract infections and calculi. High-protein foods are important in controlling decubitus ulcers, because they help to keep the tissues healthy, and they increase the ability of the tissues to heal.

Psychological Problems

As the patient begins to recover from the overwhelming physical injury, he gradually becomes aware of what has happened to him. He finds that he is unable to move part of his body. Because he can no longer feel these parts, he must look to see if they are still there. Psychological trauma is intense. The body image must be changed. Now, instead of viewing himself as a whole, healthy person, the patient must recognize that part of his body is permanently useless. At first, most patients react with depression and withdrawal. They lie and stare into space, and they show no interest in people and events around them. During this period it is better to emphasize quiet presence, empathy, and attention to physical needs, than it is to adopt a cheer-him-up campaign. It will take time for the patient to recover from the psychological as well as the physical hurt of so devastating an experience.

The patient recognizes his complete dependence on others, and he is fearful because he can no longer help himself. He wants someone near him day and night. Particularly, if he is a quadriplegic, his helplessness is extreme. He must be bathed, toileted and dressed—just like an infant. His mind is active, though, even if his body is not.

The nurse may be able to help him by being a good listener. When the patient is ready to talk about how angry or discouraged he is, he does not need advice; he does not need cheering up. He needs someone who can help to lift the burden by accepting how he feels. A patient who tells a nurse that he wishes only for death may not tell her that again if her response is, "Oh, you have lots to live for. You can read, and you have two lovely children," or if she says, "Don't talk like that. Where there's life, there's hope." The patient will still feel as hopeless as he did. He just will not discuss that subject with that nurse again.

The nurse who can reply, "You feel pretty discouraged," or "You don't see much purpose in life now," by implication is telling the patient that she understands how deeply he is discouraged, and that there is nothing wrong about feeling as he does. If his feelings are accepted by the nurse, the patient may be able to express himself further, and afterward he may be able to give the nurse some clue as to how she can help him.

Incontinence poses a tremendous problem. Very early in life human beings are taught to maintain high standards of personal cleanliness. Much is made of the shamefulness of not controlling excretory function. An adult who becomes unable to control these functions, often feels shamed and disgraced—even though intellectually he understands the reason for the lack of control. Incontinence poses a social problem, too. Patients are very sensitive to the reaction of others. Many paraplegics are constantly fearful that an embarrassing accident will occur while they are with others, or that other people will detect odors from catheters and urinals. Hence, the rehabilitation, when possible, of the bowels and the bladder is highly important, not only for physical reasons, such as preventing decubiti, but also for its effect on morale: it helps the patient

to overcome the threat of embarrassment, and so it helps him to feel more like his adult, independent self.

Many paraplegic men are impotent, and these patients suffer a severe blow to their manhood. They may feel that they are being regarded with scorn and derision. Some women patients are able to have children. Questions about sexual functioning must be answered individually by the doctor for each patient, since the degree of normal function will be determined by the particular nature and the extent of the illness. Both the patient and the wife or the husband should have an opportunity to discuss this subject with the doctor.

In addition to disturbances of the sexual and the reproductive function, the opportunities for meeting people usually are curtailed and opportunities for marriage decreased. The patient does not conform to the ideals of masculine or feminine attractiveness made fashionable by society. For instance, women must wear braces, use crutches and wear low-heeled oxfords to walk. A tall, well-built man who develops paraplegia no longer appears tall when he sits in his wheelchair.

The paraplegic is subject to a great deal of frustration. He cannot move about freely, and in many situations he must rely on others to help him. A quadriplegic may be unable to light his own cigarette, but he may have an even greater desire to smoke than he did before his injury, when his attention was absorbed by many activities.

Because of his disability he is less able than most other people to get away from situations that are irritating or frightening or to "work off steam" by physical activity. With his mobility decreased and his frustration increased, it is not surprising that the paraplegic often flies into a rage over apparent trifles. Sometimes the frustration of not getting someone to light his cigarette is just too much after all the other discouraging situations.

Rehabilitation

The aim of rehabilitation is to help paraplegics and quadriplegics to use their remaining capacities to the fullest and to avoid complications resulting from the disability. For example, decubitus ulcers seriously interfere with the program of rehabilitation. The patient who develops a large ulcer on the sacrum must return to bed and lie on his abdomen to relieve pressure on the part.

An important part of the role of the nurse in rehabilitation involves helping the patient to avoid complications, so that he can profit from the rehabilitation program. For example, she can help by:

• Giving good skin care; being alert for beginning signs of pressure sores; placing a foam-rubber cushion in his wheelchair to help to relieve pressure.

• Teaching the patient about skin care, change of position, massage, and the importance of inspecting paralyzed areas daily. Because the patient cannot feel the discomfort caused by a beginning decubitus, he must be especially observant. Patients should use a mirror to inspect parts that they cannot see.

• Maintaining good body alignment; putting joints through a full range of motion (see Chap. 19): flexion, extension, abduction, adduction, internal rotation, external rotation, pronation, supination.

• Encouraging high-fluid intake; using careful aseptic technic when irrigating catheters.

• Showing sensitivity to the emotional needs of the patient; encouraging but not forcing him toward self-care; allowing him to express his feelings concerning the disability.

Positioning. The will of the patient, plus the help of skilled therapists, can mean the difference between invalidism and independence. Paraplegics can learn to put on their own braces and to move from the bed to the wheelchair. Because of the tremendous effort required to walk (the patient must raise the entire weight of his body, plus the weight of the braces, with his arms), most paraplegics use the wheelchair most of the time and walk only short distances. However, it is important for the patient to assume upright posture at intervals during the day, whether or not he is able to walk. Quadriplegic patients who cannot stand or walk may be placed in an upright position with the aid of a tilt table or by using a CircOlectric bed. This position helps the patient to breathe more deeply, relieves pressure on the sacral region, relieves spasms, and helps to prevent urinary calculi and osteoporosis. The patient often feels dizzy and faint the first few times that he assumes an upright position. He must be watched carefully and protected, so that he does not fall. The pooling of blood in the abdominal area is a factor in causing postural hypotension. The application of an abdominal binder and elastic stockings to the legs before the patient gets up helps to prevent dizziness and faintness. When a tilt table is used, patients are strapped to it, and it is tilted gradually until the patient is standing erect.

Parallel bars help to support the patient whose upper extremities are unaffected. Therefore, he can support his own weight by grasping the bars. With the help of parallel bars, paraplegic patients can learn to balance themselves and to practice skills that later will be useful in crutch walking.

Bowel Rehabilitation. The rehabilitation of the bowels and the bladder is of crucial importance in helping the patient to move toward independence. Many patients can achieve self-controlled emptying of the bowels and the bladder, provided that they and those who care for them exert the persistent effort required to achieve this goal. Control of the bowels usually is easier to achieve than control of the bladder. The following steps are useful in helping patients to achieve self-controlled emptying of the bowel:

• Encourage the patient to drink plenty of liquid and to eat foods that produce bulk, such as fresh fruits and vegetables. Teach him not to eat foods that normally cause him to have loose stools.

• Help the patient to plan to go to the toilet at a certain time each day. Select a time that will fit later into his own schedule for self-care.

• Allow the patient privacy and sufficient time to have a bowel movement.

• As soon as he is able, encourage the patient to go to the bathroom rather than to use the bedpan. The physical activity involved in getting out of bed often helps the patient to move his bowels. Using the bathroom has psychological value, too, with its indication of self-help rather than helplessness.

Enemas and suppositories may be needed at first. For example, the patient may be given a small enema each day at the same time. He later may find that inserting a suppository just before the time for defecation will result in a normal bowel movement. Later his bowel function may become regulated so well that he has normal bowel movements without the aid of enemas or suppositories.

Giving an enema to a paraplegic patient requires skill. Here are some methods that have been developed by nurses who have had a great deal of experience in working with paraplegics:

• Be very careful in checking the temperature of the solution, and gentle in inserting the rectal tube. The inability of the patient to feel means

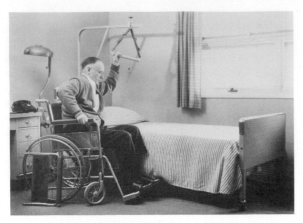

FIG. 20-5. From wheelchair to bed. The height of the bed, which is adjustable, has been made the same as the height of the seat of the wheelchair. The brakes on the wheelchair and the casters on the bed have been locked to prevent them from moving. The arm rest nearest the bed has been removed, making it easier to slide from one piece of furniture to the other. The overhead bar and the remaining arm rest are grasped firmly during the transfer. The telephone, the lamp and the light switch controlling the overhead light are within easy reach of the bed. A duplicate light switch is near the door of the room. The window can be opened and closed easily by a crank.

that he is more, not less, vulnerable to trauma.

• Because the patient cannot retain the solution during the administration of the enema, use some device to prevent the solution from running out as fast as it runs in. One device consists of a hard rubber ball with a hole in it. The rectal tube is passed through the ball, and, as the enema is given, the ball is held close to the patient's body.

• Provide ahead of time for leakage of the solution during the enema. Regardless of the technic, some leakage is likely to occur. For example, the bed can be protected by a large rubber sheet.

Bladder Rehabilitation. The control of the bladder is more difficult to establish, but many patients can achieve it. (See Chap. 18 for a discussion of rehabilitation of patients who are incontinent of urine.)

Prognosis depends upon many factors. The level of the cord injury, the occurrence of complications, the patient's motivation and perseverance, and the quality of care he receives are important influences upon prognosis. Many

paraplegics are able to go home, to care for themselves, and in some instances to resume work.

Nursing Guidelines. Helping paraplegic and quadriplegic patients to resume living that is as normal as is possible presents a tremendous challenge and equally great rewards. It is not an easy kind of nursing. Here are some suggestions on how to help the patient and how to avoid some common pitfalls:

• Let the patient do as much as he can for himself. Arrange the environment so that self-care is encouraged (feeding devices, keeping belongings handy, and so on). It will take him longer to do it himself than it will for you to do it for him. Try to arrange the schedule to allow him extra time for such activities as feeding himself.

• Avoid pushing the patient. Great sensitivity is required to know when he is ready to attempt something new. These tasks look easy to us. Activities of daily living (ADL), such as feeding, bathing and dressing, seem elementary. Do not be surprised and try not to show disappointment on days when he seems to regress.

• Encourage the patient to be up and about, to get dressed, to go to the dining room, the bathroom, the recreation rooms. Try to help him to achieve as nearly normal living as is possible. Remember that these activities are very fatiguing, especially at first, when the patient is not used to them, and plan for rest periods as well as activity.

• Rigid insistence on self-help can waste time and energy. If, for example, it would take a quadriplegic an hour to mark his menu himself, but only five minutes to do it with help, it may be wise to help him with it, so that he can use the time and energy for other things.

• Partial self-care may not be as dramatic, but it is just as important a goal as the more complete rehabilitation of a less disabled person. Think what a difference it makes to the patient and his family if he can feed himself or pick up a telephone to call for help. Learning these skills may mean the difference between having to have a family member stay with him constantly and being able to be left alone.

• All the emphasis on activity and on being with others often makes patients long for a few moments to themselves. Do not insist that the patient be busy and with other people every minute. Everyone needs a balance of solitude and companionship.

The Environment—Hospital and Home

The environment of the patient is important. Whether he is at home or in the hospital, his recovery is slow, and he is less free to move from one place to another. Some paraplegics are hospitalized four or five years. The significance of the ward environment is much greater for these patients than for those who return home after a few days.

Because physically disabled patients need special facilities, they often are grouped together in hospitals. Paraplegics, quadriplegics and amputees may share a ward. Each patient compares his disability with that of others. "I can use my arms; that poor fellow can't." "Losing a leg isn't very much. He'll be able to walk again." Envy of the amputee is common among paraplegics. Besides being able to walk with an artificial leg, amputees usually do not suffer the problems of impotence and of the loss of control of the bowels and the bladder.

Relationships among these patients affect rehabilitation. Attitudes are contagious, and the role of the nurse involves working not only with individuals, but also with groups of patients. The depression of one patient or his sarcasm may upset the whole ward. The cheerful good humor of one patient may help his buddies to laugh. Being around 20 to 30 severely disabled people can be like sitting on a powder keg: one spark, and the emotionally charged atmosphere can explode. Each individual is facing severe emotional strain. Patients find various ways of expressing their feelings about the disability.

Patients and staff get to know one another very well over the many months, and even years, in which they are together. This can be a rewarding, valuable experience—really knowing the patient and his family and home situation and having the opportunity to work with him and to see his progress over a longer period of time.

However, there are some pitfalls in caring for long-term disabled patients. Identifying some of them will help you to avoid them.

• Do not play favorites. These patients are very sensitive to any show of favoritism, and they are quick to resent it. Treat all alike in the sense that they have equal call on your knowledge and skill. Treat each differently in the sense that each patient has his own unique needs.

• Remember that you are the nurse of the patient, not a family member or a pal. (The

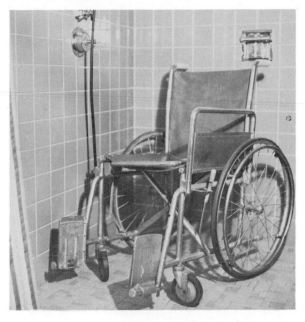

FIG. 20-6. Bathing. An extra wheelchair is stationed permanently in the shower stall. The stall is wide, allowing plenty of room for the wheelchair. One can sit in the wheelchair and bathe without assistance. Water for the shower comes through the hose seen at the left. If the water suddenly becomes too hot or too cold, the rubber hose can be directed away from the body. Some paraplegics use a chair or a stool rather than a wheelchair in the shower. Sitting under the shower is much easier than getting in and out of a bathtub.

relationship of nurse and patient sometimes tends to become confused when the nurse has cared for the patient over a long period of time.)

• Note how the patients get along with one another. Place them near those whose company they seem to enjoy.

• Avoid regimentation. For some the hospital is now the only home that they have. On special occasions let them keep the television on a few minutes after the usual "lights out."

In one way the home environment is less restricted than that of the hospital; in other ways it may be more so. At home the patient can have visitors at any hour, and he can arrange his own schedule for sleeping and waking, and so on. On the other hand, if his home does not have facilities that help him to get about, he may spend all his time in one room. One man found that he had to say in one room all day while his wife was working, because the doorways were too narrow to permit his wheelchair to pass through. No one ever came to see him, and he found life in the hospital freer and pleasanter. "There were people to talk to, and I could get around in my chair," he said. Neighbors and friends sometimes avoid the disabled. They may be curious and stare because the person looks different, or they may try to do everything for him, assuming that if he is in a wheelchair, he must be completely helpless.

Yet home is the usual environment—and usually the best one—provided that the patient has a home and a family who want him. Going home is a major step in rehabilitation. It presents the challenge of helping the disabled patient to adjust to his home and his community. What may be some of the problems that the patient faces?

- How will my family feel about me?
- Will I be a burden to them?
- Will my friends forget me?
- Will I be able to manage without the doctors and nurses around?
- What if I'm alone in the house and something happens—like a fire? In the hospital there's always someone around to help.

The patient and his family will need help in planning for his homecoming. The home situation will need to be evaluated; often a public health nurse or a social worker makes this evaluation. She notes the physical environment—the stairs, the bathroom, etc.—as well as the attitude of the family toward the return of the patient.

After the patient returns home, continued care and supervision will be needed. The patient may be seen regularly by his private doctor or at a clinic. The public health nurse may continue the teaching begun in the hospital, showing the family how to adapt care to the home situation, as well as carrying out treatments, such as injections or dressings. In some communities physical therapists are available who come to the patient's home and continue the program started in the hospital.

REFERENCES AND BIBLIOGRAPHY

BELAND, I.: *Clinical Nursing*, ed. 2, New York, Macmillan, 1970.

BERGER, S.: Paraplegia, *in* GARRETT, J. F. (ed.): *Psychological Aspects of Physical Disability*, Washington, D.C., U.S. Department of Health, Education and Welfare, (n.d.).

BUCY, P.: Paraplegia—the neglected problem, *Phys. Ther.* 99:269, March, 1969.

BURNSIDE, I. M.: The patient I didn't want, *Am. J. Nurs.* 68:1666, August, 1968.

CARINI, E., and OWENS, G.: *Neurological and Neurosurgical Nursing*, ed. 5, St. Louis, Mosby, 1970.

CHRISTOPHERSON, V. A.: Role modifications of the disabled male, *Am. J. Nurs.* 68:290, February, 1968.

CULP, P.: Nursing care of the patient with spinal cord injury, *Nurs. Clin. N. Am.* 2:447, September, 1967.

FROST, R.: *Success or Failure in the Economic Rehabilitation of Paraplegics and Quadriplegics—a Survey*, New York, Paralyzed Veterans of America and the 52 Association of New York, (n.d.).

GARDNER, E.: *Fundamentals of Neurology*, ed. 5, Philadelphia, Saunders, 1968.

HAAN, SR. M. S.: An exploratory study of the subjective experience, in hospitals, of the paraplegic patient, unpublished master's thesis, New Brunswick, N.J., Rutgers University, 1970.

HIRSCHBERG, G. G., et al.: *Rehabilitation*, Philadelphia, Lippincott, 1964.

IVERSON, S. M.: Helping a quadriplegic patient to adjust, *Am. J. Nurs.* 64:128, January, 1964.

MERRITT, H. H.: *Textbook of Neurology*, ed. 4, Philadelphia, Lea, 1967.

NAYER, D. D.: They don't notice her wheelchair, *Am. J. Nurs.* 71:1130, June, 1971.

OLSON, E. V., et al.: The hazards of immobility, *Am. J. Nurs.* 67:779, April, 1967.

SCHWAB, J., and HARMELING, J.: Body image and medical illness, *Psychosom. Med.* 30:51, Jan.-Feb., 1968.

SUDDUTH, A. L.: Comprehensive care of the traumatic paraplegic, *RN* 33:58, May, 1970.

TRIGIANO, L. L.: Independence is possible in quadriplegia, *Am. J. Nurs.* 70:2610, December, 1970.

TUDOR, L. L.: Bladder and bowel retraining, *Am. J. Nurs.* 70:2391, November, 1970.

Visual and Hearing Impairment

21

The Visually Handicapped · The Partially Sighted · The Blind
Some Eye Disorders · Nursing Considerations · Hearing
Impairment · Conditions of the Middle Ear · Disorders of the
External Auditory Canal · Disorders of the Inner Ear · Review of
Some Common Nursing Procedures

Nurses frequently are asked such questions as "Are contact lenses safe?" and "Are certain eyedrops any good?" Often, too, we are the first to be consulted after accidents at work or at home, such as when a neighbor splashes bleach into her eyes. In such situations we need to know what first aid we can give, and how to instruct others to give it in our absence. Also, we must know when to refer the patient to the doctor.

Contact lenses are tiny, almost completely invisible plastic lenses that fit directly on the cornea, separated only by the tear film from the eye itself. They are worn by people who object to the appearance of conventional glasses in frames and by those with special needs that can be met more adequately by contact lenses. (Sometimes, patients who have had cataracts removed benefit from the use of contact lenses.)

The most common dangers involved in the use of contact lenses are injury and infection of the cornea. Patients who express interest in contact lenses should be referred to the ophthalmologist. If it is decided that the patient is a suitable candidate for contact lenses, he is carefully fitted with them and is instructed by the doctor in their use. A special type of contact lens known as a scleral lens fits the entire front of the eyeball. These lenses are sometimes prescribed for treatment of certain diseases of the cornea or conjunctiva. Athletes sometimes wear scleral lenses.

Eyedrops. People who ask about the use of eyedrops to soothe the eyes can be told that such preparations approved for sale without prescrip-

tion are generally (but by no means always) harmless in themselves, but that harm can come from using any such preparation as a substitute for medical attention when the eyes are persistently irritated or uncomfortable. Allergy, the need for glasses, and even beginning glaucoma may cause discomfort. Those who experience itching, burning or other discomforts of their eyes should consult an ophthalmologist.

Professional Functions. Many people are confused by the terms *optician, optometrist, ophthalmologist* and *oculist*. An *optician*, like a pharmacist, fills prescriptions given by the doctor. In this instance the prescription is for glasses. The optician has the prescribed lenses made and sees that the glasses are properly fitted. An *optometrist* is one who has had special training in testing vision for refractive errors and in prescribing and fitting glasses to correct such errors. Because he is not an M.D., he is not permitted to prescribe medications for the eye or to diagnose or to treat eye diseases. The terms *ophthalmologist* and *oculist* are synonymous and refer to a medical doctor who has had special training in the diagnosis and the treatment of eye diseases, including refraction and the prescription of glasses.

Instruments. The physician uses an instrument called an *ophthalmoscope* to examine the interior of the eye. After the lights in the room have been turned off, the doctor holds the ophthalmoscope close to his eye and to the patient's eye, and looks through the instrument. The ophthalmoscope contains a light and is

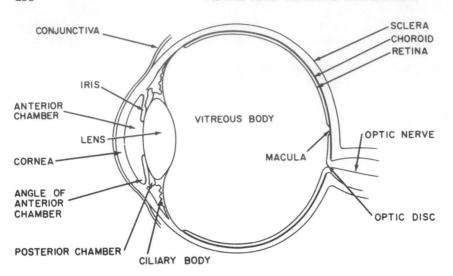

FIG. 21-1. Diagram showing the location of some of the important structures of the eye. The cornea, aqueous humor, lens, and vitreous are the refractive media.

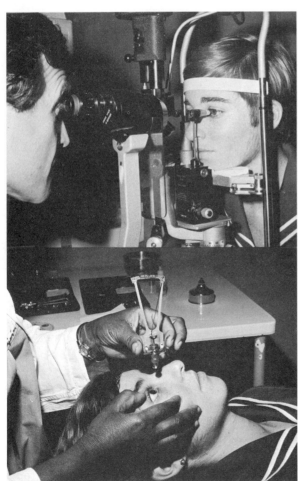

FIG. 21-2. (*Top*) Intraocular pressure measured with the Goldmann applanation tonometer. (*Bottom*) Intraocular pressure measured with the Schiotz tonometer. (Raymond Harrison, M.D.)

operated by batteries or house current. The ophthalmoscope must not be sterilized by boiling or autoclaving, because it contains many small lenses. Since the ophthalmoscope does not come into direct contact with the patient's eye, sterilization after each use is not necessary.

The doctor uses a tonometer to test the pressure within the eyeball. Increased intraocular pressure is a sign of glaucoma. Two methods of tonometry are commonly employed. With the Schiotz tonometer, the patient usually is seated in a treatment chair, and the chair is tilted to a reclining position. Drops of a local anesthetic, such as proparacaine (Ophthaine) 0.5 per cent, are administered to anesthetize the cornea. The tonometer, a small metal instrument, then is placed gently on the cornea. The moving pointer indicates the intraocular pressure. Because the footplate of the tonometer touches the eye, it must be sterilized before use with each patient. This is usually done by holding the instrument in a flame. In the past few years another method known as applanation tonometry has become increasingly used by ophthalmologists because of its greater accuracy. This instrument is the Goldmann tonometer and it attaches to the slit-lamp microscope. A drop of anesthetic solution is used, as with the Schiotz tonometer, followed by the use of fluorescein on the eye. The patient sits forward at the slit-lamp, where the instrument is placed on the cornea by the examiner who reads the pressure. Sterilization of the tonometer is carried out with an antibacterial solution.

Tonography is a recently devised method of recording intraocular tension over a period of

4 minutes, during which time a specially sensitive Schiotz type tonometer is allowed to rest on the eyeball. The tonometer in this instance is attached to an electric recording device. This test is of value for diagnosis of early glaucoma and for confirming that known glaucoma is being satisfactorily controlled by treatment.

Some simple rules for the daily care of the eyes include the following:

• Have a good light when reading, writing, sewing or other close work is being done. Place the light so that a shadow is not cast by the hands. The light source should be shielded to prevent direct glare on the eyes.

• Rest the eyes periodically when prolonged fine work is being done. Looking out of a window at intervals rests the eyes by allowing them to focus on distant objects (relaxation of accommodation). Looking continuously at small print or tiny stitches is fatiguing.

• General health is important in maintaining the health of the eyes. For example, a form of night blindness, a condition in which the individual is unable to see adequately in darkness, is related to a deficiency of vitamin A. (The adjustment of the eye to see in the dark, called *dark adaptation,* involves a complicated photochemical process in the retina.) Epithelial tissues of the eye also are affected by vitamin A deficiency, and, if the deficiency is severe, the cornea may be so damaged that blindness results.

• Get plenty of sleep. Lack of sleep is a common cause of irritation and discomfort of the eyes, as well as visual difficulties.

• Keep hands away from eyes. Rubbing the eyelids causes irritation and may introduce infection.

• Do not use eyecups (fortunately now less popular). They can spread infection or cause injury.

• Avoid direct exposure of the eyes to sun lamps. They can burn the lids and the cornea, as can excessive exposure to sunlight at the beach or on snow-covered ground. Ultraviolet rays can cause painful burns that are not apparent for several hours after overexposure.

FIRST AID

Almost everyone has suffered the exquisite discomfort of a foreign body in the eye. A cinder barely large enough to see feels like a boulder when it gets in the eye. A foreign body can be removed by the nurse if:

• It is not on the cornea.

• It has not penetrated the eyeball (for instance, a sharp splinter of metal or wood that has pierced the eyeball).

• It is removed readily by a sterile applicator. The first requisite is a good light. Remind the patient not to rub the eye. This is an urge that is hard to resist when a foreign body is present, but it may lead to further injury and irritation or to imbedding the particle, making it difficult to remove. Wash your hands thoroughly. Then, with the patient seated, examine the eye, including the inside of the upper and lower lids. To evert the upper lid, lay a toothpick swab just back from the edge of the upper lid, grasp the lashes gently but firmly with your other hand, pull the upper lid slightly outward from the eye and turn it upward, exposing the underside of the lid.

When you locate the tiny particle, touch it gently with a sterile swab moistened in clear water or sterile saline. (The latter is preferable, if it is available.) If the particle is not readily removed in this manner, avoid further attempts to remove it. Picking at it with the swab can push it into the tissues and may injure the eye. Explain to the patient that the services of an ophthalmologist are needed, and help the patient to make arrangements for further care, either in the doctor's office or at an eye clinic. Assure the patient that this referral does not necessarily mean that there is anything seriously wrong, but only that the doctor's skill is needed to remove the particle safely. A similar explanation can be made if the foreign body is on the cornea. Attempts to remove it could lead to scarring of the cornea and to diminished vision. The doctor's skill and his delicate instruments can remove the particle with the least possible injury to the cornea.

Irrigating the eye with sterile saline also is effective sometimes in removing a foreign body. An irrigating tip attached to a flask of sterile saline may be used for this purpose, in a manner similar to that used when acids or other irritants are splashed unexpectedly into the eye.

After the particle has been removed, the patient usually continues to feel some irritation. An oval eye pad applied over the closed lids with Scotch tape affords relief. Instruct him not to rub his eye, and, if it is not completely comfortable within a short time (an hour or so), to visit an ophthalmologist.

Splashing an irritating chemical, such as bleach, into the eye is another common emergency. The eye should be flushed copiously with water to remove the chemical as promptly as possible. If sterile saline is available, use it, but do not delay the irrigation to obtain it. Use plain tap water instead. If the accident occurs in the home or at work, take the patient to the nearest sink or water fountain, and have him hold his eyelids open while the water cleanses the eye. The importance of speed cannot be overemphasized, because the longer the chemical is in contact with the eye, the more damage it does. The same procedure is followed if an eye-drop is instilled into the wrong eye, or if the wrong kind of medication is used. After the eye has been irrigated, the patient is instructed to close his eye, and an eye pad is applied over the lid and held in place with Scotch tape. The patient is taken immediately to an ophthalmologist or to a hospital emergency room for further treatment. Assure the patient that everything possible is being done to avoid any further injury to his eyes.

Usually, further irrigation with sterile saline is carried out at the doctor's office or the clinic. A flask of sterile saline is hung on an infusion pole about 6 inches above the eye, and, by means of rubber tubing and an irrigating tip, copious amounts of the solution are used to flush away the harmful chemical. The patient may be draped with a plastic apron like those used in beauty parlors to prevent wetting the clothing. The return flow is caught in a large emesis basin. The patient lies on a cot or is seated in a chair that can be placed quickly in a reclining position. The flow of solution is directed from the inner canthus to the outer canthus, so that it does not flow into the opposite eye. If both eyes must be irrigated, it is preferable to have two nurses, or a nurse and an assistant, work simultaneously. If this is not possible, the person performing the irrigation switches the flow from one eye to the other frequently, so that both eyes are irrigated as quickly and thoroughly as possible. The upper lid is everted and any solid particles, such as lime, are carefully washed out.

THE VISUALLY HANDICAPPED

Visual disorders are extremely common. So many people wear corrective glasses that the need for them usually is not considered a disability. However, some individuals cannot have their vision improved by glasses or any other type of treatment. Their defective vision may have been caused by injury or by a disease,

such as glaucoma. Regardless of its cause, poor vision affects the individual's emotional, social and vocational life. The incidence of visual handicaps rises markedly with increasing age.

Visual acuity is expressed as a fraction and is based on a standard of "normal vision." For example, to the person with 20/200 vision, letters readable to the normally sighted at 200 feet are readable at distances no greater than 20 feet. If you have 20/70 vision, you must be within 20 feet of letters large enough for one with normal vision (20/20) to read at 70 feet, in order to read them.

The term *blindness* is used for many legal purposes when central visual acuity is 20/200 or less in the better eye, even when corrective glasses are worn. Those with severe restrictions in the field of vision also are referred to as "blind." For instance, the patient may be able to see only an area the size of a book page at a distance of 20 feet. Those who have visual acuity between 20/70 and 20/200 in the better eye, with the use of glasses, are referred to often as "partially sighted."

THE PARTIALLY SIGHTED

Contrary to the beliefs of many patients and families, the use of the eyes by the partially sighted does not necessarily harm or strain them. Some refuse to read with a special magnifying glass for fear of further reducing their vision. The patient should be guided by his ophthalmologist's advice concerning how much to use his eyes. Practice in using a special lens, either as a hand lens or fitted into eyeglass frames, can help the patient to make the most effective use of his remaining vision. The chief objectives in the rehabilitation of partially sighted individuals include:

• Preservation of the remaining sight by treatment, if possible, of the underlying disorder.

• Making the fullest possible use of the remaining vision by special lenses, large type, or holding the object closer to the eyes.

The patient's visual ability and the type of aids that might help him are evaluated carefully. Vocational preparation is undertaken in the light of the patient's ability to see. For example, a severe visual handicap would make the job of a bus driver a hazard for everyone concerned, whereas certain types of factory work could be performed efficiently and safely. The partially sighted individual should be assisted and encouraged to work at a suitable occupation and to help to take care of his home and his family. Ingenuity and willingness to try new ways of doing things can help the individual to maintain his independence. A diabetic patient with failing vision should not place himself in a position of dependence on a family member; instead, he can use a magnifying glass to help him to see the markings on his insulin syringe.

THE BLIND

Misconceptions

For centuries blindness has been shrouded in mystery. Many myths have developed, such as that blind people develop extraordinary powers of hearing and touch to compensate for the loss of vision. Tests of these senses among blind and sighted people have not shown the blind to have unusual perception in the other senses. It is now believed that blind people learn to make more effective use of their other senses in their effort to interpret their environment. For example, the blind person learns to be especially aware of tones of voice. This helps him to recognize changes in other people's moods, although he cannot see facial expressions. Most of us could learn to make greater use of auditory and tactile stimuli, but our ability to see makes this effort seem to be less necessary.

"Living in darkness" is another common misconception. Many blind people can perceive light. Some blind people describe blindness as being surrounded by fog, or by grayness, which is neither light nor dark.

Orientation and Aids to Self-Care

How can we as nurses help a blind person to take his place in the community? Often, the nurse works with newly blind persons. These patients, just like others who have lost a part of themselves, usually show sadness and depression, a natural reaction to loss. At this time the patient needs a feeling of support and encouragement—someone to listen when he feels like expressing his feelings, someone to guide his first faltering steps, so that his clumsiness will be less embarrassing and less dangerous.

Gradually, the patient is helped to orient himself to his room in the hospital or at home. Where is the chair? The dresser? He is helped to form a mental image of his surroundings and gradually to move about his room without assistance.

At mealtime he is told where the food is on his plate. Likening the location of the food to the hands of a clock is helpful. In Figure 21-3 the meat is at 9 o'clock, the potato at 3 o'clock and the vegetable at 6 o'clock. Placing the patient's food on his plate in the same position day after day will help him to become adept at finding it. Other articles should be kept in the same position at each meal—for example, the napkin always on the left, near the fork, and the milk always on the right, near the knife. The patient is given as much help as is necessary to avoid repeated spilling and discouragement. At first he will need help in buttering bread, cutting meat and pouring beverages. Gradually, he masters even these tasks. Many blind people can eat with little or no assistance, once they have been oriented to the location of the food and the tableware.

Remember to tell the patient when something has been moved or is different from usual. Explain that the easy chair has been placed on the other side of the room, or that he is having spaghetti instead of meat, potato and vegetable. Leave the doors open wide or completely closed. The patient is likely to bump into a partly opened door.

Let the patient gradually assume responsibility for his own grooming. Bathing, combing hair, shaving, and brushing the teeth are all activities that he can learn to do himself. Keep his toilet articles in the same place. Never move them without telling him. If his electric razor is always in the top drawer and his towel on the rack nearest the sink, see that no one moves

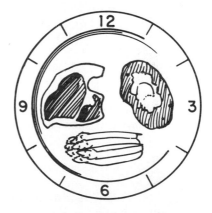

Fig. 21-3. Telling the patient that his meat is at 9 o'clock, potato at 3 o'clock, and vegetable at 6 o'clock helps him to locate them on his plate.

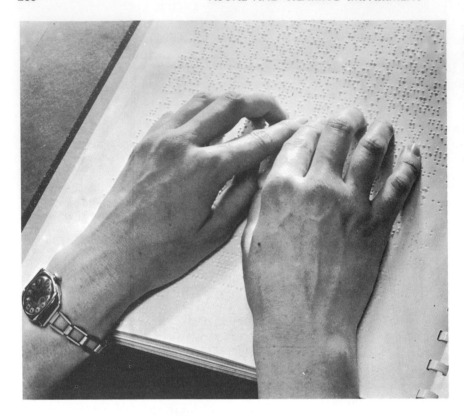

FIG. 21-4. A page of Braille. Note the raised dots and the placement of the fingers on the page. Note also the special watch with dots in place of numerals. It has no crystal, and the user can tell the time by feeling the relationship of the hands and the dots. (American Foundation for the Blind, Inc., New York, N.Y.)

them. The patient at first will require tactful assistance. If he has missed part of his whiskers, tell him so gently and help him to learn to feel his skin to make sure that his shave is complete.

Reading in an invaluable pastime for persons with all sorts of disabilities. Blind people can read, too, but methods for doing so must be adapted to their particular needs. Braille is a system of raised dots that the patient can feel with his fingertips. The dots are arranged in different ways to signify letters of the alphabet and punctuation marks. The use of Braille requires learning and a great deal of patience. Information about securing Braille books may be obtained from the Library of Congress, Washington, D.C. Agencies for the blind, such as the American Foundation for the Blind, and state agencies for the blind can provide information about teachers of Braille, many of whom go directly into the patient's home. Braille watches also are available. They have no crystal, and the blind person feels the hands and the raised characters on the face of the watch with his fingertips.

Talking books are long-playing records that allow the patient to listen to recordings of books and even some magazines. For instance, the *Review of the Week* section of the Sunday *New*

York Times is recorded each week and mailed to blind subscribers. Talking books are available for purchase or loan. Information concerning talking books is available from the Library of Congress, Washington, D.C., and from state agencies for the blind.

Special typewriters are available that type Braille, making it possible for blind people to write to one another. Blind people use a regular typewriter when they write to their sighted friends. They use the same touch system as sighted people. Also, handwriting is possible. Some blind people lay a ruler underneath the line of writing to keep it straight.

The newly blind person typically reacts with depression to the loss of his vision. Gradually, with assistance and support, he may move through this grief reaction to the point where he is ready to learn to become as independent as possible. Some patients react initially with denial of their disability; these patients are especially disadvantaged, as they must first be helped to recognize the fact of their disability.

Aiding Blind Travelers. We nurses can help and teach others to aid blind travelers by:

• Resisting the impulse to rush up and to try to help. If the blind person seems to be managing well, he will appreciate being allowed to continue to do so, rather than being whisked across the street, often opposite to where he wishes to go, by an impulsive "helper."

• Courteously asking the blind person how we can help him, if he seems lost or uncertain. If he requires directions, remember that he cannot see landmarks like "the big church on the corner." He can count the streets that he crosses and then turn left or right.

• Avoiding any fuss that would embarrass him and call attention to his disability. Unobtrusive, thoughtful help—offering him a seat in a crowded bus or preventing him from being pushed—is appreciated. When you guide a blind person, let him take your arm. Walk slightly in front of him, so that the movement of your body when you stop or step up or down will give him advance warning of what to expect. Seizing the blind person's arm and pulling him along is a common mistake. It is destructive of his dignity and is likely to throw him off balance. Encourage the blind person to walk erect and to turn his head toward the person speaking to him.

Courtesies and Attitudes

Certain courtesies smooth the way for the blind person and his sighted companions. When you address the blind person, especially when he is with a group, call him by name to save him the embarrassment of not knowing you are speaking to him. He cannot see that you are looking in his direction. Speak to him before touching him, so that he will realize you are there, and what you are going to do. For instance, the sighted hospitalized patient can observe the syringe in your hand, and he knows even before you tell him that he is about to receive an injection. The blind patient has no such way of preparing himself, and he is especially dependent on others for an explanation of what is about to happen, and what is expected of him. Tell the patient when you are entering or leaving the room, so that he is spared the uncomfortable realization that he has been talking to someone who has already left. Teach the patient to turn on the light at a certain time each evening when he is alone. This will prevent others from the startling experience of unexpectedly finding him sitting in a dark room, when they were not aware that he was there.

Some people are afraid of the blind, and avoid contact with them. Perhaps they feel a certain eeriness in the lack of normal eye contact. Some blind people have learned that a handshake helps to overcome this when they meet people for the first time. Shake the blind person's hand when he extends it, but remember that he cannot see your hand if you initiate the handshake. In the latter instance, you will have to reach for his hand.

The only thing that blind people share in common is the inability to see. They differ from one another in other ways, just as sighted people do. The patient must be helped to maintain his individuality, and he must not, because of his handicap, be expected to conform to some nebulous personality considered appropriate for "the blind." Blind people rely on us, not for pity, but for help in resuming independent lives despite the handicap. The one ingredient that often has been lacking, despite many charitable enterprises for the benefit of the blind, is true acceptance by the sighted community.

SOME EYE DISORDERS

Refractive Errors

The cornea, the aqueous humor, the lens and the vitreous body constitute the *refractive media* of the eye. Ocular refraction is the process by which rays of light are "bent" so that they will focus on the retina. Normally, all the refractive media are transparent.

Refractive errors are the commonest type of eye disorder, resulting when the refractive media do not converge light rays to a focus on the retina. Many refractive errors have a tendency to be inherited.

Myopia (nearsightedness) usually results from elongation of the eyeball. Because of the excessive length of the eyeball, light rays focus at a point in the vitreous humor before reaching the retina.

Hyperopia (farsightedness) results when the eyeball is shorter than normal, causing the light rays to focus at a theoretic point behind the retina.

Astigmatism results from unequal curvatures in the shape of the cornea or, sometimes, of the lens. Vision is distorted. For example, a straight object may appear to be slanted to the patient. Often a patient has both astigmatism and myopia or hyperopia. Astigmatism is corrected by cylindrical lenses.

Myopia, hyperopia and astigmatism can cause diminished and blurred vision. The individual

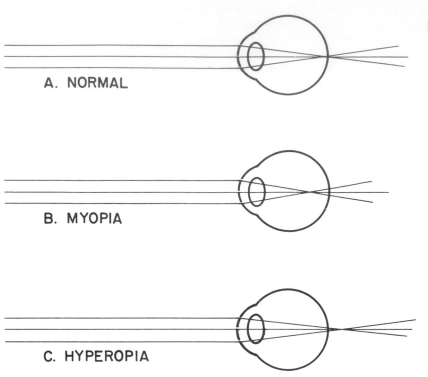

Fig. 21-5. Ocular focusing of parallel light rays.

A. NORMAL

B. MYOPIA

C. HYPEROPIA

with myopia must bring things close to his eyes to see them, whereas the person with hyperopia usually can see objects better at a distance. The conditions are corrected by lenses that bend light rays in a way that compensates for the patient's refractive error.

The shape of the lens is changed by the action of the ciliary muscle, thus providing the eye with a focusing mechanism. This process is known as *accommodation*. The lens is elastic and pliable in youth and early adult life. In middle life and old age it becomes more rigid.

Presbyopia is caused by the gradual loss of the elasticity of the lens which leads to a decreased ability to accommodate to near vision. Small objects and print must be held farther and farther away to be seen clearly, because the eye has lost the ability to adjust the shape of the lens to permit clear vision of close objects. The person trying to read may comment jokingly, "My arms aren't long enough any more." The loss of accommodation begins in youth and progresses gradually. By the time the person is in his 40's the loss is sufficiently marked to interfere with reading, sewing and other close work.

Bifocals often are prescribed. They are really two pairs of glasses in one. The lower part of the glass is for near vision; the upper part, for distance vision. The glasses permit the patient to see both near and distant objects clearly. A further refinement is the use of trifocals (3 strengths of lens in 1 glass), which some patients find even more effective for viewing objects at various distances. Some persons who have never needed glasses previously use "reading glasses" that enable them to see close objects. Bifocals with a plain upper portion are used sometimes for those who need no distance correction, so that glasses do not have to be removed and replaced constantly. Halfmoon or "half-eye" lenses attain the same purpose.

Cataract

A cataract is a condition in which the lens of the eye becomes opaque (no longer transparent). The lens is a small, transparent structure that lies behind the iris. It is enclosed in an elastic membrane called the *capsule*. The lens is one of the refractive media through which light passes. Normally, the lens is not visible; we see only the dark spot which is the opening (pupil) through which light passes. When the patient's lens becomes opaque, it becomes visible as a white or a gray spot behind the pupil.

Vision diminishes as the lens becomes opaque. The process usually advances slowly, and eventually it leads to loss of sight. If both eyes are severely affected, the patient becomes blind. Cataract is, in fact, the most common cause of blindness.

Cataracts may be congenital, they may be caused by injury to the lens, or they may be secondary to other diseases of the eye. When cataracts occur in response to injury, usually they develop quickly. Most cataracts, however, are caused by degenerative changes associated with the aging process, and they tend to develop slowly. Although some people develop cataracts in earlier life, the incidence of the condition rises steadily with advancing years. Cataracts are especially common among persons in the 7th, the 8th and the 9th decades of life. A high incidence of cataracts occurs among patients with certain diseases, such as diabetes. A family history of cataracts is often pronounced.

The treatment of cataract involves removing the lens when vision is sufficiently impaired; changing eyeglasses does not give any improvement. No way has yet been found to restore the lens to its normal transparency. Removal of the lens is necessary, because its opacity prevents light rays from reaching the retina. The lens may be removed by the intracapsular method (removal of the lens within its capsule) or by the extracapsular method (removal of the lens, leaving the posterior portion of its capsule in position). The choice of method is made by the surgeon after considering the patient's age and the degree of opacity (often called "ripeness") of the cataract. The intracapsular extraction is done usually today. The operation is often done under local anesthesia, but general anesthesia is sometimes used and has certain advantages especially in the case of a very apprehensive patient. An enzyme, alpha-chymotrypsin, is sometimes used to dissolve the lens ligaments, thus facilitating removal of the cataract. A recent development has been the use of a probe cooled to very low temperatures. The cataract is partially frozen and extracted in contact with the cold probe. This technic is know as cryosurgery. Implantation of intraocular lenses, i.e., substituting a plastic lens for the lens that has been removed, is being studied.

After his lens has been removed, the patient must wear a strong lens (eyeglass) to take its place. The correcting lens causes the patient to see objects about one third larger than a normal eye sees them. If both eyes have had the lens removed, the patient can continue to use both eyes simultaneously. However, if only one eye has had the lens removed, the patient must use only one eye at a time. Contact lenses usually solve this problem. Some patients can be fitted with a contact lens for the aphakic eye (the eye from which the lens has been removed). The use of the contact lens lessens the difference in the size of the image perceived by each eye and makes binocular vision possible.

Two major complications of cataract extraction are loss of vitreous humor and hemorrhage. Loss of vitreous humor can occur during or after surgery; it is serious, because vitreous does not regenerate, and its loss may cause serious damage to the eye. Hemorrhage can injure the delicate structures of the eye. Special care is taken during the postoperative period to prevent straining, such as straining at stool, and sudden movement or jarring of the head, which might lead to hemorrhage or opening of the incision.

Glaucoma

The *anterior chamber* of the eye lies between the cornea anteriorly and the iris posteriorly. The anterior chamber is filled with *aqueous humor,* a transparent fluid that nourishes the lens and the cornea. At the outer margin of the anterior chamber, between the iris and the cornea, lies the angle of the anterior chamber. It is at this angle that the aqueous humor drains through sievelike structures into the canal of Schlemm and, from there, into the general circulation. A balance is achieved between the amount of aqueous humor formed by the ciliary body and the amount drained out of the eye. This balance helps to maintain normal intraocular pressure.

Glaucoma is a condition that results from increased intraocular pressure due to a disturbance of the normal balance between the production and the drainage of the aqueous humor that fills the anterior chamber. Sometimes, this disturbance is caused by a narrowing of the angle leading to the drainage channels around the anterior chamber (closed-angle glaucoma). In other instances the angle appears to be open but the drainage channels are obstructed (open-angle or chronic simple glaucoma). This latter form is more common. Glaucoma may also arise as a complication of other eye disease such as injury, inflammation, tumor, or detached retina. This form is termed secondary glaucoma.

Although glaucoma can occur at any age, it is most common over 40. Anatomic abnormalities and degenerative changes play a part in causing glaucoma. Its appearance sometimes seems to be related to emotional stress. Glaucoma is much more common among people who have a family history of glaucoma.

Prompt diagnosis and treatment are of the utmost importance in preventing loss of vision. Everyone should be examined regularly for early indications of glaucoma.

Acute Glaucoma

Symptoms include severe pain in and around the eyes, blurred vision and the appearance of halos (colored circles), particularly around lights. The attack also may be accompanied by nausea and vomiting, and a steamy appearance of the cornea. Acute attacks can occur suddenly, with little or no warning.

Drug Therapy. Miotics (drugs that constrict the pupil) are given at once to pull the iris away from the drainage channels, so that drainage of aqueous can resume, thus reducing the intraocular pressure and relieving the symptoms. Acetazolamide (Diamox) or other carbonic anhydrase inhibitors are given to slow the production of aqueous fluid, thus helping to decrease the intraocular pressure. Urea and mannitol are given intravenously for the same purpose. Glycerol, given by mouth with orange or lime juice, is also effective. They are likely to be used just before and during surgery, in order to lessen intraocular pressure thus rendering the operation safe. Analgesics are given to relieve pain, and the patient is kept at complete rest.

Surgery. Early surgical intervention usually is indicated to relieve acute glaucoma and to prevent further attacks. *Iridectomy* is performed to relieve the symptoms of acute closed-angle glaucoma: a section of iris is removed, thus preventing it from bulging forward, crowding the

chamber angle and obstructing the drainage of aqueous fluid. Thus, a permanent entrance to the drainage canal is achieved. Two types of iridectomy are the *peripheral,* in which a small section of iris is removed at the periphery, and sector or *keyhole iridectomy,* in which a larger segment of iris is removed (Fig. 21-6).

Chronic Glaucoma

Symptoms. Chronic glaucoma occurs more frequently than acute glaucoma. Often, symptoms are absent, or they are not so dramatic and therefore are more readily disregarded. The patient may have occasional periods when he sees rings around lights, has blurred vision and experiences some discomfort or aching of the eyes. These mild symptoms sometimes are precipitated by prolonged watching of TV or moving pictures, or by emotional upsets. Sometimes, a reduction in the field of vision is the first indication of chronic glaucoma. The patient may fail to see things on either side and appear to be awkward or clumsy by bumping into doors or furniture. The impairment of peripheral vision is a hazard if the person drives a car, because he is unable to see pedestrians or vehicles that are off to the side. Sometimes the patient's family are the first to notice this visual defect, perhaps after narrowly escaping a highway accident.

Drug Therapy. Patients who exhibit such symptoms should seek medical attention promptly. As in acute glaucoma, miotics, such as eserine, pilocarpine, or Carbachol are used. Newer long-acting miotics include Phospholine iodine which requires instillation only once or twice in 24 hours. Epinephrine is also used as eyedrops. Carbonic anhydrase inhibitors, such as Diamox, often are prescribed. Some of these patients require iridectomy if chronic angle-

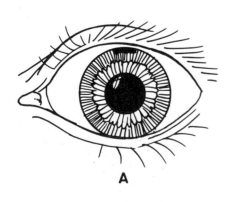 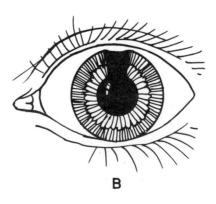

A   **B**

FIG. 21-6. (A) Appearance of the eye after peripheral iridectomy. (B) After keyhole (sector) iridectomy.

closure is present. When medical treatment is no longer effective, surgery is considered.

Surgery. Drainage operations frequently performed for chronic glaucoma include sclerectomy, trephination, iridencleisis and thermal sclerostomy.

General Measures

All patients with glaucoma (even those who have had surgery) require continued care and examinations as they are recommended by the ophthalmologist. Certain general measures also can help to control the condition. The patient should be instructed to:

• Avoid wearing a too tight collar.

• Avoid drinking too much fluid at one time.

• Maintain regular bowel habits. (Straining at stool can raise intraocular pressure.)

• Avoid emotional upsets, and especially avoid crying, which increases intraocular pressure.

• Avoid heavy lifting. (This, too, can raise intraocular pressure.)

• Limit activities that make the eyes feel strained or fatigued (for instance, prolonged reading).

• Keep an extra supply of prescribed drugs on hand for vacations, over holidays, or in case some is spilled.

• Carry a card stating that he has glaucoma, so that necessary therapy can be continued even if he is sick or hurt.

Extreme care must be taken in administering eyedrops to any patient and especially to patients with glaucoma. Usually, a miotic is ordered to constrict the pupil. If through error a mydriatic, such as atropine, is given, the resulting dilation of the pupil can further obstruct drainage of aqueous humor, precipitating an acute attack that could result in permanent blindness. *No amount of caution is too great to prevent such a tragedy.* Notice carefully which eye is to receive the medication, read the doctor's order and the label on the bottle carefully, and identify the patient before instilling the drop in his eye.

Detached Retina

The *retina,* the innermost coat of the eye, lies inside the choroid. The retina is composed of a pigmented outer layer and an inner sensory layer. The two layers are held very closely together; however, there is a potential space between them. The sensory layer of the retina receives visual stimuli that are then transmitted to the brain by the optic nerve. The pigmented layer is in close contact with the choroid, through which both layers of the retina receive their blood supply.

In detached retina the sensory layer becomes separated from the pigmented layer of the retina. The separation of the two layers of the retina deprives the sensory layer of its blood supply. Vision is lost in the affected area, because the sensory layer is no longer able to receive visual stimuli. Fluid (vitreous humor) flows between the separated layers of the retina, holding them apart and causing further separation.

Retinal separation usually is associated with a hole or a tear in the retina, which results from stretching or from degenerative changes in the retina. Often, retinal detachment follows a sudden blow, a penetrating injury, or surgery on the eye (especially cataract removal). Loss of vitreous is particularly liable to lead to retinal detachment. It may be a complication of other disorders, such as myopia or advanced diabetic changes in the retina. Retinal separation occurs more commonly among those over 40.

Symptoms. The patient often notices definite "gaps" in his vision or areas in which he cannot see. Sometimes, he has the feeling that a curtain is being drawn over his field of vision, and he commonly sees flashes of light. The sensation of spots or moving particles before the eyes is common. Complete loss of vision may occur in the affected eye. The patient has no pain, but he is usually extremely apprehensive.

Although the prognosis is guarded, patients with detached retina now have a more favorable prognosis because of the advances in surgical treatment.

Diagnosis and Treatment. Prompt diagnosis and treatment are essential. After examining the patient's retina with the ophthalmoscope and establishing the diagnosis, the doctor usually recommends prompt admission to the hospital. The physician's orders on admission usually include rest and the use of mydriatics to dilate the pupil, thus facilitating further examination.

An operation often used is called *scleral buckling.* The operation involves removal of the section of sclera overlying the detachment, diathermy, and suturing to deliberately cause inward buckling of the remaining sclera. Adhesions from the inflammation caused by diathermy help to close the retinal holes. The surgery accomplishes two objectives: draining the fluid that lies between the layers of the retina, and inducing inflammation of the choroid that overlies the hole(s) in the retina.

Another type of operation, now less commonly used, is called *retinopexy,* in which diathermy is applied to the sclera, without thinning the sclera and making it buckle inward. The subretinal fluid also is drained off, and the hole is sealed by diathermy. Cryosurgery is replacing diathermy since it is less damaging to the sclera.

When retinal holes have been detected, but the retina has not yet been detached, the holes may be sealed with a process like "spot welding." This may be achieved by diathermy, cryosurgery or using an intense light beam shone into the eye through the pupil (light coagulation).

Condition	Definition	Treatment
Uveitis	Inflammation of the uveal tract (iris, ciliary body, choroid)	Mydriatics, antibiotics, hot compresses
Conjunctivitis (pinkeye)	An inflammation of the membrane that lines the eyelids and covers the front of the eyeball, except the cornea	Depending on cause: antibiotics or avoidance of allergen, antihistamines
Keratitis	Inflammation of the cornea	Antibiotics, chemotherapeutic agents, cycloplegics
Hordeolum (sty)	An infection at the edge of the eyelid which originates in a lash follicle	Hot compresses; occasionally, surgery and antibiotics may be necessary
Chalazion	Infection and firm swelling of the gland in the eyelid that helps to maintain the normal tear-film on the eyeball	Surgical excision
Ectropion	Turning out of the eyelid	Usually surgical
Entropian	Turning in of the eyelid	Usually surgical
Ptosis	Drooping of the upper eyelid	Usually surgical

Postoperative Care. After scleral buckling the patient returns from the operating room with both eyes covered. Although doctors' specific instructions vary, many patients who have scleral buckling are permitted out of bed the next day. On the operative day they must lie very quietly in bed and keep the head as still as possible. Frequently, the patient may go home approximately one week after surgery. He is instructed to avoid jarring or bumping his head, and not to do any heavy lifting. Usually, he is advised to wear dark glasses for several weeks, thereby preventing the discomfort from bright light that occurs after treatment with mydriatics.

Sympathetic Ophthalmia

Injury of one eye sometimes results in the development of severe inflammation of the fellow eye. This rare condition is called *sympathetic ophthalmia.* Typically several weeks after serious injury to one eye, the other eye develops severe uveitis that eventually may lead to loss of sight.

The cause of sympathetic ophthalmia is unknown. It is most likely to occur after penetrating injuries of the eyeball. Therefore, it is sometimes necessary to remove a severely injured eye (enucleation) without delay, in order to avoid risk to the unaffected eye with the possibility of the loss of sight in both eyes. Recently, however, corticosteroids have proved to be so effective that enucleation often is avoided.

Often, enucleation is resisted by the patient and his family. Frequently, they feel that while the patient still has the eye, there is hope that it will heal. Removal of the eye means irreparable loss of the use of that eye, as well as the trauma accompanying the loss of a part of oneself. Such decisions in many cases are made more difficult by the fact that they follow an accident that already has caused pain and fear and has threatened loss of sight. Because the mechanism of sympathetic ophthalmia is mysterious, it is difficult for a patient to believe that such a thing could happen to the unaffected eye.

The nurse can help the patient and his family by letting them express their fears and disbeliefs and ask questions. It is essential that the nurse know just what the doctor has told the patient and his family. She then can repeat this explanation, or, if the patient seems not to understand, the nurse can talk the matter over with the doctor.

Enucleation

Removal of the eye also may be necessary when the eye has been destroyed by injury or disease. Such blind eyes sometimes develop malignant tumors. Malignant tumors of the eye fortunately are not common. However, removal of the eye is necessary when a tumor is discovered, to prevent the spread of malignant cells to other parts of the body. Sometimes, the eye is removed to relieve pain, when it has been severely damaged by injury or disease, and is blind.

The terms *enucleation* and *evisceration* have different meanings. *Evisceration* means that the contents of the eyeball have been removed, leaving the sclera in place. *Enucleation* means removal of the entire eyeball.

When enucleation is performed, a ball made of metal or plastic usually is buried in the capsule of connective tissue from which the eyeball has been removed. The eye muscles attach to this capsule and give movement to the ball that it now contains. After the tissues have healed, a glass or plastic prosthesis, shaped like a shell, is placed over the buried ball. The shell is painted to match the patient's remaining eye, and it is the part that sometimes is referred to as a "glass eye."

Depression is common after the operation. No amount of explanation or reassurance erases the fact that the patient has lost his eye, and that the loss is irretrievable. Most patients gradually are able to accept the result of enucleation, and they become interested in acquiring and learning to use the prosthesis.

After enucleation, a pressure dressing is applied for 5 days. The patient is observed carefully for any symptoms of bleeding or infection. The dressing is changed by the surgeon. Usually, the patient is allowed out of bed the day after the operation.

When healing is complete (approximately 2-4 weeks), the patient is fitted with the shell. The patient learns to insert and to remove the prosthesis himself. Usually, he removes it before going to bed at night, and he inserts it the next morning. When the patient is learning to insert and to remove the prosthesis, he should hold his head over a soft surface, such as a bed or a well-padded table, so that the shell will not be broken if it is dropped. The shell is cleansed gently after removal, and it is kept in a safe place where it will not be scratched or broken.

NURSING CONSIDERATIONS

Any eye disease, injury or operation can be upsetting and even frightening because of its possible effect on vision. The patient can be helped by careful explanation of his condition and his treatment by both the doctor and the nurse.

Some patients experience photophobia. Turning the bed so that it does not face the window and adjusting the blinds to keep out direct sunlight are important comfort measures. Often, the patient is instructed to wear dark glasses to protect his eyes from excessive light and glare.

Preoperative Care

Many patients with eye disorders come to the hospital for surgery. At the time of admission the patient may have diminished or absent vision; sometimes, as in corneal transplantation, he enters the hospital in the hope that his vision will be improved by an operation. In other instances the patient has useful vision on admission, but, because of the kind of operation to be performed, both eyes may be covered during the immediate postoperative period. Since both eyes move together, it is often necessary to cover both eyes to provide rest for the eye that has had surgery, e.g., after detached retina surgery.

Admission Procedure. The admission procedure should be modified to help both types of patient. If the patient cannot see, make a special effort to help him to become oriented to his surroundings. Introduce him to the other patients in the room. If he is able, allow him to walk about his room with assistance, noting the location of the furniture, the bathroom, and particularly the call bell, so that he knows how to call for help when he needs it. A walk about the ward, showing him the location of other rooms, nurses' station, and lounge, also helps him to form a mental picture of his new surroundings.

If, on the other hand, the patient can see and later will have both eyes covered, help him to use his sight to the greatest advantage in orienting himself to his room, his neighbors, and the ward as a whole. The next day, when his eyes are covered, he will be able to recall the layout of his new surroundings, and he will feel less lost and confused. If both eyes are to be covered, even though only one actually will have surgery, it is important to explain this to the patient, so that later he does not fear that some injury or complication has befallen his unaffected eye.

Sedation. Usually, the preoperative preparation includes sedation to ensure rest the night before surgery, and relaxation before the patient goes to the operating room. Elderly patients should be observed carefully after sedatives have been administered. Sometimes, the patient becomes disoriented and restless after the administration of sedatives, particularly the barbiturates.

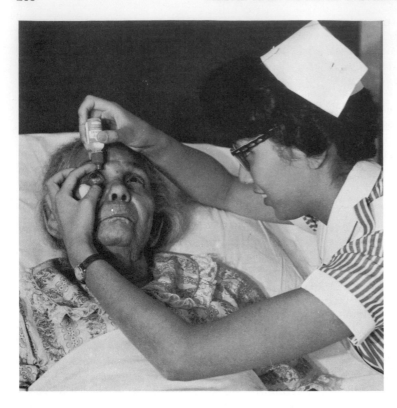

Fig. 21-7. The nurse rests her hand against the patient's forehead, thus steadying her hand and controlling the movement of the bottle. The drop is placed inside the lower lid.

Eyedrop Technic. Often, eyedrops, such as antibiotics or mydriatics, are ordered at specified intervals. When you instill an eyedrop, have the patient lying down or seated, with his head tilted backward. Rest against the patient's forehead the hand in which you are holding the dropper. (Your little finger and the side of your hand rest against the patient's forehead, while your thumb and forefinger grasp the dropper or the plastic squeeze bottle containing the medication.) This position helps to steady your hand and provides control of the dropper. The dropper never should be poked toward the patient's eye without resting the hand on the patient's forehead; if the patient moves suddenly, the dropper could be thrust into his eye. The patient is asked to look up, the lower lid is gently everted, and the drop is placed just inside the lower lid. The patient is asked to close his eye gently, allowing the medication to bathe his eye. The drop should not be allowed to fall on the cornea, which is very sensitive. Plastic squeeze bottles are often used in place of droppers. The medication is instilled into the eye directly from the bottle. The procedure for holding the bottle and inserting the drop is the same as that described in relation to the dropper.

Other Considerations. Sometimes, an enema is ordered the evening before surgery, particularly if it is desirable for the patient to avoid the exertion of moving his bowels for the first day or two after surgery.

If the patient's head must be kept very still postoperatively, it is important to plan ahead, so that as much care as possible can be given before surgery, and preparations can be made that will permit the patient to lie quietly with the least possible discomfort. For example, the male patient should shave before his operation. The woman patient should have her hair carefully combed and held back from her face. Braiding the hair helps to keep long hair neat. A contour sheet fits better than an ordinary sheet, and stays smooth longer without frequent need for pulling and tightening it.

Any respiratory condition, such as allergy or infection, that might cause sneezing or coughing is treated before the patient has surgery to minimize the possibility of sneezing and coughing after surgery. Sneezing or coughing can cause hemorrhage postoperatively.

Eye surgery on adults is often performed under local anesthesia. Preoperative sedation helps to lessen the patient's apprehension during the procedure. However, he is able to respond and to co-operate with the surgeon. For example, he can follow directions, such as "Look up." The use of local anesthesia formerly had the advantage of lessening the likelihood of postoperative nausea and vomiting. Vomiting produces strain and may cause hemorrhage or separation of the incision. With modern anesthetic technics and the use of new drugs, however, there should be no nausea or vomiting after general anesthesia. This is especially advantageous in cataract surgery.

Postoperative Care

Postoperative care is directed toward the prevention of hemorrhage or the disruption of the surgical wound. Pressure or trauma to the eye or the head, such as that resulting from jarring or suddenly turning the head, is avoided. The patient is encouraged to move his arms and his legs, but he is discouraged from raising his head or turning it suddenly.

In Bed. After surgery the patient is moved carefully and gently from the operating table to his bed. Placing him directly in his own bed means that he is moved only once, and that he does not have to be moved to a stretcher and then to his bed.

The patient is wheeled back to his room. If both eyes are covered, it is important to show him the location of his call bell and to assure him that he is back in his own room. Whether or not both eyes are covered, side rails should be kept in place. Older people, especially, are likely to become confused and to attempt to get out of bed.

Keeping both eyes covered provides rest for the operated eye. Some older people, however, become restless and disoriented when they are unable to see. It is very important to stay with the patient as much as possible. A few words spoken frequently and the touch of your hand help the patient to realize that he is not alone, and they help to keep him in contact with his environment. Many patients need frequent gentle reminders not to touch the dressing or to lift the head. Often the assurance of someone's presence can help the patient to relax enough to fall asleep. Sometimes, a family member can help by sitting quietly at the patient's bedside and assuring him that someone is there.

When a patient with both eyes covered becomes extremely excited and disoriented, attempting to climb out of bed over the side rails, the unoperated eye is uncovered as an emergency measure. Usually, the ability to see helps the patient quickly to become oriented, and it calms him enough to be able again to cooperate. Restraining the patient or giving him additional sedation often makes him more disoriented in such circumstances. It is important to check with the surgeon beforehand concerning the measures to be taken if the patient becomes disoriented.

If the patient vomits, his head should be turned gently to the side to prevent aspiration of vomitus, but the head should not be raised. Measures that help the patient to avoid vomiting, sneezing or coughing should be used. For example, do not give him anything by mouth if he feels nauseated, since this may lead to vomiting. Sometimes, taking a deep breath or sucking on an ice chip or a piece of hard candy helps the patient to avoid coughing. If he experiences nausea, report this symptom promptly to the surgeon. He may prescribe the injection of a drug, such as chlorpromazine, to relieve the nausea and to lessen the possibility of vomiting. Often a p.r.n. order for an antiemetic drug is given.

The patient who must maintain a fixed head position has to be fed. Often the diet is restricted to fluids on the day of surgery to avoid nausea, vomiting and the facial movements required by chewing. Usually, a soft diet is permitted on the day after surgery. The patient is fed until the surgeon indicates that the fixed head position is no longer necessary, and until the unaffected eye is uncovered.

Specific postoperative orders differ widely, depending on the type of operation and the preferences of the surgeon. Before you work with any patient who has had eye surgery, you should be able to answer each of the following questions. Most of the information can be obtained directly from the doctor's order sheet. Conferences with the doctor and the head nurse also will help you to know the answers.

- May the patient have a pillow?
- May the head of the patient's bed be elevated? If so, how much?
- May the patient turn? If so, to which side may he turn?
- May he brush his teeth, or should mouth care be limited to rinsing his mouth with mouthwash?
- How soon may he be shaved?

Everything must be done for the patient in a slow, gentle way. Explanation is important, particularly if both the patient's eyes are covered.

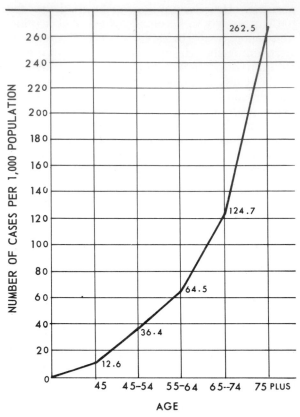

FIG. 21-8. Hearing impairments in the United States. (U.S. Department of Health, Education and Welfare, Public Health Service: *Distribution and Use of Hearing Aids, Wheelchairs and Artificial Limbs,* Washington, D.C., U.S. Government Printing Office)

Saying your name helps the patient to learn who you are by the sound of your voice. Avoid jarring the bed, because sudden movements can startle the patient and may even injure his eye.

Diversion helps the long hours to pass more quickly. It also helps to keep the patient in contact with his environment. A radio becomes a real companion to a patient who cannot see. A volunteer or a member of the family can help by reading to the patient or chatting with him.

If the patient is unable to turn for several days, certain adaptations in his care will be necessary. The sheets are kept as clean and smooth as possible without changing them. If necessary, a small disposable pad may be placed under the patient's buttocks and changed as it is necessary merely by sliding it in and out when the patient raises his hips. Assistance with the use of the bedpan and the urinal is important, so that the patient does not raise his head. Cleaning after toileting is done by nursing personnel, because the patient is not permitted to move about. The sacrum may be massaged gently by slipping the hand under the patient's back when he raises his hips slightly off the mattress. Sometimes a small, flat piece of foam rubber helps to relieve pressure on the sacrum.

Out of Bed. The length of time that the patient must remain in bed varies. Often he is allowed out of bed a day or two after surgery, and the unoperated eye is uncovered. Sometimes, he must remain quietly in bed for as long as a week or even longer. Usually, his appetite returns to normal when he is allowed up and can feed himself. He also finds it easier to move his bowels when he can assume a more normal position on a commode chair or a toilet. Sometimes, the doctor orders an enema or gentle laxative to help to re-establish regular elimination. Straining at stool must be avoided, because it may lead to hemorrhage or strain the wound in the operated eye.

The patient still needs considerable nursing assistance and supervision, even when he is permitted out of bed. He is cautioned not to stoop, to lift anything heavy, or to become excited and to laugh heartily or to cough. His movements must be slow and deliberate. Good posture helps to relieve muscle strain, and it makes the patient more comfortable.

HEARING IMPAIRMENT

Hearing loss may be divided into two types: conductive and sensorineural. *Conductive hearing loss* is caused by any disease or injury that interferes with the conduction of sound waves to the inner ear. For example, an accumulation of cerumen in the auditory canal or the failure of the ossicles to vibrate may cause conductive hearing loss. *Sensorineural hearing loss* (formerly known as *perceptive* loss and sometimes called "nerve deafness") results from the malfunction of the inner ear, the auditory nerve or the auditory center in the brain. The prognosis is better in conductive hearing loss because often its cause can be treated—for example, by removing excess cerumen from the auditory canal or by performing surgery to restore the ability of the ossicles to vibrate. Persons with conductive deafness benefit more from the use of hearing aids, since the organs that perceive sound, such as the auditory nerve and the brain, are able to function.

Sensorineural deafness is usually irreversible and, thus far, is beyond surgical correction. Unfortunately, these patients frequently have difficulty understanding speech and therefore can be helped to a very limited degree by a hearing aid.

Some patients have *mixed hearing loss,* a combination of conductive and sensorineural elements.

The Patient with Hearing Loss

Communication and Attitudes. Hearing loss can impair seriously a person's ability to protect himself and to communicate with others; thus it can keep him out of touch with his environment. Perhaps most of us do not realize how often sounds warn us of danger. For example, the failure to hear the sounds of a fire or an approaching car could lead to serious injury. Listening to what others say is a vital element in all human relationships. Everyday life is accompanied by a background of sounds that we hear without being aware of them. The sound of others moving about the house or of traffic in the distance helps us to feel part of a dynamic world and to feel more alive ourselves. The loss of this aspect of hearing has profound effect on the patient, who may describe having a feeling that "the world is dead." The loss of this auditory background is believed to contribute significantly to the depression that so commonly occurs after a patient loses his hearing. Besides serving to keep us in tune with the world, the auditory background noises serve as clues to changes that are occurring in the environment, thus helping us to become ready to meet and cope with these changes. Because he lacks these cues, the deaf person often feels vaguely insecure. While he is very keenly aware of his inability to hear con-versation, he may be unaware of the reason for his feeling of insecurity. Explanation of this relationship can help the patient to cope with this reaction.

Whereas blindness usually is obvious to others, deafness usually is not. The person with impaired hearing looks very much like everyone else, and so his quizzical expression, his frequent requests to have statements repeated, and his in-attention often are attributed to stubbornness, ill temper or eccentricity. These attitudes frequently persist even after others become aware of the individual's disability. Such comments as "He can hear when he wants to" are common.

Such attitudes are unusual in relation to people who are blind or handicapped in other ways. Just why this difference exists is not clear. The less visible nature of hearing loss may be one factor. People may become irritated when one who seems to have no disability fails to join in a conversation or talks too loudly. (The inability to hear their own voices causes some deaf people to speak too loudly or in monotonous tones.)

People with hearing impairment are very sensitive to these attitudes. Many flatly refuse to wear a hearing aid, because they feel it carries a stigma. On the other hand, glasses are well accepted by most people. Some persons with hearing loss refuse to admit that they have the disability and thereby they deprive themselves of the help that they require. For example, in addition to helping the patient hear, the hearing aid can serve useful purposes by calling attention to the disability, thus encouraging others to speak more slowly and more distinctly and indicating that problems in communication are due to hearing deficit rather than to intellectual impairment.

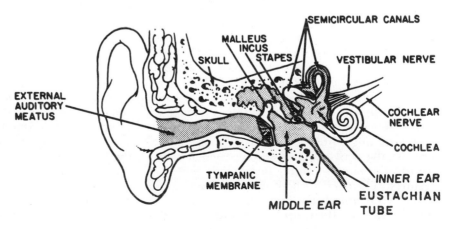

Fig. 21-9. Diagram of a section through the ear.

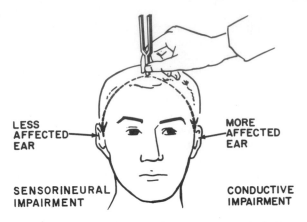

LESS
AFFECTED
EAR

MORE
AFFECTED
EAR

SENSORINEURAL
IMPAIRMENT

CONDUCTIVE
IMPAIRMENT

FIG. 21-10. When a vibrating tuning fork is placed against the forehead, to the patient with conductive hearing loss the tone sounds louder in the more affected ear; whereas to the patient with sensorineural hearing loss, the tone sounds louder in the less affected ear.

Factors Influencing Rehabilitation. The age at which hearing loss occurs, as well as the severity of the impairment, affects rehabilitation. If a person has been born deaf, his education and his opportunities for marriage, friendship and career may be jeopardized unless he has had a great deal of help in learning to compensate for the handicap. Those who become deaf later in life have the advantage of having heard normally and of being able to become educated, start a home and find a job before the onset of deafness. Older people may find it difficult to adjust to loss of hearing, especially if it occurs quite suddenly. Whereas the persons who develop hearing impairment early in life usually have become accustomed to the use of a hearing aid or have acquired skill in lip reading during childhood, the development of these capabilities entails considerable new learning and adaptation for older persons.

There are many ways of helping people with hearing loss. Many patients are taught speech reading. They learn to watch facial movements so closely and skillfully that they can understand what is said. Often the patient does not catch every word; however, he understands enough to enable him to follow the conversation. The term *speech reading* is preferred by many to *lip reading*, because the skill actually encompasses not only reading lips but also noting facial expressions and gestures. The person who uses speech reading can be helped if others face him when they speak, so that he can see their lip movements and facial

expressions. Adequate light is important. One patient appeared much deafer to the night nurse than to the day nurse, until the night nurse discovered that the patient used speech reading. Thereafter, she turned the light on before trying to talk with him.

Another way of helping people who use speech reading is to mention briefly and tactfully the topic of the conversation that he is following. For example, if a lively discussion about baseball is taking place among the patient's wardmates, turning to him and saying distinctly, "We are discussing baseball" will help him to follow the conversation. If the patient does not understand you, restate the thought in different words. Some words are more difficult to "read" than others, and changing the wording often helps the speech reader to understand what is meant. Avoid dropping your voice at the end of a sentence. Pronounce new or unfamiliar words with special care. Do not try to talk to the patient when you have something in your mouth, and avoid placing your hand over your mouth while you are speaking.

Shouting is seldom a help. Often it only confuses and embarrasses the patient. Speak somewhat more loudly, but emphasize slowness and distinctness of speech. Above all, try not to show excitement or impatience when the patient fails to understand. Treat the disability as you would any other—accept it, and do everything that you can to help the patient to compensate for it. If he speaks too loudly, tell him so tactfully, so that he can learn to modulate his voice.

Hearing Aids

Modern hearing aids are battery-operated sound amplifiers with a transistor circuit. Adjustable volume and tone controls are provided, so that the wearer can adapt the aid to changing conditions.

Although hearing aids have helped many people, they do not restore normal hearing. In general, they do not provide as good a correction for the hearing loss as glasses provide for faulty vision. And unlike glasses, hearing aids require considerable time and effort to learn to use. The failure to understand these facts has led many persons to become discouraged and to abandon the use of the aid.

Because sound is considerably modified as it passes through the aid, it will approximate—but not duplicate—the sound that the patient remembers hearing before he became deaf. The range of tones is greatly reduced. However, the sounds are sufficiently similar to be interpreted correctly by most patients. The aid has the disadvantage of amplifying background noise as well as the sounds that the patient wants to hear. Amplified background noises are distracting, particularly to patients who have not become accustomed to the aid.

Despite these disadvantages, the modern hearing aid opens new vistas to many patients with hearing loss. Constant improvements are being made in these instruments, making them not only less conspicuous but more efficient. Their very efficiency poses a problem in adjustment. Patients sometimes find that the sudden increase in their ability to hear is quite startling. They must become accustomed to the sounds of everyday experiences all over again. (However, this is an adjustment that most people are delighted to make!)

Here are some ways that nurses can help patients to obtain the best possible results from hearing aids:

• Direct the patient to an otologist or an otologic clinic for help in determining whether an aid is likely to benefit him, and if so, what type of aid would be most useful for him.

• Avoid building up unrealistic hopes about the help that a hearing aid can give. Stress the need for patience and training in the use of the aid.

• Encourage the patient to follow the directions given him by his doctor or by the manufacturer of his instrument.

• If a patient with hearing difficulty is admitted to the hospital, find out whether or not he uses an aid. If he does, ask his family to bring it to him. In the stress of illness the aid may be forgotten, and its absence can make the patient's adjustment to the hospital all the more difficult.

• Give your patient time to adjust his aid, if he needs to, before speaking with him.

• Remember that the aid is very valuable to the patient, besides being expensive. Protect it from loss or injury when the patient is unable to do so—for example, when his illness is severe, or when he is in the operating room.

CONDITIONS OF THE MIDDLE EAR

The middle ear is a small, air-filled cavity in the temporal bone. Stretched across the middle ear cavity from the tympanic membrane to the oval window lies a chain of small bones called *ossicles*—the malleus, the incus and the stapes—joined together by small ligaments and attached to the tympanic membrane by the handle of the malleus. The footplate of the stapes fits into the oval window, held in position by a ligament that allows free motion for the transmission of sound. The medial wall of the middle ear has two openings that communicate with the inner ear, the oval window (fenestra ovalis) and the round window (fenestra rotunda). Sound waves pass into the external ear and its canal and strike the tympanic membrane, causing it to vibrate. The vibrations are transmitted by way of the mechanical linkage of malleus, incus and stapes to the oval window. The motion of the footplate of the stapes in the oval window agitates the perilymph and the endolymph, thus stimulating the sensitive sound receptors of the organ of Corti, in the inner ear.

Otosclerosis

Otosclerosis is a common cause of hearing impairment among adults. It is estimated that about 5,000,000 people suffer from otosclerosis in the United States today. It results from bony ankylosis of the stapes, which interferes with the vibration of the stapes and the transmission of sound to the inner ear. Fixation of the stapes occurs gradually over a period of many years. The hearing loss usually becomes apparent to the patient during the second and the third decades of life. Otosclerosis is more common among women. Heredity is an important causative factor; the majority of patients have a family history of the disease. The underlying cause of otosclerosis is unknown.

The progressive loss of hearing is the most characteristic symptom. The patient notices this symptom when it begins to interfere with his ability to follow conversation. The patient has particular difficulty in hearing others when they speak in soft, low tones, although he can hear adequately when the sound is loud enough. *Tinnitus* (a ringing or buzzing in the ears) may appear as the loss of hearing progresses. Tinnitus, which can occur in any type of hearing loss, is noticeable especially at night, when the surroundings are quiet, and it can be very distressing to the patient.

The diagnosis is made by an otologist after noting the family history, examining the ears and testing the hearing. Although the hearing loss in otosclerosis is of the conductive type, often with progression of the disease, involvement of the cochlea supervenes and the hearing loss becomes a mixed type.

Although at present there is no cure for otosclerosis, the hearing loss can be corrected by surgery and the use of a hearing aid. The potential success of surgery, as well as the ability to wear an aid, depends greatly on the severity of the sensorineural involvement; the prognosis for each is best when the hearing loss is purely conductive. An otosclerotic patient has a choice between wearing an aid or undergoing surgery.

Fenestration Operation. The fenestration operation is seldom used today, for reasons stated below. However, because the nurse works with patients who have already undergone fenestration, the procedure is described here.

Fenestration means making a window, in this case a new window through which vibrations can pass from the external auditory canal to the inner ear. Since the fixation of the stapes renders the patient's oval window useless, a new window about the size of the head of a pin is made. The sound waves strike directly against the new *fenestra,* causing vibrations in the perilymph of the inner ear. Because the structures are so tiny, the operation is done under special magnification.

The benefit of fenestration is limited by several factors:

• The incus is removed during the surgery to allow access to the horizontal canal and this interruption of the ossicular chain makes a later stapedectomy difficult.

• The operation leaves a modified radical mastoid cavity which must be cleaned by the otologist three to four times per year. If this is not done, debris tends to accumulate in the cavity and may become infected.

• Since the ossicular chain is bypassed and since the sound vibrations are being delivered to a part of the inner ear other than the oval window, the maximum correction obtained is usually less than that possible with stapedectomy.

• The *fenestra* shows a great tendency toward partial or complete closure; the patient's improved hearing is sometimes only temporary.

Stapes Surgery. In a procedure known as stapedectomy, surgeons remove the entire stapes and replace it with a prosthetic device composed of such substances as fat or Teflon.

The surgery is carried out using very fine instruments designed specifically for minute tasks, and at its termination the patient is able to hear better. The hearing improvement is superior to that achieved by fenestration, the procedure is easier on the patient (being done under local anesthesia and in about $\frac{1}{4}$ of the time), and the postoperative diasability is far less.

At the conclusion of the stapedectomy the ear is packed and allowed to remain so for approximately 7 days. It is then unpacked and the patient is instructed to wear a piece of cotton loosely in the meatus to prevent dust and other foreign matter from getting into the canal. Occasionally the ear may ooze immediately after surgery. The nurse should notify the doctor but should not attempt to stop the bleeding by additional pressure on the canal packing as this pressure may dislocate the prosthesis. For the first 48 hours after surgery, the patient is usually instructed to remain on strict bed rest with the head of the bed elevated 30° and the operated ear up. This is to minimize the possibility of formation of a perilymphatic fistula between the inner and the middle ear.

On the third postoperative day the patient is allowed to begin walking about. He may have some vertigo for a short time postoperatively and should therefore have assistance when he begins walking. Handrails in corridors and bathrooms are important in preventing falls and in giving the patient a greater feeling of security. The total period of hospitalization is usually brief; the patient may sometimes be discharged on the fourth postoperative day. He is cautioned not to blow his nose suddenly or violently, as this action may dislodge the prosthesis or loosen the ear drum before healing has taken place, or may result in infectious matter being blown up into the eustachian tube to the middle ear. He is cautioned to keep water out of the ear as this, too, may lead to infection. He should keep a piece of clean dry cotton in the external auditory canal to help keep the canal clean. The cotton should be inserted gently and never pushed deeply into the canal. It is changed usually once or twice daily for approximately 10 days after surgery. After healing has occurred the patient may shower, swim, and engage in practically all activities. Many surgeons restrict their patients from deep-water diving and caution against flying with a head cold, because severe pressure changes may dislodge the prosthesis.

Infections

The middle ear connects with the nasopharynx by way of the eustachian tube, which serves to equalize the air pressure on either side of the tympanic membrane. Upper respiratory infections spread readily from the nose and the throat to the ear through this tube. Children are especially vulnerable because of the more nearly horizontal position of the eustachian tube during childhood. However, adults can and do develop ear infections, and in addition they suffer from the consequences of ear infections that occurred when they were children. Before the development of antimicrobial agents, ear infections often caused considerable damage before the patient's own resistance finally overcame them. Death from ear infections now is unusual, although it used to be quite common before antibiotics became available. However, antibiotics have created another problem: microorganisms are becoming resistant to them, and we are faced again with some infections for which the available antibiotics are of little benefit.

Serous Otitis Media. This condition, in which fluid forms in the middle ear, can result from obstruction of the eustachian tube. The obstruction itself may be caused by infection, allergy, tumors or sudden changes in altitude, such as sudden descents in an airplane. When due to sudden descents in an airplane, the condition is sometimes referred to as aero-otitis media. Measures that help to prevent aero-otitis media include avoidance of flying while suffering from a head cold. Chewing gum, yawning or repeated swallowing during descent open the eustachian tubes.

The symptoms of serous otitis media include a feeling of fullness, diminished hearing, and hearing one's own voice echoing in the involved ear. If allowed to remain, the fluid thickens, and scars form, with resulting permanent hearing loss.

The treatment includes aspiration of the fluid after puncturing the eardrum (*paracentesis*). The underlying cause of the condition also may be treated. For example, antibiotics may be required to treat an infection; to treat an allergy, desensitization and/or antihistamines may be necessary.

Acute Purulent Otitis Media. This acute infection of the middle ear (sometimes abbreviated O.M.P.A.) usually results from the spread of microorganisms to the middle ear through the eustachian tube during upper respiratory infections. Pus collects in the middle ear, causing increased pressure which, in turn, causes bulging of the eardrum.

The symptoms include fever, malaise, severe earache and diminished hearing. The doctor notes that the eardrum is red and bulging. Some-

times, it has perforated, and pus is present in the auditory canal. Prompt treatment usually can avoid rupture of the eardrum. Rupture often causes a jagged tear that heals slowly, sometimes incompletely, and with considerable scarring. Such scarring can interfere with the vibration of the drum, causing diminished hearing.

To prevent spontaneous rupture, the doctor may incise the drum (*myringotomy*), letting the pus escape. This eases the pressure and relieves the throbbing pain. The incision heals readily with very little scarring. At first the discharge from the ear is bloody, and then it is purulent. The doctor may order eardrops to facilitate drainage. He may ask the nurse to wipe the external portions of the canal with a dry sterile applicator. Cotton plugs should not be stuffed into the ear, because it is important for the pus to drain. The external ear must be cleaned frequently. Applying petrolatum to the skin helps to prevent excoriation. A small piece of cotton may be placed loosely at the meatus to help to absorb the drainage. It should be changed frequently. The drainage may continue for several days.

Culture and sensitivity tests are performed on specimens of the purulent material to determine which antibiotics will be effective against the organisms. Antibiotics are given to control the infection. Fluids are encouraged. Rest and the avoidance of chilling are important until all symptoms of the infection have subsided.

The complications of acute purulent otitis media include mastoiditis (the middle ear connects with the mastoid process by complex passages through which infection can travel), scarring and/or permanent perforation of the eardrum and hearing loss. The infection also may spread to the meninges, causing meningitis, or it may become chronic (chronic otitis media). Other complications include labyrinthitis, indicated by nystagmus, vertigo, nausea and vomiting; lateral sinus thrombosis (spread of the infection to the large veins at the base of the brain), causing clot formation and septicemia. Infection may injure the facial nerve and cause facial paralysis. Brain abscess may result from the extension of the infection to the brain.

Cholesteatoma can result from chronic perforation of the eardrum. The skin normally lining the external ear enters the middle ear, due to the perforation. Desquamation (shedding) of the skin occurs in this tiny space. The dead skin becomes trapped, collects, and becomes mixed with mucus. The collection gradually enlarges, grows into a ball, and becomes a medium for bacterial growth. Since it cannot escape, it causes damage by pressure on nearby structures. The cholesteatoma must be removed surgically.

Fortunately, these complications are less common than formerly, because of the prompt control of the infection with antibiotics. However, patients with perforated eardrums are prone to repeated infections throughout life. Often a chronic infection develops that is difficult to cure, and that spreads throughout the ear and the mastoid process. Patients who have perforated eardrums should avoid getting water in the ear, since this readily causes infection. Special precautions must be taken when they are bathing; swimming and diving usually are forbidden. Custom-molded ear plugs plus a bathing cap are sometimes recommended to keep water out of the ears during swimming or bathing. Some physicians advise their patients who have perforated eardrums not to swim at all, because of the risk of severe infection if water should enter the middle ear. Do not advise patients concerning this matter; refer them to the physician.

Plastic surgery (myringoplasty) usually is successful in repairing the perforated drum. In one technic the edges of the perforation are cauterized, and a patch of bloodsoaked Gelfoam is used as a scaffolding over which new tissues grow until they have completely filled in the defect.

Subsequent repeated and chronic infections, with all their risk of spreading the infection to the brain and the loss of hearing, may be avoided if the drum can be repaired.

Chronic Otitis Media. This preventable condition usually results from neglect or incomplete treatment of acute otitis media. The patient usually has a chronic discharge from the ear, a reduction of hearing and sometimes a slight fever. Treatment with antibiotics may be effective in controlling the infection. However, when it has persisted for a long time, destruction occurs in the middle ear and the mastoid process. Such patients have marked loss of hearing, and often they are in danger of spread of the infection to the brain. Surgery usually is recommended to eradicate the disease and to prevent further complications. Often, a radical mastoidectomy is necessary to remove the diseased tissue.

Mastoiditis. The spread of the infection to the mastoid process can occur in either acute or chronic otitis media. The symptoms of *acute mastoiditis* include pain and tenderness over the mastoid process, chills, fever, malaise and head-ache. The treatment includes prompt administration of antibiotics and sometimes, if there is not a favorable response to medical treatment, simple mastoidectomy. Through a postaural (behind the ear) incision, the surgeon removes the infected mastoid cells. Hearing impairment usually does not occur.

Chronic mastoiditis carries a less favorable prognosis. Chronic infection in the mastoid process leads to destruction of the tissue, causing hearing loss. The infection usually involves the middle ear also, since chronic otitis media frequently causes chronic mastoiditis. Often, radical mastoidectomy is necessary to remove the diseased tissue. Usually, the hearing is reduced markedly because of the necessity for removing important structures. The diseased mastoid cells are removed, as well as the incus, the malleus and the eardrum. The middle ear and the mastoid become one cavity. The stapes is left in position to protect the entrance to the inner ear. Just how radical the operation must be depends on the extent of the infection. The more extensive the surgery, the greater the hearing loss. Surgical procedures have been developed recently that preserve important structures. These delicate operations are performed under magnification, and they require a great deal of time, patience and surgical skill. *Tympanoplasty* is the term used to describe the plastic reconstruction of the middle ear. Tympanoplasty may be performed with or after mastoidectomy in an attempt to rebuild the middle ear structures. Results of these efforts at restoration of middle ear function have been disappointing in the more severe cases.

Principles in the Care of Any Patient After Ear Surgery

Regardless of the specific nature of the operation, certain principles are applicable to the care of any patient after aural surgery. These may be summarized as follows:

• Make sure that the external ear and the surrounding skin are meticulously clean. Excess cerumen will be removed from the canal by the doctor.

• Injury to the facial nerve may occur during ear surgery. Note whether the patient can wrinkle his forehead, close his eyes, pucker his lips and bare his teeth. Report any inability to perform these movements. If these signs appear immediately after surgery, there probably has been damage to the facial nerve. If the paralysis appears after 12 to 24 hours postoperatively, it

FIG. 21-11. Pomeroy syringe, usually used by the physician when he is removing cerumen by irrigation.

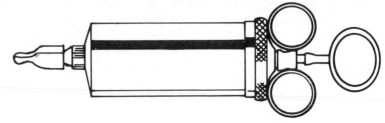

is probably due to edema; the doctor may recommend loosening the ear dressing and administering anti-inflammatory drugs. Occasionally, the nerve is damaged permanently as a result of the surgery.

• Strict adherence to aseptic technic is essential. Because the ear is so close to the brain, any infection may endanger the patient's life. Antibiotics may be ordered to help to prevent infection. Instruct the patient to keep his hands away from the dressing, which is changed only by the surgeon. Observe the dressing for drainage.

• Vertigo is common, due to the temporary effects on the body-balancing function of the semicircular canals. Special measures should be employed to protect the patient from falling. Side rails and handrails should be used, and the patient should be helped out of bed. Vertigo is very distressing. Explain that this symptom is not unusual after ear surgery, and that it will subside gradually.

• Instruct the patient not to blow his nose. During the postoperative period, nasal secretions should be wiped off the end of the nose without blowing it. Blowing the nose can permit infectious material to enter the operative area through the eustachian tube or may dislodge prostheses or grafts in the ear.

DISORDERS OF THE EXTERNAL AUDITORY CANAL

The external auditory canal extends from its own orifice in the auricle to the tympanic membrane. The canal is approximately an inch long and contains the ceruminous glands.

The external auditory canal is subject to a variety of annoying disorders. Usually, these are discomforts rather than threats to life or hearing. However, if they are not carefully and adequately treated, these disorders may involve the middle ear and become serious problems. For instance, unskilled attempts at removing cerumen or foreign bodies may perforate the eardrum and push the material into the middle ear.

The nurse never should irrigate a patient's ear without specific orders from the doctor after he has examined it. Sometimes, the nurses who work in otologic clinics are specially instructed by the physician, and they may be delegated by him to perform the irrigation after he has examined the ear. Emphasis is placed on this, because patients often ask nurses to perform ear irrigations without medical direction. The doctor examines the ear before irrigating. The nurse is not equipped to do this, and therefore she never should perform ear irrigations on her own initiative.

External Auditory Canal Disorder	Treatment
Impacted cerumen	Warm water irrigations following ear examination by physician
Furuncles (boils)	Antibiotics, local application of heat, analgesics
External otitis	Ear drops containing antibiotics, steroids or copper sulfate, glycerin and alcohol

Insects in the Auditory Canal. Insects occasionally enter the canal. Although they usually fly out again, sometimes they remain inside. Their fluttering and buzzing are agonizing. Holding a flashlight to the ear often draws the insect out by attracting it to the light. A few drops of alcohol or mineral oil may be effective in killing the insect; turning the head to the side may help the dead insect to float out of the meatus. If these measures are not successful, the patient should be taken immediately to a doctor or a hospital emergency room. Never try to remove the insect with forceps or tweezers. Sometimes the insect has fastened itself into the eardrum. Great care and skill are necessary to remove the insect without injuring the patient's ear. The procedure is carried out only by a doctor.

DISORDERS OF THE INNER EAR

The inner ear, or labyrinth, is a very complicated structure that lies deep in the temporal bone. It is surrounded, for protection, by the hardest bony substance in the body. The inner ear consists of a series of cavities and canals. The bony canals and spaces constitute the bony labyrinth. They are lined with periosteum and enclose the much smaller membranous labyrinth. The space between the two is filled with *perilymph*. The membranous labyrinth is filled with *endolymph*. The movement of this fluid stimulates the nerve endings of both branches (vestibular and cochlear) of the auditory nerve. There are two sections to the inner ear: an anterior portion, the cochlea; and a posterior portion, the semicircular canals.

Disorders of the inner ear are difficult to treat. Inner-ear deafness is of the sensorineural type, which usually cannot be helped by surgery and only occasionally by hearing aids. The auditory center in the brain, the inner ear, and the auditory nerve may be injured by drugs (for example, streptomycin can damage the auditory nerve), tumors, systemic diseases (such as measles), prolonged exposure to loud noise, and the aging process. The management involves the prevention of further injury, if this is possible, and training in speech reading.

Meniere's Disease. The cause of Meniere's disease is unknown, and the pathologic changes responsible for the symptoms are not entirely clear. Many theories have been stated.

This condition is characterized by vertigo, tinnitus and progressive hearing loss. It usually involves only one ear. An attack may last from a few minutes to weeks. The attacks occur with alarming suddenness. Often, the patient becomes afraid to leave his home lest he have an attack in public. Frequently, continued employment becomes impossible.

Symptomatic treatment includes the use of a low-sodium diet to lessen edema. Sedatives may help to relieve apprehension. Such drugs as dramamine and bonamine may lessen the symptoms. Bed rest usually is necessary during an acute attack. Vasodilating agents such as nicotinic acid are prescribed sometimes. Some patients recover spontaneously from the disorder. On the other hand, it may be so incapacitating that the labyrinth is destroyed surgically to relieve the symptoms. Ultrasonic waves have been used recently to destroy the labyrinth. Recently, another type of operation has been developed that establishes permanent drainage of excessive endolymph from the inner ear into the subarachnoid space around the brain.

The nursing care of the patient with Meniere's disease is challenging. Every effort must be made not to aggravate the symptoms or to precipitate attacks by sudden movement. The patient should not turn over quickly or be jarred in his bed. All movements must be explained carefully beforehand and then carried out slowly. Protection from falls is essential when the vertigo is severe. It is important to use side rails when the patient is in bed and to give him assistance when he is out of bed. Foods and fluids are accepted better if they are offered frequently and in small amounts, and if the patient's preferences are considered.

REVIEW OF SOME COMMON NURSING PROCEDURES

The following points will be useful in caring for patients with ear disorders.

Straightening the Canal. The canal should be straightened before attempting any procedure such as instillation of drops or irrigation, because the straightening enables you to see what you are doing and permits the medication or the solution to be directed into the canal. Pull the auricle upward, backward, and slightly outward to straighten the adult's auditory canal. Never introduce anything into the canal farther than you can see after straightening it, because the eardrum may be damaged.

Dry Wipe. If the patient has a discharge from his ear, the doctor often orders dry wipes to keep the canal clean. Take a small, sterile, dry applicator, straighten the canal with one hand, and with the other insert and gently rotate the applicator to remove the drainage. A good light is essential, so that you can see the canal, the position of the applicator when you insert it, and how many wipes are necessary to clean the canal. Usually, several applicators are required, since the canal often must be wiped several times. Discard the soiled applicators immediately, and wash your hands.

Eardrops. Have the patient lie on his side with the affected ear uppermost. Straighten the canal; adjust the light and look into the canal. If drainage is present, remove it with a dry wipe. Instill the drops, as they were ordered. Rest your hand on the patient's head, so that you have good control of the dropper if the patient should move suddenly. The amount and the strength of the solution to be used always are specified by the doctor. Warming the medication to body temperature makes the procedure more comfortable for the patient. The patient should remain on his side for 5 to 10 minutes, so that the drug will remain in the canal and produce maximum benefit. Cotton sometimes is inserted loosely into the orifice of the external canal to collect drainage.

Irrigation. When a nurse irrigates a patient's ear, she ordinarily uses a rubber bulb syringe, because it exerts only slight pressure. The solution ordered should be warmed to body temperature. Drape the patient with a plastic apron, and have him hold a large emesis basin under his ear. The irrigation usually is performed with the patient in a sitting position.

Expel air from the syringe. Straighten the canal with one hand. With the other, gently instill the solution, directing it either to the roof or floor of the canal, but not directly against the drum. Avoid obstructing the canal with the syringe; the solution should be allowed to flow back freely at all times. Failure to permit its return would cause too much pressure on the eardrum. Note the return flow. After the irrigation, have the patient lie on the affected side for a few minutes to allow all the solution to run out. Protect the pillow with a treatment rubber and a towel or with a disposable pad. Dry the ear thoroughly.

REFERENCES AND BIBLIOGRAPHY

ALDER, F. H.: *Textbook of Ophthalmology,* ed. 7, Philadelphia, Saunders, 1962.

BALLANTYNE, A. J., and MICHAELSON, I. C.: *Textbook of the Fundus of the Eye,* Baltimore, Williams & Wilkins, 1963.

BAUMAN, M. K., and YODER, N.: *Adjustment to Blindness—Re-viewed,* Springfield, Ill., Thomas, 1966.

BRANSON, II. K.: Preparing the blind for hospital jobs, *Am. J. Nurs.* 62:98, January, 1962.

BRUEGGEN, S. L.: Eye health in industry, *Am. J. Nurs.* 61:83, September, 1961.

———: Nurses' opportunities to conserve sight, *Nurs. Outlook* 10:658, 1962.

CALLAHAN, A.: *Surgery of the Eye,* Springfield, Ill., Thomas, 1956.

CHEVIGNY, H.: *My Eyes Have a Cold Nose,* New Haven, Yale University Press, 1946.

CHEVIGNY, H., and BRAVERMAN, S.: *The Adjustment of the Blind,* New Haven, Yale University Press, 1950.

CLIFTON, B.: *None So Blind,* New York, Rand McNally, 1962.

COWEN, E. L., et al.: *Adjustment to Visual Disability in Adolescence,* New York, American Foundation for the Blind, 1961.

DAVIS, H., and SILVERMAN, S. R. (eds.): *Hearing and Deafness,* New York, Holt, 1961.

DeWEESE, D. D., and SAUNDERS, W.: *Textbook of Otolaryngology,* ed. 3, St. Louis, Mosby, 1968.

DiBIASIO, A. G.: Postoperative care of patients having ear surgery, *Nurs. Forum* 4:104, 1965.

FARRELL, G.: *The Story of Blindness,* Cambridge, Harvard University Press, 1956.

FAYE, E.: Visual aids for the partially sighted, *Nurs. Outlook* 8:320, 1960.

FINESTONE, S.: *Social Casework and Blindness,* New York, American Foundation for the Blind, 1960.

FRANCIS, G. M., and MUNJAS, B.: *Promoting Psychological Comfort,* Dubuque, Wm. C. Brown, 1968.

GARRETT, J. (ed.): *Psychological Aspects of Physical Disability,* Washington, D.C., U.S. Government Printing Office, (n.d.).

GORDON, D. M.: The inflamed eye, *Am. J. Nurs.* 64:113, November, 1964.

GREISHEIMER, E. M., and WIEDEMAN, M. P.: *Physiology and Anatomy,* ed. 9, Philadelphia, Lippincott, 1970.

HADDAD, H.: Drugs for ophthalmologic use, *Am. J. Nurs.* 68:324, February, 1968.

HEVEY, L.: Vision and Aging, *Nurs. Outlook* 12:61, June, 1964.

HOGAN, M. J., and ZIMMERMAN, L. E. (eds.): *Ophthalmic Pathology,* ed. 2, Philadelphia, Saunders, 1962.

JONES, I. S., and BOSANKE, L.: The cataract extraction operation and nursing care of the patient with a cataract extraction, *Am. J. Nurs.* 60:1433, 1960.

MOORE, M.: Diagnosis: deafness, *Am. J. Nurs.* 69:297, February, 1969.

NATIONAL INSTITUTE OF NEUROLOGIC DISEASE: *Vision and Its Disorders,* Monograph No. 4, Washington, U. S. Department of Health, Education and Welfare, Public Health Service Publication No. 1688, 1967.

NILO, E. R.: Needs of the hearing impaired, *Am. J. Nurs.* 69:114, January, 1969.

OHNO, M. I.: The eye patched patient, *Am. J. Nurs.* 71:271, February, 1971.

Proposed legislation for eye safety, *Sight-Saving Review* 38:157, Fall, 1968.

SAUNDERS, W., et al.: *Nursing Care in Eye, Ear, Nose and Throat Disorders,* ed. 2, St. Louis, Mosby, 1968.

SHAMBAUGH, G. E.: *Surgery of the Ear,* Philadelphia, Saunders, 1967.

THEODORE, F. H. (ed.): *Complications After Cataract Surgery,* Boston, Little, Brown, 1964, 1965.

UJHELY, G. B.: *Determinants of the Nurse-Patient Relationship,* Part III, New York, Springer, 1968.

U.S. DEPARTMENT OF HEALTH, EDUCATION AND WELFARE, Public Health Service: *Distribution and Use of Hearing Aids, Wheelchairs and Artificial Limbs,* Washington, D.C., U.S. Government Printing Office, 1961.

WOOD, M.: *Blindness-Ability, Not Disability,* New York, Public Affairs Pamphlets, 1960.

The Patient with Disease of the Nose or the Throat

22

Disorders of the Sinuses and the Nose • Laryngitis
Cancer of the Larynx

DISORDERS OF THE SINUSES AND THE NOSE

The lateral walls of the nasal cavity are formed by three bony protuberances on either side—the superior, the middle and the inferior turbinate bones. Between the turbinates are grooves that contain the openings through which the sinuses drain. There are three pairs of openings (meatus)—superior, middle, and inferior—each beneath its respective turbinate. The entire nasal cavity is lined with a highly vascular mucous membrane, the surface of which is composed of ciliated columnar epithelial cells. Interspersed with the columnar cells are numerous goblet cells that secrete mucus which is carried back to the nasopharynx by the movement of the cilia.

The paranasal sinuses are extensions of the nasal cavity into the surrounding facial bones. The lining of these sinuses is continuous with the mucous membrane lining of the nasal cavity. These sinuses are located in the frontal, the ethmoid, the sphenoid and the maxillary bones. Their functions are to lighten the weight of the skull, and to give resonance to the voice.

The two frontal sinuses lie within the frontal bone, extending above the orbital cavities. The ethmoid bone contains a honeycomb of small spaces known as the ethmoid sinuses, or cells, located between the eyes. The sphenoid sinuses lie behind the nasal cavity. The maxillary sinuses (antra of Highmore) are located on either side of the nose in the maxillary bones. They are the largest of the sinuses, and most accessible to treatment.

The olfactory area lies at the roof of the nose; directly above is the cribriform plate which forms a portion of the roof of the nose, and the floor of the anterior cranial fossa. Trauma or surgery in this area, therefore, carries risk of injury or infection to the brain.

Sinusitis is an inflammation of the sinuses. A maxillary sinus (antrum) most often is affected. Sinusitis is caused principally by the spread of an infection from the nasal passages to the sinuses and by the blockage of normal sinus drainage. Lessened resistance to infection is an important predisposing factor. Emotional strain, fatigue and poor nutrition increase one's susceptibility to sinusitis. Sinusitis that accompanies or follows the common cold illustrates the role played by infection and obstruction. Because the mucous membrane lining of the nasal passages and the sinuses is continuous, infection spreads readily from the nose to the sinuses.

Anything that interferes with the drainage of the sinuses predisposes to sinusitis, because the trapped secretions readily become infected. Allergy frequently causes edema of the turbinates and therefore frequently leads to sinusitis. Nasal polyps and deviated septum are other common causes of faulty sinus drainage.

Sinusitis can lead to serious complications, such as spread of the infection to the middle ear or even the brain. Also, it can lead to bronchiectasis and asthma. Nurses should encourage the prompt treatment of conditions that predispose to sinusitis, such as allergy and polyps, and should emphasize the importance of early medical attention when sinusitis occurs.

TREATMENT. Acute sinusitis frequently responds to conservative treatment designed to help the patient to overcome the infection. Bed rest, ample fluid intake, and salicylates for the relief of pain often are effective. Warm compresses sometimes soothe the discomfort. The use of vasoconstrictors is of great importance, in order to shrink the edematous turbinates, thus permitting drainage from the opening under the middle turbinate. Neo-synephrine, 0.25 to 0.5 per cent, and Otrivin 0.1% nose drops commonly are prescribed. The nose drops are used only during the phase when the discharge is thick, and the turbinates are swollen. When they are used at 4-hour intervals over a period of several days, these drugs help to maintain drainage of the sinuses. Antibiotics sometimes are necessary to combat the infection.

The misuse of nose drops and other medicines can make the condition worse. When nose drops are applied too frequently or over too long a period, they provide shorter and shorter periods of relief, and are followed by "rebound" swelling of the turbinates, making the problem of obstruction worse. Many preparations may be purchased without prescription. The nurse who observes prolonged indiscriminate use of these preparations can perform a real service by advising the person to consult his doctor. Vasoconstrictors may be absorbed systemically and should be used with caution. Patients with hypertension should seek their physician's advice before using these preparations.

Many "cold tablets" contain antihistamines which thicken nasal secretions; while this action may temporarily decrease the discomfort of profuse nasal secretions it can lead to failure of the sinus to drain adequately, due to the thickened secretions. Secretions thus trapped readily form a focus for continuing infection.

If the lack of drainage has resulted in the accumulation of pus, the maxillary sinus often is irrigated to remove the purulent material and to promote drainage. Usually, a special catheter can be inserted through the normal opening under the middle turbinate. This procedure is relatively painless.

When the normal opening is so obstructed that a catheter cannot be inserted, an antrum puncture is performed in order to irrigate the sinus. An instrument called a *trocar* is used to pierce

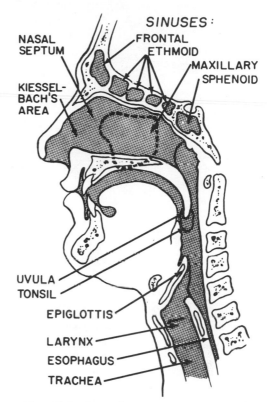

FIG. 22-1. Some important structures of the nose and the throat.

the bony wall separating the nose and the antrum, so that the irrigating fluid can be introduced into the maxillary sinus. Pain, pressure and, sometimes, faintness accompany antrum puncture and irrigation. Local application of cocaine to the nasal mucosa is used before the procedure to lessen the discomfort. It is sometimes helpful for the nurse to support the patient's head with her hands during the brief interval when the doctor is applying pressure with the trocar. Place your hands at the back of the patient's head. Supporting the head makes the pressure less distressing to him. Support of his head as a means of lessening discomfort should be briefly explained to the patient so that he does not, in the apprehension of the moment, interpret it as restraint.

Warm normal saline usually is used for the antrum irrigation. The patient holds a basin under his nose, and the irrigating fluid and pus drain into the basin. The nurse assists the doctor during the procedure. In addition to helping with the preparation and the aftercare of the

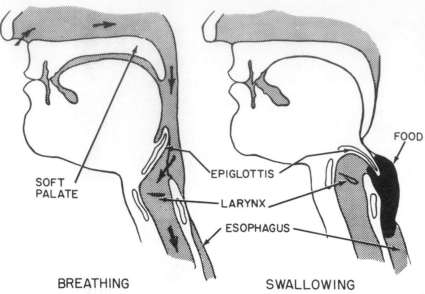

Fig. 22-2. During swallowing, the soft palate is elevated to close off air from the nose. Breathing is interrupted momentarily. The larynx rises, and its opening is shut off by the epiglottis until the food has passed down into the esophagus.

equipment, the nurse may be asked to help to explain the procedure to the patient.

After the saline is used, air is usually injected, to remove the saline. The patient should be told that he will experience a popping sensation when air is inserted. Antrum irrigation is an uncomfortable and sometimes a frightening experience for the patient. The nurse can support him by such actions as placing her hand on his shoulder, handing him tissues as he needs them, quietly reminding him to breathe through his mouth, quickly supplying him with a clean drainage basin when it is needed, and helping him to a comfortable chair or cot where he may rest for a few moments when the procedure is over. The patient treated by antrum puncture and irriga-

tion should be observed carefully for faintness and dizziness during and immediately after the procedure.

Trephine of the frontal sinus is used in treatment of refractory acute frontal sinusitis. In this procedure, a tiny tube is inserted into a drill hole made into the frontal sinus. This allows drainage of secretions from the sinus, and a route through which medications can be instilled directly into the sinus.

Surgery may be indicated in treatment of chronic sinusitis. A new opening may be made in the inferior meatus to provide sinus drainage. This relatively simple operation is called an *antrotomy*, or antrum window operation. A more radical procedure occasionally is done

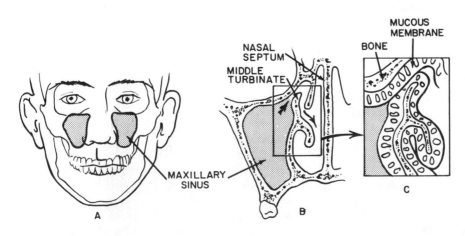

Fig. 22-3. Edema can cause obstruction of sinus drainage. (A) Location of maxillary sinuses. (B) The maxillary sinuses normally drain through the openings that lie under the middle turbinates. Note that the opening for the drainage is nearest the upper portion of the sinus. (C) Edema, such as that which commonly accompanies upper respiratory infections, can obstruct the opening and prevent normal sinus drainage.

through the mouth, above the upper teeth. This is called the Caldwell-Luc operation. The diseased mucous membrane lining of the sinus is removed, and a new opening is made into the inferior meatus of the nose, so that adequate drainage can occur. The nursing care after nasal surgery is discussed later in the chapter.

Nurses can avoid, and help others to avoid, the attitude that sinusitis is something to "put up with," and that nothing can be done about it. Modern treatment can prevent much needless misery, as well as help to avoid chronic sinusitis and serious complications such as bronchiectasis.

Polyps

Polyps are grapelike tumors that are believed to result from chronic irritation, such as that caused by infection or allergy. When polyps grow in the nose, they obstruct nasal breathing and sinus drainage. They are removed under local anesthesia. Unfortunately, polyps tend to recur, and the patient often must undergo surgery more than once for the same condition. The excised tissue is examined microscopically to determine whether it is benign or malignant.

Deviated Septum

The nasal cavity is divided into two passages by a septum consisting of bone and cartilage. Few people have an absolutely straight nasal septum, and some have a markedly crooked one. Sometimes the crookedness is congenital; often it is caused by trauma. When the septum is crooked, one nostril may be much larger than the other. Marked septal deviation can result in complete obstruction of one nostril and interference with sinus drainage. Surgical correction is necessary to restore normal breathing space and to permit adequate sinus drainage. Patients who have septal deviation due to injury should seek medical advice, so that the deformity can be corrected, and chronic sinusitis can be avoided.

The operation performed for deviated septum is called a *submucous resection*. After a local anesthetic has been administered, the surgeon makes an incision through the mucous membrane and removes the portions of the septum that are causing obstruction. When the surgery is completed, both sides of the nasal cavity are packed with gauze, which usually is left in place for 24 to 48 hours. A mustache dressing (a folded piece of gauze applied under the nostrils and held in place with adhesive tape) is applied to absorb any bloody drainage.

General Postoperative Nursing Care

Regardless of the particular operation performed on the nose, the principles of postoperative nursing care are similar.

Adequate preoperative instruction may help to allay some of the patient's fears, thus providing for a smoother postoperative course. For instance, the prospect of surgery on any part of the face may cause considerable anxiety over the possibility of a changed appearance. The doctor usually advises the patient that his appearance will return to normal after the postoperative edema subsides.

Another fear common among patients who have surgery under local anesthesia is that they will experience pain during surgery. The nurse can reassure such patients that they will receive enough local anesthesia to prevent pain but that they may feel some pressure.

The patient should also be instructed that he will have to breathe through his mouth for a day or two following surgery because he will have packing in his nose. The patient's postoperative temperature will be taken rectally for this reason.

• Be alert for hemorrhage, the major complication of nasal surgery. It is not unusual to saturate two or three moustache dressings; there is considerable bloody drainage after this type of surgery. Use a flashlight to inspect for trickling blood in the back of the patient's throat. Check blood pressure and pulse frequently and change the moustache dressings as necessary.

• Keep the patient and his environment neat. There is no need for blood-stained shirts, soggy moustache dressings or soiled tissues to be in plain sight.

• Instruct the patient to spit out drainage so that the amount and character can be noted. However, some swallowing of blood is usual after nasal surgery and the patient may even pass a tarry stool postoperatively.

• Protect the patient from falling by using side rails until the effects of sedation have worn off. Assist him the first few times that he gets out of bed.

• Elevate the head of the bed to a 45-degree angle to decrease edema and to promote more comfortable breathing.

• Encourage the patient to help himself as much as possible, for example, by applying cold compresses to his nose.

• Mouth care and oral fluids are important nursing measures. Old blood can give a foul odor and taste to the mouth, and dryness of the mouth is inevitable during mouth breathing.

• Do not force the patient to try more than liquids and soft foods until after the packing has been removed. This period lasts only a day or two, and afterward the patient quickly resumes a normal diet.

• Occasionally, nasal packing slips back into the throat causing gagging and discomfort. The surgeon should be advised of the situation. In emergency treatment for packing that has slipped back into the throat and obstructs breathing, get the patient to open his mouth, then grasp the packing with forceps and pull it out through the open mouth.

• An enema sometimes is ordered preoperatively to empty the lower bowel, so that swallowed blood will pass through the gastrointestinal tract more quickly after surgery. Cathartics may be ordered postoperatively for the same purpose.

• Sedatives and/or analgesics may be necessary during the postoperative period to control pain, apprehension and restlessness. However, nasal surgery is usually relatively painless; mentioning this to the patient preoperatively can help allay fear of pain.

Epistaxis (Nosebleed)

Most nosebleeds occur in Kiesselbach's area, a plexus of capillaries located on the anterior part of the nasal septum. Epistaxis may result from picking the nose or from local trauma, such as any kind of blow. Also it may result from diseases, such as rheumatic fever, hypertension or blood dyscrasias. Epistaxis resulting from hypertension is likely to be especially severe and difficult to control.

Nosebleed is a common occurrence and is usually not very serious, but it is often a very frightening one for both the person experiencing it and those who witness it. Every nurse should be familiar with simple first aid for epistaxis. Merely applying pressure by holding the soft parts of the nose firmly between thumb and forefinger for several minutes often is effective in controlling bleeding. Have the patient sit with his head tilted slightly forward to prevent the blood from running down his throat; instruct

him to breathe through his mouth, and then apply firm pressure. The sitting position usually is preferable, because it lessens the possibility of fainting, as well as the fatigue and the discomfort caused by standing. Also, the flow of blood to the head is lessened by keeping the head elevated while the patient is sitting. The patient can be shown how to apply pressure, and often he can control the bleeding himself if it occurs while he is alone. If the bleeding is severe, a basin must be provided to catch the blood. The patient should be instructed not to swallow blood that may run into his mouth and throat, but to spit it out. If the bleeding is slight, tissues or a handkerchief may be sufficient to prevent soiling the clothing. Applying cold compresses to the bridge of the nose sometimes is helpful.

If the bleeding is profuse, or if it does not stop within a few minutes, the doctor should be called. He may place cotton pledgets saturated with epinephrine 1:1,000 inside the nostril, as well as apply pressure. If the bleeding cannot be controlled, the nasal cavity may have to be packed with gauze to apply continuous pressure for approximately 24 hours. Sometimes, the bleeding area is cauterized. Calmness on the part of the nurse and others who are with the patient is essential.

LARYNGITIS

The larynx often is called the *voice box*. A valvular mechanism leading into the trachea, it is made of a more or less rigid framework of cartilages held together by ligaments. The interior of this boxlike structure is lined by ciliated mucous membrane that is continuous with the mucous membrane of the pharynx and the trachea. The cartilaginous framework of the larynx consists of the *thyroid*, the *arytenoid* and the *cricoid* cartilages.

On each lateral wall of the laryngeal cavity are two horizontally placed folds of mucous membrane—the ventricular folds or "false cords" and the vocal folds or true vocal cords. The latter are the lower of the two. The larynx and the air passages of which it forms a part constitute an air column that produces sounds of varying pitch. However, the larynx cannot produce words. The sounds made by the vibrating vocal cords are molded into speech by the pharynx, the palate, the tongue, the teeth and the lips.

Laryngitis is an inflammation and swelling of the mucous membrane lining of the larynx.

Laryngitis often accompanies upper respiratory infections, and it is due to the spread of the infection to the larynx. Laryngitis also can be caused by excessive or improper use of the voice or by smoking. The symptoms include hoarseness or, sometimes, the inability to speak above a whisper. A cough and a feeling of throat irritation commonly accompany laryngitis.

The diagnosis sometimes is made by the patient on the basis of the symptoms alone. If the condition persists, the individual should seek the advice of a physician. Most doctors believe that hoarseness which persists more than two weeks warrants a laryngoscopic examination, whereby the larynx can be examined visually. Indirect laryngoscopy is the visualization of the larynx by means of a laryngeal mirror held in the pharynx while a light is directed onto the mirror. In direct laryngoscopy, a laryngoscope (a hollow instrument with a light at its distal end) is passed to the larynx after the patient's throat has been anesthetized with cocaine. Nursing care before and after direct laryngoscopy is similar to that of a patient having bronchoscopy (see p. 295). The prompt investigation of the cause of persistent hoarseness is essential, because this symptom may be due to cancer of the larynx.

The treatment of laryngitis involves voice rest and the treatment or the removal of the cause. The meaning of the term "voice rest" should be explained to the patient. It means writing what he wishes to communicate rather than speaking. It must be emphasized that whispering is as bad as talking. Voice rest facilitates the healing of the inflamed mucous membranes, and, when the condition is due to an upper respiratory infection or to brief overuse of the voice, it is usually the only specific treatment required.

CANCER OF THE LARYNX

Cancer of the larynx is most common among people over 45. Men are affected much more frequently than women. Although the cause is unknown, it is believed that chronic laryngitis (caused by excessive smoking, drinking of alcohol, or habitual overuse of the voice) and heredity may predispose to the condition.

Symptoms. Persistent hoarseness usually is the earliest symptom. Often this is slight at first and is readily ignored. Also, the patient may have a sensation of a swelling or a lump in his throat, followed by dysphagia and pain when he is talking. If the malignant tissue is not removed promptly, the patient develops symptoms of advancing carcinoma, such as weakness, weight loss and anemia. The importance of consulting a doctor for any persistent hoarseness or difficulty in swallowing cannot be overemphasized. Patients who seek treatment early have a good chance of cure, because cancer of the larynx usually does not metastasize as early as cancer in some other parts of the body.

Diagnosis. The diagnosis is established by laryngoscopy, biopsy and x-ray films.

Treatment. The surgical removal of the tumor, and often of the entire larynx, is necessary. Radiotherapy also may be employed. If the tumor is discovered promptly, the surgeon sometimes can remove it without removing the entire larynx; this less radical procedure is called *laryngofissure*. Because laryngofissure does not involve a removal of the total larynx, but only a portion of it, the patient does not lose his voice. However, his voice is husky. Laryngofissure is now less commonly performed. Patients who would formerly have been treated by laryngofissure now tend to be treated by radiotherapy. In more advanced cases total laryngectomy is necessary. If the disease has spread to the cervical lymph nodes, radical neck dissection (removal of the lymph nodes and the adjacent tissues) also is performed. Patients who have total laryngectomy have a permanent tracheostomy, because after surgery the trachea does not connect with the nasopharynx. The patient no longer can speak normally. The larynx is severed from the trachea and removed completely. The only respiratory organs in use thereafter are the trachea, the bronchi and the lungs. Air enters and leaves through the tracheostomy; the patient will no longer feel air entering his nose. The anterior wall of the esophagus connects with the posterior wall of the larynx, and consequently it must be reconstructed. Tube feeding facilitates healing by avoiding muscular activity and irritation of the esophagus.

Nursing Care of a Laryngectomy Patient

Preoperative Preparation. The doctor explains the need and the expected extent of the surgery to the patient preoperatively. If total laryngectomy is necessary, the patient often is shocked and dismayed at the prospect of losing his voice. (Even the temporary loss of the ability to communicate verbally with others causes a great deal of anxiety.) A detailed explanation of the measures that will be used to help the patient to communicate with others is important before

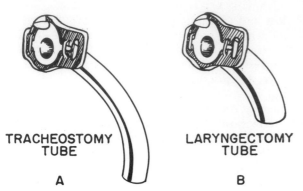

TRACHEOSTOMY TUBE

A

LARYNGECTOMY TUBE

B

Fig. 22-4. Both tubes come in different sizes.

surgery is performed. For example, the patient should know that he can write messages immediately after surgery, and that he will have a call light that will be answered promptly. As soon as he recovers from the surgery sufficiently, he can be taught *esophageal speech,* a method of speaking by regurgitating swallowed air, or the use of an electronic larynx. A visit from someone who has undergone laryngectomy and has mastered esophageal speech often does more to convince the patient that such speech is possible than all the explanations by his doctor and his nurses.

The patient should understand that he will be fed through a nasogastric tube postoperatively. It will remain in place until sufficient healing has occurred. The patient can look forward to eating normally after the tube has been removed.

The patient is told that he will have a permanent tracheostomy, and that he will be taught how to care for this opening, as well as how to camouflage it with scarves, collars and the like.

Instruction and emotional support help the patient to mobilize his defenses and to begin to learn how to cope with the effects of the operation. Many cities have Lost Chord Clubs—groups of people who have had laryngectomy and who help one another to cope with the disability. Many of the club members visit others who are hospitalized for laryngectomy, and they distribute literature that offers practical help and encouragement to others with the condition. Patients can find out about the club nearest them by contacting the American Cancer Society, 219 East 42nd Street, New York City, 10017, or by contacting their local chapter of the Society.

Care of a Patient with a Tracheostomy. The patient requires almost continuous nursing care immediately after surgery. Not only is he unable to speak, but he must breathe through a new opening in his trachea. A tube made of sterling silver or plastic material is placed in the tracheal opening. The tube used after laryngectomy is shorter than that inserted after tracheostomy for other causes. Often, it is called a *laryngectomy* tube, to distinguish it from the longer tracheostomy tubes. The principles of care are similar to those of any patient who has a tracheostomy for any reason. (Note that some surgeons do not have their patients wear a tube in the stoma after laryngectomy, in the belief that not using a tube at all produces less irritation and a better stoma. However, the use of a laryngectomy tube postoperatively is more usual than the practice of not using one.) When a tube is employed, there is now a tendency for its use to be discontinued more promptly than was formerly the case. For example, many patients now have their tubes removed after only two days.

Tracheostomy without laryngectomy may be necessitated by any condition, such as allergy or infection, that causes edema and results in obstruction of the patient's airway. In such situations the tracheostomy is performed as an emergency measure to create a new opening through which the patient can breathe. The operation may be performed at the bedside, or even outside the hospital, when the patient's condition suddenly requires it. However, in most instances it is possible and preferable to prepare carefully for this operation and to perform it in a methodical way before the patient's respiratory distress is so acute that his life is in jeopardy. Nurses can help by promptly reporting respiratory difficulty to the doctor, so that the needed care can be given immediately. Patients who have had tracheostomy without laryngectomy can speak by taking a breath, briefly covering the tube with a finger, uttering a word or two, and then removing the finger to resume breathing.

The tube (cannula) has three parts—an outer tube, an inner tube and an obturator. Before the outer tube is inserted into the tracheal opening, the obturator is placed in the tube. The lower end of the obturator protrudes from the end of the tube to be inserted. The protruding end of the obturator is smooth, facilitating insertion. Since the obturator obstructs the lumen of the tube, it is removed immediately, once the tube is in place. The parts of the tubes are not interchangeable; they fit only one particular tube. If one part is lost, the entire set is useless. Therefore, each part, including the obturator, is carefully accounted for, and accidental loss is avoided

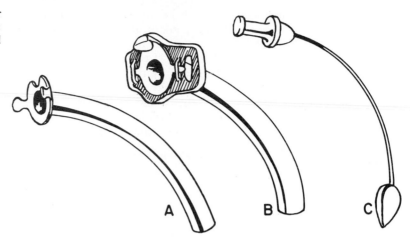

Fig. 22-5. A tracheostomy or laryngectomy tube has three parts: (A) inner tube, (B) outer tube, and (C) obturator.

carefully. The obturator usually is taped to the patient's wrist when he returns from the operating room, so that it is returned to the unit with the patient.

The inner tube slides inside the outer tube. It is removed by the nurse as often as necessary, cleaned and replaced. Always be sure that the inner tube is locked securely in position after reinserting it. Various methods are used for cleaning the inner tube. Because dried mucus sticks inside, merely rinsing the tube with water is not sufficient. The lumen must be wiped as well. Some nurses use a piece of bandage threaded through the tube to clean the inside; others prefer a small brush. Soap and cold water, plus friction applied with a bandage or a brush, remove all the secretions. The tube always should be held up and inspected to be sure that it is clean and dry before it is reinserted.

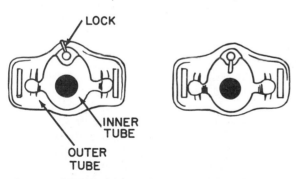

Fig. 22-6. The inner tube fits snugly into the outer tube. Turning the lock up with the finger makes it possible to remove the inner tube for cleaning. Turning the lock down keeps the inner tube securely in place. The inner tube always is locked in place after it is reinserted.

In the immediate postoperative period, the inner tube may have to be removed as often as every half hour. Before the inner tube is reinserted, the outer tube is thoroughly suctioned. The inner tube should be cleaned promptly and reinserted. Otherwise, the outer tube will collect secretions. The outer tube is left in position. The entire tube usually is changed by the doctor daily or several times a week.

An extra set always is kept at the patient's bedside, since immediate change may be necessary if the patient's tube becomes blocked with mucus that cannot be removed by suction or removal of the inner cannula. Each time that the doctor changes the patient's tube, the one that has been removed is scrubbed thoroughly with soap and water and sterilized by boiling. It is then ready for reuse. Often, the tube is placed in a jar and labeled with the patient's name. The tubes come in various sizes, and it is important that the patient always have the correct size at his bedside.

The outer tube is held snugly in place by tapes inserted in openings on either side of it and tied at the back of the patient's neck. These tapes always should be tied securely in a knot. A bow may be added if desired. If the knot is not tied

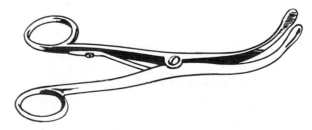

Fig. 22-7. Tracheal dilator.

securely, the patient can cough the tube out. This is a very serious occurrence if the edges of the trachea have not been sutured to the skin, as is the case in a temporary tracheotomy. If the outer tube accidentally comes out, the nurse immediately inserts a tracheal dilator to hold the edges of the opening apart until the doctor arrives to insert another tube. The tracheal dilator is kept at the bedside at all times. If the tube should come out after tracheostomy, it should never be forced back in. If force is used, the patient's trachea may be compressed (by pushing the tube alongside the trachea, thus compressing the trachea, rather than inserting the tube into the stoma). Such action could cause asphyxiation. It is essential for the nurse to try to remain calm if the patient's tube should come out, remembering to hold open the stoma with a tracheal dilator until the physician arrives, if the tube cannot be deftly and easily re-inserted by the nurse.

Many patients wear a "bib" of folded gauze or mesh over the tube as a camouflage. If the material is kept damp, it helps to humidify the inspired air. The bib never should be made of the kind of gauze that has a layer of cotton inside, since bits of cotton easily are sucked into the tube. It is important not to let any material hide the condition of the tube. Unless the nurse is alert to this possibility, a badly crusted tube much in need of being cleaned and changed may be overlooked.

A gauze dressing is placed under the tube to absorb the secretions. Gauze squares usually are used for this purpose. A slit is cut halfway through the square, so that the gauze can fit around the tube. This piece of gauze should be changed as often as necessary.

The patient's respiratory passages react to the creation of the new respiratory opening with irritation, excessive secretion of mucus, and formation of crusts of dried mucus. The inspired air passes directly into the trachea, the bronchi and the lungs without becoming warmed and moistened by passing through the nose. The copious respiratory secretions that characteristically occur immediately after the new opening has been made are a threat to the patient's life. They may clog the only remaining breathing passage—the tracheostomy—and quickly cause death by asphyxia. The patient is usually very much aware of this possibility, and often he is terrified of being left alone even for a moment. Constant vigilance and care are necessary during the immediate postoperative period to keep the tube pat-

ent and to reassure the patient. He is taught to care for the tube himself as soon as possible; the ability to care for himself is the patient's most effective defense against the fear of a blocked airway.

A suction machine is placed in readiness before the patient returns from surgery, and it is kept at his bedside at all times. Mucus is gently suctioned from the tube by a No. 14 or No. 16 (F.) sterile catheter, inserted gently into the lumen of the tube. Suction is not applied while the catheter is on the way down the trachea, because this causes unnecessary irritation of the lining of the trachea. Instead, the suction is commenced once the catheter has been passed, and suctioning is continued while the catheter is withdrawn slowly. As the catheter is withdrawn it is rotated, so that the openings in the catheter can remove mucus more effectively. This procedure may be necessary as often as every 5 or 10 minutes in the immediate postoperative period. Sometimes 1 or 2 drops of sterile saline or sterile sodium bicarbonate, 5 per cent, are introduced into the tube to loosen crusts of mucus. Cleanliness of all equipment used in caring for the tracheostomy is essential. The hands should be washed before suctioning the patient, and equipment kept at the bedside should be exchanged frequently (at least every 24 hours) for fresh supplies from the central supply room. Failure to observe these precautions results in the introduction of large numbers of harmful microorganisms each time the catheter is introduced. Poor technic may lead to postoperative pneumonia by spread of infection to the lungs. If it is necessary to suction through the nose or the mouth, another catheter (not the one used for the tracheostomy) should be used. Some hospitals provide disposable catheters, thus lessening the danger of transmitting infection via catheters.

If the airway becomes completely obstructed, the patient will become markedly cyanotic and frightened, and he will die within a few moments if the obstruction is not relieved. Therefore, first aid is of the greatest urgency, and, if the nurse is the one who happens to be with the patient, she promptly does everything in her power to remove the mucus, and simultaneously she has someone else call the doctor. The removal of the tracheostomy tube followed by suctioning may be lifesaving. This first-aid measure usually may be undertaken safely after laryngectomy when healing has sealed the tracheal opening to the surrounding skin. Consultation with the doctor

FIG. 22-8. This patient is learning to clean the inner tube by threading a piece of bandage through it. Note the gauze dressings that fit snugly around the outer tube to absorb secretions.

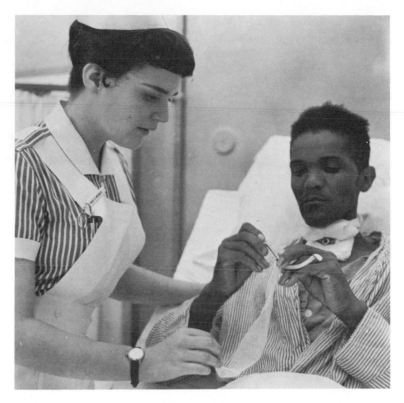

ahead of time concerning the first-aid measures acceptable for the nurse to perform for each individual patient is essential. The nurse then will know which patients may have their tubes removed as an emergency measure.

Immediate Postoperative Period. The patient is positioned on his side until he reacts from anesthesia. When he has reacted, and his blood pressure is stable, the head of the bed is elevated to a 45° angle. This position decreases edema and makes breathing easier. At first the patient is very apprehensive and restless. However, the constant presence of the nurse usually helps him to feel more secure. Frequent suctioning and cleaning of the inner tube and providing a means of communication also are reassuring. In the immediate postoperative period, writing messages is the only means of communication left to the patient. A Magic Slate is useful for this purpose, because the words can be erased promptly by raising the plastic cover, and the tablet is ready for reuse. The patient should not be left unattended during this early postoperative period, because he is unable to care for his own tube,

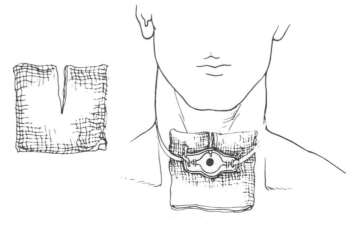

FIG. 22-9. Gauze squares, slit halfway down, are placed around the tube to catch secretions. These dressings are changed by the nurse as often as necessary. Note the tapes that hold the outer tube in place. The tapes are tied in a knot at the back of the patient's neck.

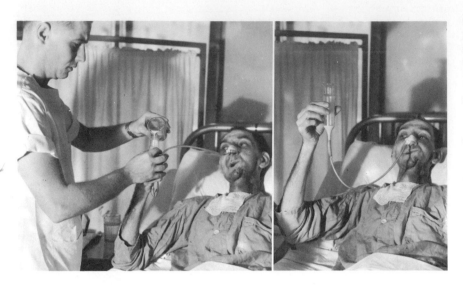

Fig. 22-10. (*Left*) The nurse is shown pouring the tube feeding into an Asepto syringe, which is being used as a funnel. The tube is kinked while the syringe is being filled. Note the damp mesh square that the patient is wearing over his tracheostomy tube. Facial deformity has resulted from the extensive surgery that was necessary to treat his condition. (*Right*) The feeding is permitted to flow through the tube by gravity. Before the syringe is empty, more of the feeding will be added. The patient is encouraged to help with the procedure.

and he could quickly experience respiratory obstruction from copious secretion of mucus. Leaving him alone may lead to panic, if not suffocation, and may frighten him so much that later rehabilitation will be difficult.

Opiates usually are ordered sparingly, because of their tendency to depress respiration. Fortunately, this type of surgery does not ordinarily cause a great deal of postoperative pain. When narcotics are given, the nurse should note carefully their effect on respiration and report any respiratory depression. The patient is observed for cyanosis and dyspnea, as well as for other postoperative complications, such as shock and hemorrhage. Often, the patient returns from surgery with a Hemovac apparatus for collection of drainage. The Hemovac device must be watched carefully and not allowed to become plugged.

Usually, the patient is allowed out of bed on the first postoperative day. By this time he can be taught to suction his own tube, aided by a mirror, so that he can see what he is doing. The patient can safely be left unattended when he is able to use his call light and to suction his own tube. He is also taught how to remove and clean the inner cannula. The patient's call light always should be answered immediately. The realization that someone will come right away if he needs help is tremendously important in helping the patient to develop enough confidence to stay alone.

After laryngectomy the patient is fed through a nasogastric tube, usually for about a week (see Fig. 22-10). However, some surgeons now discontinue the nasogastric feedings and begin oral feedings as early as the second postoperative day.

When the patient can swallow, he is allowed sips of water. When he is able to swallow fluids without difficulty, the nasogastric tube is removed. The patient is permitted soft foods and fluids. Gradually, he is permitted to resume a normal diet.

LEVIN (NASOGASTRIC) TUBE FEEDINGS. Patients unable to swallow but able to digest foods placed in the stomach may be fed liquids through a Levin tube passed through the nose to the stomach (Fig. 22-10). A patient fed this way can be kept alive for years, in good water and electrolyte regulation and well nourished. The amount and the type of tube feeding is ordered by the doctor. The food passed through the tube is a liquid form of an adequate diet. The patient does not taste the mixture (fortunately, since such mixtures are usually unpalatable). Feedings may be ordered at 1, 2 or 4 hourly intervals.

Caution must be used to avoid aspiration, especially when tube feedings are given to a comatose patient, or one who is disoriented or restless. Before feeding, the tube is checked to make sure that the end is well situated in the stomach. Some tubes are marked with black lines. When the black line is at the nose, the end of the tube is in the stomach. Even if the tube has no such line, you can tell if it has pulled out by seeing whether or not the adhesive tape that holds it in place has been disturbed. The end of the tube can be placed in a glass of water. If bubbles appear as the patient exhales, do *not* feed. The end of the tube may be in the respiratory passage.

Tube feedings are warmed to body temperature and are allowed to flow in by gravity through an Asepto syringe, a funnel, or a 50 ml. syringe. After the feeding is finished, follow it with a syringe full of clean water to rinse the tube and to prevent food particles from lodging in the tube and turning sour. Give the patient mouth care and observe for irritation of the nostril through which the tube passes.

Oral medications may be crushed thoroughly, mixed with water, and administered through the nasogastric tube. Always administer water through the tube after instilling the medication. Otherwise, the patient will not receive the entire dose, because part of the medicine will remain in the tube.

The patient is taught to administer his own tube feedings as soon as he is able. He is instructed never to let the funnel become empty during the feeding (since this would allow air to enter his stomach) and to clamp the tube carefully after administering the feeding. Many patients fold the tube over on itself, and secure it with an elastic band. A heavy metal clamp is not desirable, because its weight is uncomfortable and tends to pull the tube out.

Later Postoperative Period. The patient is allowed up and about as much as he wishes after the fourth or fifth postoperative day. He bathes himself, administers his own feedings, suctions and cleans his inner cannula. From this point on, the nurse spends less time in direct physical care and more in teaching the patient to care for himself. Besides the technics of suctioning and cleaning the inner tube, the patient must learn what foods he may eat when he returns home. (At first, soft foods and liquids are easier to swallow; gradually he resumes normal diet.) He also may learn acceptable ways of camouflaging his tube if he wishes. A scarf helps to keep dust and dirt out of the trachea, as well as to make the tracheostomy less obvious. A scarf made of smooth material, such as silk or rayon, may be worn loosely; fabrics that have fuzz must be avoided, since small fibers can be drawn into the tube.

The patient with a permanent tracheostomy must prevent water from entering the tracheal opening, since it would flow down his trachea to his lungs. He never can go swimming, and he must be careful to prevent entrance of water into the tracheostomy during his bath.

REFERENCES AND BIBLIOGRAPHY

ARNOLD, G. E.: Alleviation of a laryngeal aphonia with the modern artificial larynx, *Logos* 3:55, October, 1960.

DeWEESE, D., and SAUNDERS, W.: *Textbook of Otolaryngology,* ed. 3, St. Louis, Mosby, 1968.

FENTON, M.: What to do about thirst, *Am. J. Nurs.* 69:1014, May, 1969.

FRANCIS, G. M., and MUNJAS, B.: *Promoting Psychological Comfort,* Dubuque, Wm. C. Brown, 1968.

FRIEDMAN, R. M.: Interferons and virus infections, *Am. J. Nurs.* 68:542, March, 1968.

GARRETT, J. F. (ed.): *Psychological Aspects of Physical Disability,* Washington, D.C., U.S. Government Printing Office, (n.d.).

PITORAK, E.: Laryngectomy, *Am. J. Nurs.* 68:780, April, 1968.

SAUNDERS, W., et. al.: *Nursing Care in Eye, Ear, Nose and Throat Disorders,* ed. 2, St. Louis, Mosby, 1968.

TOTMAN, L. E., and LEHMAN, R.: Tracheostomy care, *Am. J. Nurs.* 64:96, March, 1964.

WEBB, M. W., and IRVING, R. W.: Psychologic and anamnestic patterns characteristic of laryngectomies, *J. Am. Geriat. Soc.* 12:303, 1964.

The Patient with Acute Respiratory Disorder 23

Diagnostic Tests · Pneumonia · Pleurisy · Empyema · Influenza
Common Cold · Injuries of the Chest

Respiratory disorders are the most frequent type of acute illness. Who has not experienced the "common cold"? Much of the time in the basically healthy person, milder respiratory infections result in unpleasant symptoms and the inconvenience of loss of time from work, school, or social activities. However, a similar infection which develops as a complication of another disease, or in the elderly person, or in a person with chronic respiratory impairment may make the difference between life and death. If such a patient recovers, convalescence is prolonged and costly.

One of the most vital needs of man is a continuous supply of oxygen. Severe disease in the network of the respiratory passages can interfere with the oxygen supply. Because many respiratory conditions can be prevented to a certain extent, the nurse needs to know what causes them to develop, how they are spread, how their severity can be reduced and how to care for the patient who becomes acutely ill.

DIAGNOSTIC TESTS

Roentgenography. The roentgenogram of the chest is secondary only to the physician's stethoscope in the diagnosis of acute respiratory disorders. Often, when the physical examination of the patient fails to reveal a respiratory disorder, small lesions may be noted on the chest x-ray.

The x-ray examination under normal circumstances is performed in the radiology department. When the patient is too ill to be transported to the radiology department, a chest film may be obtained at the bedside with the use of portable x-ray equipment. Modern portable x-ray equipment has reduced unnecessary patient radiation

exposure to a minimum. The nurse helps to position the patient according to the directions of the x-ray technician.

In the acutely ill patient there is no need to shut off oxygen if fire safety standards are adequate.

Fluoroscopy. This examination enables the physician to view the thoracic cavity and all its contents in motion. Usually, the patient sits or stands in front of the machine, and he may need help in moving to the machine from the wheelchair. Currently, many hospitals are equipped with special image intensifiers on their x-ray equipment which are capable of displaying a continuous motion study of the chest on a television screen.

Bronchoscopy. The physician may elect to use a bronchoscope for direct visual examination of the trachea, the two major bronchi, and multiple smaller bronchi in both the diagnosis and therapy of acute respiratory disorders. The bronchoscope is a hollow instrument which can be passed readily into the trachea under local anesthesia. Through the lumen of the bronchoscope the physician may pass suction tubes in order to obtain secretions for culture and papanicolaou cell studies. If required, special biopsy forceps can be introduced and specimens obtained for direct pathologic evaluation. In life-threatening circumstances such as when a foreign body has been aspirated or when a very sick patient with an obstructing mucous plug is too ill to be moved, bronchoscopy can be performed anywhere in the hospital. However, the location of choice is the operating room.

Before bronchoscopy the patient should have mouth care and any dentures removed. He is usually given nothing to eat or drink for 8 to 12 hours before bronchoscopy to avoid the danger of vomiting and aspiration. Lights in the bronchoscopy room are dimmed, and a towel often is placed over the patient's eyes. If the procedure has been explained to him, he may be better able to help by keeping his neck muscles relaxed and breathing through his nose.

After the procedure the patient may have increased secretions due to irritation. Because the gag reflex has been temporarily abolished, he is given nothing by mouth for several hours. The return of the gag reflex may be tested by touching the posterior pharynx with a cotton swab. Supplied with a sputum cup and tissues, the patient should be encouraged to expectorate and to clear the secretions as often as necessary. Following bronchoscopy, his throat may feel irritated for several days and he is advised to smoke and talk as little as possible. Some bloody mucus usually is expectorated after the test.

COMPLICATIONS of bronchoscopy include laryngeal edema—which may be so severe that the patient requires a tracheostomy—and bleeding, if a biopsy has been taken. Red streaks of blood may be expected after biopsy, but frank bleeding requires the immediate attention of the physician.

Bronchography. After the pharynx and larynx have been anesthetized by spray, the doctor introduces a catheter into the trachea by either the nasal or oral route and it is positioned above the bifurcation. A radio-opaque oil is then injected into the trachea via the tube and the patient is tilted in various positions so that the dye flows throughout the bronchial tree. X-ray films (bronchograms) are then taken that reveal the now radio-opaque outlines of the bronchi and bronchioles. The airways of both the right and the left lung can be studied at one session. However, the doctor usually prefers to perform a complete evaluation in two sessions because, with different views of the chest, opacified airways may overlie each other and confuse the diagnosis. If tracheobronchial secretions are profuse, postural drainage may be necessary before the examination to clear mucus and to enable better visualization of smaller bronchi. The patient should be informed of the discomfort that he may experience during the procedure and should be advised not to cough during instillation of the contrast material since this may drive the dye into the alveoli. Sedation may be ordered. Following bronchography, postural drainage may again be required to remove excess oil. The newer contrast media, however, are absorbed by the body and the lungs are usually clear

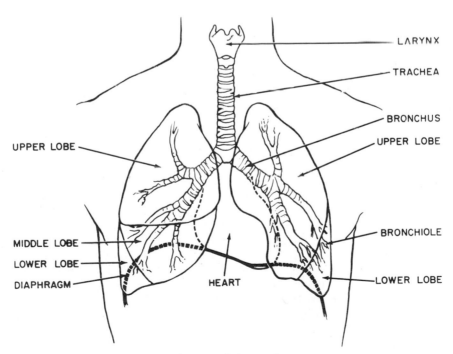

FIG. 23-1. Diagram of the respiratory tract.

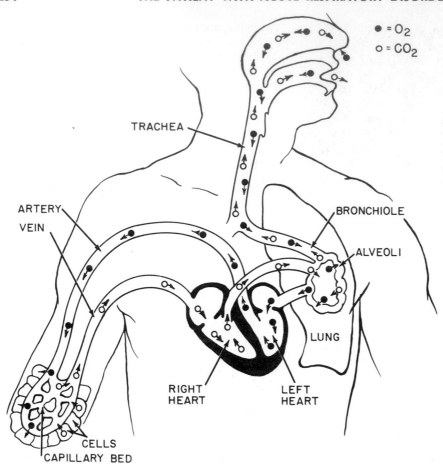

● = O_2

○ = CO_2

TRACHEA

ARTERY

VEIN

BRONCHIOLE

ALVEOLI

LUNG

RIGHT HEART

LEFT HEART

CELLS

CAPILLARY BED

FIG. 23-2. Inspired oxygen, drawn in through the nose, can be traced into the alveoli, the left heart and the capillary bed; and carbon dioxide can be traced from the capillary bed to the right heart, the lung and out of the body.

within a 12 to 24-hour period. Frequently, bronchography follows bronchoscopy, and the care of the patient is similar.

Respiratory Function Tests. These studies may be divided into two components. The first is the analysis of the physical phenomena involved with the movement of the air in and out of the chest. The second is a measure of the effectiveness of the mechanical processes. The first group includes the vital capacity, maximum breathing capacity, timed vital capacity, and the forced midexpiratory flow rate. These measurements are obtained during various respiratory maneuvers. The *vital capacity* is a measure of the amount of the air a patient can expire following a maximal inspiration. The normal range is 3500 to over 5000 ml., but is dependent significantly upon age and sex. The pattern of the vital capacity as recorded by the respirometer can then be related to time, permitting measurement of the *timed vital capacity* and the various flow rates. Edema, pain, fibrosis, and space-filling

lesions, such as cancer, can lower vital capacity. The *maximum breathing capacity* is the most air that a patient can voluntarily move in and out of the lungs within a period of one minute. This study is a measure of the airway resistance within the lungs and is reduced in patients with asthma and chronic obstructive pulmonary disease. The M.B.C., however, is a very strenuous test and many patients with acute respiratory disease perform poorly due to fatigue.

The primary tests for the assessment of the effectiveness of *ventilation* (the movement of air in and out of the lungs) are measures of the partial pressures of oxygen and carbon dioxide in the arterial blood. The analysis of arterial blood in the normal subject results in the following range of values: pH, 7.39–7.45; Pa_{CO_2}, 35–45 mm. Hg.; Pa_{O_2}, 96–100 mm. Hg breathing room air; and arterial oxyhemoglobin saturation, 96–100 per cent.

Sputum Examination. Samples of bronchial secretions frequently are collected and sent to

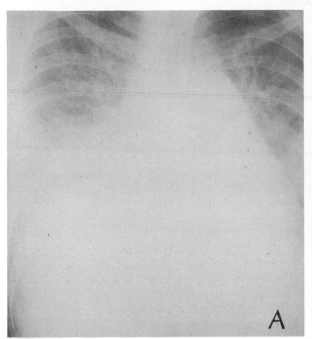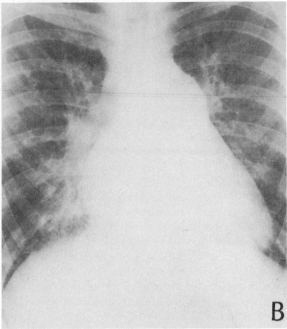

FIG. 23-3. (A) Right lobar pneumonia. Note the consolidation of the right lower lobe. The left lung field is essentially normal. (B) Complete resolution of the pneumonia after two weeks of antibiotic therapy. (Department of Radiology, Methodist Hospital of Brooklyn)

the laboratory. The microscopic examination of appropriately stained smears may reveal casts, cancer cells or pathogenic organisms. If an attempt is to be made to grow the organisms in a culture, the collecting receptacle must be sterile, and both the nurse and the patient should be careful not to contaminate the inside. Because negative smears do not indicate necessarily the absence of disease, repeated examinations may be ordered on successive days. Sometimes 24-hour specimens are collected. Sputum specimens should be raised from deep in the bronchi, such as the sputum first expectorated in the morning. The patient's mouth should be cleaned first, so that no saliva or old food particles are expectorated into the collecting receptacle. Color, consistency, odor and quantity of sputum should be noted and charted. The appearance of blood should be reported to the physician. A waterproof, waxed sputum cup or a wide-mouthed bottle should be used. Instruct the patient to keep the outside of the container free of contamination by the secretions. The cup or bottle should be covered to keep air-borne organisms and odor inside and to prevent the contents from being easily viewed. Refrigerate the specimen, if there is a delay in sending it to the laboratory.

Analysis of Gastric Contents. Because pathogenic organisms causing lung disease frequently are swallowed, the fasting contents of the stomach may be examined. This diagnostic procedure is used sometimes when tuberculosis is suspected in a debilitated or aged patient who is not expectorating sputum.

PNEUMONIA

An acute illness caused by inflammation or infection of the lungs, pneumonia is characterized by a productive cough, chest pain and fever.

Pathology

Coarse hairs at the entrance of the nose filter larger particles from the inspired air. The mucous membrane that lines the respiratory passages has an outer layer of ciliated epithelium, and its tiny, hairlike projections trap debris and microorganisms that enter with air. A sticky mucous secretion gathers these foreign bodies together. Then the motion of the cilia carries the foreign particles into the pharynx, where they either are swallowed or are eliminated through the nose or the mouth. Irritation of the respiratory passages due to noxious gases or large foreign particles stimulates additional secretions, sneezing and coughing—all of which help to expel foreign particles and accumulated mucus. The defenses of the respiratory tract against infection are so efficient that not until the body is weakened, or the noxious stimuli are overwhelming, do the lungs become infected.

When bacteria enter the alveoli they act as irritants and cause the exudation of edema fluid filling the alveolar sacs. The fluid is an excellent culture medium and, as organisms grow in the fluid-filled alveolar sac, the body responds, as it does to all infections, by pouring more fluid into the area. The previously filled alveolus spills some fluid into the adjoining sac, and pneumonia spreads. The infected fluid moves into the bronchioles, and as the patient breathes and coughs, more alveoli become filled.

The final stage of the process, consolidation, is a filling of the alveoli with thick exudate, so that an exchange of gases is impossible in these areas of the lung. When the pleura becomes infected, the patient has a severe, stabbing chest pain as the inflamed tissues rub over each other with each inspiration.

As the disease spreads, the mucous membranes of the nose, the pharynx, the trachea and the bronchi become inflamed, as are the alveoli of the lungs. Secretions containing mucus, serum, fibrin and cast-off cells exude from the membranes. As inflammation proceeds, blood oozes from the membrane and colors the sputum to the characteristic rusty color. Irritation of the mucous membrane with the collection of secretion causes coughing. At first, the cough may be dry and unproductive, but later the secretions are mucopurulent, and then they are rusty. Coughing and expectoration help to prevent clogging of the bronchi with mucous plugs.

When the inflammation is confined to one or more lobes of the lung, it is called *lobar pneumonia*. Patchy and diffuse infection scattered throughout both lungs is called *bronchopneumonia*. Pneumonia caused by the pneumococci usually leads to lobar rather than bronchopneumonia.

Etiology

Pneumonia can be caused by many different types of organisms, such as viruses, rickettsiae, streptococci, staphylococci, fungi and Friedländer's bacilli. However, the most common causative organism is the pneumococcus (*Diplococcus pneumoniae*). This bacterium is common in the air. It often can be cultured from the throats of healthy persons. It causes illness when the resistance of the individual is lowered, or when the person is exposed to an extraordinarily large concentration of the organisms or to particularly virulent organisms. *Staphylococcus aureus* is responsible for 1 to 5 per cent of bacterial pneumonias.

Pneumonia can be caused by a group of organisms called *Mycoplasma pneumoniae*. For many years bacteria could not be cultured from secretions of patients with this type of illness. The disease was then called primary atypical pneumonia or "virus" pneumonia. It is now known to be caused by the mycoplasma, one of the smallest organisms that can be grown in cell-free media. The disease is also known as Eaton's agent pneumonia.

Hypoventilation of lung tissue over a prolonged period of time—as happens when a patient lies quietly in bed, breathing with only a part of his lungs over a prolonged period—can result in the accumulation of bronchial secretions and cause hypostatic pneumonia. Pure oxygen, if inhaled for a period of several days, can result in atelectasis or collapse of the lung. The collapsed segment then becomes susceptible to bacterial invasion and can be the site of a pneumonic infiltrate. Smoke particles and other air pollutants such as nitrogen dioxide can cause irritation of the linings of the air passages and create the setting for bacterial invasion. If the epiglottis does not close completely on swallowing, and fluid or other food particles are aspirated into the bronchial tree, an acute chemical pneumonitis can result followed by bacterial infection and classical pneumonia. People who are unconscious because of anesthesia, coma, sedation, or alcoholic intoxication are prone to pneumonia because the epiglottal reflex is slowed and because hypoventilation with retention of fluid occurs.

Nursing Implications. When suctioning is indicated, it should be done promptly, before the mucus is aspirated. Levin-tube feedings to a comatose patient are dangerous if the tip of the tube should slip up above the epiglottis, or if the patient regurgitates. Oral fluids never should be poured into the mouth of an unconscious person. The thin, slippery secretions of a head cold (unlike bacteria breathed in with dusty air) are less likely to be rejected from the body by the cilia, and, therefore, they may reach the alveoli, establishing an initial infection. Likewise, oily substances are not easily passed upward by ciliary action and may fill alveoli with fluid in which bacteria can grow. This is the reason that saline nose drops are preferable to those in an oil base.

Symptoms

The onset of bacterial pneumonia is sudden. Without warning symptoms, the patient is struck with severe, sharp pain in his chest, rapid prostration that sends him to bed, and often a shaking chill that gives way to a fever going as high as 106°F.

Irritation of the tissues of the respiratory tract produces a cough that is painful, since it causes movement of the chest wall and a consequent rubbing together of the two pleural layers. The sputum often is rusty in color. Breathing also causes pain, and the patient tries to breathe as shallowly as possible.

In bacterial pneumonia the alveoli become filled with exudate. Bronchitis, tracheitis and spots of necrosis in the lung may follow. In pneumonia caused by mycoplasma there is thickening of the alveolar septa and partial filling of the alveoli with exudate. A hyaline membrane may line the alveoli. As the inflammatory process continues, there is more interference with the exchange of gases between the bloodstream and the lungs. With an increase in the carbon dioxide content of the blood, the respiratory center in the brain is stimulated, and breathing becomes more rapid and shallow. The nostrils flare with each inspiration. Often there is dyspnea, and the patient is more comfortable and better able to breathe while he is sitting up. Although the cheeks are flushed, cyanosis may appear, especially around the mouth and in the nail beds. The normal arterial oxygen saturation is 96 per cent. If it falls to 85 per cent, the patient experiences symptoms due to hypoxia, such as dyspnea, cyanosis and delirium (Morrow et al.). In an attempt to get blood to the lungs more quickly and in response to the fever, the heart rate increases.

If the disease process is not halted, the patient becomes sicker and perhaps delirious. If the circulatory system is unable to maintain the burden of decreased gaseous exchange, the patient may die from heart failure or asphyxia.

The fever of mycoplasmal or viral pneumonia resolves by lysis; that is, it slowly returns to normal. Viral pneumonia also differs from bacterial pneumonia in that the blood cultures are sterile, the sputum may be more copious, the chills are less frequent, and the pulse and the respirations are characteristically slow.

The course of viral pneumonia usually is less severe than that of bacterial pneumonia, although the patient is far from comfortable. In viral pneumonia the mortality rate is low, but it rises when bacterial pneumonia occurs as a secondary infection. Often, the patient with viral pneumonia is weak and ill for a longer time than the patient with successfully treated bacterial pneumonia.

Diagnosis

The diagnosis of pneumonia is made usually through the clinical signs and symptoms. Sputum and blood cultures are done immediately to identify the causative organism. Since the organism may not be present in early cultures, several cultures usually are ordered. Sputum for culture should be collected before antibiotics are given, since the choice of the antibiotic will depend on the positive identification of the organism. If antibiotic therapy is started before the specimen is taken, it may mask the organism. If a physician has ordered that an antibiotic be given after the collection of a sputum specimen, and difficulty is encountered in obtaining the specimen, the physician should be consulted concerning whether or not the antibiotic should be started. Cultures of the sputum require at least 24 to 48 hours to grow.

A chest roentgenogram will be ordered. The pattern and extent of pulmonary infiltration may be extremely valuable to the physician in the diagnosis and treatment of the pneumonia. A consolidated lobe of the lung may be characteristic of a pneumococcal pneumonia while the presence of multiple pulmonary abscesses is the hallmark of staphylococcal pneumonia.

The laboratory is also helpful in establishing the etiology of the pneumonia. Gram stain of a sputum smear will separate gram-positive from gram-negative organisms and frequently the specific organism can be tentatively identified on the microscope slide pending culture. The white blood cell count is useful because it is most often normal or below normal in mycoplasmal infection while the elevation may be dramatic (30,000/cu.mm.) in staphylococcal pneumonia.

Treatment

The specific antibiotics chosen for treatment depend on the sensitivity of the causative organism to their action. Sometimes, tragically, an organism will be encountered that does not respond to any available antibiotics. If the infecting organism has not been identified, broad-spectrum antibiotics, i.e., antibiotics that are effective against a large number of organisms, may be ordered.

Drug Therapy. *Penicillin* often is used in pneumococcal and streptococcal pneumonia. Penicillin is usually given intramuscularly but may also be given intravenously if the rapid attainment of high blood levels is mandatory in the treatment of the extremely ill patient. The antibiotic is usually continued for approximately one week or until the patient is afebrile for from two to three days.

Penicillin is harmless for the majority of people. However, some persons, usually those who have had penicillin previously, develop an allergic reaction that manifests itself in a mild or severe urticaria, ulcerated mucous membranes and fever. Some patients are killed by anaphylactic shock caused by allergy to penicillin. Patients should be observed closely for signs of an allergic reaction, and these signs should be reported promptly to the physician.

Pneumonia due to *Staphylococcus aureus* may be treated with methicillin (Staphcillin), oxacillin (Prostaphlin) or cephalothin (Keflin). Only oxacillin can be given orally. Methicillin is rapidly destroyed by acid solutions and by gastric secretions while cephalothin is poorly absorbed by the oral route. Toxic reactions are common, including thrombophlebitis at the site of the infusion, depression of renal function, fever and rash.

Ampicillin, a synthetic penicillin, is active against most organisms that cause pneumonia. In addition to its penicillin-like activity, it is effective against gram-negative organisms such as *E. coli* and *H. influenzae*. The usual dose for adults is 250 mg. 4 times a day. The doctor may increase the dose significantly (2 to 4 Gm. daily in divided doses) in the presence of severe infection. A contraindication to its use is a previous hypersensitivity reaction to any of the penicillins.

Streptomycin is an intramuscularly administered drug that is effective against both gram-positive and gram-negative organisms. It is particularly effective against the tubercle bacillus. Report side effects which include skin rash, fever, nausea and vomiting, loss of appetite, and pain at the site of injection. Anaphylaxis can occur. A most dangerous toxic effect is VIII cranial nerve damage resulting in dizziness, ringing in the ears, loss of equilibrium or hearing loss. The usual dose is 0.5 to 1 Gm. twice a day which is ordered reduced after one or two weeks. In tuberculosis, the medication is often ordered in low dosage for several months.

Tetracycline is effective against mixed bacterial infections of the respiratory tract, penicillin-resistant and some staphylococcal infections, and the Eaton's agent. Tetracycline is absorbed readily from the gastrointestinal tract and is excreted in feces and urine. It is usually given orally, although it may be given intramuscularly or intravenously. The dosage usually is 250 to 500 mg. 4 times a day. It is relatively nontoxic, although some patients experience nausea, vomiting, diarrhea, or pruritus of the anus or scrotum, and some may be allergic to the drug. It is not given to pregnant women in the third trimester when fetal tooth development is under way because it may cause discoloration of the teeth (yellow-grey-brownish).

Chloramphenicol (Chloromycetin) is a potent antibiotic that is effective against a wide variety of organisms. The response of patients with rickettsial infections is often dramatic. It is, however, a very toxic drug used only in serious infections for which less dangerous drugs are ineffective or contraindicated. The principal use for the drug is in the treatment of Salmonella typhi infection (typhoid fever). The adult dose is 50 mg./Kg./day in divided doses. The main toxic reaction is the development of bone marrow depression. Serious and fatal blood dyscrasias such as aplastic anemia are known to occur. It is desirable for patients to be hospitalized while on this medication in order to facilitate blood examination for signs of toxicity, although bone marrow depression may occur weeks or months after the drug treatment is completed.

Erythromycin is effective against most gram-positive organisms. It is absorbed readily from the gastrointestinal tract. The oral dose is 250 to 500 mg. every 4 to 6 hours. It has few toxic effects. This drug often is used when the patient is sensitive to penicillin.

Cephalothin (Keflin) closely resembles penicillin in its chemical structure and mechanism of action. It is useful against many gram-positive and gram-negative organisms. The value of this medication is in the treatment of infection when the organism is resistant to other agents. The drug must be given by intramuscular or intravenous route. The usual dose is 4 to 6 Gm. daily in divided doses but up to 12 Gm. daily may be ordered for severe infections. It is administered with great caution to penicillin-sensitive individuals because of partial cross-allergenicity. This drug causes a false-positive reaction for glucose in the urine with Benedict's solution or with Clinitest tablets, but not with urine sugar analysis paper (Tes-tape).

Gentamycin (Garamycin) is effective against a variety of organisms many of which are resistant to other antibiotics. This drug is administered intramuscularly in a dose of 3 to 5 mg./Kg. daily in divided doses (about 75–125 mg. 3 times a day). The patient requires close observation as it is potentially nephrotoxic and ototoxic. Observe the urinary output. Report dizziness, loss of equilibrium, ringing in the ears or hearing loss which may indicate involvement of the vestibular or auditory branches of the VIII cranial nerve.

Supportive Therapy. Other treatment of the patient is primarily supportive, including bed rest to enable the body to use all its powers for fighting the disease. Fluids in large quantities are ordered to replace those lost through increased respiration and perspiration. If the patient cannot tolerate them by mouth, intravenous fluids are given.

For cough and chest pain, codeine, 30 mg. or 60 mg., may be ordered orally or subcutaneously every 4 to 6 hours. Codeine depresses respirations less than does morphine. Toxic effects include nausea, vomiting, constipation and excitement.

If the inflammatory process is far advanced, the patient may have considerable respiratory difficulty and be cyanotic. The humidification of the inspired air is usually very helpful in liquefying secretions and is best administered by cool-mist vaporizer. A nasal catheter or cannula is usually ordered for supplementary oxygenation. In the presence of severe infection with thick, abundant secretions, the doctor may perform endotracheal intubation or tracheostomy. These technics make suctioning easier, and in addition, permit more effective ventilation by a positive pressure breathing apparatus.

If an oxygen tent is ordered, the patient should be told that it will make breathing easier, that since it is of transparent plastic, he will be able to see through it, and that the nurse will be able to take care of him through zippers in the sides. Many patients still think of an oxygen tent as a last drastic measure, and they are frightened by its use. While the nurse prepares to put the patient in the tent, she can explain briefly its use to him, emphasizing that it will make him more comfortable. Fasten the call bell near the patient's hand. Because he may have a chill, wrap a cotton blanket around his neck and his shoulders and another across his body. Some patients are more comfortable if the blanket over the shoulders is draped over their heads like a hood, so that no cold breeze from the tent can creep down their necks. The liter flow is ordered by the physician; 12 liters per minute is usual.

Intravenous fluids are ordered when the patient is vomiting or unable to eat. Antibiotic medication may be ordered by the intravenous route, into the I.V. bottle, sparing the patient repeated injections. Observe that the intravenous flow rate is at the speed ordered to maintain an adequate blood level of the antibiotic, and observe the patient carefully for side effects and toxic effects. If the combination of specific treatment, supportive measures, and the patient's own body defenses are insufficiently responding to the infection, he can go into shock. Since shock must be treated early and rapidly if the patient is to survive, report promptly to the physician any signs or symptoms of shock.

Nursing Care of Pneumonia Patients

The patient admitted to the hospital with pneumonia usually is very sick and very uncomfortable. He is likely to be frightened. He not only has fallen ill suddenly, but also may be having great difficulty in breathing. Some severely ill patients are exhausted and have to struggle through pain for every breath. Elevate the head of the bed. Place the pillow lengthwise, so that it supports his entire back and helps to expand his chest. A pillow across the upper portion of his back will tend to bend him forward and lessen the expansion of his chest.

Temperature, Pulse, Respiration. These are taken on admission and every 4 hours, except during chills and sponges, when they are recorded more frequently. An increase of temperature to over 103° or below 98.6° should be reported to the physician immediately, since these signs are warnings of a drastic change in the patient's condition. A sharp increase or a sharp decrease in pulse rate warns of circulatory complications and also is reported. The character as well as the rate of respirations is observed closely. Increasingly labored respirations indicate very rapid progress of the disease and are often a sign that more drastic treatment measures are required. It is characteristic for the patient to grunt with each expiration. Temperature is taken rectally, since coughing and oral breathing render oral readings grossly inaccurate. Alcohol sponges may be ordered for fever over 102° or 103°. Avoid exposing the patient to a draft or chilling him during a sponge.

Medications and Treatment. Plan these so that the patient is disturbed as little as possible. Antibiotics should be given on time to maintain consistent blood levels. Plan nursing care so that when you give him medication you also give him mouth care and fluids, change his position and take his vital signs, thus allowing for uninterrupted rest periods. Although the daily bath should be omitted during the acute phase to avoid tiring the patient, a back rub and fresh linens are essential. Also, to avoid chilling, change the patient's pajamas and linen every time that they become wet with perspiration.

Talking. During the early phase of the disease, keep the patient as quiet as possible. One nurse cautioned her colleagues, "Guard against heart exertion, allow little speaking, save the patient's strength, and keep [him] free from all excitement" (Gordon). This was written in 1904 and holds true today.

Some patients feel that even when they are exhausted, they must do their part to establish a relationship with their nurses through talking. If the patient attempts to make small talk while he is acutely ill, ask him to conserve his strength. It is an interesting challenge to show interest in the patient without stimulating him to excessive talk.

Food, Drink. When it is fatiguing to drink fluids, they should be offered in small quantities at frequent intervals and in variation to promote appetite. Fruit juices, broths, consommé, milk and eggnogs may be used. Since the ingestion of food may stimulate coughing, fluid should not be offered after a coughing spell. Ice chips may be used to moisten the mouth if fluids are not tolerated orally. Frequent mouth care is essential to prevent stomatitis. The lesions of herpes simplex often appear around the mouth and are a source of great discomfort for the patient. Camphor ice, cold cream or tincture of benzoin may be applied. Because the sputum is foul, always give mouth care before offering the patient anything to eat or to drink. The physician may order only fluids or a light diet for the

acutely ill patient. A regular diet is resumed when the appetite returns, and the patient's condition improves.

Excretion. Pay heed to urinary output. If it is not consistent with intake, the discrepancy should be reported to the physician. Since abdominal distention and paralytic ileus are complications of pneumonia, bowel movements should be observed and recorded, and the abdomen should be watched for distention. Distention pushes the diaphragm up, so that it presses on the base of the lungs at a time when they are especially in need of space for expansion.

Expectoration. When the patient is disturbed for medications or for treatment, encourage him to cough up mucus. Whenever he coughs, whether voluntarily or by reflex, place your hands on his chest where it hurts. Use firm pressure to splint the chest. This will decrease the pain a little and help the patient to be more willing to cough. Some patients are shy about expectorating in the view of another person, but the infected sputum should not be swallowed. Take care that the patient does not cough directly into your face; there are live organisms in the sputum. Provide a sputum cup with a cover if the sputum is to be saved for inspection or measurement. If not, disposable tissues and a paper bag in which to dispose of them may be used instead. Keep this equipment within easy reach, so that he does not have to exert himself to reach it. Change the sputum cup or paper bag at least twice a day, handling them with great care and sealing them so that the infection is not spread.

Restlessness. Observe the patient closely for signs of restlessness. If you cannot stay with a patient who is acutely ill with pneumonia, observe him at least every half-hour. Listen to his respirations, look at his color, note whether he is restless. If he is, ask him to tell you why. You may be able to relieve his pain, to help him to cough out some sputum or to change his position. Restlessness may be a prelude to delirium. Inform the physician at once if delirium should occur. Protect the patient with padded side rails and with restraints when they are ordered.

Isolation. In some hospitals patients with pneumonia (particularly staphylococcal pneumonia) are isolated during the acute phase. Some physicians believe that the spread of pneumonia is prevented by this measure; other physicians believe that hand washing and ordinary cleanliness are sufficient to prevent the spread of infection. In either case, medical asepsis is enhanced if an isolation gown is worn over the uniform when giving direct care. The patient needs to be protected from secondary infection. The nurse should wash her hands before caring for him, as well as before leaving the unit. Visitors with head colds should be excluded from his room.

The room should be well ventilated so that the air is as fresh as possible. The nurse works with the Admitting Office so that the patient acutely ill with pneumonia is placed in a room as close to the Nurses' Station as possible. If isolation is not used, care should be taken that the patient's roommates are not in a high risk group, such as the aged, postsurgical patients or those with chronic obstructive pulmonary disease.

Convalescence. With the administration of antibiotics, symptoms usually subside rapidly during the first 48 to 72 hours, and the patient feels much improved. However, he will be weak and tired. He is kept in bed for several days after his temperature has returned to normal. He then is helped gradually to resume normal routine and self-care. A follow-up roentgenogram usually is ordered to make sure that the disease process is clearing. Emphasize the importance of having this examination performed and also of following the physician's instructions about returning to work.

Complications of Pneumonia

Complications of pneumonia are seen more rarely today than previously, since antibiotics usually reverse the disease process early. Congestive heart failure is a serious complication. On occasion a patient's temperature may fall within two days, but his pulse may remain fast. Even though the fever is gone, the lung pathology and the other symptoms remain. The patient is still acutely ill.

Empyema, the collection of pus in the pleural space, and pleurisy (see below) may occur. Symptoms include continued fever and other signs of infection. The pain in the chest is usually at the site of infection. Empyema is treated with the antibiotics that are specific for the invading organism. This is determined through thoracentesis and bacteriologic examination of the fluid obtained.

The invasion of the bloodstream by organisms, which occurs during periods of septicemia while the patient is having a chill, makes all the body accessible to the organisms. A secondary focus of infection may be established, resulting in endocarditis, meningitis or purulent arthritis.

Atelectasis, or the collapse of the lung, is caused by the plugging of a bronchus with mucus. Encouraging the patient to cough and changing his position frequently will help to prevent this complication.

Otitis media, bronchitis or sinusitis may complicate recovery, especially from atypical pneumonia, by the spread of the organisms to these organs.

Prevention of Pneumonia

Because colds can lower resistance and lead to more serious infections, such as pneumonia, patients in hospitals should be isolated promptly at the first signs of a cold. It is especially important that colds be treated promptly and carefully in people with increased susceptibility—for example, alcoholics and older persons. Health personnel with colds, including nurses, should remain at home.

Nurses have a particular responsibility to prevent hypostatic pneumonia. Every patient on bed rest is a candidate for this disease, especially the heavily sedated, comatose and elderly patients. All patients should move or be moved regularly, and they should take several deep breaths at least every hour during the day.

PLEURISY

Pathology

Pleurisy is an inflammation of the *pleura,* the membrane that covers the lungs in two layers. Pleurisy occurs as a complication of pulmonary disease. Two forms are seen: acute fibrinous or dry pleurisy, in which only small amounts of exudate are formed during the inflammatory process; and *pleurisy with effusion,* in which large amounts of fluid are secreted and collect in the space between the pleural layers. There may be so much fluid that the lung is collapsed partially on that side, and there is pressure on the heart and the other organs of the mediastinum. Dry pleurisy is seen most commonly in pneumonia, in which the inflammatory process spreads from the lung to the parietal pleura. Pleurisy with effusion may result from tuberculosis, carcinoma of the lungs, cardiac and renal disease, systemic infections, pneumonia and pulmonary embolism. The pleura becomes thick, swollen and rigid. The visceral pleura has no pain fibers, but the parietal pleura does. Very sharp pain occurs when the two surfaces of the pleura rub over each other during respiration. As fluid is formed, this pain gradually subsides; but the patient has a dry cough, fatigues easily and may get out of breath.

Treatment and Nursing Care of Pleurisy Patients

The care of the patient with pleurisy is similar to that of the patient with pneumonia. Bed rest is required. The room should be warm and well ventilated. The patient needs encouragement to cough. The nurse can help by firm pressure at the painful spot. Positioning the patient on the side of the effusion helps to splint the painful area and also encourages the expansion of the other side of the rib cage. A heating pad or hot-water bag to the painful area may be ordered for comfort.

If there is a great deal of fluid with respiratory embarrassment, the fluid may be removed by thoracentesis. The nurse prepares the equipment, including that needed for the collection of specimens. She watches the patient closely during the thoracentesis for signs of weakness, excessive diaphoresis, increased respirations or dyspnea, pain, chill, nausea, coughing or shock. Any symptoms are reported to the physician, who then proceeds more slowly or discontinues the treatment. It may be necessary for the nurse to

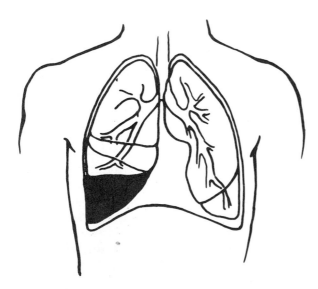

FIG. 23-4. Fluid in the pleural space can compress the lung.

support the weakened patient in position. He should be comfortable so that he can remain immobile during the procedure. Leaning forward over a pillow-padded bed table is generally a helpful position.

EMPYEMA

Empyema, pus in the pleural space, is a rare complication of pneumonia or chest trauma since the introduction of antibiotic therapy. Its presence is characterized by chest pain, fever and evidence of a pleural effusion. The doctor confirms the diagnosis by a diagnostic thoracentesis with culture of the withdrawn fluid. Usually he inserts a surgical drain in order to empty the empyema cavity. (If this cavity is not emptied, fibrosis of the pleural linings can occur which may require surgical removal at a later time.) The care of the patient is similar to the care of any patient with an infection and a draining, infected wound. Observe him for signs of pneumothorax.

INFLUENZA

Influenza is an acute respiratory disease of short duration caused by one of several related and yet distinct viruses.

Influenza occurs chiefly in epidemics, although sporadic cases appear between epidemics.

Epidemics can be predicted, and vaccines are available, but significant protection against influenza epidemics is not yet a reality.

Most patients recover. Fatalities usually are due to bacterial complications, especially among pregnant women, the aged or debilitated and those with chronic conditions, such as cardiac disease. During an epidemic, the death rate from pneumonia and cardiovascular disease rises.

Symptoms

The incubation period is 2 to 3 days, and the onset is sudden, with considerable individual variation in symptoms. The patient looks acutely ill and complains of chilliness, severe headache, muscular aching and fever. There may be anorexia, weakness and apathy, as well as respiratory symptoms, sneezing, sore throat, dry cough, nasal discharge and herpetic lesions of the lips and the mouth. Severe disease causes prostration and may lead to vasomotor collapse. Fever, 100° to 103°, persists about 3 days, but other symptoms usually continue for 7 to 10 days. Cough may persist longer.

The return to normal activities should be gradual, because of the amount of prostration typical of influenza. Overexertion and chilling should be avoided. The patient should not return to work until all symptoms have subsided, including the cough.

Complications include tracheobronchitis, caused by damage to the ciliated epithelium of trachea and bronchi; bacterial pneumonia; and cardiovascular disease. Staphylococcal pneumonia is the most serious complication, exhibiting a fulminant, often fatal course.

Treatment and Nursing Care of Influenza Patients

Bed rest in a warm, well-ventilated room is recommended until the temperature is normal and for 1 or 2 days afterward. Temperature, pulse and respirations are taken every 4 hours during the elevation. Copious amounts of fluid, given frequently, may include fruit juices, milk and egg drinks and broths; a regular diet is given as soon as the patient's appetite returns. Sponges and back rubs promote the patient's general comfort and may help him to sleep. Acetylsalicylic acid (aspirin), 0.3 to 1.0 Gm., may be given every 4 to 6 hours for headache and muscular aching. Steam or cool vapor inhalation eases a dry cough. The physician may order codeine 30 to 60 mg. every 6 hours, as needed, to control the coughing.

The patient should be taught to use paper handkerchiefs once, to fold them carefully to avoid spreading infection and to discard them in a paper bag. The viruses that cause influenza are transmitted through the respiratory tract. Hospitalization is not recommended in uncomplicated cases, because of the possibility of exposing the patient to a secondary bacterial infection.

The patient is observed carefully for signs of increasing fever, elevated pulse rate, chest pain, difficulty in breathing, change in the amount and the quality of the sputum—particularly, whether it is purulent or rusty—and for marked pain anywhere. A prompt report of any of these symptoms is made to the physician.

COMMON COLD

A large number of filterable viruses cause colds. Immunity is of very short duration, and incubation is short. Extraneous factors, such as fatigue, chilling, emotional upset, exposure to irritating gases or allergens—all of which affect the nasal mucosa—are believed to lower the natural resistance, facilitating invasion by the virus.

Symptoms. Although there is considerable individual variation in the symptoms, they may include sneezing, chilliness, headache, watery eyes and a dry scratchy throat, followed by copious nasal discharge, sore throat, hoarseness and cough. There may be a slight fever. The cold lasts from 4 to 14 days, with symptoms gradually subsiding.

Treatment. Bed rest is perhaps the most important aspect of the treatment, since it restricts contact with others and limits the spread of the cold. It is particularly important for the individual who may be susceptible to complications—infants, aged and debilitated individuals, and those whose temperature is elevated. Ordinarily, the otherwise healthy adult does not remain confined to bed, although he should get extra rest and avoid contact with others. Fluids in large amounts are helpful. Petroleum jelly around the nose and the mouth will relieve chapping. Visitors should be restricted, and the patient should be instructed in the proper use of paper handkerchiefs and in hand washing.

Individuals who have a tendency to develop a secondary bacterial infection may benefit from prophylactic antibiotic therapy. In this group are patients with asthma, chronic obstructive pulmonary disease and other chronic lung ailments. Aspirin, 0.3 to 0.6 Gm., may be given every 4 to 6 hours for the relief of general discomfort. Although nose drops or inhalers obtained commercially may help to relieve some of the nasal congestion, indiscriminate use of them is harmful. Many of them contain drugs that affect the body systemically, or they cause local irritation of the mucous membrane of the nose. Work is in progress to develop vaccines that would offer protection against at least some of the viruses that cause colds.

INJURIES OF THE CHEST

Fractured ribs are a common form of injury to the chest. They may be caused by a hard fall or by a blow on the chest. Automobile accidents are a frequent cause. Although rib fractures are very painful, they usually are not serious unless injury to other structures results. For example, the sharp end of the broken bone may tear the lung or blood vessels. If the injury involves fractured ribs without other complications, the patient often is permitted to return home after treatment. The usual treatment includes supporting the chest with an Ace bandage or adhesive strapping to minimize the pain, and the administration of analgesics. Sometimes a regional nerve block is necessary to relieve the pain. If the patient is treated on an outpatient basis, it is important for him to understand that:

1. He should breathe as deeply as possible; his natural inclination will be to take very shallow breaths to minimize pain.

2. He should take the analgesic as ordered, in order to minimize the pain, to promote rest, and to permit more normal breathing.

3. He will probably breathe more comfortably in a sitting position than when he is lying flat.

4. If he experiences sudden, sharp chest pain or difficulty in breathing, he should call his doctor at once.

Blast injuries, such as those that result from compression of the chest by an explosion, cause serious injury to the lungs by rupturing the alveoli. Death often results from hemorrhage and asphyxiation. The treatment includes the provision of complete rest and the administration of oxygen.

Penetrating wounds of the chest are also very serious. An open wound may permit air to enter the thoracic cavity, causing *pneumothorax*. If the wound is large, it may cause a sucking noise as air enters and leaves the chest cavity. Applying an airtight dressing is an important first-aid measure to prevent the entrance of more air into the chest cavity. Air also may enter the pleural space from an injury to the lung tissue. For example, the sharp end of a broken rib may tear the lung tissue, permitting air to enter the pleural space. Many chest injuries involve both pneumothorax and *hemothorax* (blood in the pleural space).

When medical aid has been obtained, the air and the blood are aspirated from the pleural space by thoracentesis. Sometimes a chest catheter is inserted and attached to closed drainage (see p. 321). Later it may be necessary to perform a thoracotomy to repair or to remove injured tissues. Foreign bodies that have entered the chest should be removed only by the doctor. Their presence in the wound may prevent the entrance of air, and their removal without medical aid may cause pneumothorax.

REFERENCES AND BIBLIOGRAPHY

AHLSTROM, P.: Raising sputum specimens, *Am. J. Nurs.* 65:109, March, 1965.

Asian variant influenza, *Public Health Rep.* 73:99, 1958.

DAVENPORT, F. M.: Prospects for the control of influenza, *Am. J. Nurs.* 69:1908, September, 1969.

GOODMAN, L. S., and GILMAN, A.: *The Pharmacological Basis of Therapeutics,* ed. 3, New York, Macmillan, 1965.

GORDON, E. C.: Pneumonia—the nursing of pneumonia, *Am. J. Nurs.* 4:924, 1904.

HARRISON, T. R., *et al.* (eds.): *Principles of Internal Medicine,* ed. 5, New York, McGraw-Hill, 1966.

HINSHAW, H. C.: *Diseases of the Chest,* ed. 3, Philadelphia, Saunders, 1969.

HOLINGER, P. H.: Laryngoscopy, bronchoscopy, and esophagoscopy, *AORN* 4:61, May-June, 1966.

HUNTER, D.: *The Diseases of Occupations,* ed. 4, Boston, Little, Brown, 1969.

HUSE, W.: The least you should know about chest injuries, *Consultant* 8:42, September, 1968.

Influenza Surveillance, Communicable Disease Center, U.S. Department of Health, Education and Welfare, Report No. 77, June 14, 1963.

LEWIS, H. E.: *Pneumonia—A Symposium on the Occurrence, Etiology, Diagnosis, Prognosis and Treatment of Pneumonia,* New York, American Medical Publishing, 1910.

RODMAN, M., and SMITH, D.: *Pharmacology and Drug Therapy in Nursing,* Philadelphia, Lippincott, 1968.

SARTWELL, P. E.: *Maxcy-Rosenau Preventive Medicine and Public Health,* ed. 9, New York, Appleton-Century-Crofts, 1965.

TURNER, H. C., JR.: The anatomy and physiology of normal respiration, *Nurs. Clin. N. Am.* 3:383, September, 1968.

The Patient with Chronic Respiratory Disorder 24

Allergic Rhinitis • Bronchial Asthma • Bronchitis • Chronic Obstructive Pulmonary Disease • Bronchiectasis • Empyema Lung Abscess • Pneumoconiosis • Cancer of the Lung Postoperative Care of Chest-Surgery Patients • Nursing Care of Patients with Chronic Respiratory Disorders

Any change in the size, shape, or function of the body is apt to stir up anxiety. When the usual automatic function of breathing enters awareness and becomes a struggle, a vicious cycle often ensues. The dyspneic patient is anxious because he can't breathe normally, and the more anxious he becomes the more difficult it is for him to breathe. When the nurse uses measures which facilitate the patient's breathing (such as mechanical devices and drugs), she reduces his anxiety and her own anxiety as well.

The incidence of serious chronic respiratory disease is increasing. Between 1962 and 1966 the

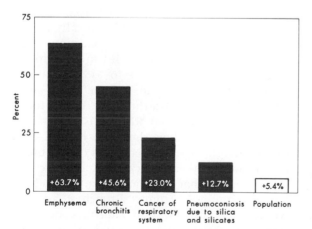

FIG. 24-1. Per cent increase in deaths from selected respiratory diseases compared with population change between 1962 and 1966, United States. (National Center for Health Statistics, Washington, D.C.)

increase in death rate from respiratory diseases as a group was greater than that for any other cause of death. Although all factors leading to this increase are not understood, two important factors are smoking and air pollution.

The nurse demonstrates her concern with the contributing factors to chronic respiratory disease by participating in programs and other educational efforts to eradicate or minimize personal air pollution (smoking) as well as environmental air pollution.

ALLERGIC RHINITIS

Definition. Allergic rhinitis is a term used to describe the reaction of the nasal mucous membrane to various allergens commonly found in the environment. The allergic response is characterized by swelling of the nasal mucous membrane, sneezing, and increased nasal secretions. Other terms such as hayfever or rosefever have been used to describe the allergic response secondary to specific allergenic substances. Allergic rhinitis may occur seasonally and be specifically related to pollens or on a perennial (nonseasonal) basis where the reaction is due to other environmental antigens such as dust or feathers.

Etiology and Pathology. The condition is caused by allergy to a specific antigen (see Chap. 6 on allergy). When the symptoms are seasonal, allergic rhinitis usually is caused by pollens from weeds, trees, or grasses. Perennial allergic rhinitis may be caused by dust, feathers, and animal danders. The allergen-antibody reaction occurring in the nose causes immediate release of histamine that affects the local tissues of the nose by causing edema, itching, and a watery discharge. The eyes and the pharynx also may be affected.

Incidence. Allergic rhinitis is common in persons who have an allergic background. Often there is a family history of allergy, although the specific allergen may vary between different members of the same family. Allergic rhinitis can occur at any age. Although it tends to recur in the same individual for an indefinite period, its course over a lifetime is variable. One person may have the onset of symptoms at puberty; another may develop symptoms for the first time in middle life. It is possible for the symptoms to subside without apparent cause or to subside and be replaced by other allergic manifestations such as asthma.

Symptoms. The patient usually experiences itching of the nose, eyes, throat, and roof of the mouth. This is accompanied by sneezing, a profuse watery discharge, and tearing of the eyes. Marked swelling of the nasal mucosa may cause complete obstruction of the nasal airway, making breathing difficult. During a full-blown episode of allergic rhinitis a feeling of malaise accompanies the episode. Symptoms due to pollen are more severe on clear, windy days and during early morning and evening hours.

Diagnosis. Allergic rhinitis is diagnosed by securing a careful history concerning the events related to the attacks. Symptoms may appear only a few weeks at the same season each year, leading the doctor to suspect pollen, or they may have their onset when a new pet or a new feather pillow is acquired. Skin testing is helpful in determining which substance is causing symptoms and, frequently, the patient may be allergic to several different substances. Physical examination and microscopic examination of nasal secretions are also helpful in diagnosis. The nasal mucous membrane usually appears edematous and pale. An abundance of eosinophils is found typically in nasal secretions.

Treatment. The most effective treatment is avoidance of the allergen. For the person who can afford it, an ocean voyage during the season when the symptoms occur may provide a delightful solution. However, for the majority of patients, treatment centers around desensitization, antihistamines, and diminishing contact with the allergen.

Contact with pollen can be diminished by remaining indoors, away from open windows on windy days, and by using an air conditioner. Should the allergic rhinitis be of the perennial type and due to animal danders or feathers, the use of a foam rubber pillow and a new home for the pet may result in complete remission of symptoms. For those persons whose interest in the outdoors or love of a pet outweighs the desire for total relief, desensitization will often diminish the symptoms. Antihistamines frequently give temporary relief. ACTH and cortisone are not used except under life-threatening circumstances such as laryngeal edema. Symptoms are lessened by maintaining good general health.

Course and Prognosis. Allergic rhinitis is most severe when exposure to the allergen is at its height. Fatigue and emotional strain tend to aggravate the symptoms. Because the edema may block the drainage of the sinuses, sinusitis sometimes complicates allergic rhinitis. Obstruction of the eustachian tube results in middle ear infection, a common finding in allergic rhinitis. Should infection of the nasal mucosa intervene during an acute episode, nasal polyps may develop. These polyps further tend to obstruct the nasal air passages, resulting in difficult breathing. Some patients may go on to develop asthma as a consequence of their disease. Although allergic rhinitis is not a threat to life, it is a major cause of discomfort. Effective treatment, usually desensitization, cannot eradicate the condition, but can greatly add to the patient's comfort and decrease the likelihood of sequelae.

BRONCHIAL ASTHMA

Definition. Asthma is derived from the Greek word for panting and is used clinically to mean shortness of breath. Many conditions which have as their main clinical feature shortness of breath have been referred to as asthma. Coal miners' asthma, cardiac asthma, and allergic asthma or bronchial asthma are but a few examples. Since "all that wheezes is not asthma," the diagnosis of asthma should be limited strictly to the allergic type. Other forms of shortness of breath would then be called congestive heart failure, not cardiac asthma, and anthracosilicosis, not coal miners' asthma. Bronchial asthma is typified by paroxysms of shortness of breath, wheezing, cough, and the production of thick tenacious sputum. The onset and the duration of the acute episode vary markedly between individuals. The duration may be brief, lasting less than one day, or extend into prolonged periods of several weeks.

Symptoms and Pathophysiology. The triad characteristic of the acute asthmatic state consists of spasm of the smooth muscle of the bronchi and larger bronchioles, swelling of the mucosal lining, and thick bronchiole secretions. The degree of airflow obstruction is directly related to the severity of the above mechanisms. Once the air has entered the alveoli, air trapping takes place since the bronchioles and bronchi narrow during the expiratory effort. The attempt to move air across a narrowed orifice results, as in the playing of any reed instrument, in the production of musical tones. This is the classical wheezing that the physician hears on auscultation of the chest and which may be audible without the stethoscope to a nurse. The patient is often aware of the wheezing and reports it as one of his symptoms. Every breath becomes an effort and during the acute episode the work of breathing is greatly increased. The patient may suffer from a sensation of suffocation. Frequently, a classical sitting position is assumed with the body leaning slightly forward and the arms at shoulder height. This position facilitates expansion of the chest as well as more effective excursions of the diaphragm. Because life depends on the power to breathe, fear accompanies the symptoms. Unfortunately, fear and anxiety tend to intensify the symptoms and not to relieve them. The effort to move trapped air within the alveoli is accompanied by a marked prolongation of the expiratory phase of respiration. Coughing commences with the onset of the attack, but is ineffective in the early stage and only as the attack begins to subside is the patient able to expectorate large quantities of thick, stringy mucus. Usually, the patient's skin is pale; however, if the attack is very severe, mild cyanosis of the lips and nailbeds may be noted. Perspiration is usually profuse during an acute attack. Following spontaneous or drug-induced remission of the episode, examination of the lungs commonly reveals normal findings and it is frequently impossible to diagnose bronchial asthma by physical signs without observation during the acute attack. Occasionally, however, the acute state can intensify and be resistant to all therapy, progressing into "status asthmaticus."

Etiology. Prominent among the causes of asthma are antigen-antibody reactions as seen in allergy, infection, and emotional stress. These factors vary in importance in different patients, but with careful observation all three components may be found active at the same time.

Bronchial asthma has been divided into two separate groups. The first is extrinsic asthma which occurs chiefly in response to allergens such as pollen, dust, spores, or animal danders. Intrinsic asthma is the second type and has been associated with upper respiratory infection or emotional upsets.

Incidence and Course. Asthma may occur at any period in life. Approximately 50 per cent of all asthma occurs prior to the age of 10. A significant relationship between bronchiolitis in the first year of life and the development of bronchial asthma in early childhood has been noted. When the illness starts in early childhood, the symptoms tend to become less severe as the child grows older. Extrinsic asthma is the most common form noted in the childhood and young adult types. Intrinsic asthma due to recurrent infection frequently related to chronic sinusitis or chronic bronchitis is most frequently seen beyond the age of 40. Asthma may be limited to occasional attacks and the patient is usually symptom free in the interim. Extensive long-term studies have been conducted that reveal normal pulmonary function studies during remission in asthma. For the average individual, other than the occasional acute episode, there is no progression of the disease and pathologic examination of the lung during the asymptomatic state reveals normal structure. Occasionally, however, frequent and prolonged attacks, particularly those related to recurrent infection, tend to lead to chronic bronchitis and, if inadequately treated, may progress to emphysema.

Treatment of Patients with Bronchial Asthma

Symptomatic treatment is given at the time of the attack. The long-term care of the patient involves measures to control the cause of the illness. Thus, treatment of allergy, infection, and emotional disorders may all play a part in the therapy.

Oxygen Therapy. Oxygen is usually not necessary during an acute attack. This is because most patients with bronchial asthma are actively hyperventilating. Rarely, particularly after a long bout of asthma, some patients may develop cyanosis. Oxygen may then be given by nasal catheter, mask, or preferably intermittent positive pressure breathing. Thus, the nurse does not automatically reach for oxygen for the patient in the acute asthmatic state unless cyanosis is present. Oxygen administration should be prescribed for each patient, as drugs are prescribed.

The nurse can play a negative part in the patient's care if she does not insist on the physician prescribing what is to be done in the event of an acute attack and if oxygen is to be given, what technic and liter flow are to be used.

The nurse should explain to the patient the reason for the mask or the catheter. This explanation, as well as remaining with the patient initially until he gets adjusted to the oxygen and equipment, is necessary to allay the patient's anxiety and reduce the fear of suffocation. Intermittent positive pressure breathing employing equipment such as the Bird or Bennett Respirator may greatly aid the patient by taking over the work of breathing and by promoting better alveolar ventilation.

Bronchodilators. The bronchodilator preparations are usually divided into two groups: the sympathomimetic drugs and the theophylline preparations. The sympathomimetic medications are those most commonly used in the treatment of acute bronchial asthma and include such drugs as epinephrine (Adrenalin), isoproterenol (Isuprel), and ephedrine. These agents tend to reduce bronchospasm by causing relaxation of the smooth muscle lining the bronchi and larger bronchioles.

Epinephrine is usually administered to the adult in a subcutaneous dose of 0.3–0.5 ml. of a 1:1000 solution. The dose may be repeated at 30-minute intervals if required. The drug, however, is a potent stimulant and affects not only the smooth muscle of the tracheobronchial tree, but the entire body. The side effects of the drug are common and include tachycardia, palpitation, tremors, pallor, and anxiety. Frequently, a sedative medication such as phenobarbital may have to be administered concurrently in order to reduce the side effects.

The nurse observes the patient for drug toxicity and side effects, and especially the anxiety and tachycardia accompanying the use of epinephrine. There is a great need for nursing judgment when epinephrine is ordered on a p.r.n. basis. The doctor should be consulted if the patient is becoming more anxious and tachycardic, has chest pain, trembling or other systemic effects of epinephrine. Patients vary greatly in their response to this drug and need close observation. When in doubt about a further dose, call the physician.

Epinephrine and isoproterenol are extremely effective bronchodilators when given by nebulizer in solutions of 1:100 and 1:200. The ad-

vantage of delivering the bronchodilator by nebulizer directly into the lung is that the effect is maximal on the bronchial musculature and although side effects do occur, they are limited as compared with the subcutaneous injection. Since the effectiveness of the nebulized bronchodilator is dependent on the dose and proper delivery of the drug into the lung, specific instructions must be given to the patient. The usual dose is 0.5 ml. of the drug placed in the nebulizer reservoir. This should not be diluted by the addition of water or any other agent. It has been shown that the effectiveness of the nebulized bronchodilator is dependent solely on its concentration. Therefore, if the 0.5 ml. of drug is diluted with 2 ml. of saline, the overall effectiveness of the therapy will be one-fifth of that expected. It is important that the nurse understand the rationale of drug administration. Otherwise she may unwittingly reduce the effectiveness of a drug by carrying out an institutional routine (such as unwarranted dilution of a drug) without question. If the nurse receives an order to dilute the drug, she should discuss this with the physician.

When delivered by a hand-bulb nebulizer, it will take approximately 15 minutes to deliver the bronchodilator drug. In order to simplify delivery, many drug companies now prepare the bronchodilator in pressurized aerosol form. The pressurized container is small and can be carried everywhere with the patient. It is an urgent nursing concern that the patient have his own nebulization equipment, that it be cleaned thoroughly between use, disinfected daily, and sterilized between patients. Otherwise, bacterial contamination of the patient's lungs with resultant infection can occur. Hospital policy and surveillance committees should reflect this concern.

The usual dose of the aerosol is one or two sprays delivered to the tracheobronchial tree every 4 hours. The tip of the nebulizer, whether hand-bulb or aerosol type, should be placed into the open mouth. The nurse instructs the patient not to close his lips around the nebulizer. Then, while breathing in, the patient should squeeze the bulb or press on the aerosol can. In this manner, the nebulized material will be carried with the airstream into the trachea, bronchi, and bronchioles. If not so instructed, many patients will close their mouth around the mouthpiece and while breathing through their nose, deliver the drug. This results in deposition of the bronchodilator in the oral cavity and absorption by the mucosa of the mouth. The principal effect will then be on the cardiovascular system with very little relief of respiratory symptoms. Because the pressurized aerosol form is so readily available, overmedication can become a problem. Obviously, these agents must be used with great caution in individuals who have cardiac disease.

The nurse explains to the patient and family the purpose of the drug, when and how it should be used, and why it should not be overused. They should be aware of the harmful, systemic side effects of the drugs and when to report these to the physician. The physician should also be informed when the usual dose of the aerosol seems to be ineffective. The public health nurse can give overall health supervision and specific instruction in the use of drugs at home to the patient. Especially when the patient is elderly or has other handicaps, the family needs both instruction and support to assist him.

Ephedrine acts similarly to epinephrine, but its effects are not as strong. Its principal usefulness is that it can be given orally in doses of 25 mg., repeated every 4 hours as needed. Sedatives may be required to counteract unpleasant side effects such as nervousness, trembling, and insomnia.

Aminophylline is the most effective of all the theophylline derivatives in reducing bronchospasm. It is most useful when administered intravenously in a dose of 0.25–0.5 Gm. The doctor injects the drug slowly over a period of approximately 10 minutes in order to avoid a sudden drop in blood pressure, with dizziness, faintness, palpitation, and headache. If given rapidly, death may ensue. To avoid the risk of complications, aminophylline is often given as a small infusion consisting of 100 ml. of normal saline into which the dose of medication has been added. This may be given over a period of one-half hour. The risk of hypotension is minimized, but the patient should be carefully observed and his blood pressure checked frequently. For prolonged in-hospital use, the dose of aminophylline may be given over an 8-hour period in 500 ml. to 1000 ml. of intravenous fluid. The use of aminophylline as a rectal suppository is valuable and effective. Most patients develop anorectal irritation, however, if the dose exceeds 0.5 Gm. every 12 hours. The nurse observes whether and to what extent symptoms are relieved and whether there is anorectal irritation. While the oral administration of theophyl-

line and its derivatives would be the route of choice, to the present date, the oral preparations have not been effective.

Humidification of the inspired air is extremely important in the therapy of the bronchospastic state. It has been shown that dehydration of the respiratory mucous membrane may by itself lead to attacks of bronchial asthma. The use of steam or cool vapor humidifiers has proved effective. The value of humidification becomes evident as the attack subsides and the patient brings up thick, stringy sputum. The liquefaction of the secretions promotes more effective clearing of the airways and a rapid return to normal.

A large daily intake of fluids also helps the patient to bring up secretions and serves to replace fluid lost by the profuse perspiration during the acute attack. The initiative for increasing fluid intake rests with the nurse. She must keep going to the patient and offering fluids. The exhausted dyspneic patient often cannot reach for and take them himself.

Expectorants are not effective in the therapy of acute bronchial asthma. They may be used during the convalescent stage to raise the thick respiratory secretions that are further obstructing respiration. Saturated solution of potassium iodide (SSKI), 10 drops, diluted in milk or water, frequently is given several times daily. Terpin hydrate, though not as effective as SSKI, may prove useful in some patients.

Sedatives and Tranquilizers. These drugs are frequently used to control anxiety during the acute attack. However, care must be taken to avoid depression of respiration and the cough reflex. The anxiety that accompanies the acute attack is related to the patient's inability to breathe. To sedate the patient simply to relieve anxiety prior to relieving the respiratory distress may intensify the symptoms and, if the respiratory center is sufficiently depressed, death may occur. Narcotics, because of their respiratory depressant effects, are not used unless preparations have been made for mechanical support of respiration.

There is a great need for nursing judgment in the carrying out of p.r.n. orders for sedatives and tranquilizers for the dyspneic, asthmatic patient. The nurse should be aware that there can be a very human tendency to want to calm the patient down for one's own benefit and comfort, or out of kindness for the patient, and thus administer sedation unnecessarily. The nurse who works with dyspneic patients needs to develop an awareness of her own reactions to the patient's condition. If severe dyspnea makes her fearful, she can readily increase the patient's anxiety.

Nursing measures that help to lessen the patient's apprehension include:

- Simply staying with the patient, if possible.
- Listening to his concerns.
- Indicating by words and actions that his condition does not unduly alarm those caring for him.
- Providing him with a way to signal for help. answering calls promptly, and observing him when he does not call.
- Doing nothing to indicate within the patient's hearing that his attack is unusually severe or not responding to treatment.
- Checking with the doctor if there is doubt requiring administration of sedatives for securing mental and physical rest so that anxiety resulting from the nurse's indecision is not transferred to the patient.

Steroids are not generally used in the treatment of the patient with uncomplicated bronchial asthma. Medical opinion holds that bronchodilators, when used promptly, can be as effective as steroids but without the serious side-effects. Should the disease progress, the doctor may order steroids by the oral route. During status asthmaticus intravenous steroids in massive doses greater than 3 Gm. of hydrocortisone daily in divided doses have occasionally been effective and life saving.

Antibiotics. If the acute asthmatic state is complicated by an infection, the doctor orders antibiotics. Because most infections of this type are gram-positive, penicillin or one of the penicillin derivatives is the drug of choice. Many allergists believe that all bronchial asthma is always complicated by infection and now prescribe antibiotic therapy even in the absence of clinical signs and symptoms of infection.

Environment. The asthmatic patient's environment should be as free as possible of factors which contribute to respiratory infection. Nurses or visitors with upper respiratory infection should avoid contact with the patient. The patient's living quarters should be damp-dusted daily and he should be protected from exposure to allergens that may have set off his attacks or that may continue to perpetuate them. Thorough cleanliness of all inhalation therapy equipment is urgent.

Long-term Care

Efforts to determine the cause of the attacks are essential. If the patient's history and his diagnostic tests indicate that allergy is an important causative factor, treatment by the avoidance of the allergen, by desensitization or by antihistamines may be used.

Common inhalants that may cause asthma are dust, feathers, pollens and animal danders. It is important to keep the patient's environment as free as possible from substances to which he is allergic. Careful damp-dusting of his room daily helps to keep dust at a minimum. The use of draperies, rugs and upholstered furniture is unwise, since they can be cleaned less readily. Careful attention should be given to the removal of dust from less obvious places, such as the mattress and the rungs of the bed and the chairs. Air conditioners are very helpful in eliminating pollen as well as in controlling temperature and humidity. Feathers and down frequently cause symptoms. Pillows made of synthetic fibers or foam rubber are preferable. Flowers also may aggravate the symptoms. When family or friends express a desire to send gifts to the patient, the nurse often may suggest tactfully that the gift be something other than flowers.

The control of infection plays a major role in the care of patients with asthma. Frequently, the patients are susceptible to respiratory infections, and these infections tend, as the patients say, "to go to the chest." Patients should avoid factors that predispose to respiratory infections, such as exposure, fatigue and contact with persons who have colds.

Respiratory infections, when they do occur, should be treated promptly. Antibiotics are often necessary. Sometimes patients who acquire repeated respiratory infections with serious consequences are given daily prophylactic doses of antibiotics, particularly during the winter.

Emotional stress is often a causative factor in asthmatic attacks. Adjustments in home or job situations may be helpful in relieving stress. Psychotherapy may help the patient to understand and to handle his emotional reactions better and may be suggested by the doctor, if the patient's attacks seem closely related to emotional factors.

The maintenance of good general health is important in reducing the frequency of attacks and in helping the patient to achieve the maximum benefit from his treatment. Rest, optimum diet and a balance of work and recreation are important.

Nursing Care of Asthmatic Patients

Seeing a patient in extreme respiratory distress may be a frightening experience for the nurse. The patient is very anxious and looks to those who care for him for support and reassurance. Since it is the nurse who spends the greatest amount of time with the hospitalized patient, a large measure of this support and this reassurance become her responsibility.

Although the extreme dyspnea, the wheezing and the struggle for breath make it appear that the patient will not survive, most patients who have acute asthmatic attacks do recover from them. Most attacks are temporary and short; thus the nurse on the basis of this understanding may help the patient to feel that his attack will subside. Occasionally, however, asthmatic attacks are very prolonged or recur in rapid succession. This condition is called *status asthmaticus*. Although most patients do not die during an asthmatic attack, nevertheless it is true that death sometimes occurs. The patient often fears that each breath will be his last. He may describe a feeling of suffocation or of drowning. Through her understanding that the spasm of the patient's bronchi is causing marked interference with a vital function, the nurse will avoid giving glib and superficial reassurance. She will recognize that, although emotional factors may precipitate attacks in some patients, the patient who is having an attack is very ill, regardless of what may have caused the symptoms. Such attitudes as "It's all in his mind—he could snap out of it if he wanted to," betray a gross misunderstanding, and they seriously interfere with the nurse's ability to care for patients with asthma.

Let us consider the general principles in the nursing care of patients with asthma.

Initial Care. The nurse must recognize that the patient's entire concern is with his breathing, and that nursing care must involve nothing that would increase the patient's difficulty in breathing. Measures should be taken, before the doctor arrives, to make him more comfortable. Routine admission procedures may need to be modified temporarily. For instance, it would be most unwise to place an oral thermometer in the patient's mouth for an admission T.P.R., since the patient needs to breathe through his mouth. Recognizing that a sitting position makes breathing easier during an asthmatic attack, the nurse

would not insist that the patient lie in bed, but she would assist the patient to assume the position that is most comfortable for him.

Because she recognizes the patient's anxiety during the attack, the nurse should stay with him, if possible, and by her manner and her actions convey to the patient that someone is there to help him. There are many small ways in which the nurse can demonstrate this, e.g., replacing the moist nightgown with a dry one, showing the patient the call bell, and assuring him that, when he rings, someone will come.

Since most patients with asthma already feel closed in, it is important to avoid intensifying this sensation by drawing curtains around the bed or closing the doors and the windows. It is wise not to ask the patient to answer any unnecessary questions, because respiratory difficulty is made worse by an attempt to talk. The nurse should observe and chart: rate and character of respirations; pulse, color, cough, sputum, emotional state and diaphoresis.

Continuing Care. What nursing care will be needed after the doctor leaves? Since he has been frightened, and since he is now in a strange environment, it would be wise to leave a dim light in the patient's room at night and to encourage him to signal the nurse whenever it is necessary. Rest and adequate fluid intake are important. As he becomes assured that his breathing has improved, he probably will be comfortable with the head of the bed elevated. If plenty of fluids are provided within easy reach, and the patient is encouraged to drink them, the increased fluid intake will help his secretions to become less tenacious and will help to replace the fluids lost through perspiration. Tissues and a sputum cup should be provided, and the patient should be encouraged to expectorate the mucus.

It is not unusual for the patient with asthma to signal the nurse repeatedly often for apparently insignificant requests. Frequent use of the call bell is particularly likely at night or when the patient has had a recent attack and usually indicates that he is anxious and wants someone to stay with him. It is true that in many situations the nurse has many patients to care for and cannot spend as much time with the patient as might be desirable. Regardless of how much time the nurse has, she can spend it more effectively by devoting her care to what the patient really seems to need. Spending 10 or 15 minutes with the patient, allowing him to express some of his fears and to ask questions concerning his condition may require no more time than answering the call light a dozen times to adjust the window, and is often much more effective in helping the patient to rest.

Observation for Toxic Effects of Drugs. This is an important nursing function. It is especially necessary when the patient is receiving repeated doses of epinephrine, which may cause palpitation, nervousness, trembling, pallor and insomnia.

BRONCHITIS

Acute bronchitis is a disease characterized by inflammation of the mucous membranes lining the major bronchi and their branches. Frequently, the inflammatory process also involves the trachea, and is then referred to as tracheobronchitis. The most common cause of acute bronchitis is viral infection. Frequently starting as an upper respiratory infection (URI), the inflammatory process extends into the tracheobronchial tree, with direct involvement of the mucous linings. This involvement takes the form of inflammatory change with the production of increased amounts of mucus by the secretory cells of the mucosa. Usually the disease is self-limiting, lasting approximately 3 to 4 days, with symptoms that initially include a dry, nonproductive cough that later becomes productive of a mucopurulent sputum, fever, and malaise. It is treated simply by bed rest, salicylates, and a light, nourishing diet with plenty of liquids. Humidifiers are used, because dry air aggravates the cough. Occasionally, secondary bacterial invasion takes place and the previously mild infection may now become a serious bacterial infection with the production of a thick purulent sputum and a cough that may persist for several weeks. While antibiotics are not generally ordered for the treatment of acute bronchitis of viral etiology, the doctor usually interprets the establishment of the secondary invader in the tracheobronchial tree as an indication for culturing the sputum and starting antibiotic therapy. A period of 2 to 3 days will be required prior to the sputum culture report. During this time period, the doctor may order a broad-spectrum antibiotic such as tetracycline. He may change the antibiotic medication later depending on the sputum culture report. Acute bronchitis may be complicated by laryngitis with hoarseness and occasionally loss of voice, and sinusitis. These secondary areas of infection will usually subside as the bronchitis subsides.

Although acute bronchitis is most often related to an infectious process, chemical irritation due to noxious fumes (sulfur dioxide, nitrogen dioxide, smoke, and other air pollutants) can also cause acute bronchitis. The disease may be further complicated by the development of bronchial asthma. Nursing care of the patient with acute bronchitis is similar to that in any acute respiratory infection with emphasis on rest and prevention of the secondary infection, as well as on preventing the spread of infection to others.

Chronic Bronchitis

Chronic bronchitis is the disease characterized by the hypersecretion of mucus by the bronchial glands as well as a chronic or a recurrent respiratory infection. It is a serious health problem with symptoms that develop gradually and go untreated for many years until the disease is well established. A chronic cough, often attributed to smoking, may persist and gradually grow worse. The cough is frequently disregarded and early treatment delayed.

Etiology and Incidence. Multiple factors in the causation of chronic bronchitis have been recorded. The development of the disease may be insidious or may follow a long history of bronchial asthma or an acute respiratory infection, such as influenza or pneumonia. Air pollution is a major cause of chronic bronchitis, as evidenced by the extremely high incidence of disease in Great Britain. The role of cigarette smoking cannot be overemphasized. In one study of 150 patients with chronic obstructive pulmonary disease, it was found that 143 were cigarette smokers (Mitchell). In fact, the advanced stages of chronic bronchitis are usually never seen except in smokers. Smoking characteristically causes hypertrophy of the mucous glands and hypersecretion. The mucosal surface of the tracheobronchial tree is lined by uncountable numbers of small hairs called cilia. These cilia play a significant role in clearing the air passages of the lung of mucus and secretions. Their function is specifically to propel excess secretions to the trachea, where a cough or other method of clearing the throat will rid the body of this material. Many air pollutants, such as sulfur dioxide and smoke, have been shown to significantly alter cilial activity with retention of secretions the end result. These secretions form plugs within the smaller bronchi and are excellent culture media. Infection readily ensues. A chronic infection of the airway can then result in further increases in mucus secretion and ultimately areas of focal necrosis and fibrosis.

Those individuals who are exposed to large amounts of irritating dusts and chemicals are very likely to develop chronic respiratory diseases such as bronchitis. For instance, coal miners are especially prone to develop chronic bronchitis. Although the disease may occur at any age, it is most frequently seen in middle age and is usually the result of many years of untreated, low-grade bronchitis.

Symptoms. A cough is usually the earliest symptom, and is accompanied by the expectoration of thick, white, stringy mucus that is usually attributed to cigarette smoking. The cough is ordinarily most marked on arising in the morning and just prior to going to bed. Acute respiratory infections are frequent during the winter months and all colds tend to "settle in the chest" and may persist for several weeks or more. As the disease progresses, the sputum may become purulent, copious and occasionally streaked with blood after a severe paroxysm of coughing. Although the patient may have a sensation of heaviness in the chest, dyspnea is usually not a symptom of uncomplicated chronic bronchitis. In fact, pulmonary function tests are frequently normal. The general health is usually maintained and the physical examination may be remarkably normal.

Diagnosis. The patient's history is very important and the doctor can usually make the diagnosis by evaluation of the duration of symptoms, circumstances under which they started, type of employment, previous respiratory diseases, and smoking history. Physical examination, x-ray films of the chest, fluoroscopy, and pulmonary function tests may all be normal. Examination of the sputum, particularly the volume expectorated per day, may be helpful in assessing the severity of the disease. Sputum culture may be of therapeutic interest. All the above studies must be obtained in order to exclude other diseases such as bronchogenic carcinoma, bronchiectasis, tuberculosis, and other diseases where cough is a predominant feature.

Treatment. Management of patients with chronic bronchitis requires long-term planning and infinite attention to detail. Patients may be disappointed to learn that there is no miracle drug that can wipe out chronic bronchitis. If chronic infection is present, all treatment is usually palliative in nature. However, careful treatment can do much to minimize symptoms and prevent complications.

In general, the essence of treatment is directed toward the prevention of recurrent irritation of the bronchial mucosa either by infection or chemical agents. The smoking of tobacco in any form should be immediately discontinued as it is virtually impossible to prevent exacerbation and progression of the disease during active smoking. The patient must be helped to realize that even one cigarette may cause marked irritation of the mucosa and can by itself lead to bronchospasm.

With only slight readjustment in the diet, most individuals do not gain any additional weight following cessation of smoking and the anxiety that accompanies the discontinuation of tobacco usually diminishes with substitution of other appropriate outlets for tension relief, such as small but repetitive motor actions. If the patient's work involves exposure to dust and chemical irritants, a change of occupation may be necessary. It is impossible to escape from the air pollution of our urban areas. However, in the patient's home, air conditioning with filtration of incoming air often can result in marked reduction of sputum production and cough. The maintenance of optimal general health and the avoidance of other respiratory infections are very important in maintaining the patient's resistance. A diet that contains adequate protein, vitamins, and other nutrients is important as well as adequate rest and the avoidance of emotional strain. There is usually no need for any change of climate and, although some individuals may derive relief from living in a warm, dry climate, it is better that the patient live in an area where the relative humidity is maintained at a moderate level so as to assist in the liquefaction of secretions and prevention of mucus plugs. In fact, the maintenance of a high relative humidity between 40 and 50 per cent in the home is considered a prerequisite for good treatment, especially in the winter months.

The specific therapy is directed toward the prevention of recurrent infection and the suppression of chronic infection. In the late stages of chronic bronchitis the infection is usually persistent and antibiotic therapy may become a life-long therapeutic measure. It has been shown that it is impossible, once chronic infection has set in, ever to eradicate the bacteria from the lung. The suppression of infection is therefore of paramount importance and can be done by several technics. The preferred method is to give antibiotics, usually tetracycline, on any two consecutive days of the week at a dose level of 250 mg. q.i.d.

This intermittent therapy has proved highly successful because effective suppression of the bacterial growth occurs on the two days of therapy, followed by a period of five days of slow bacterial growth, and then resuppression. In this manner the level of infection is always held at a low point and an acute exacerbation of the disease does not occur unless an overwhelming bacterial infection takes place. Should this occur, the antibiotic dosage may be increased to a daily program or a different antibiotic may be given as treatment for the acute infection.

Course and Prognosis. Although the disease commences with the hypertrophy in the mucous glands in the bronchi, it frequently progresses to chronic inflammatory changes with fibrosis and structural damage. If adequate treatment is not requested or given, chronic bronchitis may progress into a more severe form of chronic obstructive pulmonary disease with progressive destruction of the alveolar linings of the lung and the capillary bed. With adequate control many patients can be maintained for the rest of their lives without further progression of the illness. The aim of the treatment is to arrest the disease and to prevent the further destruction of tissue.

CHRONIC OBSTRUCTIVE PULMONARY DISEASE (COPD)

Emphysema

Definition. The term "pulmonary emphysema" has been used for many years to define the *clinical* triad characterized by marked shortness of breath with persistent breathlessness even at rest, a chronic cough productive of large quantities of mucoid sputum that may be purulent, and intermittent episodes of expiratory wheezing. This triad of symptoms is nonspecific and can be seen in patients suffering with bronchial asthma as well as chronic bronchitis. By contrast, however, the term "emphysema" refers to a specific morphologic change in the lung that is characterized by overdistention of the alveolar sacs, rupture of the alveolar walls, and the destruction of the alveolar capillary bed. Currently, any patient presenting the above symptoms is diagnosed as having chronic obstructive pulmonary disease (COPD). This title was selected in order to provide a more suitable term for the clinical labeling of this group of patients. Chronic obstructive pulmonary disease can be subdivided into two groups: (1) chronic bronchitis, and (2) generalized obstructive lung disease. The latter is further subdivided into reversible obstructive lung disease, such as asthma, and irreversible or persistent obstructive pulmonary disease of the type pathologically described as pulmonary emphysema. Since the symptoms in asthma, chronic bronchitis, and other obstructive disease may all be present concurrently, the term COPD can encompass the symptoms of all three disease states. Further subdivision is unnecessary for the treatment of the disease and a definitive diagnosis must often await thorough morphologic examination.

Etiology. The exact cause of chronic obstructive pulmonary disease is unknown. The frequent association of chronic bronchitis with the development of severe COPD suggests more than a casual relationship. Those factors previously listed in the section on chronic bronchitis are of obvious importance. These include smoking, respiratory infection, air pollution, and allergy. Although a direct relationship between cigarette smoking and chronic obstructive pulmonary disease has not been established, over 90 per cent of all individuals with this disease are heavy smokers. The constant irritation of the tracheobronchial tree and the suppression of normal ciliary function in the respiratory airways predisposes the respiratory tract to chronic infection. The repeated pulmonary infection can result in alteration of lung structure and destruction of pulmonary tissue. Inner pollutants such as nitrogen dioxide and sulfur dioxide result in chronic irritation of the tracheobronchial linings and may cause permanent changes. The industrial exposure to coal dust, asbestos, cotton fibers, and molds and fungi has resulted in COPD. Hereditary factors have also been incriminated in the causation of COPD. The disease is more prevalent and of greater morbidity and mortality in men than in women. Aging may play a role in the causation of this group of diseases. A normal manifestation of the aging process is overaeration of the lung and enlargement of the alveolar sacs. The destruction of alveolar walls and change in the pulmonary capillary bed has not been noted, however, as part of the aging process.

Pathology. The lungs in chronic obstructive pulmonary disease are large and do not collapse when the thorax is opened. Large air sacs or bullae may be seen over the surface of the lung.

The cut surface of the lung reveals large air spaces everywhere, giving a moth-eaten appearance. On microscopic examination, the walls of the alveoli are broken down, resulting in one large sac rather than multiple small air spaces. The capillary bed previously located within the alveolar walls is destroyed and much of the tissue replaced by fibrous scarring.

Symptoms. Exertional dyspnea is usually the first symptom of COPD. As the disease progresses, the breathlessness may continue even at rest. A chronic cough is invariably present and is productive of mucopurulent sputum. Inspiration is difficult because of the rigid chest cage and the patient must use the accessory muscles of respiration to maintain normal ventilation. Expiration is prolonged, difficult and often accompanied by wheezing. In advanced emphysema, respiratory function is markedly impaired. The appearance of the patient is quite characteristic. He looks drawn, anxious, pale, and speaks in short, jerky sentences. He sits up, often leaning slightly forward, and appears markedly dyspneic. Often the veins in his neck distend during expiration.

In advanced COPD, the patient may have loss of memory, drowsiness, confusion, and loss of judgment. These changes are due to the marked reduction in oxygen reaching the brain, and the increased amount of carbon dioxide in the blood. If untreated, the level of carbon dioxide in the blood may reach toxic levels, resulting in lethargy, stupor, and finally coma. This is called carbon dioxide narcosis.

Diagnosis. A thorough history will usually reveal many of the symptoms of chronic obstructive pulmonary disease. The disease can be diagnosed on the basis of the history alone. Physical examination may reveal classical signs that can be confirmed on x-ray films and fluoroscopy. Tests of pulmonary function may indicate characteristic changes.

Blood gas studies, including the measurement of arterial pH, P_{O_2} (partial pressure of oxygen), P_{CO_2} (partial pressure of carbon dioxide), plasma bicarbonate concentration (HCO_3^-), and arterial oxyhemoglobin saturation, are useful in assessing the state of blood gas exchange across the lung. The more severe the chronic obstructive pulmonary disease, the higher will be the Pa_{CO_2} and the lower the Pa_{O_2} and arterial oxyhemoglobin saturation.

Prevention, Treatment, and Control. The prevention of COPD is directly related to the control of cigarette smoking as well as more effective public health measures against air pollution. Prompt and effective treatment of conditions that predispose to pulmonary obstructive disease is essential. The education of the public in the necessity for medical evaluation of minor respiratory symptoms, such as "morning cough" or "smoker's cough," is important in breaking the chain of events leading to emphysema.

Symptomatic treatment is similar to that in chronic bronchitis. Efforts to increase pulmonary ventilation by reducing bronchospasm include the use of such medications as epinephrine, ephedrine, and aminophylline. Unfortunately, as patients develop advanced states of the disease, the bronchospastic component may be negligible and not responsive to bronchodilator therapy. The use of expectorants, humidity control, and postural drainage is necessary to remove the excess respiratory secretions. The control of infection is important. This may be achieved by measures to increase the individual's resistance, by the avoidance of contact with those suffering with respiratory infection and by the use of antibiotics. It must always be remembered that the lung in COPD is chronically infected. Attempts to eradicate the infection by continuous long-term antibiotic therapy in single or multiple drug combinations are useless. As described in the section on chronic bronchitis, some physicians prefer to give antibiotics on only two consecutive days of the week for suppression of the infection. Because of its broad spectrum nature, tetracycline has been found to be extremely effective for chronic therapy at a dose level of 250 mg. q.i.d. During acute exacerbations of the illness continuous therapy, daily, with tetracycline alone or with additional drugs may be ordered following culture of the sputum. Oxygen may be necessary in severe obstructive disease if the arterial oxyhemoglobin saturation is significantly reduced. However, the use of oxygen in high concentrations can be dangerous if the level of carbon dioxide in the patient's blood has increased. The respiratory center of the brain is usually sensitive to a level of carbon dioxide in the blood and if the level increases slightly, the respiratory rate and the depth increase so as to eliminate the carbon dioxide. If, however, the carbon dioxide level is chronically elevated, the respiratory center becomes insensitive to carbon dioxide changes. Under these circumstances the level of oxygen in the blood becomes a regulatory factor—the hypoxic drive to respiration.

As long as the oxygen saturation of the blood is at a low level, the patient will tend to breathe effectively in order to maintain oxygenation. Should the patient suddenly be given 100 per cent or any other high concentration of oxygen by mask or other means, the hypoxic drive to respiration is lost and the respiratory rate will drop. This leads to the further retention of carbon dioxide, apnea, and death. The safest method for the administration of oxygen for the patient with COPD is either by nasal catheter or cannula, with the oxygen flow rate set at no more than 2 or 3 liters per minute. There is danger in the routine administration of oxygen to patients whose medical history is unknown. If the patient's color improves but he becomes increasingly somnolent, he may be approaching respiratory arrest. (See Chap. 52.)

Intermittent positive pressure with compressed air or oxygen is frequently used to provide a more adequate aeration of the lungs. The many different types of equipment available are divided into two groups. Pressure-cycled equipment is regulated by a gauge on the face of the machine which registers the pressure developed by the on-rushing air in the trachea and the major airways. When the inflow pressure equals the pressure set at the machine, the machine shuts off and expiration starts. The volume of air delivered to the patient is dependent on the generated pressure and may vary from minute to minute in a very sick patient. The volume-cycled respirators do not rely on pressure as a sensing device and are not pressure regulated. The physician simply decides the volume of air to be delivered during each respiratory cycle. This technic insures the continued delivery of a known quantity of air under all circumstances. While the pressure-cycled apparatus may be used with either mask or mouthpiece, volume-cycled equipment can only be effectively applied via a tracheostomy or an endotracheal tube. It is important for the nurse to become familiar with the equipment before undertaking the care of the patient. Information concerning the particular type of equipment in use may be obtained from the physician, the inhalation therapy department, the head nurse, the hospital procedure manual or from information supplied by the manufacturer. (See Chap. 52 for care of the patient on assisted or controlled ventilation.)

As the disease progresses, the patient is forced to curtail more activities, may have to retire early with less pay, and often the male patient may have to relinquish his role as breadwinner to his wife. Impotence due to physical inability or loss of self-esteem or both occurs often in the male, and the femal loses interest also in sex. Fears of death and fear of the unknown predominate. If the patient is not helped by competent medical and nursing care, there is progressive failure of sleep and appetite, loss of weight and physical strength, and lack of interest in activities. These symptoms of depression, a heightened degree of somatic complaints, and diffuse anxiety based upon fear of suffocation are the type of psychopathology manifested by the emphysema patient (Nett and Petty).

Nursing Care of Emphysematous Patients

Nursing care of patients with severe pulmonary emphysema demands a great deal of judgment and skill. These patients have severe limitations on their physical activity. Even moving from bed to chair can cause extreme dyspnea. In contrast with asthmatic patients, whose attacks usually are interspersed with periods of relative well-being, patients with far-advanced pulmonary emphysema receive little respite from their respiratory distress. For many of these patients the severe curtailment of their daily activities and their enforced dependence on others are made more difficult by the realization that their condition is not likely to undergo marked improvement. Helping such patients to live with their disability without resorting to false promises such as, "You'll be fine in a month or two— spry as ever," demands sensitivity and tact. It is essential that the nurse understand what the physician has told the patient concerning his condition and prognosis, so that the patient is spared the added anxiety of receiving conflicting information.

An approach that emphasizes the day-to-day progress, however slight, often helps these patients to continue to follow their treatment. For example, noting that the patient walked to the bathroom this week, whereas last week he found it impossible to do so, can be a point of encouragement. Patients who are highly motivated are better able to profit from whatever treatment is available and, despite their severely damaged lungs, are able to make the best possible use of their remaining pulmonary function.

Because the illness is a discouraging one and one that is believed to be closely linked to smoking, it is essential for the nurse to guard particularly against:

• Adopting an attitude that implies that the patient has, by his smoking, willfully brought the condition on himself.

• Becoming enveloped in the patient's discouragement and, therefore, becoming unable to help him.

Many of these patients express sadness and bitterness at not having been able to stop smoking before illness became incapacitating. Helping such patients to believe that there is some use in trying to stop smoking now and that it is worthwhile to follow the physician's recommendations concerning other aspects of treatment can, in some instances, result in greater symptomatic relief than was originally thought possible.

Therapeutic breathing exercises emphasize the effective use of the diaphragm, thus relieving the compensatory burdens on the muscles of the upper thorax. The patient is taught to let his abdomen rise as he takes a deep breath and to contract the abdominal muscles as he exhales. He can feel whether he is doing the exercise correctly by placing one hand on his chest and the other on his abdomen. During abdominal breathing his chest should remain quiet, and his abdomen should rise and fall with each breath. Other exercises include practice in blowing out candles at various distances and blowing some small object, such as a pencil or a piece of chalk, along a table top. Patients are encouraged to exhale more completely by taking a deep breath and then letting the body bend forward at the waist while they exhale as fully as possible.

Postural drainage helps to remove secretions by gravity. The exact position of the patient during the treatment will depend on the location of the lesions to be drained and will be ordered by the physician. Usually recommended is 5 to 15 minutes three times a day in each prescribed position while inhaling slowly and blowing the breath out through the mouth.

For some patients postural drainage may require the headdown jackknife position but a number of other positions in bed are designed to drain a specific bronchopulmonary segment. For example, the upper lobes are drained in the sitting position. Leaning 30° forward drains the posterior upper lobe segments. A backward lean of 30° drains the anterior segments. If the bed is gatched in the center or two pillows are placed under the patient's hips so that his head is about 30–45° from the general body axis and the

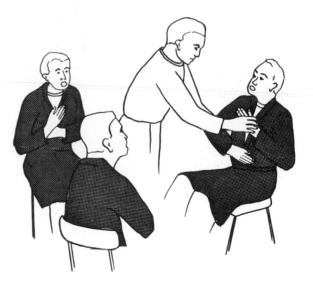

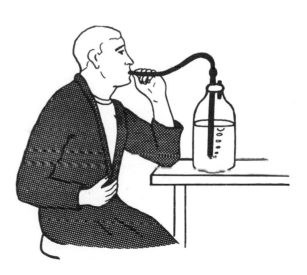

FIG. 24-2. Breathing exercises help to improve the patient's respiratory function. (*Top*) The physical therapist teaches patients abdominal breathing. Placing one hand on his chest and the other on his abdomen helps the patient to recognize when he is doing the exercise correctly. During abdominal breathing the movement of the abdomen is felt with each breath, whereas the chest remains quiet. (*Bottom*) A blow bottle like this one can be prepared easily for use at home or in the hospital. The long glass tube extends below the water and is connected to rubber tubing, through which the patient blows. By taking deep breaths and exhaling, the patient causes the water to bubble vigorously.

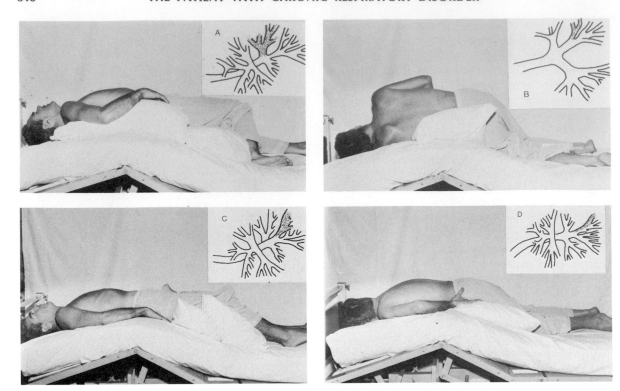

FIG. 24-3. (A) Postural drainage of the right middle lobe of the lung. (B) Postural drainage of the lateral basal segment of the right lower lobe. The patient is placed on the unaffected side. (C) Postural drainage of the anterior basal segment of the right lung and the anterior and medial basal segments of the left lung. (D) Drainage of the posterior segments of the right or left lower lobe bronchi. (Ayers, S. M. and Giannelli, S.: *Care of the Critically Ill,* New York, Appleton-Century-Crofts)

patient is positioned on his abdomen, the posterior lower lobe segments can be drained. Lying on the back in this position drains the anterior lower lobe segments, and lying on either side drains the lower lateral segments.

Patients are assisted as necessary to assume each position and are encouraged to cough between positions. A sputum cup, tissues, and a call bell should be available. Pulmonary physiotherapy measures by a prepared nurse or therapist include gentle shaking or vibrating during expiration over the segment being drained and gentle but firm clapping or percussion with cupped hands on the chest wall over the segment. These measures help to loosen secretions which are then moved by gravity to the trachea where they can be coughed up or suctioned (Rie).

Patients vary in their tolerance for postural drainage. Aged and debilitated patients may need the procedure modified, so that the head is not placed too low, and the length of time that the position is maintained is shorter. Special care and observation of elderly or weak patients is important during and after postural drainage. Observe the patient very frequently, assist him to resume normal position when the treatment is over, and encourage him to rest afterward. Dizziness and falling are especially likely to occur if the patient gets up and if these precautions are not taken. Younger, more vigorous patients may be able to carry out the procedure with little or no assistance after they have done it a few times with the nurse's help.

Mouth care is important after the treatment, because sputum leaves an unpleasant taste and an odor in the mouth. Note the amount and the type of sputum that the patient expectorates during and immediately after the treatment.

Postural drainage should not be attempted after meals, because nausea and vomiting may result from the position and the coughing.

BRONCHIECTASIS

Bronchiectasis is a chronic infectious disease in which structural changes in the bronchial walls result in saccular dilatations of the bronchi. Purulent material collects in these dilated areas. The expulsive power of the affected areas is diminished, and the purulent material tends to remain in the dilated bronchi.

Etiology. Infection is the principal cause. Bronchopneumonia and chronic sinusitis may be precursors of bronchiectasis. Congenital weakness of the bronchi may be a contributing factor. The disease often begins in early adulthood and frequently has a long slowly progressive course.

Symptoms. Patients with bronchiectasis cough and expectorate foul, greenish-yellow sputum. Coughing is most severe when the patient changes position, as on arising in the morning or lying down at night. The amount of sputum produced in one paroxysm varies with the stage of the disease. It may be 200 ml. or more. The expectoration of the foul sputum leaves an unpleasant odor in the mouth and on the breath, making frequent oral hygiene especially necessary. Fatigue, loss of weight and anorexia are common. *Hemoptysis* may occur. Usually, the symptoms develop gradually.

Diagnosis. The diagnosis of bronchiectasis requires bronchography.

Treatment. The treatment of bronchiectasis includes drainage of the purulent material from the bronchi. Antibiotics are used to control infection.

If bronchiectasis is confined to a relatively small portion of the lung, a cure may be achieved by surgical removal of the diseased portion. Medical treatment is palliative, since the damaged bronchi do not return to normal. For patients with extensive disease of both lungs, this is the only treatment possible.

EMPYEMA

Empyema is a general term used to denote pus in a body cavity. However, it usually refers to pus within the thoracic cavity (thoracic empyema). Empyema results from infection, which causes the formation of pus. Infection may follow trauma or pre-existing diseases, such as pneumonia, tuberculosis or lung abscess. Before the introduction of antibiotics, empyema was a frequent complication of pneumonia. Symptoms of empyema include fever, pain in the chest, dyspnea and malaise. Diagnosis is made by roentgenogram and by aspiration of purulent fluid during thoracentesis.

Initial treatment often consists of antibiotics, given both parenterally and into the pleural space, and aspiration of pus by thoracentesis. Sometimes closed drainage of the empyema cavity is used. Open drainage may be used when pus is very thick, and when the walls of the empyema cavity are strong enough to keep the lung from collapsing during the time that the chest is opened. One or more soft rubber tubes may be placed in the opening to promote drainage. The wound then is covered by a large absorbent dressing that is changed as it is necessary. The drainage of the pus results in a fall in temperature and general symptomatic improvement.

If empyema is inadequately treated, it may become chronic. A thick coating may form over the lung, preventing its expansion. Decortication (removal of the coating) allows the lung to re-expand.

LUNG ABSCESS

An abscess, a localized area of suppuration, may occur in the lung as a result of the aspiration of a foreign body or of respiratory secretions after surgery. Lung abscesses also may follow pneumonia or a mechanical obstruction of the bronchi, such as that due to cancer. The prevention of lung abscess involves the avoidance of the aspiration of secretions by patients who are unconscious and the avoidance and the prompt treatment of obstructions and infections in the respiratory tract.

Symptoms of lung abscess include chills, fever, weight loss and cough productive of purulent or bloody sputum. Clubbing of the fingers often occurs in chronic cases.

The treatment of lung abscess involves the drainage of the abscess, the control of infection and measures to increase the body's resistance. Sometimes, postural drainage and the use of antibiotics prove sufficient; in other instances, surgical drainage of the abscess may be necessary. The portion of the lung containing the abscess may be removed surgically.

PNEUMOCONIOSIS

Pneumoconiosis is an inclusive term used to describe any disease of the lung caused by the inhalation of dust. It usually refers to diseases caused by inhalation of silica (silicosis) or asbestos (asbestosis). Pneumoconiosis is common among persons who work in industries in which exposure to these substances is prolonged, such as mining, stonecutting and manufacture of products using asbestos.

Only the tiny particles of dust reach the lung; the larger ones are trapped in the respiratory passages. Therefore, the tiny particles are the most hazardous; they cause irritation and gradual fibrosis of lung tissue. The lung tissue loses its elasticity: reduced vital capacity, with dyspnea and cough, results. Tuberculosis has a very high incidence among persons who have silicosis. The diagnosis of pneumoconiosis is based on the history of exposure (usually over a prolonged period), roentgenography and pulmonary function studies.

CANCER OF THE LUNG

Incidence. Carcinoma of the lung has shown marked increase in incidence during the last several decades. More accurate diagnosis may be partly responsible; increasing numbers of older persons in the population, the popularity of cigarette smoking, and increasing air pollution in industrial centers may be other factors contributing to increased incidence. Carcinoma of the lung is approximately 6 times more common in men than in women. Most patients are over 40 when the disease is discovered. It has been noted that the incidence of carcinoma of the lung is especially high among those who suffer from chronic bronchitis, and that many of these chronic bronchitis sufferers have been heavy smokers for many years.

Pathology and Symptoms. Bronchogenic carcinoma, a malignant tumor arising from the bronchial epithelium, is the most common type of lung cancer. The tumor usually produces no symptoms at first; however, as it enlarges, the patient may experience cough productive of mucopurulent or blood-streaked sputum. The cough may be slight at first and be disregarded or attributed to smoking. As the disease advances, the patient experiences fatigue, weight loss and anorexia. Dyspnea and chest pain occur late in the disease. Hemoptysis is not uncommon.

Diagnosis. An early diagnosis of cancer of the lung is difficult, since symptoms often do not appear until the condition is well-established. Routine chest roentgenograms, particularly in persons over 40, are recommended as part of the physical examination to detect carcinoma of the lung in the early, asymptomatic stage. Other diagnostic measures include bronchoscopy, biopsy, examination of sputum and surgical exploration.

Treatment. Surgical removal of the malignant tissue offers the only type of cure and usually is successful only in the early stages of the disease. Depending on the size and the location of the tumor, lobectomy or pneumonectomy may be performed. Radiation therapy may be helpful in slowing the spread of the disease and in providing symptomatic relief. Chemotherapy is used to slow the course of the disease and to alleviate symptoms.

Course and Prognosis. The prognosis is poor unless the condition is treated early. Since cancer of the lung presents few warning symptoms during the period when cure is possible, the mortality rate is high. Metastasis occurs to the mediastinal and cervical lymph nodes, the esophagus and the opposite lung. The patient with advanced carcinoma of the lung with metastases is very ill. Marked wasting of tissues, pain, dyspnea and cough are present.

POSTOPERATIVE CARE OF CHEST-SURGERY PATIENTS

Special Postoperative Nursing Measures

In addition to the general principles of postoperative care that apply to any patient who has had surgery, the opening of the thoracic cavity requires certain special postoperative nursing measures. Preoperative care of this group of patients is similar to that of other preoperative patients. However, because of the specialized procedures that the patient experiences postoperatively, and because his participation is essential to the success of his postoperative regimen, giving careful instruction to the patient concerning what to expect postoperatively is especially important. The array of special equipment required for postoperative care can be very frightening if the patient does not understand its purpose, and that its use after chest surgery is usual and does not indicate the development of complications.

One particularly significant problem in relation to chest surgery is the interference with normal pressure relationships within the thoracic cavity. When the chest is opened, the air from the atmosphere rushes in, due to the negative pressure which normally exists in the thoracic cavity. The entrance of air under atmospheric pressure collapses the lung, causing serious impairment of respiratory function. By administering anesthesia and necessary oxygen through an endotracheal tube, collapse of the lung is prevented in spite of the opening of the chest.

Chest Drainage

After chest surgery it is usually necessary to drain secretions and blood continuously from the thoracic cavity. Accumulation of blood and other fluids within the chest would prevent the necessary re-expansion of the lung. Drainage ordinarily must be carried out by the closed (underwater) method. An open drainage system would allow air to enter the thoracic cavity, for the air would be sucked in every time the rib cage expanded. The air entering from the atmosphere would collapse the lung further. Open drainage of the thoracic cavity, which permits air to flow back into the chest, is used only when adhesions have formed that prevent the collapse of the lung.

Closed drainage of the thoracic cavity is accomplished by means of a catheter placed in the pleural space during surgery. Postoperatively it is allowed to drain under water into a bottle. By keeping the end of the drainage tube always under water, air is prevented from being drawn up through the catheter to the pleural space. A sterile drainage bottle, into which a measured amount (usually 500 ml.) of sterile water has been poured, is used for this purpose. The drainage bottle is connected by rubber tubing with a control (trap) bottle, used to regulate the amount of suction being applied. The trap bottle is connected by rubber tubing with a suction device, such as a wall suction outlet. The doctor regulates the amount of suction being applied by adjusting the position of a tube in the control (trap) bottle. The length that this tube is submerged under water in the trap bottle determines the amount of suction applied. The trap bottle is used because usually the amount of suction applied by the ordinary suction device is too great to be applied to the chest catheter. Therefore, the trap bottle lessens to the desired extent the degree of suction applied. The water in the trap bottle (in contrast with that in the chest drainage bottle) need not be sterile.

Any break in the system, either from the tubing becoming loose or from the bottles being broken, would present the hazard of air entering the tubing and being drawn up to the pleural space. All connections of stoppers and tubing are taped carefully to minimize the possibility,

for instance, of having the end of a catheter slip off a glass connecting tip. Placing the drainage bottle in a holder is another precaution. The holder helps to protect the bottles from being knocked over and broken. More elaborate devices also are available to hold the bottles. A clamp always must be in readiness so that, if any break in the system occurs, the chest tube immediately can be clamped as close to the chest wall as possible. The clamp is placed where it can be easily seen.

Preventing fluids from flowing up through the catheter and entering the pleural space also is essential. While connected for drainage, the chest drainage bottle **never** is raised from floor level. Raising the bottle could result in a flow of fluid to the pleural space.

Often 2 chest catheters are used—1 anteriorly and 1 posteriorly. In this instance 2 bottles are used into which the chest drainage flows, and each is labeled *anterior* or *posterior*. Two clamps are kept in readiness in case of any break in the drainage systems—1 for each chest catheter. The amount and the character of the drainage in each bottle is noted and recorded separately.

The principles illustrated here are essentially the same even though the nurse may see different kinds of chest drainage apparatus. Commercial products are becoming available which are safer for the patient because they are designed to prevent backflow of air into the chest space.

The drainage tube must be patent to allow for the necessary escape of fluids from the pleural space. Clogging of the catheter, which may occur if a blood clot lodges in it, or if it becomes kinked, will cause the drainage to stop. This will prevent the lung from re-expanding normally, and it may cause the position of the heart and the great vessels to shift (mediastinal shift). In the first hours immediately after surgery the nurse is constantly alert to the functioning of the drainage system so that, if a malfunction should occur, precious minutes will not be lost in correcting it.

The fluid in the long glass tube in the drainage bottle will fluctuate with each respiration, and bubbling will occur in the drainage bottle if the system is working properly. Failure of the fluid to fluctuate in the long glass tube may mean that the catheter is clogged, or that the lung has completely re-expanded. During the early postoperative period the former possibility is more likely. In some hospitals, milking the drainage tube from the patient toward the drainage bottle to remove an obstruction is considered a nursing responsibility. If drainage is not resumed by milking the tube, notify the doctor at once. A roentgenogram (made by a portable machine) may be ordered to determine whether the failure of the fluid to fluctuate is due to re-expansion of the lung.

It is important to check the color and the amount of the chest drainage frequently and to note the condition of the dressings over the operative area. Although some bloody drainage is expected through the catheter postoperatively, it should not appear bright red or be copious. In some hospitals, measuring and emptying the drainage bottles is a nursing function; in others, the doctor assumes this responsibility. If the nurse is to empty the drainage bottle, she first should clamp the chest catheter close to the patient's chest. The stopper then is removed from the bottle and the contents measured.

It is important to subtract from the total amount of drainage the amount of sterile water originally placed in the bottle. A sterile bottle to which sterile solution has been added to cover the end of the drainage tube is placed in position, the stopper inserted and the clamp removed from the chest catheter. Drainage must be re-instituted promptly, so that the catheter does not become clogged or the necessary drainage delayed.

Effect on the Patient

What does the patient see when he regains consciousness? Usually he sees a transfusion running, several drainage bottles beside his bed, suction equipment, and oxygen. He has a tube running into his nose (for oxygen), tubes running out of his chest, and a tube carrying fluids into a vein in his arm. Many other types of equipment also may be in use, such as monitoring devices which continuously record his ECG on a screen, hypothermia equipment, and a monitoring device which indicates his rectal temperature.

Patients who have had chest surgery need nurses who are familiar with the equipment, who have operated it enough to be at ease with it, and who can center their attention on the patient, using the machines as tools rather than concentrating so narrowly on operating the machines that the patient is forgotten. The nurse's manner of sureness and confidence as she performs necessary tasks can convey a feeling of confidence to the patient which no words, in the absence of such sureness of technical skill, can convey.

NURSING CARE OF PATIENTS WITH CHRONIC RESPIRATORY DISORDERS

The nursing care of patients with chronic respiratory disorders requires patience, attention to detail and the ability to maintain interest and hope when progress is slow.

The patient's *general health* is important in his struggle with chronic respiratory illness. It is important to teach him and his family the principles of optimum nutrition and to help them to plan for rest, recreation and suitable work. Often these patients feel there is little use in trying these measures, and an important aspect of nursing care involves communicating the belief that treatment is worthwhile. Most of the gains will come about slowly, as a result of prolonged and painstaking effort in the maintenance of general health, regular visits to the doctor or the clinic and faithful following of instruction concerning medications, breathing exercises, rest, activity and avoidance of infection. Helping the patient to establish a regular routine, whether he is cared for in the hospital or at home, is important in helping him to maintain therapy over long periods. It is not unusual for these patients to follow the treatment carefully for the first few days or weeks and then gradually to abandon it when dramatic improvement does not ensue.

Smoking is contraindicated in chronic respiratory disease.

Observation of the patient for changes in symptoms is necessary. It is important to note the amount of coughing, the amount and the character of sputum, the degree of dyspnea and/or wheezing, as well as the patient's color, weight and appetite. Instructing him in oral hygiene and helping him to carry this out before meals may improve his appetite, particularly if he is raising considerable sputum.

The patient's *attitude* is very important in his improvement. Sometimes, emotional factors have played an important part in causing the disease. Whether or not this is the case, prolonged breathing difficulty often causes feelings of helplessness and despair. Patients who have formerly been active and self-sufficient often feel severely crippled by their inability to walk up a flight of stairs without gasping for breath. The fact that the disability is less immediately obvious than the amputation of a limb makes it no less distressing to the patient.

In collaboration with the physician and others who care for the patient, the nurse may help him *to adjust his activities* within the framework of his tolerance. Although it is undesirable for the patient to undertake strenuous exertion, neither is it wise for him to abandon all his interests and his activities. The latter course rapidly leads to invalidism. Adjustments in the patient's schedule can help him to continue his accustomed activities.

For example, one man with chronic bronchitis arranged to work from 10 A.M. to 6 P.M. rather than from 8 A.M. to 4 P.M., because the early morning hours were especially difficult for him. He almost invariably experienced prolonged, severe coughing and some dyspnea for an hour or two after arising. Starting work later gave him an opportunity to recover from these symptoms before going to work. Had he not been able to adjust his hours of work, he could have gone to bed earlier, and arisen an hour or two earlier each morning, to allow time to get over the coughing.

The nurse must carefully observe the patient for *complications and progression of his illness.* Increased dyspnea, cough and sputum are important, as are symptoms of respiratory infection, such as chills and fever. Right heart failure (cor pulmonale) may occur because of the increased resistance in the pulmonary vascular bed, which in turn increases the work of the right ventricle. Symptoms of heart failure include edema and cyanosis, as well as dyspnea, orthopnea and cough.

REFERENCES AND BIBLIOGRAPHY

AMERICAN THORACIC SOCIETY, COMMITTEE ON THERAPY: Principles of respiratory care, *Am. Rev. Resp. Dis.* 95:327, February, 1967.

ASHENBURG, N. J.: The effects of air pollution on health, *Nurs. Outlook* 16:22, February, 1968.

BASS, H., *et al.*: Exercise training: therapy for patients with chronic obstructive pulmonary disease, *Chest* 57:116, 1970.

BELINKOFF, S.: *Introduction to Inhalation Therapy,* Boston, Little, Brown, 1969.

BENDIXEN, H. H., *et al.*: *Respiratory Care,* St. Louis, Mosby, 1965.

BLOCK, V. C.: Helping the patient to ventilate, *Nurs. Outlook* 17:31, October, 1969.

EGAN, D.: *Fundamentals of Inhalation Therapy,* St. Louis, Mosby, 1969.

FOLEY, M. F.: Pulmonary function testing, *Am. J. Nurs.* 71:1134, June, 1971.

FRIEDMAN, A.: The patient with chronic obstructive lung disease and his care at home, *Nurs. Clin. N. Am.* 3:437, September, 1968.

GIBBON, J. H., JR., *et al.*: *Surgery of the Chest,* ed. 2, Philadelphia, Saunders, 1969.

HARGRAVES, A.: Emotional problems of patients with respiratory disease, *Nurs. Clin. N. Am.* 3:479, September, 1968.

HELMING, M.: Nursing care of patients with chronic obstructive lung disease, *Nurs. Clin. N. Am.* 3:413, September, 1968.

KINNEY, M.: Rehabilitation of patients with COLD, *Am. J. Nurs.* 67:2528, December, 1967.

KURIHARA, M.: Postural drainage, clapping, and vibrating, *Am. J. Nurs.* 67:76, November, 1965.

LEVINE, E. R.: Inhalation therapy—aerosols and intermittent positive pressure breathing, *Med. Clin. N. Am.* 51:307, 1967.

MASFERRER, R.: Role of patient instruction in improving IPPB treatments, *Inhal. Therapy* 14:17, 1969.

MUSHIN, W., *et al.*: *Automatic Ventilation of the Lungs,* ed. 2, Philadelphia, Davis, 1969.

NETT, L., and PETTY, T. L.: Why emphysema patients are the way they are, *Am. J. Nurs.* 70:1251, June, 1970.

PETTY, T. L., *et al.*: A comprehensive care program for chronic airway obstruction, *Ann. Intern. Med.* 70:1109, June, 1969.

————: A new, simple IPPB device for hospital and home use, *JAMA* 203:871, March, 1968.

Pulmonary care unit, *Am. J. Nurs.* 70:1255, June, 1970.

RIE, M. W.: Physical therapy in the nursing care of respiratory disease patients, *Nurs. Clin. N. Am.* 3:463, September, 1968.

SAFER, P. (ed.): *Respiratory Therapy,* Philadelphia, Davis, 1965.

SCHWAID, M.: The impact of emphysema, *Am. J. Nurs.* 70:1247, June, 1970.

Smoking and Health, United States Department of Health, Education, and Welfare, Public Health Service, Public Health Service Publication No. 1103, U.S. Government Printing Office, 1964.

TRAVER, G.: Patients, nurses, and chronic respiratory diseases. The nursing assessment, New York, NLN Publication No. 45-1334, 18, 1968.

The Patient with Pulmonary Tuberculosis 25

Incidence and Predisposing Factors • Attitudes Toward Tuberculosis
Etiology • Protection of Personnel • Pathology • Signs and
Symptoms • Diagnosis • Treatment • Complications • Care in
General Hospitals • Rehabilitation • Casefinding and Control

INCIDENCE AND PREDISPOSING FACTORS

The number of people who react positively to tuberculin has declined sharply in this country. It has been estimated that 13 per cent of the population of the United States has a positive reaction to tuberculin; the majority of these positive reactors are over 45 years old (NTRDA).* In contrast, widespread infection with the tubercle bacillus, starting early in life, used to exist in many areas of the United States, and still exists in many of the underdeveloped nations, and in the poverty-ridden sections of large cities in industrialized countries.

Dramatic improvement in the mortality rate from tuberculosis has taken place within the lifetime of people still alive. In 1902 tuberculosis was the leading cause of death in the U.S.; in 1966 it ranked 20th as a cause of death (NTRDA). The death rate from tuberculosis has declined markedly in recent years. For example, there were 10,866 deaths from tuberculosis reported in the U.S. in 1960. In 1967 the figure was reduced to 6,901 (NTRDA). This marked reduction in mortality has led some people to the false assumption that tuberculosis is no longer an important health problem. Although progress has been made in fighting tuberculosis, the disease is by no means conquered. Case rates have declined much more slowly than death rates.

Resistance to the disease varies considerably with age. Infants and very young children have poor resistance to the infection, and with the onset of puberty there is a marked rise in the incidence of tuberculosis. However, since an increasingly high incidence of tuberculosis is being found among older people, tuberculosis can no longer be considered a disease primarily of adolescents and young adults. As age advances, men have a higher death rate from the disease than do women. Men also have a higher case rate; of all reported cases, 66 per cent are men (NTRDA). The reasons for these differences are not clear. However, it has been suggested that, because the disease is closely linked to health practices, homeless men and men who live alone may be especially vulnerable to the illness because of poor dietary habits. It also has been postulated that men have greater exposure to the disease than do women because of their greater incidence of employment outside the home.

In the United States, nonwhite persons have a case rate of tuberculosis more than four times that of white persons (NTRDA). This difference usually is attributed to less advantageous social and economic conditions among nonwhite persons.

The fact that tuberculosis is more common among persons of low social and economic status reflects the effects of poorer living standards. Overcrowding and poor hygienic conditions make the spread of the disease more likely.

Tuberculosis morbidity and mortality differ widely in different sections of the country. The highest incidence tends to occur in the most densely populated areas.

* National Tuberculosis and Respiratory Disease Association.

324

Diabetics have a higher incidence of tuberculosis than do nondiabetics, presumably due to their diminished resistance to this infection.

The incidence of tuberculosis is especially high among alcoholics because of health and social problems associated with alcoholism—for example, malnutrition. In recent years there has been a considerable shift in the incidence of tuberculosis in relation to social and economic status. There has been a decline in the incidence of tuberculosis among those who are socially and economically advantaged, and a high incidence among the socially and economically deprived—so much so that tuberculosis is now often described as a "social disease with medical overtones."

ATTITUDES TOWARD TUBERCULOSIS

Fear and shame were common reactions to tuberculosis in the past, as were feelings of being "unclean," and of guilt over the possibility of spread of the disease to others. While such reactions still occur, they are not as widespread today. These changes in attitude stem from the vastly improved outlook for tuberculosis patients, and from changes in therapy. For instance, it is no longer necessary for most patients with tuberculosis to have extended care in a sanatorium, nor is it common nowadays for them to give up their usual jobs. Most patients can resume their accustomed activities and relationships promptly enough to avoid the major upheaval in personal and vocational life which used to be common among patients with tuberculosis, who were sometimes confined to a sanatorium for several years. Changes in protective technics have had an effect, too, on attitudes toward this disease. No longer are most patients cared for by staff swathed in cap, mask and gown, nor do they see the letters they have written and the books they have read placed on a window ledge to air for several days!

Nevertheless, the recollection of older forms of treatment and of a less hopeful outlook for recovery remains vivid among some older people, who in turn influence attitudes of younger people. It is not unusual, therefore, for the nurse to find that her patients' and their families' attitudes toward tuberculosis may be related more to past experiences (either their own, or those of others) than to current realities. An important task of the nurse involves listening to the views of patients and their families concerning tuberculosis, and helping them obtain up-to-date information about the disease and its treatment. A similar appraisal of her own attitudes is necessary for the nurse, too, so that she does not unwittingly convey to patients an attitude of unwarranted pessimism, and an over-concern with future restriction of life patterns and goals, which may not become necessary, and so that she does not burden herself with exaggerated fears of contracting the disease.

ETIOLOGY

The presence of *Mycobacterium tuberculosis,* the tubercle bacillus, is a necessary cause of the disease, but usually it is not the only cause. In contrast with the number of people who have at some time been infected with the tubercle bacillus, only a very small proportion ever become ill from tuberculosis.

Many factors predispose to the development of tuberculosis. When the body's resistance is lowered, such as through inadequate rest and poor nutrition, or when the organisms are sufficiently virulent and numerous, the clinical disease may develop.

Emotional factors also may play an important part in lowering the body's resistance to disease. Anxiety, tension and unhappiness may contribute to the development of tuberculosis by upsetting the body's metabolic and physiologic balance.

Although predisposing factors in the physical and the emotional life of the individual are important, it is still true that infection with the tubercle bacillus is necessary to the development of the disease. Some understanding of this organism and of the ways of controlling its spread is essential to the nurse in protecting herself and others. Tubercle bacilli are aerobic, gram-positive and acid-fast. They are rod-shaped and can be identified by microscopic examination of sputum and other body substances. Although tuberculosis occurs in many species, including birds, cattle and swine, the types of organisms that are imporant sources of human infection are the bovine and the human.

Infection with the bovine type was once quite common, but it is now relatively rare in many countries, including our own, due to the eradication of tuberculosis in cattle and to the pasteurization of milk and milk products. Infection with the human-type tubercle bacillus occurs most commonly from prolonged close contact with persons who have active tuberculosis. Ordinarily, tuberculosis is not contracted from brief exposure (as measles can be, for example). Particular danger exists in family groups in which one member has undiagnosed active tuberculosis and, also, in work settings where a co-worker has active but undiscovered disease. The danger is intensified if ventilation and sanitation are poor and if crowding exists.

Although the bacilli can live in the dark for months in particles of dried sputum, exposure to direct sunlight kills them in a few hours. The organism is difficult to kill with ordinary disinfectants. Tubercle bacilli are killed by pasteurization (30 minutes at 62° C.), a process widely used in preventing the spread of tuberculosis by milk and milk products. Boiling for 5 minutes destroys the bacilli. Although organisms are found most commonly in the sputum, they may be found also in the feces and the urine, in pus from tuberculous osteomyelitis and in milk from tuberculous cows.

Tuberculous infection is spread most commonly by direct contact with a person with active disease, through the inhalation of the droplets from coughing, sneezing and spitting. By far the most important means of spread is inhalation of organisms. The disease is primarily airborne, a point of relevance for protective technics.

Bacilli are borne on tiny particles called "droplet nuclei" that remain suspended in the air after being discharged in respiratory secretions of an infected person. The droplet nuclei circulate in the air, where they can be inhaled by a heretofore uninfected individual, and become implanted in his lung.

PROTECTION OF PERSONNEL

Various technics have been established for protecting hospital personnel from infection. It is important for the nurse to familiarize herself with the details practiced in each particular setting, since protective technics are ineffective unless they are consistently practiced by all personnel. In medical as well as in surgical asepsis each practitioner, whether doctor, nurse, orderly or maid, depends on the others for meticulous attention to such matters as hand washing and handling of sputum cups. Knowing whether the patient's sputum or excreta contain tubercle bacilli forms the rational basis for the use of precautions. No protective technic is required, other than the usual hygienic measures employed with any patient, when the patient's body is not discharging organisms. Therefore, patients

with arrested disease may mingle freely with others both within the hospital and later when they resume living in the community.

Protective Technics

Patient Education. Teaching patients with positive sputum to cover their noses and mouths while they are coughing or sneezing, to expectorate into sputum cups and to wash their hands afterward is highly effective in preventing the spread of droplet infection to nurses and other hospital personnel.

Chemotherapy. Also, modern drug treatment greatly reduces the risk of infection among hospital personnel. By controlling the patient's disease the chance of the spread of the organisms to others is lessened. It has been found that effective chemotherapy promptly (within weeks or even earlier) reduces the hazard of spread of the disease, even before smears and cultures become negative.

Face masks are being considered less necessary in protection of personnel. When face masks are used (as may be the case, for instance, when a seriously ill, newly admitted patient is being cared for, who cannot "cover his cough" and who is just commencing drug therapy) plastic masks are considered safer than cotton masks. If a mask is used, it should cover the wearer's nose and mouth, and it should be discarded immediately after use. In some instances, when staff are working closely with a patient who has positive sputum, a mask is placed over the patient's nose and mouth during the period of close contact.

Gowns are used much less frequently now in care of patients with tuberculosis. Since the infection is primarily air-borne, protective measures are aimed at preventing contamination of the air, and decontaminating infected air. Linen and other fomites are no longer considered significant sources of infection (NTRDA).

Combating Airborne Infection. The air, both in the immediate vicinity of the patient and at some distance from him, is the greatest source of danger in spread of tuberculosis.

The air becomes contaminated by tubercle bacilli when the patient with active tuberculosis, who has positive sputum, coughs, sneezes, laughs and talks. These tiny droplets of moisture emanate from the noses and mouths of all persons, but, in the case of the patient with tuberculosis, these droplets contain tubercle bacilli. The tiny drops of moisture dry, and become droplet nuclei, which are so small and light that they remain suspended and travel about in air currents. The tubercle bacilli, thus suspended in the air, can be breathed into the lungs of another person, where they initiate infection.

Replacing contaminated air with fresh air by ventilation, exposure of the air in the vicinity of infectious patients to ultraviolet light, which kills the tubercle bacilli, and teaching the patient to cover his nose and mouth when sneezing or coughing, all serve to counter the spread of infection by contaminated air. The National Tuberculosis and Respiratory Disease Association recommends that ultraviolet light be used in rooms where newly admitted patients with active tuberculosis are being treated, and in areas where patients whose conditions have not yet been diagnosed are treated (such as the emergency room).

Disposal of Sputum. Safe disposal of sputum is an important consideration. In many instances the patient is taught to expectorate into tissues, and to place them in a special container. These containers of contaminated tissues are later collected and burned. When it is necessary to observe the amount and color of sputum, the patient is provided with a sputum cup. When the sputum is disposed of, an absorbent material such as sawdust is first placed in the cup. Then the disposable sputum cup is wrapped and put into a separate container until it is burned.

Hand Washing. Although hand washing is important in the care of all patients, it is especially necessary when caring for patients with tuberculosis. Hands should be thoroughly washed after touching the patient or any of his equipment, to provide for the mechanical removal of the organisms from your skin. Such habits as putting the hands in the mouth or chewing on tips of pencils should be avoided. Effective hand washing is facilitated by keeping the nails short and clean and by not wearing jewelry on the hands when giving care.

Other Measures for Preventing Spread. Fomites are not now considered to be significant sources of infection, and routine procedures for airing fomites (such as books the patient has read) on a window ledge for several hours are being discarded (NTRDA).

The practice of using paper dishes for patients with tuberculosis is now considered unnecessary (Ream). Particularly in hospitals, but in all public eating places, careful technics of food service are important to prevent spread of infection. When safe technics, such as the proper tempera-

ture of wash and rinse water in dishwashing machines are used, there is no necessity for elaborate special precautions for food service of patients with tuberculosis (Ream).

Variations in Protective Practices. In many hospitals, protective technics have not changed in accordance with current knowledge about the transmission of tuberculosis (Ream). Reliance on caps and masks for protection, overconcern about the hazards of fomites, and insufficient attention to more effective methods of control, such as decontamination of air, are common (Ream). Remember that the disease is primarily *air-borne,* and that therefore the protective technics used must be aimed at lessening the problem of contaminated air. The air at some distance from the patient (such as at the nurse's station) is not necessarily safe, since droplet nuclei travel on air currents. See that good ventilation is used, and work with others in promoting use of ultraviolet light in areas where newly admitted infectious patients are being treated. Wash your hands thoroughly after contact with these patients, as with all others.

Changes in protective technics have important advantages for patients as well as for staff. The decreasing use of gowns and masks helps patients to feel more accepted, as does the growing practice of permitting ambulatory patients to use attractively furnished lounges. Eliciting the patient's cooperation in preventing spread of infection, such as "covering his cough" conveys greater respect for him than measures which deny him a role in helping to provide a safe environment for others.

PATHOLOGY

Tubercle bacilli are inhaled into the respiratory passages, or they may be ingested and travel by way of blood and lymph to the lungs. Transmission of the human-type tubercle bacillus is primarily through the respiratory passages; transmission of the bovine-type tubercle bacillus mainly by ingestion of contaminated food, such as milk from infected cows. Tuberculosis most frequently affects the lungs, and sometimes the organisms may be carried by the circulatory system to other organs, such as bones, kidneys or fallopian tubes. Tissue sensitivity or allergy, manifested by a positive tuberculin reaction, develops about 6 weeks after the initial infection. Although the intensity of the allergic response is not a measure of immunity, these two factors are believed to be related closely.

When the tubercle bacilli enter the lung, they set up a small focus of infection often referred to as a *primary infection*. Usually, healing occurs by fibrosis and calcification; subsequent roentgenograms may reveal such calcified nodules. The individual may experience no symptoms during this process, or he may experience briefly malaise, chills and fever. The fact that primary infection has occurred may be discovered later by a routine tuberculin test or a roentgenogram.

Unlike many other infections, which result in prompt symptoms and subsequent elimination of the infection, infection with the tubercle bacillus may remain dormant for many years. Organisms may remain within the body and, for reasons not fully understood, later cause active disease. It is thought that activation of a dormant infection may be related to stress. A person with an inactive infection may develop active tubeculosis years later, perhaps in response to fatigue, malnutrition or emotional strain.

If individual resistance is low, if the organisms are very virulent or numerous, or if contact is repeated and prolonged, the focus of infection may enlarge and undergo *caseation,* a form of necrosis with a cheeselike appearance. This area of caseation may slough away, leaving a cavity in the lung. The caseating focus may rupture into a bronchus, causing acute tuberculous pneumonia, or into a blood vessel. In the latter instance massive infection of the bloodstream may result in the spread of many small foci of infection throughout the lungs (a phenomenon called *miliary tuberculosis*) as well as spread, via the blood, to distant parts of the body. Bronchial dissemination of the infection results from the inhalation of the bacilli into healthy alveoli during breathing. The more the disease spreads, the more difficult and prolonged the treatment is, and the more uncertain the prognosis. Lesions of tuberculosis heal slowly.

Reinfection, or *secondary infection,* may occur from a new infection entering the body from outside (*exogenous*), or it may result from the reactivation of a previous infection within the body (*endogenous*). It is possible for live tubercle bacilli to continue to exist within an apparently healed lesion for long periods. A patient who has seemed to recover from the disease may have another outbreak if his resistance is decreased.

SIGNS AND SYMPTOMS

The onset of tuberculosis is insidious, and early symptoms vary somewhat from person to person. For a long time the patient may have no symptoms at all; indeed, he may feel well. The problem of early diagnosis is made more difficult by the widespread belief that people with tuberculosis always look sick—thin, pale, gaunt. Actually, these symptoms often do not appear until the disease is well advanced. This fact further emphasizes the need for routine examinations for the detection of tuberculosis.

The early symptoms of tuberculosis are often vague, and they may be readily dismissed. Fatigue, anorexia, weight loss and slight, nonproductive cough are all symptoms that can be attributed to overwork, excessive smoking or poor eating habits; however, they are also early symptoms of tuberculosis. Elevation of temperature, particularly in the late afternoon and the evening, and night sweats are frequent as the disease progresses. The cough often becomes productive of mucopurulent and blood-streaked sputum. Hemoptysis, the coughing up of blood, may occur. Occasionally, it is the first symptom of the disease. Marked weakness and wasting are characteristic of later stages of the illness; dyspnea may be a late symptom. Chest pain may result from the spread of infection to the pleura.

DIAGNOSIS

Diagnostic tests for tuberculosis consist chiefly of tuberculin tests, chest roentgenograms and examinations of sputum and other body substances.

Tuberculin Tests

The use of tuberculin tests is based on the fact that, after the body has been invaded by the tubercle bacilli, tissue sensitivity or allergy develops gradually in about 6 weeks. A positive tuberculin test is evidence that a tuberculous infection has existed at some time, somewhere in the body. In relation to tuberculosis the word *infection* is used to indicate that the organisms have entered the body and the body has reacted to them. This may or may not lead to active disease. Since most such infections with the tubercle bacillus do not result in disease, a positive test is not necessarily an indication of the development of active clinical disease.

The chief value of tuberculin testing lies in case finding and control of tuberculosis. By means of tuberculin tests it is possible to discover which persons have been infected by the tubercle bacillus and to perform further tests on them to determine whether clinical disease is present. Tuberculin tests are also of value in prevention of active clinical disease, because those persons who have had recent conversion from a negative to a positive tuberculin reaction are now usually given isoniazid to help to prevent the development of clinical tuberculosis.

The Mantoux Test. Tuberculin may be administered in several ways. The most accurate, since an accurately measured dose can be given, is the Mantoux test. Two types of tuberculin are in use: old tuberculin (OT), which contains some impurities; and purified protein derivative (PPD), a substance made by a newer process that produces a purified, stable substance. Purified protein derivative is used most frequently today. Given intracutaneously, 0.0001 mg. of PPD (often referred to as "intermediate strength") is used widely.

The intracutaneous injection usually is given into the palmar surface of the forearm. The tip of the needle is inserted between the layers of the skin, and a small amount (usually 0.1 ml.) of solution is injected. A whitish raised area appears as the solution is injected. The test is read 48 to 72 hours after the injection. The diameter of the area of induration (firmness) is measured and recorded in millimeters. An area of induration of 10 mm. or more in diameter constitutes a positive reaction. Standard procedures for administering the test and interpreting the result are very important.

The administration of the test should always be preceded by an explanation of its significance; in the period between the administration of the test and its reading, the patient often is separated from medical personnel. If during this period a positive reaction develops, and the patient believes that this is certain evidence of active clinical disease, he may become extremely and unnecessarily apprehensive.

Other Tuberculin Tests. Other methods of performing tuberculin tests are the *patch test* (Vollmer) and the *scratch test* (Von Pirquet), neither of which is now in common use. Formerly, they were used rather commonly in mass tuberculin testing, particularly of school children.

Tuberculin tests using *multiple-puncture technic* have largely replaced the patch and the scratch tests. Various companies manufacture equipment for multiple puncture tests. Some of those commonly used in this country include the tine, the Sterneedle, and the Monovacc tests. The advantage of these tests is that the equipment comes individually sterilized, packaged and ready for use. No syringes or needles are necessary. The tine test is administered by pressing a small disk firmly against the palmar surface of the patient's forearm. Tiny tines, or prongs, that have been impregnated with tuberculin pierce the skin. The test causes scarcely any discomfort. Other multiple-puncture tests employ similar technic. Multiple-puncture tests are read after 48 to 72 hours. The area of induration is measured in millimeters. These tests, although frequently used for mass screening, are regarded as less accurate than the Mantoux test. For this reason, the Mantoux test is used to verify results of multiple puncture tests used in mass screening.

Roentgenography

Chest roentgenograms are used to determine whether the disease is present in persons who have a positive tuberculin test and to follow the course of the disease in those who do develop tuberculosis. They also are used sometimes without prior tuberculin testing to discover new cases of tuberculosis; however, it is recommended that the tuberculin test be used as a preliminary

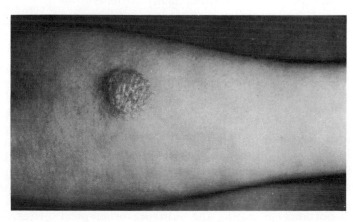

Fig. 25-1. A positive reaction to tuberculin following a Mantoux test. (Medichrome— Clay-Adams, Inc., New York, N.Y.)

screening device, particularly in children and young adults, to avoid unnecessary exposure to radiation.

Sputum Examination

Microscopic examinations of sputum to detect acid-fast bacilli are often carried out when tuberculosis is suspected. The patient is instructed to cough deeply, so that the specimen will not consist merely of saliva. Most patients find that they are most likely to expectorate sputum when they first get up in the morning; therefore, this is the best time for them to obtain a specimen. A wide-mouthed specimen bottle is used for this purpose. It is important to see that the outside of the bottle is free from contamination and to avoid contamination of the specimen with other organisms. Specimens of sputum are often obtained for culture of the organism (growing it on a suitable laboratory medium). This test takes 4 to 8 weeks to complete.

Since it is possible that tubercle bacilli, although present, may not be recovered in a single specimen, serial tests of sputum are often ordered by the doctor. A frequent order reads: "Sputum for acid-fast bacilli × 3." It is important to explain to the patient the necessity for repeated tests, so that he will not become irritated or apprehensive by the request for more than one test.

Gastric lavage or gastric aspiration may be used to determine the presence of the organisms, particularly among patients who have difficulty raising a sputum specimen for examination. It is believed that the mechanism whereby tubercle bacilli reach the stomach from the lungs is that sputum is raised and is not expectorated but swallowed.

Gastric aspiration is used less commonly than it was previously. Instead, many patients who have difficulty producing a sputum specimen are asked to inhale a heated vapor (aerosol) of saline or saline mixed with propylene glycol. After inhaling the vapor for 10 minutes, the patient is asked to cough. The vapor helps to loosen secretions, making it easier for the patient to produce sputum for the examination. A variety of cytochemical tests are performed to identify the organisms and to note its characteristics (including atypical forms). Of particular importance in relation to therapy is the sensitivity of the organism to various chemotherapeutic agents.

Increasing recognition is being given to the importance of noting the existence of atypical forms of acid-fast bacilli. Often these atypical forms are resistant to drug therapy.

TREATMENT

Chemotherapy is the most important aspect of treatment for tuberculosis. Occasionally, advanced disease or the failure to respond to medical treatment may indicate the need for surgery. Rest and a nutritious diet are important also in the therapeutic regimen.

While prolonged bed rest used to be typical, it is no longer considered necessary for most patients. Bed rest is usually prescribed only for seriously ill patients and for those who have had recent hemoptysis. Others are permitted to go to the bathroom, and to be out of bed for gradually increasing periods. Rest, in the sense of relief from worry and strain, continues to be important. If the patient is tense and anxious, worried about his prognosis or his family, he will be unable to rest.

If the patient is not accustomed to accepting responsibility for his own health, it is difficult, but extremely important to help him learn how to follow his treatment, and to assist him in adapting his mode of life as necessary in order to carry out his treatment. All the drug discoveries are of no use unless the patient can be helped to realize the necessity for taking prescribed medications over a long period.

Chemotherapy

Drugs have made recovery more rapid, and they have provided a chance for the arrest of the disease for those with advanced lesions, but drugs do not provide a guaranteed cure. Their usefulness lies in their ability to decrease the growth and the multiplication of the tubercle bacillus, thus giving the patient's body a chance to overcome the disease. Two factors make drugs less than ideal: toxicity and the tendency of the tubercle bacillus to develop resistance to the drugs. Combined therapy with two or more drugs decreases the problem of drug resistance, increases to some extent the tuberculostatic action of the drugs, and lessens somewhat the toxicity of the drugs for the patient.

Streptomycin was the first antibiotic to be employed against tuberculosis. Initially, the physician may prescribe 1 Gm. of streptomycin intramuscularly daily. However, as soon as the most severe symptoms become controlled, the dose is usually reduced to 1 Gm. 2 or 3 times a week, in order to minimize toxic effects of the drug. Toxic reactions may include vertigo, ataxia, deafness, nausea, vomiting, fever, and rash.

Isoniazid (INH) is another important drug in the treatment of tuberculosis. It has the added advantage of oral administration and relatively low toxicity. Isoniazid may be given orally and parenterally; the oral route is most common. The usual dose is 300 mg. per day, although higher dosage often is used. Toxic symptoms include peripheral neuritis, muscular twitching, constipation, and difficulty in voiding. Since toxic symptoms associated with the administration of large doses often are related to pyridoxine deficiency, supplementary doses of pyridoxine (50 to 100 mg. daily) often are prescribed when large doses of isoniazid are administered. Streptomycin and isoniazid are sometimes referred to as primary drugs in the treatment of tuberculosis. Therapy with each of them is combined frequently with para-aminosalicylic acid.

Para-aminosalicylic acid (PAS) is used primarily in combination with streptomycin or isoniazid to increase their effectiveness and to delay drug resistance. Para-aminosalicylic acid is not as effective a tuberculostatic agent as isoniazid and streptomycin. PAS is given in doses of 12 to 15 Gm. daily, usually in 3 doses of 4 Gm. each. Toxicity includes diarrhea, nausea and vomiting, and some patients show allergy and fever. The drug is tolerated better when given after meals.

Other Chemotherapeutic Agents. Several other drugs are used in the treatment of tuberculosis. These drugs are often called secondary or second-line drugs. So far, none of these agents has proved more effective than the primary drugs discussed above. These secondary drugs are used when patients have adverse reactions to the primary drugs, and when the patient's organisms become resistant to the primary drugs. Use of secondary drugs is limited by their tendency to cause toxic symptoms. Bacterial resistance also occurs when secondary drugs are used. However, because of the growing number of persons whose organisms are resistant to primary drugs, the secondary drugs are of increasing importance. These secondary drugs include: viomycin, Pyrazinamide, cycloserine, kanamycin, ethionamide, and ethambutol. A frequent dosage schedule for viomycin is 2 Gm. I.M. twice weekly. Toxic symptoms include disturbances of kidney function. The usefulness of Pyrazinamide is limited by toxic effects on the liver. The drug is sometimes given in doses of 0.5 Gm. 3 times daily.

Cycloserine is given in doses of 0.5 Gm. daily. It may produce toxic effects on the central nervous system, such as convulsions or psychoses. Kanamycin is given in doses of 1 Gm. daily or 3 times weekly. Kanamycin sometimes causes kidney damage. Ethionamide is given in doses of 500 to 1,000 mg. daily, orally. Toxic effects include liver damage, deafness, and gastrointestinal symptoms, such as anorexia, nausea, and vomiting. Ethambutol is a more recently introduced drug which is being used as a secondary drug for patients whose organisms are resistant to first-line drugs. It is also used sometimes instead of PAS. For example, sometimes ethambutol is used along with INH to initiate therapy of tuberculosis. Ethambutol can be given in lower dosage than PAS and does not cause the gastrointestinal distress sometimes associated with the large doses required for PAS therapy. Ethambutol occasionally causes headache, dizziness, nausea, and reduction of visual acuity. If the latter symptom occurs, the drug is discontinued. The average dose of ethambutol is 400 mg. to 1 Gm. daily, given in a single dose.

All of the tuberculostatic drugs should be given for long periods without interruption, since healing is slow and resistance to drugs may be increased by interrupted treatment. Lapses in the administration of these drugs can be serious, and the patient should understand the importance of taking his drugs regularly. If he refuses or is unable to take the prescribed medication, the nurse should consult the physician. For example, if for some reason a patient becomes nauseated and is unable to take isoniazid, the physician frequently will ask the nurse to give the medication parenterally.

Corticosteroids have been used, in some instances, in the treatment of tuberculosis, since these drugs provide symptomatic relief; for example, fever may decline and appetite may improve. The dosage is gradually decreased and then discontinued altogether. These drugs are not given for extended periods, as are such drugs as isoniazid. There is a difference of medical opinion as to whether corticosteroids help to clear the disease process more promptly. As is true whenever corticosteroids are administered, the patient must be observed for toxic symptoms. Corticosteroids are likely to be used in treating tuberculous meningitis and advanced pulmonary tuberculosis. When therapy with corticosteroids is used, it is used in combination with tuberculostatic drugs.

Usually, the greater period of drug therapy (and in some instances, the entire period) is carried out while the patient is at home. It is important to emphasize to the patient the necessity for returning regularly to the physician's office or clinic for follow-up care. In addition to other aspects of treatment and assessment carried out at these periodic visits, tests of the sensitivity of the patient's organisms for the drugs he is taking must be performed, and the toxicity of the drugs for the patient must be evaluated.

Surgical Treatment

Surgical treatment may be required for patients with advanced disease or for those who do not respond to medical treatment. Resistance of organisms to chemotherapeutic agents is an important factor in lack of response to medical treatment.

Radical surgery, such as pneumonectomy, is done less frequently than formerly, and there is increasing use of operations that remove only a portion of the lung. When the disease is located primarily in one section of the lung, that portion may be removed by *segmental resection* (removal of a segment of a lobe) or by *wedge resection* (removal of a wedge of diseased tissue). If the diseased area is larger, *lobectomy* (removal of a lobe) may be done. In some cases the entire lung is so diseased that a pneumonectomy is necessary.

COMPLICATIONS

Hemorrhage

Hemorrhage may begin with streaking or staining of sputum, or it may occur without warning. Patients may be restless and anxious before hemorrhage from any part of the body; however, these changes may be so slight as to be noted only in retrospect. The amount of bleeding may vary from a few drops to several ounces. Copious bleeding is extremely frightening to the patient and to the family if they are present. The nurse will need no reminder to report severe bleeding to the physician, since her first inclination is to seek help.

The nurse can be of greatest help to the patient by staying with him and signaling for someone else to call the doctor. If the nurse is the only staff member on the ward, she should explain to the patient that she must leave to call the doctor, but that she will return promptly. She can reassure her patient better if she herself realizes that hemorrhage is seldom fatal. Death, when it occurs, is due more often to asphyxia than to actual blood loss.

The nurse's first action when hemoptysis occurs usually is to provide a receptacle into which the patient may expectorate and to help him to assume a position that prevents aspiration of the blood. The nurse's presence is a potent factor in reassurance, since being left alone at this time increases the patient's fear. Although she may not feel calm, an assured and confident manner will help to lessen the patient's apprehension.

It is important to note the amount of bleeding, the patient's color, pulse and blood pressure and to be ready to report these to the doctor. Blood that is expectorated, as well as the receptacles used, should be handled with careful medical aseptic technic.

The doctor often will order sedation only sufficient to decrease coughing and not sufficient to abolish it or to permit the retention of blood in the respiratory passages. Frequently, complete bed rest and nothing by mouth are ordered immediately after the hemorrhage. If fluids are permitted, sips of cold beverages are refreshing. Lying on the unaffected side should be avoided (the doctor will determine the site of the bleeding and advise you), since it may increase the likelihood of spreading the disease. All aspects of nursing should encourage rest and avoid factors that might lead to renewed bleeding.

Assisting with personal hygiene should be carried out with discretion; morning care should not become an automatic routine. For example, even though it may be time for the bath, it may be better for this patient to be allowed to rest. A little later a partial bath may be given. It is advisable to be very gentle when giving back care; this precaution may help to prevent further bleeding. Careful mouth care is important to remove the disagreeable taste and the odor of old blood.

Sometimes transfusions and infusions are necessary if the bleeding has been severe. Care must be taken to administer intravenous fluids slowly, so that bleeding is not reactivated. Occasionally, pneumothorax or an emergency lobectomy or pneumonectomy is used to help to stop the bleeding.

Spontaneous Pneumothorax

Occasionally, during the disease process air escapes from the lung and enters the pleural space, causing the lung to collapse. The collapse of the lung interferes with respiration and may lead to empyema. Spontaneous pneumothorax may occur in a variety of pulmonary conditions, including emphysema. It occurs infrequently in association with tuberculosis.

The first symptoms of spontaneous pneumothorax are a sudden sharp pain in the chest, dyspnea and severe apprehension. Other symptoms include faintness, profuse perspiration, fall in blood pressure and weak, rapid pulse. The color usually is pale or slightly cyanotic. As in the nursing of a patient with hemorrhage, it is desirable, if possible, for one nurse to remain with the patient to help to lessen his apprehension, while another nurse notifies the doctor and prepares equipment for him to use in treatment.

The patient should be placed in a sitting position, since this makes it easier for him to breathe. Oxygen may be ordered. A thoracentesis is performed in order to remove air from the pleural space and to permit the re-expansion of the lung. If air continues to enter the pleural space, a catheter may be inserted and closed drainage of the chest instituted. After spontaneous pneumothorax, the patient should be allowed to rest and instructed to avoid physical exertion. Lessening the patient's apprehension will help him to breathe quietly and to avoid gasping and coughing. Re-expansion of the lung is checked by roentgenography and fluoroscopy.

CARE IN GENERAL HOSPITALS

Relatively short-term care of patients with tuberculosis in general hospitals is becoming more common. This practice could be increased if greater attention were given in general hospitals to use of safe and effective procedures for preventing the spread of tuberculosis. Too often patients with tuberculosis are unnecessarily transferred to a chest hospital many miles from home, when they do not require extended hospitalization or highly specialized procedures. Nurses can, by their own attitude of rational concern about measures to prevent spread of infection, and by careful adherence to protective measures, foster care of patients with tuberculosis in general hospitals.

Nurses have a key role in helping the tuberculosis patient in the general hospital to have a positive experience which enables him to learn more about his illness, to understand the ways he can participate in protecting others from infection, and to establish a treatment regimen which he can later carry out at home.

Fostering the patient's participation, by instructing him in such measures as "covering his cough," and disposing of sputum can help increase his feelings of self-esteem and responsibility toward himself and others.

REHABILITATION

One of the earliest measures in rehabilitation is helping the patient and his family to accept the reality of the diagnosis. Unless the patient can accept the fact that he has tuberculosis, he will be unable to perceive the need for instruction and treatment. It may take the patient some time to accept the fact that he has tuberculosis; the nurse's supportive attitude may help him in this adjustment.

The nurse can find many ways of helping the patient to bridge the gap between dependence on care during illness and independent living. The gradual resumption of independence as the illness improves is important. The opportunity to go to the dining room, rather than having a tray brought to the bedside, the wearing of street clothes rather than night clothes and the opportunity to participate in group activities are all part of rehabilitation and help to restore self-confidence.

The period of disability from tuberculosis is considerably shorter now than was the case a few years ago. It is therefore especially important to help the patient and his family participate in the plan of treatment as soon as they are able. The objective is to avoid, as much as possible, the interruption in the patient's life due to tuberculosis, which was until recently so common. Although drug therapy must be continued for an extended period, most patients are able to resume their usual activities within a relatively short period.

Positive relationships between the patient and the staff are extremely important. The patient naturally will seek the approval of those whose care is so important to his recovery. It is essential that the staff, by their own attitudes and their relationships with the patient, encourage his independence, self-respect and self-reliance.

CASEFINDING AND CONTROL

Since tuberculosis in the early stages is frequently asymptomatic, screening devices such as tuberculin tests and roentgenograms are used to discover the disease in apparently healthy people. It is recommended that all children and adults have tuberculin tests as part of the yearly physical examination, and that roentgenograms be taken of those who show a positive reaction.

Early diagnosis is essential to bring the patient's illness under control, for his own welfare and for that of his associates and the community as a whole.

BCG. and Isoniazid as Prophylaxis

For people who are exposed to the disease frequently or who may be particularly vulnerable to it, BCG. (bacille Calmette Guérin) vaccine is sometimes recommended. This vaccine is made from living, attenuated tubercle bacilli and is given to those who react negatively to tuberculin. Although it offers some protection, BCG. cannot be relied on for the complete prophylaxis of the disease.

The ultimate goal is a population completely tuberculin-negative, which would indicate eradication of tuberculosis. Rapidity of progress toward this goal varies widely in different parts of the world and is closely related to social and economic conditions. In countries or sections of countries where tuberculosis is widespread the use of BCG. is prevalent. Because those who receive BCG. develop a positive tuberculin reaction, the use of the vaccine interferes with the usefulness of tuberculin testing. Those who receive BCG. are given periodic x-ray examinations to detect possible development of tuberculosis. However, in areas where the incidence of tuberculosis is high and where a considerable segment of the population is tuberculin-positive, interference by BCG. with the use of tuberculin testing often is viewed as less important than the conferring of some degree of protection.

Isoniazid is being used as prophylaxis against development of active tuberculosis among those in whom the tuberculin reaction recently has changed from negative to positive. For example, in one program of prophylaxis, all persons whose tuberculin reaction has changed from negative to positive within the past 6 months are advised to have treatment with isoniazid for one year. Also, isoniazid is being given prophylactically to persons with silicosis and to some patients who are receiving long-term therapy with corticosteroids for other diseases such as rheumatoid arthritis.

Further Prophylactic Measures

The education of the public and improved living and working conditions have helped to reduce the incidence of tuberculosis. People in our country are better clothed, fed and housed than they were at the turn of the century, when tuberculosis was a leading killer. Hours of work are shorter, and, as more active cases are detected and treated, fewer sources of infection exist within the community.

REFERENCES AND BIBLIOGRAPHY

BARHAM, V. Z.: Changing the attitudes of hospital nurses, *Nurs. Outlook* 19:538, August, 1971.

BURKE, R. M.: *An Historical Chronology of Tuberculosis,* ed. 2, Springfield, Ill., Thomas, 1955.

Chemoprophylaxis for the Prevention of Tuberculosis, "A Report of the Ad Hoc Committee on Chemoprophylaxis, New York, National Tuberculosis and Respiratory Disease Association, 1967.

COMMISSION ON CHRONIC ILLNESS: *Chronic Illness in the United States,* Vols. 1 and 2, Cambridge, Harvard University Press, 1956-57.

CREIGHTON, H., and TAYSIEN, D. P.: The enigma that was Annabelle, *Am. J. Nurs.* 60:987-989, 1960.

CUMMINS, S. L.: *Tuberculosis in History,* London, Bailliere, 1949.

GARRETT, J. F. (ed.): *Psychological Aspects of Physical Disability,* Washington, D.C., U.S. Department of Health, Education, and Welfare, U.S. Government Printing Office, (n.d.).

The indispensable laboratory: *Nat. Tuberc. Assoc. Bull.* 54:3, June, 1968.

Infectiousness of Tuberculosis, Report of the NTRDA Ad Hoc Committee on Treatment of TB Patients in General Hospitals, New York, National Tuberculosis and Respiratory Disease Association, 1967.

Introduction to Respiratory Diseases, ed. 4, New York, National Tuberculosis and Respiratory Disease Association, 1969.

KELLY, H. B.: Patient population and treatment choices, *Nurs. Outlook* 19:541, August, 1971.

KOONZ, T.: Nursing in tuberculosis, *Nurs. Clin. N. Am.* 3:403, September, 1968.

NATIONAL TUBERCULOSIS AND RESPIRATORY DISEASE ASSOCIATION: Information supplied for use in this chapter by the National Tuberculosis and Respiratory Disease Association, New York, 1969.

PFUETZE, K., and RADNER, D.: *Clinical Tuberculosis: Diagnosis and Treatment,* Springfield, Ill., Thomas, 1966.

PHILLIPS, S.: *Current Problems in Tuberculosis,* Berkeley, University of California Press, 1964.

REAM, C. R.: Tuberculosis in the general hospital, *Public Health News* 50:182, August, 1969.

RILEY, R. L.: Airborne infections, *Am. J. Nurs.* 60:1246-1248, 1960.

SOUTH, J.: *Tuberculosis Handbook for Public Health Nurses,* New York, National Tuberculosis Association, 1965.

SPARER, P. J. (ed.): *Personality, Stress, and Tuberculosis,* New York, International Universities Press, 1956.

U.S. DEPARTMENT OF HEALTH, EDUCATION AND WELFARE: *The Future of Tuberculosis Control,* Washington, D.C., U.S. Government Printing Office, 1964.

WEG, J. G.: Tuberculosis and the generation gap, *Amer. J. Nurs.* 71:495, March, 1971.

The Patient with a Blood or Lymph Disorder

26

Common Diagnostic Tests • Anemia • Leukemia • Purpura
Hemophilia • Polycythemia Vera • Agranulocytosis
Lymphosarcoma • Hodgkin's Disease • Infectious Mononucleosis

Many people with blood dyscrasias or related disorders are chronically ill. The chronically ill have fears based on fact and reality. Among these are the fear of death, incapacitation, abandonment, economic bankruptcy, and the fear of spreading disease to others.

When the patient's disease carries a fatal prognosis, as in leukemia, the nurse can provide support in many ways. Physical care and various therapies such as the use of chemotherapeutic agents exert heavy demands on knowledge, skills,

and time. However, the emotional drain on the nurse who supports the patient during the experience is taxing. She becomes vulnerable to feelings of helplessness, frustration, anger, and sadness.

It would be wise for the nurse who works with patients who have blood dyscrasias to seek help with her own feelings. This can be done, for example, through a hospital sponsored inservice program. (See Chapter 11 for care of the dying patient.)

Part 1: Blood Disorders

The term *blood dyscrasias* often is used to describe a large group of disorders affecting the blood. (*Dyscrasia* is derived from Greek words meaning *bad* and *mixture*.) Although all blood dyscrasias affect the blood in some way, the disorders themselves are manifestations of many different pathologic processes. For instance, leukemia is believed to be due to malignant changes; anemia may be due to a variety of causes, such as blood loss, inadequate formation of red blood cells, or increased destruction of red blood cells. However, regardless of the pathology, disorders of the blood lead to many similar symptoms and nursing problems, and they necessitate many similar kinds of diagnostic tests. For instance, many of these patients exhibit a bleeding tendency that may be due, for example, to reduction in the number of

platelets (as occurs in leukemia) or a disturbance of the coagulation of blood (as in hemophilia). Whether bleeding is due to leukemia or hemophilia, nursing problems involving care and observation of the patient with a bleeding tendency are similar.

COMMON DIAGNOSTIC TESTS

Samples of the blood often are examined for the number of cells and the amount of hemoglobin. The number of white blood cells, platelets and red blood cells per cubic millimeter is compared with the normal values. Frequently, the relative number of the different types of white cells is of diagnostic importance, and a differential count of white blood cells is ordered. The size and the shape of the cells, as well as their number, may be significant. Red blood cells of normal size are called *normocytic*, abnormally small ones are called microcytic, and abnormally large ones are called *macrocytic*. The amount of hemoglobin contained in the erythrocytes may be contrasted with the normal, using the terms *hypochromic* (less hemoglobin than normal) and *hyperchromic* (more hemoglobin than normal). Samples of the blood are examined also for the clotting time.

Since many patients with blood dyscrasias have a bleeding tendency, the site of the puncture should be inspected frequently to make sure that there is no oozing. The patient usually is instructed to apply firm pressure to the site for a few minutes after the blood has been withdrawn, preferably with a sterile dry gauze after alcohol sponge.

Because the nurse frequently is not actually present when a specimen of the blood is drawn, she must make a special effort to remember the patient's need for explanation and reassurance. Often patients comment jokingly, "You know, if you keep on taking my blood, I won't have any left." For some patients this is merely a joke, but for others it reflects real apprehension, which is increased by a lack of understanding of the relationship between the amount of the blood drawn and the total amount in the body, as well as the body's constant formation of new blood cells.

Sternal Puncture. Specimens of bone marrow are very useful in studying the formation of blood cells. Although these specimens can be obtained from the sternum or the iliac crest, sternal puncture is performed most frequently. The patient lies on his back, either in bed or on the treatment table. The skin over the sternum is cleansed and anesthetized with procaine. A needle is inserted into the marrow of the bone. A dry, sterile 5 to 10 ml. syringe is attached, and specimens are withdrawn. The patient may feel discomfort when the specimen is taken, as well as apprehension and a feeling of pressure when the needle is inserted. (A special needle is used that is short and strong; there is generally a guard on the needle that will prevent it from being inserted too far.)

The nurse has two important functions during this procedure: assisting the physician and making the patient as comfortable as possible. The necessary equipment is outlined in your hospital procedure manual. After preparing the equipment and assisting with the explanation of the procedure, the nurse positions and drapes the patient, and she assists the doctor by handing him equipment, adjusting the lighting and labeling the specimens. As with any test or treatment that is uncomfortable or upsetting, a few words or a smile of encouragement help the patient.

Capillary Fragility Test. This test is done to determine how easily the capillaries rupture. In some blood dyscrasias, capillary fragility is increased, leading to tiny hemorrhagic spots (*petechiae*) under the skin. The doctor wraps a blood-pressure cuff around the patient's arm, inflates it to a point between the patient's diastolic and systolic blood pressure, and leaves the cuff inflated for 15 minutes. After he removes the cuff, the doctor examines the skin distal to the area where pressure was applied. Normally, only 1 to 2 petechiae per square inch are noted. If the patient's capillaries are abnormally fragile, many petechiae will be found. The doctor explains the test to the patient; the nurse may or may not be asked to assist. Usually, the patient is not told how many petechiae normally appear, since this information might cause him additional worry. Usually, the doctor explains that the development of some tiny red spots on the skin is to be expected when the cuff is removed.

Changes in the blood often accompany other disorders. Anemia may be the first warning of cancer, or it may be the first clue to the discovery of a peptic ulcer that has been causing the persistent loss of small amounts of blood. Finding an abnormal blood count is only the beginning. In order to treat the patient effectively, the doctor must first discover the cause of the condition.

Patients can be helped by explaining the need for medical care, encouraging them to have whatever diagnostic tests are necessary, and showing them the folly of succumbing to the lures of advertising and trying remedies that can waste their money or provide false assurance while a serious disease continues to be undiscovered.

ANEMIA

The term *anemia* means that the patient has a decrease in the number of red blood cells and a lower than normal hemoglobin level. The number of red blood cells normally present varies with age, sex and altitude. Infants have more red blood cells per cubic millimeter than adults. Women have fewer erythrocytes per cubic millimeter than men; normally women average about 4,500,000 red blood cells per cubic millimeter of blood; men average 5,000,000 per cubic millimeter. The difference between men and women in the number of red blood cells is most noticeable during the reproductive years. People who live at very high altitudes have an increased number of red blood cells.

Erythrocytes perform the important function of carrying oxygen from the lungs to the tissues, and carbon dioxide from the tissues to the lungs. The red color of the blood is caused by hemoglobin, which is contained in the erythrocytes. Hemoglobin combines with oxygen to form oxyhemoglobin. The average amount of hemoglobin is 14.5 to 15.0 Gm. per 100 ml. of blood. Men have slightly more hemoglobin than women. As the blood passes through the lungs, oxygen is taken up and carbon dioxide is released. Oxygenated blood is bright red and is carried by arteries and capillaries to all tissues of the body. After the oxygen has been released from the hemoglobin for use by the tissues, the hemoglobin is called "reduced hemoglobin." The blood at this time looks dark red and is returned by the veins to the heart and to the lungs, where the carbon dioxide is released and the blood reoxygenated.

Anemia can be caused by loss, destruction or faulty production of red blood cells and hemoglobin. Blood loss can occur suddenly and copiously, as in severe hemorrhage from a severed artery, or it may result from slow but persistent bleeding from hemorrhoids or a peptic ulcer. Conditions that can lead to chronic blood loss, such as hemorrhoids or uterine tumors, should be treated promptly to avoid the development of anemia. Bleeding also results in the loss of iron from the body, since iron is contained in the hemoglobin. Normally, the body saves and reuses the iron for the production of new hemoglobin after the worn-out red blood cells have been broken down. By increasing its production of erythrocytes, the body can compensate for some degree of loss or destruction of erythrocytes; anemia becomes manifest only when the body is unable to increase its production of erythrocytes sufficiently to compensate for these losses.

Hemolysis (the destruction of red blood cells) leads to a reduction of their number. It is believed that, normally, each red blood cell survives for about four months. Old red blood cells are destroyed in the spleen, the bone marrow and the liver. The body constantly is making new red blood cells and destroying old ones, so that the number is kept fairly uniform. In hemolytic conditions the red blood cells do not survive as long as they normally do. They may survive only two weeks. The increased destruction of red blood cells leads to anemia. Hemolysis may be caused by infection, abnormal red blood cells, transfusion of incompatible blood or exposure to harmful chemicals.

Inadequate production of red blood cells can be due to an injury to the bone marrow (for example, by toxic effects of drugs) or to the lack of necessary materials (such as iron, folic acid, vitamin B_{12}) for the formation of red blood cells and hemoglobin. Anemia also may be caused by other diseases, such as cancer and rheumatoid arthritis.

Symptoms of anemia are similar, regardless of the cause, and are due largely to the inability of the blood to transport sufficient oxygen to the tissues. Fatigue, anorexia, faintness and pallor are typical.

Iron-Deficiency Anemia

Iron is necessary for the production of hemoglobin. Iron-deficiency anemia is frequent among persons whose need for iron is increased. Less than 10 per cent of the iron obtained from food is absorbed. During periods of rapid growth, at the onset of the menses and during pregnancy there is increased need for iron, which often results in anemia unless additional iron is obtained. It is sometimes difficult to provide for these increased needs by dietary measures alone, although correction of a faulty diet, if it exists, is an important aspect of treatment. Iron-deficiency anemia is characterized by red blood cells that are microcytic and hypochromic.

The treatment involves the administration of extra iron, usually given after meals to lessen the likelihood of gastrointestinal irritation, the most common side-effect of iron administration. Some physicians now recommend that iron be given before meals, in the belief that better absorption results. Iron causes the stools to appear black, and patients are always informed of this fact, so that they will not fear that the color indicates gastrointestinal bleeding. Iron is given occasionally in liquid form. It should be taken through a straw, otherwise it will stain the teeth. Iron is given occasionally by injection, particularly when the patient has some intestinal disturbance, such as colitis, that impairs the absorption of iron from the gastrointestinal tract. A preparation for intramuscular use is iron-dextran complex (Imferon). Foods high in iron are important in the diet. The patient may have to force himself to eat at first, because the anemia causes anorexia.

Pernicious Anemia

An intrinsic factor normally present in the stomach secretions is necessary for the absorption of vitamin B_{12} found in food. Vitamin B_{12} is necessary for the normal maturation of red blood cells. Patients with pernicious anemia have a lack of the intrinsic factor, which normally is contained in the gastric juice.

The body requires such small amounts of vitamin B_{12} that most people have an adequate supply in their food. Animal proteins, such as meat, milk, eggs and cheese, contain vitamin B_{12}, and even a small daily intake of these foods ensures an adequate supply of the vitamin.

This point is stressed, because some patients mistakenly believe that pernicious anemia can be cured by diet, and that medication will no longer be necessary. Patients with pernicious anemia do need an adequate diet to maintain general health, and instruction in what constitutes such a diet is indicated if the patient's nutrition is poor. Yet dietary treatment alone is not sufficient. Everyone must help the patient to understand this. Probably, the crux of the problem lies in helping the patient to understand that different types of anemia require different kinds of treatment. The patient with pernicious anemia may have a neighbor with iron-deficiency anemia, whose condition responded quickly to the administration of iron and an improved diet, and who therefore could stop taking the medication.

In contrast, patients with pernicious anemia must have regular injections of vitamin B_{12} to control the disease, because their lack of the intrinsic factor in gastric secretions prevents the adequate absorption of vitamin B_{12} from food.

Diagnosis of pernicious anemia is established by the patient's history and symptoms and by studies of his blood and bone marrow.

Treatment. Vitamin B_{12} (cyanocobalamin) is given intramuscularly in a dosage that is adequate to control the disease. No toxic effects have been noted from the use of vitamin B_{12}. Occasionally, oral treatment is given, in the form of capsules or tablets containing both vitamin B_{12} and gastric mucosa (containing the intrinsic factor) obtained from animals.

Other Considerations. In addition to the usual symptoms of anemia, patients with pernicious anemia occasionally develop a sore tongue and mouth, digestive disturbances and diarrhea. The anemia may be so severe that the patient experiences dyspnea on the slightest exertion. Jaundice often occurs. Personality changes are not unusual, especially when the disease is severe. Often the patient is irritable, confused and depressed. Such changes are most likely to be noted by the patient's family, who often observe that "He just isn't himself lately." Fortunately, personality changes usually disappear promptly with treatment.

If the condition is not treated promptly, the patient develops degenerative changes in the nervous system, sometimes referred to as *combined system disease*. Numbness and tingling of the extremities and ataxia are common. Vibratory and position sense may be lost. Symptoms of neurologic damage may improve somewhat, but permanent damage sometimes occurs before treatment is begun. The earlier the diagnosis and the more prompt the treatment, the greater is the likelihood of escaping permanent neurologic damage. Physical therapy may be of benefit.

Nursing Care. During the severe phase of the illness, nursing care involves keeping the patient warm and at rest. Despite anorexia, the patient is encouraged to take easily digested, nutritious foods and fluids. Soft foods that are not highly seasoned are preferable, especially if the patient's mouth is sore. Eggnog, gelatin and creamed chicken are examples. Appetite usually returns promptly after treatment is begun. Gentleness and patience are important, because the patient is often irritable and apprehensive.

Neurologic symptoms should be watched for and reported if they occur. The prevention of falls is particularly important if the patient is ataxic. Refer questions concerning the possibility of recovery from neurologic symptoms to the patient's doctor. Some of these symptoms may subside or improve after treatment, but the patient may need help in accepting some permanent residual disability. Because the patient is ill and weak, he does not have normal resistance to other illnesses and infections. He should be protected from contact with those who have any type of infection.

Some patients are more likely to take the injections with the frequency recommended by the doctor if a member of the family is taught to administer the medication. If such instruction cannot be arranged, the patient must return to the doctor's office or clinic or have the injections given by a public health nurse. Some patients require the injections once a week. Others require them less often. If the patient has been hospitalized, plans for continued treatment should be made before he leaves the hospital. It is of paramount importance that he and his family understand the necessity for continued therapy. If the medicine is skipped, the patient will at first feel no ill-effects and may, unless instructed otherwise, believe that the injections are no longer necessary. Teaching the family is particularly important because one of the symptoms of this disease is mental confusion and apathy. The patient who neglects his therapy (visits to the physician; following treatment at home) may begin to have mental changes that make it impossible for him to recognize the need for treatment.

Anemia Due to Blood Loss

Blood contains cells and liquid (plasma) in approximately equal volume. It has been estimated that the total blood volume is approximately one thirteenth of the body weight. An adult weighing 154 pounds has about 6 quarts of blood. Normally, the quantity of blood circulating in the body is kept relatively constant at all times.

Blood loss, either acute or chronic, causes anemia. Sudden severe bleeding leads to *hypovolemia* (diminished volume of circulating blood) and shock. The most effective treatment involves the replacement of lost blood by transfusions. If blood loss is chronic, as may be the case in uterine tumors or hemorrhoids, the main treatment is that of the underlying condition causing the bleeding. Depending on the amount of the blood lost, the treatment may include transfusion and/or administration of iron to help the body to compensate for the blood loss. Continued care and observation are necessary for any patient who has experienced blood loss. Sometimes, the patient does not understand the reason for continued care, and, once the emergency is over, he continues to experience fatigue and weakness due to anemia that might have been readily corrected had he realized the importance of returning to his doctor's office or to the clinic.

Anemia Due to Destruction of Red Blood Cells

A reduction in red blood cells and hemoglobin may be caused by hemolysis. The life span of the red blood cells is shortened; the cells die more rapidly than they normally should. An example of hemolytic anemia due to an abnormality of the red blood cells is *sickle cell anemia*. This hereditary disease occurs chiefly in Negroes. In addition to the classic symptoms of anemia, the patient with this condition may develop chronic leg ulcers and attacks of fever and pain in the abdomen or the extremities. There is no cure for sickle cell anemia. Transfusions are given as palliative treatment, but life expectancy usually is decreased.

Acquired hemolytic anemia (sometimes called autoimmune hemolytic disease) is due to the development within the patient's body of substances harmful to his erythrocytes. These patients are treated by corticosteroids. In some patients the steroid can be withdrawn after several weeks; in others, not for several months. Sometimes splenectomy is performed. Tranfusions may be necessary.

One group of hereditary hemolytic anemias is referred to generally as *thalassemia*. Thalassemia major, or Cooley's anemia, has a high incidence in the Po valley (Italy) and on islands of the Mediterranean. Treatment of the various forms of thalassemia is symptomatic. Transfusions may be required frequently.

Hemolysis often accompanies severe infections, such as malaria and subacute bacterial endocarditis. Rapid hemolysis is accompanied by chills, fever, prostration, headache and gastrointestinal disturbances. Jaundice follows, due to the rapid destruction of erythrocytes and the escape of hemoglobin into the plasma. Hemolysis can be caused also by transfusions of incompatible blood and by administration of certain drugs, such as quinine.

The treatment of hemolytic anemia is that of the underlying condition—for instance, stopping the transfusion or the drug and giving supportive treatment, such as oxygen, or treating whatever infection may be present. Transfusions may be necessary to replace red blood cells and hemoglobin.

Aplastic Anemia (Bone Marrow Failure; Aregenerative Anemia)

Erythrocytes, granular leukocytes (granulocytes) and platelets are formed in the bone marrow. *Aplastic anemia* is the term used to describe a condition in which the activity of the bone marrow is depressed, and red blood cells, white blood cells and platelets are not adequately produced. The formation of one or all of the three elements may be impaired, with varying degrees of severity.

Aplastic anemia is a serious toxic manifestation of certain drugs, such as streptomycin, Chloromycetin (chloramphenicol) and nitrogen mustard. This condition also occurs without known cause. It is believed sometimes to have a hereditary basis.

Anemia, leukopenia (decreased leukocytes) and thrombocytopenia (decreased platelets) result in fatigue, weakness, exertional dyspnea, lowered resistance to infection and a bleeding tendency. Patients with aplastic anemia are very ill, and the death rate is high.

In treating the condition, every effort must be made to prevent infection. The patient should be in a private room. Meticulous hand washing and a clean gown worn over the uniform while caring for the patient help to prevent the transmission of organisms to him via the hands or the clothing. The use of a face mask also is recommended occasionally.

The causative agent, if it is known, is removed; for instance, the administration of a toxic drug is discontinued. Repeated transfusions are given to supply erythrocytes and hemoglobin. Usually, antibiotics are given to help to prevent infection. The objectives of treatment are to supply the missing elements of the blood and to prevent or to treat the infection or the bleeding, in the hope that the patient will recover his ability to produce the blood cells. If the bone marrow has been so damaged that this recovery is impossible, death will result. The nursing care and the observation of patients with a bleeding tendency are discussed below.

LEUKEMIA

There are three types of leukocytes (white blood cells): *lymphocytes, monocytes* and *granulocytes*. Normally, there are between 5,000 and 7,000 leukocytes per cubic millimeter of blood. Fighting infection is one important function of the leukocytes, and they increase in number during most infections. This increase is called *leukocytosis*.

Lymphocytes are produced in the lymphatic tissue; granulocytes are produced chiefly in the bone marrow. It is believed that the different types of leukocytes survive varying lengths of time. Much remains unknown concerning the life span of various kinds of leukocytes. At the end of their life span the leukocytes die and are replaced by the new white blood cells that are constantly being formed.

Blood platelets (*thrombocytes*) are concerned with the clotting of the blood. Normally, there are about 300,000 platelets per cubic millimeter of blood. It takes blood about 5 minutes to clot in a test tube. This laboratory test is often referred to as "coagulation time" or "clotting time."

Leukemia is a fatal disease characterized by a marked increase in the number of the leukocytes. This rampant increase in the white blood cells is not useful to the body. The patient is less, rather than more, able to cope with infections. Although he has more leukocytes, they are immature and therefore are not effective in fighting infections. The rapid proliferation of the leukocytes and of the tissues that produce them results in the diminution of the number of erythrocytes and platelets. The patient eventually suffers from severe anemia, and the reduction in platelets leads to bleeding.

The cause of leukemia remains unknown. Some researchers believe that, rather than being one disease with one cause, leukemia may be a group of diseases of varied etiology. There are two main theories regarding the etiology of leukemia. One is that the disease is caused by infection; the other is that it is essentially a malignant neoplasm causing the unruly proliferation of the white blood cells. Recent studies concerning the role of a virus in the etiology of cancer could prove eventually that both theories are correct. Heredity and excessive exposure to radiation are other factors that are believed to play a part in causing leukemia.

Acute Leukemia

Symptoms. In acute leukemia, symptoms begin abruptly. The onset often coincides with an acute upper respiratory infection. Ordinarily, attention is directed at first to the symptoms of sore throat, fever or rhinitis, whereas the seriousness of the underlying illness is unsuspected. Sometimes, the patient is admitted to the hospital for the treatment of the respiratory infection, and the discovery of an unusually large number of leukocytes in the routine-admission blood count is the first clue to the existence of the disease. Sometimes unusual pallor, weakness, fatigue or bleeding warn that the illness involves more than a cold or tonsillitis, and examination of specimens of blood and bone marrow confirms the diagnosis. The leukocyte count can reach 30,000 or even 50,000 per cubic millimeter.

Anemia is usually severe and causes pallor, weakness and fatigue. The number of the platelets is reduced, causing a tendency to bleed. Bleeding may be internal or external. Common sites from which bleeding occurs include nose, mouth, gastrointestinal tract and vagina. The bleeding tendency also may be reflected by the persistent oozing of blood after such a minor injury as the administration of an injection. Usually, fever is present, particularly as the disease advances. Occasionally, the patient will develop a spontaneous temporary remission of symptoms, perhaps lasting several months. More often, the symptoms grow progressively and steadily worse.

Treatment. Although there is no cure, treatment gives respite from the symptoms. The patient is given repeated blood transfusions to increase his red blood cells and his hemoglobin. Antimetabolites, such as aminopterin, methotrexate (Amethopterin) and 6-mercaptopurine, are given. Arabinosylcytosine and 6-Thioguanine is one of the most effective drug combinations in the treatment of the adult acute leukemia patient (Gee). These drugs interfere with the multiplication of cells, particularly of cells undergoing rapid proliferation, such as the leukocytes of patients with leukemia. They are highly toxic and can impair the formation of all blood cells, including erythrocytes and platelets. Other toxic effects include anorexia, nausea, vomiting and diarrhea. The patient's blood picture is watched very carefully while these drugs are being administered. Vincristine sulfate is currently being used and is a useful drug in acute lymphoblastic leukemia, but is more effective when used in combination with a corticosteroid like prednisone. Toxic effects include neurologic and neuromuscular disorders such as paralysis, confusion and nervousness, as well as moderate to severe constipation. Patients should be cautioned to maintain normal bowel habits, with the aid of laxatives if necessary. If constipation occurs, the patient should be advised to let his physician know. Vincristine may also cause severe partial or total alopecia (hair loss). This side-effect generally causes a psychological depression and patients should be reassured that if their hair does fall out, the hair will re-grow after the drug is stopped. The regrowth will take three to four months. Since wigs are currently in vogue, the selection of one may help the patient feel better during the regrowth period.

Vincristine is carefully administered intravenously generally once a week. If the drug is accidentally infiltrated subcutaneously, a painful inflammation and subsequent ulceration may appear at the injection site. Dosage is individualized; the smallest therapeutically effective amount is utilized.

Antibiotics are given to treat the secondary infections that so commonly are the complications of the illness. ACTH and cortisone provide temporary relief from the symptoms of leukemia.

The patient eventually becomes resistant to all forms of treatment, and he becomes severely ill with weakness, fever, bleeding and, often, secondary infections such as pneumonia. Often death occurs within a few weeks after the patient develops resistance to treatment.

Chronic Leukemia

Onset and Symptoms. The two most common types of chronic leukemia are lymphocytic and granulocytic. Both conditions have an insidious onset. In chronic lymphocytic leukemia the total leukocyte count is increased, with the largest proportion of the increase in the lymphocytes. Often the disease commences with the painless enlargement of one or several lymph nodes in neck, axilla or groin. The patient develops anemia, characterized by fatigue, palpitation, pallor and dyspnea. A decrease in platelets is reflected in a bleeding tendency. Often the spleen is enlarged (*splenomegaly*).

Marked splenomegaly is often the earliest symptom of chronic granulocytic leukemia. The patient may notice a swelling in his left upper quadrant and a sense of heaviness in his abdomen. The largest proportion of the increased leukocytes consists of granulocytes. The patient develops anemia and thrombocytopenia (symptoms arising from these conditions were discussed previously).

In both types of chronic leukemia the patient may, with treatment, live five years or longer. However, eventually he no longer responds to treatment, and he becomes very weak, has a tendency to bleed and develops fever. Secondary infections such as influenza or pneumonia are common.

Treatment. The treatment of chronic leukemia includes radiotherapy, 6-Mercaptopurine, transfusions and antibiotics for the treatment of secondary infections, and corticosteroids, which provide some relief of symptoms. Chlorambucil (Leukeran) is used, particularly in chronic lymphocytic leukemia. It is a derivative of nitrogen mustard, a drug that is toxic to all tissues and especially so to rapidly growing cells. Severe depression of bone marrow may result from its use, causing aplastic anemia. Nausea and vomiting also may occur. Busulfan (Myleran), which resembles nitrogen mustard, is used, particularly in chronic granulocytic leukemia. Busulfan acts particularly on the cells of the bone marrow. It can cause severe depression of the bone marrow and the development of aplastic anemia. Chlorambucil and busulfan are administered orally. The usual dose of each drug is 2 to 6 mg. Radioactive phosphorus also is used in the treatment of chronic leukemia. The rapidly growing cells—those in the bone marrow particularly—take up the phosphorus. Its radioactivity helps to slow their unruly growth. Radioactive phosphorus is excreted in the urine; special precautions are necessary in the disposing of the urine. Cyclophosphamide (Cytoxan), another drug sometimes used in treatment, inhibits multiplication of cells. Toxic effects include depression of bone marrow, leading to aplastic anemia, nausea, vomiting and diarrhea. The usual dose is 2 to 3 mg. per Kg. of body weight, daily, orally. The medication may be given intravenously, but generally the oral medication is more convenient and equally effective.

Nursing Care of Patients with Leukemia

Caring for patients with leukemia makes particular demands on the nurse's insight and adaptability. Newer drugs can cause dramatic changes in the course of the disease. A patient admitted to the hospital with acute leukemia may appear moribund—pale, weak, bleeding and feverish. Two weeks later, as a result of treatment, he may be up and about and ready to go home. Often he continues to feel well for months or even years after the original diagnosis.

Long-range planning is important. When the patient feels well, he is encouraged to continue his usual activities—at school, at work, or at home. The disease has been temporarily checked, but it has not been overcome. Sometimes, the patient is aware of his diagnosis and prognosis; in other situations, the family knows, but the patient does not.

The remission of symptoms in leukemia is often quite dramatic and poses somewhat different problems from those of the patient with cancer. For instance, a 20-year-old who feels well is usually active, busy and very much involved in planning for his career and establishing his own home and family. If he has acute leukemia, such plans and activities will be short-lived. Most people who work with these patients believe that they should be helped and encouraged to live as full, normal lives as possible. Activity in itself is not harmful, and staying at rest will neither slow the course of the disease nor alter the eventual outcome. The patient should take every precaution to avoid infections, such as colds, and he should seek medical care promptly if he develops the symptoms of any illness. Sufficient rest and an adequate diet are important in preventing secondary infections.

To advise the patient to live as fully and as normally as possible gives no recognition of the agonizing decisions that face patients who know they have leukemia. If the patient is engaged, he may wonder whether going ahead with the marriage would be fair to his fiancée.

The patient and others intimately affected by his illness must make these decisions after learning as much as they can about the disease and its prognosis. For every patient, as long as he lives, there is the hope and the possibility that a cure will be found before death occurs.

Life expectancy is longer for patients with chronic leukemia. Because they tend to be older when the disease appears, concern is more likely to be with helping them to maintain their usual occupations and home life than with making decisions concerning career and marriage. Nevertheless, with both types of patients, there is the tremendously important need to help the patient to maintain his will to live and his determination to keep on trying despite an uncertain future.

The patient must understand the importance of returning regularly to the doctor's office or clinic. Frequent examinations of the blood and sometimes of the bone marrow are essential, both in the light of his disease and of the treatment that he is receiving. Emphasis should be placed on the importance of these examinations in helping him to stay well rather than on the possible complications from drug therapy.

Usually, the patient is admitted to the hospital several times over a period of a few years. Each time that he leaves, he is improved, although often he is not as strong as he was in the early phase of his disease. However, the time comes when his illness strikes for the last time—this time to win. Usually, the patient and his family are well aware when this time has come.

During the Final Illness. Sometimes the patient is cared for at home, so that he can remain with his family and in familiar surroundings. Private-duty or public-health nurses help to provide care in the home.

The nurse's role involves helping the family to endure the emotional and the physical strain of the patient's illness. Frequently, the family appreciates the opportunity to do things that help the patient or add to his comfort. Feeding him or bringing in a dish of his favorite food gives the family opportunities to express their love and their concern. The sensitive nurse can encourage such participation without giving the family any less support and help and without pushing them to become involved in the aspects of the care that are too upsetting or too emotionally taxing for them.

The death of a young person is usually harder to accept than that of an older person. Young people with acute leukemia are often surrounded by family members who are deeply grieved and shocked. The staff, too, feel the helplessness of watching a young person die. Usually, the doctor and often the nurses have worked with the patient for several years and know him well. The care during the patient's last illness demands of them a high degree of compassion and an awareness and a control of their own feelings.

Everything possible is done to help the patient and his family. Does a member of the family want to stay all night? Move a lounge chair into the room and give him a pillow and a blanket. The quiet, reassuring presence of a loved one may mean more to the patient than anything else and should be permitted whenever it is possible. Ordinarily, the patient is permitted diet as desired. However, if his mouth is sore and bleeding, it is best to exclude rough or highly seasoned foods.

The patient's clergyman often provides comfort and help, both for the patient and his family. Show him by your courtesy and your helpfulness that you recognize his important contribution.

PHYSICAL CARE. The physical care of the patient is demanding. *Bleeding* may occur suddenly and severely. Develop the habit of watchfulness. Always look at the contents of the bedpan, the urinal and the emesis basin before emptying them. You may find a large, tarry stool, indicating gastrointestinal bleeding, or bloody urine, or blood-streaked saliva from the mouth and the gums. Epistaxis (bleeding from the nose) is common. Report bleeding promptly. Whenever it is possible (as in the case of epistaxis), try to stop the bleeding by applying pressure and elevating the part. Pulse and blood pressure are important indicators of internal bleeding. Watch for a rapid, weak pulse and a sudden drop in the blood pressure. Observe the patient's color, and watch for purpuric spots.

Keep the patient's nostrils clean with moistened applicators in order to limit the patient's need to manipulate them. Instruct the patient to blow the nose gently if this is necessary so as not to rupture a fragile vessel.

Extreme caution should be taken if cuticle scissors, a blade razor, or other sharp instruments are used.

Note his *temperature* frequently. Because an accurate reading is so important, the temperature should be taken rectally, unless this method is contraindicated by some rectal pathology. If fever is high, the doctor may order alcohol sponges or salicylates to help to reduce the temperature and to make the patient more comfortable.

The patient's *skin* will bruise easily, and the administration of injections may cause the oozing of blood and ecchymoses. Never give two injections when one will suffice. (Check with the doctor to determine which drugs prescribed for the patient may be combined in one syringe.) Never use any larger gauge needle than is necessary to inject the medication. Apply firm pressure over the site of the injection after the withdrawal of the needle to control bleeding. Handle the patient with extreme gentleness when you are bathing or turning him. Frequent turning and skin care are important in preventing decubitus ulcers.

Disorientation may develop quite suddenly. Be alert for this, and keep side rails on the bed whenever you believe that the patient is confused and might try to get out of bed. Falls are serious, because they may precipitate internal or external bleeding.

Protect the patient from *infection* as carefully as you would a newborn infant. Wash your hands before caring for him. Often it is desirable to wear a clean gown over your uniform to protect the patient from organisms that may be carried on your clothing. Staff members and visitors who have any kind of infection, such as colds or boils, should not enter the patient's room.

Frequent, gentle *mouth care* is important. If the gums bleed easily, avoid using a toothbrush. Cotton swabs are less likely to cause bleeding and can be used for cleansing. Allowing the patient to rinse his mouth frequently and cleansing the mouth with moistened cotton applicators help to avoid the distressing odors and taste caused by old blood around the mouth and the lips. Frequent oral hygiene also helps to prevent infection of the raw, oozing mucous membranes of the mouth. Make sure that your technic is scrupulously clean when you are giving mouth care—clean hands, clean applicators and fresh solution. Mouthwash, saline or glycerine may be used.

Report symptoms of infection promptly. Be alert for a sudden rise in temperature and for chills, cough and purulent exudate from the sores around the mouth.

Watch for *toxic effects of drugs*. Often the patient is being given powerful and potentially dangerous drugs to stem the tide of the disease. The doctor must steer a narrow course between helping and hurting the patient. The nurse can help by watching for the toxic effects of the drugs and reporting them promptly.

Transfusions are often necessary. When you are assisting with a transfusion, be sure to check the label on the blood carefully, to prevent the administration of incompatible blood. Observe the patient frequently during the transfusion. See that the blood runs at the rate recommended by the doctor. If the patient shows any symptoms that might indicate an allergic reaction to the blood, or that possibly he is receiving the wrong blood, clamp off the flow of blood immediately and notify the doctor. Watch especially for chills, cyanosis, rise in temperature, dyspnea, orthopnea, pain in the lumbar region, restlessness or urticaria.

Sometimes it is noted that family members, once they learn that death is inevitable, gradually withdraw their emotional involvement with the ill person, probably as a way of attempting to cope with a situation that makes overwhelming demands on them. It is especially important for physicians and nurses to recognize the burdens that families face in such situations. By helping the family to cope with the experience, doctors and nurses may make it more possible for the family to contribute to the patient's comfort during his last days, as well as to provide the family with support that can aid them, not only during the final days of illness, but afterward, as well, in dealing with their grief. Some ways in which such help can be given include:

• Providing an atmosphere in which the family members can discuss, if they wish, some of their feeling and concern, and providing this opportunity not only in the patient's presence, but away from the bedside, as well.

• Making it possible for the family to participate in some aspects of the patient's care, but avoiding exposing them to situations (such as massive bleeding or care of incontinence) which can add greatly to their anguish.

• At all times demonstrating concern and compassion as well as skillful care of the patient.

PURPURA

The term *purpura* refers to small hemorrhages in the skin, the mucous membranes or the subcutaneous tissues. The hemorrhagic area may be tiny, as when petechiae occur, or it may be larger and result in ecchymoses of various sizes. Purpura results either from lack of platelets or from abnormality of the blood vessels. For example, certain diseases (leukemia) or the administration of x-ray therapy or certain drugs can depress the formation of platelets. Lack of ascorbic acid can damage the blood vessels, thus leading to bleeding. The treatment of all of these conditions involves discovering and treating the cause of the purpuric lesions. Often the purpuric spots are only one symptom of a bleeding tendency. The patient may suffer severe or even fatal hemorrhages in other parts of his body.

Idiopathic thrombocytopenic purpura is characterized by a reduction in platelets, the development of purpuric lesions (petechiae and ecchymoses) and bleeding from other parts of the body, such as the nose, the oral mucous membrane and the gastrointestinal tract.

Patients with idiopathic thrombocytopenic purpura often recover spontaneously. ACTH and cortisone are used frequently to provide symptomatic relief until the patient recovers from the disease. Transfusion of platelets as well as blood may be necessary to supply additional platelets in a hemorrhagic emergency, but generally are of limited usefulness. (Platelets cannot survive in stored blood.) If the patient does not recover spontaneously, splenectomy may be performed. This operation is useful, because the spleen (for reasons not fully understood) may be destroying too many platelets. The removal of the spleen often results in a rise in the platelet count and relief of the symptoms. The patient is observed carefully postoperatively for any symptoms of hemorrhage.

Nursing Care. The nursing care of the patient with purpura is essentially the same as that for any patient with a bleeding tendency and has been discussed in relation to leukemia.

HEMOPHILIA

Hemophilia is a hereditary disease characterized by prolonged coagulation time, which results in persistent and sometimes severe bleeding. It results from deficiency of the antihemophilic factor normally present in blood plasma. The disease is transmitted from mother to son as a recessive sex-linked characteristic. Although women do not develop the disease, they can inherit the trait, which, when it is passed on to a male infant, results in the development of the disease.

Hemophilia occurs with varying degrees of severity. Mild forms sometimes go unrecognized for years, until unusual bleeding is noted after an injury. Usually, however, bleeding is noted in infancy and childhood. There is persistent oozing of blood after slight injuries, such as a pin prick or a tiny cut. Often, bleeding occurs into joints, eventually damaging the joint and leading to deformity and limitation of motion. Relatively minor surgical procedures, such as tooth extraction, carry considerable risk and must be performed in a hospital. Transfusions usually are necessary even when minor surgery is performed.

Life expectancy is considerably shortened by the disease; many patients do not reach adulthood. On the other hand, those with mild hemophilia may lead full and productive lives despite the illness. Treatment includes avoidance of injury, transfusions of fresh blood or frozen plasma, and the application of thrombin to the bleeding area. Other measures to help to control the bleeding include direct pressure over the site of the bleeding and sometimes the use of cold compresses. Presently a cold precipitated concentrate of antihemophilic factor is available on a limited scale. This preparation would enable hemophiliacs to control accidental bleeding by obtaining an intravenous injection of the concentrated factor, similar to the control of diabetes mellitus by insulin injection.

POLYCYTHEMIA VERA
(Primary Polycythemia)

Polycythemia vera is a disease characterized by the excessive production of red blood cells and hemoglobin. The number of white blood cells also is increased. Its etiology is unknown. The patient may have 10 million red blood cells per cubic millimeter rather than the normal 5 million. The increased number of cells in the blood makes it more viscous than normal and leads to increased blood volume and to a tendency to develop thrombi. When clots cut off the blood supply to the tissues, areas of infarction result. The thrombosis of cerebral vessels is common.

Polycythemia vera, fortunately, is quite uncommon.

Often the color of the face, and especially of the lips, is a reddish-purple. Fatigue, weakness, headache and dizziness are common. The patient may bleed excessively after minor injuries, perhaps because of the engorgement of his capillaries and his veins. Splenomegaly commonly occurs. The condition usually has an insidious onset and a prolonged course.

The treatment involves measures to reduce the volume of the circulating blood, to lessen its viscosity, and to curb the excessive production of the red blood cells. Frequent medical examinations are important to determine the course of the disease and the patient's response to therapy.

Venesection (*phlebotomy*) may be performed at intervals. Usually 500 ml. of blood are removed from the vein at a time. This is one instance in which bleeding the patient still has a legitimate place in modern medical treatment.

Radioactive phosphorus and roentgen rays are sometimes administered to decrease the production of the blood cells in the bone marrow. Antineoplastic drugs, such as nitrogen mustard and busulfan may be administered to curb the excessive activity of the bone marrow.

The patient is encouraged to continue his usual activities as long as he is able. He is observed carefully for symptoms of thrombosis. The patient is advised to limit his dietary intake of iron, since this limitation may lessen to some degree the production of the red blood cells.

AGRANULOCYTOSIS

Agranulocytosis is a condition characterized by a decreased production of the white blood cells. Agranulocytosis may result from the toxic effects of drugs, such as sulfonamides, tranquilizers, aminopyrine and barbiturates.

The symptoms of agranulocytosis include fatigue, fever, chills, headache and the appearance of ulcers on the mucous membranes of the mouth, the throat, the nose, the rectum or the vagina.

The prognosis is related to the cause of the condition. When the cause can be determined and promptly removed, and when the treatment can be commenced immediately, the patient usually recovers.

The treatment includes removing the causative factor—for example, stopping the drug that is producing the toxic effect. Infection usually occurs promptly and severely, and the patient, if he is untreated, is powerless to fight the pathogens. Antibiotics are given to control infection. Careful medical aseptic technic is important in preventing the spread of pathogenic organisms to the patient. Meticulous hand washing and the wearing of clean gowns and masks while caring for the patient are necessary. The removal of the drug usually results in the resumption of the normal production of the white blood cells.

Self-medication. A particular hazard is self-medication. It is not unusual to find a patient who has been taking tranquilizers for months without medical supervision. Often a person whose doctor has prescribed the drug for him has with misplaced generosity kept a friend supplied with the medication. One man commented: "I didn't think it could do him any harm. After all, I take it, and it helps me to sleep, and so I thought it might help Joe, too."

When such sharing of prescriptions comes to your attention, explain the necessity for medical supervision in the use of medications and the importance of accurate, individualized diagnosis. Remember that the people involved are trying to be helpful to one another. Factual explanations are likely to be more effective in encouraging people to seek medical advice than scolding or blaming.

Part 2: Related Disorders

LYMPHOSARCOMA

Lymphosarcoma is characterized by overgrowth of lymphocytes in lymph nodes, spleen and lymphoid tissues in other parts of the body. As is true in other forms of neoplastic disease, the overgrowth of tissue (in this instance of lymphocytes) is unruly and, unless it can be completely eradicated, ultimately fatal. Lymphosarcoma is more common in later life than in the young.

Symptoms depend on the site of lymph-node involvement. Lymph-node enlargement typically occurs in cervical, axillary and inguinal regions. For example, if cervical lymph nodes are enlarged, dyspnea and dysphagia can result from pressure on nearby structures. In the final stages of illness the patient develops fever, cachexia, bleeding and vulnerability to infection.

Treatment includes primarily irradiation, corticosteroid and chemotherapy with such agents as nitrogen mustard. Surgical removal of involved lymph nodes may be performed. The objectives of therapy are to control the growth and the spread of the disease and to provide symptomatic relief during the course of the illness, which may last from several months to several years. It is questionable whether patients are ever cured of this disease; it is considered likely that even patients who experience unusually long remissions will eventually succumb.

HODGKIN'S DISEASE

Hodgkin's disease is characterized by the painless enlargement of the lymph nodes. Usually, the cervical nodes are involved first; inguinal and axillary nodes usually are affected later.

The cause of Hodgkin's disease is unknown. One theory states that the disease is due to infection; another states that it results from a malignant neoplasm of the lymphatic tissue. Hodgkin's disease is more common among men than women. It occurs most frequently during young adulthood. Like acute leukemia, Hodgkin's disease is a particularly tragic condition, because it so often claims the lives of young people.

Although some patients survive ten years or longer, most succumb in four or five years. It has been stated that patients whose disease is localized to one section of the body may occasionally be cured with present treatment methods, such as irradiation.

The diagnosis of Hodgkin's disease is established by a biopsy of an affected lymph node. The pathologist notes the changes that are typical of Hodgkin's disease, including the presence of a particular type of abnormal cell called a *Reed-Sternberg cell*.

Symptoms. The early symptoms of Hodgkin's disease include the painless enlargement of one or several lymph nodes. As the nodes enlarge, they often press on adjacent structures. Enlarged retroperitoneal nodes can cause a sense of fullness in the stomach and epigastric pain. Marked weight loss, anorexia, fatigue and weakness occur. Chills and fever are common. Sometimes the patient develops marked anemia and thrombocytopenia, which results in a bleeding tendency. The resistance to infection is poor, and staphylococcal infections of the skin and respiratory infections often complicate the illness. Pruritus is a common symptom. Patients who receive treatment usually have remissions that may last months or even years. However, symptoms recur, and eventually they cause death from respiratory obstruction, cachexia or secondary infections.

Treatment. The treatment of Hodgkin's disease includes x-ray therapy, steroids, and such antineoplastic drugs as nitrogen mustard and chlorambucil. Antibiotics are given to fight secondary infections. Transfusions may be necessary to control anemia. Nitrogen mustard is highly toxic. Nausea and vomiting commonly occur. The depression of the formation of the blood cells may result in severe anemia, leukopenia and thrombocytopenia. Nitrogen mustard is given intravenously. Usually, the drug is introduced into the tubing of an infusion that is already running, since this method helps to prevent the irritation of the vein from the contact with the drug.

Rubber gloves are worn during the preparation and the administration of nitrogen mustard, because contact of the drug with the skin is irritating and harmful. Sometimes, sodium phenobarbital and chlorpromazine are given with nitrogen mustard to lessen the nausea and the vomiting caused by the drug. Frequently, nitrogen mustard is given in the evening, and sedation is given to help the patient to sleep through the night. By morning the most severe gastrointestinal symptoms may have subsided. In any case, never take a meal tray to the patient who is experiencing severe nausea after the administration of nitrogen mustard. Let the patient rest quietly until the symptoms subside. Because the drug is so toxic, it usually is prepared and administered by the patient's doctor.

The nodes may be subjected to intensive x-ray therapy to reduce their size. Although irradiation of a node may be followed by a remission, the disease usually returns and continues its progressive course.

The nursing care of patients with Hodgkin's disease is similar to that of patients with leukemia.

INFECTIOUS MONONUCLEOSIS

Infectious mononucleosis is a condition that affects lymphoid tissues primarily. Lymph-node enlargement is typical, accompanied by malaise, fever, sore throat and headache. The cause of the disease is unknown, although viral etiology is suspected. Infectious mononucleosis seems not to be very contagious, since members of the same family and other close associates usually do not contract the disease, even when no special precautions are taken.

Infectious mononucleosis occurs most commonly among college students and students in medical and nursing schools. There has been a steady rise in the incidence of the disease since 1948 (Shapiro). The designation "kissing disease" is occasionally used as a synonym for infectious mononucleosis, due to the mode of transmission suggested by some investigators. Besides kissing, other forms of rapid indirect oral contact such as passing a soft drink or beer bottle from mouth to mouth are thought by some to spread the disease. The incubation period is about six weeks.

Diagnosis is based on the symptoms, the presence of lymphocytosis and a positive heterophil agglutination test. The latter two diagnostic tests are performed on samples of the patient's blood.

There is no specific treatment for this disease which, fortunately, is usually self-limited. Rest, optimal diet, and prevention of secondary infection are important. Secondary infections, if they occur, may be treated with antibiotics. The average course of the disease is four weeks, after which most patients experience a period of weakness and fatigue of variable duration. Nursing care involves provision of rest and quiet recreation, measures to avoid secondary infection and guidance in gradual resumption of activities after recovery. Young people who have missed school work need help in planning their return to a full schedule gradually, instead of trying to resume school and make up what they have missed while still feeling below par.

REFERENCES AND BIBLIOGRAPHY

AGLE, D., and MATTASON, A.: Psychiatric and social care of patients with hereditary hemorrhagic disease, *in* RATNOFF, O., *et al.: Treatment of Hemorrhagic Disorders,* New York, Harper, 1968.

ALEXANDER, L.: New hope for patients with Hodgkin's disease, *RN* 29:50, September, 1966.

ARNOLD, P.: Total body irradiation and marrow transplantation, *Am. J. Nurs.* 63:83, February, 1963.

BAINTON, D. F., and FINCH, C. A.: The diagnosis of iron-deficiency anemia, *Am. J. Med.* 37:62, 1964.

BEESON, P. B., and McDERMOTT, W. (eds.): *Cecil-Loeb Textbook of Medicine*, ed. 12, Philadelphia, Saunders, 1967.

BERLIN, N. I.: Determination of red blood cell life span, *JAMA* 188:375, April, 1964.

BEUTLER, E.: Drug-induced blood dyscrasias, *JAMA* 189:143, July, 1964.

Closing In—Research on Leukemia, New York, Leukemia Society of America, 1967.

CROUCH, M. L., and GIBSON, S. T.: Blood therapy, *Am. J. Nurs.* 62:71, March, 1962.

DAMESHEK, W., and DUTCHER, R. (eds.): *Perspectives in Leukemia*, New York, Grune, 1968.

DAMESHEK, W., and GUNZ, F.: *Leukemia*, ed. 2, New York, Grune, 1964.

DRAPEAU, J.: The nurse and the hemophiliac patient, *Canad. Nurse* 63:38, July, 1967.

Fact and fancy about infectious mononucleosis, *Pt. Care* 2:102, July, 1968.

FRANCIS, G.: Cancer, the emotional component, *Am. J. Nurs.* 69:1677, August, 1969.

GEE, T. S., *et al.*: Treatment of adult acute leukemia with arabinosylcytosine and thioguanine, *Cancer* 23:1019, May, 1969.

GURSKI, B.: Rationale of nursing care for patients with blood dyscrasias, *Nurs. Clin. N. Am.* 1:23, March, 1966.

HOAGLAND, R. J.: Infectious mononucleosis, *Am. J. Nurs.* 64:125, October, 1964.

KLAGSBRUN, S. C.: Cancer, emotions and nurses, *Am. J. Psych.* 126:1237, March, 1970.

KÜBLER-ROSS, E.: *On Death and Dying*, New York, Macmillan, 1970.

LEAVELL, B. S., and THORUP, O. A.: *Fundamentals of Clinical Hematology*, ed. 2, Philadelphia, Saunders, 1966.

LUNCEFORD, J. L.: Leukemia: disease process, chemotherapeutic approach and nursing care, *Nurs. Clin. N. Am.* 2:635, December, 1967.

MANGAN, H.: Care, coordination and communication in the life island setting, *Nurs. Outlook* 17:40, January, 1969.

MEINHART, N.: The cancer patient: living in the here and now, *Nurs. Outlook* 16:64, May, 1968.

O'KELL, R. T.: Understanding the hemophilias—a, b, and c, *Am. J. Nurs.* 62:101, March, 1964.

PAPPAS, A. M., *et al.*: The problem of unrecognized mild hemophilia, *JAMA* 187:772, March, 1964.

PARETS, A.: Emotional reactions to chronic physical illness, *Med. Clin. N. Am.* 51:1399, November, 1967.

PETITCLERC, C.: Hemophilia, *Canad. Nurse* 63:36, July, 1967.

Progress Against Leukemia, U.S. National Cancer Institute, Bethesda, National Institutes of Health, Publication No. 960, 1968.

QUINT, J.: The dying patient: a difficult nursing problem, *Nurs. Clin. N. Am.* 2:763, December, 1967.

ROBERTS, H. R., *et al.*: Intensive plasma therapy in the hemophilias, *JAMA* 190:546, November, 1964.

RODMAN, M.: Drug therapy today. Drugs that affect blood coagulation, *RN* 32:59, June, 1969.

SHAPIRO, S. L.: Some unsolved problems concerning infectious mononucleosis, *Eye Ear Nose Throat Mouth* 48:594, October, 1969.

VERNICH, J.: Milieu design for adolescents with leukemia, *Am. J. Nurs.* 67:559, March, 1967.

VILTER, R. W.: Nutrition in relation to the anemias, *Med. Clin. N. Am.* 48:1169, September, 1964.

VOTAW, M., and BULL, F.: Drug therapy for neoplastic disease in adults, *Med. Clin. N. Am.* 53:1265, May, 1969.

The Patient with Heart Disease: Anatomy; Diagnostic Tests

27

Epidemiology • Structure (Anatomy) of the Cardiopulmonary System • Observation of Signs and Symptoms • Diagnostic Tests

The diagnosis of heart disease causes fear and anxiety in most people. The heart has always been thought of as the central and most vital organ. This attitude is reflected in such expressions as "the heart of the matter." Somehow, to most people, it never sounds quite so grave to have gallbladder disease or a broken hip as it does to have heart disease. Nevertheless, an individual may live quite comfortably with heart disease for 20 years and then succumb to a seemingly less serious condition.

People often have intense reactions to the diagnosis of heart disease. They may be frightened out of all proportion to the seriousness of the condition and become helpless invalids, when all that the doctor has suggested is a slowing down of the hectic pace of their lives. Other people may verbally acknowledge the doctor's recommendations and yet drive themselves all the harder, getting less sleep than ever and smoking twice as much. Such patients seem to be saying by their actions—and often they express the thought in words when they are given an opportunity—"What's the use? Nothing can be done for it anyway. When your heart goes, that's it, and I may as well get as much fun as I can out of life in the time that I have left."

It is true that tremendous advances have been made in the treatment of heart disease; particularly spectacular have been the advances in heart surgery. Not quite so dramatic, but just as important in helping cardiac patients to live more comfortably are some of the new drugs. For instance, the newer diuretics are helping to relieve edema, thereby enabling many cardiacs to live longer and more comfortably. Despite these modern advances anxiety over heart disease persists, and it is not likely to be dispelled by such pat reassurances as "Oh, they can do wonderful things for heart disease nowadays."

All too often the patient is discouraged from talking about his condition—particularly his feelings concerning it. Nor are such discussions easy for those who minister to the patient. Being able to listen to him without catching some of his anxiety demands the utmost in skill, tact and self-understanding. We may tell patients, "Now don't you worry about your heart! Just let us do the worrying." Such comments will not relieve anxiety and may even intensify it by preventing its expression. Instead of denying the patient's natural concern, we should allow the patient to discuss his worries and to learn more about his condition and his treatment.

Fear of Sudden Changes. What are some of the things that patients and those who care for them fear most about heart disease? Sudden death or even a "sudden turn for the worse" is one. Such sudden changes are by no means limited to heart disease; nevertheless, almost everyone has heard and read about a person who was apparently in excellent health and

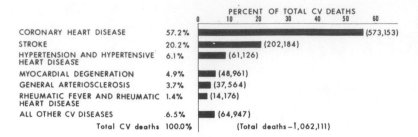

FIG. 27-1. Percentage breakdown of total cardiovascular deaths by specific cause, United States, 1967. (*Cardiovascular Diseases in the United States, Facts and Figures,* New York, The American Heart Association)

suddenly of a "heart attack." (The term "heart attack" has no precise medical meaning, but it is often used to refer to myocardial infarction. The very unpredictability of some types of heart disease forms a basis for fear and uncertainty. Fear of sudden and dire symptoms may make the patient afraid to go on a trip or to continue with his job—even though the doctor has assured him that his condition does not warrant curtailments of these activities.

The Value of Accurate Knowledge and Reporting. When the doctor anticipates certain complications, he often will leave specific written orders to guide the nurse until he arrives. For example, a patient who is likely to develop dyspnea and cyanosis may have an order on his chart for oxygen as necessary.

In reporting a sudden change in the patient's condition, try to select and to report clearly the significant points. "Mr. Brown suddenly has sharp pain in the left side of his chest. He is very pale and frightened. His blood pressure is 95/60, and his pulse is 100 and weak" is more helpful than "Come right away. Mr. Brown has gone bad." Concise, relevant observations clearly reported save time, and often make it possible for the doctor to give directions for the patient's care until he arrives. To give accurate information saves seconds that can be vital.

Meeting Different Needs. Despite the sudden onset of some types of heart disease, by far the largest proportion of patients find that their disease has become a lifetime companion. Many of these people continue to lead active, useful lives, though chronically ill, while others become incapacitated.

The care of chronically ill cardiac patients is difficult and, in a different way, demanding, too. Teaching the patient to care for himself and guiding him in planning his activities and following his treatment require patience and understanding. The nurse must be willing to work with a situation that may improve slowly and almost imperceptibly, or possibly not at all.

Despite rapid progress in the treatment of heart disease, there are still some patients who cannot be helped by present medical knowledge. Some of them are older people whose failing hearts no longer respond to treatment. Others are young people whose hearts have been functioning under great handicap, such as the severe damage that results from rheumatic fever. These patients need our support and care as their independence and well-being gradually diminish. All too often the attitude of doctors and nurses in working with patients who do not respond to treatment is pessimistic if not fatalistic. At such times our patients need us the most. Caring for the patient does not stop even when there seems little likelihood of cure.

EPIDEMIOLOGY

In this country heart disease is the leading cause of death. The number of people succumbing to heart disease mounts steadily as age increases. So much emphasis has been placed on mortality from heart disease that its importance as a cause of disability is sometimes not fully understood. It has been estimated that there are 16,421,000 people in the United States suffering from heart and circulatory disturbances (National Health Education Comm.).

Sometimes these alarming figures are viewed as evidence that "nothing can be done for it," and that people's hearts merely are growing weaker. Actually, these dire predictions are not true. Heart disease is an especially serious problem among the aged, and because of the increased life-span more and more people are living long enough to develop it. Improved diagnosic methods have indicated that deaths once attributed to "old age" now may be classified as deaths from heart disease. When old age has greatly weakened the body, and the time of death draws near, some one organ of the body must give way first, precipitating death. Often this organ is the heart. However, death at the age of 88, precipitated by a failing heart, does

Fig. 27-2. Diagram illustrating the flow of the blood through the heart and the lungs. The path can be observed by starting at the vena cava and following the arrows through the right atrium, the right ventricle, the pulmonary artery, the lungs, the pulmonary vein, the left atrium, the left ventricle and into the aorta.

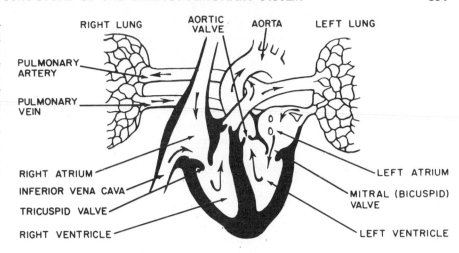

not mean the same thing in terms of life goals as sudden death from coronary occlusion at the age of 50 or disability from rheumatic heart disease during the entire span of an adult life.

STRUCTURE (ANATOMY) OF THE CARDIOPULMONARY SYSTEM

The heart is a four-chambered muscular pump about the size of a man's fist. It can be viewed as a master pump to which is attached a system of tubes for outflow and inflow, namely, the aorta and pulmonary arteries, and the vena cavae and pulmonary veins.

The heart is anchored in the mediastinum, under and a little to the left of the midline of the sternum. (The part of the heart directly under the sternum is the right ventricle and this is significant for the dynamics of external cardiac compression.) The heart's lower border lies on the diaphragm, and forms a blunt point extending to the left, which is called the apex of the heart.

Three distinct layers of tissue make up the heart wall. The bulk of the heart consists of specially constructed muscle tissue known as the *myocardium*. Covering the myocardium on the outside and adherent to it is the *pericardium*. Lining the interior wall of the heart is a delicate layer of endothelial tissue known as the *endocardium*. This is the layer that the blood directly contacts.

The term cardiac cycle means a complete heartbeat, consisting of contraction (systole) and relaxation (diastole) of both atria plus contraction and relaxation of both ventricles. The two atria contract simultaneously; then as they relax, the two ventricles contract and relax, instead of the entire heart contracting as a unit; this gives

a kind of "milking" action to the movements of the heart.

Though having different kinds of work to do, and working under different pressures, both sides of the heart work in unison. The left atrium receives newly oxygenated blood from the lungs via four pulmonary veins. This oxygenated blood flows during diastole into the left ventricle through the mitral valve and during atrial systole, there is a squeezing down of additional blood into the ventricle before the valve closes.

Attached to the mitral valve are cord-like structures known as chordae tendinae which in turn attach to two major muscular projections from the left ventricle known as papillary muscles. During contraction of the left ventricle these muscles also contract, thereby providing tension on the mitral valve and preventing prolapse or invagination of the mitral valve back into the left atrium. If this were to happen as it sometimes does when the papillary muscles are involved in a myocardial infarction, then blood would flow not only forward into the aorta but also backward into the left atrium through an incompetent mitral valve (mitral regurgitation).

During ventricular systole, the blood is pumped through the aortic valve into the aorta from which it then flows under pressure into many smaller arteries, thence to arterioles. Arterioles branch into capillaries which permeate the tissues of each individual organ and are in intimate contact with the cells of those tissues. Oxygen and metabolic foods are delivered to the cells through this complex circulatory network. The thin walls of the capillaries, their tremendous surface area, and their tiny size, all allow for rapid exchange of gases and metabolic substances between the blood and cells. After this exchange takes place, deoxygenated venous blood is transported back to the heart under low pressure by the veins.

Veins from all organs of the body drain into the superior or inferior vena cava, and along with blood from the coronary veins, empty into the right atrium of the heart. Then this venous blood is pumped into the right ventricle through the tricuspid valve. From this chamber it is pumped through the pulmonary artery into the pulmonary or lesser circulation. This smaller circulatory unit is responsible for the exchange of oxygen and carbon dioxide. Blood leaving the right ventricle flows through the pulmonary artery to the pulmonary capillaries. Here, carbon dioxide which has built up in the venous blood because of its release from the tissue as a metabolic end product, is transferred from the blood into the lung spaces (alveoli) and is exhaled. The venous blood takes on oxygen by coming in contact with inspired air. After this exchange of oxygen and carbon dioxide has taken place, the oxygenated blood is transported through four pulmonary veins to the left side of the heart.

Though the structure of the pump itself, and the complex lengthy system of arteries and veins is impressive, the entire cardiopulmonary system is designed to serve as a transport system to provide oxygen and other nutrients and to remove metabolic end products from the *individual cells*. It is at the cell level where the critical action is.

OBSERVATIONS OF SIGNS AND SYMPTOMS

In any situation the more the nurse knows of the condition of her patient, the more astute her observations will be. Because prompt and accurate reporting and recording of these symptoms help to keep the doctor informed of the patient's condition, they facilitate the patient's treatment. Physical activity and emotional upset further increase the work of the heart. If you observe the appearance or the increased severity of symptoms, place the patient at rest, and stay with him as much as possible, providing reassurance and support.

Insufficient blood supply to the heart is an important factor in some kinds of heart disease. It is often indicated by chest pain, pallor, apprehension and sweating. Note the location, the intensity and the duration of the pain; place the patient at rest, and report the symptoms immediately.

A variety of symptoms appear in congestive heart failure (the condition in which the heart is unable to keep pace with the demands made on it). Inefficient pulmonary circulation can lead to congestion in the lungs. The left side of the heart cannot pump the blood out efficiently; fluid accumulates in the lungs, causing congestion. Insufficient oxygenation of the blood may be reflected in a variety of respiratory symptoms, such as cyanosis, cough, dyspnea, and orthopnea (difficulty in breathing in a flat position). Watch for cyanosis around the lips and the nailbeds. If your patient becomes dyspneic, place him at rest, with his head elevated.

Observation of temperature, pulse, respiration and blood pressure is particularly important. Sometimes we are hesitant to make and record observations. Perhaps we assume that the doctor already has noted the symptom, or that if he wanted us to observe for a particular symptom, he would have ordered it specifically. This assumption is nowhere more false than in the care of cardiac patients. Their symptoms often change suddenly. Significant symptoms, such as changes in heart rate and rhythm, may manifest themselves only at brief intervals. If the nurse who is with the patient fails to note and to report them, important information may be lost.

Temperature. Fever is characteristic in some types of heart disease, particularly in acute myocardial infarction, rheumatic fever and subacute bacterial endocarditis. Patients with these conditions should have their temperatures taken rectally, since this method provides the most accurate reading. Though a rectal temperature is more accurate, oral temperatures might be ordered in order to avoid vagal stimulation from the insertion of the rectal thermometer. Vagal stimulation can produce slowing of the heart (bradycardia) and other cardiac arrhythmias such as heart block, especially in the patient with acute myocardial infarction. If the more accurate rectal temperature is still desired, care should be taken that the thermometer is well lubricated and inserted gently. An eye on the electrocardiographic monitor or a finger on the patient's pulse will give evidence of excess vagal stimulation. This should be reported.

Pulse. When you take the pulse, note not only its rate but also its rhythm and its quality. Is the rhythm regular? If not, does the irregularity have a pattern? (For example, you may note an unusually long interval after every 4th beat, or that weak and strong beats alternate.) Is the

FIG. 27-3. (*Top*) Technician taking an ECG. Leads have been placed on arms, legs and chest. (*Bottom*) A sample of the graphic record obtained by electrocardiography.

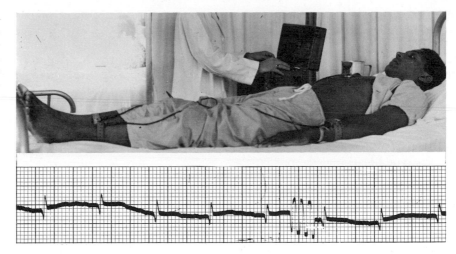

pulse strong, or does it seem weak and hard to detect? Can it be easily obliterated by the pressure of your fingers? Is the pulse bounding and perky, so that it seems to be striking forcefully against your finger?

The pulse rate is not always the same as the heart rate. Some of the beats may be too feeble to produce a pulsation in the radial artery. Counting the radial pulse of such a patient is equivalent to counting only the strong beats. Listening to his heart with a stethoscope may show you that his heart is beating 90 times a minute rather than the 60 beats per minute you counted when you were taking the radial pulse. The difference between heart rate and pulse rate is known as *pulse deficit*. It can be detected by taking an apical-radial pulse. One nurse counts the beats as she listens over the apex of the patient's heart with a stethoscope. (The apex of the heart is the lowermost point of the left ventricle. Usually, it is easiest to hear the heartbeat over the apex (5th intercostal space in the left midclavicular line). Place the stethoscope near the left nipple or, in mature women, under the left breast.) Simultaneously, another nurse counts the radial pulse. Both nurses count for at least a full minute, leave the patient's bedside and compare results. Both figures are charted (for example, $\frac{A90}{R60}$). Remember that if a pulse deficit exists, the number of beats at the radial artery is fewer than the number heard at the apex. If your results indicate that the radial rate is more rapid than the apical rate, you have made a mistake! The apical rate is most significant in a patient with pulse deficit. For example, when you count the pulse prior to administering

digitalis, do not report that the pulse is below 60 until you have checked the apical rate.

Today many hospitalized cardiac patients receive continuous electrocardiographic monitoring. This monitor will indicate the patient's heart rate and rhythm but not the quality of the beat. The quality of the beat can be ascertained by feeling the pulse. Correlating pulse quality with the cardiac monitor provides useful information. The cardiac rhythm on the monitor, for example, can look normal but the cardiac output, reflected in a weak, thready pulse, can be low. Also, the monitor pattern might be irregular but the pulse and other data show that the patient can maintain sufficient cardiac output. By correlating cardiac monitor data with the feel of the patient's pulse while the patient is on the monitor, the nurse is better able to detect arrhythmias by feeling the pulse when the patient is off the monitor.

Blood pressure readings are important, because diseases of the heart often are closely associated with changes in blood pressure. For instance, a drop in blood pressure frequently follows acute myocardial infarction. Be sure that the patient is sitting or lying in a comfortable position, and note carefully and record the systolic and diastolic readings. Take the blood pressure in both arms on admission and once a day. Report any discrepancy.

Respirations. Careful observation of the rate and character of respiration is important. Some nursing studies have shown that inaccuracy in reporting respiration is so widespread that the results of the procedure are of little value. Too often, also, the nurse focuses only on rate, although other observations are equally significant.

While counting the rate for a full minute, observe the quality of respiration. Is the patient's breathing easy or labored (dyspneic)? Are his respirations deep or shallow, wet or dry, wheezing or quiet? Does he use his neck muscles or abdominal muscles to help him breathe? Is the rate faster than normal (tachypnic)? Is he restless or confused? (This can indicate oxygen lack.) Does he have late signs of hypoxia, such as cyanosis or orthopnea? Does he have Cheyne-Stokes type breathing (see p. 359)?

Edema. Note edema, particularly in dependent parts of the body such as the feet and the ankles, and over the sacrum. Edema often accompanies congestive heart failure. The blood is not pumped efficiently, and venous blood that is being returned to the heart by the large veins cannot be received promptly and pumped by the right side of the heart. As a result the venous blood being returned to the heart dams up in the veins. The inefficient return of the blood to the heart causes congestion in the veins and the collection of extra fluid in the tissues.

Fluctuations in weight are important indications of edema. A gain in weight often means that edema is increasing, and not that the patient is growing "fatter," in the usual sense of the term. Loss in weight often reflects the desirable and needed loss of excess fluid that has collected in the tissues. If a daily weight is ordered, weigh the patient at the same time each day and with the same amount of clothing. The recording of weight should be as accurate as possible. A pound more or less may indicate that edema is increasing or decreasing.

DIAGNOSTIC TESTS

Electrocardiogram (EKG)

The scalar electrocardiogram is a graphic record of electric currents generated by the heart muscle. The record is made by a special instrument, called an *electrocardiograph,* which measures and records these currents. The 12-lead EKG is especially useful in determining the nature of myocardial damage and in interpreting arrhythmias. Connections are made between the machine and the patient by means of electrodes that are placed at various points in the patient's body. A special conducting jelly is rubbed on the points of contact. The electrodes are placed on the outside of the skin, usually on the wrists, the ankles and the chest, in a number of combinations. The leads that go to the extremities

are strapped in place. The chest lead is held in position by the technician using a suction cup.

No special preparation for the test is needed other than explaining it to the patient, but since the test does involve the heart the explanation should be individualized to prevent undue anxiety. The nurse should explain that the test is completely painless, and that it merely records the electrical currents of the heart. Otherwise, patients who are having it done for the first time may feel uneasy, when they see wires being attached to them, and wonder whether they are about to receive some kind of electric shock.

The role of the nurse in relation to an EKG involves:

• Helping the patient to understand what to expect. (For example, the patient should know that the EKG is often repeated in order to aid the physician in following the course of the patient's illness.)

• In addition to the usual information, such as the patient's name and ward location, the request slip should state whether or not the patient is receiving digitalis or quinidine; these drugs produce changes in the electrocardiogram that resemble those seen in disease.

• Introducing herself or the technician to the patient and making sure that the patient is comfortable and ready for the test.

• Staying with the patient, if he is very ill, during the test. This is especially important if the patient is anxious, dyspneic, or in pain. If the patient is in an oxygen tent, make a hood around the patient's head with the tent during the brief period of the test. If you have any doubts about the electrical integrity of the machine, don't use it. A spark in the presence of oxygen quickly becomes a fire. Also, faulty wiring or improper grounding of equipment can lead to electrocution of the patient!

• There usually accompanies the tracing and the detailed explanation of the findings a brief summary statement of the results of the test. For example, the statement may indicate recent damage to the myocardium that has resulted from coronary occlusion, or it may describe a disturbance in heart rhythm. All nurses should develop the habit of reading the written summary. The findings may significantly affect the nursing care plan.

Vectorcardiogram

Spatial vectorcardiography is a type of electrocardiography in which the heart's forces are represented by arrows and loops, rather than by waves and complexes.

Heart damage can sometimes be inferred from the oscillographic loop when it is inapparent or questionable in the conventional electrocardiogram.

The vectorcardiogram is obtained by a specially trained technician and interpreted by a cardiologist. Preparation of the patient is similar to that for the electrocardiogram.

X-ray and Fluoroscopy

Fluoroscopy is frequently helpful in the examination of the heart, because the doctor can observe the heart in action. X-ray examination of the chest has the advantage of providing a permanent record. For example, it is often useful in determining the extent of cardiac enlargement. (When heart function is inefficient, the heart enlarges—a mechanism that helps the heart to compensate or to keep up with the circulatory load.) No special care other than an explanation is required before or after the taking of x-ray films or before or after fluoroscopy.

Angiocardiogram

An intravenous angiocardiogram is a record of a test in which a radiopaque dye is injected into a vein, and its course from the right heart to the lungs, back to the left heart and out the aorta is recorded by a rapid series of x-ray pictures. The pictures reveal not only the size and the shape of these structures but also the sequence and the time of their filling with blood. Magnetic tape recordings provide a permanent record. The angiocardiogram is used particularly in diagnosing certain congenital abnormalities of the heart and the great vessels. This test, which is uncomfortable but rarely dangerous, is used only when simpler diagnostic measures fail to provide the necessary information. Breakfast is omitted the morning of the test, and sedative and antihistaminic drugs are administered $\frac{1}{2}$ to 1 hour before the patient is taken to the x-ray department.

Arteriograms

Aortogram. Dye is injected into the aorta, and x-ray films are taken to outline the abdominal aorta and the major arteries in the legs; dye also may be injected into other vessels to help to visualize them in the x-ray pictures.

Peripheral Arteriogram; Coronary Arteriogram. Dye is injected into the femoral or the popliteal artery, and x-ray films are taken to diagnose occlusive arterial disease. In deciding whether or not a patient is a candidate for surgery for the relief of myocardial ischemia, a catheter is passed through an artery, such as the right femoral artery, to the heart, dye is injected through the catheter into various coronary arteries, and serial films are taken. The physicians look for localized blockage of a coronary vessel which may be amenable to surgery. After the test there is a greater chance for bleeding than after a venipuncture. A pressure dressing is applied. Patient activity is restricted for 12 hours. The nurse observes for bleeding, arrhythmias, and peripheral circulation.

Allergic Reactions and Other Complications. During and after such tests as the three immediately above, in which a dye is used, the nurse watches for allergic reactions to the dye, including urticaria, flushing of the skin, fall in blood pressure, nausea, vomiting and, less commonly, respiratory distress and anaphylactic shock. Before the test a skin test may be performed to determine possible allergy to the dye, so that severe allergic reactions can be avoided.

For 5 or 10 minutes after the injection of the dye the patient experiences a feeling of intense heat throughout his body. Due to sudden blood vessel dilation he may develop a headache. Systemic allergic reactions are most likely to occur shortly after the dye has been administered, while the patient is in the x-ray department. However, when the patient returns to the ward, the nurse should observe him for any symptoms of delayed systemic reaction. Watch for adequate urinary output when dye has been injected into an artery or a vein, as the dye may cause a temporary renal insufficiency.

The treatment of allergic reactions includes epinephrine, antihistamines, and oxygen for respiratory distress. Drugs to combat allergic reactions, such as epinephrine and antihistamines, and equipment for giving oxygen should be available.

Other emergency resuscitation equipment such as a defibrillator, an "Ambu" or other breathing bag, and a tracheostomy set, likewise is kept available for immediate use. The patients undergoing the tests are likely to have cardiac impairment. A continuous ECG is usually taken during the tests to monitor the patient's condition. Frequent check is kept of the patient's pulse. Cardiac arrhythmia—ventricular fibrillation is the most common—and cardiac arrest may occur.

Thrombosis and irritation of the vein into which the dye was injected also may occur, and the dye may cause irritation if it leaks beneath the skin. Check the pulse distal to the site of injection in the search for a clot or spasm of the vessel. The absence of a pulse on that side requires the immediate attention of the physician. The vein used for the injection should be observed for pain and swelling. Tenderness over the vein is usual and disappears in one or two days.

The tests are tiring. For example, an angiocardiogram may take 2½ hours. On returning from the x-ray department the patient should be given the opportunity to rest in a quiet atmosphere.

Operative permits are required for most of these procedures.

Cardiac Catheterization

Cardiac catheterization involves passing a long flexible catheter into the heart and the great vessels. As the catheter enters the various chambers, the pressures are measured, and samples of the blood are obtained and analyzed for the content of oxygen and carbon dioxide. For example, the oxygen content of the blood in the right atrium is higher than normal when there is an atrial septal defect—a hole in the septum that separates the atria. The test usually is performed to aid in the diagnosis of congenital defects.

A team, usually comprising several physicians, a nurse and technicians, performs the test. During the test the nurse functions as an assistant to the physician, and she reassures the patient, making him as comfortable as possible. The patient lies supine on a table in a special room equipped with x-ray machines and fluoroscopy machines. The procedure usually takes from 1 to 3 hours; the table is covered with a foam rubber pad, and the patient is positioned carefully, so that he will be as comfortable as possible.

Usually, the room is darkened at intervals during the test to facilitate the use of the fluoroscope. However, a new device, called a *fluoroscopic image amplifier,* or image intensifier, sometimes makes it possible to perform this test in a lighted room.

Ordinarily, the adult patient is not anesthetized (the walls of blood vessels have no fibers that transmit pain), but he is given a sedative before the test. Breakfast is withheld on the morning of the test. The procedure is usually quite painless. The patient may have some slight discomfort at first from the cutdown and the insertion of the catheter. As the catheter enters the chambers of the heart, he may experience some irregularity of heart rhythm that resembles a feeling of fluttering or "butterflies in the chest." If this should occur, the patient is reassured that the sensation will pass, and that there is no cause for alarm. The patient may cough when the catheter is passed up the pulmonary artery. If so, he is told that the sensation will pass quickly. However, despite sedation the patient often is alert and apprehensive, and he is very much aware of the slightest sensation that is out of the ordinary.

When the procedure is over, the catheter is withdrawn gently, and the patient returns to the ward with a small sterile dressing over the site of the cutdown.

Cardiac catheterization is not without danger, although most patients experience no complications, except possibly transient arrhythmia during the actual procedure. The patient's pulse is checked frequently after the catheterization has been performed. If the pulse is rapid or irregular, report this information to the doctor. The site of the cutdown should be watched afterward for any tenderness or inflammation. Pulmonary edema and air embolism are rare complications. Sometimes the patient's temperature is elevated for a few hours after the test. Some doctors permit the patient to resume his usual activities after cardiac catheterization. Others advise that the patient remain in bed, except for bathroom privileges, for the rest of the day.

REFERENCES AND BIBLIOGRAPHY

ELLIOTT, F. C., and WINCHELL, P.: Heart catheterization and angiocardiography, *Am. J. Nurs.* 60:1418, 1960.

Facts on the Major Killing and Crippling Diseases in the United States Today, New York, The National Health Education Committee, 1966.

GEORGE, J. H.: Electronic monitoring of vital signs, *Am. J. Nurs.* 65:68, February, 1965.

HURST, J., and LOGUE, R.: *The Heart,* New York, McGraw-Hill, 1966.

KELLY, A. E., and GENSINI, G. G.: Coronary arteriography, *Am. J. Nurs.* 62:86, February, 1962.

MIGNAULT, J. DE L.: Cardiac catheterization, *Canad. Nurse* 60:340, 1964.

ROY, P.: Angiography, *Canad. Nurse* 60:243, 1964.

WHALEN, R., and STARMER, C. F.: Electric shock hazards in clinical cardiology, *Mod. Conc. Cardiovasc. Dis.* 37:7, February, 1967.

ZIMMERMAN, H. A. (ed.): *Intravascular Catheterization,* Springfield, Ill., Thomas, 1959.

The Patient with Heart Disease

28

Congestive Heart Failure • Nursing Care • Acute Pulmonary Edema

CONGESTIVE HEART FAILURE

The term "heart failure" usually implies to the lay person that the heart has stopped beating. ("She nearly had heart failure when she found out that her brakes wouldn't hold.") When the term is used medically, it has a quite different meaning. It describes the condition of a patient whose heart is unable to keep up with the job of pumping blood, and who therefore develops symptoms due to the derangement of the circulation. For example, the heart muscle may not be able to cope with the added burden placed on it by a damaged valve. The term *congestive* is often used in describing heart failure, because the inefficient circulation leads to the congestion of many organs with blood and tissue fluid.

Heart failure can occur with varying degrees of severity. When symptoms are slight, the patient may be able to be up and about without having any marked symptoms. In contrast, the patient in severe heart failure is critically ill. A patient can go through varying degrees of heart failure, and with treatment he often can recover from it. When the patient shows symptoms of heart failure, his condition is described as *decompensated*—that is, his heart is not able to compensate or to make up for the demands placed on it. When the treatment succeeds in enabling the heart to keep up with the circulatory load, the symptoms disappear, and the condition is described as *compensated*. Often, however, the abnormality of the heart that led to heart failure remains, and unless the patient has continued treatment, he may again develop the symptoms of congestive heart failure.

Causes of Congestive Heart Failure

Congestive heart failure may result from many different forms of heart disease. This condition usually develops gradually, as the result of strain placed on the heart by congenital defects, diseases of the heart and blood vessels, or other diseases that overburden the heart. For example:

• Rheumatic fever can damage the heart valves, and the strain of pumping a sufficient amount of blood through the damaged valves may cause heart failure.

• A branch of a coronary artery may become occluded and cut off the blood supply to a portion of the heart muscle (myocardial infarction). The efficiency of the heart as a pump is impaired and congestive heart failure may develop.

• The pericardium may become inflamed, and later scarred and constricted. Constriction can interfere with heart action by pressing on the heart and so lead to heart failure.

• Hyperthyroidism, if it exists for many years, can cause a normal heart to fail because of the excessive demands placed on the heart by the very rapid heart action that occurs in hyperthyroidism.

The treatment of congestive heart failure involves locating the cause and, if possible, correcting it. Sometimes, cure of the underlying condition is impossible, and treatment consists entirely of measures designed to help the heart to continue to function as efficiently as possible despite the underlying disease. Thus, an abnormality of a valve damaged by rheumatic fever may be corrected surgically. If surgery is not possible, medical treatment designed to help the heart to function despite the valvular lesion would constitute the treatment. The treatment of hyperthyroidism can cure congestive heart failure due to the overactive thyroid.

Particularly in older age groups congestive heart failure frequently is brought about by a combination of factors. The blood vessels may gradually lose their elasticity (a condition called *arteriosclerosis*), and the lumen of the arteries may slowly grow smaller due to the fatty deposits in the walls of the arteries (*atherosclerosis*). The elevation of the blood pressure is common among older persons. In time, these vascular changes can lead to congestive heart failure by interfering with the blood supply to the heart muscle and by causing the heart to pump blood through vessels that have become narrowed and inelastic. The heart itself is not exempt from the process of aging. Gradually, with advancing age, cardiac reserve is lessened, and the heart becomes less able to withstand the effects of injury or disease. Congestive heart failure, then, is not a separate disease; rather it is a pathologic state resulting from a variety of conditions that impair heart function. Although the immediate treatment of congestive heart failure is the same regardless of the cause, the treatment of the underlying condition can involve a variety of measures, both medical and surgical, designed to relieve or to cure the underlying disorder.

The Process of Congestive Heart Failure

Disturbances of one part of the heart, if they are severe enough or last long enough, eventually affect the entire circulation. Let us examine the process of congestive heart failure from mitral stenosis as one example of the process of congestive heart failure:

• The narrowing of the mitral valve impedes the flow of the blood from the left atrium to the left ventricle.

• The left atrium, because it cannot empty normally, becomes enlarged, and the pressure within it increases.

• This increased pressure, in turn, causes the lungs to become congested with fluid, because the distended left atrium cannot effectively receive the oxygenated blood coming to it from the lungs.

• Lung congestion results in the inefficient oxygenation of the blood. The patient develops dyspnea, cough, orthopnea and sometimes hemoptysis. These are symptoms of left-sided heart failure.

• Because of the congestion in the lungs, it becomes harder for the right ventricle to pump blood to the lungs. The right ventricle must pump more forcefully to overcome the resistance of the lungs to the blood coming from this ventricle.

• The right ventricle eventually becomes unable to keep up with its work. It cannot pump the blood effectively, and the right side of the heart becomes congested with blood.

• Venous blood returning to the right side of the heart cannot be pumped to the lungs quickly and efficiently enough because of the failure of the right side of the heart. Congestion develops in the large veins leading to the heart and eventually in other organs and tissues of the body as the result of inefficient venous return.

• Dependent edema, such as that of the feet and the ankles on standing, appears. The abdomen may become distended with fluid (ascites). The liver, too, becomes edematous and enlarged. Presacral edema may be present in the patient on bed rest. The veins in the neck become distended. These are symptoms of right-sided heart failure.

This is only one example of the process of congestive heart failure. In each type of heart disease the process is somewhat different, depending on the location of the heart damage and its severity. Yet the process is similar in that, although one part of the heart and the circulation are primarily affected at first, the process, if it continues, eventually affects the entire circulation. The sequence in which symptoms appear reflects the sequence of physiologic disturbance. Symptoms of either right-sided or left-sided heart failure may appear first; eventually, symptoms of failure in both sides usually will be present.

Patients with congestive heart failure retain excessive amounts of sodium. This excess sodium contributes to the problem of edema by holding water in the tissues.

Symptoms of Congestive Heart Failure

Often the patient notices that he is unusually tired after work that previously had not caused fatigue. Some patients find that dyspnea on exertion is their first symptom. For instance, a patient who lives on the second floor may find that he becomes short of breath and has to rest on the landing before he attempts the second flight of steps. He may notice that he has difficulty breathing while he is lying flat, and he begins to use two or even three pillows. Cough, occasionally productive of blood-streaked sputum, may occur.

The patient may notice that his feet and his ankles are swollen, particularly at the end of the day, when he has been standing and walking.

Fig. 28-1. (*Left*) Pitting edema of feet and lower legs. (*Right*) The same patient after treatment relieved the edema. (CIBA Pharmaceutical Company)

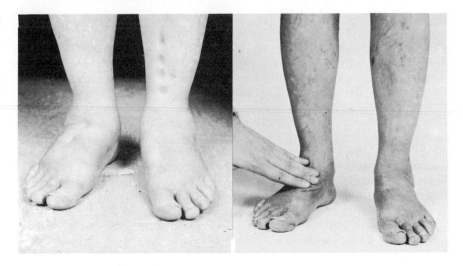

This swelling usually disappears during the night when his feet and his legs are elevated but the fluid can shift to the lungs or sacral region.

Actually, the edema does not really disappear. It is just distributed differently due to the patient's posture and is therefore less noticeable. When he stands, his ankles gradually will swell again. By the time that the edema becomes noticeable, the patient usually has retained 10 or more extra pounds of fluid in his tissues. These extra pounds, which actually are due to the retained fluid, show up on the scale when the patient is weighed. His apparent gain in weight is not in the usual sense of increased fat or muscle tissue. Although the patient's weight gradually increases, he usually is losing rather than gaining fat and muscle tissue. When this process has continued for a time, the patient often looks strangely out of proportion. The lower parts of his body (the ankles, the legs and eventually the thighs and the abdomen) become swollen and heavy, whereas his face and the upper parts of his body look thin and wasted. When edema is relieved by treatment, his family and friends often are amazed at how thin and frail he looks.

Edema of the feet and the legs rarely causes pain, but it makes the patient's legs feel heavy, clumsy and tired. It is described usually as "pitting edema," because, when pressure is exerted, the part that has been pressed will become indented. The indentation gradually disappears after the pressure has been released. Edema of other areas, though it is less visible, often causes symptoms of the dysfunction of the organs involved. For example, the distention of the liver

and the other abdominal viscera may cause flatulence, anorexia and nausea. The collection of fluid within the lungs and the pleural space leads to dyspnea and sometimes to persistent cough.

Some patients with congestive heart failure experience Cheyne-Stokes respirations. This symptom is believed to be due to poor circulation to the brain, causing the respiratory center in the brain to become less sensitive to the amount of carbon dioxide in the blood. Irritability, restlessness and decreased attention-span may occur when the condition is very severe. These symptoms are due to impaired cerebral circulation, and they may progress to stupor and coma before death.

Diagnosis

Because congestive heart failure is a disorder that can be produced by a variety of diseases of the heart, any test or combination of tests used for cardiac patients may be ordered in an effort to discover the underlying cause of congestive heart failure. For example, in addition to the history and the physical examination, the patient may have electrocardiograms, x-ray examination and fluoroscopy of his chest, or cardiac catheterization.

Two tests—measuring the venous pressure and the circulation time—are done especially to determine the congestion and the slowing of the circulation so typical of congestive heart failure.

Measuring Venous Pressure. The technic of measuring arterial pressure, which we usually refer to as "taking the blood pressure," is a familiar one. Measuring venous pressure is done less often, and it may be less familiar. The doctor performs this test, and the nurse may assist when it is performed. First, the patient's arm is positioned at the same level as his heart by supporting the arm with a pillow or a rolled blanket. The doctor performs a venipuncture, and to the needle and the syringe he attaches a water manometer that has had sterile normal saline placed in it. A 3-way stopcock connects the syringe, the needle and the manometer. When the manometer is in place, the stopcock is adjusted to allow the saline from the manometer to flow into the patient's vein. The pressure in the vein will permit only a certain amount of the saline to run in. When the saline stops entering the vein, the level of the saline left in the manometer is read. The normal venous pressure ranges from 7 to 14 cm. of water. It is increased in congestive heart failure.

Measuring Central Venous Pressure. The most accurate measurement of venous pressure is obtained when a catheter is inserted into a peripheral vein and threaded into the vena cava or right atrium. This is called central venous pressure. The catheter is connected via a three-way stopcock to a water manometer and an intravenous infusion bottle and serial readings are taken. Central venous pressure is recorded as the height of the fluid column in the manometer when it is filled with fluid from the infusion bottle. When the venous pressure is not being read, the three-way stopcock is adjusted so that the intravenous fluid runs through to keep the catheter patent. Since venous pressure decreases slightly on inspiration and increases slightly with expiration, oscillations of the fluid level in the manometer occur with the patient's breathing. Right atrial venous pressure is about 0-4 cm. of water. Vena cava pressure is about 4-10 cm. of water. Central venous pressure is increased in congestive heart failure. (See p. 629 for use of central venous pressure in shock.)

Normally the external jugular veins in the neck are collapsed above the level of the suprasternal notch when a person sits or stands. Distention of these veins indicates that the pressure within them is elevated.

Measuring Circulation Time. The circulation time is determined by the intravenous injection of a substance that can be tasted by the patient when it reaches his tongue. Decholin, which causes a bitter taste, or sucrose, which causes a sweet taste, may be used. The substance is injected into a vein in the arm, and the time interval between the injection and the patient's tasting the substance is called the *arm-to-tongue time*. Normally, this is less than 15 seconds. The test is timed by a stopwatch, after careful instruction of the patient to signal as soon as he tastes the substance. In congestive heart failure the circulation time is prolonged.

Treatment

The treatment of congestive heart failure involves measures to help the heart to function as effectively as possible and to relieve the symptoms produced by the inefficient circulation:

• The patient is helped to rest. His heart may be able to meet the demands of the body at rest, but be unable to cope with the demands placed on it by physical or emotional stress. Sedatives are sometimes necessary to help the patient to rest.

• The abnormal retention of sodium is combated by limiting the patient's intake of sodium, whether in food or drugs.

• Digitalis is given to slow the heart rate and to strengthen its beat. These two actions help the weakened overburdened heart to pump blood more efficiently.

• Diuretics are given to rid the body of the excess fluid and the sodium that have been stored in the tissues. Paracentesis sometimes is necessary to relieve ascites.

• Oxygen is ordered to improve ventilation when oxygenation is impaired by congestion and sluggish circulation through the lungs.

We sometimes mistakenly think that all the dramatic recoveries are reserved for surgical treatment. Actually, most patients with heart disease are treated medically, and many of them have spectacular relief of symptoms.

NURSING CARE

Nursing care involves a variety of abilities. When the patient is admitted with acute congestive heart failure, nursing care involves speed, assurance, and technical skill in quickly providing oxygen and medications. The nurse has the responsibility for observing the critically ill patient and for notifying the doctor of changes in his condition. The nurse conveys to the patient and family a feeling that she knows what she is doing and that she will respond quickly and capably to the patient's nursing needs. When a patient is suddenly admitted to the hospital in a critical condition, the need for reassurance is especially great. Because the situation demands speed and action, the nurse, rather than drawing up a chair and talking with the patient, reassures by her competence and her kindliness as she quickly assists the doctor with emergency treatment.

Detailed explanations are deferred until the patient improves. At first he is too sick to take in complicated explanations, and care must be given quickly. For example, instead of giving a detailed explanation of why oxygen is necessary, the nurse assures the patient that it will help his breathing, deftly applies it, and stays with the patient. A quiet, "All right, now just breathe in and out," until the patient becomes accustomed to the oxygen mask or other device, conserves the patient's energy and helps him to realize that it really does help him to breathe and will not smother him. Seeing prompt, competent, compassionate care given to a loved one gives the family assurance that they are leaving the patient in the hands of people who know enough and care enough to help him, and that whatever happens, they will do their best for him. For example, a family member who is sitting at the bedside can be told, "Now, if you want anything at all, just press this light switch, and I'll be right in." In this way, even when the nurse cannot be present all the time, the family feels her continued concern and support.

The nurse has to be alert for possible complications and their prevention. Because she recognizes the danger of thrombophlebitis in patients who are confined to bed, she does not roll up the knee gatch to hold the patient up in bed and leave the gatch that way for days. A footboard is used so that by placing the feet against it the patient is kept from sliding down in bed. A covered supply box is a simple method of extending a footboard to keep the short patient from sliding down in bed. Maintain the feet and legs in good alignment. Massage and a foam-rubber pad or sheepskin can be used to prevent decubiti.

If it is necessary for the nurse to open an oxygen tent, such as for feeding, turn the liter flow up to maintain the concentration of oxygen. Matches and electrical appliances are excluded from the environment to minimize the fire hazard.

Intake and output are carefully recorded. If the patient has an order for daily weights preferably the same person should perform the procedure at the same time daily (before breakfast). Similar clothing or bed clothing should be incorporated each time the patient is weighed.

Rest is very important. The nurse does not fall into the trap of assuming that her patients receive poor care if they do not have a complete bath every day. The nurse selects aspects of care that are most important at the time. Provision for rest at intervals during care is important.

Careful note is taken of the degree of the ankle edema, the dyspnea or the cyanosis, and of the quality and the rate of both apical and radial pulse. The pulse is checked before administering digitalis. If signs of digitalis toxicity are present, such as an apical pulse below 60 per minute, increasing P-R interval, dropped beats, or premature ventricular contractions, notify the doctor before giving the drug.

Know the predicted time of effect of the diuretic given the patient. For example, with a newer diuretic such as sodium ethocrynate (Lyovac Sodium Edecrin) given intravenously, diuresis can be observed in 15 minutes with the peak volume in 30-60 minutes. After a similar drug (Ethacrynic acid, Edecrin) is given orally, the peak urinary volume occurs in about 2 hours. Patients, especially elderly ones, may be given sedation along with the diuretic on admission. Sudden diuresis can result in bed wetting or in acute urinary retention. Offer the patient the bedpan or urinal and check the bladder for distention. Urinary frequency and urgency is very tiring especially on the first day of hospitalization so assist female patients to get on and off the bedpan. Keep a close check on the male patient so that he has an empty urinal when he needs it. Watch the patient for signs of electrolyte depletion.

Each time the patient's activities are increased, or when supportive therapy is withdrawn, be especially watchful. For example, when the patient eats his first meal out of the oxygen tent, unobtrusively observe his reactions while replenishing the solution in the thermometer holder. New activities are taken gradually. A few steps to the chair and staying up only until fatigued the first time is sufficient. In addition to checking the pulse, the nurse can choose this time to make the patient's bed, so that she will be nearby if the patient becomes fatigued and needs to go back to bed. The first trip to the bathroom can be reserved for another day.

As a result of data gathered from clinical studies some physicians believe that chair rest, rather than bed rest, is more beneficial for the patient

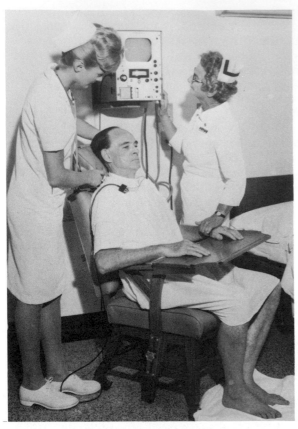

Fig. 28-2. The patient in a bedside cardiac chair. (Tampa Tracings, Oldsmar, Fla.)

in congestive heart failure (Levine). The principle involved is that the heart works less in the sitting position than in the recumbent position. The patient in the chair does not engage in any more activity than he would if confined to bed. Only bradycardia or hypotension sufficient to interfere with cerebral circulation are contraindications to chair rest. The patient is assisted to sit in bed, then to touch the floor, and pivot into a chair. He is not lifted. He is returned to bed in the same manner. Because the legs are dependent, critics of chair-rest treatment state that increased incidence of thrombophlebitis is a sequela. However, proponents of chair rest deny this. The use of Ace bandages and foot and ankle exercises prevent stagnation of blood, whether the patient rests in bed or in a chair. A lounge-type chair in which the pelvis is lower than the patient's legs is not a recommended cardiac chair because blood can pool in pelvic veins (see Fig. 28-2).

Teaching

As soon as the patient recovers from his most acute symptoms, the nurse begins to use opportunities for teaching. For instance, when the patient first asks for salt, the nurse explains that many foods in their natural state contain some salt. Later, when the patient feels better, he is taught that the sodium contained in the salt makes it necessary for him to limit his intake of salt, and that many foods, as well as medications, contain large amounts of sodium. The sodium helps to hold fluid in the body.

If the patient asks, "I have no pain in my heart, but my ankles swell. Why is that?" the reply can be, "Your circulation gets slowed down when your heart isn't pumping as efficiently as it should, and fluid tends to stay in your tissues. It usually shows up most in the lowest part— for instance, in your feet and your legs when you're standing up."

Diet

Low Sodium Diets. The dietitian can talk with the patient or family member several times about the sodium content of various foods, the kind and the amount of food that he could have each day without exceeding the amount of sodium permitted, and the variety of other seasonings that can be used. The nurse can help the patient to understand that many foods in their natural state contain sodium. Some contain relatively large amounts, and these must be eliminated from the diet. Depending on the amount of sodium specified in the doctor's prescription, foods containing moderate amounts of sodium may have to be used in very small amounts. Try to help the patient to understand that it is the sodium rather than the salt per se that has to be limited. This distinction will help him to recognize that drugs containing sodium must be excluded also unless the doctor has been consulted about the use of the medication. The patient whose sodium intake is restricted cannot take a teaspoonful or two of sodium bicarbonate to relieve indigestion.

The amount of sodium allowed varies from about 500 mg. to 3 Gm. daily. Patients on very low sodium intake should be watched, especially in hot weather, for symptoms of sodium deficit. When the patient perspires a great deal, he may need more sodium than his diet provides and as a consequence develop weakness, dizziness, headache, abdominal cramps and diarrhea. If these symptoms appear, the doctor increases the allowance of sodium. The patient should consult his doctor before using any salt substitute, such as potassium chloride. The nurse can recommend the use of other seasonings, such as lemon juice or onion juice.

A good many prepared foods have salt added to them in the process of canning or freezing. Help the patient to cultivate the habit of reading labels on all prepared foods. Other forms of sodium, such as sodium benzoate, baking powder and sodium propionate, are contained in many prepared foods.

When the patient asks for a snack between meals, it is easy to forget that the amount of sodium must be considered. Discuss this addition to the daily diet with the dietitian and consider the amount of sodium in the snack as part of the patient's daily allotment. Give only foods that you know to be virtually free of sodium, such as fresh fruit. Encourage the family to munch their pretzels out of sight of the cardiac patient. When carried to extremes, this practice may interfere with the rights of others, but in moderation it is a kind help to the person on a diet, especially in the beginning.

The following common foods are high in sodium and usually are excluded completely: ham, bacon, salted fish, salted nuts, potato chips, salted crackers, ketchup, mustard, peanut butter and cheese (except washed cottage cheese).

The following foods also contain considerable sodium and may be excluded or restricted in amount: ordinary bread, butter and milk (special preparations of all these are available that limit the sodium content), cake and cookies, most shellfish, frozen peas, lima beans and some frozen fish.

Staying on a special diet, be it reducing, low purine or low sodium, is not a moral issue but a complicated medical problem. The nurse who gives her patient a low-sodium diet and discusses with him what he is allowed to eat once he goes home, will be most constructive when her attitude is light in touch and sympathetic in nature. She will be *most* helpful if she can be *least* like a punitive mother who denies her naughty child candy.

Restriction of diet may be a true loss to a patient. Only anger and rebellion will be aroused in a patient whose overbearing nurse says or implies: "This is your diet. You had better stick to it if you know what's good for you. If you don't and get an attack, don't come crying to me."

The nurse can find out the patient's favorite foods in order to help to preserve as many as possible in the patient's diet. The nurse works also with the doctor to clarify the order. ("Just how many grams of sodium may he have, doctor?") She keeps the doctor and the dietitian informed about how the patient is eating and reacting to the diet.

Often special diets are thought of as modifications of our own American diet. But, Spaniards, Egyptians and Japanese go on special diets in their own countries. The special diet should be an adaptation of a normal diet for that patient. Unfortunately, attempting to change food patterns often seems like saying to the patient, "You must get over being Italian and be American."

• The patient needs to know how and where to get help with his diet after he leaves the hospital and how to get his questions answered. The American Heart Association (11 East 23rd Street, New York City, 10010) and the United States Public Health Service (write the Government Printing Office, Washington, D.C. 20025) have pamphlets available that describe the uses of sodium in the body, sample diets and recipes in "Your 500 mg. Sodium Diet," "Your 1,000 mg. Sodium Diet" and "Your Mild Sodium Restricted Diet." Some communities have diet counseling services.

Dietary Potassium. Some patients are instructed to increase their dietary intake of potassium. Foods high in potassium include fresh fruit juices, except apple and cranberry, most whole fruits such as bananas, but only if they are fresh or dried, nuts, high protein foods such as meat or fish, nonstarchy vegetables such as spinach, milk solids, and whole grain cereals. Foods low in potassium include fats, carbohydrates including starchy vegetables, apples and cranberries, and products made from them, and canned fruits.

Hypokalemia. In severe potassium deficiency with digitalis intoxication (hypokalemia) potassium may be given intravenously. The usual rate of administration is 40 mEq. every 8 hours. The maximum rate is 40 mEq. every 2 hours.

Drugs

Digitalis preparations vary in dosage from grams to milligrams. Digitalis is a very powerful drug, and in incorrect dosage it is a very dangerous one. Read the label very carefully and know the average dose of the particular preparation that you are giving. Relatively large doses of these preparations are given at the beginning of therapy in order to accumulate therapeutic amounts of the drug in the body. This is called *digitalization*. A daily, smaller dose is then given that is sufficient to maintain therapeutic amounts of digitalis in the body. This is called the *maintenance dose*. Many patients take digitalis for years. It has helped many cardiac patients to control their disease and to live comfortably. Patients especially need to know that they should not discontinue their digitalis when they feel well, or take more than the prescribed dose when they don't feel well.

Toxic effects can occur from digitalis. They tend to appear gradually. The patient is generally instructed to consult the physician if he experiences sudden loss of appetite for 24 hours, unexplained nausea or vomiting, unusual palpitation or change in pulse, or sudden disturbance in vision (LaDue and Burckhardt). If early symptoms are noted and reported to the doctor, more serious toxic effects usually can be avoided. Postdischarge instruction of the patient is discussed with the physician early in the hospital stay so that the patient and family have the opportunity to ask questions.

Examples of teaching points for a patient with congestive heart failure might be:

• He cannot add any salt to his food, either when it is prepared or when it is served; naturally salty foods like ham and bacon are to be omitted.

• He is to weigh himself every morning before breakfast, always wearing similar clothing when he is weighed. Daily weight is to be recorded and shown to the doctor each time that he visits his office.

• Digitalis is to be taken once each morning. Any loss of appetite, any nausea, or any vomiting or irregular heart action should be reported to the doctor.

• Chlorothiazide should be taken once daily. A large glass of orange juice is to be taken every morning to guard against the development of hypopotassemia, a complication of chlorothiazide therapy.

• Any recurrence of symptoms is to be reported to the doctor—for example, edema of the ankles, dyspnea, unusual fatigue.

ACUTE PULMONARY EDEMA

Pulmonary edema represents an acute emergency for the patient and often is associated with heart disease. The weakening of the left ventricle, which may be caused by such conditions as acute myocardial infarction, arteriosclerotic heart disease, or rapid cardiac arrhythmias, makes the left ventricle incapable of maintaining sufficient output of blood with each contraction. However, the right ventricle continues to pump blood toward the lungs. The pulmonary capillaries and the alveoli become engorged, because blood continues to flow to the lungs and is not adequately and promptly pumped into the systemic circulation by the left ventricle. Sometimes, the lungs become rapidly inundated with fluid. This inundation of the lungs can occur in patients who have congestive heart failure; it may be triggered by some unusual exertion or by slipping down in bed during sleep. (Lying flat may cause edema to settle in the lungs, which are then lower than the rest of the body.) Acute respiratory distress develops. This is termed paroxysmal nocturnal dyspnea.

Acute pulmonary edema can result also from injury to the lung tissue, such as blast injuries, causing many small hemorrhages within the lung, and from conditions in which the drainage of the pulmonary secretions is impaired. For example, chronic pulmonary diseases, such as emphysema, may lead to the obstruction of the respiratory passages when the patient is unable to cough up secretions. Pulmonary edema also may be caused by the inhalation of irritants, such as ammonia.

Patients with acute pulmonary edema experience prodromal anxiety, restlessness, sudden dyspnea, wheezing, orthopnea, cough (often productive of pinkish, frothy sputum), cyanosis and severe apprehension. Respirations sound moist or "gurgling."

The relief of these symptoms is urgent. The patient literally can drown in his own secretions during an attack of acute pulmonary edema. Every effort is made to relieve the congestion in the lungs as quickly as possible.

The doctor's orders may include measures to provide physical and emotional relaxation, to relieve hypoxia, to retard venous return to the heart, and to improve cardiovascular function.

• Provide physical and emotional relaxation. Morphine or Demerol often is ordered intravenously to lessen apprehension. Morphine, particularly, seems to help to relieve the attack by depressing higher cerebral centers, thus relieving anxiety and slowing the respiratory rate. In addition, morphine promotes muscular relaxation to reduce the work of breathing. Very importantly, morphine dilates peripheral veins thus reducing venous return by a so-called internal or pharmacologic phlebotomy (Hultgren). The patient should be permitted to stay in the position most comfortable for him, usually sitting up. Avoid anything that would increase his feeling of breathlessness and choking. Do not pull curtains around his bed or close the window if the patient indicates he wants it open. If it is possible, have someone else talk to the doctor, so that you do not have to leave the patient. If you must leave, tell the patient you will be right back, and be right back.

- Relieve hypoxia and improve ventilation.

To raise the rate of oxygen diffusion across the fluid barrier of edema in the alveoli, 100 per cent oxygen through a positive pressure, non-rebreathing type of mask, may be ordered initially. This helps to prevent further engorgement of the lungs with fluid. Later, a nasal catheter, nasal cannula, or tent may be substituted. Apply the mask quickly, but do not forget a brief word of explanation and reassurance to the patient, who is already afraid of suffocation, and who may be made more so by the sudden application of the mask. Be sure there is a firm seal between the mask and the patient's face, but guard against pressure damage to the patient's skin. Frequent drying of the skin will minimize this risk.

Oxygen must always be humidified to prevent the drying of secretions and further impairment to ventilation.

Aminophylline may be administered intravenously to dilate the bronchi and to make breathing easier, and to lessen pulmonary-capillary transudate. An intravenous drip of the drug in solution not to exceed a rate of 20 mg. per minute may be ordered.

- Retard venous return to the heart.

Measures may be taken to decrease the volume of circulating blood, thus helping to relieve the congestion of blood and fluid in the lungs. These measures consist of wet or dry phlebotomy, the use of an intermittent positive pressure ventilator, and the use of morphine. Wet phlebotomy of approximately 500 ml. of blood may be performed, or rotating tourniquets may be used to trap blood in the extremities, so that it is not returned to the already overburdened and congested heart and lungs, a so-called "dry" phlebotomy.

When rotating tourniquets are used, they may be applied clockwise or counterclockwise, pro-vided that the tourniquets are always rotated in the same direction throughout the treatment. The tourniquet is applied tightly enough to interfere with venous return and not tightly enough to cut off arterial circulation. If a rubber tourniquet is used, check the pulse in the extremity after applying the tourniquet. If the pulse has been obliterated, the tourniquet has been applied too tightly, and it should be loosened. If blood-pressure cuffs are used, inflate each cuff to a point between the patient's systolic and diastolic blood pressure.

The exact procedure to be used varies, and it will be specified by the doctor. Tourniquets may be rotated every 15 minutes, although in some instances the doctor may order more frequent rotation. If 15-minute intervals are used, each extremity will have had the tourniquet on it for 45 minutes and will have been free of the tourniquet 15 minutes. (See Table 28-1 and Fig. 28-3.)

The patient's extremities will become swollen, mottled and uncomfortable due to engorgement with venous blood. Explain to the patient that the swelling will disappear when the tourniquets are removed. Check the pulse in the extremity frequently, to be sure that the circulation to the part is adequate.

When the tourniquets are to be removed, follow the same rotation already established and remove one tourniquet every 15 minutes, so that by the end of 45 minutes all tourniquets will have been removed. Never remove them all at once. To remove them all at the same time would cause a sudden increase in the amount of circulating blood, with a return of more blood to the heart and the lungs than they can handle, causing another attack of pulmonary edema. If the extremities do not return promptly to their normal appearance when the tourniquets have been removed, notify the doctor.

Several models of electrically operated automatic rotating tourniquet machines are currently available. The use of this machine saves nursing

TABLE 28-1. PLAN FOR ROTATING TOURNIQUETS

TIME A.M.	RIGHT LEG	LEFT LEG	LEFT ARM	RIGHT ARM
9:00	off	on	on	on
9:15	on	off	on	on
9:30	on	on	off	on
9:45	on	on	on	off
10:00	off	on	on	on

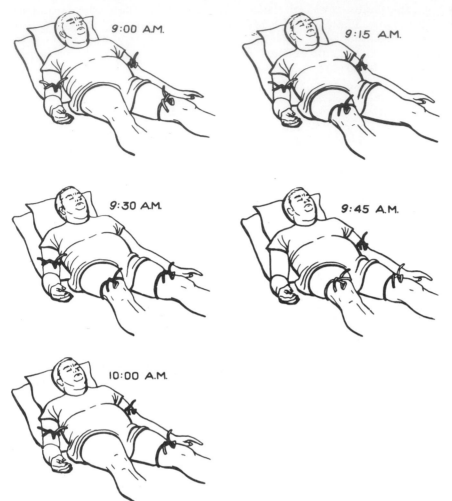

time since there is no need to change the velcro-fastened blood pressure cuff-type tourniquets once they are applied. Inflation and deflation time is automatically cycled. The machine is more efficient since it eliminates the variability in technic and cuff pressure which results when more than one person manually applies rubber tourniquets. Human failure resulting from "forgetting" to rotate the tourniquets or not being able to get back to the patient on time is eliminated.

Blood pressure can be taken easily using the pressure gauge on some machines or, on others, by disconnecting an arm cuff from the machine and attaching a syphgmomanometer to it. The same observations relative to arterial circulation and discontinuance of therapy are necessary.

Some physicians advocate mechanical positive pressure breathing during inspiration (IPPB) to reduce venous return to the heart in the treatment of acute pulmonary edema. Normally, the intrathoracic pressure of spontaneous respiration is negative. When this negative pressure is replaced by positive pressure, venous return to the heart is reduced. The doctor determines flow-rate, pressure, and inspiratory/expiratory ratio in order to arrive at an intrathoracic net positive pressure which will impede venous flow. (If the patient is hypotensive, further reduction of venous return to the heart is contraindicated.) IPPB has the additional benefit of assisting ventilation in all lung segments and is an effective means of administering oxygen. (See Chap. 52 for care of the patient on a respirator.)

Morphine sulfate, because of its property of pooling blood in peripheral vascular beds, is

Fig. 28-4. Patient receiving treatment with automatic rotating tourniquets. (Jobst Institute, Inc., Toledo, Ohio)

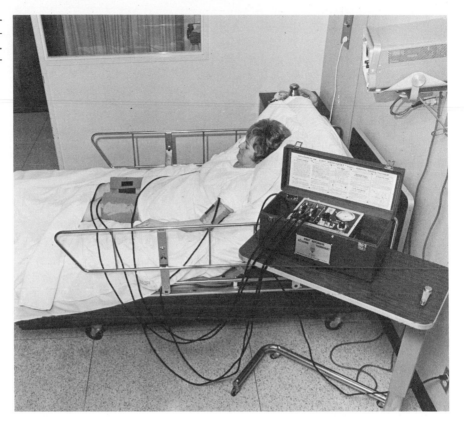

used to retard venous return as well as to decrease anxiety and relieve dyspnea.

• Improve cardiovascular function.

When the attack of pulmonary edema is due to congestive heart failure, other measures for the treatment of this condition may be begun promptly, if the patient has not already been receiving them. For example, digitalization with a rapidly acting preparation, like ouabain, and the injection of a rapid-acting, potent diuretic such as sodium ethacrynate (Lyovac Sodium Edecrin) may be ordered.

REFERENCES AND BIBLIOGRAPHY

BETSON, C., and UDE, L.: Central venous pressure, *Am. J. Nurs.* 69:1466, July, 1969.

BROWSE, N.: *The Physiology and Pathology of Bed Rest,* Springfield, Ill., Thomas, 1965.

EGAN, D.: Management of acute pulmonary edema, *Hosp. Med.* 2:20, February, 1966.

GUYTON, A.: *Textbook of Medical Physiology,* ed. 3, p. 601, Philadelphia, Saunders, 1966.

HANCHETT, E., and JOHNSON, R.: Early signs of congestive heart failure, *Am. J. Nurs.* 68:1456, July, 1968.

HULTGREN, H., and FLAMM, M.: Pulmonary edema, *Mod. Conc. Cardiovasc. Dis.* 38:1, January, 1969.

HURST, J., and LOGUE, R.: *The Heart,* New York, McGraw-Hill, 1966.

LARSON, E.: The patient with acute pulmonary edema, *Am. J. Nurs.* 68:1019, May, 1968.

LEVINE, S.: Chair rest versus bed rest, *Hosp. Med.* 2:2, January, 1966.

LADUE, J., and BURCKHARDT, D.: Digitalis intoxication, *Hosp. Med.* 23, 1967.

MACGREGOR, E.: *Social Science in Nursing.* Chap. 6, Psychosocial aspects of physical disabilities and rehabilitation, New York, Russell Sage, 1960.

MCINTYRE, H.: Clinical nursing and the congestive heart failure patient, *Cardiovasc. Nurs.* 3:19, September-October, 1967.

OLSEN, E., et al.: The hazards of immobility, *Am. J. Nurs.* 67:779, April, 1967.

Potassium imbalance: Programmed instruction, *Am. J. Nurs.* 67:343, February, 1967.

SCHWARTZ, D., et al.: *The Elderly Ambulatory Patient,* New York, Macmillan, 1969.

The Patient with Inflammatory or Valvular Disease of the Heart

29

Rheumatic Fever and Rheumatic Heart (Valvular) Disease
Active Rheumatic Fever • Rheumatic Heart (Valvular) Disease
Bacterial Endocarditis • Pericarditis

Patients with cardiac diseases such as rheumatic fever or rheumatic valvular disease, bacterial endocarditis, or pericarditis share certain commonalities besides the often overwhelming awareness that they have been struck down by dreaded heart disease. These disorders are inflammatory and often follow infection elsewhere in the body which has left the patient in a weakened condition to cope with additional physical and psychosocial threats. The treatment process is not dramatic but rather slow and tedious. The diseases are frequent among young adults who must forego their usual job, civic, and family and social responsibilities for a long period, sometimes with loss of income. All of the diseases carry an uncertainty about the future.

The extent of the damage often is not fully manifest during youth, but may lead to symptoms later in life when the individual experiences additional stressors, such as another illness, childbearing, or the aging process.

RHEUMATIC FEVER AND RHEUMATIC HEART (VALVULAR) DISEASE

Rheumatic fever is found most among those who are between the ages of 5 and 15. It sometimes occurs in late adolescence and young adulthood, particularly in persons with a history of the disease in childhood; it is rare after the age of 25 except when crowded living conditions favor streptococcal infections.

Rheumatic fever often leads to permanent damage to the heart and valves with subsequent chronic valvular heart disease. *Rheumatic heart disease* refers to the cardiac manifestations of rheumatic fever, either in the acute phase or the later stage of chronic damage. This is the major reason that the condition is important among adults. In caring for adults we are concerned primarily with rheumatic heart disease, but it is important to understand something about its original cause, rheumatic fever. At one time rheumatic heart disease was the commonest form of organic heart disease in persons under 50 in the United States. Between 1944 and 1965, however, the death rate from acute rheumatic fever in the United States showed a decline of 90 per cent, primarily due to vigorous treatment with penicillin (National Health Education Committee).

Cause

The precise cause of rheumatic fever is unknown, but it is believed to be related to streptococcal infection. Rheumatic fever is a systemic response found in 3 per cent of persons infected with group A hemolytic streptococci (Erb and Wilson). Why 3 people are affected and 97 escape is an unsolved mystery. A previous attack increases the risk of recurrent attack following streptococcal infection from 30/1,000 (3 per cent) to 500/1,000 (50 per cent) or higher (Stamler). It often follows such conditions as pharyngitis, tonsillitis and scarlet fever. Some investigators have noted a strong familial tendency, but this is sometimes attributed to the spread of streptococcal infection within a family.

Rheumatic fever is most prevalent during cool, damp weather, and its incidence is greater in the northern sections of our country than in the southern regions. The changes in incidence may be related to the higher incidence of streptococcal infections during cold, damp weather. Poor living conditions, such as crowding and poor diet, seem to increase the incidence of rheumatic fever by lessening the individual resistance to infection and increasing the likelihood of the spread of the streptococcal infection from one person to another.

Some doctors believe that rheumatic fever occurs in persons who have a hypersensitivity to the streptococcus or its products, and that rheumatic fever is essentially an allergic reaction to streptococcal infection.

Diagnosis

No single diagnostic test proves that a patient has rheumatic fever. The doctor makes the diagnosis after he has carefully evaluated the patient's personal and family history, his symptoms, and certain physical and laboratory findings that have been found to be especially useful in the diagnosis of rheumatic fever. In the last group are the following:

• Subcutaneous nodules. These appear as small round or oval lumps under the skin. Not all patients with rheumatic fever have these nodules. When they occur, they are considered characteristic of the disease.

• Increased sedimentation rate. The rate at which the red blood cells settle to the bottom of a tube is increased in rheumatic fever. The particular usefulness of this test in rheumatic fever lies in the tendency of the increased sedimentation rate to persist even after other evidences of active disease have subsided. The sedimentation rate is more useful in determining whether the patient's disease is still active than it is in indicating whether the disease is rheumatic fever.

• Leukocytosis and anemia. These are characteristic during an acute rheumatic infection.

• C-reactive protein. This protein substance, which is not present normally in the blood, appears in the blood in a variety of infections, including rheumatic fever.

• Abnormal electrocardiogram. During the course of rheumatic fever the ECG frequently shows rhythm disturbances and other cardiac changes and is an aid in assessing the presence and the severity of cardiac damage.

• Abnormal heart sounds. An example is heart murmurs. Murmurs can indicate a change in valve configuration or myocardial dilatation.

• Epidemiologic studies show the association of group A hemolytic streptococci with pharyngitis preceding rheumatic fever by 1 to 3 weeks. An immunologic response is seen in the antigen-antibody reaction to streptococcal infection. The antibody response in the patient's blood can be measured as the antistreptolysin-O titer (ASO titer). The level of the antibody response, or a rising antibody titer, gives some indication as to the intensity of tissue reaction and is an aid to diagnosis of rheumatic fever. With the measurement of antibodies it is now possible to demonstrate preceding streptococcal infection in 95 per cent of patients with acute rheumatic fever if they are studied within 2 months of onset (Stamler).

The nurse can help the patient and his family during the diagnostic tests by encouraging the continuation of the tests recommended by the doctor. Often it is hard for the patient to understand that there is no single definite test for rheumatic fever, and that varied and repeated tests are necessary to establish the diagnosis. Also, the nurse participates in the explanation of the various diagnostic procedures, and sometimes she assists with the collection and the labeling of specimens.

ACTIVE RHEUMATIC FEVER

Symptoms

Rheumatic fever affects the connective tissue in many different areas of the body. Therefore, symptoms often are widely distributed, involving, for example, joints, heart and nervous system. In one patient most of the symptoms may be related to the nervous system, whereas in another patient the inflammation of the joints may be severe. Sometimes, the disease is so mild that it escapes detection, or it is so atypical in its symptoms that many and repeated tests, plus very careful observation of the patient, are necessary to confirm the diagnosis.

The disease may appear 1 to 4 weeks after a

streptococcal infection. It may be gradual in onset, with slowly increasing fatigue, anorexia, weight loss, lassitude and slight fever, or it may begin suddenly with acute swelling and inflammation of one or many joints, moderate fever and malaise and pallor. Joint symptoms often are described as *migratory polyarthritis,* meaning that the condition moves from one joint to another, eventually involving many joints in the body. The joints later heal completely; even those that were very swollen and painful have no permanent deformity.

Epistaxis (nosebleed), abdominal pain, a rash resembling giant hives but which does not itch, and subcutaneous nodules may be part of the patient's symptomatology.

Cerebral lesions can be associated with neurologic symptoms such as chorea. Chorea occurs in childhood, especially in girls, and it is characterized by uncontrollable, uncoordinated, purposeless movements. These symptoms usually disappear entirely after a period of rest and supportive care. Children who have chorea should be observed carefully for symptoms related to cardiac function.

Pulmonary and pleural lesions can also occur.

The amount of the cardiac involvement is of great concern in rheumatic fever, because the heart can develop permanent deformity as a result of the disease. The involvement of the heart varies from patient to patient. Typically, patients with rheumatic fever have tachycardia out of proportion to the degree of the fever. Some experience palpitation associated with rapid heart action. Pain over the heart sometimes occurs. Myocarditis (inflammation of the heart muscle) and pericarditis (inflammation of the sac enclosing the heart) account for most of the cardiac symptoms that occur during the acute phase of the disease. If the involvement of the heart is severe enough, the function of the heart will be impaired, and the patient with active rheumatic fever may show symptoms of congestive heart failure or cardiac arrhythmias.

The endocardial involvement consists of inflammation of the endocardium and valve leaflets. Characteristic vegetations (verrucae) appear in the valves. There is edema and inflammation of the valve ring which heals with scar formation. This can seriously deform the delicate valve structures and result later in chronic valvular disease manifested by cardiac enlargement, congestive heart failure and rhythm disturbances.

As a result of clots or a piece of valve breaking off and entering the general circulation, cerebral emboli or peripheral arterial occlusions can develop. (Valvular heart disease due to rheumatic fever is discussed below.)

Treatment

Rest is very important during the active stage of rheumatic fever. The patient is kept in bed. Some doctors allow bathroom privileges if the disease seems mild. In recent years a few doctors are allowing more flexibility than others in the strictness of bed rest after the second week of the onset of the disease, provided that there has been no evidence of carditis. If cardiac involvement occurs, it does so within the first two weeks of the illness in 80 per cent of the patients who develop this complication. However, the effects of activity beyond strict bed rest during acute rheumatic fever have not yet been well studied, and most doctors prefer that bed rest be maintained until all signs and all symptoms of active disease have subsided. The patient's emotional reaction is considered, too. If he becomes extremely restless and discontented after many weeks of strict bed rest, the doctor may permit him to be taken to the bathroom once daily in a wheelchair. The chance to get out of bed, carried out in such a way that it entails as little exertion as possible, may boost the patient's morale and help him to comply with the order for extended rest.

Rest is both facilitated and made more difficult by other aspects of treatment. Salicylates and/or steroids promptly and effectively relieve the symptoms, but they do not cure the underlying disease. The patient feels better, and although the lessening of the joint pain and the fever helps him to rest more comfortably, it also makes him wonder why he needs to rest at all. It is hard for him to understand that feeling well is not necessarily indicative of being well.

Medication. The first principle in the treatment of active rheumatic fever is said to be the eradication of the Group A beta hemolytic streptococcus from the patient. Penicillin is the drug of choice. Erythromycin may be used if the patient is sensitive to penicillin. Throat cultures may be ordered at various times after the onset of treatment to confirm eradication of the organism.

Salicylates are very effective and have been used for many years for the symptomatic relief of rheumatic fever. Usually, fairly large doses are necessary to control the symptoms.

ACTH and cortisone promptly and effectively relieve the symptoms of rheumatic fever; like salicylates, they do not cure the disease. Their effectiveness in decreasing the damage to the heart is being studied. It has been suggested that the prompt administration of these steroids, by decreasing the inflammation, may lessen the damage to the heart.

Diet is important in helping the patient to overcome the disease. Because patients with rheumatic fever tend to have poor appetites, frequent small meals may be tolerated better than three large ones. A liberal fluid intake is important. Sodium may be restricted to prevent edema due to steroids, or if the patient develops congestive heart failure.

Nursing Care

Skillful nursing care can make the difference between a fretful, restless patient who tosses and turns, one who seems to delight in finding new ways to defy the doctor's recommendation of rest, and a patient who is able to tolerate the restricted activity.

Here are a few brief reminders of ways in which the nurse can help:

• Smooth, sure, unhurried movement by the nurse prevents any additional pain in the patient's swollen, painful joints. Reduction of the possibility of sudden jerky motions may be accomplished through the use of temporary supporting splints or pillow support of the extremities, especially when the patient is turned.

• Do not insist on unnecessary restrictions, or carry out in a punitive manner those that are necessary. Most patients with rheumatic fever are young people. They are accustomed to activity, and they need gradually increasing independence.

• Find out from the doctor what kind of activity and what kind of diversion the patient may have. Reading and television help to while away the hours, as do hobbies, such as painting or handwork.

• Add your efforts to those of the doctor in helping your patient to understand the reason for the restriction of activity. Encourage the patient to keep up with his studies, if the doctor permits.

• Never underestimate the importance of pleasant, cheerful surroundings. If the patient is in the hospital, try to place him near others who are congenial.

• Remember all the devices for keeping bed patients comfortable: the extra long back rub; placing his feet in the basin when you wash them; a bottom sheet so tightly tucked in that it stays smooth all day; attention to details of personal grooming. Make sure that the patient's gown and his bedding are dry. If he perspires freely, several changes a day may be needed. Massage carefully over bony prominences, and encourage a frequent change of position.

• Be prepared for your patient's ups and downs. Any young person who has to curtail so many pleasures and so many of the normal experiences of growing up is bound to become discouraged and angry at times.

• If your patient is allowed out of bed for a short time each day, make these precious moments count by giving him a change of scene, perhaps wheeling him to a window or a porch. This is the time to strip and to air the bed and to turn the mattress, so that everything is fresh and clean when the patient returns to bed.

• Help the young person to develop self-discipline and concern for others. A prolonged illness can interfere with the development of these abilities and attitudes, and as a consequence the patient's relationships with others may suffer.

The nursing care of patients with chronic rheumatic heart disease involves observation for the symptoms of congestive heart failure (dyspnea, cough, orthopnea, edema, fatigue) and for those symptoms that might indicate the recurrence of rheumatic infection or any streptococcal infection (fever, sore throat, swollen painful joints, malaise).

RHEUMATIC HEART (VALVULAR) DISEASE

A series of thin but strong valves ensures that the blood in passing through the heart does not seep back and reverse its direction of flow. A valve separates the atrium from the ventricle on each side of the heart, preventing blood from passing back into the atrium each time the ventricle contracts. Valves also prevent blood that is pumped into the aorta and the pulmonary artery from flowing back toward the heart. The name of the artery is used to describe its valve; these valves are the *pulmonary* valve and the *aortic* valve.

Endocarditis (inflammation of the lining of the heart, including the lining of the heart valves) is the type of the rheumatic involvement of the heart that leads to permanent scarring and deformity. As an end-result of endocarditis, heart valves, particularly the mitral and the aortic valves, become scarred, and they function inefficiently. Damage to the valves can be found even after attacks of such mildness that the patient does not recall having had the disease. Often such lesions are detected by the doctor many years later during a routine physical examination. If the deformities of the valves are slight, these patients may continue to be asymptomatic, requiring no treatment and no limitation of their physical activity. If the deformity of the valves is considerable, the patient's heart function may in time become sufficiently impaired that the heart can no longer keep up with the circulatory load, and the patient will develop symptoms of congestive heart failure. These symptoms may appear first when the patient encounters some unusual strain, such as a pregnancy, an infection, or an unusual physical exertion. Atrial fibrillation is another disorder that may occur in patients with rheumatic heart disease.

Mitral Stenosis. The mitral valve lies between the left atrium and the left ventricle (see Fig. 27-2 on p. 351). It has two leaflets. In the healthy heart these open with each pulsation of the atrium to allow the blood to flow from the left atrium into the left ventricle, and then they close as the ventricle fills.

The most common cause of stenosis (narrowing) of the valve is the inflammation and the scarring of the leaflets as a result of rheumatic fever. The leaflets stick together and are prevented from opening all the way, as a valve should. They tend to become progressively thicker. The opening narrows, so that the blood in the atrium does not have time to flow into the ventricle. The atrium cannot then empty to receive a new full load of blood from the pulmonary artery and veins. To compensate, the atrium contracts harder. It enlarges. Pressure is exerted backward through the blood vessels of the lungs. Pressure builds up in the pulmonary artery (pulmonary hypertension), which carries blood from the right ventricle to the lungs. Eventually, pressure also increases in the right ventricle. Because it usually takes less force to pump blood through the lungs than through the rest of the body, the walls of the right ventricle are thinner than the walls of the left ventricle. In long-standing mitral stenosis the walls of the right ventricle get thicker. When hypertrophy of

the muscular walls no longer meets the demands of the increased work caused by the narrowed mitral valve, pressure is passed to the right atrium, and to the entire venous system of the body. The liver and the lungs become congested; edema of the legs appears. Because the ventricles are not receiving a normal amount of blood to pump through the body, the organs are not getting sufficient nourishment. The patient tires easily and becomes dyspneic. He suffers the progressive disability of cardiac failure.

Another symptom of this condition is lowered systolic blood pressure. When you are taking the blood pressure of a patient with mitral stenosis, do not report immediately that he is in shock if you get a reading of 80/60! By checking the patient's chart to see what previous readings have been, you probably will find that this is the usual blood pressure for this patient. The patient often appears emaciated. Although he may gain weight due to edema, he has poor appetite, and is chronically tired and listless.

Mitral stenosis is the most common vascular aftermath of rheumatic fever. Two-thirds of all patients with mitral stenosis are females.

TREATMENT. The symptomatic relief of congestive heart failure forms a very important part of the treatment of some patients with mitral stenosis. Surgical treatment is possible. However, not all patients with mitral stenosis are suitable candidates for surgery. Usually excluded are those whose condition is so slight that it does not cause symptoms, or so severe or of such long duration that profound changes in the heart and the lungs have occurred. The earlier the operation, the greater is the likelihood of cessation of symptoms. Patients who have had one episode of cerebral or peripheral embolization from a piece of clot or valve but are in good condition nonetheless are candidates for surgical correction.

The usual operative treatment of mitral stenosis is commissurotomy, valvuloplasty, or valve replacement.

Mitral Insufficiency. Insufficiency of a valve means that it does not close completely, consequently allowing blood to regurgitate back through it. A hole remains when the valve is supposed to be completely closed. Any heart valve may become insufficient.

Insufficiency of the mitral valve is caused most commonly by rheumatic fever. The left ventricle becomes overfilled with blood, because each contraction of the ventricle fails to empty the cham-

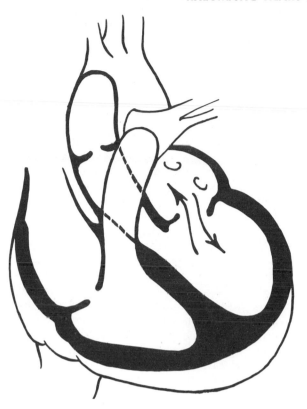

FIG. 29-1. Mitral insufficiency. The inadequate valve allows blood to return to the left atrium.

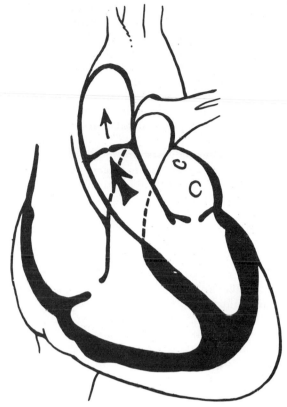

FIG. 29-2. Aortic stenosis.

ber through the aorta. Instead, some blood is pushed back through the mitral valve into the left atrium, and then leaks back into the ventricle. The walls of the ventricle become distended, and the patient may suffer from left ventricular failure.

The surgery for mitral insufficiency has a higher mortality rate and a poorer prognosis than the surgery for mitral stenosis. Frequently, patients with mitral insufficiency are disabled to a greater degree before the operation. Among the operations performed to correct mitral insufficiency are the suturing of loose valves and the implanting of a prosthetic valve to restore unidirectional blood flow. (See Chap. 55.)

Aortic Stenosis. The 3-leaf aortic valve is between the aorta and the left ventricle. The cusps may be thickened, stiffened and eventually calcified after rheumatic fever, although the aortic valve is affected less commonly than the mitral valve. In older patients aortic stenosis may be caused by arteriosclerosis.

When there is stenosis of the aortic valve, the work of the left ventricle is increased. More force

is needed to push blood through the narrowed opening. A sufficient supply of blood may not be passing through the narrowed valve to nourish adequately the brain and the muscles of the heart. In this instance the patient will present symptoms of dizziness, fainting and anginal pain from insufficient blood in the coronary arteries. Instead of being full, the radial pulse is weak. It seems to crawl against the finger rather than to hit it. Characteristically, angina and syncope occur before heart failure. Surgery should be considered before the patient reaches the late stages of the disease and suffers dyspnea, a congested liver and dependent edema, as the left ventricle enlarges, and heart failure occurs.

Aortic Insufficiency. Aortic insufficiency can be caused by rheumatic heart disease, by subacute bacterial endocarditis (especially when it is superimposed on a valve already damaged by rheumatic fever) and by syphilis. When the aortic valve is incompetent and does not close tightly, blood flows through it during systole, dropping back into the ventricle instead of moving forward through the aorta. This backflow results in a decrease in the amount of circulating blood and an increase in the amount of blood in the ventricle. The patient may have a "pistol-shot" pulse, which consists of a pronounced pulsation and then an extraordinarily long interval before the next sharp beat. The left ventricle hypertrophies and goes into failure. The patient is aware of palpitation, a throbbing sensation in the head, and dyspnea related to the failure of the left ventricle.

Aortic insufficiency is the most serious of the valvular diseases. It can cause sudden death, even before left ventricular failure, due to ventricular fibrillation.

Prevention of Rheumatic Fever

Mass throat culture programs and appropriate antibiotic therapy result in a decreased incidence of acute rheumatic fever. The nurse acts as a case finder and also gives leadership to community efforts to prevent the spread of streptococcal infections such as in throat culture programs underwritten by voluntary or state funds. Financial support is also given by various health agencies for rheumatic fever prophylaxis. Cost, then, is not a deterrent to prevention. Find out what resources are available within your own or your work community.

To take a throat culture, the swab should be brought down across the tonsil on one side, the tip should touch the posterior pharyngeal wall as it crosses the throat to the other side, and then the swab should touch the other tonsil as it comes up. This is the "down-across-up" maneuver (Watson).

Every possible measure is taken to prevent further streptococcal infections in patients who have had rheumatic fever, because every such infection carries with it the high possibility of recurrence. Each new attack carries the threat of heart damage. Some doctors recommend that the siblings of patients with rheumatic fever also have prophylactic treatment. The prevention of this disease is extremely important, because there is at present no cure. It causes serious heart disease among many young people, often interfering with their plans for a career, marriage and family life; and sometimes it results in severe illness and death during what should be their most productive years.

The following measures have been recommended for the prevention of rheumatic fever:

• Prophylactic medication. Oral penicillin (200,000 to 400,000 U.) or sulfadiazine (1.0 Gm.) is given daily to protect the patient from streptococcal infection. An injection of repository benzathine penicillin G (one that is slowly liberated from the tissues after the injection) may be given once a month, particularly if the patient is not reliable in carrying out his daily oral treatment. Most doctors agree that prophylactic medication should be taken for at least five years following the most recent attack of rheumatic fever and be reinstituted prophylactically if the patient has to undergo dental surgery or other kinds of stressful experiences where the risk of streptococcal infection is increased.

• Avoidance of contact with persons who have upper respiratory infections. Although this cannot always be accomplished, the person who has had rheumatic fever should take reasonable precautions.

• Reporting to the doctor any symptoms, such as sore throat and fever, that might indicate a streptococcal infection.

• Following the physician's recommendations concerning regular visits to the doctor's office or clinic for careful cardiac follow-up after the attack is over. The regimen for rheumatic fever prophylaxis has been outlined succinctly by the Inter-Society Commission for Heart Disease Resources: Prevention of Rheumatic Fever and Rheumatic Heart Disease, established by the American Heart Association.

Prognosis and Rehabilitation

Many people recover from attacks of rheumatic fever with little or no permanent heart damage. However, the prognosis grows less favorable with each repeated attack. When death occurs, it is due usually to severe cardiac damage resulting in congestive heart failure. The later in life the first attack occurs, the better is the prognosis, since the likelihood of repeated attacks diminishes with age, and recurrence after the age of 25 is very unlikely. It has been estimated that approximately 25 to 50 per cent of the patients who have had rheumatic fever develop some degree of permanent heart damage (Beeson and McDermott).

Although the lack of medical care and unawareness of the symptoms of rheumatic fever still exist, particularly among the underprivileged, greater recognition of the problem has led to earlier diagnosis and more thorough treatment for many children whose illness might once have been dismissed as "growing pains." Because of improved diagnosis and treatment, the outlook for people with rheumatic fever is more favorable than it was a generation or two ago. Recurrences of rheumatic fever have decreased markedly due to the prophylactic use of antibiotics among those who have had an attack.

Continuing nursing care for the patient involves:

• Education of the patient concerning his abilities and his limitations, in the light of the degree of heart damage, and helping the patient to learn to live within his limitations.

• Teaching the patient what symptoms to watch for and to report, if they should occur (for example, fever, sore throat, ankle edema, fatigue).

The plan of rehabilitation depends on the degree of heart damage and the patient's reaction to his experience with the illness. Those patients who do not develop heart disease after rheumatic fever are encouraged to live active lives. Their only reminder of the disease is the need for preventing further attacks. Because rheumatic fever so frequently results in heart disease, it is hard for some of these patients to believe that their hearts can tolerate normal activity.

Invalidism can become a way of life, especially in an illness like rheumatic fever and rheumatic heart disease that imposes prolonged restrictions on the patient's living. Some patients through fear are unable to break away from this pattern even when their physical condition no longer makes it necessary.

BACTERIAL ENDOCARDITIS

Bacterial endocarditis (inflammation of the membrane that covers the heart valves and lines the cavities of the heart) used to kill almost all its victims. The recovery of a large proportion of patients through the use of antibiotics is one of the most dramatic achievements of modern medicine. Although the prognosis has improved markedly, bacterial endocarditis continues to be a serious and a relatively common health problem among adults.

Bacterial endocarditis may be acute or subacute. The acute condition has a more abrupt onset and a more rapid course, whereas the subacute form has a gradual onset, and the duration of the illness is usually longer. In subacute bacterial endocarditis the infecting organisms are usually less virulent, whereas the organisms causing acute bacterial endocarditis are usually more virulent. When the infecting organisms are sensitive to antibiotics, the prognosis of the patient usually is good. With other organisms the mortality rate is approximately 50 per cent (Mandell), and the disease often is crippling for those who survive. Modern therapy, with emphasis on prompt diagnosis and the control of the infection, has so altered the course of the disease that the terms "acute" and "subacute" are now less frequently used to describe this disease.

Incidence

People whose heart valves have been damaged are most vulnerable to bacterial endocarditis. The majority of patients who develop it have had rheumatic fever. The relationship between rheumatic heart disease and bacterial endocarditis is so marked that bacterial endocarditis often is considered a complication of rheumatic heart disease. The condition also occurs in those who have congenital defects of the heart. Although it may occur at any age, bacterial endocarditis is most common during young adulthood and early middle life.

Etiology and Pathology

Transient bacteremia occurs fairly commonly in the lives of most people—for example, after tooth extraction. In most instances the organisms are quickly overcome by the body's own defenses. However, patients with damaged heart valves are especially prone to develop bacterial endocarditis after such relatively safe experiences as the pulling of a tooth, cystoscopy, childbirth, or an upper respiratory infection. Organisms that invade the bloodstream after such occurrences tend to settle on damaged heart valves, where they multiply and produce vegetations (verrucae)—clumps of material composed of bacteria, necrotic tissue and fibrin, which accumulate on the affected heart valves. These vegetations are *friable* (easily broken). Pieces of the vegetation tend to break off and travel in the bloodstream. They are then called *emboli,* and they may damage other organs by occluding blood vessels, thus interfering with the organ's blood supply.

A variety of bacteria can cause bacterial endocarditis. *Streptococcus viridans* is one of the organisms most frequently responsible (50 per cent of cases).

Today the pattern of bacterial endocarditis is changing somewhat. An increased incidence is evident in such populations as those undergoing heart surgery with cardiopulmonary bypass and heroin and morphine addicts who use the intravenous route of injection. A fungus or staphylococcus can be the causative agent.

Maintenance of strict surgical asepsis is an essential task of the team involved in insertion of cardiac pacemakers, cardiac catheterization or cardiac surgery if the complication of bacterial endocarditis is to be avoided (Rabinovich).

Signs and Symptoms

Often the disease has an insidious onset, with slight fever, malaise and fatigue. The patient may ignore the early manifestations of the illness, attributing them to "a touch of the flu" or overwork. Early diagnosis and treatment are very important. Patients—particularly those with rheumatic or congenital valvular defects—should report promptly to their doctors any fever, malaise or other symptoms of infection, because they may have bacterial endocarditis or a recurrence of rheumatic fever.

As the condition advances, the patient often develops a muddy, sallow complexion, sometimes described as the color of *café au lait*. His fever becomes more marked and more frequent, and often it is accompanied by chills and sweats. Pronounced weakness, anorexia and weight loss are common. Petechiae, tiny reddish-purple hemorrhagic spots on the skin and mucous membranes, are characteristic. Anemia and slight leukocytosis are common. Heart murmur is present in the vast majority of patients.

Embolism, resulting in the occlusion of a blood vessel by a clump of vegetation that has broken away from the heart valve, may cause sudden disturbances in many organs of the body. One patient with bacterial endocarditis suddenly developed excruciating pain, pallor, and coldness of one leg below the knee. An embolus had cut off circulation to his lower leg. Had it not been for the speed and the teamwork of his doctor, his nurse, and the surgeon who was immediately called, the patient would have developed gangrene and therefore would have lost his leg by a necessary amputation. Another patient suddenly became dyspneic, coughed and expectorated bloodly sputum. She had suffered pulmonary embolism. An embolus to the spleen may cause sudden pain in the left flank, whereas an embolus to a kidney may result in hematuria and flank pain. Emboli may affect the brain, causing neurologic symptoms, such as paralysis and aphasia.

Clubbing of the fingers and the toes may appear later in the course of the illness. The symptoms of congestive heart failure may appear, either during the active infection or afterward as a result of the damage to the valves during the illness. Often this development is best described as further damage to the heart valves, because many of the patients already have some valvular damage.

Diagnosis

The doctor carefully evaluates the patient's history, particularly in relation to rheumatic heart disease or congenital defects and in relation to any recent operation, injury or illness. He orders blood cultures in an attempt to discover the organism circulating in the blood. Often several blood cultures are required before the organism is found. Occasionally, no bacteria are found despite repeated blood cultures, although the patient has a history and symptoms that are typical of the disease. In these instances the diagnosis is made as carefully as possible on the basis of other evidence, but the treatment with antibiotics cannot be as precisely planned when the sensitivity of the organism to various drugs is not known. Persistent negative blood cultures are found in 15 to 20 per cent of autopsy-proved cases of bacterial endocarditis (Rabinovich).

Treatment and Nursing Care

Large doses of the antibiotic to which the organism is sensitive are given. For example, a patient may receive 4 to 20 million units of penicillin daily in divided doses intramuscularly or via a continuous intravenous infusion. Treatment is continued for 3 to 4 weeks.

Be sure to give the drugs on time, exactly as ordered, so that a sufficient amount of the drug will be maintained continuously in the patient's blood. Observe the patient carefully for any toxic reactions to the drugs, and report them if they occur. Good technical skill in giving injections helps to minimize the patient's feeling of being a "dart board." Rotating the site is essential when so many injections are given, so that one area does not become traumatized from repeated injections. Even the most stoical patients grow weary of repeated injections. Your skill, patience and encouragement can help them to continue with the treatment that is lifesaving.

If the patient is receiving his antibiotics intravenously, he will have an intravenous line inserted for the duration of treatment to avoid frequent venipunctures. The antibiotic may be given either in divided doses with a "keep-open" infusion running between doses, or the drug may be given by continuous drip. Observe the venipuncture site for signs of infiltration or inflammation. Check that the level of fluid in the bottle is sufficient to keep it from running out and that the flow rate is that ordered for achievement of drug blood level. Often patients fear that air will enter their veins if the fluid is all absorbed. They also dread the necessity of needless needle reinsertion. Since the patient may become ambulatory after 7 to 10 days of therapy, his I.V. pole should have casters incorporated.

In some institutions with progressive nursing care services the patient may be discharged home after 7 to 10 days and the nurse supervises his daily care. This involves preparation in intravenous technics since the infusion may need to be restarted.

Supportive care is important in helping the patient to overcome the infection. Usually, bed rest is ordered at first. When the patient begins to improve, he is permitted gradually to go to the bathroom and later to be up and about. While the patient is on bed rest, do everything that you can to spare him exertion and to make him as comfortable as possible. Promptly change bedding that becomes damp from perspiration, as it often does when the patient's fever abates. Encourage the patient to eat, and particularly encourage him to drink fluids; fluids are especially important because of the fever and the sweating.

Observe the patient carefully. Note fluctuations in temperature. The temperature usually is taken rectally every 4 hours. Be alert for changes in the rate and the quality of the pulse and for the appearance of any new symptoms, such as petechiae. Watch especially for symptoms of embolization.

Without drugs, patients with bacterial endocarditis almost surely die. The patient needs you, too, to help him through the attack. As his symptoms subside, gradually he will be allowed increased activity. See that he does not overdo, and that new activities are stopped short of fatigue.

When the antibiotic treatment is discontinued, observe him for any recurrence of the symptoms. Sometimes, although the infection seems to be conquered, it flares up again after the drugs have been discontinued. Then the treatment has to be resumed and continued until the infection has been eradicated.

No drug, however dramatic be its effect, renders skilled nursing care unnecessary. Nowhere is this need more evident than in the care of patients with bacterial endocarditis, who are seriously ill and subject to a variety of complications that may appear without warning.

Prognosis

It has been estimated that about 90 per cent of patients with bacterial endocarditis can recover from the infection. Much depends on the sensitivity of the organism to available drugs. The amount of heart damage that existed before the attack, as well as that which may result from the endocarditis, also affects the prognosis. Some patients have the infection controlled by drugs, but not before heart damage or embolization has occurred. These patients may be incapacitated by or succumb to congestive heart failure or damage inflicted on the vital organs by the emboli.

Prevention

Any patient with damaged heart valves should have antibiotics just before and for a short time after any event that might cause bacteremia, whether it be a tooth extraction or childbirth. The patient must understand that this precaution is a lifelong necessity. Unfortunately, bacterial endocarditis does not provide immunity to further attacks. The patients who develop the condition are usually those whose previous valvular damage predisposes them to it. They will continue to be vulnerable to this disease as long as they live.

PERICARDITIS

Covering the myocardium on the outside is a loose fitting inelastic sac known as the *pericardium*. The outermost layer is the fibrous pericardium. The innermost layer, or that adhering to the myocardium, is the visceral layer or epicardium. The pericardial space contains a few drops of pericardial fluid which lessens the friction between the myocardium and the pericardium. Since the pericardium does not stretch, overdilatation of the heart during diastole cannot take place.

Inflammation of the pericardium (pericarditis) can result from infection, trauma, or neoplasms. Blood, excess fluid, or pus can accumulate in the pericardial space and produce partial or complete cardiac tamponade with fall in cardiac output or death. Sections of the epicardium and

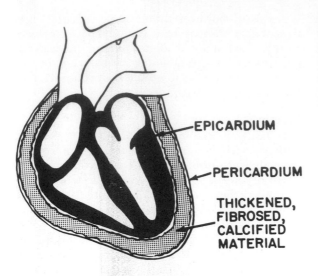

EPICARDIUM

PERICARDIUM

THICKENED, FIBROSED, CALCIFIED MATERIAL

FIG. 29-3. Pericarditis. Normally, the epicardium and the pericardium slide over each other easily. They are lubricated by a small amount of fluid, which in pericarditis is replaced by thicker material that can cause the surfaces to adhere.

pericardium can adhere and cause chronic constrictive pericarditis.

Acute Pericarditis

Pericarditis can be caused by an infection with any organism. For example, tubercle bacilli and streptococci can cause a purulent pericardial exudate. Infection from a virus or pneumonia or a lung abscess can spread to the pericardium. Myxedema and uremia can produce a nonbacterial, serofibrinous pericarditis. In acute pericarditis there may be sharp pain aggravated by moving and breathing due to the rubbing together of the two inflamed surfaces. A pericardial friction rub can usually be heard with a stethoscope and is the most striking sign.

The pain of acute pericarditis is very similar to the pain of acute myocardial infarction—sudden, severe, beginning over the sternum and radiating to the neck and left arm. However, the pain of the patient with pericarditis is usually increased by rotating the chest or deep breathing and is relieved by sitting up and leaning forward. In contrast, the pain of acute myocardial infarction is not usually influenced by position, movement, or breathing. Acute pericarditis is a disease of the younger age group (15 to 35 years) and is generally preceded by an upper respiratory infection or hay fever.

X-ray may show dilatation of the heart with pericardial effusion. Serum enzyme changes are confusing in that they are similar to those of acute myocardial infarction.

If there is sufficient fluid in the pericardial space to compress the heart (*tamponade*), there may be signs of congestive heart failure and a pulse that is weaker on deep inspiration (*paradoxical pulse*).

The patient with acute pericarditis is generally treated with coronary precautions until myocardial infarction is ruled out.

Treatment depends on the underlying cause. Rest, analgesia, antipyretics, and other supportive treatment is given. Antibiotics and steroids may be ordered.

Chronic Constrictive Pericarditis

Patients may have no symptoms and no disability, even when there is some adherence of the two linings. However, as scar tissue forms in chronic constrictive pericarditis, there is compression of the heart (as there is when fluid is present in the pericardial sac) that prevents the **ventricle from filling fully.** The cardiac output of blood is decreased, even though the heart rate increases to compensate. The patient tires easily and eventually shows such signs of cardiac failure as hepatomegaly, dyspnea, edema and distention of the superficial veins, especially of the neck.

Treatment. When there is fluid in the pericardial sac, the surgeon may aspirate it (pericardial paracentesis), or if there is pus in the sac, he may incise the pericardium and insert a drain. A chronic accumulation of fluid may be treated by making a pericardial opening (window), thus allowing the fluid to drain into the pleural space. Constrictive pericarditis is treated surgically by removing the binding pericardium (pericardectomy or decortication) to allow more adequate filling and contraction of the heart chambers.

The surgical nursing care of the patient having pericardectomy is similar to that of other patients undergoing cardiac surgery. Nursing care may also include keeping the patient prone for several hours at a time to allow dependent drainage if surgical drainage of the pericardium was performed for the management of purulent pericarditis.

Postpericardiotomy (postcardiotomy) Syndrome

A febrile illness with symptoms and signs characteristic of acute pericarditis may develop one to three weeks after the pericardium has been surgically opened. It is thought to be due to reaction to the presence of fibrin and blood in the pericardial sac. In most patients the episode resolves spontaneously in 1 to 3 weeks. Analgesics and antipyretics may be ordered as well as steroid therapy.

REFERENCES AND BIBLIOGRAPHY

BAILEY, C. (ed.): *Rheumatic and Coronary Heart Disease,* Philadelphia, Lippincott, 1967.

BEESON, P. B., and McDERMOTT, W. (eds.): *Cecil-Loeb Textbook of Medicine,* ed. 12, Philadelphia, Saunders, 1966.

BISHOP, L. F.: Pericarditis vs. myocardial infarction, *Hosp. Med.* 3:9, 1967.

BRINSFIELD, D.: Rheumatic fever, *J. Miss. Med. Assoc.* 4:538, 1963.

ERB, B., and WILSON, G.: Rheumatic heart disease, *Cardiovasc. Nurs.* 4:1, January-February, 1968.

Facts on the Major Killing and Crippling Diseases in the United States Today, New York, The National Health Education Committee, 1966.

FEINSTEIN, A., *et al.:* Rheumatic fever in children and adolescents, cardiac changes and sequelae, *Ann. Intern. Med.* 60:87 (Suppl. 5), 1964.

HARRISON, T., and REEVES, T.: *Principles and Problems of Ischemic Heart Disease,* Chicago, Yearbook Publishers, 1968.

MANDELL, G.: Enterococcal endocarditis, *Arch. Int. Med.* 125:258, February, 1970.

MOTOCK, E.: A patient with sarcoma of the pericardium, *Nurs. Clin. N. Am.* 1:15, March, 1966.

RABINOVICH, S., *et al.:* The changing pattern of bacterial endocarditis, *Med. Clin. N. Am.* 52:1091, September, 1968.

STAMLER, J.: *Lectures on Preventive Cardiology,* New York, Grune, 1967.

WANNAMAKER, L. W., *et al.:* Prevention of rheumatic fever, Circulation 31:948, 1965.

———: Prevention of bacterial endocarditis, *Circulation* 31:953, 1965.

WATSON, H. T.: The role of the school nurse in the support of children with certain cardiovascular disorders, *Nurs. Clin. N. Am.* 1:35, March, 1966.

WOOD, P.: *Diseases of the Heart and Circulation,* ed. 3, Philadelphia, Lippincott, 1968.

The Patient with Heart Disease: Coronary Heart Disease; Functional Heart Disease

30

Coronary Artery Disease • Pathophysiology • Angina Pectoris
Functional Heart Disease • Myocardial Infarction

CORONARY ARTERY DISEASE

Coronary Circulation

Contrary to what might be expected, blood does not pass directly from the chambers of the heart into the heart muscle. Rather, the myocardium has its own blood supply through a system of coronary arteries. Blood flows through these vessels and through branches over the outer surface of the heart, then into smaller arteries and capillaries in the cardiac muscle and finally back to the systemic circulation through the coronary veins which empty into the coronary sinus in the right atrium.

Usually there are two main coronary arteries, a right and left, and these originate from the aorta immediately above the aortic valve. Thus the coronary arteries get the first supply of the rich, oxygenated blood leaving the left ventricle. The myocardium is nourished with very little overlap of vessels from one region to another. Thus, if a coronary artery is acutely blocked, few other vessels can take over the blood supply to the area served by the blocked artery and the viability of the myocardial tissue is threatened. During the course of slowly advancing atherosclerotic disease of the coronary arteries, or with time, after an acute coronary occlusion, pre-existing anastomotic channels open up and grow into the involved area. In the person with coronary heart disease the rate of development and the extent of this new collateral circulation is of critical importance in the survival and viability of myocardial tissue.

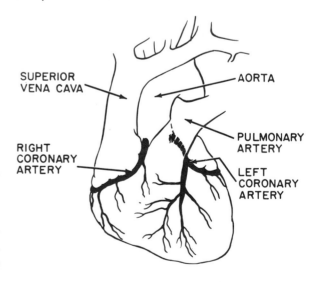

FIG. 30-1. Anterior view of the heart, showing the right and the left coronary arteries that supply the myocardium with blood.

380

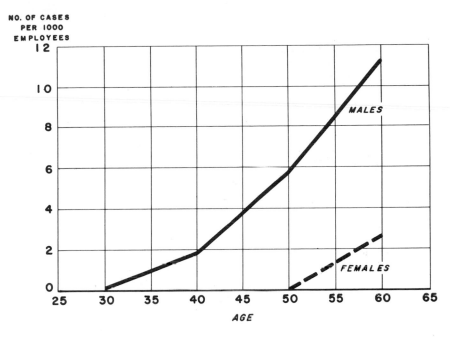

FIG. 30-2. Age at the time of the initial myocardial infarction. (Rosenbaum, F. F., and Belknap, E. L. (eds.): *Work and the Heart,* New York, Hoeber)

Hypoxia, or diminished oxygen supply to cells, is one of the best stimulants to myocardial blood supply. Thus the person with slowly progressive coronary atherosclerosis may have developed some collateral vessels over the course of time which may hold him in good stead in the event of a sudden occlusion of a major vessel. However, the young man who never had the need or opportunity to develop collaterals, has a greater chance of dying instantly following a coronary occlusion due to the sequelae of overwhelming oxygen lack to a critical portion of the myocardium.

Like other arteries in the body, the coronary arteries may develop degenerative changes or disease. The pathologic change most responsible for coronary artery disease is atherosclerosis—the gradual deposition of substances, such as lipids and calcium, within the walls of the arteries, making them narrower. Cholesterol is one of the lipid substances believed to be implicated. The lipid deposits are often called *plaques.* Coronary artery disease is more common among people over 50, but it may occur in younger people. A familial tendency toward early development of the condition has been noted. During early middle life men are affected much more frequently than women.

In man at rest, a normal myocardial blood flow may be maintained despite considerable coronary artery narrowing; however the ability to increase this flow sufficiently during exer-cise in order to meet the increased metabolic needs of the heart may be markedly impaired. Beyond the narrowed segment, the vessels supplied by the artery dilate. Because of this vasodilation and the development of a good collateral circulation, patients with significant coronary atherosclerosis may be fairly asymptomatic and their disease may go unrecognized during their lifetime particularly if they lead a sedentary existence. During exercise, or emotional stress with increased cardiac workload, however, the normal coronary arterial vasodilatation which usually allows myocardial blood flow to increase proportionately can no longer occur since the local capillary bed is already in a maximally dilated state. Under these circumstances the myocardial demand for oxygen and metabolic nutrients exceeds the ability of the coronary circulation to supply them and clinical manifestations of coronary heart disease such as chest pain of cardiac origin (angina pectoris) may then ensue.

Epidemiology

Coronary heart disease in epidemic proportions continues to rage in this country. Approximately 600,000 people die each year from this, the leading cause of American deaths. Many of these deaths are premature in the sense that the victims are young or middle-aged adults with basically sound myocardiums. For each fatality, there are two nonfatal but disabling events. The disease is most serious because its ravages affect the prime productive years of life. The patient, his family, and society as a whole suffer from the loss of productivity. Of the 600,000 fatalities from CHD (coronary heart disease) in 1965, 165,000 were among persons under age 65 and 76.5 per cent of the fatalities were men (Stamler *et al.*). Lown notes that close to two-thirds of the victims die before reaching a hospital. Of the one-third who reach the hospital, mortality has been reduced from about 30 to 20 per cent in coronary care units, which is conceded to be about the maximum contribution that in-hospital care can make to reduction in CHD mortality for the foreseeable future. Thus, the data compel the conclusion that *prevention* of CHD should be a primary national goal.

As with other epidemic diseases, coronary artery disease is considered to be due to multiple causative factors rather than to a single cause. Considerable study is being directed toward the discovery of measures to diagnose coronary artery disease before an acute myocardial infarction occurs and to develop ways of decreasing, or at least arresting, the process of atherosclerosis before damage occurs to the muscle of the heart.

Factors which when present are thought to increase the risk of coronary artery disease are:

Age

Sex (The incidence of coronary artery disease in women rises after the menopause and becomes similar to that among men. It has been suggested that estrogens may protect younger women from coronary artery disease).

Family history of coronary disease

Hypertension

Blood lipid abnormalities involving serum cholesterol and triglycerides

Obesity

Cigarette smoking

Lack of physical activity

Personality-behavior patterns

Emotionally stressful situations

Electrocardiographic abnormalities

Other diseases, such as gout and diabetes mellitus

A number of pamphlets explaining risk factors for the lay public, as well as for the professional, are available from the local affiliates of the American Heart Association.

PATHOPHYSIOLOGY

The symptoms of coronary heart disease result from an insufficient supply of blood to the myo-cardium. Like other muscles, the myocardium requires more blood when it works hardest—as is the case during physical exertion or emotional stress. Blood supply through narrowed arteries may be sufficient for a body that is at rest, but not adequate for some of the more strenuous activities of daily living.

If the normal vessels, or collateral circulation are not adequate for the needs of the heart during exertion, symptoms of *myocardial ischemia* develop.

Coronary occlusion, or the closing of an already narrowed coronary artery can occur from a variety of mechanisms. Usually a clot lodges in the vessel (coronary thrombosis). Occlusion can also result from subintimal hemorrhage of a coronary artery or from a gradually increasing build-up of atheromata. A sudden loss of blood supply to a portion of the myocardium from an occluded coronary artery often leads to necrosis (death) of that portion of the muscle of the heart. The area of necrotic tissue is called a *myocardial infarction.* This condition is usually accompanied by persistent, severe pain and clinical evidence of dead heart tissue. *Coronary insufficiency* is a term used to describe a clinical condition in which cardiac pain is frequently more severe than typical angina pectoris, but death of heart muscle does not take place.

Coronary occlusion does not necessarily result in myocardial infarction. A small coronary vessel may be occluded, but collateral circulation may be adequate to prevent infarction. On the other hand, myocardial infarction may occur in conditions other than coronary occlusion; for example, drastic curtailment of the blood supply to the myocardium during shock or general anaesthesia can result in myocardial infarction.

ANGINA PECTORIS

The chief symptom of myocardial ischemia is pain. When ischemia and the resulting pain are fleeting, as is often the case during periods of stress when the blood supply is briefly inadequate for the heart's increased needs, the condition is called *angina pectoris.*

Characteristics. Attacks of angina pectoris are characterized by sudden chest pain or pressure, which may be most severe over the heart under the sternum (substernal). Sometimes, the pain radiates to the shoulders and the arms, especially on the left side, or to the jaw, neck, or teeth. Some patients may deny that they have "pain," but will describe other sensations such as tightening in the chest, a squeezing, choking feeling in the upper chest or throat, indigestion, or burning in the epigastric region.

The patient may experience dyspnea, pallor, sweating and faintness. Although the intensity of the pain and the apprehension that it arouses may make minutes seem to be hours, the attack usually lasts less than five minutes. Sometimes, the patient seems to "freeze"—the pain makes him suddenly stop whatever he is doing, and he waits, tense and motionless, for it to subside. The attacks characteristically occur during periods of physical or emotional stress. Sometimes, a particular activity almost invariably brings on an attack. For one patient this might be the morning walk to his train; for another, an argument with his wife.

In some patients the severe pain comes without any apparent relation to meals, activity, rest, excitement or anything that is under the patient's control. These patients are prone to a particularly helpless feeling, because there seems to be little that they can do to lessen the frequency of the attacks.

The pain usually subsides as soon as the patient rests, thus lessening the need of the heart for blood. Most patients quickly discover this, and they need no further urging to stop their activity. Occasionally, a patient may feel that if he just ignores it and refuses to "give in to it," the pain will disappear. The pain is a warning that the heart is not receiving enough blood.

Heeding the warning may help the patient to avoid serious illness or even sudden death. The possibility of the sudden death of patients who have angina pectoris is very real. The underlying problem of atherosclerosis and diminished circulation makes the heart especially vulnerable to serious arrhythmias and myocardial infarction (see Chaps. 62 and 63), which may cause sudden death.

The patient need not lie down to rest. In fact, having him lie down often increases his sensations of breathlessness. Merely stopping the activity and standing or, if it is possible, sitting quietly for a few minutes usually suffices. Some patients with angina learn to cease their activity quite inconspicuously—for example, by pausing in a walk and appearing to look in a store window or by merely sitting down quietly and waiting for the attack to subside. If you are with a patient who often has had attacks in the past, take your cues from him. Help him to find a place to rest, locate any medication that the doctor has prescribed, and stay quietly and calmly with him, assuring him by your presence and your manner that the attack soon will be over. If the pain does not subside within 10 to 15 minutes, keep the patient at rest and call his doctor.

Treatment

Drugs. Nitroglycerin often is used to relieve attacks that do not disappear quickly with rest and also to prevent attacks. Nitroglycerin is thought to act by relieving spasm of the coronary arterioles, thus permitting vasodilation. Another theory is that nitroglycerin causes peripheral vasodilation, thus reducing the amount of blood returning to the heart and, in effect, temporarily reducing the cardiac workload so that the heart has a chance to rest.

Nitroglycerin is given sublingually in doses of 0.3 to 0.6 mg. (gr. 1/200 to 1/100). Do not be misled if the bottle is labeled "hypo tablets." They are prepared in such a way as to dissolve quickly under the patient's tongue. Nitroglycerin relieves the pain within two or three minutes. The duration of its effect is also brief, lasting only about half an hour. Sometimes nitroglycerin causes throbbing headache, flushing and nausea; usually these side-effects can be minimized by decreasing the dose. A patient who is not accustomed to taking nitroglycerin should remain seated for a few minutes after taking the medication since some people experience a feeling of faintness. If they take the drug while they are seated, fainting and injury due to falls can be prevented.

When a patient is about to undertake an activity that usually causes anginal pain, taking a nitroglycerin tablet a few minutes beforehand often will prevent the attack. Nitroglycerin is a safe drug; many patients take it for years without ill effect. If the drug has been taken repeatedly for a prolonged period, it may lose its effectiveness temporarily, but cases of this sort are rare. Stopping the use of the drug for a short time usually restores the patient's susceptibility to its effects.

Amyl nitrite works faster, has a similar action, but it is used much less commonly than nitroglycerin. It comes in perles or ampules that are broken into a handkerchief and inhaled. Most patients find the nitroglycerin more convenient, less conspicuous and cheaper than the amyl nitrite.

Drugs such as aminophylline and Peritrate, Isordil or Cardilate, sometimes are given in an effort to produce prolonged dilation of the coronary arteries, thereby preventing attacks of angina. Aminophylline may be given orally in doses of 0.1 to 0.2 Gm. or in rectal suppositories. Peritrate (pentaerythritol tetranitrate) is given in doses of 10 to 20 mg. several times daily. Side-effects of Peritrate include weakness, palpitation, flushing and headache. Some patients find these drugs helpful; others experience little relief from their use.

Papaverine, or the long-acting preparation Pavabid, a non-narcotic alkaloid obtained from opium, may be ordered to relax the smooth muscles of the coronary arteries thus permitting increased blood flow.

A newer drug, the beta-adrenergic blocking agent, propranolol (Inderal) has been found effective in some patients. Reflex coronary vaso-constriction may be blocked with this drug. Also cardiac energy requirements and therefore coronary blood flow need are reduced.

Surgery. Surgical attempts to correct the pathology caused by the diseases of the blood vessels that serve the muscle of the heart have been directed mainly toward improving vascularization, because the basic problem of coronary artery disease is insufficient blood supply to the muscle of the heart. There are several approaches.

In the Vineberg procedure or its modifications, a single or double mammary artery implant into the left ventricle is performed to supply blood to the heart muscle. The blood runs into the sinusoids that are characteristic of the myocardial muscle, and this eventually encourages the development of new coronary circulation to the ischemic left ventricle. Anastomoses form between the implanted artery and the left coronary arterioles. The heart-lung machine is not necessary for this operation.

In one report, it was found that the implanted arteries were supplying blood to the heart muscle in more than 92 per cent of patients a year or more after the surgery. The surgical mortality risk was less than 10 per cent (Effler).

Some surgeons resect the diseased portion of the coronary artery and anastomose the normal ends, or they cut into a thrombosed vessel and remove the obstructing material (coronary endarterectomy). This operation is effective for those few patients whose obstruction is limited to a single vessel.

In another procedure, the surgeon cuts out the diseased portion of the coronary artery and replaces it with a section of vein taken from the patient's groin. In a gas endarterectomy, a jet of high-pressure carbon dioxide is injected with a special needle between the layers of the arterial wall. This causes atheroma to become loosened and to separate from the wall of the artery. The artery is then surgically opened and the atheroma coaxed out in one piece thus restoring patency. Patients are selected for these operations who have incapacitating anginal pain together with a threat to life from massive myocardial infarction. For example, the operations are not applicable to a patient with severe, generalized atherosclerosis. Localization of the obstruction must be diagnosed by a coronary arteriogram. During the surgery the heart beat is stopped, and the heart-lung machine is used. When the operation is successful, the relief of pain is dramatic.

Often the doctor advises the patient to stop smoking, because of the association of smoking with the increased risk of coronary artery disease.

Patients with angina are advised to eat small meals rather than large ones, as large meals increase cardiac output and so may precipitate attacks of angina. Regular exercise, such as walking out of doors, often is beneficial in promoting collateral coronary circulation, thus lessening the frequency and the severity of attacks. Overweight patients in most instances benefit from weight reduction.

Daily Activities. Many patients continue to live active, productive lives despite attacks of angina pectoris. Vasodilators and careful regulation of activity may decrease the frequency and the severity of the attacks. For instance, the patient who has attacks of angina every morning while he is walking to the railroad station may find that leaving the house earlier, walking more slowly and taking a nitroglycerin tablet will prevent the attack.

Some patients find that their symptoms remain the same for years. In others the atherosclerosis advances rapidly, and anginal attacks become more frequent and severe despite treatment. These patients are crippled by such severe interference with blood supply to the heart that everyday activities must be curtailed.

The patient with angina faces the problem of finding what is his level of tolerance for activity and then learning to live within that level. Data obtained from the patient's performance on various tests in a cardiac work evaluation clinic is most helpful to the physician.

The patient also has to learn to live with the ever-present possibility of an attack. For some patients the fear aroused by the attack is worse than the pain. Some feel each time that an attack comes, "Well, this is it." Some patients react to this illness by being more angry at the necessary curtailment of their activity than by being afraid. All who care for the patient must strive to relieve and, if it is possible, to prevent the symptoms. They will need to help the patient to strike a reasonable compromise with his condition: to avoid the one extreme of giving up all activity and allowing his entire life to revolve around the possibility of an attack and to avoid other extreme of refusing to acknowledge that his heart places some definite restrictions on the amount of exertion that he can undertake safely. Because the prognosis is so variable—the patient may live for years, or he may die suddenly because of the poor circulation to his heart—he is encouraged to live each day as it comes, to take reasonable precautions, and to continue with his prescribed activities, provided that they do not precipitate attacks of angina.

FUNCTIONAL HEART DISEASE

Anxiety can produce a variety of physical discomforts (see Chap 8). Symptoms associated with heart disease also can be produced by anxiety, and they are referred to as functional heart disease.

Careful examination of the patient is essential to rule out organic heart disease and to assure the patient that his heart is normal. Regular, complete physical examinations are especially important. Because the patient is known to have had a functional disturbance, early symptoms of organic disease may be ignored or attributed to the functional disorder.

The treatment of functional heart disease involves:

• Carefully evaluating the factors, both in the patient's personality and in the environment, that seem to be related to the attacks.

• Providing symptomatic relief while the underlying causes of the condition are investigated. In functional heart disease, relief might be obtained by a vacation or by the use of sedatives or tranquilizers.

• Gradually helping the patient to understand that his symptoms may be due to anxiety, and that treatment involves helping him to recognize and to deal with his emotional problems, and sometimes modifying his environment.

New and taxing situations often provoke symptoms, such as dyspnea, fatigue and chest pain. Treatment involves a gradual and lifelong process of re-education, in which the patient is helped by his doctor and, hopefully, by his family, his employer and his friends. Referral to a psychiatrist may be necessary.

MYOCARDIAL INFARCTION

For a presentation of the care of the patient with acute myocardial infarction, see Chapter 54.

REFERENCES AND BIBLIOGRAPHY

Conference on Coronary Heart Disease: Preventive and Therapeutic Aspects, New York, New York Heart Association, 1968. Reprinted from *Bull. N.Y. Acad. Sci.* 44:899, August, 1968.

DAWBER, T., and EMERSON, H.: Risk factors in coronary heart disease, *Cardiovasc. Nurs.* 6:29, January-February, 1970.

EFFLER, D.: Surgery for coronary disease, *Sci. Am.* 219:36, October, 1968.

ELEK, S.: Emotional tension as a factor in coronary disease, *Hosp. Med.* 6:15, February, 1970.

ELLIOTT, W., and GORLIN, R.: The coronary circulation, myocardial ischemia, and angina pectoris (I), *Mod. Conc. Cardiovasc. Dis.* 35:111, October, 1966.

———: The coronary circulation, myocardial ischemia, and angina pectoris (II), *Mod. Conc. Cardiovasc. Dis.* 35:117, November, 1966.

FOX, S., and HASKELL, W.: The coronary spectrum: physical activity and health maintenance, *J. Rehab.* 32:89, March-April, 1966.

HARRISON, T., and REEVES, T.: *Principles and Problems of Ischemic Heart Disease,* Chicago, Year Book, 1968.

HELLERSTEIN, H.: Exercise therapy in coronary disease, *Bull. N.Y. Acad. Med.* 44:1028, August, 1968.

HINKLE, L., *et al.:* Occupation, education, and coronary heart disease, *Science* 161:238, July, 1968.

INGELFINGER, F. (ed.), *et al.: Controversy in Clinical Medicine,* Philadelphia, Saunders, 1966.

KAGAN, A., *et al.:* The Framington Study: a prospective study of coronary heart disease, *Fed. Proc.* 21:52, 1962.

KERSHBAUM, A., and BELLET, S.: Cigarette, cigar, and pipe smoking; some differences in biochemical effects, *Geriatrics* 23:126, March, 1968.

LOWN, B.: Intensive heart care, *Sci. Am.* 219:19, July, 1968.

MASTER, A. M.: The spectrum of anginal and non-cardiac chest pain, *JAMA* 187:894, March, 1964.

Risk Factors and Coronary Disease—A Statement for Physicians, New York, American Heart Association, 1968.

ROSENMAN, R.: Emotional factors in coronary heart disease, *Postgrad. Med.* 42:165, September, 1967.

SHAPIRO, S., *et al.:* The H.I.P. study of incidence and prognosis of coronary heart disease. Preliminary findings of incidence of myocardial infarction and angina. *J. Chron. Dis.* 18:527, June, 1965.

STAMLER, J.: Cigarette smoking and atherosclerotic coronary heart disease, *Conference on Smoking and the Heart,* New York, New York Heart Association, 1969. Reprinted from *Bull. N.Y. Acad. Med.* 44:1471, December, 1968.

STAMLER, J., *et al.:* Detection of susceptibility to coronary disease, *Conference on Automated Multiphasic Health Screening,* New York, New York Heart Association, 1970. Reprinted from *Bull. N.Y. Acad. Med.* 45:1257, December, 1969.

The Patient with Hypertension

31

Arterial Blood Pressure · Hypertensive Disease

The lack of certainy about the future is a condition of life—particularly so for patients with hypertension, in which the development of complications is to some extent unpredictable. Hypertension hastens the onset of atherosclerotic coronary and cerebrovascular disease. The patient may be fortunate and live comfortably for many years, or he may be less fortunate and suffer a cerebrovascular accident or cardiac failure. In either case he and his family may need nursing help in living each day as fully and as hopefully as possible, avoiding, on the one hand, the extremes of ignoring the illness and failing to follow treatment and, on the other hand, dwelling on its possible consequences to the point that there is no joy in living.

The term *hypertension* may be used in a general sense to describe any condition of elevated tension or tonus and, as such, is a sign. However, it commonly refers to a disease entity characterized by sustained elevation of arterial pressure. The systolic, diastolic, and mean arterial pressure may be elevated.

ARTERIAL BLOOD PRESSURE

Systolic blood pressure is determined by the rate and volume of ventricular ejection and the distensibility of the aorta. Normally the walls of the aorta are elastic and yield to the volume of blood which bursts into it on ventricular contraction. In older persons with a rigid, atherosclerotic aorta, however, systolic blood pressure may be quite elevated due to loss of this elasticity. Systolic hypertension is a response to change in central hemodynamics.

Diastolic blood pressure is the pressure recorded during the period of ventricular relaxation. It depends on the peripheral resistance and the diastolic filling interval. If arterioles are constricted, blood will have to be at an increased pressure to flow through the constriction. On the other hand, if the arterioles are wide open, then there will be brisk blood flow and diastolic pressure will fall rapidly. Diastolic hypertension is a response to change in peripheral hemodynamics.

The mean arterial pressure is the average pressure tending to push blood through the system's circulation. It is usually slightly less than the average of the systolic and diastolic pressures, however, since arterial pressure is nearer to diastolic level during the greater portion of the pulse cycle. Mean arterial pressure is important from the point of view of tissue blood flow since it takes into account systemic resistance, blood flow, and blood pressure. A high mean arterial pressure can be produced by a high systolic pressure and a normal diastolic pressure, or a normal systolic pressure and an elevated diastolic pressure, or when both pressures are elevated.

Pulse pressure is the difference between the systolic and diastolic pressures. The magnitude of the pulse pressure largely determines the forcefulness and the volume of the radial pulse felt at the wrist. Factors which *increase* the systolic pressure, such as a rigid, atherosclerotic aorta, or factors which decrease the diastolic pressure, such as a slow heart rate, will increase the pulse pressure. A strong bounding pulse reflects a wide pulse pressure.

Factors which *decrease* the systolic pressure and increase the diastolic pressure will decrease the pulse pressure. A rapid, weak, and thready pulse reflects a decreased or narrowed pulse pressure. This is the case in shock.

Physiologic Control of Arterial Pressure

Arterial pressure is regulated by the autonomic nervous system, the kidneys, and the endocrine glands. Normal blood pressure for adults ranges from about 100/60 to 140/90. Although a progressive increase in blood presssure with age has been frequently noted in the United States, this is not invariably true. The reasons for the changes in blood pressure in advancing age are not fully understood.

Blood pressure normally fluctuates with changes in posture, exercise and emotion. It is lowest when an individual is sleeping, slightly higher when he is awake but lying down, higher still when he is sitting up, and elevated even further when he is standing. Exercise and emotional stress cause elevation of blood pressure. These normal fluctuations show the importance of measuring blood pressure under similar conditions. For example, the patient's blood pressure should not be taken before he has been out of bed one morning, and the next morning while he is sitting in a chair immediately after he has taken a shower. Record on the nursing care plan the designated circumstances for taking the patient's blood pressure so that conditions are most nearly duplicated.

HYPERTENSIVE DISEASE

A person having a sustained blood pressure of 150/90 or above is usually considered to be hypertensive. This is a serious condition because it causes increased workload of the heart and damage to the arteries by excessive pressure brought about by increased resistance of the arterioles to the flow of blood. Congestive heart failure, myocardial infarction, stroke and renal failure are serious sequelae of hypertension.

When cardiac abnormality (such as electrocardiographic or x-ray evidence of enlargement of the left ventricle) is present with the elevated blood pressure, the term *hypertensive heart disease* is used. When extracardiac vascular damage is present without heart involvement, the term *hypertensive vascular disease* is used. When both heart and extracardiac pathology are present with hypertension, the appropriate term is *hypertensive cardiovascular disease* (Stamler *et al.*).

Hypertension is divided into two main categories: primary (essential) and secondary. The cause of *primary hypertension* is unknown. About 90 per cent of hypertensive patients have the primary or essential type.

Secondary hypertension is a term used to describe a variety of conditions in which elevation of blood pressure is secondary to some known cause. Pheochromocytoma (a tumor of the adrenal gland) is an example of a condition causing secondary hypertension. The condition is corrected by the removal of the tumor. The Regitine (phentolamine) test, histamine test, and determination of catecholamines in the urine or blood are diagnostic aids.

Secondary hypertension is also associated with such conditions as toxemia of pregnancy, increased intracranial pressure, congenital blood vessel and heart malformations, and diseases of the kidney such as glomerulonephritis, pyelonephritis, and polycystic disease. Only 10 per cent of persons with hypertension are estimated to have the secondary type. Treatment is directed at relief of the underlying cause.

Primary (Essential) Hypertension

Primary hypertension is characterized by sustained elevation of the diastolic pressure. A diastolic pressure of 95 mm. Hg or greater is generally accepted as a cut-off point for diagnosis (Stamler *et al.*). Many believe that sustained diastolic pressure over 90 mm. Hg requires treatment. Mean arterial pressure and systolic pressure may be elevated as well.

Symptoms

The onset is very gradual; usually, it is first discovered during a routine physical examination.

Women are affected more often than men. Because of the insidious onset, it is hard to say when the disease begins. Persons in their 30's and 40's may be discovered to have a sustained elevation in their blood pressure without any symptoms. Often the condition is present for 10 or 15 years before the patient experiences any discomfort or complications.

One patient may experience no discomfort, whereas another with a similar blood-pressure reading may complain of headache, dizziness, fatigue, insomnia and nervousness. Headache often is described as throbbing or pounding. The person may have nosebleeds (epistaxis), blurring of vision or spots before the eyes. Angina pectoris or shortness of breath may be the first clue to hypertensive heart disease.

Hypertensive disease, unfortunately, may not be diagnosed until the patient becomes ill from its complications. The heart may enlarge, and eventually the patient may develop congestive heart failure. Many of the complications arise from hemorrhage or occlusion of blood vessels supplying important organs. The atherosclerotic process is increased by hypertension. Hemorrhage from the tiny arteries in the retina may cause marked visual disturbance or blindness. Cerebrovascular accident may result from hemorrhage or occlusion of a blood vessel in the brain. Myocardial infarction may result from occlusion of a branch of a coronary artery. Impaired circulation to the kidney is believed to be related to the frequency of degenerative kidney disease among hypertensive patients.

The term *malignant hypertension* is used to describe the condition when it has an abrupt onset and is followed rapidly by severe symptoms and complications. The prognosis is poor. Most untreated patients live only a few months to one or two years. Death frequently is caused by damage to heart, brain or kidneys, resulting from the very high blood pressure which may rise rapidly into the range of 250/150.

Theories about Etiology

Among the many theories concerning the cause of primary hypertension are these:

Heredity. Many investigators have noted a strong familial tendency toward the development of primary hypertension.

Fluid-Electrolyte Metabolism. A disturbed relationship among salt intake, body fluid-electrolyte metabolism, and renal-adrenal function has been observed in many studies, but the results are inconclusive.

Emotional Stress. Patients with hypertension are described sometimes as those who have particular difficulty expressing and dealing with their aggressive impulses. Although they are outwardly calm and composed, inwardly they may be in a turmoil.

Obesity. It has been noted that overweight persons have a higher incidence of hypertension than those of normal weight.

Bacteruria. Higher prevalence rates of bacteria in the urine have been found in hypertensive persons (Stamler *et al.*).

Incidence

Hypertension is presently estimated to affect 17,000,000 adults in the United States. In 1960-62 the National Health Survey estimated that over 1,000,000 Americans in the age group 35-44, of a total population of about 24,000,000 in this age range, had definite hypertensive heart disease. Almost 170,000 were Negro men and almost 170,000 Negro women, showing a markedly higher proportionate incidence among Negroes than whites. Hypertensive heart disease is the major health problem of American Negroes today. More recent studies demonstrate the same age-sex-race patterns. On the basis of several studies, sporadic elevated blood pressure readings in young adulthood indicate increased risk for the later development of sustained hypertension (Stamler *et al.*).

Prevention

Despite the lack of knowledge concerning the etiology of primary (essential) hypertension, the information available from current epidemiologic studies affords a useful basis for its prevention. Factors that increase the risk of hypertensive disease, according to Stamler *et al.* are:

- Race
- Obesity
- Positive family history
- Blood pressure lability in young adulthood
- Family and/or personal history of diabetes mellitus
- History of urinary tract infection

Measures to decrease the risk in susceptible populations may help to forestall the development of symptoms or curtail advancement of the disease.

People with a family history of hypertension or those who have shown transient elevations of blood pressure (often considered to be indicative of a tendency to the disease) may be helped by:

- Having a periodic health examination at least annually
- The correction of obesity and the direction of efforts to remain lean and trim through a nutritious diet and physical exercise
- Moderation in salt intake—about 5 Gm. per day instead of 15-20 Gm.
- Routine midstream urine cultures for the early detection and treatment of urinary tract infections
- Learning to deal more effectively with problems at work, home, or in other circumstances. Some people may need professional assistance. If, for some reason, the patient doesn't learn to cope better, it may become necessary for him to avoid certain stress-producing situations.
- Improving general health habits, if the patient has been taking them lightly. Plenty of sleep, rest and relaxation may prove to be a tremendous help in controlling the condition.

Treatment and Nursing Care

Because the cause is not definitely known, it has not been possible to develop a cure for primary hypertension. However, many forms of treatment are available that often help to lower the blood pressure and to prevent, or at least to delay, discomfort and complications.

The objective of medical care is sustained nutritional-hygienic-pharmacologic management in order to prevent major complications. For example, weight reduction and moderate salt restriction suffice to lower blood pressure in a significant number of patients although the reason is not clear. Some patients find the degree of salt restriction unpalatable and drug therapy is also prescribed by the physician.

Drugs. Drugs do not counteract the cause of the pressure elevation. Rather, they relax constricted arterioles so that the high arterial peripheral resistance is reduced. In general, the doctor prescribes the weakest drug which will keep the pressure at a near normal level. Combinations of drugs may be used. The more potent drugs have more serious side-effects and are reserved for patients with severe, sustained hypertension.

Nursing Implications. When hypotensive drugs are administered, observe the patient carefully for side-effects, and promptly report them if they occur. Since some drugs may cause orthostatic hypertension, if your patient feels faint or weak when he stands up, instruct him to get up slowly. When he arises in the morning, he first should sit on the edge of the bed a few moments and then stand. Teach him to sit or, preferably, to lie down promptly if he feels faint. Getting off his feet will help the feeling to subside, as well as prevent injury from fainting and falling.

Some patients, especially those who are receiving very potent hypotensive drugs, are taught by the nurse or physician to record their own blood pressure, usually sitting and standing while they are at home. A family member may be taught to take the patient's blood pressure. Then therapy can be planned and adjusted according to multiple blood pressure recordings made in the patient's usual surroundings. Make sure that the patient is in the desired position when you are taking the blood pressure. For instance, some doctors will ask you to check it each morning before the patient arises; others will ask you to take it with the patient standing.

Often the patient seeks repeated reassurance and explanation from the nurse. Find out what the doctor has told the patient about his particular condition, so that you can be as helpful to your patient as possible. Avoid the pitfalls of

ANTIHYPERTENSIVE DRUGS

DRUG	WHEN USED	USUAL DOSAGE	ROUTE	SIDE EFFECTS
Thiazide diuretics (Diuril)	Mild hypertension May be used in combination	250 to 500 mg. 1 to 3 times daily	Oral	Fatigue, weakness, gastrointestinal upsets, hypopotassemia
Rauwolfia alkaloids	Mild to moderate hypertension	0.25 mg. to 1 mg. daily	Oral or parenteral	Nasal congestion, obstruction, and nosebleed; diarrhea, somnolence, mental depression
Hydralazine (Apresoline)	Moderate to severe hypertension	10 to 100 mg. several times daily	Oral; I.V. in crisis	Tachycardia, palpitations, headache, nausea, edema, fever, psychosis, lupus-like syndrome
Methyldopa (Aldomet)	Moderately severe hypertension	.5 Gm. to 1.5 Gm. daily	Oral; I.V. in crisis	Postural hypotension, drowsiness, arthralgias, myalgias, grippe-like illness
Ganglionic blocking agents (Arfonad)	Hypertensive crisis	1 to 4 mg. per minute	Titrated by I.V. microdrip	Severe hypotension; damage from renal, myocardial, or cerebral ischemia
Guanethidine (Ismelin)	Severe hypertension	10 to 25 mg. daily	Oral	Marked postural hypotension, worsening of previously stable renal insufficiency; diarrhea, impotence, peptic ulcer, muscular weakness, bradycardia

For further nursing implications of drug therapy, see Chapter 23, Rodman, M., and Smith, D.: *Pharmacology and Drug Therapy in Nursing*. Philadelphia, J. B. Lippincott, 1968.

giving your patient information for which he is not prepared or of withholding information that he has long considered necessary for self-care.

For example, a patient who has been admitted for diagnosis, and who asks you his blood pressure, should not be told blithely, "It's 160/120." Such information, in the absence of a definite diagnosis and an explanation from his doctor, could be very upsetting to him. On the other hand, a patient who has had the condition for years, and who has been taking and recording his own blood pressure at home may be justifiably irritated if you refuse to tell him his blood pressure reading. There is no substitute for knowing what the doctor has told the patient about his condition.

When the patient learns that he has hypertension, he needs a great deal of explanation and reassurance concerning its possible consequences. Almost everyone has heard of people who have had strokes or heart attacks that were attributed to high blood pressure. Often the patient's first thought is that such a catastrophe is about to befall him. The doctor usually helps the patient to understand the course of the disease, and he explains how the patient can help himself.

Here is a sample of what one doctor told his patient, who had just been found to have hypertension:

Patient: "People with high blood pressure usually get strokes, don't they?"

Doctor: "Some do, and many do not."

Patient: "My mother has had high blood pressure for years. Is it hereditary?"

Doctor: "Often there does seem to be a family tendency to it."

Patient: "I guess I should cut out exercise and really take it easy."

Doctor: "Well, that depends. If the exercise is something you enjoy, and it is not too strenuous, you needn't stop it. What kind of exercise do you mean?"

Patient: "I like to play golf and work in the garden on weekends."

Doctor: "Fine! Just don't overdo it. In fact, it probably will be good for you—especially, if it helps you relax."

Patient: "If my blood pressure goes down, that will keep me from getting a stroke, won't it?"

Doctor: "No one can predict the future. None of us knows for sure what lies ahead. This is true of everyone—not just people with high blood pressure. We have found, though, that treatment can lower blood pressure, and we believe this will help to keep you in good health."

Working with hypertensive patients gives the nurse an opportunity to participate in long-term care that may help the patient to live longer and more comfortably. This care places a premium on the nurse's ability to teach, to listen and to guide the patient in following his treatment. The treatment in a sense becomes a way of life for the patient. It continues for years, with gradual adaptations, according to the patient's condition.

REFERENCES AND BIBLIOGRAPHY

ARMSTRONG, M.: Progress in the diagnosis of secondary hypertension, *Med. Clin. N. Am.* 52:1213, September, 1968.

BEESON, P. B., and McDERMOTT, W. (eds.): *Cecil-Loeb Textbook of Medicine,* ed. 12, Philadelphia, Saunders, 1966.

BELAND, I.: *Clinical Nursing,* ed. 2, New York, Macmillan, 1970.

BREST, A., and MOYER, J.: *Cardiovascular Disorders,* Philadelphia, Davis, 1968.

Facts on the Major Killing and Crippling Diseases of the United States Today, New York, National Health Education Committee, 1966.

GORDON, T., and WATERHOUSE, A. M.: Hypertension and hypertensive heart disease, *J. Chron. Dis.* 19:1089, 1966.

GUYTON, A. C.: *Textbook of Medical Physiology,* ed. 3, Philadelphia, Saunders, 1966.

GUYTON, A. C., *et al.*: Physiological control of arterial pressure, *Bull. N.Y. Acad. Med.* 45:811, September, 1969.

HABER, E.: The renin-angiotensin system in curable hypertension, *Mod. Conc. Cardiovasc. Dis.* 38:17, April, 1969.

HARRINGTON, P.: The nurse, the cardiac patient, and his diet, *Cardiovasc. Nurs.* 2:31, Fall, 1966.

KIMBALL, J. T., *et al.*: Circulatory emergencies, Part III. Hypertensive crisis, in Meltzer, L., *et al.*: *Concepts and Practices of Intensive Care for Nurse Specialists,* Philadelphia, Charles Press, 1969.

LEVY, R., *et al.*: Transient hypertension—the relative prognostic importance of various systolic and diastolic levels, *JAMA* 128:1059, 1945.

LEWIS, C. E., *et al.*: Nurse clinics and progressive ambulatory patient care, *New Eng. J. Med.* 277:1236, December, 1967.

RAY, C. T., *et al.*: Nutrition in relation to cardiovascular disease, *Med. Clin. N. Am.* 48:1189, 1964.

RODMAN, M.: Drug therapy today: drugs for managing high blood pressure, *RN* 32:73, May, 1969.

RODMAN, M., and SMITH, D.: *Pharmacology and Drug Therapy in Nursing,* Philadelphia, Lippincott, 1968.

STAMLER, J.: *Lectures on Preventive Cardiology,* New York, Grune, 1967.

STAMLER, J., *et al.*: *The Epidemiology of Hypertension,* New York, Grune, 1967.

THOMAS, C. B.: Developmental patterns in hypertensive cardiovascular disease: fact or fiction? *Bull. N.Y. Acad. Med.* 45:831, September, 1969.

THOMAS, J., and HOLIDAY, E.: Detecting secondary hypertension, *Am. J. Nurs.* 64:94, February, 1964.

TUCKER, R., and HUNT, J.: Recent advances in the medical and surgical treatment of hypertension, *Med. Clin. N. Am.* 52:1227, September, 1968.

WOLF, S., *et al.*: *Life Stress and Essential Hypertension,* Baltimore, Williams & Wilkins, 1955.

The Patient with Peripheral Vascular Disease: Thrombosis and Embolism

32

Ischemia • Arteriosclerosis and Atherosclerosis • Raynaud's Disease • Thromboangiitis Obliterans (Buerger's Disease) Varicose Veins • Thrombophlebitis and Phlebothrombosis Lymphedema • Thrombosis and Embolism • Surgical Conditions of the Blood Vessels

The term *peripheral vascular disease* (PVD) refers to diseases of the blood vessels that supply the extremities. Whether the disease involves the veins, arteries or lymphatics, or all of these, patients with peripheral vascular disease experience a number of similar problems. Pain is common but the kind of pain may vary. For example, the patient with an ulceration often experiences constant and severe pain, which interferes with his ability to sleep as well as to carry on his usual life activities. While the pain of varicosities may not be as acutely intense, nevertheless, the heaviness and burning interfere with the patient's ability to concentrate, and restrict his activities. Constant pain undermines morale and affects the patient's response to his surroundings, his associates, and his medical treatment.

The long-term nature of peripheral vascular diseases is discouraging. Treatment is tedious, and often painful, and healing is slow. A small ulceration that may be looked upon by the hospital staff as relatively "minor" compared with more dramatic patient conditions is a tragedy to the patient if he loses his ability to walk. It may require months of treatment for healing to take place. Worry about finances, loss of job, and

suspension of family and civic responsibilities compound the patient's burden.

Peripheral vascular disease is especially common among older people. Many of the disorders are chronic and tend to be progressive with advancing age. Often, only palliative treatment is possible. Care consists of a multitude of detailed measures to control the disease, to halt its progress and to prevent complications.

The nurse must have a great deal of patience and willingness to carry out the detailed care that can mean the difference between invalidism or continued ability to carry out daily activities. Often, the patient requires treatment for the rest of his life. He is faced with the management of a condition that usually necessitates changes in his mode of living for years, not merely for weeks or months.

Many of these patients have multiple diagnoses. Peripheral vascular disease is often only one manifestation of a widespread vascular disorder affecting many different organs. For instance, the patient may have suffered myocardial infarction due to atherosclerosis of coronary vessels, and he may have failing vision due to vascular changes in the tiny blood vessels of the retina. Diabetics are especially prone to arteriosclerosis and atherosclerosis. Plans for the nursing care must encompass not only the peripheral vascular disease, but also any other disorders from which the patient is suffering.

Patients with peripheral vascular disease often are obliged to change the type of work they do. Among the types usually contraindicated are those involving considerable outdoor exposure to cold or prolonged standing or repeated trauma to the feet. Indoor, sedentary occupations are the most suitable. However, a change of job is frequently difficult or impossible for the older person. Often, illness carries the threat of prolonged disability, loss of earning power and, as a consequence, lessened personal independence. Retirement from active work may be necessary earlier than had been anticipated.

Although the patient may require hospitalization for acute exacerbations of his illness or for complications arising from the condition, the bulk of his care usually is carried out at home. Therefore, the teaching of self-care and the arranging for continued medical and nursing supervision through the doctor, the clinic and the public health nurse are of special significance.

Helping the patient to stop smoking is an important aspect of nursing care (Chap. 9).

Understanding the factors that may hamper or facilitate peripheral circulation is essential in caring for patients with peripheral vascular disease. It is important to know whether the arteries, veins, lymphatics or all three are involved in the disease process, and what pathologic changes are responsible for the symptoms. For instance, the idea that elevating the legs always improves circulation is erroneous. Elevating the legs promotes venous and lymphatic return; it does not improve—it actually reduces—the blood supplied by the arteries.

Errors in positioning the patient can be avoided by:

- Basic understanding of the dynamics of circulation to the extremities
- Understanding the patient's particular disease
- Frequent conferences with the patient's doctor, so that specific procedures concerning important details, such as positioning the patient, can be fully discussed.

If you are in doubt about positioning the patient, it is best to have him keep his legs flat on the bed rather than elevated or dependent until you have opportunity to discuss the matter with the doctor.

ISCHEMIA

Ischemia is the term used to describe a lack of blood supply to meet the needs of the tissues. At one time or another almost everyone has had the experience of "pins and needles" in his foot or his leg, perhaps from sitting on the leg or with the legs crossed for a long time, causing pressure that interferes with blood supply. When the leg is first moved, it feels heavy, numb and awkward. However, these sensations quickly vanish when change of position and exercise improve the circulation to the leg.

What would happen to the leg if circulation were impaired for a long time? What kinds of pathologic change can cause diminished blood supply? A blood clot (embolus) can lodge in an artery, quickly reaching its destination. Excessive vasoconstriction can result in diminished flow of blood. Gradual occlusion of the lumen of the artery by fatty deposits (atherosclerosis) can slowly and inexorably reduce the amount of blood that the arteries can deliver. Such occlusion may be speeded by formation of a blood clot at the atherosclerotic site (thrombosis). Regardless of the particular pathology responsible for the decreased blood flow, certain changes in the affected part will occur if the diminished blood supply is severe and persistent.

- Coldness. Ordinarily, the body feels warm to touch, because of the presence of warm blood. When the blood supply is markedly decreased, the part is cold to touch and also feels uncomfortably cold to the patient.
- Pallor. The normal pink hue of the skin is due to the blood in superficial vessels. Diminished arterial blood supply causes pallor.
- Rubor (redness). Redness—usually a reddish-blue color—results when the superficial blood vessels have been injured by anoxia or coldness and remain dilated. The extremity is both blue-red and cold, rather than pink and warm, as it normally should be.
- Cyanosis (blueness). Cyanosis indicates that the blood in the part contains less than the normal amounts of oxygen. Cyanosis usually results from a blood supply that is diminished and yet not diminished sufficiently to cause blanching.
- Pain. Pain is characteristic when the blood supply is not adequate for the requirements of the tissues. Pain that occurs only after a certain amount of exercise is called *intermittent claudi-*

cation. The patient may walk a block and then have to stop because of severe aching in his calf muscles. His arteries are not able to deliver the amount of blood required by his legs during this exercise. The pain disappears when the patient rests, but it promptly returns when he repeats the same amount of exercise. Pain occurs even at rest (rest pain) when sudden occlusion of an artery by an embolus occurs, because there is not sufficient blood supply to sustain the tissues even when no exercise is undertaken.

• Trophic Changes. The term refers to abnormal changes in the skin and the nails due to impaired circulation. The skin becomes smooth, shiny, taut, dry and hairless. It has very little resistance to infection.

Measures to Increase the Blood Supply

In what general ways can the blood supply to an extremity be increased? How may these measures be utilized in the care of patients with diminished blood supply to an extremity?

• Position. The flow of arterial blood to the limb is improved when the part is dependent (lower than the heart) or at least flat, rather than raised. Raising the limb will further diminish the amount of blood reaching the part.

• Warmth. The kind of warmth that merely insulates the extremity from a cold environment may be safely used. Warm gloves and socks are examples. Extra heat provided by hot-water bottles, hot foot soaks or heating pads never should be used. Often, the patient has diminished sensation in the part, making him less able to note when excessive heat is applied and therefore placing him in even greater danger of being burned.

Heat sometimes is applied to the abdomen to cause reflex dilation of the blood vessels in the extremities. Warm (95° F.) baths or thermoregulated cradles are recommended sometimes.

• Interrupting sympathetic stimuli. Interruption of sympathetic stimuli to the extremity prevents vasoconstriction. Sympathetic stimuli may be removed temporarily by sympatholytic drugs or by injecting the vertebral sympathetic ganglia with alcohol.

Permanent interruption of sympathetic stimulation is achieved by cutting the nerve (sympathectomy), with resultant decrease in vasoconstriction.

• Vasodilators. In order to be effective, vasodilators must have more than a fleeting action. Alcohol and papaverine are examples of drugs

used to cause vasodilation. The usefulness of vasodilators is limited by the fact that organic changes, such as arteriosclerosis, often make the vessels incapable of dilating. Thus, diseases characterized by spasm of vessels or vasoconstriction respond best to vasodilators.

• Dissolving and/or preventing clot formation. If clots are impeding circulation, such anticoagulants as heparin and Dicumarol may be given to prevent further clot formation. Enzymes, such as streptokinase and thrombolysin, are sometimes used to dissolve clots. Their usefulness in the treatment of vascular disease is being studied.

• Avoidance of vasoconstriction. Nicotine leads to vasoconstriction; therefore, smoking or the use of tobacco in any form is contraindicated in any patient with diminished arterial circulation. Exposure to cold causes vasoconstriction and should be avoided whenever possible. The constriction of vessels by pressure also must be avoided. For instance, sitting with the knees crossed causes pressure on popliteal vessels and lessens further the blood supply to the legs.

• Exercise. If exercise does not cause greater demand for blood than the body can supply to the extremity, it is beneficial. Mild exercise with frequent rest periods is usually recommended. Pain is a warning that the patient has exercised more than his blood supply will allow; he should stop and rest.

• Replacement or by-pass of diseased arteries using synthetic vessels or veins (grafts). When successful, surgery of this type produces the most rapid and dramatic improvement possible.

ARTERIOSCLEROSIS AND ATHEROSCLEROSIS

Arteriosclerosis and atherosclerosis commonly accompany the aging process. *Arteriosclerosis* refers to the hardening and the loss of elasticity of the arteries. *Atherosclerosis* refers to the deposition of fatty plaques (composed chiefly of cholesterol) inside the artery and is the most common cause of peripheral arterial disease. These plaques gradually reduce the size of the lumen, resulting in partial or complete obstruction of the artery and in impairment of the blood supply to the part of the body served by the artery.

Arteriosclerosis and atherosclerosis affect many different parts of the body. Heart, brain and kidneys, as well as extremities, may be involved.

Frequently, one extremity is affected more severely than the other, although the circulation to both legs and both feet usually is impaired.

It is believed that the loss of elasticity and the deposition of fatty substances occur gradually over many years. The process usually is not advanced enough to cause symptoms until late middle life or old age.

The rate at which the changes occur varies in different persons. Patients with diabetes mellitus suffer these changes quite early in life. Other factors that may influence the age of onset and the severity of the condition are heredity and diet. Some authorities assert that a diet high in fat, and particularly in cholesterol, may contribute to the occurrence of atherosclerosis. Patients with a family history of vascular disease may be especially prone to develop the condition.

Symptoms. The symptoms are those of ischemia of the feet and the legs. These symptoms have already been discussed and can be briefly summarized as follows:

- Color changes (pallor, rubor, cyanosis)
- Coldness
- Absent or diminished pulse
- Trophic changes in skin and nails
- Susceptibility to infection, lessened ability to fight infection, tendency to develop ulcers and gangrene
- Pain—intermittent claudication and rest pain. Cramping pain may occur at night, particularly in the calf muscles.
- Numbness and tingling.

Treatment. Treatment may be summarized as follows:

- Keeping the parts warm, such as by wearing warm clothing, but avoiding excessive warmth and taking special precautions to avoid burns
- Cleanliness; prompt medical care of even minor cuts or infections
- Avoiding factors, such as exposure to cold and smoking, that cause vasoconstriction
- Moderate exercise, provided that it does not exceed the patient's tolerance
- Avoidance of prolonged standing or sitting in a position that places pressure on the legs, particularly pressure in the popliteal space
- Resting with the legs somewhat lower than the rest of the body. Elevating the head of the bed on shock blocks accomplishes this and facilitates the flow of blood to the legs.

- The oscillating bed stimulates circulation by providing a frequent change of position. The bed is operated electrically. The amount of position change can be adjusted according to the needs of the patient. The bed provides a smooth, continuous, seesaw motion. The head is raised, and the feet are lowered; then the feet are raised, and the head is lowered. Many patients who have pain at night find the oscillating bed especially helpful in relieving pain and promoting sleep. Although some patients say that the constant motion makes them feel "seasick" at first, most become quite accustomed to the movement and do not find it uncomfortable. The patient feels more secure if he is given the switch and shown how to stop the movement of the bed when he wishes (for example, during meals or for use of the bedpan)
- Buerger-Allen exercises involve elevating the feet and the legs until the feet blanch, lowering them until they appear red, and then resting with the legs and the feet in a horizontal position. The patient performs the exercises while he is lying on a bed or sofa, first raising the legs, then dangling them over the side of the bed; and finally resting with his legs flat on the bed. The length of time that the patient is to spend in each position and the number of times the exercise is to be repeated are ordered by the doctor. The patient is instructed to watch the color of his legs and feet and to lower them as soon as they turn white. Blanching indicates an inadequate blood supply. The maintenance of this position could harm the tissues. Walking and active foot exercises may be prescribed by the physician instead of Buerger-Allen exercises
- Measures to lessen vasoconstriction. Because vasoconstriction often is not a prominent factor in causing the symptoms, the use of these measures frequently gives disappointing results. However, sympatholytic drugs like tolazoline and azapetine phosphate (Ilidar), vasodilators such as cyclandelate, nylidrin, alcohol and nicotinyl alcohol, and sympathectomy may be tried.
- Treatment of ulcers and infections by cleansing, use of antibiotics, and all the measures previously mentioned to improve circulation

- Surgical procedures, such as endarterectomy (removal of an atherosclerotic plaque from the lumen), bypass operations and the replacement of diseased vessels with prostheses made from such materials as nylon are sometimes effective in increasing the blood supply to the part
- Possibly resorting to amputation if gangrene occurs.

There is no cure for arteriosclerosis. Such measures as meticulous attention to personal cleanliness and avoidance of injury and exposure often can preserve the limb, as well as lessen the patient's discomfort.

Care of Leg Ulcers

Ulcers often complicate peripheral vascular disease, and they require a great deal of care. Because the ulcers tend to heal very slowly, the patient and those who care for him may become discouraged. Meticulous technic is especially important when carrying out prescribed care, such as the application of ointments and dressings. Sometimes, the patient (and, alas, occasionally the staff, too) grow so accustomed to the lesion that they use technic that would be considered unthinkable in the care of a surgical incision. The patient may apply ointment with his hands, often without even washing them first! No care is too great in preventing further infection.

Patients with peripheral vascular disease are especially vulnerable to infection. They develop infection readily, and their ability to control it and to heal wounds is so lessened by poor circulation that gangrene and amputation are not unusual. Use the most careful technic possible, and teach the patient to do so. Washing the hands thoroughly before starting to care for the lesion, applying prescribed medication with a sterile tongue blade to sterile gauze, and then laying the gauze and medication against the ulcer are examples of simple technics that can lessen the problem of infection. Teach the patient not to touch the side of the gauze that he places next to the ulcer.

When the patient has a leg ulcer, he often must stay off his feet for weeks or even months. Part or all of this time may be spent in the hospital. Diversion is very important. Hours and weeks pass slowly, and the patient often worries about his finances, his family and his job. Take the time to listen, when he expresses some of his worries and fears—perhaps of amputation or of losing his job.

Helping to Lessen the Patient's Pain

Pain may cause restless days and agonizing nights. The pain tends to be chronic, but it occurs with special severity at certain times of the day. Narcotics usually are avoided, if possible, because of the long-term nature of the condition and the consequent danger of addiction. Salicylates may give relief, particularly when they are used in combination with measures to improve circulation, such as position, exercise, warmth and vasodilators. Sometimes, codeine is given with the salicylates.

Remember that the reluctance to use narcotics stems from the danger of addiction; it does not mean that the pain is trivial. As much concern and zeal to relieve pain are required for these patients as for any others on the ward. All too often the patient senses a slackening of interest, and he may have the impression that his pain is not so dramatic or given as careful consideration as that of a postoperative patient. Its chronicity makes the pain harder to bear rather than easier. The pain itself is added to the fatigue from many sleepless nights and the uncertainty about when the symptoms will abate. Prolonged pain can set nerves on edge and make the patient seem to be cranky or demanding.

What can the nurse do to help to lessen the patient's pain?

- Use any measures that are approved by the doctor to improve circulation. For example, placing the legs in a dependent position often helps. Let the patient put his legs over the side of the bed, and be careful that this position does not also cause pressure from the edge of the bed against the popliteal space, since this pressure could further impair circulation. Give him a stool or a chair on which to support his feet, so that the pressure behind his knees is relieved.
- Make sure that his feet do not become chilled. If he gets up at night to put his legs over the edge of the bed or to sit in a chair, be sure that he wears his warm socks and has a blanket over his legs and his feet.
- Give "p.r.n." analgesics promptly when they are needed. A dose given about one-half hour before a dressing change or soak may make the pain of the treatment easier to bear.

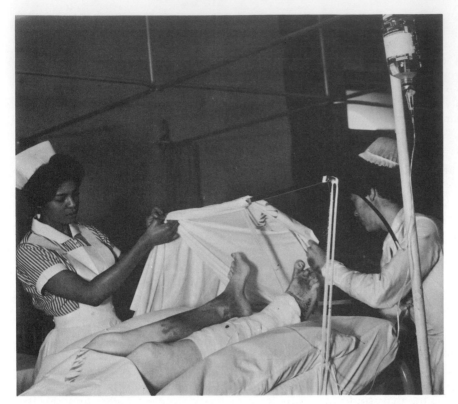

FIG. 32-1. A bed cradle keeps the weight of the covers off the patient's feet. Note the discoloration of the skin and the thickening of the nails that occur typically in patients with peripheral vascular disease. The pillows under the patient's legs have been protected with plastic covers. The dressing is being kept wet with enzymes used to dissolve clots and fibrinous exudates. The enzymes pass through the tubing to the dressing.

- Flexibility in carrying out the care is important. If the patient was awake most of the night and has just gone to sleep, do not waken him for his bath just because it is 8 A.M. If he is restless at night, try to place him where he will be least likely to disturb others, so that the emphasis can be on helping him to rest rather than on scolding him, "Sshh, you'll wake everyone up."

- Place a foam rubber pad under the heels to help to prevent necrosis—a frequent complication in patients with peripheral vascular disease

- Nurses carry major responsibility for the patient's safety as well as his comfort. Patients with peripheral vascular disease are especially prone to burns. A thermoregulated cradle to warm the patient's foot is far safer than an ordinary cradle, in which a light bulb has been placed. The temperature in thermoregulated cradles can be set according to the doctor's directions (95° F. is usual), and it can be maintained constant as long as it is desired. The Aquamatic pad is another

example of a device that can be used to apply heat safely.

- A bed cradle or a footboard may be used to keep the weight of the bedclothes off the feet

- Test the temperature of the bath water with a bath thermometer before having the patient place his feet in the bath basin or the bathtub (95° F. is a safe temperature). Instruct him to do the same when he goes home. Placing the feet in bath water that is too hot may result in a severe burn or even the loss of a leg.

- Use external heat only as it is approved by the doctor. In some situations it has been customary to permit the application of a hot-water bottle to the feet without a doctor's order. Patients with peripheral vascular disease should never have a hot-water bottle applied—especially not to their feet—without the doctor's specific order.

The patient will see your concern for his welfare reflected in your promptness, in your measures concerning warmth and position and in your manner, which conveys your feeling of caring.

Foot Care

If the patient is feeble, has poor vision or has an unsteady hand, someone else must assume the responsibility for inspecting his feet regularly, bathing them and trimming the nails. A member of the family may give this care, or, if the patient lives alone, a weekly visit from the public health nurse can provide this important care, as well as continued instruction and encouragement in the care that the patient can still perform himself.

The services of a chiropodist are valuable in managing such problems as the cutting of thickened, brittle nails. The patient should explain that he has peripheral vascular disease and give the name of his physician. These measures enable the chiropodist to carry out treatment with consideration of the patient's impaired circulation, as well as to confer with the patient's physician concerning particular needs and problems.

Teaching the Patient and His Family

The nurse has an important role in teaching the patient and his family. The following instructions are applicable to most patients with peripheral vascular disease:

• Keep your feet clean. Wash them once a day, and inspect them regularly for cuts or bruises. Wear clean socks or stockings daily.

• Avoid having your feet constantly moist, because constant moistness predisposes to infections, like athlete's foot.

• Trim your nails regularly, at least once a week. Nail clippers and emery board are safer to use than pointed scissors. *Never* use a razor blade for this purpose. Cut the nails straight across, and not too short.

• Don't treat cuts, corns or calluses yourself. Ask your doctor's advice. If you accidentally cut your foot, cleanse the wound with 70 per cent alcohol, apply a dry sterile dressing and see your doctor. Never apply any medication, such as corn plasters, to your feet without first consulting your doctor.

• If your feet are dry, apply lotion or cream after bathing. Applying alcohol and prolonged soaking increase dryness and should be avoided.

• Wear comfortable shoes that fit. Heels that are too high cause pressure on the toes. Sneakers make the feet perspire and are not advisable.

A comfortable shoe with good support and a leather sole is preferable. Shoes made of soft leather with rounded rather than pointed toes help to prevent pressure and friction.

• Socks and stockings should be large enough to avoid any tightness or pressure. Avoid bulky darns that could cause pressure and irritation of your foot.

• Never wear circular garters. Use a girdle or a garter belt to hold up stockings.

• Avoid garments that cause constriction around the thigh. Some girdles are in this category.

• Never go barefoot, even at home. There is too much chance of cutting or bruising your feet. "Thong" sandals do not give adequate protection to the feet.

• Avoid positions that cause pressure on your legs. Do not curl your legs under you when you are sitting, or cross your knees. The edge of the chair should not come right behind your knees.

• Follow your doctor's directions concerning exercise. If walking causes pain, learn to judge distances, so that you stop and rest before pain occurs. Walking slowly will enable you to walk farther without experiencing pain.

• Avoid prolonged standing. Unless your doctor has advised otherwise, alternate rest with mild exercise, such as walking.

• Keep your feet warm, and avoid excessive heat. An extra blanket at the foot of your bed, warm socks and fleece-lined boots are examples of safe ways to keep your feet and your legs warm. Bath water should be tested with a thermometer. Never use an electric heating pad, hot-water bottle or hot foot soak without the advice of your doctor. Ask him before using an electric blanket, too.

These general instructions are modified and supplemented in the light of each patient's particular program of treatment. Most patients are advised to stop smoking; many are on special diets, such as reducing diets, low cholesterol diets (in atherosclerosis) or diabetic diets. Instruction concerning diet forms an important part of the teaching program for such patients. The patient is encouraged to follow his doctor's directions concerning medications.

If a sympathectomy has been performed, the patient should understand that the affected extremity will no longer perspire. Dryness of the skin can be prevented by applying cream or lotion frequently. If Buerger-Allen exercises have been prescribed, be sure that the patient

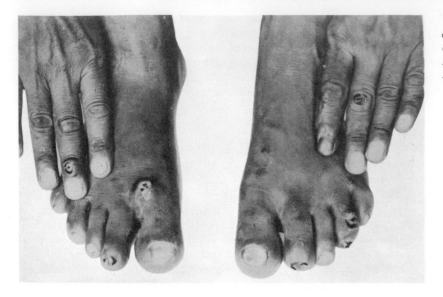

Fig. 32-2. Thromboangiitis obliterans, with gangrenous ulcers. (Vakil, R. J., and Golwalla, A.: *Clinical Diagnosis,* Bombay, Asia Publishing House)

understands how often to do them, how long the legs are to remain in each position, and how to support his legs when they are elevated. He can rest them against the wall beside his bed or against the back of a sofa.

RAYNAUD'S DISEASE

Raynaud's disease is characterized by periodic constriction of the arteries that supply the extremities. The digital arteries of the hands and the feet commonly are affected. Nose, ears and chin are involved less commonly.

The underlying cause of Raynaud's disease is not entirely clear; however, it is believed to be related to emotional stress and exposure to cold. The condition is much more common among women than men, and it usually occurs in young adults. Familial predisposition may play a part in causing the disease.

Symptoms. The attacks occur intermittently and with varying frequency, but especially with exposure to cold. The hands become cold, blanched, wet with perspiration, and they feel numb and prickly. Awkwardness and fumbling are noted, especially when fine movements are attempted. After the initial pallor, the hands, and especially the fingers, become deeply cyanotic. The cyanosis often is accompanied by aching pain. Usually, the patient learns that the attack can be relieved by placing the hands in warm water or by going indoors, where it is warm. The warmth relieves the vasospasm, and blood rushes to the part. The skin in the deprived areas becomes flushed and warm, and the patient has a sensation of throbbing.

In the early stages of the disease, the hands usually appear perfectly normal between attacks. The disease does not necessarily progress to cause severe disability. In many instances the symptoms are mild, and they may even improve spontaneously. However, when the disease is severe and of long duration, cyanosis of the fingers may persist between the attacks, and trophic changes gradually may occur. Ulcers and superficial gangrene may appear at the fingertips and are exquisitely painful. The fingers are especially vulnerable to infection. Healing of even minor lesions is often slow and uncertain.

Treatment. The treatment of Raynaud's disease involves avoidance of the factors that precipitate attacks. The patient is instructed to avoid chilling. Electric blankets are helpful. It is important to encourage the patient to dress warmly without sacrificing style and attractiveness. Smoking is absolutely contraindicated since it causes vasoconstriction.

The patient also should be helped to recognize situations that cause emotional upset. Often, counseling is effective in helping the patient to change her environment and/or her ways of reacting to it, in order to minimize stress.

Sympatholytic drugs, such as tolazoline (Prescoline) and phenoxybenzamine (Dibenzyline) often are prescribed to relieve spasm of the arteries, thus providing greater blood supply to the tissues. Vasodilators, such as alcohol or papaverine, are also useful in preventing or relieving the attacks. Nylidrin (Arlidin), cyclandelate (Cyclo-spasmol), or nicotinyl alcohol (Roniacol) may also be prescribed.

Sympathectomy is performed occasionally when the disease is severe and progressive, and when medical treatment fails to relieve the condition. The areas from which sympathetic stimuli have been removed will no longer perspire. The patient is instructed to apply cream frequently to prevent excessive dryness of the skin.

THROMBOANGIITIS OBLITERANS (BUERGER'S DISEASE)

The name of this disease describes the pathology—inflammation of blood vessels associated with formation of clots and with fibrosis of arteries. This condition leads to the obstruction of the blood vessels. The disease affects primarily the arteries and the veins of the lower extremities. The upper extremities occasionally are involved.

The cause of thromboangiitis obliterans is not established definitely; however, some believe it to be an allergic response to tobacco. It is far more common among men than women, and it usually has its onset during young adulthood.

Symptoms. The patient notes that one foot or both feet are always cold. Intermittent claudication is a common symptom. Usually, the symptoms fluctuate in severity. Attacks of acute distress often are followed by remissions, during which the disease is quiescent.

Cyanosis and redness of the feet and legs are noted often. Frequently, the color is a mottled purplish-red. Ulcers that heal slowly or progress to the development of gangrene may occur, particularly at the toes and the heel. Trophic changes in the skin and the nails are characteristic when circulation has been impaired for a considerable period. Phlebitis is common. Rest pain occurs when circulation has been impaired seriously, and particularly when ulcers have formed. Although the disease usually is most pronounced in one leg and foot, both legs usually are affected to some degree.

Treatment. The use of tobacco in any form is contraindicated, and it never should be resumed, even if the symptoms of the disease abate. The resumption of smoking leads to an exacerbation of the disease. The patient is instructed to avoid chilling. Warm socks, boots and gloves are essential in cold weather. Prolonged standing should be avoided. Sometimes, these requirements mean that the patient must change his job. The prevention of injury and of infection of the extremities is very important.

Exercise is helpful in stimulating circulation, provided it is not excessive and does not cause pain. *Buerger-Allen exercises,* walking, and active foot exercises may be prescribed by the physician. The oscillating bed may be used.

Sympatholytic drugs, such as tolazoline and phenoxybenzamine, may be ordered. Analgesics often are required to lessen pain. Since the disease is chronic, the doctor attempts to control the pain without narcotics because of the danger of addiction.

The vasodilating effect of heat may be utilized, provided that the heat is properly applied. The heat is not set above body temperature, and no appliance should be used in which the amount of heat cannot be reliably regulated. (The optimum temperature is 95° F.) Some doctors permit their patients to use electric blankets, provided that the blankets are in good condition, and the temperature can be regulated safely. Thermoregulated heat cradles also may be used, if they are kept at body temperature or slightly below it.

The patient's legs are kept horizontal or dependent, except during Buerger-Allen exercises, or while on the oscillating bed, if these have been prescribed. Elevating the legs increases the ischemia, and therefore it causes or increases pain.

Sympathectomy is performed sometimes to relieve vasospasm. If lesions occur on the extremity and become infected, antibiotics are ordered to help to control the infection. Enzymes, such as streptokinase-streptodornase, are ordered sometimes to débride the lesion. If the circulation becomes so impaired that gangrene results, amputation may be necessary.

VARICOSE VEINS

Veins serving the extremities have valves that keep the blood flowing in one direction only. The closure of successive sets of valves along the veins keeps the blood moving up toward the heart and prevents it from seeping down toward the feet.

Varicose veins are dilated, tortuous veins. Blood collects in these veins and cannot be returned efficiently to the heart. The valves of the veins are incompetent. They close incompletely or not at all, and blood is permitted to seep backward, rather than being propelled always onward toward the heart. This seepage causes

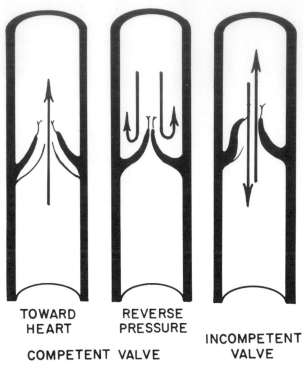

TOWARD HEART

REVERSE PRESSURE

INCOMPETENT VALVE

COMPETENT VALVE

Fig. 32-3. Competent valves in the veins permit the blood to flow toward the heart and prevent the flow of the blood in the opposite direction. Incompetent valves, by failing to close tightly, permit the blood to flow in both directions.

further congestion of the part with venous blood and further distention of the veins. The saphenous veins of the legs commonly are affected. However, varicose veins occur in other part of the body, such as the rectum (hemorrhoids) and the esophagus (esophageal varices).

Some people have a familial tendency toward varicose veins. The valves of the veins become incompetent early in life, resulting in the development of varicosities. Men as well as women suffer from varicose veins—a point sometimes overlooked because men's trousers conceal their legs. Often, the condition first manifests itself when other factors impair venous return. For example, pelvis tumors or pregnancy may exert pressure on the veins, causing interference with venous return. Prolonged standing aggravates the condition, because the venous return is impaired further by the force of gravity. The action of the leg muscles during exercise, such as vigorous walking, aids venous return. Anything that causes constriction or pressure on the legs makes varicosities worse. Circular garters are a familiar example. Obesity contributes to inefficient venous return by placing excess weight on the legs. Thrombophlebitis (discussed later in this chapter) sometimes leads to the development of varicose veins, because the valves of the veins may be damaged during the inflammatory process. Often several of these factors combine to produce varicose veins.

Symptoms. When blood is not returned efficiently from the legs, it tends to collect in the saphenous veins. Because these veins are superficial and less well supported by surrounding tissues, they are especially prone to distention. The deeper veins of the legs are better supported by muscles. The veins become swollen and tortuous. They can be seen under the skin as dark blue or purplish swellings. The patient's legs feel heavy and tired and often become edematous, particularly after prolonged standing. There may be cramping pains. Inefficient venous return causes congestion of the tissues of the leg and the foot. This congestion leads to diminished arterial blood supply and results in impaired nutrition of the tissues with consequent reduction in their ability to resist infection and to allow wounds to heal. Minor injuries readily become infected and ulcerated. The healing of such lesions is slow and uncertain.

Treatment. The treatment of varicose veins usually is surgical. One frequently used procedure is called *ligation and stripping.* The affected veins are ligated, severed from their connections and removed. The entire great saphenous vein, which extends from the groin to the ankle, usually must be removed. In the course of stripping, numerous small incisions are made on the leg. These incisions are covered with sterile dressings, and then elastic bandages are applied firmly from the foot to the groin. The operation may be performed under local or general anesthesia.

The patient returns from the operating room with the elastic bandages in place. The foot of his bed usually is elevated in the immediate postoperative period to aid venous return. Elevation can be accomplished by using shock blocks or, with some of the newer beds, by merely turning a crank or pushing a foot pedal. The standard knee gatch is not satisfactory for this purpose, because it causes a bend in the knee and pressure behind the knee. The operative sites are observed for bleeding. If any is noted, manual pressure is applied over the bleed-

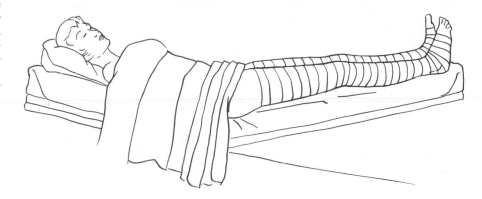

FIG. 32-4. Postoperative positioning in surgery for varicose veins. Feet and legs are elevated to aid venous return. Elastic bandages from feet to groin were applied in the operating room.

ing area, the limb is elevated, and the doctor is notified.

Early ambulation is an important aspect of postoperative treatment. It stimulates circulation and helps to prevent venous thrombosis. If the patient asks how the blood will be returned from the leg "now that my veins have been removed," explain to him that the blood will be returned by the deep veins of his leg, which are still working efficiently.

Help the patient to understand that walking is a part of his postoperative treatment. Often, he is startled to learn that he is expected to take a walk shortly after he recovers from anesthesia. Unless he understands the reason, this treatment may seem like unmitigated cruelty to him. Be sure to stay with him the first few times that he gets up. His legs will feel clumsy and painful. This, plus the effect of preoperative medications and anesthesia, makes it especially important to protect the patient from falls.

As a rule, the patient remains in the hospital only 2 or 3 days. After the immediate postoperative period, nursing care involves helping the patient to plan his activities so that he takes frequent short walks, alternating with periods of rest in bed and in the chair. Often, the patient is instructed to elevate his legs when he is sitting in a chair. However, the foot of the bed usually is elevated only during the immediate postoperative period. Elastic bandages must be checked regularly and reapplied as it is necessary, because they tend to become loose when the patient walks about. At first these bandages are changed and reapplied by the surgeon; later they are changed by the nurse.

Before his discharge from the hospital the patient is instructed in the correct procedure for applying the bandages, because he ordinarily is advised by the physician to continue their use at home. After returning home, the patient is instructed by the doctor concerning how long to wear elastic bandages, and when to begin to wear elastic hosiery.

The postoperative period provides an excellent opportunity for the patient to learn how to minimize the possibility of the recurrence of varicosities or (if only one leg was affected) their development in the other leg. The patient has already found that he has a tendency to varicose veins and therefore must make every effort to control and, if it is possible, to prevent them in the future. Unfortunately, many patients cherish the belief that the operation will make further precautions unnecessary. Emphasize the importance of follow-up care at his doctor's office or clinic. Encourage him to follow the doctor's directions concerning future care.

General instructions given by most doctors include:

• Whenever possible, the patient should elevate the legs when he is sitting.

• He should avoid prolonged standing. For example, it is better to walk about at the bus stop than to stand still.

• Circular garters or tight girdles should not be worn.

If the patient is obese, the doctor usually recommends a reducing diet.

Varicose Ulcers. Varicose ulcers usually appear on the lower leg over a vein. It is believed that the ulcer is usually caused by inflammation of the vein and the surrounding tissues. This inflammatory process impairs the blood supply to the overlying skin and leads to the development of an ulcer.

Varicose ulcers are painful and disabling, since elevation of the leg usually must be maintained in order to facilitate venous repair and promote healing. The treatment involves primarily the treatment of the varicose veins that have led to the formation of ulcers. Every effort should be made to persuade patients to have treatment before ulcers develop. The ulcers are slow to heal and have a tendency to recur. Sometimes a gelatin paste boot (Unna's paste boot) is applied, and the patient is permitted to walk about. The principle is similar to that of an elastic bandage or stocking. The boot, which consists of a circular gauze bandage saturated with a special paste, is applied while the patient's foot is elevated. It dries and "sets" after about 20 minutes, and it provides firm support, compressing the superficial varicose veins and facilitating the return of the venous blood through the deeper veins of the leg.

Careful technic is important in the application of dressings or local medications, because the tissues have poor ability to combat infection. Antibiotics often are ordered to treat infection locally if it occurs.

THROMBOPHLEBITIS AND PHLEBOTHROMBOSIS

Thrombophlebitis means inflammation of a vein accompanied by clot formation. *Phlebothrombosis* refers to the presence of clots in a vein that has little or no inflammation.

Avoiding Venous Stasis. Venous stasis predisposes to the development of both conditions. The factors contributing to venous stasis are inactivity after surgery or any illness, heart failure and pressure on the veins in the pelvis or legs.

Unless leg exercises are contraindicated by the patient's condition, all patients who are unable to walk about should have leg exercises while they are in bed. Preferable are active exercises, such as bending the knee, rotating the foot at the ankle and wiggling the toes. However if the patient is unable to carry out these active exercises, passive exercise may be given by the nurse. Pressure should not be applied to the legs. For example, pillows and blanket rolls should not be placed behind the knees, and the knee gatch should not be elevated for prolonged periods. Prolonged sitting is inadvisable, because the chair may cause pressure behind the knees. Con-

valescent patients should alternate sitting with walking about the room or lying on the bed. The vague instruction, "Move your legs often," or "Don't sit in the chair too long" is not effective in motivating patients who are in particular danger of developing thrombophlebitis—for example, fresh postoperative or aged patients. Specific instructions, such as, "Bend your knee this way [demonstrate] five times," is far more likely to result in the paient's actually performing the exercise. Remember to observe and to encourage him in this exercise throughout his period of inactivity. Brief instruction given only once is easily overlooked or forgotten, especially when a patient is tired or in pain. The activity plan should be recorded on the nursing care plan so that all who care for the patient will carry it through.

Elderly patients and those with heart disease, infections or dehydration are susceptible to thrombophlebitis. And it does not occur only in hospitals. Prolonged sitting on airplane flights, on bus rides, or in front of TV has led to thrombophlebitis. The importance of changing position frequently and of exercising the legs at intervals cannot be overemphasized.

Wrapping the legs with elastic bandages or wearing elastic stockings or support hose may help to prevent thrombophlebitis in susceptible persons by giving added support to the veins and facilitating venous return from the legs. Sometimes, anticoagulants are given to patients who are especially susceptible to thrombophlebitis in an effort to prevent the development of thrombi. Elevating the foot of the bed on 6-inch blocks aids venous return, and this measure is sometimes used to help to prevent thrombophlebitis when illness necessitates bed rest.

Symptoms. The symptoms of thrombophlebitis include pain, heat, redness, and swelling in the affected region. Usually, the legs are involved. If there is marked interference with deep venous return, the leg becomes markedly swollen and may have a mottled bluish color. Often, the patient has systemic symptoms of fever, malaise, fatigue and anorexia.

Phlebothrombosis produces few if any symptoms, since inflammation is slight or absent. Sometimes, the limb suddenly becomes swollen and cyanotic, calling attention to the condition. The patient may experience pain in the calf on dorsiflexion of the foot (Homan's sign).

Treatment. The treament of thrombophlebitis usually includes complete rest of the limb and promotion of venous return by elevating the foot of the bed on 6-inch blocks. Keeping the leg at rest and avoiding massage help to prevent clots from being dislodged and traveling in the bloodstream. The affected part *never* is rubbed since rubbing might dislodge a clot and result in embolism.

Some difference of opinion exists among physicians concerning the advisability of elevating the leg, and keeping it at complete rest. Specific orders concerning the position of the part and the amount of activity permitted should be obtained.

Warm (95° F.) wet packs are ordered sometimes to lessen pain and to decrease inflammation. After she has gently applied petrolatum to the skin to lessen the danger of burning, the nurse should wring out the warm towels as dry as possible, either by hand or with a mechanical wringer. Thorough wringing is very important because burns may result if the towels are soppy. Sometimes, the doctor orders hot-water bottles to be placed on top of the towels to keep them warm longer. If hot-water bottles are used, they should be placed against the side of the leg, so that the weight of the bottle is supported by the mattress. Be sure that the foundation of the bed is covered with plastic material, so that it does not become wet. The pack should be kept warm during the entire time ordered for its application. The foot should be incorporated in the pack. A thermoregulated cradle or a pad, such as the Aquamatic pad, which provides accurate and constant temperature control, is used sometimes instead of the hot water bottle to apply heat to the limb.

Frequently, anticoagulants are ordered to prevent further clot formation. Such enzymes as fibrinolysin and streptokinase may be used to dissolve clots that have already formed. However, the use of such drugs to dissolve clots is relatively new and is still being studied. Sometimes, the clot is removed surgically, or the vein is ligated in order to prevent embolism.

When symptoms have subsided, the patient gradually is permitted more activity. The limb is elevated for only part of the day, and the patient is allowed to walk about. Usually, elastic bandages or elastic stockings are advised at first to give support and to promote venous return. The condition frequently subsides completely, and the patient may resume his accustomed activities. The illness and the convalescent period often last several weeks or even several months.

The patient requires encouragement to continue his treatment as long as it is necessary. Diversion helps the time to pass more quickly and lessens the restlessness and the impatience that so often accompany restricted physical activity.

LYMPHEDEMA

Lymph is similar in composition to tissue fluid and plasma. A system of vessels called *lymphatics* carries tissue fluid from the body tissues to the veins. Obstruction to lymph vessels causes accumulation of tissue fluid in the affected part. Edema (often massive) occurs, resulting in deformity and poor nutrition of the tissues. This condition is called *lymphedema*.

Lymphedema occurs usually in the legs and the genitalia. It also occurs quite frequently in the arms, particularly in patients who have had radical mastectomy.

Lymph vessels can be damaged in a variety of ways. For example, filarial worms may invade lymph channels, causing a condition known as *elephantiasis*.

Burns and excessive radiation can damage the lymphatics and cause lymphedema. Some children are born with inadequate lymph channels, although the edema may not manifest itself until puberty. Carcinoma often spreads by way of the lymph channels. Often, the lymphatics are damaged, either by the malignancy or by the extensive surgery required to cure it. The infection of lymph channels by such organisms as the streptococcus also can lead to lymphedema. Lymphedema can also follow repeated bouts of phlebitis and supervening streptococcal (erysipeloid) infection. With each attack more permanent scar accumulates and edema fluid becomes trapped in small "fibrous" lakes (Oschner).

The symptoms of lymphedema include enlargement due to edema of the limb and tight, shiny skin. Sometimes, the skin becomes thickened, rough and discolored. Because nutrition of the tissues is impaired, ulcers and infection are common.

The treatment of lymphedema consists of removing the cause, if it is possible. Rest, prevention of reinfection and a drug such as diethylcarbamazine citrate (Hetrazan) are used to combat filarial worms. Such antibiotics as penicillin may be given to treat streptococcal infections of the lymphatics. The obstruction of lymphatics caused by injuries, such as burns, can be corrected sometimes by surgery. The Kondoleon operation, a radical excision of involved tissue, is occasionally performed for severe, disabling lymphedema.

Mild cases of lymphedema may respond to symptomatic treatment. The limb is elevated at intervals to promote lymphatic drainage. Elastic bandages or an elastic stocking is worn when the part is dependent. Massage starting at the toes or the fingers and moving up toward the body may be helpful.

THROMBOSIS AND EMBOLISM

When an embolus reaches a blood vessel that is too small to permit its passage, the vessel is occluded, and blood is prevented from flowing through the rest of the vessel. The tissues lying beyond the obstruction are deprived of their blood supply. Thrombosis of a blood vessel means that a clot has formed within the vessel. Often, the clot enlarges, causing partial or complete obstruction of the vessel. Clots form relatively easily in arteries whose lining has become roughened and narrowed from the deposition of fatty plaques (atherosclerosis).

Symptoms. The symptoms of an embolism affecting the extremities are due to ischemia of the tissues that depend on the obstructed vessel for their blood supply.

If the curtailment of blood supply is drastic, the extremity suddenly becomes white, cold and excruciatingly painful. Normal arterial pulse is absent below the area of the obstruction. The patient may feel numbness, tingling or cramps. Surrounding vessels go into spasm. These symptoms are followed by a loss of sensation in the affected area of the limb and a loss of the ability to move the part. Unless the obstruction is promptly relieved, necrosis of tissue occurs and necessitates amputation. Symptoms of shock frequently occur if a large vessel has been obstructed. When a small vessel is occluded, symptoms of ischemia, such as pallor and coldness, occur, but they are less severe.

Initial Care. To save the limb, the treatment must be immediate. Patients who already are hospitalized have a better chance for cure, since treatment is available immediately. The symptoms usually occur suddenly.

Place the extremity in a dependent position to facilitate some possible blood flow to the part. Keep the part at complete rest. Keep the patient warm, since chilling may lead to further vasospasm, thus further decreasing the blood supply to the extremity. Wrap the extremity in cotton to prevent radiation of heat and pressure necrosis. Direct heat never is applied to ischemic tissues, because it may burn the skin and accelerate the development of gangrene. Call the doctor immediately, and describe the symptoms as accurately and concisely as you can. Assure the patient that the doctor is coming, and that meanwhile you will stay with him.

The doctor may order an immediate injection of heparin to help to prevent the development of further clots or the extension of those already present. An attempt may be made to improve the circulation by relaxing the vasospasm. Such drugs as papaverine may be used for this purpose. A block of the sympathetic nerves, usually by injecting procaine into the sympathetic ganglia, may relieve vasospasm. A narcotic, such as Demerol, may be ordered to relieve the pain and to lessen the patient's apprehension.

Surgery. If, as a result of this treatment, the limb does not regain normal color and warmth, surgery is performed. Prepare the patient for the operating room as quickly as possible. However, avoid giving him the feeling of haste or confusion.

Surgery may be done under local anesthesia, except when a clot has become stuck at the bifurcation of the aorta into the iliac arteries (saddle embolus). In an embolectomy the vessel is cut above the clot, the clot is suctioned out, and the vessel sutured together (arteriorrhaphy). In an endarterectomy the intima also is resected. When it is necessary, a temporary bypass shunt is created to maintain circulation while the diseased segment is repaired. Sometimes the problem is solved surgically by a permanent bypass graft.

Nursing Care. Both preoperatively and postoperatively, the patient with an acutely occluded vessel needs to be constantly attended. The pain is severe, and the patient is apprehensive. Postoperative observations include blood pressure and continued observation of the extremity. The blood pressure should not vary widely, as fluctuation tends to increase clotting. Is the leg warmer, and has its normal color returned? Does a pulse reappear? Watch for signs of ischemia. The vessel that was operated on may become plugged again due to clot formation from surgical trauma. When normal circulation has been reestablished, the part becomes warm, normal in color and sensation. It is no longer paralyzed. The pulses can be felt again.

Watch, also, for bleeding on the bandage, a drop of blood pressure and a rapid pulse. The patient may have been given anticoagulants, such as heparin or Dicumarol. Hemorrhage, if it occurs, may be severe. Apply pressure over the wound while waiting for the doctor. The patient may have to be returned to the operating room in order to stop the bleeding. Transfusions are given to replace lost blood.

Exercise of the affected limb is not given postoperatively without the direction of the surgeon. Avoid chilling and pressure. The knee gatch should not be elevated, pillows should not be placed under the knees unless the surgeon specifically orders them, because pressure on the legs may impair circulation and lead to thrombosis.

Pulmonary Embolism

An embolus is any foreign substance, such as a particle of fat or a clot, that travels in the bloodstream. A clot becomes dislodged from a vein and is carried back toward the heart and the lungs. Often, the clot occludes one of the pulmonary vessels, causing infarction. If the blood vessel is large and the area of infarction is extensive, the patient may go into acute cor pulmonale (right heart failure). Complete cardiovascular collapse (cardiac arrest) may follow and the patient may die despite resuscitative attempts.

Predisposing conditions to pulmonary embolism, in addition to thrombophlebitis and phlebothrombosis, are recent surgery, confinement to bed rest, fracture or trauma of the lower extremities, the postpartum state and debilitating diseases. Studies are presently being conducted to determine the relationship between thromboembolic disorders and the use of oral contraceptives.

If the occluded blood vessel is small, the patient may experience chest pain, dyspnea, wheezing, tachypnea and tachycardia, cough, hemoptysis and cyanosis.

An ECG and chest x-ray may be ordered. Their results are suggestive but not specifically diagnostic. They are used in conjunction with the results of a lung scan and angiogram. A pulmonary radioisotope scan would show an area of hypoperfusion, but the physician needs to distinguish this from other causes such as tumor or pneumonitis.

The patient is treated with heparin and other measures such as complete rest, oxygen, and analgesia. Heparin prevents the extension of the thrombus in the pulmonary artery and prevents the development of additional thrombi in the veins from which the embolus arose. Heparin is preferably given intravenously, initially in higher doses than usually recommended for anticoagulation since there is evidence that high initial dosage decreases mortality.

Other forms of therapy include the use of fibrinolytic agents such as urokinase. For massive embolus, embolectomy may be performed using cardiopulmonary bypass to support the circulation, while the embolus is being removed.

Since the embolus to the lungs passes through the inferior vena cava, it can be interrupted by various means if pulmonary embolus is recurrent. Because of the problem of severe venostasis and edema in the lower extremities following ligation of the inferior vena cava, methods which attempt to stop large emboli without blocking blood flow have been devised. These include plication of the inferior vena cava (stitching folds between the walls), creation of a suture filter, or application of a smooth or serrated plastic clip around the vessel.

Pulmonary embolism is a greater danger in phlebothrombosis than in thrombophlebitis, because the absence of inflammation makes clots less likely to adhere to the vein and more likely to be dislodged and to travel in the bloodstream.

SURGICAL CONDITIONS OF THE BLOOD VESSELS

It is a good rule to assume that the patient with a vascular disease has other circulatory problems. A thrombus in the leg may precede a coronary occlusion.[8] Anything that affects one blood vessel may have repercussions throughout the entire cardiovascular system, and patients should be cared for with this in mind. For example, observations of the blood pressure and of the rate and the quality of the pulse may give important clues to pathology elsewhere in the system.

Aneurysms

The middle layer, or *media,* of the walls of arteries is elastic, allowing for pulsation with every heartbeat. When the elasticity is weakened by disease or trauma, an outpouching, called an *aneurysm,* of the wall is created. The aneurysm grows progressively larger under the pressure of the blood. Some aneurysms become very large, and they exert relentless pressure on surrounding structures. Untreated, some few aneurysms lay down layer on layer of clots, but the overwhelming majority become larger and larger

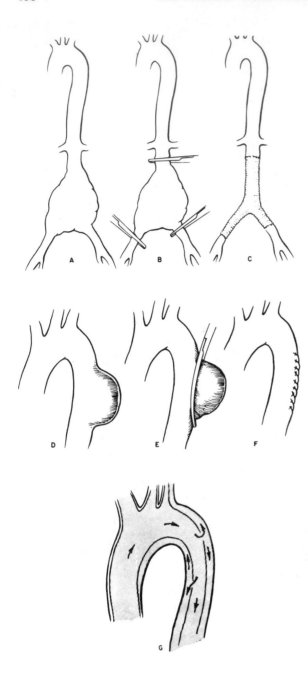

FIG. 32-5. Aneurysms. (A) A fusiform aneurysm of the abdominal aorta. (B) It is clamped off before removal. (C) Replacement with a graft. (D) Sacciform aneurysm. (E) Clamping before suturing. (F) The sutured vessel. (G) Dissecting aneurysm. In this instance blood is seeping between the layers of the vessel wall through two holes.

until they burst, and then the patient bleeds to death.

When the walls of the aneurysm contain deposits of calcium, the exact location of the outpouching can be seen on a roentgenogram. Aortography may be done.

Aneurysms may cause pain. Other symptoms may be related to pressure on nearby structures. For example, a thoracic aortic aneurysm can cause bronchial obstruction, dysphagia or dyspnea. An abdominal aortic aneurysm can produce nausea and vomiting from pressure exerted on the intestines, or it may cause back pain from pressure on the vertebrae. Sometimes it can be felt as a pulsating mass. Sometimes an aneurysm of a superficial vessel can be seen as a pulsating bulge. Sometimes aneurysms go undetected, producing no symptoms until the patient has a massive hemorrhage.

Aneurysms are treated surgically whenever it is possible; there is no other cure. Heparin is used during these procedures to control the formation of thrombi. The diseased vessel is clamped off above and below the aneurysm while surgical repair is in progress. If the heart of the aortic arch is involved, the situation may call for, or the surgeon may elect, to divert the bloodstream from the work site temporarily by the use of a heart-lung machine. Bypass also may be used when the surgery would interrupt the circulation to important organs, especially the kidneys.

Atherosclerosis

When calcified plaques of atherosclerosis ulcerate and cause thrombosis, a vessel can become completely filled, so that no blood flows through it. The discovery of the location of the site of the occlusion is aided by an arteriogram or an aortogram. The surgical treatment includes an endarterectomy, a bypass graft, a shunt, and a replacement graft.

Trauma

The surgical treatment of direct trauma to a blood vessel includes simple closure of the laceration, resection and closure, and graft replacement. A patient entering the hospital with vessel damage—for example, after he has been injured in an automobile accident, or after he has been shot—usually will have multiple injuries that will complicate both his treatment and his nursing care.

Nursing Care Following Revascularization Procedures. The preoperative and postoperative care of a patient undergoing vascular reconstructive surgery is similar to that of a patient who has heart surgery. When the surgery involves opening the thoracic cavity, preoperative and postoperative care are similar to the nursing care of any patient who has chest surgery.

The correction of an aneurysm or other reconstructive vascular procedure frequently necessitates a long incision. The abdominal aorta is reached through a midline abdominal incision, and the intestines are retracted to one side. To reach the thoracic aorta, the chest cavity must be entered. The aneurysm may not have been easily accessible, and the surgery may have been long and taxing. Consequently, expect the patient to have considerable incisional pain, which may interfere with his willingness to turn from side to side and to cough. Support the incisional area with the palm of your hand while the patient coughs. Apply an abdominal binder, when ordered, for an incision in that area.

Postoperatively, the nurse should maintain careful observation of the pulses, especially during the first 24 hours. She may be ordered to take the apical-radial pulse. She should take also the pulses distal to and fed by the vessel operated on (see Fig. 32-6). If the pulse cannot be detected, she should inform the surgeon. A thrombus may have formed. Sometimes a reflex spasm will prevent pulsation. The area where the pulse can be felt may be marked with ink preoperatively. When in doubt, another person can count the radial or precordial pulse simultaneously with the uncertain observer.

The patient is positioned flat in bed or with his head elevated, or the revascularized part may be ordered to be positioned above the level of the heart (perhaps 15°) in order to improve venous and lymphatic drainage, reduce the formation of edema, and facilitate fresh arterial blood flow.

Change the patient's position at least every two hours, and encourage him to move his legs frequently. Any pain or cramping in a leg should be reported immediately, as it may indicate the occlusion of an artery or a thrombosis in a vein.

When an abdominal aortic aneurysm has been repaired, the appearance of back pain may be serious. It may indicate a hemorrhage or a thrombosis at the graft site. Abdominal distention may be an uncomfortable complication, but

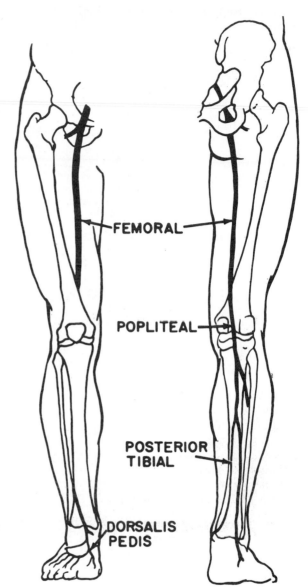

FIG. 32-6. Major arteries of the leg that can be palpated for pulsation where they come close to the surface, such as in the popliteal area and immediately below the ankle.

it is less serious. Distention may occur, because the intestines were handled during surgery. A Levin tube may be passed and attached to suction apparatus.

Patients who have had successful surgery may look forward to complete or partial relief from symptoms. The return to full activity should be scheduled according to the doctor's orders. The nursing measures for the protection of the extremity from tissue damage, including teaching the patient and family, are continued.

REFERENCES

ADAMS, J., and DE WEESE, J.: Partial interruption of the inferior vena cava with a new plastic clip, *Surg. Gynec. Obstet.* 123:1087, November, 1966.

AJEMIAN, S.: Bypass grafting for femoral artery occlusion, *Am. J. Nurs.* 67:565, March, 1967.

AMERY, A., *et al.:* Recent progress in thrombolytic therapy, *J. Clin. Path.* 22:371, May, 1969.

BEESON, P. B., and McDERMOTT, W. (eds.): *Cecil-Loeb Textbook of Medicine*, ed. 12, Philadelphia, Saunders, 1966.

BRESLAU, R.: Intensive care following vascular surgery, *Am. J. Nurs.* 68:1670, August, 1968.

CANNON, J. A.: Endarterectomy, *Am. J. Nurs.* 58:995, 1958.

CROW, T., and BRAK, M.: Aortic aneurysm: a patient study, *Nurs. Clin. N. Am.* 4:131, March, 1969.

DALE, W. A.: Ligation, stripping and excision of varicose veins, *Surgery* 67:389, February, 1970.

DALEN, J., and DEXTER, L.: Pulmonary embolism, *JAMA* 207:1505, February, 1969.

DE WEESE, M., and HUNTER, D.: A vena cava filter for the prevention of pulmonary embolism, *Arch. Surg.* 86:852, 1963.

EASTCOTT, H.: *Arterial Surgery*, Philadelphia, Lippincott, 1969.

ELIZABETH, SR. M.: Occlusion of the peripheral arteries: nursing observations and symptomatic care, *Am. J. Nurs.* 67:562, March, 1967.

FEEGAN, W. G.: Continuous compression technique of varicose vein ligation, *Lancet* 2:109, 1963.

ISRAEL, H. L., *et al.:* Fibrinolysin treatment of thromboembolism, *JAMA* 188:628, May, 1964.

KRAUSE, G. L., and VETTER, F. C.: Varicose veins, *Am. J. Nurs.* 53:70-72, 1953.

LATHAM, H. C.: Thrombophlebitis, *Am. J. Nurs.* 63:122, September, 1963.

LOFGREN, K. A.: Pitfalls in vein surgery, *JAMA* 188:17, April, 1964.

LONG, J. M.: Target: stroke. Carotid thromboendarterectomy, *Am. J. Nurs.* 66:1969, September, 1966.

McKUSICK, V. A., *et al.:* Buerger's disease: a distinct clinical and pathologic entity, *JAMA* 181:5-12, July, 1962.

MILES, R., *et al.:* A partial occluding vena caval clip for prevention of pulmonary embolism, *Am. Surg.* 30:40, 1964.

MILLER, R., and KNOX, W.: Colon ischemia following infrarenal aortic surgery, *Ann. Surg.* 163:639, April, 1966.

OSCHNER, A.: The sequelae of phlebitis, *Postgrad. Med.* 45:103, April, 1969.

POWERS, M.: Emotional aspects of cardiovascular surgery, *Cardiovasc. Nurs.* 4:7, March-April, 1968.

QUINT, J. C.: Nursing the patient with endarterectomy, *Am. J. Nurs.* 58:996-998, 1958.

RODMAN, M., and SMITH, D.: *Pharmacology and Drug Therapy in Nursing*, Philadelphia, Lippincott, 1968.

ROSE, O.: Thrombophlebitis, *Hosp. Med.* 5:6, May, 1969.

SABISTON, D., and WAGNER, H., JR.: The diagnosis of pulmonary embolism by radioisotope scanning, *Ann. Surg.* 160:575, 1964.

SASAHARA, A., and FOSTER, V.: Pulmonary embolism: recognition and treatment, *Am. J. Nurs.* 67:1634, August, 1967.

SCULLY, N.: A new look at pulmonary embolism, *Surg. Clin. N. Am.* 50:343, April, 1970.

SENSENIG, D. M., and MORSON, B.: Buerger's disease, *Am. J. Nurs.* 57:337-340, 1957.

SILVER, D., *et al.:* Management of pulmonary embolism, *Med. Clin. N. Am.* 54:361, March, 1970.

VESSEY, M., *et al.:* Investigation of relation between use of oral contraceptives and thromboembolic disease, *Brit. J. Med.* 2:199, April, 1968.

WESOLOWSKI, S. A., *et al.:* Artificial arteries, *AORN* 7:35, January, 1968.

WOOD, J. E.: Oral contraceptives, pregnancy, and the veins, *Circulation* 38:627, October, 1968.

WILSON, S.: Chronic leg ulcers. Nursing management, *Am. J. Nurs.* 67:96, January, 1967.

WINSOR, R., and HYMAN, C.: *A Primer of Peripheral Vascular Diseases*, Philadelphia, Lea, 1965.

Rehabilitation of Patients with Heart Disease

33

Functional and Therapeutic Classification • Measuring Functional Capacity and Prescribing Energy Expenditure Levels • Some Overall Points in Rehabilitation

The rehabilitation of the cardiac patient presents some particular problems and challenges. Heart disease is not an obvious disability. In some ways this aspect helps the patient to resume his previous relationships and activities; on the other hand, it may make it harder for others to recognize his limitations.

Specific, knowledgeable advice helps the patient guide himself back to health in an orderly fashion. To return to his job and recreation successfully, he and the physician, nurse, family, employer and other team members need to know what the goals are each step of the way. If the patient understands the goals, and they are his goals, and if he receives guidance in achieving them, he is likely to have a high level of motivation. When family and health team members are more certain about the plan of rehabilitation, they are less apt to advise the patient to restrict his activities unnecessarily. This lessens the tension and worry which sometimes can be far worse than the sickness and it also can help promote more positive relationships among the patient, the family, and health team.

All who care for the patient—doctors and nurses, as well as family members—must guard against the insidious temptation to protect themselves by overprotecting the patient. (It is so easy to think: "If I don't let him do anything, it won't be my fault if something happens to him.") They may have a tendency to assume total responsibility for anything that may happen to the patient, forgetting that there are many unpredictable events over which human beings have no control. For the cardiac patient, rehabilitation means evaluating how much and what kind of activity the patient's heart will allow him to do and helping him to live as fully and contentedly as possible within these limitations.

Helping the cardiac patient extend his physical independence benefits him emotionally and socially as well. The earlier physical rehabilitation is initiated, the less likely is the patient to develop satisfaction in the secondary gains of illness such as overdependence or disability income benefits.

Physical rehabilitation of the cardiac is concerned with:

• Achieving maximal physical capacity through a program of physical training and conditioning. This is especially applicable to those patients with coronary artery disease.

• Balancing the energy costs of the activities the patient will engage in with his energy capacity.

• Decreasing the energy cost of various activities so that he can negotiate the physical environment in which he functions; for example, reorganizing the cardiac homemaker's kitchen so that the facilities require a minimum of energy expenditure in reaching and using them.

FUNCTIONAL AND THERAPEUTIC CLASSIFICATION

The functional and the therapeutic classifications developed by the New York Heart Association have helped to establish a precise definition of what the patient is physically able to do (functional classification) and what he should do as part of his treatment (therapeutic classification). These two are not always the same in degree of restriction. For example, a patient with active rheumatic fever may be physically able, so far as cardiac function is concerned, to be up and about. However, to derive maximum value from treatment, it may be necessary for him to remain on bed rest to protect his heart. Such a patient might be classified IIE.

THE CLASSIFICATION OF PATIENTS WITH DISEASES OF THE HEART*

Functional Capacity

CLASS I. Patients with cardiac disease but without resulting limitation of physical activity. Ordinary physical activity does not cause undue fatigue, palpitation, dyspnea or anginal pain.

CLASS II. Patient with cardiac disease resulting in slight limitation of physical activity. They are comfortable at rest. Ordinary physical activity results in fatigue, palpitation, dyspnea or anginal pain.

CLASS III. Patients with cardiac disease resulting in marked limitation of physical activity. They are comfortable at rest. Less than ordinary activity causes fatigue, palpitation, dyspnea or anginal pain.

CLASS IV. Patients with cardiac disease resulting in inability to carry on any physical activity without discomfort. Symptoms of cardiac insufficiency or of the anginal syndrome are present even at rest. If any physical activity is undertaken, discomfort is increased.

Therapeutic Classification

CLASS A. Patients with a cardiac disease whose ordinary physical activity need not be restricted.

CLASS B. Patients with cardiac disease whose ordinary physical activity need not be restricted, but who should be advised against severe or competitive physical efforts.

CLASS C. Patients with cardiac disease whose ordinary physical activity should be moderately restricted, and whose more strenuous efforts should be discontinued.

CLASS D. Patients with cardiac disease whose ordinary physical activity should be markedly restricted.

---

* This classification was developed by the New York Heart Association and is used here with permission.

CLASS E. Patients with cardiac disease who should be at complete rest, confined to bed or chair.

MEASURING FUNCTIONAL CAPACITY AND PRESCRIBING ENERGY EXPENDITURE LEVELS

The physician employs one or more of the following methods, depending on available resources, to arrive at a work prescription which is both beneficial and safe.

• The patient's own account of how much and what type of activity he can perform without experiencing symptoms, and what kinds of activity are associated with discomfort, such as dyspnea, palpitation or chest pain, serves as a helpful guide to the physician.

• Standardized tests, giving the patient a definite amount of exercise and evaluating his response, also are used. The Master "2-step" exercise test is an example. (The test involves a specified number of trips up and down 2 steps, each 9 inches high, within a definite time interval.)

This test requires approximately 8.5 calories per minute, which is higher than almost all kinds of work except the extremely heavy. The pulse and blood pressure response of the patient, as well as the ECG, can allow the physician to estimate what the heart might do under actual job conditions.

• More sophisticated equipment, such as the treadmill or ergometer (an apparatus such as a bicycle equipped for measuring the amount of work done by a human or animal subject) may be used to obtain a more exact appraisal of the patient's response to various exercise loads. Because of the potential for cardiac emergencies to occur if the patient is inadvertently overstressed, each cardiac evaluation unit should be equipped with a "crash cart" containing cardiac emergency drugs and equipment.

• An actual trial work situation often is used to determine how well the worker can tolerate a certain type of activity. Knowing this is of great value, because the ability to perform a certain task comfortably depends on many factors other than sheer physical exertion. Some of these factors are:

Temperature
Humidity
O_2 content of air
Toxic exposures

Rate of work
Skill and coordination
Self confidence
Rest periods—length and environment
Shift changes (biologic rhythms)
Anxiety over type of work, quality of work,
    effects of work on self and others
Interpersonal relations with supervisors and
    co-workers
Physical condition
Food habits
Smoking

Recently it has become possible to monitor a person's electrocardiogram throughout his daily activities by use of a portable, magnetic tape recorder. Electrodes are placed on the chest and connected to a recorder contained in a small bag carried over the shoulder or attached to the belt. The patient carries out his usual daily functions and keeps a diary of his activities and his subjective response to them. The physician replays the ECG tape and notes the effects of various activities such as work, recreation, sexual intercourse, or emotional stress on heart rate, rhythm, and metabolism as denoted in any ST-T wave ischemic changes. A special rapid scanning device enables the physician to review an entire 10-hour ECG record in 10 minutes and to stop it when necessary to study irregularities.

Another type of physiologic monitoring is through a biotelemetry system. This is being used more and more frequently as the patient increases his physical activity in the hospital. The patient goes through his usual activities with chest electrodes connected to a small radio transmitter attached to his belt. This sends his ECG to a radio receiver not more than 1,500 feet away. The physician or nurse views the transmitted radio signal (ECG) directly on an oscilloscope screen, or it can be printed on standard ECG equipment for study at a later time.

• By using the functional classification of heart disease along with the energy expenditure of common activities expressed in calories per minute, the doctor can initiate a progressive energy-expenditure prescription for the patient. The final plan would depend on a real or simulated work trial.

For example, from a physical rehabilitative standpoint the patient with a myocardial infarction who has an uncomplicated course of healing may have the following level of energy expenditure:

• In the coronary care unit (1 to 3 days), from 1 gradually up to 2 calories per minute.

• During remainder of hospital stay (about 2 weeks), up to 3 calories per minute.

• During convalescence at home (8 to 12 weeks) up to 4 to 5 calories per minute.

• After recovery (12 weeks), dependent upon the functional classification of the patient (see Table 33-1).

• After 12 weeks and indefinitely, a program of graded activities under medical supervision merged into a regimen of physical conditioning that becomes a lifetime program of regular exercise as strenuous as the patient is able to perform with safety. According to the functional classification of the patient, energy expenditure would be prescribed for

Class I patients—eventually from 6.6 to 11–12 calories per minute or higher.

Class II patients—eventually from 4 to 6–7 calories per minute.

Class III patients—possibly only a slight increase, up to 3–3.5 calories per minute.

Class IV patients—probably no practical physical rehabilitation possible.

When the level of permitted energy expenditure is established, the patient can be assisted by the doctor, nurse and other team members to live within his limits by using a table of approximate energy requirements of common activities. Examples of the energy requirements of common activities are given below. More complete charts can be obtained from the local chapters of the American Heart Association.

• Cardiac Work Evaluation Units have been set up in various parts of the country to evaluate the capacity of cardiac patients for employment. Patients are referred to these units by their own doctors or by their employers. Often, the staff consists of a physician, nurse, and technician. Evaluation and consultation services are available on a part- or full-time basis with other team members such as a psychologist, psychiatrist, social worker or vocational counselor. Each state in the United States has a Rehabilitation Commission which can provide such specialized services. These units help to educate patients, doctors and employers concerning the employment of patients with heart disease, as well as to evaluate workers' capacity for specific kinds of jobs.

For example, three to four months after myocardial infarction a patient is tested at increasing workloads. If the electrocardiogram being taken reveals no abnormal response, the level is believed to be safe. The goal is to raise the pulse rate high enough to gain a stressful enough response to help strengthen the myocardium. This will vary according to age, with younger people able to attain higher rates. If there is ECG evidence of ST segment depression or arrhythmia, the effort is considered to be too much and activities of lower output are used.

Exercise tests are not done on patients with congestive heart failure, impending myocardial infarction, angina at rest (angina decubitus), uncompensated arrhythmias, general disability, or on patients within three months after myocardial infarction.

The fact that maximum heart rate declines with age is very important. This is often overlooked by potential cardiacs who self-prescribe their physical conditioning program (such as jogging) without benefit of a physical examination and stress ECG. (See Table 33-1.)

From the data made available through a Cardiac Work Evaluation Unit, the physician can plan a more strenuous rehabilitative exercise program. Gradually the level of activity can be raised as the heart improves its efficiency. Most physicians believe that a 30 to 40 minute workout to a prescribed pulse rate level three times a week is required to maintain fitness. The supervised workout includes calisthenics followed by games or other activities such as cycling, swimming, walking, or jogging. Once the person learns how to manage his prescription, he can substitute other activities such as gardening, cycling, running, or just continue walking, which is probably the one best, most practical activity. Patients are encouraged to walk stairs rather than ride elevators and to walk a number of blocks rather than park their cars immediately adjacent to their place of work. The eventual goal is to be as physically active as possible.

Some Overall Points in Rehabilitation

For many cardiacs, especially those men with atherosclerotic coronary artery disease, the concept of cardiac rehabilitation—returning to as near normal as possible—may well mean doing more physically after a "heart attack" than before. Lack of regular physical exercise could have been one of the major factors leading to the illness. Exercise is of extreme importance in reconditioning the heart muscle. Its efficiency improves just as any other muscle which is made

to work harder. Exercise is prescribed on a regular basis with gradually increasing loads. The danger is to move ahead too rapidly with the possibility of overload. Thus, specific graded programs are essential for safety.

Though patients with compensated congestive failure and those following cardiac surgery require rehabilitation, the vast majority of patients today requiring conditioning programs are those with coronary artery insufficiency or myocardial infarction. In addition to a prescribed physical conditioning program, the patient is strongly urged to cease smoking since smoking results in increased catecholamine secretion (epinephrine and norepinephrine) which causes the myocardium to use more oxygen. Many studies have indicated that smoking is associated with increased pulse rate and some deviation of blood pressure.

Avoiding or correcting obesity is important, since overweight can increase strain on an already damaged heart. Diets that limit calories often are prescribed. Restrictions in sodium and cholesterol are frequently necessary. The nurse can work with the dietitian in teaching the patient the rationale of the diet, as well as helping him to plan appetizing menus that conform to the diet prescription.

Rehabilitation also involves learning how to minimize emotional tension, or if the kind of assistance needed for the patient to learn this is lacking, then it may be necessary for him to avoid certain stress situations. Emotional tension leads to catecholamine excretion, which is oxygen wasting and can result in serious cardiac arrhythmias.

The same principles are used in the rehabilitation of the cardiac homemaker. After an assessment of functional capacity, and the energy costs of various household activities are learned

TABLE 33-1. RELATIONSHIP OF PULSE TO DEGREE OF WORK*

AGE	100% (CAPACITY)	50% (HEAVY)	30% (MODERATE)	10% (LIGHT)
20 Yrs.	198	130	102	70
30 Yrs.	188	125	98	70
40 Yrs.	180	120	96	70
50 Yrs.	170	116	92	70
60 Yrs.	160	110	90	70
70 Yrs.	152	108	86	70

* Derived from Communications from the Testing and Observation Institute of the Danish National Association for Infantile Paralysis, Hellerup, Denmark, 1959.

from the charts, a matching of "cost" and "capacity" can be carried out. The patient and doctor decide what activities are most essential in the light of the patient's welfare and that of her family. The nurse can assist by evaluating methods used in an activity and helping the patient to adopt methods that will produce a satisfactory result with a minimum of strain and fatigue.

Although housework is important, it is not the only consideration in the rehabilitation of the cardiac homemaker. The strains of pregnancy, childbirth and child rearing may present special problems for the woman with heart disease. Social activities and jobs outside the home have to be considered, too.

On the other hand, doing various household tasks can actually help in rehabilitation. Housework can be viewed as a form of exercise and doing routine things may serve as a tension reliever. Most housework is not too heavy in terms of caloric expenditure and the problem is lessened if labor-saving devices such as a clothes washer and a dryer are available. The American Heart Association has several pamphlets depicting energy costs of household activities and methods of conserving energy expenditures. Advice regarding community resources for homemaker services for the cardiac is also available.

A summary of the experience of individuals engaged in the placement of cardiac patients indicates that between 70 and 75 per cent of cardiac patients can return to their former employment; that the emotional impact of cardiac disease is as important or even more important than the disease itself in roughly one-half of the patients; and that the absentee rates of cardiac patients who return to their former jobs are significantly lower than the general absentee rate of the company (Feldman).

The need for a broader viewpoint in relation to the employment of cardiacs has been highlighted by the more widespread use of careful physical examinations, x-ray examinations and even electrocardiograms before employment. Many persons who have slight cardiac abnormalities and few, if any, symptoms are being discovered. This is a good trend, since treatment can be initiated in the early stages of heart disease, with the possibility of preventing serious illness. However, this trend could work a hardship for some people, if employment is denied or discontinued without considering the worker's capabilities.

The person with heart disease who lives and works within the limits of his capacity is usually healthier and happier than is the person who gives up his accustomed pursuits. Idleness is no guarantee of long life, and in fact, may hasten the person's death.

Nursing Implications

Nurses in many fields of practice can assist in the cardiac's rehabilitation program throughout all its phases by doing the following:

● Watching for danger signals accompanying increased activity such as anginal pain, palpitation, dyspnea, dizziness, undue fatigue, arrhythmias, inordinate rise in pulse rate or prolongation of its return to its resting level at the end of a period of activity. Discussing these with the doctor before the patient repeats the activity is necessary.

● Listening to the patient as he talks about his illness—what led up to it, what the acute illness means to him, and what he thinks about the future. Helping the patient to establish realistic goals and to assess his strengths and assets as well as his losses and liabilities can assist him in a realistic way to make the most of what he has.

● Using a positive though realistic approach to the patient. For example, when asking the hospitalized patient to move his legs and feet, emphasize the need to maintain the muscles in good condition since these will have to carry him when he starts to walk again, rather than placing emphasis on the prevention of venous thrombosis and emboli.

● Working with the vocational counselor, psychologist, physicians, nurses and other team members in various settings so that the best program for the individual cardiac patient can be achieved.

● Being aware of the facilities available in the community for vocational evaluation, job retraining, and placement, such as the State Rehabilitation Commission.

● Recognizing that the patient is the driving force for his own rehabilitation. The team makes his potential evident and provides encouragement and continued support.

REFERENCES AND BIBLIOGRAPHY

BISSONNETTE, G.: The rehabilitation of the employee with heart disease: a challenging responsibility of the occupational health nurse, *Am. Ass. Indus. Nurs. J.* 14:6, June, 1966.
BUGG, R.: They're mending hearts with exercise, *Today's Health*, 45:50, October, 1967.

CAIN, H. D. *et al.*: Graded activity program for safe return to self-care after myocardial infarction, *JAMA* 177:11, July, 1961.

The coronary spectrum. Part II: Rehabilitation, *J. Rehab.* 32:48, March-April, 1966.

FELDMAN, D.: Rehabilitation of the cardiac patient, *Mod. Treatm.* 5:93, September, 1968.

FISHER, S.: The coronary spectrum: the cardiac homemaker, *J. Rehab.* 32:74, March-April, 1966.

FRASHER, W., *et al.*: Office procedures as aids to work prescription for cardiac patients (I) (II), *Mod. Conc. Cardiovasc. Dis.* 32:769, 32:776, January and February, 1963.

GRIFFITH, G.: Home care of the aged cardiac patient, *Geriatrics* 22:140, June, 1967.

GIBSON, T. C., *et al.*: Community nursing visits to patients with cardiovascular disease, *Am. J. Public Health* 57:1004, June, 1967.

HALL, L., and ALFANO, G.: Incapacitation or rehabilitation, *Am. J. Nurs.* 64:7-20, November, 1964.

HELLERSTEIN, H.: Exercise therapy in coronary disease, *Bull. N.Y. Acad. Med.* 44:1028, August, 1968.

———: Sexual activity and the post-coronary patient, *Med. Aspects Human Sexuality*, 3:70, March, 1969.

KOHN, R. M.: Physical reconditioning after myocardial infarction, *N.Y. Med. J.* 70:516, 1970.

LEMBRIGHT, K.: The coronary spectrum: role of the occupational health nurse, *J. Rehab.* 32:81, March-April, 1966.

REMBERG, J.: Motivating people to stop smoking, *Nurs. Clin. N. Am.* 4:385, June, 1969.

SIEGEL, W.: Prescription for middle-aged sedentary men: exercise, *Circulation* 41:19, 1970.

WRIGHT, B.: *Physical Disability: A Psychological Approach*, New York, Harper, 1960.

ZOHMAN, M. D., and TOBIAS, J. S.: *Cardiac Rehabilitation*, New York, Grune, 1969.

Introduction, Diagnostic Tests, Functional Disorders

34

Diagnostic Tests • Gastrointestinal Decompression • Functional
Disorders: Interaction of the Psychological and the Physical

INTRODUCTION

Patients with disorders of gastrointestinal
functions have a wide variety of health problems. The commonalities among these patients'
conditions involve disturbances in ingesting,
digesting, and absorbing nutrients, and eliminating waste products from the gastrointestinal
tract.

The patient's condition may be caused predominantly by emotional factors, or by physical
factors. There are many patients with gastrointestinal disturbances whose conditions cannot
be neatly classified as emotional or physical in
origin; their illnesses seem to have origins both
in psychological and physiologic malfunction,
with each of these spheres constantly interacting
with the other.

The functions of eating and eliminating are
important in the emotional development of the
child, and in his relationship with his parents.
Food is usually associated with love, as the infant
nurses, and as the child receives from his parents
the food he needs and enjoys. Toilet training
comes as a restraint or curbing of the young
child's impulse to defecate when his rectum is
full, regardless of time and place. Learning to
control defecation is necessary for the child in
order to please his parents. Later, of course, it
becomes a social expectation when the youngster
leaves home to attend school and to play. The
emotional significance of eating and eliminating
does not cease when an individual has matured
physically. Instead, these functions remain areas
of emotional expression and gratification, as well
as necessary physiologic functions. Disturbance
of these functions, from whatever cause, has important psychologic as well as physiologic repercussions. The patient who has a colostomy (opening of his colon onto the abdomen, for expulsion
of feces) typically experiences considerable anxiety over the fecal soiling which occurs postoperatively, since one firm expectation adults
have of themselves (and which others have of
them) is ability to control bowel movements.

When working with patients with gastrointestinal disturbances it is especially necessary to be
sensitive to patients' emotional responses, as well
as to their physiologic reactions. Both aspects
require the nurse's expert care and observation.
No matter how concretely "physical" the condition, remember that it has an emotional component; no matter how obvious an association there
is between emotional disturbance and physical
symptoms, remember that the patient's physical
symptoms require care and relief. The patient
who has a peptic ulcer needs his Gelusil on time,
as well as your concerned "listening ear."

Another area of concern in care of patients
with gastrointestinal problems is nutrition. The
patient's nutrition may be affected only slightly,
or so severely that he is in danger of death.
Inadequate intake of foods (as in patients with
cancer of the esophagus and anorexia nervosa),
and problems in absorption of nutrients (as in
patients with ulcerative colitis) can result in
severe emaciation. A great deal of effort is necessary to provide necessary nutrients in whatever

form the patient can tolerate them. Observation of what nutrients the patient actually receives is essential.

Accurate observation of stool is also important. A tarry stool indicates bleeding into the intestinal tract, as may occur when the patient has a peptic ulcer. Bright red blood mixed with stool is indicative of bleeding near the rectum, as can occur from hemorrhoids. Consistency of the stool, whether hard, formed, very soft, or liquid, is important, as is the color. The normal brown color may be replaced with a greyish color (the so-called "clay-colored stool") in various conditions affecting the liver and gallbladder.

Knowledge of normal physiology and microbiology is essential in making judgments about how to proceed with nursing care.

Normally, the digestive tract contains many microorganisms. The food and the fluids that we ingest are not sterile; the feces are laden with bacteria. This consideration is important when caring for patients with gastrointestinal dis-

orders, because it is the rationale for using clean rather than sterile technic in certain nursing procedures. Nevertheless, the equipment for the procedures that do not require aseptic technic must be meticulously clean. Clean technic is not merely a careless way of using asepsis; it is a way of performing a procedure with a recognition of the characteristics of the part of the body that is being treated.

Normally, the walls of the digestive organs prevent the gastric and the intestinal contents from escaping outside the lumen of the digestive tract. Since this material contains many microorganisms, any perforation that allows material to seep out of the digestive tract is a serious event, because it will cause severe infection of surrounding tissues—particularly of the *peritoneum,* the sac that lines the abdominal cavity.

DIAGNOSTIC TESTS

The diagnostic tests commonly used in disorders of the gastrointestinal tract include the col-

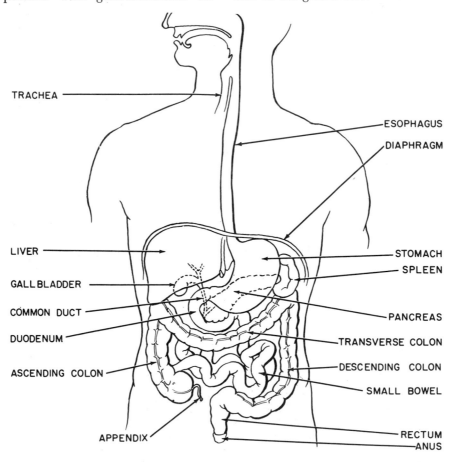

FIG. 34-1. Diagram of the gastrointestinal tract.

lection of specimens, such as feces and gastric contents, endoscopy, and x-ray studies.

Gastric Analysis

Specimens of gastric contents may be collected from vomitus or, more commonly, by passing a nasogastric tube and aspirating the stomach contents with a syringe.

Gastric analysis is useful to the physician in determining the:

1. Ability of the patient to secret hydrochloric acid.

2. Level of secretory activity in a patient with a peptic ulcer.

3. Possible presence of the Zollinger-Ellison syndrome in an ulcer patient. (This is a syndrome in which a pancreatic tumor produces a gastrin-like hormone that causes the stomach to secrete astronomical quantities of acid juice. The usual medical and surgical treatment of peptic ulcer fails and the patient requires a total gastrectomy.)

4. Completeness of vagotomy.

5. Effectiveness of therapy on secretory activity. Gastric analysis is of no value in the routine diagnosis of duodenal or gastric ulcer. It is of some value in conjunction with other tests in attempting to determine if a gastric ulcer is benign or malignant.

Food and fluids are withheld eight hours before the test is done. Usually, the patient is instructed to take nothing by mouth after midnight, and the test is performed early the next morning. A nasogastric tube is passed, and specimens of gastric secretion are obtained by attaching a syringe with an adapter to the end of the tube and drawing back on the plunger. The number of specimens and the intervals at which they are withdrawn vary in different hospitals and with different doctors. Each specimen is placed in a separate bottle. The time the specimen is taken and the number of the specimens in the series are indicated on the label. (The first specimen is marked #1, the second #2, and so on.) The end of the tube is kept clamped between the withdrawal of specimens to prevent air from entering the stomach. The tube is taped to the patient's face.

There are two methods used at the present for gastric analysis: (1) The basal secretion method whereby specimens are collected for four 15-minute periods, and (2) the stimulated secretion method using histamine 0.04 mg./Kg. preceded by intramuscular antihistamine to minimize un-desirable cardiovascular effects or using betazole hydrochloride (Histalog) 1.5 mg./Kg. or 100 mg. empirically. (One action of histamine is to stimulate gastric secretion.) This is called the Maximal Histamine Test. The insulin (Hollander) test is another stimulated secretion test used to determine the completeness of a vagotomy in inhibiting acid output of the stomach. A dose of 0.2 unit of regular insulin/Kg. is given intravenously and the acid output after insulin is compared with the preceding basal secretion.

Always check with the doctor to make sure that the part of the test requiring histamine is to be carried out. The use of histamine is not without danger, because some patients are sensitive to it. A sudden fall in blood pressure, weakness, pallor, sweating, rapid, weak pulse, and the clouding or the loss of consciousness are indications of shock after the use of histamine. Emergency treatment of the shock includes the prompt administration of epinephrine. A fleeting sensation of warmth and a flushing of the skin commonly occur and are no cause for alarm.

The three most important points to remember in relation to the use of histamine during gastric analysis are:

1. The drug never is given routinely; it is to be used only when specifically requested by the doctor.

2. Whereas it is harmless to most people, histamine occasionally causes serious reactions. The patient should be carefully observed after an injection of histamine.

3. Epinephrine should be available for immediate use; the availability of this drug should be checked before the histamine is given.

Some doctors specifically order a dose of epinephrine (0.3 to 0.5 ml. of a 1:1,000 solution is commonly used) to be given subcutaneously by the nurse in case a reaction occurs. The doctor is notified promptly of the patient's condition, and of the fact that epinephrine has been given.

When the required number of specimens has been obtained, the nasogastric tube is withdrawn, mouth care is given, and, as soon as the patient feels hungry, breakfast is served.

Gastric analysis sometimes is performed without passing a nasogastric tube. A dye called azuresin (Diagnex Blue) is administered orally. When it is acted on by hydrochloric acid, the dye gives the urine a blue color. This change in the color of the urine indicates the presence of hydrochloric acid in the gastric juice.

Stool Specimens

Stool specimens often are examined for occult blood (blood not visible to the naked eye), for fat, for intestinal parasites and eggs, and for various pathogens, such as the typhoid bacillus. Usually, only a small piece of stool is needed. A tongue blade is used to place it in a disposable waxed container. Then it is labeled and sent to the laboratory. If the stool is being examined for occult blood, the patient is permitted to eat no red meat for 24 hours before the specimen is taken. The guaiac or the benzidine test commonly is used to detect occult blood. If the stool is to be examined for parasites, it should be taken to the laboratory while it is warm and fresh, so that the motion of the parasites can be seen through a microscope.

Whether or not stool specimens are specifically ordered, it is important to save a sample of any fecal material that is unusual in appearance. For example, streaks of blood or large amounts of mucus may be noted. Sometimes, the nurse is the first to observe worms in the stool. When you are in doubt, it is best to save the specimen. If the material is not found to be significant, or if the doctor already has observed it, no harm has been done, whereas discarding it may mean the loss of a valuable clue to the patient's diagnosis.

Sometimes, it is necessary to give an enema in order to obtain a stool specimen. The solution ordered is normal saline or tap water, so that no other substance, such as soap, will be mixed with the stool.

Roentgenography and Fluoroscopy

The use of roentgenograms and fluoroscopy is very valuable in diagnosis, because they permit the visualization of the entire gastrointestinal tract. For example, tumors and ulcers may be noted by x-ray examination. The area to be examined should be as empty as possible, so that the contrast medium can outline clearly the entire area that is being studied. Barium sulfate is the contrast medium (radiopaque substance) used most often.

X-ray studies of the upper gastrointestinal tract often are called a "G.I. series." The patient swallows barium, and fluoroscopic and x-ray studies are made. The speed with which the barium passes through the tract and the appearance of the organs themselves are noted. Normally, the barium that the patient has swallowed leaves the stomach within six hours. Additional x-ray films often are taken six hours after the ingestion of barium to note whether any barium still remains in the stomach.

A major discomfort caused by this test is hunger. The patient fasts after midnight, omits breakfast, and often has a late lunch. Always check with the x-ray department to find out whether the series has been completed before giving the patient anything to eat. Sometimes, he must return to the department for additional films. When the series has been completed, see that the patient promptly receives an appetizing meal. If lunch is delayed, cold foods should be kept in the refrigerator and hot ones reheated before the tray is served.

The taste of the barium is chalky and unpleasant. Some hospitals have barium that is flavored to make it more palatable. The series of x-ray examinations is quite tiring, especially for weak and aged patients. Besides fasting, they must assume various positions on the x-ray table while the series of films is being taken. Many of the patients return quite exhausted, and once they have eaten, they enjoy an opportunity for uninterrupted rest.

Roentgenography and fluoroscopy of the large intestine are carried out after barium has been introduced into the bowel by means of an enema. The procedure usually is referred to as a barium enema. The barium is administered in the x-ray department. The patient is asked to retain the barium while the films are taken. He then expels the barium, and additional films are taken. Air is instilled rectally as additional contrast when polyps are suspected.

A laxative and enemas are given by the nurse prior to the x-ray examination to cleanse the bowel of feces. The number of enemas, the type of solution, the times specified for their administration and the type of laxative vary in different hospitals. Sometimes two or three enemas are given. In some institutions one commercially prepared enema, such as a Fleet, is given, and it is considered adequate preparation.

Whenever barium is introduced into the gastrointestinal tract, provision must be made for its prompt elimination. Often, a cathartic is ordered after a G.I. series. Retained barium can become a hard mass that could cause an intestinal obstruction or an impaction in the anus or rectum. Always note, after barium has been used, whether the barium has been passed, and whether the patient is having regular bowel movements.

Endoscopy

Endoscopy refers to the examination of certain organs through a hollow instrument passed through one of the body openings. The doctor looks through the lumen of the instrument and, aided by the electric light attached to the instrument, he is able to inspect the organ into which the scope has been passed. A significant advance in recent years has been the development of flexible endoscopes made of fiberglass. These are more readily and comfortably passed than the former rigid instruments. They also have the unique advantage of providing color photographs of the areas visualized. Flexible esophagoscopes and gastroscopes are now in use in many hospitals and an experimental sigmoidoscope has been receiving clinical trials. It can be passed almost twice the distance of the rigid scope and will probably be of significant help in early diagnosis of carcinoma of the colon. Biopsies also may be performed through the lumen of the instrument. The following endoscopic procedures frequently are used in examination of the gastrointestinal tract:

- Esophagoscopy—visualization of the esophagus
- Gastroscopy—visualization of the stomach
- Sigmoidoscopy—visualization of the sigmoid, the rectum and the anus
- Proctoscopy—visualization of the rectum and the anus
- Anoscopy—visualization of the anus

The instruments are named according to the procedure for which they are used. The doctor inspects all areas through which the scope passes, which is the reason that sigmoidoscopy includes examination of the anus and the rectum, as well as the sigmoid. The area of the gastrointestinal tract being examined must be as empty as possible to permit effective visualization of the tissues.

Helping with Endoscopy. Passing a scope into any body cavity is uncomfortable, and sometimes it is quite painful. Usually, it causes apprehension, and tenseness and fear tend to increase the discomfort of the examination. Not only are these reactions distressing to the patient, but they make it more difficult for the doctor to complete the examination quickly and successfully. After the doctor has discussed the need for the examination with the patient, the nurse can help to allay the patient's fears by explaining further what will be required of the patient.

ESOPHAGOSCOPY AND GASTROSCOPY. Nothing is given by mouth eight hours prior to esophagoscopy and gastroscopy, so that the visualization of the organs will not be obscured by the presence of food, and so that the patient will not regurgitate as the gastroscope is being passed down his esophagus. Usually, this procedure is carried out in the operating room, and the preparation of the patient is similar to that of any patient going to the operating room. For example:

- Morning care is completed before the patient leaves the ward.
- Dentures, jewelry and hairpins are removed.
- Patients usually wear turbans; hospital clothing is worn. Since the examination entails only the upper part of the body, patients are permitted to wear both shirts and trousers.
- The patient is given the opportunity to void just before going to the operating room, so that he will not be uncomfortable or embarrassed by this need during the procedure.
- The patient signs written permission for the examination.
- Sedation is given, as ordered by the doctor. A barbiturate, such as phenobarbital, and Demerol often are ordered approximately one hour before the patient leaves the ward.

Usually, sedatives are sufficient for adults. Occasionally, if the patient is very apprehensive and unable to hold still, general anesthesia may be required.

When the patient returns to the ward, he is permitted nothing by mouth until his gag reflex returns. The return of this reflex, which may take three or four hours, can be tested by touching the back of the patient's throat with a tongue blade. Usually, the patient is very tired and needs an opportunity to rest. Note any expectoration or vomiting of blood, since this may indicate injury to the esophagus. However, the expectoration of a small amount of blood-tinged mucus is not unusual. When the local anesthesia wears off, the patient's throat will feel sore. Assure him that this soreness will disappear gradually over a period of several days. Any severe pain should be reported to the doctor.

SIGMOIDOSCOPY, PROCTOSCOPY and ANOSCOPY. Usually these are performed in the ward treatment room, the clinic or the doctor's office. Enemas are given, as ordered by the doctor, before the examination is carried out, since the presence of feces in the lower bowel prevents adequate visualization during the examination. If the

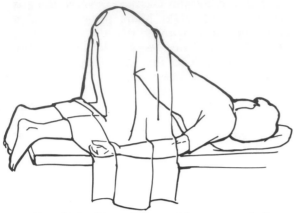

Fig. 34-2. Knee-chest position assumed for proctoscopy. Note that the patient is resting on her chest (not on her elbows) and her knees. Her feet are over the edge of the table, and her thighs are at right angles to the table. Because many people find the knee-chest position embarrassing, the nurse should be especially careful to drape the patient so that only the anus is exposed.

enemas are not effective, or if all the solution is not expelled, the doctor always should be notified before the examination is begun. Disposable, commercially prepared enemas now are used often in cleansing the lower bowel. Sometimes, the patient is instructed to limit his supper on the evening before the test to foods low in residue; for example, raw fruits and vegetables and whole-grain cereals would be excluded. Usually, the patient is permitted a light breakfast on the morning of the examination.

Of course, explanation prior to the test and support during it are indicated.

The patient is placed in the knee-chest position on the treatment table, and he is draped with a fenestrated sheet. It is helpful to show the patient how to assume this position before the test is begun, since the position is awkward, and some patients make the mistake of resting on their elbows instead of the chest (see Fig. 34-2). Some doctors prefer that the patient lie on his left side with the head of the table elevated approximately 15°; the thighs are flexed on the abdomen, and the legs are extended. As the scope is advanced, the patient is asked to extend his thighs and legs to an almost straight position. It has been claimed that this position facilitates visualization of the rectum and low sigmoid and is more comfortable for the patient.

The doctor first performs a digital examination of the anus and the rectum, using rubber gloves and a lubricant. The scope is then lubricated and inserted. To facilitate the examination with the lighted instrument, the lights are turned off, and the shades are drawn. While the sigmoidoscope is in place, the doctor uses long, cotton-tipped swabs to remove any particles of feces or mucus that may interfere with visualization. The swabs are passed through the scope and discarded immediately after use in a waste container. Also, a suction tip may be inserted through the scope to remove fluid. A suction machine should be available.

The details concerning the preparation of the equipment vary in different hospitals. For example, the doctor may bring his own equipment with him, or it may belong to the hospital. In the latter case, the nurse is responsible for preparing the equipment ahead of time. The scope should be plugged in to make sure that the light goes on. Plenty of cotton swabs should be available, as well as biopsy forceps and a container for any tissue removed for biopsy. A wastebasket lined with a paper bag is needed for discarding soiled swabs.

The nurse's role in these tests involves the following preparative and supportive measures:

- Preparation of the patient—giving the enemas, explaining the procedure, and showing him how to assume the knee-chest position
- Positioning and draping the patient for the test; observing and encouraging him during it
- Preparing the equipment and assisting the doctor (for example, turning the lights on and off, handing him swabs)
- Cleansing the anal region after the test is completed, and assisting the patient back to bed
- Caring for used equipment; discarding waste, sending specimens to the laboratory, as ordered

GASTROINTESTINAL DECOMPRESSION

Gastrointestinal decompression refers to emptying or draining the contents of the stomach or the intestines. A tube is passed through the nose and down the esophagus to the stomach. If intestinal decompression is necessary, a special tube is used that is longer and has a device facilitating its passage along the intestinal tract.

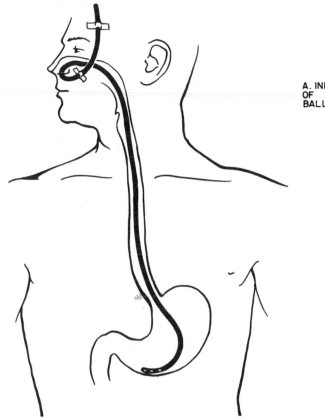

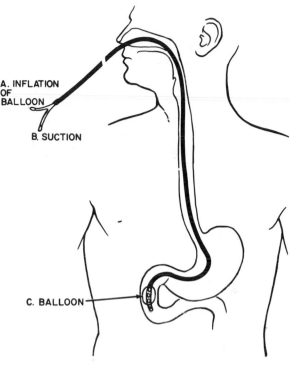

FIG. 34-3. A Levin tube in place. The Levin tube is used to aspirate gastric contents or to convey liquids to the stomach.

FIG. 34-4. A Miller-Abbott tube in place. It is advanced through the intestines to the prescribed point. The Miller-Abbott tube has a double lumen. (A) Portion of the metal tip leading to the balloon. (B) Portion of the metal tip leading to the lumen that can be suctioned. (C) Balloon inflated with air.

The contents of the gastrointestinal tract are withdrawn by suction. Because the suction usually must be continued for extended periods, a mechanical device is used that can be adjusted to provide continuously the amount of suction specified by the doctor. An electric device, such as the Gomco suction machine, often is used. Suction also may be provided by devices that create a vacuum by allowing fluid to flow from one reservoir to another. The Wangensteen suction apparatus is an example. Wall suction outlets also are used. If the withdrawal of the gastric contents is to be carried out over a brief period, as is the case when specimens are being obtained for diagnostic purposes, the suction is applied by attaching a syringe to the end of the tube and drawing back on the plunger.

The indications for gastrointestinal decompression will be discussed throughout this unit. Some of the more common of these may be summarized as follows:

- Withdrawal of specimens of gastric contents for diagnostic purposes
- Prevention and treatment of postoperative distention, particularly after surgery on the gastrointestinal tract
- Removal of accumulated contents of the gastrointestinal tract when there is obstruction in the tract
- Emptying the stomach before emergency surgery or after the swallowing of poisons

Kinds of Tubes

Because gastrointestinal decompression often is continued for several days, you may be assigned to care for patients receiving this treatment without having assisted with or observed the passing of the tube.

The type of tube most commonly used is the *nasogastric tube,* often referred to as a *Levin tube.* This is a rubber or plastic tube that has holes or "eyes" in several locations near its tip

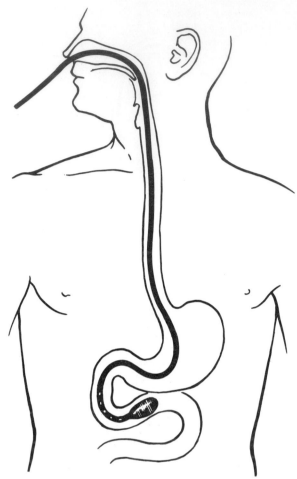

FIG. 34-5. A Cantor tube in place. This intestinal tube ends in a bag that is filled with mercury to help it to pass along the gastrointestinal tract to the point prescribed by the physician. Intestinal tubes are not taped in place until they have advanced fully. The holes for suctioning are behind the balloon.

to permit the withdrawal of the stomach contents.

The Miller-Abbott and the Cantor tubes are used often for intestinal decompression. They are longer than the nasogastric tube, and they contain devices that facilitate the passage of the tube along the intestinal tract.

The *Miller-Abbott tube* has a double lumen (a tube within a tube). One tube connects with a rubber balloon at the tip. The other connects with the eyes, or holes, near the tip of the tube. When the tube has passed through the pylorus, the balloon is inflated with air, and then pro-

pelled along the intestinal tract by peristalsis, carrying the rest of the tube with it. The intestinal contents are sucked back through the holes.

Because the Miller-Abbott tube has two lumina, each with a separate opening, it is very important to differentiate them. The end of the tube that remains outside the patient's body has a metal adapter on it. The adapter has two openings—one for suction (it is marked "suction") and the other leading to the balloon. The latter is used by the doctor for inflating the balloon with air. Labeling this opening will help everyone to remember its purpose and to understand that it never should be connected to suction or have irrigating solutions instilled into it. Some nurses place tape on this part of the adapter and write on it, "Don't use" or "Doctor only."

The *Cantor tube* has just one lumen and a bag on the end, into which mercury is inserted. The weight of the mercury helps to propel the tube along the intestinal tract. The mercury is injected directly into the bag with a needle and syringe before the patient is intubated. The mercury remains in the bag because the needle does not make an opening that is large enough to permit the escape of the mercury. The bag is elongated when the tube is inserted, so that it can be passed more easily and with less discomfort to the patient. Since the Cantor tube has only one lumen, there is only one opening at the end outside the patient's body, and therefore no confusion can result concerning which opening to use for suction and which for irrigation.

Nursing Care

Positioning the Patient. After the doctor has inserted a tube for intestinal decompression, he follows its course through the tract by x-ray films and fluoroscopy. The doctor orders that the patient be placed in various positions to facilitate the passage of the tube through the pylorus and into the intestine. For example, he may request that the patient be placed in Trendelenburg's position on his right side, and then on his back in Fowler's position, and then on his left side with the bed flat. After the tube has passed through the pylorus, the doctor may recommend that the patient walk about at his bedside to increase peristalsis and to help to pass the tube along the intestinal tract. The specific time intervals and the desired positions are ordered by the doctor in accordance with his observations of the position of the tube by x-ray and fluoroscopic examinations.

The intestinal tube never is taped to the patient's face or pinned to his bedding while it is being advanced through the intestinal tract, because these fastenings would prevent the tube from being carried along the tract. The extra length of tubing is left coiled on the bed. When the tube has reached the desired location in the intestinal tract (for example, when it has passed to the point just above an obstruction), it then may be taped to the face.

Sometimes, the doctor asks the nurse to advance the tube through the patient's nose a specified distance (perhaps 3 inches) at stated times. If the peristalsis is not adequate to propel the tube, a condition that occurs in paralytic ileus, the weight of the mercury on the end of the Cantor tube helps it to pass through the intestines by gravity.

Giving Support to the Patient. Gastrointestinal intubation is done so often that to the nurse it may seem commonplace. However, some patients describe the technic as the most upsetting and uncomfortable aspect of their entire hospital experience. The mere thought of swallowing a rubber tube is repugnant to most people. Intestinal tubes that have a balloon on the end are especially uncomfortable to swallow. While the tube is in place, the patient constantly is aware of a foreign body that partially obstructs his nose and makes his nostril and his throat feel irritated and sore. Most patients treated by intubation are permitted nothing by mouth. This restriction, plus the mouth breathing to which the patient often resorts, make his mouth feel parched.

You can minimize the patient's discomfort in many ways. Before preparing the equipment, make certain that the patient understands what is to be done. Most patients respond much better if they know what to expect, and what is expected of them. The instruction should be carried out ahead of time. Merely repeating, "Swallow, now swallow," insistently while the tube is being passed is not adequate. The patient may become so tense that he is unable to swallow the tube, and he gags and vomits.

When the doctor arrives, the patient usually is placed in a sitting position. Screening him is very important in preventing embarrassment, since some gagging and expectoration are likely to occur. A large towel or plastic apron should be used to protect the gown and the bedding, and plenty of tissues should be available for wiping the nose and the mouth. An emesis basin should be kept in readiness. Instruct the patient to relax as much as possible and to swallow when the doctor asks him to. Usually, the patient is allowed to have a few sips of water by mouth while the tube is being passed. Swallowing the water while the tube is being passed helps it to go down more easily. Try to stand and move in such a way that the patient does not feel overpowered or that something is being forced on him. Two people standing very close to the patient and passing a tube through his nose sometimes can make the patient feel like a trapped and helpless victim rather than a responsible adult who knows what is expected and tries, with the physical and emotional support of his doctor and his nurse, to do it.

Care of the Tube. Once the tube is in place, the patient usually relaxes somewhat. Taping the tubing to his face helps to support the tube and makes its presence less uncomfortable for the patient. (Remember, though, not to tape intestinal tubes until they have advanced to the desired point.) The tubing also can be supported by placing tape around it and pinning the tape to the sheet. The pin never should be placed around the tubing itself, since it might compress it and interfere with drainage. The tubing should be long enough to allow the patient to turn and to move about in bed. At first he may lie quite motionless, because he is afraid that any movement may dislodge the tube. With your help he soon will find that he can turn and move. Of course, he will need to be careful not to lie on the tubing or to kink it.

Mouth Care. Careful, frequent mouth care greatly lessens the patient's discomfort. This care helps so much to relieve the parched, dry feeling and to get rid of unpleasant tastes and odors that the mouth-care equipment should be kept within easy reach in the patient's unit. The availability of the equipment makes it easier (and therefore more likely) for busy staff members to give this care. If the patient is able, he may rinse his mouth frequently with mouthwash, if this is kept handy. Cream applied to the lips and the edge of the nostril helps to prevent dryness and cracking. A small amount of lubricant, such as K-Y jelly, can be applied to the tube where it emerges from the nose, to prevent crusts of dried secretions from forming. Such crusts are very irritating to the nostril.

Suction; Irrigation; Records. After the tube is in place and attached to the desired amount of suction, it is your responsibility to make certain that the suction is continued. The tube is attached to suction by a glass adapter. Develop the habit of noting whether fluids are being drawn out of the patient's gastrointestinal tract by watching them flow through the adapter to the drainage bottle. Also, drainage dripping into the collection bottle can be noted. If the suction does not seem to be operating satisfactorily, check the equipment for proper functioning. If there still is no suction, the doctor should be notified. Distention caused by failure of the suction can have very serious consequences; for example, it may cause strain on the suture line in postoperative patients. Vigilance in noting the suction is especially important during the night, when fewer personnel are observing the patient.

Often, the doctor orders irrigations of the tube to keep it patent. Before you irrigate the tube, find out:

- Whether the doctor has ordered the irrigations. They are not done routinely.
- How much solution is to be used, and how often the irrigation is to be done
- What solution is to be used
- Whether the procedure requires clean or aseptic technic

Great harm can be done by improper irrigations. Injecting too much solution can cause distention, with strain on sutures. Normal saline, 30 ml., frequently is ordered. The solution is injected with an Asepto syringe, or with a syringe that has been fitted with an adapter, so that it can be inserted tightly into the tube. After the fluid has been injected, it is aspirated with the syringe. The amount returned, as well as the amount injected, should be noted. The irrigating solution that is not aspirated will be suctioned later into the drainage bottle. The amount of irrigating solution that is not removed immediately should be noted on a slip of paper at the patient's bedside. At the end of the day this amount is totaled and then subtracted from the total amount of fluid in the drainage bottle.

Aseptic technic usually is advised for surgical patients during the immediate postoperative period. If the patient has not had surgery, clean technic usually is considered acceptable, because the fluid is entering an area that is not normally sterile.

The large quantities of fluids and electrolytes lost during gastrointestinal decompression must be replaced parenterally. The doctor relies on all nursing personnel to keep an accurate record of intake and output, so that the patient's needs

for parenteral fluids can be accurately determined. The total amount of fluids administered, as well as the amount of urine output and the amount of drainage obtained by decompression, are recorded every 24 hours. The type of drainage should be noted and recorded, and specimens of any unusual drainage should be saved for the doctor to see. For example, the drainage might be described as "greenish-yellow fluid containing shreds of mucus" or as "dark, brownish red and granular, resembling coffee grounds." The drainage bottle must be washed thoroughly each time that it is emptied.

Withdrawing the Tube. When the decompression is terminated, the tube is withdrawn gently. The nasogastric tube can be withdrawn quickly. However, the intestinal tubes are removed gradually, several inches at a time. Some resistance to the removal of the tube usually is felt, and it should never be forced. When the end of the tube reaches the pharynx, the balloon or the bag of mercury is removed through the patient's mouth. The remainder of the tube then is withdrawn through the nose.

Usually, a great deal of mucus is secreted, due to the irritation caused by the tube. Be sure that tissues are handy, so that the patient can blow his nose and expectorate. Mouth care is given after the tube has been removed. Soreness of the throat may persist for several days, but it grows steadily better once the tube has been removed.

FUNCTIONAL DISORDERS: INTERACTION OF THE PSYCHOLOGICAL AND THE PHYSICAL

The functioning of the gastrointestinal tract is affected greatly by the autonomic nervous system, which in turn is affected by the patient's emotions. For instance, it has been demonstrated that frustration and repressed anger are associated with hyperemia and with increased secretion and motility of the stomach. A variety of social, psychological and physiologic factors cause the gastrointestinal tract to be a common area for functional disturbances. These disturbances can cause distressing symptoms, and yet they may not be accompanied by permanent pathologic changes in the affected organs.

Almost everyone at one time or another has experienced some of these functional disorders. Commonplace are an attack of indigestion before an examination, a sudden loss of appetite before an important date, constipation or diarrhea during the first day or two at a new job. Usually these disorders disappear promptly when the tension and the anxiety are relieved. Some people are chronically anxious, or they become involved in situations that make excessive demands on their emotional resources, and the symptoms continue unabated. These individuals need a doctor's help in differentiating the condition from organic disease, in providing symptomatic relief, and in helping them to cope with their tensions.

Nausea and Vomiting

Nausea and Anorexia. These are common problems, and if they continue long enough, they may cause weakness, weight loss and nutritional deficiency. Vomiting, particularly of breakfast, may occur.

Anorexia nervosa is a severe disorder in which the patient has an aversion to food. The condition is most often found in women, and usually it has its onset during young adulthood. It is believed that anorexia nervosa is related to profound emotional problems, and that it may be associated with difficulties in assuming the adult role. Emaciation often is extreme, and it is accompanied by a variety of symptoms, such as nausea, abdominal pain and amenorrhea. The treatment of anorexia nervosa includes psychotherapy and painstaking help in restoring normal nutrition. Treatment often takes many years, and it is not always successful.

Here are some suggestions for working with patients who have functional anorexia, nausea or vomiting:

• Help the patient to avoid emotional upsets at mealtime. Make a special effort to avoid scheduling any painful or upsetting procedures at this time.

• Avoid focusing constant attention on how much the patient eats. Observe unobtrusively what he eats, so that you can keep the doctor informed, and yet avoid making the patient feel that someone is counting every mouthful.

• If the situation permits, arrange for the patient to eat with others who are up and about, perhaps by setting a table in the solarium.

• Avoid blaming the patient for not eating. When he is having particular difficulty with meals, make a special effort to spend time with him, and let him express some of his feelings.

• Work with the dietition in seeing that the patient has the kind of foods that tempt his ap-

petite, and that they are served attractively and in very small portions.

• If you know that a particular food or meal may be especially difficult for the patient (for example, a patient who has difficulty swallowing, and who is trying to eat solid food for the first time in days), remain nearby, so that the patient knows you are ready to help if he needs it.

• Avoid suggesting to the patient that any particular kind of food makes him sick. In most cases it is not the food, but the patient's reaction to it that is causing the difficulty.

Heartburn and Belching. These are also common. Regurgitation of gastric contents into the esophagus causes a burning sensation. It may follow eating too large a meal or emotional stress. The patient often is advised to eat smaller meals and to avoid hurry and worry. Some doctors recommend antacids, such as aluminum hydroxide gel or sodium bicarbonate, for symptomatic relief. Some people swallow large gulps of air when they become frightened or upset. Belching of this air from the stomach follows. Nervous tension may cause excess gas to accumulate in the large bowel, causing pain, distention and flatulence. If the patient who swallows air is made aware of what he is doing, often this awareness helps him to avoid the habit.

Overeating. Just as some people lose their appetites when they are under emotional stress, others overeat.

Some people who feel nervous and jittery find that eating helps them to relax, and they often eat too much. Others by overeating may strive to make up for the lack of certain pleasures and satisfactions. Of course, some people overeat from habit. Huge servings and frequent snacks may be customary in the family, and all its members may betray this custom by the size of their waistlines.

All too often, obese patients alternate between stringent, nutritionally inadequate reducing diets and overeating. One of the most difficult therapeutic problems is helping the patient to learn to eat only as much as his body requires and to realize that this type of diet will need to be followed for years rather than days.

Diarrhea and Constipation

Diarrhea and constipation often are related to emotional stress. Although one individual may respond characteristically with one or the other of these symptoms, the same patient may alternately have diarrhea and constipation. The terms "diarrhea" and "constipation" may be used rather loosely by the patient, and it is important to have him describe just what he means by these terms. Diarrhea to one patient may mean having two or three formed stools daily, whereas another may use the term to describe six to eight liquid bowel movements per day.

Individuals differ greatly in their bowel habits. Just as some women menstruate only three days a month, and others five or six, some people normally move their bowels every other day, whereas others have two or three movements a day. Differences in diet play a part, too. The ingestion of large quantities of fresh fruits and vegetables causes more stool. The terms "diarrhea" and "constipation," when they are used by doctors, are used to describe these symptoms:

Diarrhea—loose, watery stools, usually occurring frequently

Constipation—hard, dry stools, usually occurring infrequently

The material that moves down the large intestine is composed of food residues, microorganisms, digestive juices and mucus, which is secreted in the large intestine and aids in moving the feces toward the anus. Water normally is absorbed from the stool while it is in the colon. When the feces are propelled unusually rapidly through the tract, less water is absorbed, and the stool is softer or even liquid. When the feces are retained in the sigmoid because of spasm, or in the rectum because of inattention to the defecation reflex, too much water is absorbed, and the stool is hard and dry. In differentiating normal from abnormal function, the consistency of stools usually is considered to be more reliable than their frequency.

Constipation sometimes results from emotional stress or from poor diet or bowel habits. Frequently, the patient is not actually constipated; he just defecates less frequently than he believes is normal. Too much emphasis on the importance of moving the bowels once daily can lead the patient to develop dependence on laxatives. Instead of a normal movement every other day, he may induce a very loose stool with a cathartic, which is followed the next day by no bowel movement, leading the patient to take another dose of cathartic. These patients need to be assured that a daily evacuation is not necessary, provided that the stool is not very hard and dry, and that avoiding laxatives will allow the bowels to function normally again.

The major emphasis is placed on helping the patient to maintain habits that foster normal elimination. Eating plenty of raw fruits and vegetables and whole grain bread and cereal, a high fluid intake, and regular rest and exercise are important. Allowing sufficient time for evacuation at a definite time each day is also very helpful in restoring normal function. The program of therapy is designed to help the patient to return to normal patterns of elimination with the least possible use of enemas and cathartics.

Irritable Colon. This is one of the most common functional disorders of the gastrointestinal tract. It may also be called mucous colitis or spastic colitis. The patient has hypermotility of the large intestine, leading to diarrhea, cramps, and, if the condition continues for long, weight loss and dehydration. The stools are watery and may contain large amounts of mucus. Attacks may be mild and occur very infrequently in response to some unusual stress, or the condition may recur so frequently that the patient has few if any periods of normal bowel function. Sometimes, sudden, severe flatulence, accompanied by a feeling of churning and unrest in the abdomen, warns that an attack is starting. Some patients who have the condition are troubled alternately by constipation and diarrhea. Cathartics often further irritate the bowel and make the symptoms worse.

Treatment includes measures for symptomatic relief, as well as helping the patient gradually to recognize the relationship between the symptoms and the emotional states that precipitate them.

Many differences exist among doctors concerning the type of diet that these patients should eat. Some restrict milk; others encourage it. Some advise the patient not to restrict his diet in any way, in the belief that he gradually will be able to tolerate all foods, and that the symptoms are not significantly affected by the type of food eaten.

Preparations, such as Kaopectate (kaolin and pectin) or bismuth and paregoric, sometimes are given for symptomatic relief. Antispasmodics, such as tincture of belladonna, sedatives and tranquilizers, sometimes are prescribed.

In working with a patient who has irritable colon try to:

• Avoid occupying a great deal of the patient's time and attention with counting and describing his bowel movements. Sometimes overemphasis on detailed reporting by the patient can make him concentrate too narrowly on his elimination.

- Encourage the patient to establish one regular time for bowel movement (such as after breakfast) and to keep busy and to divert his attention from moving his bowels at other times.
- Encourage the patient to sit down after meals or during the morning rather than to do prolonged standing or walking. Since symptoms are most likely to appear at these times, being more quiet may help to relieve the symptoms.
- Encourage the patient to follow the diet recommended by his doctor.

Importance of Medical Treatment

Patients who have functional disorders of the gastrointestinal tract should seek medical advice and not decide themselves that the condition is due to fatigue or "nerves." The symptom may indicate serious disease, such as cancer, and only the doctor can carry out the necessary examinations in differentiating minor functional disturbances from early signs of organic disease.

REFERENCES AND BIBLIOGRAPHY

BEESON, P. B., and McDERMOTT, W. (eds.): *Cecil-Loeb Textbook of Medicine*, ed. 12, Philadelphia, Saunders, 1967.

DAVIS, L.: *Christopher's Textbook of Surgery*, ed. 9, Philadelphia, Saunders, 1968.

DELEU, J., and TYTGAT, H.: Diarrhea associated with pancreatic islet cell tumors, *Am. J. Dig. Dis.* 9:97, 1964.

DRUMMOND, E. E., and ANDERSON, M. L.: Gastrointestinal suction, *Am. J. Nurs.* 63:109, December, 1963.

DUNBAR, F.: *Emotions and Bodily Changes*, ed. 4, New York, Columbia University Press, 1954.

EISENBERG, S., *et al.*: Proctosigmoidoscopy, *Am. J. Nurs.* 65:113, January, 1965.

ELLISON, E. H.: Zollinger-Ellison syndrome, *Ann. Surg.* 160:512, 1964.

FUERST, E. V., and WOLFF, L.: *Fundamentals of Nursing*, ed. 4, Philadelphia, Lippincott, 1969.

HALLENBECK, G. A.: The Zollinger-Ellison syndrome, *Gastroenterology* 54:426, 1968.

HOROWICZ, CLARA: Profiles in OPD nursing: a rectal and colon service, *Am. J. Nurs.* 71:114, January, 1971.

LEVINE, M. E.: *Introduction to Clinical Nursing*, Philadelphia, Davis, 1969.

NODINE, J. H., and MOYER, J. H.: *Psychosomatic Medicine*, Philadelphia, Lea, 1962.

ROBINSON, C.: *Proudfit-Robinson's Normal and Therapeutic Nutrition*, ed. 13, New York, Macmillan, 1967.

RODMAN, M. J., and SMITH, D. W.: *Pharmacology and Drug Therapy in Nursing*, Philadelphia, Lippincott, 1968.

ROVELSTAD, R. A.: Gastric analysis, *Gastroenterology*, 45:90, 1963.

SPARBERG, M., and KIRSNER, J. B.: Gastric secretory activity with reference to HCl. Clinical interpretations, *Arch. Int. Med.* 114:508, 1964.

The relationship between acid output of the stomach following maximal histamine stimulation and the parietal cell mass, *Clin. Sci.* 19:147, 1960.

WAHL, C. W. (ed.): *New Dimensions in Psychosomatic Medicine*, Boston, Little, Brown, 1964.

WILLIAMS, LESTER F.: An acute abdomen, *Am. J. Nurs.* 71:299, February, 1971.

WOLF, S., and WOLFF, H. G.: *Human Gastric Function*, London, Oxford University Press, 1947.

The Patient with Ulcerative Colitis or a Peptic Ulcer

35

Ulcerative Colitis • Peptic Ulcer

ULCERATIVE COLITIS

The term *ulcerative colitis* refers to inflammation and ulceration of the colon. The mucosa of the colon becomes hyperemic, thickened and edematous. The ulceration is sometimes so extensive that large areas of the colon are denuded of mucosa.

Etiology. The cause is obscure. Many who have studied this disease comment that the illness seems more prevalent in those who have certain kinds of emotional problems. Patients who develop the disease are sometimes described as being inwardly hostile and yet outwardly submissive and as having strong needs for dependence. Patients with this disease often exhibit a hopeless, helpless attitude. It has been suggested that an altered blood supply to the mucosa of the colon may occur in response to emotional influences and eventually lead to ulceration of the mucosa. Others point out that functional disorders, such as attacks of diarrhea when a patient is frightened, rarely progress to ulcerative colitis, and that emotional factors may have little to do with the disease. Usually, no pathogenic organisms or parasites can be demonstrated. The possibility that symptoms are caused by infection seems slight, although it has been suggested that organisms are present that cannot be demonstrated. Some physicians believe that ulcerative colitis is a disease of multiple causative factors, which may include infection, allergy, auto-immunity and emotional stress. The term *idiopathic* (no known cause) often is used to describe ulcerative colitis.

Incidence. Ulcerative colitis is most common during young adulthood and middle life, but it can occur at any age. Both men and women are affected.

Symptoms. The condition may have an abrupt or a gradual onset. The patient experiences severe diarrhea (12 to 20 bowel movements per day), and he expels blood and mucus along with fecal matter. Weight loss, fever, severe electrolyte imbalance and dehydration, anemia and cachexia may follow. Often diarrhea is accompanied by cramps, and the patient may experience anorexia, nausea and vomiting, as well as extreme weakness. The urge to defecate may come so suddenly and with such urgency that the patient is incontinent of feces. Some patients have particular problems with incontinence while they are asleep; they are unaware that defecation has taken place until they awaken.

The condition may continue in fairly mild form for years, or it may run a rapid, fulminating course and cause death from hemorrhage, peritonitis or profound debility. Some patients have sudden, dramatic recoveries. They may remain free of the disease for years or have a recurrence of the illness.

Diagnosis. In addition to the history and the physical examination, the doctor uses x-ray examination, proctoscopy, sigmoidoscopy, and examination of the stool in diagnosing the disease. A careful search is made for other conditions that could be responsible for the symptoms, such as cancer, amebic dysentery, or diverticulitis. The nurse assists with diagnosis by preparing the patient for roentgenograms of the lower gastrointestinal tract, proctoscopy and sigmoidoscopy and by giving the doctor any necessary assistance. Cathartics are contraindicated in the preparation of colitis patients for a barium enema when the disease is at all acute. If the diagnosis can be made by sigmoidoscope, the physician may postpone the barium enema until the more acute phase is passed. Even then he may elect to have the patient on a liquid diet for a few days before, and give some gentle tap water enemas the morning of the x-ray examination.

Treatment

Medical treatment is supportive, and it is designed to provide rest for the bowel, opportunity for healing, and correction of anemia and malnutrition. About three-fourths of patients can be managed medically and helped into remission. The remainder usually come to a total colectomy and permanent ileostomy when medical treatment fails or an acute complication occurs such as perforation or severe hemorrhage.

Diet and Supplements. The patient usually is given a bland diet. Any substances that might further irritate the bowel, such as raw fruits and vegetables or highly seasoned foods, usually are eliminated. The patient is encouraged to eat as nourishing a diet as is possible. Protein foods, such as meat and eggs, are important. Often, small, frequent meals are necessary, because the patient feels too ill to eat large meals. The quantity and the type of food that the patient eats are carefully noted, as are the fluid intake and output and the number and the character of bowel movements. Some physicians advocate greater flexibility in the diet prescription for the patient who is not acutely ill, advising restriction only of those foods which the patient finds cause an increase of symptoms. The rationale behind this approach to diet therapy is that at present there is no clear evidence that certain categories of food make the condition worse.

Transfusions and iron are given to correct anemia. Parenteral fluids and electrolytes may be needed. Because the patient's diet often lacks essential nutrients, such as vitamin C, found in raw fruits and vegetables, and because the disease itself may interfere with absorption of nutrients, supplementary vitamins often are given.

Rest in bed is important during the acute phases of the illness; it is continued until the severe symptoms subside, and the patient begins to gain weight and to feel stronger. The prevention of pressure sores is important, particularly if the patient is very thin.

Drugs. A variety of drugs may be given. Although they do not cure the disease, they may lessen the symptoms and promote healing of the diseased bowel.

Sedatives and tranquilizers often help the patient to relax and to rest. Drugs that slow peristalsis, such as atropine or tincture of belladonna, or drugs used to coat and to soothe the mucosa, such as kaolin and pectin, may be ordered. Antispasmodics must be given with great caution as they may be precipitating factors in producing toxic megacolon—a marked dilatation of the colon sometimes leading to perforation and death. Any rather sudden onset of abdominal distention in a patient with acute ulcerative colitis is an ominous sign and should be reported at once.

ACTH and cortisone may be given when the disease does not respond to other measures. A dramatic relief of symptoms often follows their use. In the acutely ill patient with severe diarrhea, fever and abdominal pain, these steroids are often given intravenously for a few days until the patient can take them orally. To maintain a remission, the patient may remain on the drug for weeks or months in as low a dose as possible. The use of these potent drugs is not without hazard. The symptoms of peritonitis may be masked, and the patient may develop other undesirable reactions to the drug, such as moon face and edema. Although they are potentially dangerous, corticosteroids have helped many patients with this disease, as well as other diseases for which no certain cure is available, to live longer and more comfortably, and they have helped some to recover who otherwise might have succumbed to the disease. They have probably played a major role in reducing the operative mortality of elective colectomy by providing a better risk patient who is not as debilitated by his disease as those of the presteroid era. If a patient does not realize the drug's toxicity, he may not understand why he should not take a larger dose than the physician has prescribed, because the drug usually imparts a feeling of well-being. The patient should have ample opportunity to discuss his therapy with his physician. Because corticosteroids are not curative, they should be viewed as one aspect of treatment rather than as a replacement for other types of therapy.

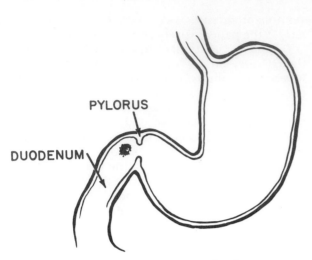

FIG. 35-1. A peptic ulcer in the duodenum.

Antibiotics, especially nonabsorbable sulfonamides, penicillin or streptomycin may be given. Antibiotics are particularly apt to be used in preparing the patient for surgery in order to decrease the number of bacteria in the bowel and thus to lessen the possibility of infection as a complication of surgery on the bowel.

Psychotherapy is often helpful when it is largely of a supportive nature. It is harmful to the patient when he is acutely ill for any deep probing to be done. Very gradually and gently, as his symptoms improve, the patient may be helped to recognize some of the emotional problems that seem related to his illness. The understanding and the aid of the family are important, but members of the family will require a great deal of assistance from physician and nurse in understanding the patient's illness and their role in helping him.

Surgery is sometimes necessary when the disease does not respond to other treatment, or when complications occur. For example, perforation of the colon is an acute, surgical emergency, because it promptly leads to peritonitis. The surgical treatment of severe, intractable ulcerative colitis usually includes total colectomy (removal of the entire colon and rectum) and a permanent ileostomy (opening of the ileum onto the abdomen for the passage of fecal matter). Many patients adjust well, once the diseased colon has been removed. Others have considerable difficulty in adjusting to the ileostomy. The fecal matter is very liquid because it does not go through the colon where water normally

is absorbed, and it is discharged immediately from the ileum.

Nursing Care

The care of patients with ulcerative colitis is a challenge to the most skillful nurse. Supportive care, both physical and emotional, can do a great deal to lessen symptoms and to assist the patient in overcoming the disease.

Any illness that is associated with fecal incontinence is physically and emotionally distressing to the patient. Our culture emphasizes cleanliness in habits of elimination. The importance of not soiling oneself is stressed from earliest childhood, and finding that he has soiled his bedding or his clothing can cause the patient a profound sense of shame and embarrassment.

Help the patient to minimize soiling by keeping a clean bedpan within easy reach, so that it is available if he needs it in a hurry. Assist him to clean himself and to wash his hands after using the bedpan. This care is important, not only for aesthetic reasons, but also because the skin around the rectum easily becomes excoriated. Applying petrolatum after the area has been cleansed helps to prevent irritation of the skin. If incontinence cannot be controlled (for example, if the patient defecates while he is sleeping), the use of perineal pads and disposable bed pads under the buttocks helps to control the extent of soiling and makes it easier to cleanse the patient.

When the patient is allowed up and about, he may at first need the extra protection and assurance provided by wearing a disposable pad; otherwise, he may be so afraid of having an accident that he refuses to go more than a few yards away from his bathroom.

Helping the patient to maintain an adequate dietary and fluid intake is essential. Serve small portions of food that the patient enjoys in an environment that is clean and odor free. His appetite often improves when his morale does.

Some patients with ulcerative colitis appear to be both emotionally and physically ill. They may show this state by being excessively dependent on the nurse, by seeming apathetic, or by constantly criticizing whatever is done for them. The patient may become extremely frightened by symptoms that seem commonplace to the nurse. It is important to realize that emotional problems do not rule out physical illness. The patient has a serious, possibly a fatal illness that may or may not be related to emotional disturbances.

The period of acute illness is not the time to expect the patient to conquer his emotional problems—even those that seem extreme, or those that present difficulties in relationships with the staff. Later, when the patient has improved physically, the combined efforts of the doctor, the nurse and the family may help the patient to deal more effectively with his emotional problems. Sometimes the physician refers the patient to a psychiatrist for treatment.

PEPTIC ULCER

Physiology. The opening between the stomach and the esophagus is called the *cardiac orifice;* that between the stomach and the duodenum is called the *pyloric orifice.* Both these openings are controlled by sphincters which, when contracted, close the orifice. When the sphincters relax, the orifice opens, permitting the contents to flow to the next organ.

The stomach stores food and prepares it by mechanical and chemical action to pass in semiliquid form into the small intestine. Gastric juice containing digestive enzymes is secreted continuously. However, the amount of secretion is increased when food is eaten. Gastric juice is acid due to the presence of hydrochloric acid. The contractions of the stomach mix the food with the gastric juice and carry the mixture of semi-liquid food and digestive juice to the small intestine. The stomach becomes empty after an ordinary meal in about 5 to 7 hours. The length of time required depends on the amount and the composition of the food eaten. For example, fats tend to delay stomach emptying.

The small intestine is divided into three portions: the *duodenum,* the *jejunum* and the *ileum.* The duodenum is the first region, extending from the pylorus to the jejunum. The greatest amount of digestion and absorption of nutrients takes place in the small intestine.

A peptic ulcer is a circumscribed loss of tissue in an area of the gastrointestinal tract that is in contact with hydrochloric acid and pepsin. Most peptic ulcers occur in the duodenum (duodenal ulcers). However, they may occur at the lower end of the esophagus, the stomach (gastric ulcer), or in the jejunum after the patient has had an anastomosis between the stomach and the jejunum.

Etiology. The immediate cause of peptic ulcer is the digestive action of acid gastric juice and pepsin on the mucosa. The underlying cause, which would explain why some people develop the lesion and others do not, is unclear.

Incidence. Peptic ulcer is a common disease among adults. Much has been written about the relationship of peptic ulcer to the stress and the strain of modern life, and it is sometimes assumed that peptic ulcer occurs chiefly in executives, salesmen, and others who do competitive work in an industrial society. Actually, peptic ulcer occurs widely throughout the world, in all societies, ranging from the primitive to the highly industrialized. Bedouins who live a nomadic desert life develop peptic ulcer, and in our own country the condition exists among all social and all economic groups. Men are affected more frequently than women. The highest incidence occurs during middle life, but the condition can occur at any age.

Symptoms. The symptoms are due largely to the irritation of the ulcer by hydrochloric acid. Pain, which may be described as "burning" or "gnawing," occurs in the epigastric region. The pain has a definite relationship to eating. It usually occurs one to several hours after meals, and it is often relieved by the ingestion of protein foods, such as milk. Sometimes the pain is accompanied by nausea, and the patient may find that vomiting relieves the pain. Patients who are severe hypersecretors of acid may experience night pain disturbing their sleep and back pain indicating pancreatic irritation by the ulcer. About 20 per cent of patients may have bleeding as the first sign of their ulcer, and hematemesis and/or melena. Protracted vomiting secondary to scarring and resultant obstruction is also seen as the first symptom in patients who have ignored their "indigestion."

Diagnosis. The diagnosis is usually suggested by the history with confirmation in the majority of patients by the G.I. series. In some patients the x-ray studies are not helpful and a trial of therapy may help make a presumptive diagnosis. Duodenal ulcers are always benign, but gastric ulcers may either be benign or malignant. It is in the differentiation between benign and malignant ulcer that the combined use of roentgenography, gastric analysis, gastric washing for cytologic examination and gastroscopy comes into play. Even if all these parameters indicate benignity, a trial of therapy in the hospital must be the next step. Failure to show significant healing by x-ray examination and gastroscopy after three weeks is usually reason to operate for suspicion of malignancy as is the occurrence of healing and then recurrence of the ulcer a few months after therapy.

Medical Treatment and Nursing Care

Medical treatment of peptic ulcer is designed to provide the optimum conditions for healing the lesion. The neutralization of acid, so that it does not further irritate the ulcer, and the reduction of hypermotility and secretion are objectives of therapy.

Neutralizing the Acid. Protein foods, which combine with acid, and alkalis are both useful in neutralizing acid. Frequent small feedings of such foods as milk, milk and cream, custard, and eggs are given. Cream is mixed with milk, because the fat in cream is digested more slowly, thus delaying the emptying of the stomach. Cream is used sparingly, if at all, for patients in whom consumption of generous amounts of fat is contraindicated, such as in arteriosclerosis or obesity. Such patients often are given plain whole milk instead of milk and cream.

During acute illness a common regimen is to alternate a glass of half milk and half cream with hourly doses of a liquid antacid for about 24 hours.

As the patient's condition improves, soft foods, such as jello, custard, and soft cooked egg, are added to his diet. Hourly feedings of milk and cream may be continued, and in addition the patient gradually becomes able to tolerate six small meals daily. Substances that might irritate the ulcer, cause excess secretion of acid, or be hard to digest or gas-forming usually are eliminated. The patient usually is not allowed any raw fruit and vegetables, highly seasoned foods, fried foods, meat broths or gravies, coffee, or alcoholic beverages. Smoking is usually prohibited, because it appears to irritate the ulcer. Diluted fruit juices often are permitted. The usual procedure is to give the small meals between 7 A.M. and 7 P.M. and to discontinue feedings during the night, to allow the patient to rest. If the patient has pain during the night, medications and hourly milk and cream may be continued during the night.

Hourly milk and cream feedings are discontinued when the patient's condition permits. Sometimes, he is able to return rather promptly to three or four meals daily, while he continues to eliminate irritating or hard-to-digest foods, or foods that cause increased gastric secretion. Some patients better tolerate smaller and more fre-

quent meals; these patients continue with a six-feeding schedule for several months or longer. Supplementary vitamins may be added. Constipation may be a problem, due to the lack of roughage in the diet, and gentle laxatives, such as Dulcolax suppositories, may be needed.

Some physicians now recommend a more liberal dietary regimen in the treatment of peptic ulcer. They advise the patient to eliminate foods that he has found cause him distress. Emphasis is placed on more flexibility in the type of foods that the patient is permitted and on encouraging him to return to a normal diet as soon as he can tolerate it. The rationale underlying the more liberal approach to diet is that there is no conclusive evidence that certain foods, such as coarse-grained cereals, either lead to the development of peptic ulcers or retard their healing.

Antacids are given to neutralize hydrochloric acid. Aluminum hydroxide gel (Amphojel) may be given orally, 5 to 30 ml. at intervals of 1 to 4 hours. A combination of magnesium trisilicate and aluminum hydroxide gel (Gelusil) is another commonly used antacid. At intervals of 1 to 4 hours 4 to 8 ml. are given. Maalox, a combination of aluminum hydroxide gel and magnesium hydroxide, is given in doses of 8 ml. Each of these antacids should be given mixed with a small amount of milk or water, or milk or water should be swallowed after the medication. These preparations are not absorbed from the gastrointestinal tract, and therefore they do not produce alkalosis even when they are given in large doses. Although sodium bicarbonate neutralizes acid, it is readily absorbed from the gastrointestinal tract, and may, if it is given in large doses, produce alkalosis.

Reduction of Hypermotility and Secretion. Antispasmodics, such as tincture of belladonna and atropine, often are given to decrease gastric motility and acid secretion. Tincture of belladonna is given in doses of 0.6 ml. (10 drops); atropine, in doses of 0.4 to 0.6 mg. The side-reactions include dryness of the mouth, dilation of the pupils, blurring of the vision, and difficulty in voiding. Banthine (methantheline) and Pro-Banthine (propantheline) are newer preparations with effects similar to those of atropine and belladonna. The side-effects also are similar, but they may not be as marked. Banthine is given in tablets of 50 mg., and Pro-Banthine in tablets of 15 mg., several times daily.

These drugs are given usually 30 minutes before meals to suppress the increased acid secretion that follows food ingestion; they are usually administered also at bedtime. In patients with partial obstruction these drugs are contraindicated since they further decrease the motility of an atonic stomach and add to the obstructive symptoms.

Rest and relaxation are of prime importance in the treatment of peptic ulcer. In the absence of complications this aspect of treatment may not necessarily entail rest in bed. In most instances the patient may be permitted to use the bathroom and to relax in a chair as he reads or watches television. Sedatives may be prescribed to promote rest.

The long-term management of peptic ulcer includes avoiding fatigue and stress, and sometimes it involves maintaining a diet in which substances that might cause irritation and excess secretion of hydrochloric acid are eliminated. Patients are advised to avoid smoking, to avoid drinking alcoholic beverages, coffee and tea, and to take medications as they are ordered. Peptic ulcer tends to recur, and each recurrence brings the possibility of complications.

Surgical Treatment and Nursing Care

Peptic-ulcer patients who do not respond to medical treatment, who have frequent recurrences, or who develop complications may require surgery. Various surgical procedures are used in the treatment of peptic ulcer, depending on the location of the ulcer and the degree and the location of the deformity that the ulcer may have caused.

Subtotal Gastrectomy; Gastroenterostomy; Vagotomy. Subtotal gastrectomy with gastroenterostomy is an operation in which the lower one-half to two-thirds of the stomach is removed, and the remaining portion of the stomach is joined to the jejunum. The surgical joining (anastomosis) of the stomach and the small bowel is called *gastroenterostomy*. The operation removes the ulcer and the portion of the stomach that stimulates the secretion of acid; the food passes directly from the upper portion of the stomach to the jejunum. (Sometimes the terms *subtotal gastric resection* and *hemigastrectomy* are used rather than *subtotal gastrectomy*.) The stomach may be joined to the duodenum (Billroth 1) or to the jejunum (Billroth 2). A patient whose duodenum is deformed from duodenal ulcer may have the remainder of his stomach joined to his jejunum, whereas a patient with a gastric ulcer whose duodenum is normal may have the remainder of his stomach joined to his duodenum.

Sometimes, in patients who are too infirm to tolerate such extensive surgery, a gastroenterostomy alone without gastrectomy is performed. The jejunum is drawn up close to the stomach, and an opening is made between the stomach and the jejunum. This opening allows the food to pass directly from the stomach to the jejunum, bypassing the duodenum, in which obstruction due to the ulcer may have developed.

Vagotomy (division of the vagus nerves) sometimes is performed in the treatment of peptic ulcer. When the impulses traveling down the vagus nerves are prevented from reaching the stomach, the secretion of hydrochloric acid and gastric motility are lessened. It is always used in conjunction with a resection of part of the stomach or gastroenterostomy, because when it was formerly used as a sole procedure in the treatment of ulcer, there was a significant incidence of recurrent ulcer. There is good evidence that the nutritional problems that follow gastric resection are related to the amount of stomach removed. Consequently, the trend has been to lesser resections, e.g., hemigastrectomy particularly in thin patients.

Preoperative and Postoperative Nursing Care. Preoperatively, careful attention is given to water and electrolyte regulation. Whether fluids are given orally or parenterally, care is taken that the patient is well hydrated. Usually a Levin tube is inserted and connected to suction before surgery, to empty the stomach of food and secretions.

The patient returns from the operating room with the Levin tube in place. It is attached to suction, as ordered by the doctor. The tube is left in place as long as it is necessary—usually two or three days. Its purpose is to promote healing by keeping the operative area clean and free of pressure. Although at first a small amount of bright red blood may be mixed with drainage, this promptly disappears. If large amounts of bright red blood appear, or if the drainage should continue to be streaked with it, the doctor should be notified immediately. The drainage usually is dark red or brownish at first, indicating the presence of old blood, and then it changes to the normal greenish-yellow color of gastric secretion plus bile. The amount, as well as the color of the drainage, is carefully noted. Usually, the doctor orders irrigation of the Levin tube, so that it will remain clean and patent. It is important to use only the amount and the type of solution specified by the doctor, since it is being introduced into the operative area. Too much fluid could cause strain and pressure and might injure the incision.

Nothing is given by mouth for one or two days. Mouth care greatly relieves the discomforts of the dryness and the unpleasant taste and odor from the anesthesia, the inability to take oral fluids, and the presence of the Levin tube. Usually, the patient is given 30 ml. of water orally, starting on the second day. If this is well tolerated, the amount is increased, first to 60 ml. and then to 90 ml. The patient gradually progresses to a soft diet and then, in most instances, to a normal diet. However, feedings are small and frequent.

The patient is observed carefully for any feeling of fullness or distention, and for vomiting. Repeated vomiting of small amounts of food usually indicates that the feedings are not progressing normally through the gastrointestinal tract. Sometimes this condition is due to edema near the incision. The Levin tube may have to be reinserted for one or two days, and the oral feedings may be temporarily reduced or discontinued.

The patient is encouraged to breathe deeply and to cough up mucus. Both are especially important, because the incision is high in the abdomen, and the patient tends to take shallow breaths to avoid pain. In most cases he is allowed to take a few steps and to sit in a chair for a short period on the day after surgery. This position change can be achieved without dislodging either the infusion needle or the Levin tube (both of which may still be in place), provided that the tubing is long enough, and the patient is helped slowly and carefully. When these treatments have been discontinued, and the patient feels stronger, he is helped to walk about, and he is allowed to carry out more of his own personal hygiene.

Often, by the time that the patient returns home, he is able to eat six small meals daily. Most patients who have had subtotal gastrectomy are able gradually to eat larger meals and to eat less frequently, because their bodies gradually adjust to the loss of a large portion of the stomach.

Dumping Syndrome. A few patients experience the "dumping syndrome," a complication of gastric surgery, which includes a sensation of weakness and faintness, frequently accompanied by profuse perspiration and palpitations. It is believed that these symptoms may be due to the rapid emptying of large amounts of food and fluid through the gastroenterostomy into the jejunum. (Normally, the food would pass through the entire stomach and the duodenum before reaching the jejunum.) The presence of this hypertonic solution in the gut draws fluid from the circulating blood volume into the intestine, thereby reducing the effective blood volume and producing a syncope-like syndrome.

Patients who experience the "dumping syndrome" are instructed to:

- Eat small, frequent meals.
- Avoid drinking fluids with meals. Fluids are taken later.
- Follow a low carbohydrate, high protein, moderate fat diet.
- Lie down for about a half-hour after eating.

Complications of Peptic Ulcer

Complications are common, and their symptoms may be responsible for the patient's seeking medical care. The complications that are found most frequently are as follows:

Hemorrhage is the most frequent complication of peptic ulcer. Bleeding occurs when a blood vessel is eroded by the ulcer. If the vessel is large, massive hemorrhage results. If the vessel is small, even unnoticed blood loss occurs. (An examination of stool for occult blood is helpful in detecting this type of bleeding.) Continuous bleeding may be noted only when the loss of blood has been sufficient to cause faintness, weakness and dizziness.

Vomiting of blood (hematemesis) or passing of tarry stools may occur. Blood that is vomited may appear bright red or as dark material that resembles coffee grounds. Although the tarry stool may not be as frightening to the patient as the vomiting of bright red blood, it is equally ominous, and treatment should be sought immediately. (When bleeding occurs high in the gastrointestinal tract, the material passed looks black and sticky. Bleeding near the anus, such as that which may occur with hemorrhoids, causes bright red blood to be mixed with stool.)

If the blood loss is severe, the symptoms of hemorrhage are acute: pallor, rapid, weak pulse, thirst, faintness, sweating and collapse. Treatment includes complete rest, transfusions, and sometimes opiates or sedatives to relieve restlessness. Usually, nothing is given by mouth, and the patient is given intravenous fluids until the bleeding has stopped. Occasionally, small, frequent feedings of milk and cream are given while the patient is bleeding, provided that he is not vomiting. When bleeding cannot be controlled by these measures, the patient is taken to the operating room, and the bleeding vessel is ligated; sometimes a subtotal gastrectomy is performed.

Usually every effort is made to control the bleeding without immediate surgical intervention, because it is preferable that patients who undergo surgery have supportive treatment beforehand, such as transfusions to replace lost blood. Often, surgery is necessary later to treat the underlying disease and to prevent future episodes of bleeding.

The patient is observed very carefully. Pulse, respiration and blood pressure are taken at frequent intervals, as they are specified by the doctor. Restlessness, apprehension and pallor are important to note, because they often indicate hemorrhage. The patient is kept as quiet as possible, and only the most essential aspects of personal hygiene are cared for until his condition has stabilized.

The patient is usually aware that he is bleeding, and he is very frightened. Assure him that measures are being promptly taken to control the bleeding and to replace the lost blood. Explain the importance of resting quietly in bed. Administer sedatives, as they are ordered by the doctor, to control restlessness. Keep the environment as neat as you can, and whenever it is possible, do not allow the patient to see the amount of blood lost. Remove soiled linen and utensils immediately. Nursing care should be carried out in a way that minimizes any exertion or fatigue.

GASTRIC HYPOTHERMIA. Gastric cooling has been used for many years in treating hemorrhage, and its usefulness for this purpose is generally accepted. Because it controls blood loss, it is particularly useful in providing time for instituting other therapeutic measures. For example, while bleeding is being controlled by gastric cooling, time is made available to give the patient a transfusion and to prepare him for surgery.

The patient who because of bleeding is to be treated by gastric cooling is placed first on a warming blanket (set at 97° to 100° F.) so that the treatment, which can last many hours (24 to 36 hours often is necessary), will not cause him discomfort due to chilling or lower his general body temperature. As with any patient who is bleeding, his vital signs are checked frequently.

A sedative and topical anesthesia of the oropharynx are administered before the treatment is begun, the former to lessen apprehension and the latter to lessen the discomfort caused by passage of the tube and the balloon. A nasogastric tube is passed, and the stomach is gently lavaged with cool saline by the physician to remove accumulated blood and clots.

The lavage tube then is withdrawn, and a nasogastric tube connected with a balloon shaped like the patient's stomach is passed by the physician through the patient's mouth and swallowed by the patient. When the balloon is in place in the stomach, the physician slowly inserts a cooling solution, until the amount required to distend the balloon and fill the stomach is reached (approximately 600 ml.). The distended balloon applies both pressure and cooling to the bleeding area.

The temperature of the cooling solution is determined by the physician, and the machine is set to maintain this temperature. The cooling solution runs into the balloon and then out again, thus assuring an evenly cool temperature throughout the treatment. During the procedure the patient's position should be changed, so that complications such as pneumonia and decubiti do not occur. Care must be taken, however, not to dislodge or kink any of the tubing. If the patient bites on the tube which passes through his mouth, the tube should be padded with gauze.

When bleeding has stopped, the balloon is gradually deflated. Gradualness is important, since sudden removal of the pressure might result in resumption of bleeding. The empty balloon is left in place for approximately 12 hours in case bleeding should resume. If no further bleeding occurs, the balloon is removed. The patient continues to be observed for any resumption of bleeding.

Obstruction. Edema, spasm, inflammation and scar tissue surrounding the ulcer may interfere with the passage of food, causing retention of food in the stomach for longer than normal periods. Obstruction commonly occurs in the pyloric region. The degree of interference with the normal flow of gastric content varies. If it is slight, the patient may notice that after eating he has a feeling of fullness, distention and nausea. If the obstruction is severe, the patient has nausea and vomiting, pain and distention.

Physical examination, x-ray study of the gastrointestinal tract, and aspiration of the stomach contents help the doctor to determine the location and the severity of the obstruction. If obstruction is present, large amounts of food and secretion are obtained when a Levin tube is passed, and the contents of the stomach are withdrawn by gentle suction.

Obstruction that is due to edema and inflammation often subsides when the patient has careful medical treatment for the ulcer. In addition to other forms of medical treatment, gastric intubation and decompression are used to drain retained food and secretions. Feedings of milk and cream are administered sometimes by slow, continuous drip to help to neutralize gastric secretions, as well as to supply fluids and nourishment. The physician orders the amount and the type of feeding and the length of time that it is to be administered. Sometimes, antacids are added to the feeding.

The care of patients who have gastric intubation and decompression has already been discussed. If the obstruction is treated surgically, preoperative and postoperative measures are similar to those discussed above for any patient having gastric surgery. Measures to evaluate water and electrolyte regulation and nutritional status are especially important, because nausea and vomiting may have persisted for some time. The nurse participates in this evaluation by accurately reporting intake and output, weighing the patient, and assisting with the collection of specimens of blood and urine.

Perforation. The ulcer may penetrate the tissues so deeply that perforation occurs, allowing the contents of the gastrointestinal tract to seep out and causing peritonitis.

The symptoms of perforation and ensuing peritonitis usually are dramatic; once seen, they are unforgettable. The patient experiences sudden, excruciating pain in his abdomen, his face becomes ashen and drawn, and he perspires profusely. The patient's temperature at this time may be normal or subnormal. His abdomen becomes hard as a stone. It is extremely painful and tender, and the patient resists having it touched no matter how gentle the touch. Usually the patient lies with his knees flexed to lessen the pain. The extreme hardness of the abdomen, often described as "boardlike," is due to the rigidity of the abdominal muscles. His breathing is rapid and shallow. After an hour or two, usually the patient's face becomes flushed, and he develops fever. The abdomen becomes very distended and less rigid. Respirations be-

come even more rapid and shallow. The pulse becomes rapid and weak, and the patient dies unless treatment is given promptly.

Perforation is an emergency condition. The treatment includes immediate surgical closure of the perforation, so that no further leakage can occur; suction during surgery to remove the gastric contents from the peritoneal cavity; and the administration of large doses of antibiotics. Every moment counts. The longer the perforation goes untreated, the less likely is the patient's recovery.

When the patient returns from the operating room, he will have a Levin tube in place, which is connected to suction. After he has reacted from anesthesia, he is placed in low sitting position. Nothing is given by mouth, and parenteral fluids are administered. Antibiotics are given to combat the infection in the peritoneal cavity. The patient is observed carefully. Usually, his fever subsides, his abdomen becomes less distended, he breathes more easily and deeply, and his pulse is stronger and slower. Continued elevation of temperature, distention, weak, rapid pulse, and shallow, rapid breathing should be reported to the doctor, since they may indicate that peritonitis is not responding to treatment, or that the patient has developed an abscess. The patient should be observed also for symptoms of paralytic ileus, such as distention and failure to pass flatus or stool. When the patient recovers from surgery, the treatment of the underlying condition of peptic ulcer is continued.

Occasionally, patients who have a small perforation that is diagnosed promptly are treated medically. Continuous suction is used to keep the stomach empty, and intravenous fluids and electrolytes are administered. Antibiotics are used to combat infection. The purpose of this therapy is to facilitate the healing of the perforation and to prevent and to treat infection.

REFERENCES AND BIBLIOGRAPHY

BELAND, I. L.: *Clinical Nursing*, ed. 2, St. Louis, Mosby, 1970.
GIVEN, B., and SIMMONS, S.: Care of a patient with a gastric ulcer, *Am. J. Nurs.* 70:1472, July, 1970.
GOODMAN, L. S., and GILMAN, A.: *The Pharmacological Basis of Therapeutics,* ed. 3, New York, Macmillan, 1970.
PURINTUN, L. R., and NELSON, L.: Ulcer patient—emotional emergency, *Am. J. Nurs.* 68:1930, September, 1968.
ROBINSON, C.: *Proudfit-Robinson's Normal and Therapeutic Nutrition,* ed. 13, New York, Macmillan, 1967.
RODMAN, M. J., and SMITH, D. W.: *Pharmacology and Drug Therapy in Nursing,* Philadelphia, Lippincott, 1968.
RYNBERGEN, H.: Fewer diet restrictions in gastro-intestinal disease, *Am. J. Nurs.* 63:36-89, January, 1963.

The Patient with Cancer of the Gastrointestinal Tract

36

Symptoms • Associated Conditions • Diagnosis • Treatment
Nursing Care • Cancer of the Mouth • Cancer of the Esophagus
Cancer of the Stomach • Cancer of the Colon
Cancer of the Rectum

Cancer of the digestive tract is a major cause of illness and death. It occurs commonly in every major area of the gastrointestinal tract except the small intestine, where it is unusual. Cancer of mouth, esophagus, stomach or rectum is more common in men than women, whereas cancer of the colon is slightly more common in women.

SYMPTOMS

Cancer of the digestive tract causes the same general symptoms as cancer elsewhere in the body: for example, weakness, weight loss, fatigue and anemia. As is the case in cancer of other organs, pain is often a late symptom. Cancer of mouth and tongue has the advantage of being visible usually to the patient and his doctor relatively early in the disease. Frequently, it appears as a lump or as an ulcer or a sore that persists.

Cancer of esophagus, stomach or colon often causes few, if any, early symptoms, making the problem of prompt diagnosis difficult. Patients with cancer of the esophagus may notice a slight difficulty in swallowing solid food and a sensation of pressure or fullness under the sternum. Usually, these symptoms are so mild when they are first noted that they may be overlooked or attributed to "nerves" or indigestion. As the malignant tumor grows, the esophagus becomes obstructed gradually, and yet relentlessly. The inability to swallow solid food and the prompt vomiting of food after it is eaten are typical. Pain may be severe late in the course of the ill-

ness. The patient becomes extremely emaciated, because food cannot pass beyond the obstruction.

Cancer of the stomach usually produces vague symptoms at the outset. Slight indigestion, loss of appetite, flatulence, and a distaste for certain foods that previously were enjoyed may occur, or the patient may experience no symptoms until late in the disease, when he may have severe pain, vomiting of blood, or passage of tarry stools.

A slight change in bowel habits often is the earliest warning of cancer of the large intestine. As the lumen of the bowel becomes gradually obstructed by the tumor, the patient often develops alternating constipation and diarrhea. Diarrhea results when the intestine attempts to push the material past the obstruction by very forceful peristalsis. General symptoms, such as anemia, may appear before any symptoms referable to the intestinal tract are noted. Later in the illness the patient may have tarry stools, or if the lesion is near the anus, frank blood in the stool. Symptoms of intestinal obstruction appear when the tumor has become large enough to prevent the normal passage of intestinal contents through the colon.

The symptoms of rectal cancer may attract attention more promptly. The patient often passes bright red blood with his stool, or his stool may emerge pencil- or ribbon-shaped, due to passing through a narrowed opening. Constipation or diarrhea may occur. A feeling of fullness or discomfort in the rectum sometimes is noticed; however, severe pain is usually a late symptom.

ASSOCIATED CONDITIONS

Leukoplakia, patches of white, thickened tissue in the mouth, often is considered to be a fore-runner of cancer. Leukoplakia is most common among heavy smokers. If the white patches do not disappear when the patient stops smoking and gives careful attention to mouth hygiene, their surgical removal may be recommended to prevent the development of cancer.

Patients with *ulcerative colitis* have a higher incidence than the normal population of cancer of the colon.

People who have polyps in the bowel also may be predisposed to the development of cancer of the colon. The prompt and the effective treat-ment of conditions that often seem to precede cancer is important. The annual follow-up of patients with polyps found on sigmoidoscopy or by barium enema is important in detecting early malignancies which may supervene. Similar pro-grams are followed in patients with ulcerative colitis despite inactivity of the colitis.

DIAGNOSIS

Cancer of the digestive tract, like cancer else-where, is diagnosed by careful history and physi-cal examination, by special tests to reveal the presence of a tumor, and by biopsy. For exam-ple, a roentgenogram of the esophagus after the patient has swallowed barium may reveal a tumor that is obstructing the esophagus. Proctoscopy, sigmoidoscopy and gastroscopy also are employed. Cytologic examination of exfoliated cells (Papani-colaou test) sometimes is performed. For exam-ple, a specimen of esophageal or gastric washings can be collected from the esophagus or the stom-ach by means of a saline lavage through a naso-gastric tube; the cells in the specimen are exam-ined for malignancy.

Although the appearance of a tumor may sug-gest cancer strongly, the final diagnosis is estab-lished by an examination of a piece of the tissue itself, to determine whether or not it is malig-nant. When the lesion is readily accessible, as in the mouth, biopsy may be performed very easily. Areas that are less accessible may have biopsies taken through the instrument used for visual examination. For instance, a biopsy of a rectal tumor may be performed through the procto-scope. Some tumors are so inaccesible that tissue for examination can be obtained only by surgery.

An awareness of danger signals is most impor-tant. If patients report even minor symptoms to the doctor, there is greater opportunity for early diagnosis, and cure is more likely.

TREATMENT

If the disease is discovered in time, malignant tissue may be removed surgically or destroyed by radiation. If the malignant tissue can be eradi-cated completely, the patient is cured. When the disease has metastasized, surgery, radiation or chemotherapy may be used as palliative measures.

Supportive treatment includes the maintenance of nutrition, the use of drugs to relieve pain, and the correction of anemia by the use of trans-fusions.

NURSING CARE

In order to remove malignant tissue, it is often necessary to perform radical surgery that alters the appearance of the patient or the way in which his body functions. Extensive surgery of the mouth and the adjacent structures can be very disfiguring. A patient who cannot swallow, one who must be fed through a gastrostomy, can-not eat normally. The threat of cancer, the fear that all malignant tissue has not been removed, and the necessity for radical surgery have a tre-mendous emotional impact on the patient and his family. Preparation for surgery involves help-ing the patient to understand what it will entail, and how he can care for himself afterward. After surgery the patient is taught how to care for him-self. If complete recovery is not expected, the family may need to assume a large measure of responsibility for the patient's care when he re-turns home. Referral to the public health nurse is often very helpful in assisting the patient and family with home care.

Regardless of the site of the primary lesion, the nursing needs of patients with cancer are in many respects similar. A brief discussion of spe-cific points in the treatment and the nursing care of patients with common types of gastrointestinal cancer follows.

CANCER OF THE MOUTH

The surgical excision of malignant tissue in the mouth may result in complete cure, provided that it is performed early. Sometimes, surgery is so extensive that not only is it mutilating, but also it may interfere with normal breathing and swallowing. For instance, considerable edema may occur postoperatively, leading to obstruction of the respiratory passages. A tracheostomy may be necessary during the postoperative period until edema subsides. (Care of patients with tracheostomy is discussed in Chap. 22.) The patient may have to be fed through a nasogastric tube until healing is sufficient to allow him to swallow.

Postoperative Care

When the patient returns from the operating room, ordinarily he is positioned flat, either on his abdomen or on his side, with his head turned to the side to facilitate drainage from the mouth. Suction is carried out as it is necessary to prevent aspiration of secretions postoperatively.

When the patient recovers from the effects of anesthesia, he is often more comfortable with the head of his bed elevated. This position usually makes it easier for him to breathe deeply and to cough up secretions, and it helps to control edema. Coughing and deep breathing are important to prevent postoperative pneumonia and atelectasis. Firm support of the patient's head and his neck helps to lessen pain when he coughs. At first the nurse provides this support for the patient; later he is taught to do it himself. Place your hands gently but firmly on either side of the patient's head, supporting his head to prevent excessive movement when he coughs.

Note and report bleeding on the dressings, rapid pulse, fall in blood pressure, or the coughing up of bright red blood. Expectoration of some dark blood is to be expected in the immediate postoperative period. Note the patient's breathing. Call the doctor immediately if the patient experiences respiratory difficulty or cyanosis. Equipment for suction, administration of oxygen, and care of, or performance of, a tracheostomy should be kept at the bedside during the immediate postoperative period.

A great deal of care and judgment are necessary in the administration of narcotics postoperatively, since they can cause respiratory depression.

Old blood and mucus tend to collect in the mouth during the postoperative period. Unless the mouth is kept scrupulously clean, infection is likely to occur, and very unpleasant odors and an offensive taste in the mouth are distressing to the patient and those who are near him. Cleansing must be done frequently, and with great care not to cause trauma or to introduce infection.

Sterile technic is used in some hospitals. Others use clean technic, on the theory that sterile technic is not necessary, because the mouth normally harbors bacteria and cannot be kept sterile.

Usually, the mouth is gently irrigated to keep it clean. The frequency of irrigations and the type of solution to be used are ordered by the doctor. Normal saline is commonly used. Turn the patient's head to the side, allow the solution to run in gently and to flow out into the emesis basin. A soft rubber catheter is useful for this purpose, because it does not cause trauma. The mouth should not be irrigated until the patient regains consciousness after surgery, because he might aspirate the solution. Be very careful not to get the dressings or the patient's bed or gown wet during irrigations. Place the emesis basin carefully in position to catch the return, avoid allowing too much solution to run in at a time, and use plastic material to protect dressings and linen.

Because the postoperative patient often is unable to swallow, he is given parenteral fluids immediately, followed by feedings through the nasogastric tube. When the patient is able to swallow, he is given at first small amounts of liquid, and gradually he progresses from liquids to soft foods as they are tolerated. The patient should be observed carefully when he first attempts to swallow small amounts of liquid. If he coughs and has difficulty in swallowing, suction him immediately. Do not give further oral feedings without checking with the doctor. Some patients have had such extensive surgery that they continue to require tube feedings. These patients learn to carry out the feeding themselves.

Problems

Communication with others presents a real problem to patients who have had extensive oral surgery. The patient's ability to tell others about his discomfort, to express fears, to ask questions, or to call for help is impaired at the very time when he badly needs the opportunity to communicate with others. The "Magic Slate" is so useful that many nurses consider it standard equipment at the bedside of a patient who is unable to speak and yet able to write. Merely lifting the plastic cover erases the writing, and the slate is ready for reuse. Special care should be taken that the patient's call bell is within reach at all times, and that his call light is answered promptly.

Specific points that may be helpful in minimizing the patient's distress over his appearance after oral surgery are:

• Providing privacy during his first attempts to swallow and to eat.

• Helping the patient to minimize the problem of drooling. See that he has plenty of tissues, and that he tilts his head at intervals, so that the saliva is directed back, where it can be swallowed. Sometimes a small catheter attached to low pressure suction is used to remove excess saliva from the mouth.

• Helping him to pay extra attention to personal cleanliness and grooming. Clean pajamas, hair neatly combed, and a shave as soon as the doctor permits, all help the patient to feel more presentable.

• Allowing dressings to be left in place longer than is absolutely necessary to cover gross defects until they can be corrected by plastic surgery. (This is sometimes done; often the decision to do it is reached after consultation between the doctor and the nurse concerning the patient's reaction.)

Complications

Hemorrhage. Large blood vessels, such as the carotid arteries, are nearby. Serious hemorrhage may result when an artery is invaded by cancer and becomes ulcerated, or when necrosis follows radiotherapy. The doctor advises the nurse which patients are most likely to develop hemorrhage. These patients should be placed near the nurse's station, so that they can be observed frequently.

If hemorrhage should occur, the nurse applies direct digital pressure over the bleeding point until the doctor arrives. Another nurse, or even another patient, should be asked to report the emergency, so that the nurse who first applies digital pressure can remain with the patient and continue to apply pressure until the doctor arrives.

The doctor usually orders a narcotic to relieve the patient's apprehension and transfusions to replace lost blood. Ligation of the bleeding vessel often is necessary. The nurse's role involves assisting the doctor quickly with the control of the bleeding and assuring the patient by her swift, calm competent care that everything possible is being done to control the bleeding. After the bleeding has stopped, the patient is not only exhausted but also very apprehensive that it may recur. Visiting and observing him frequently are important in detecting any further bleeding and in assuring him that his condition is being checked carefully. The frequent observation of pulse and blood pressure is important.

Respiratory Obstruction. If respiratory obstruction should occur, it may necessitate an emergency tracheostomy. Labored breathing and cyanosis should be noted and reported promptly. Pneumonia and atelectasis may be caused by aspiration of secretions or blood. Suction, avoidance of oversedation and depression of the cough reflex, and encouraging the patient to cough up secretions are important in preventing pneumonia and atelectasis.

CANCER OF THE ESOPHAGUS

The treatment of patients with cancer of the esophagus has advanced rapidly in recent years. Since surgical treatment of the esophagus involves entering the thoracic cavity, major progress had to await the development of modern chest surgery. It is now possible through the use of such technics as endotracheal anesthesia and closed chest drainage to operate on structures within the thoracic cavity without causing collapse of the lung or decreased oxygenation of the blood. The care of the patient after esophageal surgery is essentially that of any patient after chest surgery.

Preoperative Nursing Care

The patient who enters the hospital for the treatment of cancer of the esophagus often has become emaciated from inability to swallow and regurgitation of the food that he attempts to eat. Preoperative preparation involves improving his nutrition and restoring water and electrolyte regulation. The patient receives parenteral fluids as they are required, and if he is able to swallow liquids, he is given a high calorie, high protein liquid diet.

Privacy is important when the patient is eating, because he very often regurgitates his food. The patient needs two emesis basins, so that one can be removed and emptied while the other one is left for use, if it is needed. Frequent opportunity to rinse his mouth helps to relieve unpleasant taste and odor.

An explanation of what to expect postoperatively is especially important because of the array of special equipment that the patient will find at his bedside when he recovers from anesthesia. In addition to the equipment for closed drainage of his chest (see Chap. 24), administration of oxygen, suction, and parenteral fluids, the patient may have a nasogastric tube for drainage of secretions from his stomach. Some patients are fed through a gastrostomy for several days postoperatively.

Surgical Treatment

The aim of surgery is to remove all the malignant tissue and to restore the continuity of the gastrointestinal tract, so that the patient can eat normally. Sometimes, cure is possible when the disease is treated early. Even when the disease has metastasized, surgery often can be performed that will enable the patient to eat normally for the remainder of his life; thus he is spared death by starvation or the need for a gastrostomy.

One type of operation involves removing the portion of the esophagus containing the tumor, as well as regional lymph nodes to which the disease has spread. The stomach then is drawn up into the thoracic cavity and joined to the remaining portion of the esophagus. This operation may be curative or palliative, depending on the stage of the disease. Portions of the patient's intestine also can be used to re-establish a passageway for food. For example, if the tumor cannot be removed, a piece of intestine sometimes is placed from the point above the obstruction to the stomach, thus providing a way for food to reach the stomach. Sometimes, a piece of the jejunum is used to join the stomach and the remaining portion of the esophagus. A tube constructed from a section of the gastric wall also has been used to form a passageway for food when the esophagus is obstructed. Plastic prosthetic devices that replace the excised portion of esophagus are being used.

If the patient is too ill to withstand surgery, a gastrostomy sometimes is performed, permitting food to be introduced directly into the stomach through an opening on the patient's abdomen. Sometimes the gastrostomy is a temporary measure that will be used until the patient's nutritional status has improved sufficiently to permit surgery. The gastrostomy opening then is closed. Sometimes, and now less often than formerly, the patient must be fed through the gastrostomy until death from generalized carcinoma overtakes him.

Postoperative Nursing Care

After surgery for cancer of the esophagus, the patient is given intravenous feedings and nothing by mouth for several days to allow time for the healing of the tissues. The drainage from the nasogastric tube is watched carefully for any evidence of bleeding. Although a small amount of blood may drain through the tube when the patient first returns from the operating room, the drainage should return promptly to the yellow-green color of normal gastric secretions.

Measures pertaining to the care of any patient who has had chest surgery will include:

- Care of closed chest drainage
- Particular emphasis on deep breathing and coughing
- Administration of oxygen

Often the patient is allowed to take a few steps and to sit in a chair the day after surgery to stimulate deep breathing and to improve circulation. Closed chest drainage and drainage from the nasogastric tube are continued even when the patient is out of bed. Special care is required to see that the tubing is long enough to permit the patient to move a step or two to his chair. Some patients are fed postoperatively through a temporary gastrostomy for four to seven days. In these patients the gastrostomy tube rather than a nasogastric tube is used to decompress the stomach.

After several days the patient is permitted small amounts of water frequently. He is observed carefully for regurgitation of the fluid and for such symptoms as dyspnea and fever that might indicate seepage of the fluid through the operative area to the mediastinum. Sitting up during and just after the ingestion of water helps to prevent regurgitation.

The patient gradually progresses to swallowing other liquids, soft foods and, finally, a normal diet. If the stomach has been drawn up into the thoracic cavity, the patient may have a feeling of pressure in his chest and dyspnea after eating. These symptoms can be minimized by eating frequent small meals and by not lying down for several hours after eating.

Care of a Patient with a Gastrostomy

Gastrostomy is not as common now as formerly, thanks to advances in the surgical treatment of injuries or diseases that cause obstruction of the esophagus. Cancer and stricture of the esophagus from swallowing chemicals are examples of conditions that cause obstruction of the esophagus, and that may necessitate either a temporary or a permanent gastrostomy. Gastrostomy is a relatively minor procedure. It can be performed under local anesthesia, and it can be carried out even if the patient is very weak and debilitated.

Usually, it is very hard for the patient to face the prospect of gastrostomy. Eating is one of the very basic pleasures of life. Although the patient's nutrition can be maintained by gastrostomy, thereafter he is denied during meals the physical satisfaction of taste and the emotional satisfaction of companionship. The patient feeds himself by means of a funnel and a catheter inserted into his stomach through the gastrostomy. It is the unusual patient who does not prefer privacy during this procedure.

When the gastrostomy is performed, a catheter is inserted into the opening and secured to the abdominal wall by either a suture or adhesive tape. To prevent the leakage of gastric contents, the end of the catheter is clamped except for the time that the patient is being fed. The leakage that may occur around the tube is extremely troublesome, because the gastric contents are very irritating to the skin. Dressings are applied to absorb any drainage that occurs around the tube; they must be changed frequently. The skin must be washed often with mild soap and water to prevent excoriation. Ointments, such as zinc oxide or petrolatum, may be applied to the skin to help to prevent irritation.

Initial feedings through the tube usually consist of small amounts of tap water, which are gradually increased to larger amounts as they are tolerated. The amount of fluid and the frequency of its administration are specified by the surgeon. After the patient is able to take clear liquids through the tube, the feedings are started.

When sufficient healing has taken place, the gastrostomy tube is removed and inserted only for feedings. The patient learns to insert the catheter approximately four inches into the gastrostomy and to pour the feedings into a funnel that has been attached to the end of the catheter. Usually, about 300 to 500 ml. is given at a time. Some patients feel uncomfortably full and even nauseated unless the feedings are given in small amounts. Therefore, they must take their feedings more frequently, so that the total amount ordered by the doctor is received. The tube and the funnel are washed and rinsed thoroughly after each use. A permanent plastic "button" sutured to the abdominal wall, with a screw-in plug, keeps the stoma closed between feedings.

Many doctors recommend that the patient's normal diet be converted to a form suitable for tube feeding by the use of a food blender. This method is considered desirable if tube feedings must be continued for a long period, because the patient's normal nutrition can be maintained, and the patient's family can prepare his meals readily at home.

CANCER OF THE STOMACH

The number of persons developing cancer of the stomach in the United States seems to be decreasing. The reason for this change is not understood.

The treatment of cancer of the stomach often involves total gastrectomy. The entire stomach is removed, and the continuity of the gastrointestinal tract is restored by joining the jejunum and the esophagus. Depending on the location and the size of the tumor, it may be possible to perform a subtotal rather than a total gastrectomy, thus preserving a more normal digestive function. The spleen is removed when part or all of the stomach is removed because of cancer, since metastasis to the splenic lymph nodes is common.

The care of the patient after total gastrectomy differs from that of a patient after subtotal gastrectomy in that:

• The thoracic cavity, as well as the abdominal cavity, must be entered to remove the entire stomach. The patient therefore requires care similar to that of any patient who has had chest surgery.

• Very little drainage returns through the nasogastric tube, because the stomach, which normally forms the secretions, has been removed.

• Oral feedings are started several days postoperatively with small amounts of tap water given at frequent intervals. Gradually, the patient progresses to frequent, small feedings of bland foods.

• The patient continues to eat small meals very frequently. Because of the removal of his entire stomach, he is unable to tolerate large meals, and often he experiences difficulty in digesting his food. He should be given easily digested foods, eat slowly, and chew his food thoroughly.

• Injections of vitamin B_{12} are sometimes necessary for the rest of the patient's life, because once the stomach has been removed, the intrinsic factor necessary for absorption of vitamin B_{12} is no longer produced. If therapy with vitamin B_{12} is not administered, the patient will develop symptoms of pernicious anemia.

CANCER OF THE COLON

Treatment of cancer of the colon is primarily surgical. Sometimes a combination of surgery and radiotherapy is utilized. Depending on the location of the tumor and the time that treatment is instituted, it may be possible to remove completely the malignant tissue of the affected section of bowel and to restore the normal continuity of the tract by joining the remaining portions of the intestine. If this treatment is not possible because of the size and the spread of the tumor or because of the patient's general condition, a temporary or a permanent colostomy may have to be performed to relieve the obstruction caused by the tumor. Sometimes, a temporary colostomy is carried out to relieve obstruction, and more radical surgery to remove the malignant growth and to re-establish the continuity of the bowel is performed when the patient's physical condition has improved.

CANCER OF THE RECTUM

The location of the tumor will help the surgeon to decide whether rectal cancer may be treated by an abdominoperineal resection or a "pull-through" operation that removes the diseased area of the rectum but preserves the anus. In some instances it has been found beneficial to give radiotherapy before undertaking surgical treatment.

Surgical Treatment

In an abdominoperineal resection, the anus, the rectum, and part of the sigmoid colon are removed. The operation is a major and a lengthy procedure. First, an abdominal incision is made; through it the sigmoid is divided, and the prox-

imal portion of the sigmoid is brought out onto the abdomen to form a permanent colostomy. Then the patient is placed in lithotomy position, and the anus, the rectum, and the lower portion of the sigmoid are removed through the perineal incision. The operation actually involves two major procedures, and in some instances it is performed by two teams of surgeons working simultaneously.

When the tumor is located higher in the rectum near the sigmoid, it is sometimes possible to remove the tumor and the involved portion of the rectum, to leave the anal sphincter intact, and to pull the sigmoid colon down to the anus, thus enabling the patient to continue to evacuate through the anus.

Because abdominoperineal resection involves such extensive surgery, it is especially important to observe the patient for shock after he returns from the operating room. The doctor's orders concerning the observation of pulse, respirations and blood pressure are followed carefully; an increased pulse rate and a fall in blood pressure are reported immediately, if they occur.

Nursing Care

Nursing the patient after abdominoperineal resection involves the preparation for and the care following a permanent colostomy. In addition to the abdominal incision and the colostomy, the patient returns from the operating room with a perineal wound. Dressings over the perineal wound must be checked carefully for bleeding. Usually, there is profuse serosanguineous drainage, and sometimes the dressings must be reinforced a short time after surgery to prevent soiling. Placing small disposable bed pads

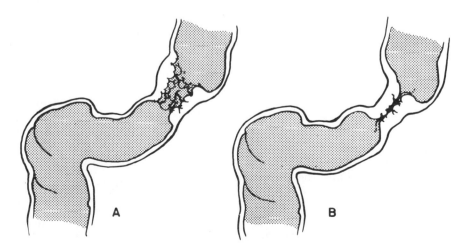

Fig. 36-1. Cancer of the colon. (A) The new growth proliferates. (B) As the malignancy grows, it can occlude the lumen of the colon and cause obstruction.

under the patient's buttocks helps to protect the bedding. The pads can be changed easily and quickly whenever they become soiled. When sufficient healing has taken place, the doctor may request that the entire rectal dressing be changed by the nurse whenever it becomes soiled.

Patients who have undergone abdomino-perineal resection usually are acutely uncomfortable during the first few days after surgery. Most surgical patients have one operative area to cause pain; these patients have two—one on the abdomen and one in the perineal region. These patients commonly require more frequent administration of narcotics than patients who have had less extensive surgery.

Measures that help to prevent respiratory complications and thrombophlebitis are especially important, because patients who have had abdominoperineal resection usually are kept in bed longer than most other surgical patients to permit the healing of the extensive perineal wound. If the patient stands and walks about before the pelvic floor has healed sufficiently, a hernia may develop in the perineal region.

Careful positioning helps to minimize pain. The patient often is most comfortable on his side, a position that avoids pressure on either of the operative areas. In the early postoperative period he is turned frequently from one side to the other, and he is encouraged to breathe deeply, to cough, and to exercise his legs. When the most acute discomfort has subsided, the patient frequently finds that he can lie on his back as well as on either side. Supporting the perineal dressings firmly with a T-binder is important in encouraging the patient to move about in bed. Unless the dressings are held snugly in place, the patient often is reluctant to turn and to move his legs for fear of dislodging the dressing.

Because a distended bladder is more subject to injury during operation, an indwelling catheter (Foley) is usually inserted just prior to surgery to keep the bladder empty. It is left in place for several days after the operation, because most patients have difficulty voiding immediately after abdominoperineal resection. The catheter also helps to prevent the soiling of perineal dressings with urine during the immediate postoperative period. When the catheter has been removed, the time and the amount of each voiding are carefully noted to determine whether the patient is able to empty his bladder satisfactorily. If the perineal dressings become soiled with urine, they should be changed promptly.

Gastrointestinal decompression ordinarily is carried out for several days postoperatively. Intravenous fluids and transfusions are given as they are necessary during this period. The patient then begins taking oral fluids, and he progresses gradually to a regular diet. Antibiotics are usually given to prevent infection.

The length of time that the patient must remain in bed varies. Often he is permitted out of bed three days after the operation. Because of the extensive surgery and the longer period of bed rest, he is usually quite weak and needs considerable assistance. Placing a rubber ring or foam rubber pad on the seat of his chair helps to lessen discomfort while he is sitting.

The surgeon sometimes packs the perineal wound to promote healing from the inside out (rather than healing of superficial tissues before deeper tissues have healed). The packing is removed gradually as the wound heals. Irrigation of the wound may be ordered. The surgeon will specify the type of solution to be used and the frequency of the irrigations.

When the patient is allowed out of bed, sitz baths often are ordered to promote healing of the perineal wound. Because the patient is weak and may become faint, it is important not to leave him alone in the sitz bath the first few times that he has this treatment. Depending on the patient's condition and the distance between his bed and the sitz bath, it is often advisable to take him to the bathroom in a wheelchair. A rubber ring is placed in the bottom of the tub to lessen the discomfort caused by sitting in the hard tub and to permit the warm water to circulate freely around the operative area. Most patients find that the sitz baths are a great help in relieving discomfort, as well as in promoting healing.

Dressings are worn over the perineal wound until healing occurs, and drainage ceases. Later in the postoperative period, when healing has progressed, and the patient is stronger, he learns to change the perineal dressings as well as the colostomy dressings or appliance. Perineal pads often are used instead of perineal dressings during convalescence. The patient is taught to continue taking sitz baths at home, using either the bathtub or a large basin.

REFERENCES AND BIBLIOGRAPHY

BARNES, M.: Clean colons without enemas, *Am. J. Nurs.* 69:2128, October, 1969.

BEESON, P. B., and McDERMOTT, W. (eds.): *Cecil-Loeb Textbook of Medicine*, ed. 12, Philadelphia, Saunders, 1967.

BELAND, I. L.: *Clinical Nursing,* ed. 2, St. Louis, Mosby, 1970.

DAVIS, L.: *Christopher's Textbook of Surgery,* ed. 9, Philadelphia, Saunders, 1968.

DIETRICH, R. A., *et al.:* Clinicopathologic study of carcinoma involving the esophagogastric junction, *Surg. Gynec. Obstet.* 118:1223, 1964.

FRAZELL, E. L., STRONG, E. W., and NEWCOMBE, B.: Tumors of the parotid, *Am. J. Nurs.* 66:2702, 1966.

GOODMAN, L. S., and GILMAN, A.: *The Pharmacological Basis of Therapeutics,* ed. 3, New York, Macmillan, 1970.

HALLBERG, J. C.: The patient with surgery of the colon and rectum, *Am. J. Nurs.* 61:64, March, 1961.

KAY, S.: A ten-year appraisal of the treatment of squamous cell carcinoma of the esophagus, *Surg. Gynec. Obstet.* 117:167, 1964.

KRAMER, P.: Progress in gastroenterology. Esophagus. *Gastroenterology* 54:1171, 1968.

LUMPKIN, W. M., *et al.:* Carcinoma of the stomach, a review, *Ann. Surg.* 159:919, 1964.

MING, S. C., and GOLDMAN, H.: Gastric polyps, a histogenetic classification and its relation to carcinoma, *Cancer,* 18:721, 1965.

RAPHAEL, H. A., *et al.:* Primary adenocarcinoma of the esophagus, *Ann. Surg.* 164:785, 1966.

ROBINSON, C.: *Proudfit-Robinson's Normal and Therapeutic Nutrition,* ed. 13, New York, Macmillan, 1967.

SHERLOCK, S.: Gastrointestinal carcinoma, *Gastroenterology* 32:434, 1957.

WILSON, J. P.: Cancer of the colon and rectum, *Nurs. Forum* 4:59, 1965.

WOLFMAN, E. F., JR., and FLOTTE, C. T.: Carcinoma of the colon and rectum, *Am. J. Nurs.* 61:60, March, 1961.

ZUIDEMA, G. D., and KLEIN, M. K.: A new esophagus, *Am. J. Nurs.* 61:69, September, 1961.

The Patient with an Ileostomy or a Colostomy

37

Planning the Patient's Care • Attitudes • Explanation and Assistance • Immediate Postoperative Care • Changing the Appliance • Control of Odor and Gas • Blockage • Patient with a Colostomy • Cecostomy

Ostomy as used here refers to an opening of the bowel onto the skin. There are two main types: *ileostomy* in which the ileum is opened onto the skin, and *colostomy* in which the colon is opened onto the skin. Fecal material drains from both of these openings, which are called stomas.

Stomas are created in the treatment of such conditions as ulcerative colitis, multiple polyposis, cancer or other obstructive lesions, and injury. Other types of stomas may be created, for example, when a ureter is brought out onto the skin, (ureterostomy) or when the ureters are implanted into a loop of ileum and one end of this ileal loop (ileal conduit) is brought out onto the skin. The patient need not be disabled; he does, however, have a change in his body which he must learn to manage and control. Teaching him to achieve this control is an important nursing role. Equally important is the nurse's role in supporting the patient during his preoperative and postoperative experience, so that he is assisted to accept the stoma.

The stoma may be temporary or permanent. At times it is not possible for the surgeon to determine the extent of surgery required. However, regardless of whether the ostomy is temporary or permanent, the patient requires assistance to learn to manage it.

The care of a patient with an ostomy should be patient-centered and living-oriented. It begins when the patient seeks care, and continues throughout the therapeutic phase and the period of recovery after discharge. The ostomate (one who has had ostomy surgery) continues to need medical and nursing care after hospitalization until he has gained security and competence in the management of the ostomy.

PLANNING THE PATIENT'S CARE

Each patient requires a care plan adapted to his individual requirements that considers not only the patient's surgical experience, but also his preparation for surgery, his recovery from it, and his learning to live with the ostomy.

The patient may be given instruction about the ostomy, and about equipment and general principles of care prior to surgery. Some patients are taught to apply the device even before surgery. Others, too ill or too bewildered to learn care of the ostomy preoperatively, are taught later.

The overall plan for caring for the patient who has an ostomy is adapted to the individual. For example: the plan includes instruction, but just how this instruction is carried out varies according to such factors as the patient's previous knowledge regarding ostomies and his emotional reaction.

A large selection of literature is available from the ostomy groups as well as from manufacturers of ostomy supplies. Reprints of articles which have appeared in professional nursing journals are available from the journal companies, local cancer societies, and some manufacturers. Excellent visual aids such as slides, charts, mini-guides and models are available and helpful in teaching the patient. A small plastic model of a stoma which has a belt attachment can be used for demonstration by the nurse, and the patient can also use these models in learning self-care technics. Preparing the patient for the appearance of the stoma by use of models and diagrams can decrease his anxiety when he first looks at his own stoma.

The patient with a stoma has no sphincter, thus no sphincter control; he is left with a problem of incontinence for the rest of his life. Therefore, efforts to assist him to regain the continent state are imperative. Every effort is made to help the patient reach the stage of recovery in which he feels a mastery over the stoma.

Attitudes

The patient who for any reason is unable to control his bowel movement frequently experiences a great deal of anxiety concerning possible rejection by others. The patient looks upon those who care for him as a reflection of the world at large. The nurse's acceptance of the patient's stoma can help him to accept it. The reactions of friends and family also influence the degree of acceptance that can be expected from the patient. The family may be very upset, wondering whether the odor of fecal drainage will permeate the home, whether relationships with friends can be maintained, and whether or not they can successfully conceal their fear or repugnance from the patient. The nurse can help the family as well as the patient by maintaining a supportive attitude, by assisting the family to learn about the stoma and to deal with their feelings concerning it, and by serving as an example to both the patient and his family in her attitude toward the stoma, and its care and in her care of the equipment being used.

It is essential to work with the patient at his stage of acceptance of the stoma, rather than to imply that he must meet certain inflexible standards set by the nurse. For example, the nurse may set expectations for her own performance in the care of the stoma, such as not wrinkling up her nose, or not carrying out the care hastily with an avoiding type touch. However, she should not imply that the patient must perform in this way. If initially, he shows reluctance or distaste for carrying out the care, the nurse should convey patience and accept his reaction rather than criticize it. This approach usually helps the patient to deal with his own reactions to the stoma care, and thus resolve them.

Attitudes and Reactions

The patient's reaction will guide you in helping him to learn to change his own dressing. You may notice that he does not look at the stoma the first few times that the dressing is changed. Many patients look away, or they cover their eyes with an arm as they lie quietly in bed. It is better not to force such a patient to look by a comment like, "You'd better watch what I'm doing, because soon you'll be doing this yourself." Instead, carry out the dressing deftly and promptly, doing everything, such as controlling odors and disposing of waste, in a way that makes the procedure as smooth as possible. Be especially careful to insure the patient privacy. Many patients dread having the stoma and the drainage exposed, even to the nurse, and they become very distressed if other patients or visitors see it. Make a special effort to show the patient that he is acceptable and clean. Keep everything in his unit spotlessly clean and neat so that his visitors will not be repelled by odors or soiled equipment. Having members of the staff and convalescent patients drop by often for a chat helps the patient to feel that his stoma is not objectionable and that others do not avoid him.

Allow the patient an opportunity to express his feelings about the stoma. It is not unusual for a patient who appeared very brave and eager to learn before the surgery to become depressed and withdrawn after the operation. Usually, however, if those who care for him show patience and support, the patient soon begins to look at the stoma and to develop interest in its care. Sometimes a casual and yet factual comment like, "The drainage is more formed today," helps the patient to begin observing and taking part in the care of his stoma. If he continues avoidance, however, his doctor should be consulted, so that further help with the patient's emotional reaction can be planned. Sometimes the nurse's attention is focused quite narrowly on the stoma and its care. It is important for the nurse to spend some time with the patient when she is not busy with his dressing—time when she can listen and show her concern for the patient, without the stress (for the patient) engendered by the care of the stoma. Particularly if the patient is experiencing difficulty accepting his stoma, such periods can be of special importance in assisting the patient to cope with his feelings.

EXPLANATION AND ASSISTANCE

As soon as the patient begins to observe and demonstrate interest in caring for his stoma, explain each step as you proceed. After several periods of observation, encourage him to help. Ask him to hold the equipment and hand you supplies as you need them. Give the patient an opportunity to wash his hands after he has helped with his bag or dressing change. Too often this important detail is forgotten even though it is taken for granted that the nurse will wash her hands.

Every patient needs to know that his nurse cares about him and understands some of his problems. He needs to know too that she has the knowledge and the ability to help him resolve these problems. The nurse demonstrates this concern and knowledge in caring for her patients by her manner, her skill, and by her attitude with which the care is given. Choice of words and tone of voice are important when the nurse discusses the ostomy with the patient. For example the nurse who gushingly refers to the ostomy as a "rosebud" may impress the patient as insincere and unrealistic; this approach may interfere with the patient's ability to express his feelings (especially negative ones) concerning the ostomy. It is preferable for the nurse to use terms which are neutral, terms which are not always laden with her own emotional reactions or with efforts to cover up her reactions. The word "rosebud" may be usefully employed as a way of describing the appearance of the stoma. If it is used, however, the nurse's tone should convey that this is a factual description of the appearance of the stoma.

When the patient has help with his stoma care a few times and is regaining his strength, he is usually ready to begin to carry out the procedure himself. Stay with him the first few times. Help when needed. Sometimes the nurse thinks that the patient who carries out the procedure correctly for the first or second time needs no further help. This often gives the patient the feeling that the nurse is eager to be rid of the task of caring for his ostomy. Even though the patient can carry out the technic of his stoma care adequately, arrange to be with him sometimes when he changes the dressing. This will enable you to observe how he is applying what he has learned. It will also give you an opportunity to note the condition of the skin, and the type and the amount of fecal drainage, and it will convey to the patient your continued interest and willingness to help.

For many patients this change in body function constitutes a loss. The nurse can help by exploring with the patient what the loss means to him. For example, one patient described it as loss of a diseased body part which endangered his health and even his life. By losing the diseased part, he gained freedom from disease and an opportunity to regain his normal health and a chance to return to living a useful, productive life.

Most patients view this experience as a loss and will go through a grieving process. This cannot be hurried. It takes time and patience and a sincere sustained concern and interest for the patient in order to help him at this time. The patient may experience a period of disbelief, denial, anger, discouragement or despair before he finally accepts the situation.

He may even be suicidal. The nurse's and doctor's presence, their concern and their helpfulness are essential here not only in accepting the patient in his grief, but also in helping him to see what progress he has made (however slight). Recovered ostomates can also provide help and encouragement. Some patients require psychiatric help to progress through stages of grief and to begin to cope with the ostomy.

The nurse and the physician should discuss each patient and his care as it evolves. The nurse should initiate the instruction necessary after consultation with the physician. Decisions about who will teach the patient the various aspects of his care must be made promptly and definitely lest the patient be discharged before he is able to care for himself. The physician informs the patient what surgery is required and why and explains the pathology to the patient. The nurse reviews this with the patient as necessary. The plan of who teaches what must be definite and agreed upon by the nurse and physician. The nurse teaches what is necessary for self care, appliance, skin care, etc., as detailed elsewhere in this chapter. The patient should *receive the equipment and instruction in its use and care while hospitalized, and should have an opportunity to demonstrate his ability to manage the ostomy prior to discharge.* Referral to the visiting nurse service or a stoma clinic for nursing care should be made upon discharge.

Visitors From Ostomy Groups

It is often beneficial to have a member of the visiting committee of the local ostomy group visit the patient. A visit from a person who has successfully mastered the care of his stoma and who has resumed his work and family life can convey to the patient a sense that it is possible to be well-groomed, attractive and successful despite an ostomy.

The nurse or doctor can find an ostomy visitor by contacting the local ostomy group (see listing in local telephone directory). Plans for the visit must first be discussed with the physician. His agreement that the visit would be beneficial is necessary before the visit is planned. It is helpful to give the person from the ostomy club who arranges visits the following information: type of visit (preoperative or postoperative), patient's age, occupation, language barrier, physical handicaps, or any other pertinent factor significant to rehabilitation.

The club's chairman of visiting arrangements will try to select a visitor with a background similar to that of the patient. The visitor may bring literature which he will leave with the patient. The visitor checks with the nurse so that he can be escorted and be introduced to the patient. This protocol provides the nurse with an opportunity to meet the visitor and discuss with him any special purposes in the visit.

THE PATIENT WITH AN ILEOSTOMY

An ileostomy is a surgically formed opening into the ileum for the drainage of fecal matter. A loop of ileum is brought out on the lower right quadrant of the abdomen, slightly below the umbilicus, near the outer border of the rectus muscle, and a stoma is formed. The stoma is "matured" at the time of surgery by everting the bowel and suturing the cut end of the ileum to the skin. The rationale for maturing the stoma is that it provides a seal at the base of the stoma. This technic promotes healing and provides a smooth peristomal area, thus permitting the application of the permanent appliance much sooner than is permissible in the nonmatured stoma. Serositis is prevented from developing as this technic eliminates the ileal flow over the serosal surface.

Fecal drainage from the ileostomy is of a liquid consistency at first since it is discharged before it passes through the colon where water absorption normally takes place. Therefore, an ileostomy requires the immediate application of a collecting appliance over the stoma to collect this fecal matter. The surgeon applies a temporary disposable plastic pouch to the skin over the stoma at the time of the operation. This pouch should be of the drainable type and may have an adhesive facing or a karaya gum seal with or without an adhesive facing.

Indications for Ileostomy. Ulcerative colitis is a common indication for ileostomy. It has been found that when a temporary ileostomy is performed, the disease process in the colon persists despite the diversion of the fecal stream. The removal of the diseased colon (colectomy) is necessary to halt the disease. When the colon has been removed the ileostomy is permanent. The procedure may be done in one, two, or three stages.

IMMEDIATE POSTOPERATIVE CARE

The principles of postoperative care are the same as those for any patient who has had surgery on the gastrointestinal tract. The use of a Levin tube and suction and the administration of parenteral fluids are usual in the immediate postoperative period. Within several days these treatments usually are discontinued, and oral feedings of easily digested foods are begun. The patient is encouraged gradually to resume a normal diet, excluding only those foods that he has found cause him to have gas or diarrhea.

Electrolyte imbalance due to large output of fluid through the ileum is a particular problem for the patient with an ileostomy. The patient is cautioned to observe for weakness, trembling and confusion especially when the ileal output is profuse. He may require administration of intravenous fluids for fluid electrolyte replacement; therefore, these symptoms should be reported to the doctor when they occur. The nurse should have a *thorough understanding* of fluid requirements and fluid therapy replacement within the context of the nursing role.

The patient returns from the operating room with a stoma and a surgical incision through which the operation has been performed. The stoma is usually covered either with a plastic disposable pouch or with fluffy gauze dressings. Sometimes the close proximity of the stoma to the surgical incision makes it especially difficult to avoid fecal contamination of the surgical incision. The plastic pouch which can be fitted snugly around the stoma and secured with adhesive, helps to prevent the fecal drainage from seeping into the surgical incision. Collodion may be used to seal the dressing over the incision, so that liquid feces cannot run in. Wide strips of adhesive may be applied tightly over the entire dressing covering the incision to protect it from fecal drainage.

Often when a colostomy is performed, the stoma is matured at surgery. That is, the stoma is everted and sutured down, and thus is open. If the stoma is not matured at surgery, a loop of bowel is brought out onto the abdomen. About 24 to 36 hours after the operation, the loop of bowel is opened, by cutting or cautery, to form the stoma. In this way the initial healing of the incision takes place without danger of contamination. The latter procedure is not physically painful, since the bowel is not sensitive to pain as the skin is. The opening of the colostomy usually is carried out at the patient's bedside or in the treatment room. The bed should be well protected, and a temporary ostomy pouch rather than a basin is used to receive the initial flow of liquid feces. The initial gush of fecal material from the stoma can be upsetting to the patient even when he understands what to expect. The patient should be prepared for the pungent odor of the cauterized tissue which will disappear shortly.

Dressings may be used over the stoma immediately after the operation. Fluffed, clean gauze is shaped into rings or doughnuts, and several of these are placed around the stoma. The stoma itself then is covered with several gauze fluffs. A similar result may be achieved by cutting holes the size of the stoma in several cellulose pads and placing them, one by one, over the stoma; several pads, left whole, are placed over the top of the stoma. This method of applying the dressing helps to absorb and to control the leakage around the stoma. Depending on the amount of the drainage, the entire dressing may be covered with several combination or "abd" pads. Montgomery straps are used to hold the dressings in place. Their use makes the application and the removal of the adhesive less frequent, and thus irritation of the skin is lessened.

Moving about in bed, coughing and early ambulation may be made more difficult by the patient's fear of soiling his clothing and his bedding. Apply the dressing snugly, and change it frequently enough, so that the patient is more willing to move about. Above all, give him the feeling that some soiling is inevitable in the immediate postoperative period, and that the changing of dressings and even of bedding is both accepted and expected by the nursing staff. Promptness in changing the soiled dressings and proceeding in a matter-of-fact manner with a sure touch do more than words to assure the patient that his condition is accepted.

Nursing measures for deep breathing, coughing, turning, exercising the toes and legs are carried out as for other surgical patients. Medication for relief of pain and discomfort should be given as required. Nursing care should be planned to provide the patient with adequate time to rest. Some surgeons advocate the use of elastic bandages to both legs (to prevent thrombophlebitis) for several days until the patient is ambulating well. If used they should be rewrapped at least once each eight-hour period. If the newer disposable cohesive bandage (3M) is used, caution should be taken not to apply the wrap too tightly (approximately $\frac{1}{3}$ of the stretch capacity will suffice for most patients). These can be reused several times if care is taken when removing them.

Temporary Bag. A temporary bag or pouch usually is placed over the stoma during the immediate postoperative period. The stoma is measured and a hole is cut in the top of the pouch that is just the right size to fit around the stoma. Some of the bags already have a hole in the top; however, this hole often has to be enlarged so that it will fit over the stoma. A commonly used type is made of plastic and has a square of double-faced adhesive at the top. One side of the adhesive sticks to the skin around the stoma; the other adheres to the plastic material. The lower end of the plastic pouch is folded securely and held closed with elastic bands. When the pouch is emptied, a large emesis basin is placed to catch the return, and the elastic bands are removed, allowing the drainage to flow out the bottom of the pouch into the emesis basin. The entire appliance is disposable, and a fresh one is used if leakage occurs.

The temporary plastic pouch is used for a variety of conditions in which drainage occurs from a stoma. Because of edema, the stoma is larger immediately after surgery than it will be later. The size of the stoma changes considerably during the initial postoperative period. The temporary appliance is especially useful because fresh ones can be cut to fit the stoma as often as they are necessary. After healing has occurred and the

FIG. 37-1. The permanent ileostomy appliance. A variety of permanent ileostomy appliances are available from the manufacturer. The features of these appliances vary as to pouch size, pouch length, pouch shape and faceplate (disk) design. (United Surgical Corp.)

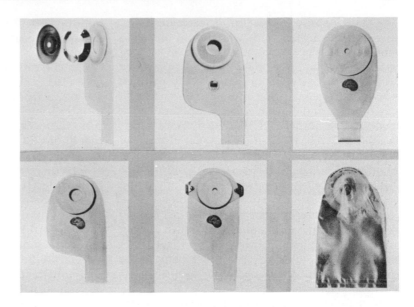

stoma has reached its permanent size and shape, a permanent appliance is fitted.

APPLICATION OF THE TEMPORARY POSTOPERATIVE APPLIANCE.

Adhesive Type. Prepare the skin by cleansing with soap and water. Pat dry. Apply one or two coats of tincture of benzoin on wet skin and dust on karaya powder or apply surgical cement. Permit cement to dry five minutes if used. Tincture of benzoin should be tacky and dry before applying the appliance. If temporary bag does not have exact size opening, measure stoma and add ⅛-in. clearance around stoma to allow for stomal size change. A karaya ring can be placed around base of stoma before applying bag. Secure end of bag with bands or barrette-type clamp.

Karaya Gum Ring with Adhesive Facing. Prepare skin as above. Peel off protective backing from adhesive facing and align carefully to guide over stoma evenly. Karaya gum ring should fit snugly around stoma. Secure closure as above.

Karaya Gum Ring. Prepare skin as above. Remove protective covering from karaya ring and guide over stoma. Secure closure as above. The karaya ring can fit snugly around the base of stoma without injuring stoma. Care should be taken not to use hard surface rings close to stoma to avoid injury to stoma.

The three basic features of the *permanent* appliance are:

1. A disk (faceplate) which surrounds the stoma and usually is adhered to the body

2. A pouch for collecting the feces, usually oblong with a spout for emptying

3. Accessories: such as a belt, belt attachments, spout closures, bands or clips

The permanent appliance may be adhered with surgical cement, a karaya gum ring or a double-faced adhesive disk.

Considerations for choosing a permanent appliance are concerned with the disk and its design. Therefore, the location of the stoma, the characteristics of abdominal contour and texture and the characteristics of the stoma must be analyzed for each individual. The material and size of the disk will depend upon individual specifications and patient preferences.

The pouch is that part of the appliance which collects the feces. If there is no fitting problem, pouch size may be the deciding factor in choosing the appliance. There is a wide variety of types of plastic and quality of rubber used with respect to odor permeability. This may be the decisive factor for some patients. Allergy to rubber or other materials may be a factor.

ALLERGY TO RUBBER AND LIQUID OR CREAMS. For those individuals allergic to rubber, patch-testing can be done with small bits of rubber (worn on the skin for 24 hours) obtained from the manufacturers of rubber appliances. A simpler solution is to wear an all-plastic appliance or a two-piece appliance with plastic disk and synthetic rubber pouch or rubber pouch with a cloth cover to avoid irritating contact.

To test for allergy to liquid, saturate ½-in. square of gauze (band-aid) with liquid or cream to be tested. Apply to inner surface of arm or leg and leave in place for 24 hours. A positive reaction (sensitivity) to the material is signified by a burning sensation. Remove test material immediately and clean with soap, water or alcohol. The absence of redness after 24 hours usually indicates no sensitivity. Delayed reaction may occur even after periods of a week in some individuals.

Belts. The belt is an accessory to the appliance. However, it is usually worn for 24 hours just as is the appliance—bathing and sleeping are no exceptions. It may occasionally be omitted when a snugly fitted girdle is worn or if disk edge is reinforced with adhesive. A rubber belt can be used while bathing or swimming as the elastic tends to stretch when wet.

The belt is used for several reasons: it holds the appliance in place when cement is not used, or it provides pressure for a good bond when cement is used. It may be used to support the weight of the appliance and filled pouch and thus prevent the disk from being pulled away from the abdomen by the weight of the liquid fecal material. It provides the new ostomate with the assurance that the appliance will not fall off.

Reston, gauze or flannel padding can be used under a belt which cuts into the flesh. Care should be taken to avoid upward or downward pull on the stoma. The belt should be placed at the level of the stoma, or double belts can be used to equalize pull on the top and bottom of the disk.

Cement is a combination of latex, a hydrocarbon solvent and usually some prophylactic additives. It is used to stick the appliance onto the body and it must be applied to a clean, dry surface. Always apply cement in thin coats and permit each coat to dry thoroughly before applying the next one. This technic permits adequate evaporation of the solvent. Allow five minutes for drying of the cement and evaporation of the solvent. This prevents excoriation of the skin and permits the bond to form. Two thin coats of cement applied to the appliance and the skin will insure a complete covering of the area without excess cement building up. Finding the right cement is a trial and error procedure. The skin should be tested for sensitivity before a cement is used because sensitivity is common. It is not necessary to remove all paste from the disk each time the appliance is changed. Slight paste

buildup provides for better adherence. However, the skin beneath the disk must be left as clean as possible.

Cement can be rolled off the skin and appliance after several days of wearing. If it does not roll off, a little solvent applied with a medicine dropper can be used *gently* with a gauze pad to rub off traces of cement. A *little* solvent is all that is necessary; wipe off the area with water after solvent has been used.

Solvent is a hydrocarbon which is highly inflammable. It is also very irritating and therefore should be applied sparingly between the body and the bag using a medicine dropper. *Excessive* rubbing will cause skin irritation. *Never* use carbon tetrachloride in place of ileostomy solvent. Carbon tetrachloride is the most toxic of all commonly used solvents and is highly dangerous. *Benzine* can be used in an emergency but *not benzene,* which is a hydrocarbon and also hazardous.

Karaya Gum Powder, Karaya Gum Rings and Neo-karaya. Karaya gum powder is made from the resin of the *Sterculia urens* tree in India. It is a useful product in that it protects the skin while it permits healing underneath and it also serves as an adherent for the ostomy appliance. Karaya gum is used by many in place of cement. Karaya gum powder becomes gelatinous when brought in contact with moisture* and can be used in this gummy state. It can be resealed by applying pressure. Rings of karaya gum are also available commercially. One manufacturer supplies ostomy drainage bags with the karaya gum ring already attached. These rings can be cut, pulled or pushed into any shape desired and therefore can be used as a protection at the base of the stoma to correct the problems created by an ill-fitting appliance.

Neo-karaya is karaya gum powder mixed with aluminum hydroxide gel. The watery portion of the aluminum hydroxide gel is poured off and only the thick part is used. This mixture is helpful in reducing the burning sensation of an excoriation and in increasing the healing potentialities of the karaya. However, it is not tacky but leathery and when pulled off it will not restick on itself under renewed pressure as do karaya and water. In severe cases of skin break-

---

* To prepare karaya gum paste: for each one level teaspoonful of karaya add two teaspoonfuls of water. Stir until smooth and tacky and apply to skin. Increase proportions according to amount needed.

down, alternating layers of aluminum hydroxide and karaya are recommended.

CHANGING THE APPLIANCE

The important factors in regard to changing the appliance are time and frequency.

There are two factors to remember. The first and the cardinal rule for changing the appliance is that when there is a burning or itching sensation underneath the disk or pain around the stoma the appliance should be removed immediately. This should be done regardless of whether the appliance has been on one hour or several days. The stoma and skin should be examined carefully to determine the cause of the difficulty. Excoriation of the skin is to be avoided at all costs. Resorting to the use of a temporary postoperative appliance may be advisable until the cause is identified and eliminated. The most frequent cause is leakage of fecal drainage or reaction to solvent or cement. (Stinging, tingling or itching may be experienced immediately after an appliance change, and will subside quickly. If the sensation is prolonged or intensified, remove the appliance.)

Second, the appliance should be changed at a time when the bowel is relatively quiet. For most ostomates this time is early in the morning, before eating or two to three hours after mealtime. However, it is best to check the patient to note the times of least bowel activity. A record of these times should be made on the patient's chart in order to coordinate plans for the patient's care. The patient will be very much aware and even concerned about the frequency of bowel activity in the beginning. However, he should be assured that as the bowel adjusts to its new state, the activity lessens. Usually, it is most active after eating and relatively quiet at other times. The patient should have quiet and privacy when making the appliance change.

A few surgeons believe that the first appliance change should be made in 24 hours. Most other surgeons think that the first change should be made in 48 hours unless there is evidence of difficulty such as burning, itching, pain or a tendency for the patient's skin to become irritated. In this case, the appliance is removed so the skin and stoma may be inspected. Too frequent changes are thought to be inadvisable, because, in removing the appliance one may remove the protective layers of epithelium and cause it to become raw and excoriated. However, if the skin and stoma appear intact, wearing time can gradually be increased to a week or longer. The two-piece appliances permit inspection of the stoma by removing only the pouch while the disk remains cemented to the body.

CARE OF THE SKIN

It is imperative that meticulous care be given the circumstomal area to prevent excoriation and skin breakdown. Time and expense should not be spared, because ileal discharge contains digestive enzymes and acids which undermine the skin; the resulting excoriation may take weeks to heal. The nurse should be aware of such problems so that they may be prevented or treated early should they occur. The nurse should be especially careful to protect the circumstomal area from ileal drainage by placing a tissue cuff around the stoma or using something to collect the drainage (a small paper cup) while caring for the skin.

CONTROL OF ODOR AND GAS

Odor is an individual matter. There are two kinds of odor that the ostomy patient is concerned about. The odor that is present when emptying the ileostomy pouch and the odor which occasionally envelopes an ileostomate and follows him about. Personal cleanliness is essential; however, the ostomate must cope with special problems, such as care of his pouch, to lessen odors.

The really serious odor problem is the particularly identifying smell that occasionally clings to the person. Leakage, the pouch, inadequate changing of the pouch, certain foods or an impending complication may be responsible. Try to ascertain the cause so it can be remedied.

There are a large number of deodorants and deodorizers on the market. These include tablets to be taken orally, such as charcoal, chlorophyll, bismuth subcarbonate, and Derifil (these must be prescribed by the doctor). There are tablets which are inserted in the pouch after each emptying, such as charcoal, chlorophyll, ordinary aspirin, oxychinol or Dis-Pel, and Odo-Way tablets. Others are in liquid form. These include Nilodor (only one drop is needed), Deo-Drops, Banish and isopropyl alcohol. A paper tissue sprayed or saturated with alcohol can be placed in the pouch. There are also aerosol deodorant sprays, such as Turgasept, Ozone and Lysol. In an emergency, aerosol underarm deodorant sprays can be used to clear the odor from the room.

To deter odor in warm weather, try slipping a plastic bag or saran wrap over the appliance. Keep the appliance clean.

To control odor at its source, a restricted diet of tea, toast and marmalade and the addition of one food at a time may be tried. Foods containing condiments, fish, eggs, onions, and cheese should be omitted. These frequently cause odors that linger. However, the patient must do this under medical supervision and work up to an adequate diet.

Medications, especially antibiotics and anti-tuberculous drugs, may cause particularly strong odors which cling to the appliance. The use of an old pouch or disposable pouches while taking these medications is helpful.

Intestinal gas is often as much as 85 per cent swallowed air. Sighing, chewing, gulping down food, and breathing with the mouth open all contribute to this component of intestinal gas. Eating slowly and chewing food well with the mouth closed help to reduce gas formation.

Some foods are gas producing and should be avoided temporarily, such as cabbage, onions, pork, beans and peppers. Later some individuals find they can add small amounts of these foods to the diet.

Both charcoal tablets and Mylicon tablets or Mylicon liquid are prescribed sometimes to relieve distress due to gas. They break up the gas bubble at its source and reduce the discomfort of bloating.

BLOCKAGE

A blockage is a serious complication. It may be due to a twisted, strangulated, or incarcerated bowel, an internal hernia, or a bolus of food caused by poorly chewed, inadequately digested, stringy, pasty or fibrous foods. A liquid ileal flow or no ileal flow will signify an obstruction. *The doctor should be consulted.*

The permanent appliance should be removed and a temporary postoperative appliance with a larger disk opening than normally worn should be used to allow for stoma swelling and to permit observation of the stoma. The stoma may become edematous and cyanotic.

Careful irrigation by the physician may relieve the obstruction if due to a food blockage. The patient may need to have surgical intervention if the bowel is twisted or strangulated.

Stenosis, tightening, and narrowing of the stoma may eventually require surgical revision. The surgeon may wish to have the patient dilate the stoma daily for a while to prevent further difficulty. The patient inserts a well lubricated index finger into the stoma for a few minutes. This should be done only on the surgeon's advice. The nail should be cut short to prevent injury to the bowel.

Prolapse or protrusion of the ileostomy is fairly common, and if it is of moderate degree (2–3 inches) it can be disregarded. Even longer prolapses might be symptomless and harmless. A truss type of support can be worn on the advice of the patient's physician. *However, should there be a sudden prolapse of the stoma, the permanent appliance should be removed immediately and a temporary appliance used and the physician should be notified.* A prolapse should be replaced by the physician as soon as possible. Edema may occur and lead to obstruction from restriction of blood supply and necrosis may result if the prolapse is not promptly and skillfully managed. Once prolapse of the stoma has occurred, its recurrence is more likely. Occasionally the prolapse occurs when the patient is far from medical help. In this instance either the patient or a companion replaces the prolapse and medical care is sought as quickly as possible.

PATIENT WITH A COLOSTOMY

A colostomy is an artificial opening of the large bowel brought out to the abdomen and fashioned into a stoma. The stoma is a small round structure which is pink in color and moist, velvety and smooth in texture. Changes in size and color of stoma vary with activity and emotional status. Anger or extreme annoyance may produce a very red or purplish color. Small beads of blood may ooze from the surface. Fright may cause blanching of the stoma. These are normal reactions and are insignificant in that the tissues will revert to their normal state when the cause is alleviated. It is important for the nurse to explain to the patient that these are normal reactions.

The presence of a cancerous lesion, an ulcerative inflammatory process, multiple polyposis or injury can be indications for a colostomy.

Types of Colostomies

A colostomy may be described in a number of ways depending upon its purpose, duration or location. It may be temporary or permanent. If described by location, it may be ascending, transverse, descending or sigmoid. It may have a single loop or a double loop (double-barreled). It may be described in terms of its therapeutic

FIG. 37-2. Single- and double-barreled colostomy. (A)
One type of single-barreled
colostomy. The distal portion of the bowel has been
removed, and the colostomy
is permanent. (B) One type
of double-barreled colostomy,
showing proximal and distal
loops. This type of colostomy
may or may not be per-
manent.

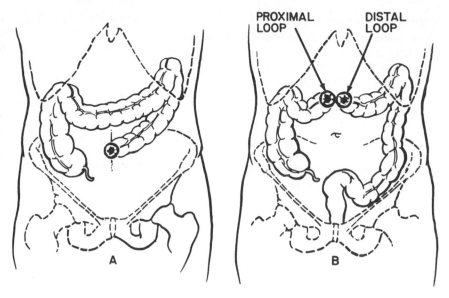

PROXIMAL LOOP   DISTAL LOOP

A   B

effect on the patient and be either curative or
palliative.

The type of colostomy the patient has will tell
you not only the location of the stoma but will
also help you to anticipate the needs of the
patient. When speaking of a colostomy in general terms, it usually relates to a sigmoid location.
Problems experienced by the patients who have
this procedure depend to a large extent upon the
type of colostomy which has been created.

Single- and Double-barreled Colostomies.
Colostomies may be double-barreled or single-
barreled. A double-barreled colostomy connects
with both the proximal and the distal portions
of the bowel. The portion of the bowel leading
from the small intestine to the stoma, through
which the feces pass to the outside, is called the
proximal portion, and its opening is called the
proximal opening or *loop* of the colostomy. The
distal portion of the bowel leads from the stoma
to the anus. Because the fecal drainage has been
diverted, the distal portion of the bowel does not
pass feces by way of the anus. However, mucus
often collects in this portion of bowel. Sometimes, the double-barreled colostomy is a temporary procedure and, after disease or injury in the
distal portion has been treated, the continuity of
the bowel is restored.

A single-barreled colostomy consists of one
opening through which fecal matter is passed.
The opening is that of the proximal portion of
the bowel. The distal portion of the bowel usu-

ally has been surgically removed, and the colostomy is permanent.

When a double-barreled colostomy is irrigated,
it is important to distinguish between the proximal and the distal loops. Often the irrigation is
ordered only for the proximal portion of the
bowel. At other times, the doctor requests that
both the proximal and the distal portions be irrigated. Ask the doctor to show you which opening is proximal and which is distal. Draw a diagram, and place it on the chart to guide all who
do the irrigation. If this diagram has not been
drawn and you are not sure which opening is
which, inspect them both for a few minutes. The
one from which the feces is flowing is the proximal loop.

The transverse double-barreled colostomy is
usually temporary. The interval before the continuity of the bowel is re-established may be from
one month to sixteen months or longer. When
the diseased portion of the bowel is removed or
healed the bowel is reconnected by anastomosis.
This is a much simpler procedure and there is
less discomfort to the patient than from the original procedure. Most physicians will insert a
nasogastric tube and give intravenous fluids for
a few days. As soon as bowel function returns,
these measures are discontinued. The patient
occasionally will experience some distress with
gas-producing foods for the bowel may narrow at
the anastomotic site. Rarely is it necessary for
the patient to be hospitalized because of this
distress.

Keeping the Patient Clean

The content of the large bowel is liquid in the ascending colon, semiliquid to pasty in the transverse colon, semisolid in the descending and solid in the sigmoid colon. The functions of the large bowel are to reabsorb water and to serve as a storage space for the feces until evacuated.

Control of fecal evacuation, therefore, is based upon the location of the stoma and the function of that portion of the bowel. An ascending type colostomy will need a carefully applied temporary appliance or an ileostomy type permanent pouch.

The patient will need more frequent emptying of the appliance. This should be done promptly to maintain the seal and to protect the patient from soiling. Observe the patient to determine the frequency with which the appliance must be emptied.

At first, the stoma constantly exudes soft and liquid feces. Frequent emptying of the plastic pouch day and night is necessary to keep the patient as clean as possible, to control odors and to prevent excoriation of the skin around the stoma from leakage.

The transverse colostomy (although some surgeons do not consider its irrigation strictly necessary) will be more manageable if irrigated daily to reduce the number of movements and to help eliminate odor. Discuss the need for irrigation with the surgeon. The use of a temporary ostomy bag will protect the skin and prevent contamination of the surgical wound. The descending and sigmoid colostomy are easier to manage because the content of the bowel is semisolid to solid. Scheduled daily irrigation to establish regularity will help the patient achieve control more rapidly. When control is obtained on a once-a-day basis, the patient is ready to try an every-other-day schedule of irrigations.

Clean rather than sterile technic is used because the opening is into the bowel, which normally contains many bacteria, and because the fecal drainage is laden with bacteria. Wash your hands carefully before and after caring for the stoma. If you have a cut on your hand, it is wise to wear a clean rubber glove during the procedure, and then it is essential to explain the reason for the glove to the patient. Otherwise he might interpret the use of the glove as reluctance or distaste on your part to care for his stoma. Collect all the needed equipment first so that you will not have to obtain supplies from cupboards or dressing supply cart while the dressing change is in progress. If you should require additional supplies, wash your hands thoroughly before leaving the patient's unit.

It is convenient to keep all necessary supplies at the patient's bedside, replenishing them as they are needed. The supplies include newspapers or paper bags for wrapping soiled dressings, extra dressings or plastic pouches, and any medication that has been ordered for the patient's skin.

Remove the plastic pouch, empty it if necessary, and wrap it in newspaper. Gently wash the skin around the stoma with mild soap and water. Gauze fluffs or disposable washcloths usually are used for cleansing. If the skin is inflamed, use only water without any soap. Wash gently and yet thoroughly; avoid rubbing because the skin is very easily irritated.

Work neatly. Avoid leaving soiled articles within the patient's view. Wrapping the soiled dressings in newspaper as soon as they are removed helps to control odor as well as to make the entire procedure more acceptable to the patient. Provide adequate ventilation, but do not chill the patient. Room deodorizers may be helpful or an aerosol deodorant spray may be used.

Various preparations may be ordered by the doctor to treat or to prevent excoriation of the skin. Whatever preparation is used it is important to remove it periodically and to observe the condition of the skin underneath. Apply the dressings or the plastic pouch snugly to minimize leakage. The adhesive that holds the plastic pouch against the skin will not stick unless the skin is clean and dry. (If ointment is used it is used sparingly and the excess is wiped off.) Apply the bag smoothly to avoid wrinkles.

Change everything that is soiled, including gowns or bedding as it is necessary.

Try to empty the pouch at least a half-hour or so before meals. Changing it close to mealtime or during the serving of trays interferes with the patient's appetite.

Methods of Colostomy Management

There are three popular methods of colostomy management—irrigation by standard method, irrigation by bulb syringe, and nonirrigation.

The first method and the most widely advocated one for irrigation is the standard method. This method consists of a daily scheduled irrigation with 1000 to 2000 ml. normal saline or tap water. The schedule gradually progresses to every other day, every third day or even twice a week. Equipment used is the standard irrigation setup: receptacle for solution (can or bag) attached to tubing and catheter, and irrigation sleeve or sheath for the fecal return. The amount of fluid instilled varies from 500 ml. to 2000 ml. The patient may be free of spillage from one to three days with effective results.

The second method employs the use of a bulb syringe* of soft rubber and a short rubber catheter. The equipment consists of the syringe, a quart container for solution, and an emesis basin or plastic sheath or apron. This method calls for several instillations of 250 to 500 ml. of solution at a time. Few patients have found this method effective for freedom of spillage for 24 hours or more. Some patients use two instillations a day. It may be an alternate choice when the standard method cannot be used for irrigation. Further investigation of this method is needed.

The nonirrigation or natural method is the third method. With this method, the patient may use a variety of devices to stimulate an evacuation. Prune or orange juice on arising or before bedtime, liquid breakfast, coffee, mild exercises, a mild laxative (Haley's MO or milk of magnesia), or lemon juice in warm water are a few measures which have been effective. The patient usually does not know when the evacuation will occur.

Another device used by nonirrigators is the suppository—glycerine or Dulcolax. It was found that at least seven days lapsed before a pattern began to be established. The movements occurred three to four times daily. Each day the movements became less and less and the time lapse was greater until the patient had two movements a day—one in the morning and one in the evening—but neither at a scheduled time.

Some patients use the suppository in addition to the irrigation method. This method is worthy of further investigation.

The Irrigation Procedure

It is essential that the colostomy patient be assisted with the irrigation procedure, because the effectiveness of the irrigation is the basis for establishing control. It can be easily and simply taught so that the patient can begin to do his own irrigation after it has been demonstrated by the nurse.

Once the equipment is assembled, irrigation solution prepared and air removed from tubing, the patient is seated on the toilet seat or on a chair in front of the toilet with the irrigation sheath directed into the toilet bowl. He is then ready to begin the irrigation. The bottom of the bag containing the irrigating solution is hung approximately at shoulder height. (The size of the catheter lumen and height of the bag determine the rate of flow. The catheter size may vary from size 18 to 28 Fr.)

The catheter is inserted through the plastic cup or through the irrigation sleeve, lubricated and then inserted into the stomal opening. The belt can then be secured after the catheter is inserted into the stoma. The catheter or irrigation tube should be inserted *slowly* and *gently* two to three inches by rotating the catheter. Difficulty inserting the catheter may be due to a hard piece of stool or to a fold of tissue. If there is difficulty inserting the catheter, withdraw the catheter and reinsert or permit water to flow during insertion. *Never* force the catheter. Once the catheter is in place it can be advanced four to ten inches as desired. However, it is necessary only that the catheter be introduced far enough for water to be retained in the bowel. Allow the water to enter the bowel slowly and gently because too rapid an instillation of fluid will result in painful cramping and an ineffective irrigation. If water returns as it is being introduced, clamp off the tubing until the flow ceases. Do not remove the catheter because the return will flow around the catheter; also, difficulty may be encountered during reinsertion. Then release clamp and continue irrigation until desired amount of solution has been used. Remove the catheter and permit the return to flow into the irrigation sleeve. The patient may remain seated on the toilet seat or may close off the edge of the sleeve and walk about to help stimulate an evacuation. Shaving or other personal care can be done while awaiting a fecal return. (Music or reading help relax the patient.)

It requires 20 to 30 minutes for the return to be completed. This time varies from individual to individual and even in the same person at first. The patient will get to know when the irrigation is sufficiently effective and the bowel is clean of feces by a spurt of gas or just a feeling which he has learned indicates that sufficient

---

* For a detailed account of the bulb syringe method see Postel, A. H., *et al.*: Simplified method of irrigation of the colonic stoma, *Surg. Gynec. Obstet.* 121:595-598, 1965.

evacuation has occurred. A clue to the effectiveness of the irrigation can be made by observing the return. If the return is watery and slightly colored and contains no stool, the bowel is probably clean. If the return is heavy with stool or thick, the bowel is not clean and an additional instillation of 500 or 1000 ml. of fluid may be necessary. Use as a guide the amount of water which returns. If what is instilled is returned, you can safely put in more. If what is instilled is not returned, you may need to siphon back the fluid or discontinue the irrigation at that point. Fluid which is not returned at time of irrigation is absorbed by the blood stream and is later voided. Patients should be discouraged from using more than two quarts of water at a time lest water intoxication result. Soap is not recommended. MacFee found that soap causes tiny hemorrhages in the bowel; therefore it should be avoided for general use. Some surgeons may advise addition of salt or soda bicarbonate to the water for individual patients. As a general rule this is not necessary. Ordinary tepid tap water will suffice (Temp. 105° F.).

Cramping may be a problem to some patients during the irrigation. A slight cramp may simply be a signal that the bowel is ready to empty. Water which is too cold or introduced too rapidly or failure to release air from tubing before inserting the fluid may cause cramping. If cramping occurs, merely pinch off the tubing, have the patient sit up straight, take a few deep breaths and relax. Cramping usually will last about a minute. When the cramp is gone, release the tubing and continue the irrigation.

Failure of the water to return may occur occasionally, even in experienced individuals. This may be caused by the catheter being inserted too far and the water remaining in the bowel temporarily, or water, trapped behind a hard stool, may be absorbed. To encourage the return of fluid material more promptly one or several of the following activities is suggested to the patient: gentle massage of the lower abdomen, tightening the abdominal muscles, taking several deep breaths and relaxing, gently twisting the body (at waist) from side to side, standing up or sitting more erect. If these measures are not effective and the patient is uncomfortable or distressed, notify the physician.

Flushing the bag from below or through a small opening made near the top of the bag will help to eliminate odors from drainage. The irrigation set can be used to flush the bag. The opening at the top of the bag should be covered with a small piece of adhesive tape to prevent leakage.

After the irrigation is completed, remove the irrigation sheath, rinse in cool water to reduce odor and discard, or clean in warm soapy water if it is to be reused.

It is the irrigation of the proximal loop that has been discussed above. If the distal loop is to be irrigated, the patient should sit on a bedpan or on the toilet seat because the solution will be expelled through the rectum. Usually mucus and, sometimes, necrotic tissue are expelled along with the solution. Examine the return carefully before discarding it. Sometimes, to decrease the number of bacteria in the bowel, an order is given for one of the sulfa drugs or neomycin to be instilled into the distal loop after the irrigation has been completed. The drug is dissolved in water and is instilled through the catheter into the distal loop of the bowel. Ask the patient to retain this solution as long as possible. Having him lie down while the medication is inserted helps him to retain it. Make sure that the bedding is well protected, and that a bedpan is handy.

Stomal Covering

The stoma may be covered with a gauze pad or temporary postoperative ostomy bag. If a gauze pad is worn, apply a small amount of lubricating jelly over the area which will come in contact with the stoma to prevent irritation of the stoma. An adhesive drainable bag or a karaya seal drainable bag is recommended for those individuals who continue to have drainage problems between irrigations. A permanent bag is not recommended.

Scheduling Irrigations

There should be uninterrupted use of the bathroom for at least one hour for the irrigation. Select a time convenient to the patient to fit into his schedule of activities. Other members of the household should be considered when setting the time for irrigation.

Katona studied the effect of normal rhythmic patterns in obtaining control and found that if the irrigation was done approximately around the time of previous bowel activity the control was effected more readily. She advises that a regularly scheduled time for the irrigation should be adhered to in the beginning. Later when control is established the time can be varied, and she suggests the following: a daily irrigation at first until control is established for 24 hours; then observe the patterning of bowel activity. When there is little or no fecal return at the time of irrigation, the irrigation can be done every other day; by observing the same pattern it can be extended to every third day. Some patients who have a tendency to have gas prefer to irrigate daily. This is a personal preference rather than a necessity.

Travel can be undertaken as soon as the patient receives his doctor's permission. Upsets can be avoided by planning in advance and by sticking to established routine. Remember water that is not drinkable is not desirable for irrigation either. Boiled or bottled water can be used. The local public health service will advise about specific concerns regarding water or foods to avoid in traveling. The local ostomy society can help with available physicians in places to be visited. Take along any supplies or equipment which may be needed in a special bag or suitcase. Carrying this bag personally will prevent needless worry over possible loss of the bag during travel.

Diet

Occasionally the physician may prescribe a special diet to help if there are irregular bowel movements or excessive gas. Otherwise a regular diet (unless there is a particular problem) can be taken with special attention to avoiding gas-forming foods such as dry beans, cabbage, uncooked onions, cheese and fish. When trying new foods, introduce one new food at a time to determine if it can be tolerated. Allow at least one day to lapse between adding new foods.

Adjustment in the diet can be made if diarrhea or constipation is a problem. Elimination of distressing food items will help to control diarrhea. Increasing the amount of bulk, water or eating laxative type foods will aid in correcting constipation. The physician should be consulted on these problems should they continue to persist after temporary measures have been used. Attention to eating slowly with mouth closed and chewing food well will reduce gas which is caused chiefly by swallowing air rather than by processes of digestion.

Clothing

With the exception of too tightly fitted items, no adjustment needs to be made regarding type of clothing worn. Women are advised to wear girdles without bones or stays lest the stoma be injured. Those of light weight expandable material such as lycra or spandex are suggested. It is *not* advisable to cut a hole in the garment for the protrusion of the stoma as this defeats the purpose of the garment. Those individuals who require a firm support (such as patients who have back problems and who wear braces) may find a stoma shield helpful in preventing undue pressure or irritation of the stoma.

CECOSTOMY

An opening made in the cecum for the drainage of intestinal contents is called a cecostomy. Usually, this is a temporary measure performed to relieve intestinal obstruction. When the patient's physical condition has improved, further surgery may be carried out. The performance of the cecostomy is a relatively minor procedure, usually done under local anesthesia. An opening is made into the cecum through a small incision in the lower abdomen, and a large catheter is placed in the cecostomy to drain feces. The catheter is connected with a drainage bottle that collects the liquid feces, and is sutured to the skin to prevent displacement.

Although the fecal material draining from the cecum is usually liquid, small clumps of formed stool also may be present and may clog the catheter. Irrigations of the catheter usually are ordered to prevent clogging. The frequency of the irrigations and the amount and the type of solution to be used are ordered by the physician. Normal saline commonly is used for the irrigation. It is allowed to run into the cecostomy tube by gravity, through an Asepto syringe. The glass portion of the syringe without the rubber bulb is used as a funnel through which the normal saline flows into the cecostomy tube. It is important not to exert any pressure (such as by using the rubber bulb) when you are doing the irrigation, because this might injure the bowel. If the fluid will not run into the tube by gravity, the physician should be consulted. The tube may be obstructed, and another tube may need to be inserted.

Fecal material may leak around the tube onto the skin. Dressings, if used,* are applied to absorb the drainage and are changed frequently to control soiling and odor and to prevent excoriation of the skin. The principles of caring for

---

* Temporary postoperative bags are preferred to dressings.

any patient who has an opening of his bowel onto the skin are similar to those for a patient with a colostomy or an ileostomy.

REFERENCES AND BIBLIOGRAPHY

ALEXANDER, E. L., BURLEY, W., ELLISON, D., and VALLERI, R.: *Care of the Patient in Surgery Including Techniques*, pp. 642-663, St. Louis, Mosby, 1967.

BACON, H. E., and OCHSNER, A.: *Ulcerative Colitis*, Philadelphia, Lippincott, 1958.

BELAND, I. L.: *Clinical Nursing*, pp. 920-1004, New York, Macmillan, 1965.

BROOKE, B. N.: *Ulcerative Colitis and Its Surgical Treatment*, Chap. 6, Edinburgh, Livingstone, 1954.

BRUNNER, L. S., EMERSON, O. P., JR., FERGUSON, L. K., and SUDDARTH, D. S.: *Textbook of Medical-Surgical Nursing*, ed. 2, Philadelphia, Lippincott, 1970.

CHERESCAVICH, G.: *A Textbook for Nursing Assistants*, ed. 2, Chaps. 28 and 29, St. Louis, Mosby, 1968.

DAVIS, L.: *Christopher's Textbook of Surgery*, ed. 9, Philadelphia, Saunders, 1968.

DENNIS, C., and KARLSON, K. E.: Cancer risk in ulcerative colitis; formidability per year in late disease, *Surgery* 50:568, 1961.

DERRICKS, V. C.: Rehabilitation of patients with ileostomy, *Am. J. Nurs.* 61:48-51, May, 1961.

DISON, N. G.: *American Atlas of Nursing Techniques*, pp. 165-174, St. Louis, Mosby, 1967.

ELLISON, E. H., FRIESEN, S. R., and MULHOLLAND, J. H.: *Current Surgical Management, III*, pp. 409-424, Philadelphia, Saunders, 1965.

HILL, L. D., STONE, C. S., and BAKER, J. W.: One-stage abdominoproctocolectomy and ileostomy, *AMA Arch. Surg.* 83:98, 1961.

HILL, L. D., STONE, C. S., and BAKER, J. W.: One-stage aspects of ulcerative colitis, *AMA Arch. Surg.* 72:968, 1956.

INGLES, T., and CAMPBELL, E.: The patient with a colostomy, *Am. J. Nurs.* 58:1544-1546, 1958.

KATONA, E. A.: Learning colostomy control, *Am. J. Nurs.* 67:3, March, 1967.

————: Patient centered living oriented approach to the patient with artificial anus or bladder, *Nurs. Clin. N. Am.* 2:623-634, December, 1967.

LINDER, J.: Inexpensive colostomy irrigation equipment, *Am. J. Nurs.* 58:1544-1546, 1958.

Manual for Ileostomy Patients, ed. 5, Boston, Q.T., Inc., 1965.

POSTEL, A. H., GRIER, W. R., and LOCALIO, S. A.: A simplified method of irrigation of the colonic stoma, *Surg. Gynec. Obstet.* 121:595-598, 1965.

SHAFER, K., SAWYER, J., McCLUSKEY, A., and BECK, E.: *Medical Surgical Nursing*, ed. 3, St. Louis, Mosby, 1964.

SIEGEL, R., and PAPUSH, H.: *The ABC of Ileostomy*, p. 90, Jamaica, N.Y., Custom Service, 1963.

SUTTON, A. L.: *Bedside Nursing Techniques in Medicine and Surgery*, ed. 2, Philadelphia, Saunders, 1969.

TURNBULL, R. B., JR.: Management of the Ileostomy, *Am. J. Surg.* 86:617, 1953.

Your Ileostomy: A Guide for the New Patient, Q.T., Inc. (c/o The Medical Foundation, Inc., 29 Commonwealth Ave., Boston, Mass. 02116), 1962.

ZIMMERMAN, L. M., and LEVINE, R.: *Physiologic Principles of Surgery*, ed. 2, Chap. 22, Philadelphia, Saunders, 1964.

Manufacturers and Distributors of Ostomy Products and Literature

Atlantic Surgical Co., Inc.
2287 Babylon Turnpike
Merrick, L.I., N.Y. 11566

Hollister Incorporated
211 East Chicago Avenue
Chicago, Ill. 60611
(Karaya gum rings and disposable appliances)

John F. Greer Co.
5335 College Avenue
Oakland, Calif. 94618
(Nuova and others)

United Surgical Corporation
Division of Howmet Corporation
11775 Starkey Road
Largo, Fla. 33540
(Binkley, Universal, Bruschwig, Featherlite, Stoma models and teaching materials)

Literature containing product information and articles on care

Ostomy Quarterly
1111 Wilshire Boulevard
Los Angeles, Calif. 90017

United Ostomy Association, Inc.
1111 Wilshire Boulevard
Los Angeles, Calif. 90017
(List of United Ostomy Associations and component organizations)

The Patient with an Intestinal or Rectal Disorder

38

Appendicitis • Peritonitis • Hernia • Diverticulosis and Diverticulitis • Hemorrhoids • Pilonidal Sinus

APPENDICITIS

Appendicitis is one of the most common surgical emergencies. The appendix—a narrow, blind tube located at the tip of the cecum—may become inflamed, for reasons that are not entirely clear. It is believed that obstruction occurs, making it difficult or impossible for the contents of the appendix to empty normally. Since the intestinal contents are laden with bacteria, an injury to the tissues in contact with the contents will often result in an infection. A hard mass of feces, called a *fecalith,* may obstruct and mechanically irritate the appendix. Inflammation and infection quickly may follow. The pressure from the fecalith and the edema of tissues that occurs during the inflammation may interfere with the blood supply, making the tissues more vulnerable to infection and leading sometimes to gangrene and perforation. Perforation is a dreaded complication, because if the intestinal contents flow into the peritoneal cavity, they can cause generalized peritonitis or, if the peritonitis is localized, an abscess.

Incidence and Symptoms

Appendicitis can occur at any age. However, it seems to be more common among adolescents and young adults.

An attack of severe abdominal pain is the most common symptom of appendicitis. Often, the pain is generalized throughout the abdomen at first, or it is localized around the umbilicus. Later in the attack, the pain typically occurs in the lower right quadrant of the abdomen. *Mc-*

Burney's point, midway between the umbilicus and the right iliac crest, is usually the site of the most severe pain. Often, the pain is most severe when manual pressure over McBurney's point is suddenly released. This is called *rebound tenderness.*

Slight or moderate fever and moderate leukocytosis often occur. Nausea and vomiting may

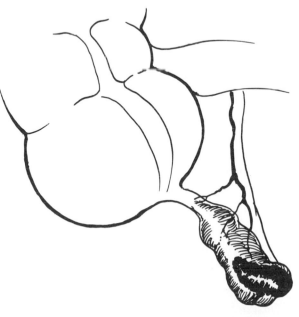

FIG. 38-1. Appendicitis. The entire appendix is red and swollen, and the tip is gangrenous. The gangrenous portion is likely to rupture, spilling its contents into the peritoneal cavity.

be present. The symptoms among the very young and the very aged are often atypical.

Diagnosis

The doctor performs a physical examination, noting especially the location of the pain and the tenderness in the abdomen. A white blood count usually is taken, and additional tests and examinations may be ordered as they are necessary to rule out other conditions that might be causing the symptoms.

Treatment

The appendix is removed surgically, resulting in complete cure. The appendix has no known function within the body, and its removal causes no change in body function. Parenteral fluids may be administered preoperatively or postoperatively. On the day after surgery the patient usually is permitted food and fluids as tolerated, and he usually is allowed out of bed on this day. Convalescence is usually rapid, but it depends on the patient's age and general physical condition. A healthy young adult usually is able to return to his regular activities within two to four weeks. He is advised to avoid heavy lifting or unusual exertion for several months.

Nursing Care

The nurse's role involves the early reporting of symptoms that may indicate appendicitis, the preparation of the patient for emergency surgery, and the postoperative nursing care required by any patient who has had abdominal surgery. Preparations for emergency surgery and postoperative care are discussed in Chapter 12.

Prevention of Complications. Early diagnosis and modern surgical treatment have made death from appendicitis a rarity in our country. Nevertheless, death can and does occur. Severe illness and death result all too often from a delay in seeking medical attention and from attempts to relieve the symptoms with home remedies.

Who has not at some time felt pain in the abdomen, whether after eating green apples or perhaps from gas after eating some baked beans? Nausea and vomiting occur from time to time, too, in the lives of most people. It is easy to understand why self-medication and delay in calling the doctor occur.

The nurse can help to reduce complications and death from appendicitis by instructing families in what to do (and especially what *not* to do) when abdominal pain occurs:

• Consult a doctor for any abdominal pain that is severe, or that does not disappear promptly.

• Do not take a cathartic or an enema. Either of these increases peristalsis, which may result in perforation of the inflamed appendix and in peritonitis.

• Take nothing by mouth. Eating may aggravate the condition, and if surgery should be necessary, it is best that the stomach be empty.

• Lie quietly in the position that is most comfortable until the doctor arrives.

PERITONITIS

The term *peritonitis* means inflammation of the *peritoneum,* a serous sac lining the abdominal cavity. The intestines, normally filled with bacteria, are among the organs enclosed in the peritoneum. Any break in the continuity of the intestines that causes a leakage of the intestinal contents can lead to inflammation and infection of the peritoneum. Two of the most common causes of peritonitis are perforation of the appendix and perforation of a duodenal ulcer. In both instances the intestinal contents escape into the peritoneal cavity, causing peritonitis. The infection may be widespread within the peritoneum (generalized peritonitis), or it may be localized and lead to abscess formation. Initial chemical inflammation of the peritoneum often follows the rupture of various organs; however, chemical inflammation usually is followed promptly by bacterial invasion.

Diagnosis

The most severe pain and tenderness usually occur over the area of the greatest peritoneal inflammation. The location of the pain helps the doctor to determine, for example, whether the peritonitis is due to a perforation of the appendix or of the duodenum. A leukocyte count and a roentgenogram of the abdomen are other important aids in the diagnosis.

Symptoms

The symptoms of peritonitis include severe abdominal pain and tenderness, nausea and vomiting. Fever may be absent initially, but the temperature rises as the infection becomes established. The pulse becomes rapid and weak, and the respirations are shallow. The patient avoids movement of the abdomen when he breathes, because such movement increases his pain. He often lies with his knees drawn toward his abdomen, because this position seems to lessen the pain. *Paralytic ileus* (paralysis of intestines), a condition in which peristalsis fails, and flatus and intestinal contents accumulate in the bowel, typically accompanies peritonitis. The patient's abdomen is rigid and boardlike at the onset of peritonitis. As the condition progresses, the abdomen becomes somewhat softer and very distended with the gas and the intestinal contents that cannot pass normally through the tract. Marked leukocytosis commonly occurs in peritonitis.

If the infection is uncontrolled, the patient becomes very weak; his pulse becomes even more rapid and thready; his abdomen is distended further, leading to even more shallow breathing; and his temperature falls. The patient is moribund.

Prevention, Treatment and Nursing Care

Modern treatment has saved many patients who would have died from peritonitis in years past and has prevented its occurrence in many other patients. The early diagnosis and treatment of such conditions as appendicitis have decreased the incidence of peritonitis. Strict surgical asepsis and the use of antibiotics before performing surgery on the intestines have diminished the number of patients who develop peritonitis as a complication of surgery.

Preventing further leakage of intestinal contents into the peritoneal cavity is an important measure in treatment. If the duodenum has perforated due to peptic ulcer, the area of perforation is closed surgically, so that no further escape of the intestinal contents can take place. If the intestinal contents are leaking from a ruptured appendix, the appendix is removed. Gastrointestinal decompression is used to drain the accumulated gas and the intestinal contents that are prevented by intestinal paralysis from passing normally through the tract.

The replacement of fluids and electrolytes is also important. The patient can take nothing by mouth, and water and electrolytes are being lost in vomitus and in the drainage from the gastrointestinal intubation. Large quantities of body fluids and electrolytes collect in the peritoneal cavity instead of circulating normally throughout the body, thus increasing the problem of water and electrolyte imbalance.

Large doses of antibiotics are given to combat infection. Analgesics, such as meperidine (Demerol), are often necessary to relieve pain and to promote rest. The head of the patient's bed is elevated to allow drainage to settle in the pelvic region, where, if abscesses occur, they may be drained more readily.

All of these measures are designed to aid the body in its fight against the infection, thereby providing favorable conditions for healing.

Nursing Care. The patient with peritonitis is very ill, and he requires detailed care and observation. His symptoms often change rapidly, and the nurse must be ready to answer and to record information about such questions as:

• Is his abdomen more distended? Is it softer, or more rigid?

• Is the pain growing less? Where does the patient feel the most severe pain?

• Is gas being passed rectally? Has the patient had a bowel movement?

• Is he vomiting? What is the character of the vomitus?

• Is the pulse weaker, more rapid? Is his temperature rising?

• How much has he voided? How much drainage has been returned through the tube which has been passed to the stomach or the intestines? How much parenteral fluid has he received?

The patient is usually in great pain. Make him as comfortable as possible in the position ordered by the doctor. Usually, the head of the bed is kept elevated, and a footboard against which the patient can brace his feet helps to keep him from sliding down in bed. Administer analgesics as ordered for the relief of pain.

Mouth care is very important. Often the patient is vomiting. The inability to take anything by mouth, the presence of a gastrointestinal tube, and fever make the patient's mouth feel dry and parched and cause an unpleasant taste and odor.

Cleanliness and an orderly environment help the patient to rest. Linen that has become wet with perspiration or soiled by vomitus should be changed. Bedside equipment, such as infusion poles and drainage bottles, should be arranged neatly.

Sometimes the patient becomes disoriented. Side rails on the bed are important to prevent him from harming himself, and he should be observed frequently.

The patient with peritonitis requires *gentleness* above all else. Every movement causes him added pain. Every unnecessary jolting of his bed or stretcher adds to his agony. If the patient must be removed from his bed to a stretcher for roentgenography or for surgery, have plenty of assistance and lift him as gently and as smoothly as possible. Guard carefully against placing any accidental pressure on the patient's fiercely tender abdomen.

HERNIA

Although the term *hernia* may be used in relation to the protrusion of any organ from the cavity that normally confines it, it is used most commonly to describe the protrusion of intestines through a defect in the abdominal wall. The word *rupture* is used sometimes by lay persons to describe this condition. When a hernia occurs, a lump or swelling appears on the abdomen underneath the skin. The swelling may be large or small, depending on how much of the viscera has protruded. Because hernia occurs frequently and sometimes causes no symptoms other than a swelling, its potential seriousness often is overlooked.

Types of Hernia. The most common types of abdominal hernia are the inguinal, the umbilical, the femoral, and the incisional. Certain

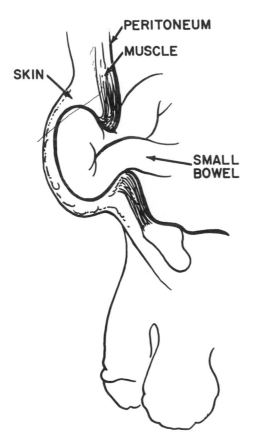

Fig. 38-2. Inguinal hernia, demonstrating how the small bowel can become caught in the herniated sac.

points on the abdominal wall are normally weaker than others, and they are more vulnerable to the development of hernia. These points are the *inguinal ring,* the point on the abdominal wall where the inguinal canal begins; the *femoral ring,* at the abdominal opening of the femoral canal; and the *umbilicus.*

Incisional hernias occur through the scar of a surgical incision when healing has been impaired. Incisional hernias often can be prevented by careful surgical technic, with particular emphasis on the prevention of wound infection. Obese or aged patients and those who suffer from malnutrition are especially prone to the development of incisional hernia.

If the protruding structures can be replaced in the abdominal cavity, the hernia is said to be *reducible.* Lying down and applying manual pressure over the area often serves to reduce the hernia. An irreducible hernia is one that cannot be replaced in the abdominal cavity. Edema of the protruding structures and constriction of the opening through which they have emerged make it impossible for them to return to the abdominal cavity. This condition is called *incarceration.* If this process continues without treatment, the blood supply to the trapped viscera can be cut off, leading to gangrene of the trapped tissues. This condition is called a *strangulated hernia* and constitutes an emergency.

Etiology. Congenital defects account for a large proportion of hernias, including those that appear after childhood. The hernia may be apparent in infancy, or it may appear in young adulthood in response to increased intra-abdominal pressure, such as that which occurs during heavy lifting, sneezing, coughing or pregnancy. Obesity and the weakening of muscles may be responsible for the development of hernia in later middle life and old age.

Incidence. Inguinal hernias are the type that occurs most commonly. Men are more likely to develop inguinal hernia; women are more likely to develop umbilical and femoral hernias.

Diagnosis usually can be made by physical examination. Occasionally, x-ray films of the intestinal tract are ordered.

Symptoms. Often, the hernia causes no symptoms other than the appearance of a swelling on the abdomen when the patient coughs, stands or lifts something heavy. Sometimes, the swelling is painful; the pain disappears when the hernia is reduced. Incarcerated hernias cause severe pain, and if they are not treated, they may become strangulated. The symptoms of strangulated hernia are discussed under complications.

Complications of Hernia

When a hernia first occurs, the defect in the abdominal wall is usually small. However, as the hernia persists, and the organs continue to protrude, the defect grows larger, making surgical repair more difficult. The hernia may become incarcerated or even strangulated. *Strangulation is an acute emergency.* The patient suffers extreme abdominal pain, and the severe pressure on the loop of intestine that is protruding outside the abdominal cavity causes intestinal obstruction. Unless surgery is performed promptly, the patient may die. If a portion of the bowel has become gangrenous due to the curtailment of its blood supply, that part of the intestine must be excised, with anastomosis of the remaining portions of the intestine.

When a hernia is neglected for many years, the tissues in the area become weakened and do not heal as readily. Obese persons who have put off surgical repair of the hernia for years are especially prone to recurrence of the hernia. Usually, the doctor advises the obese patient to lose weight before the surgery is undertaken to lessen the possibility of recurrence.

Hernia Treatment and Nursing Care

Herniorrhaphy is an operation performed for the repair of a hernia. The protruding structures are replaced in the abdominal cavity, and the defect in the abdominal wall is repaired. Herniorrhaphy may be performed under spinal or general anesthesia.

Importance of Early Treatment. The nurse can help patients to understand the importance of seeking medical care for hernias that are not painful. It is very hard to seek care (especially when one is quite sure an operation is needed) for something that causes little discomfort. It is so much easier to say, "It's not bothering me, so I won't bother it." But by the time the hernia does bother the patient, an operation that might have been relatively simple may be complicated by the poor condition of his tissues or even by strangulation. Therefore, most doctors advise patients to have hernias repaired promptly to avoid years of possible discomfort and the threat of complications.

Nursing Care. Before and after herniorrhaphy nursing care usually presents no special difficulties. Usually, the patient is permitted out of bed on the day after the operation. If he has difficulty voiding, he may be permitted to stand at the bedside, with assistance, while he uses the urinal. If possible, an orderly or a male nurse should stay with the patient if it is necessary for him to stand to void on the day of surgery. If this help is not available, evaluate by noting the patient's color and pulse, and whether or not he feels dizzy or faint, whether it is safe to step outside the curtain for a moment to afford the patient some privacy.

Usually, the patient can tolerate food and fluids on the day after surgery. However, some patients, either because of the type and the extent of the necessary surgery or because of the existence of such complications as strangulation, are permitted nothing by mouth for several days postoperatively. These patients receive parenteral fluids, and a nasogastric tube connected to gentle suction frequently is used to prevent postoperative distention and vomiting.

Every effort is made to prevent conditions that might impair healing, since impairment of healing could lead to a recurrence of the hernia. Strict aseptic technic is important in preventing infection. An increase in intra-abdominal pressure, such as that which occurs when the patient is lifting or coughing, must be avoided. If the patient has a chronic cough, its cause is investigated, and treatment is given to relieve it before the herniorrhaphy is performed. The patient is observed carefully postoperatively for the development of any sneezing or coughing. These symptoms, if they occur, are reported promptly to the physician. The patient is instructed to splint the incision with his hand if he coughs or sneezes.

Walking about and breathing deeply are important in preventing postoperative complications. The patient is encouraged to move, provided that he does not strain the operative area. Some patients are afraid to move or walk lest the hernia reappear. If the height of the bed is adjustable, place it in the lowest position before the patient gets up, to avoid strain. If the bed is not adjustable, a footstool will help the patient to step easily from the high bed to the floor. The patient is instructed not to lift any heavy objects.

Male patients sometimes develop pain and swelling of the scrotum due to inflammation and edema after the repair of an inguinal hernia. Ice bags may be ordered for the relief of the pain and the swelling, and the scrotum often is supported with a suspensory. The patient often

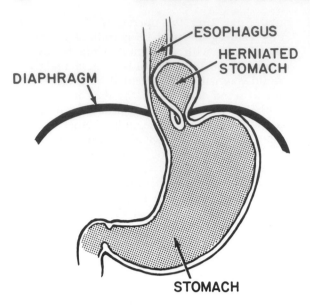

DIAPHRAGM

ESOPHAGUS

HERNIATED STOMACH

STOMACH

FIG. 38-3. Esophageal hiatus hernia—para-esophageal type. The herniated portion of the stomach protrudes through the diaphragm into the chest cavity.

finds it easier to report pain, inflammation and swelling of the scrotum to one of the men on the staff. If the patient seems to be having unusual pain and is reluctant to move after the first 24 to 48 hours postoperatively, when the most severe pain near the incision has usually subsided, provide an opportunity for him to talk with a male nurse or an orderly. If painful swelling of the scrotum has developed, the doctor should be notified.

Because the operation is usually in the inguinal region, many men feel embarrassed when the nurse checks the dressing postoperatively. Careful arranging of bedding, or giving the patient a towel to use as a drape will prevent exposing him.

Restriction of Activities. Postoperative recovery for most patients is rapid. The patients who are in good health preoperatively often go home within a week. When the patient returns home, he is instructed to avoid strenuous exertion or heavy lifting until his doctor feels this can be undertaken safely. Many factors are considered in determining how much and for how long the patient's activities must be restricted. The location and the size of the defect that was repaired, the condition of the patient's tissues, his age and whether or not he is obese are examples. The patients who always have performed heavy physi-

cal labor may have to change the type of work that they do, whereas those who perform sedentary or light physical work usually can return to full employment within a few weeks. Healthy young persons who have had repair of an uncomplicated hernia often have no restrictions on their later activity.

Esophageal Hiatus Hernia

An esophageal hiatus hernia is a protrusion, usually of a part of the stomach, through a defect in the wall in the diaphragm at the point where the esophagus passes through the diaphragm. The condition may be caused by a congenital weakness in the diaphragm or by trauma. Factors which cause increased intra-abdominal pressure, such as multiple pregnancies, contribute to the development of hiatus hernia. The loss of muscle strength and tone that occurs with aging contributes to the condition; many persons who develop hiatus hernia are in older age groups, and the condition is especially common among older women.

The symptoms include heartburn, belching, and a feeling of substernal or epigastric pressure after eating. These symptoms are more severe when the patient lies down. The diagnosis is suggested by the history and confirmed by roentgenography. The majority of patients can be managed medically by weight reduction if obese, an ulcer type diet, antacids and elevation of the head bedpost on six-inch blocks. This prevents the stomach acid from refluxing and chemically attacking the esophageal mucosa. Patients with reflex esophagitis secondary to hiatus hernia may bleed acutely, especially in the uncommon paraesophageal type. They may have melena or even hematemesis. At times occult bleeding for long periods of time produces a typical iron deficiency anemia. Patients who do not respond to a rigid medical regimen are treated surgically.

Surgical treatment involves replacing the stomach or other protruding organs into the abdominal cavity and repairing the defect in the wall. The surgery involves entering the thoracic cavity. The postoperative care is similar to that of any patient who has chest surgery (see Chap. 24). Continuous gastric suction usually is ordered postoperatively to prevent distention of the stomach and pressure on the surgical repair.

Sometimes, pneumoperitoneum (injecting air into the abdominal cavity) helps to relieve the symptoms by elevating the diaphragm, thus helping the stomach to remain below the diaphragm and not to bulge through the defect. After pneumoperitoneum the patient may feel distended. Small meals usually are recommended.

Mechanical Intestinal Obstruction

Cancer is the most common cause of intestinal obstruction, particularly in older persons. The tumor gradually becomes larger until it completely obstructs the bowel. Changes in bowel habits may be noted by the patient while an obstruction is partial. Often, he has alternating constipation and diarrhea. The diarrhea results from very forceful peristalsis, which is the body's way of pushing the intestinal contents through the narrowed lumen of the bowel. If the patient receives prompt diagnosis and treatment, complete obstruction may be averted.

Volvulus, a twisting or kinking of a portion of the intestines, is another condition causing a sudden obstruction of the intestine. *Strangulated hernia* is a third common cause of acute intestinal obstruction.

Symptoms. The symptoms of a severe intestinal obstruction may arise suddenly in a previously healthy individual. When the bowel is obstructed, the portion proximal to the obstruction becomes distended with intestinal contents, while the portion distal to the obstruction is empty. If the obstruction is complete, no gas or feces are expelled rectally. However, one or two bowel movements may occur soon after the obstruction has occurred, because the material already past the obstruction can be expelled normally.

Peristalsis becomes very forceful in the proximal portion, as the body attempts to propel the material beyond the point of the obstruction. These forceful peristaltic waves cause severe cramps, which tend to occur intermittently.

When an obstruction occurs high in the gastrointestinal tract, the patient usually vomits whatever contents are in the stomach and the small bowel. On the other hand, if the obstruction is low—for example, in the colon—vomiting usually does not occur at all.

The patient becomes very dehydrated. He is unable to take oral fluids, and he loses water and electrolytes through vomiting. The failure of the mucosa to reabsorb the secretions that are poured into the intestine contributes to the water and the electrolyte imbalance.

The increasing pressure on the bowel due to severe distention and to edema often impairs circulation, and leads to gangrene of a portion of the bowel. Perforation of the gangrenous bowel

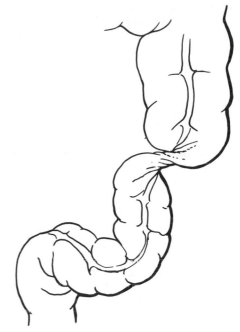

Fig. 38-4. Volvulus of the colon. The twisting can cause complete obstruction.

(which results from pressure against weakened tissue) causes the intestinal contents to seep into the peritoneal cavity, causing peritonitis. Intestinal obstruction is extremely dangerous and can be rapidly fatal if prompt treatment is not forthcoming.

Diagnosis. The doctor studies the patient's history and performs a careful physical examination. Roentgenography of the intestinal tract is usually necessary.

Treatment. Mechanical obstruction usually must be relieved surgically. The obstruction is relieved by a relatively minor surgical procedure, such as a temporary colostomy or cecostomy. After the patient's condition has improved, as a result of the relief of the obstruction and the supportive therapy described later in this section, more extensive surgery may be undertaken. Sometimes, because of the location and the extent of the malignant process, a permanent colostomy is necessary.

Intestinal decompression, parenteral therapy and antibiotics are used preoperatively to help to improve the patient's condition, so that he can withstand surgery better and make more rapid progress during the postoperative period. To permit the intestinal decompression a long tube, such as the Miller-Abbott tube, is passed into the intestine. Large amounts of accumulated secretions and gas are drawn out through the tube by gentle suction, greatly relieving distention and vomiting. Parenteral fluids and electrolytes are administered to correct fluid and electrolyte imbalance. Antibiotics may be ordered to combat infection.

DIVERTICULOSIS AND DIVERTICULITIS

Diverticula are sacs or pouches caused by herniation of the mucosa through a weakened portion of the muscular coat of the intestine or other structure. Diverticula are common in the esophagus and the colon and are especially likely to occur in the sigmoid.

The cause of diverticula is unknown. It is believed that some diverticula are congenital, though most are thought to be due to weakness in the muscular coat associated with aging. Diverticula are most common in people over 50. The term *diverticulosis* refers to the presence of

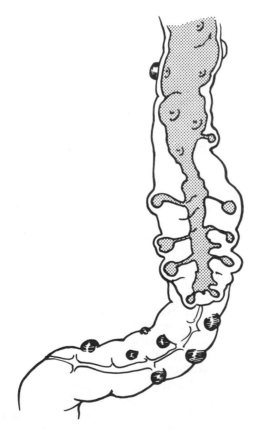

Fig. 38-5. Diverticulitis. Note the numerous small out-pouchings of the intestinal wall.

multiple diverticula; *diverticulitis* means inflammation or infection of the diverticula.

Symptoms. Diverticulosis is often asymptomatic and may be noted only when x-ray films are taken for some other condition, or at autopsy. However, the contents of the gastrointestinal tract often become trapped in these pouches, causing irritation and leading to inflammation and infection. For example, fecal material may accumulate in the pouches of the sigmoid, leading to irritation and infection of the diverticula. The patient may experience constipation, diarrhea or flatulence. Also, pain and tenderness in the left lower quadrant, fever, leukocytosis and rectal bleeding may occur. Intestinal obstruction or a perforation leading to peritonitis occasionally results from the inflammatory process.

Food that is on its way to the stomach often becomes lodged in diverticula of the esophagus, where it remains and stagnates. The patient's breath may be very unpleasant because of food decomposition in the diverticula, and he may regurgitate food eaten several days previously. Difficulty in swallowing (*dysphagia*) commonly occurs, and the patient may become seriously malnourished. Cough sometimes occurs because of irritation of the trachea.

Treatment. Diverticula noted during routine examinations require no treatment if they are not causing any symptoms. Diverticulitis with resultant stricture formation may be difficult to differentiate from carcinoma except at surgery.

Diverticulitis of the colon often responds to medical treatment. During a very acute episode with pain and local tenderness the patient may be maintained on intravenous fluids for a few days with no oral intake. As the inflammation subsides under antibiotic therapy, the diet is increased to a low residue diet. Constipation is to be avoided in these patients by good fluid intake, encouraging a regular evacuation, and the use of mineral oil (or other medications prescribed by the physician) at bedtime. If the condition does not respond to medical treatment, or if such complications as perforation, intestinal obstruction or severe bleeding occurs, surgery is necessary. The portion of colon containing the diverticula is removed, and the continuity of the bowel is re-established by joining the remaining portions of the colon. Depending on the location and the extent of the disease and on the presence of intestinal obstruction, a temporary colostomy sometimes must be performed. The continuity of the bowel is restored at a later operation, and the colostomy is closed.

Diverticula of the esophagus usually are excised, if they are symptomatic. The resulting opening in the esophagus is closed, thus restoring normal function and giving complete relief of symptoms. If a diverticulum is located in the upper portion of the esophagus, the postoperative patient may take a liquid, followed by a bland diet, soon after surgery. General postoperative nursing care is required. If a diverticulum is lower in the esophagus, the operation must be performed through an incision into the thoracic cavity.

Polyposis

Small tumors called *polyps* occur commonly in the colon and the rectum. They easily become ulcerated and bleed. Although only one or several polyps may occur, patients rarely have hundreds of them—a condition known as *familial polyposis*.

The cause of the condition is unknown, but a strong hereditary tendency has been noted. Sometimes, the polyps cause no symptoms. However, they may cause rectal discharge of blood and mucus, or changes in the bowel habits. Since the incidence of malignancy is high in familial polyposis, colectomy is the treatment of choice.

Polyps of the colon and the rectum sometimes are found in association with a separate malignancy. For this reason a barium enema with air contrast is ordered after a polyp is found on sigmoidoscopy. It is widely believed that the polyps undergo malignant changes, though some claim that benign polyps do not become cancerous, and that the growths from the beginning are composed of either benign or malignant tissue. Although surgical excision with pathologic examination is the only way to differentiate between benign and malignant tissue, some authorities would not recommend abdominal surgery in pedunculated polyps less than one centimeter in diameter found on barium enema.

Regional Enteritis

Regional enteritis (inflammation of the small intestine) is a disease of unknown cause occurring most commonly among young adults. The disease often has a patchy distribution throughout large portions of the duodenum, ileum and the jejunum.

The symptoms usually include pain in the right lower quadrant, fever and diarrhea. The patient also may have leukocytosis and tenderness of his abdomen. Often, the condition is confused with acute appendicitis. Usually, the disease has an insidious onset and a variable course. Some patients have a gradual increase in symptoms, whereas others may have acute exacerbations alternating with remissions of the disease. Sometimes, the condition subsides spontaneously. Intestinal obstruction, perforation or the formation of abscesses and fistulas may occur. For instance, fistulas may form between the loops of the intestine.

Supportive treatment usually is given. Rest, relief of emotional stress and a bland diet high in proteins and calories often are prescribed. Parenteral therapy with fluids, electrolytes and whole blood may be necessary to correct anemia and to restore the fluid and electrolyte balance. Supplementary vitamins and iron often are given. Corticosteroids are used often. None of these treatments is curative. Steroids may tide the patient over an acute exacerbation and induce a remission.

Surgical treatment is usually reserved for those who develop such complications as intestinal obstruction or perforation. The affected sections of the small bowel may be removed or bypassed and anastomosis of the remaining segments performed. The surgical treatment is made more difficult because the disease frequently is scattered widely. Often, measures are taken to divert the flow of the intestinal contents from the diseased area by joining the proximal healthy portion of the ileum with the colon (ileocolostomy), thus bypassing the diseased area of the ileum. Sometimes, the diseased portion of the ileum is removed later. However, if the patient progresses satisfactorily, it often is considered unnecessary to remove the diseased segment. Regardless of the type of treatment that is used, a recurrence of the disease is common. Surgical treatment is frequently followed by an exacerbation within a year and is therefore recommended only when absolutely necessary.

Malabsorption

Many conditions interfere with normal intestinal absorption of nutrients, water and vitamins. Malabsorption results in general symptoms of weight loss, weakness, wasting and the passage of abnormal stools. The stools are usually quite bulky, frothy, pale in color and foul smelling due to the high content of fat, i.e., steatorrhea. The cause for malabsorption may reside in the wall of the small intestine itself as in adult celiac disease or may be secondary to deficiency of digestive enzymes as in pancreatic disease, e.g., chronic pancreatitis. Symptoms are related to the particular type of malabsorption experienced by the patient. For example, deficient absorption of vitamin B complex can cause glossitis, tenderness of muscles, dermatitis and peripheral neuritis. Vitamin K loss leads to hypoprothrombinemia and easy bleeding; loss of calcium causes tetany and bone demineralization.

Patients with adult celiac disease are unable to metabolize gluten, a protein which is contained in wheat, rye and barley. In some way not fully understood, ingestion of gluten damages the intestinal musoca, thus interfering with absorption of nutrients, vitamins and water. Symptoms improve dramatically with administration of a gluten-free diet, which must be continued indefinitely, because symptoms recur if the diet is discontinued. A marked familial tendency toward this disease has been noted.

Pancreatic insufficiency with secondary malabsorption is treated by ingestion of pancreatic extract with meals. Cotazyme is one of the newer pancreatic extracts.

The diagnosis of malabsorption is not always apparent in patients who do not have a severe

form and are not malnourished individuals. Therefore, an accurate description by the nurse of the character of the stool seen in a patient with diarrhea may be critical in leading the physician to a diagnosis of malabsorption.

HEMORRHOIDS

Hemorrhoids are varicose veins of the anus and the rectum. They may occur outside the anal sphincter (external hemorrhoids) or inside the sphincter (internal hemorrhoids). These sphincters keep the orifice closed except during defecation. External hemorrhoids appear as small, reddish-blue lumps at the edge of the anus.

Etiology. Pregnancy, intra-abdominal tumors, chronic constipation and hereditary factors are believed to predispose to the development of hemorrhoids.

Symptoms. Thrombosed external hemorrhoids are painful lumps appearing near the anus. One or two such swellings may appear and disappear spontaneously within a few days. The pain and the swelling are caused by cloted blood within the vein. Thrombosed external hemorrhoids rarely cause bleeding. However, they may become large and numerous, causing a great deal of pain as well as embarrassing itching. The pain is especially severe when the patient has a bowel movement, causing him to put off defecation as long as possible. Constipation results, or if it is already present, it is aggravated. Constipation and straining at stool make the hemorrhoids worse.

Internal hemorrhoids often cause bleeding, but they are less likely to cause pain unless they protrude through the anus. The bleeding may vary from an occasional drop or two of blood on toilet tissue or underwear to a chronic loss of blood that leads to anemia. Internal hemorrhoids usually protrude each time that the patient defecates. At first, he is able to push them back inside the sphincter with his finger. Gradually, as the masses grow larger, they remain permanently outside the sphincter and often cause a chronic discharge of blood and mucus.

Diagnosis. The doctor notes the presence of external hemorrhoids merely by inspection. Unless internal hemorrhoids protrude through the anus, an anoscope or proctoscope must be used to see them. Since the symptoms may be similar to those of cancer, a very thorough examination of the anal and the rectal areas is nec-

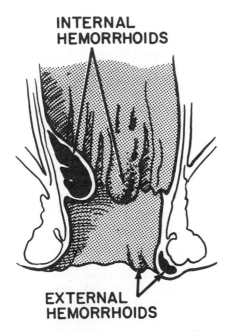

INTERNAL HEMORRHOIDS

EXTERNAL HEMORRHOIDS

FIG. 38-6. Internal and external hemorrhoids.

essary. The patient who experiences rectal bleeding may have hemorrhoids or cancer, or both.

Anyone who experiences pain, bleeding or swelling in the anal region should consult his doctor promptly, so that the cause of the condition can be determined.

Treatment and Nursing Care

A small external hemorrhoid often disappears without treatment, or it may be relieved by taking warm sitz baths. A variety of ointments containing local anesthetics are available and may be recommended by the doctor for the relief of discomfort. Ointments containing dibucaine (Nupercaine) frequently are used for this purpose. The correction of constipation is important both in relieving the condition and in preventing its recurrence. Often, mineral oil is recommended to soften the stool.

Surgical excision of the dilated veins (*hemorrhoidectomy*) frequently is necessary to cure the condition. This procedure is the most common rectal surgery among adults. Occasionally, sclerosing solutions are injected into the dilated veins.

What are the patient's particular needs for nursing care? How can the nursing staff help the patient?

• The location of the operative area causes embarrassment. It is important to drape and to screen the patient during the treatments and the examinations.

• The patient, and sometimes the staff as well, may assume that the pain and the discomfort will be minimal, since the operation itself is not considered a major procedure. But it is important to recognize that pain after a hemorrhoidectomy is likely to be severe at first, and to provide for its relief. Narcotics, careful positioning and explanation concerning what to expect, all help to lessen the discomfort.

• Although cleanliness of the operative area is essential, the anal region cannot be kept sterile. For instance, although the tub used for the sitz bath must be kept very clean, the procedure itself is not sterile.

• Gentleness is as important as cleanliness. A rubber ring should be provided for the patient to sit on, and the local cleaning should be done gently.

• Some patients have difficulty voiding following hemorrhoidectomy. Often, with the doctor's permission, the male patient is permitted to stand at the bedside to void. Women may find it easier to void if they use a commode, or if a bedpan is placed on the seat of a chair next to the bed.

• The sitz bath provides considerable relief from pain, as well as a cleaning of the area. It is a good idea to give the sitz bath when the patient is especially likely to experience pain—for example, after bowel movements.

• The first bowel movement is dreaded by most patients who have had rectal surgery. The patient needs explanation of how he is being prepared for the bowel movement (for example, by the use of mineral oil). When the movement occurs, he needs the assurance that someone is nearby to help him if he needs assistance with cleaning and measures for the relief of pain afterward.

• Plans must be made for continued care when the patient returns home. He is shown how to take sitz baths and instructed in the use of medications, such as mineral oil, to soften the stool. Any problems that predisposed to the hemorrhoids must be corrected if they can be. For instance, treatment and instruction may be necessary to overcome constipation.

The principles in the care of any patient after rectal surgery are similar, regardless of the type of surgery performed. Although hemorrhoids are the most common indication for rectal surgery, the following conditions also are encountered frequently among adults.

PILONIDAL SINUS

Pilonidal is a term which means "a nest of hair." The words *sinus* and *cyst* are both used to

COMMON RECTAL CONDITIONS

CONDITION	DESCRIPTION	TREATMENT
Anal fissure	Ulcer involving the skin of the anal wall	Sitz baths, local anaesthetics, surgery
Anal abscess	Localized infection of tissues near the anus	Incision and drainage
Anal fistula	Abnormal tunnel or passageway within the tissues often caused by anal abscess	Fistulotomy

describe the condition. However, studies indicate that the lesion is not a cyst but a sinus (Mulholland). In other words, rather than being a sac filled with fluid, the lesion is believed to be a canal underneath the skin with a narrow opening or openings onto the skin. The condition typically occurs after puberty, when the hair in the anogenital region becomes thick and stiff. The skin deep in the cleft in the sacrococcygeal region becomes macerated. Predisposed are persons with a deep cleft in this region and those who are hirsute. Inadequate personal hygiene, obesity and trauma to the area also predispose to the development of pilonidal sinus. (During World War II soldiers called pilonidal sinus "the Jeep disease." Jeeps now have cushions.) Stiff hairs in the sacrococcygeal region irritate and pierce the soft macerated skin, becoming imbedded in it. The hairs then are foreign bodies and cause inflammation of the tissues. Infection readily follows, due to the break in the skin which permits the entrance of microorganisms. Several channels lead from the sinus to the skin; their openings on the skin are called *pilonidal openings*. Often, hair protrudes from them.

Usually, the patient is unaware that he has a pilonidal sinus until it becomes infected. The patient experiences pain and swelling at the base of his spine, and he may note purulent drainage on his clothing.

The treatment of pilonidal sinus involves an operation in which the sinus and all its connecting channels are laid open; drainage of purulent material, removal of the hair and cleaning facilitate healing with normal, healthy tissue. Antibiotics may be administered.

Nursing Care. Particular points in the nursing care after the surgical treatment of a pilonidal sinus include:

• Care must be taken not to soil the dressings. Women void while lying on the abdomen.

• Moving the bowels is avoided for the first few days. Mineral-oil and oil-retention enemas may be used before the first bowel movement.

• After the first few postoperative days the nurse may be asked to change the dressing.

During the immediate postoperative period the patient lies on his abdomen. The length of time that he is kept in bed varies from one to several days. When he is first permitted out of bed, he is instructed to take short steps and to avoid prolonged sitting, so that strain will not be placed on the incision. The height of the bed should be adjusted, or a footstool should be used, when the patient gets in and out of bed to prevent strain on the operative area.

REFERENCES AND BIBLIOGRAPHY

BARNES, M.: Clean colons without enemas, *Am. J. Nurs.* 69:2128, October, 1969.

BARRETT, N. R.: Achalasia of the cardia, *Brit. Med. J.* 1:1135, 1964.

BEESON, P. B., and McDERMOTT, W. (eds.): *Cecil-Loeb Textbook of Medicine,* ed. 12, Philadelphia, Saunders, 1967.

BELAND, I. L.: *Clinical Nursing,* ed. 2, St. Louis, Mosby, 1970.

BOCKUS, H. L.: *Gastroenterology,* ed. 2, Philadelphia, Saunders, 1964.

CALABRO, J. J.: Hereditable multiple polyposis syndromes of the gastrointestinal tract, *Am. J. Med.* 33:276, 1962.

CASTLEMAN, B., and KRICKSTEIN, H. I.: Do adenomatous polyps of the colon become malignant? *New Eng. J. Med.* 267:469, 1962.

————: Current approach to the cancer-polyp controversy, *Gastroenterology* 51:108, 1966.

DAVIS, L.: *Christopher's Textbook of Surgery,* ed. 9, Philadelphia, Saunders, 1968.

DERISI, L. I.: Starving in the midst of plenty: adult celiac disease, *Am. J. Nurs.* 70:1048, May, 1970.

GOODMAN, L. S., and GILMAN, A.: *The Pharmacological Basis of Therapeutics,* ed. 3, New York, Macmillan, 1970.

HALLBERG, J. C.: The patient with surgery of the colon, *Am. J. Nurs.* 61:64, March, 1961.

HARMER, B., and HENDERSON, V.: *Textbook of the Principles and Practice of Nursing,* ed. 5, New York, Macmillan, 1955.

HOROWICZ, C.: Profiles in OPD nursing: a rectal and colon service, *Am. J. Nurs.* 71:114, January, 1971.

MARSTON, A.: Mesenteric arterial disease, *Gut* 8:203, 1967.

MULHOLLAND, J. H., *et al.*: *Current Surgical Management, II,* Philadelphia, Saunders, 1960.

NANSON, E. M.: Treatment of achalasia of the cardia, *Gastroenterology* 51:236, 1966.

Proceedings of the World Congress of Gastro-Enterology, vols. I, II, Baltimore, Williams & Wilkins, 1959.

RAPHAEL, H. A.: Primary adenocarcinoma of the esophagus, *Ann. Surg.* 164:785, 1966.

ROBINSON, C.: *Proudfit-Robinson's Normal and Therapeutic Nutrition,* ed. 13, New York, Macmillan, 1967.

RODMAN, M. J., and SMITH, D. W.: *Pharmacology and Drug Therapy in Nursing,* Philadelphia, Lippincott, 1968.

ROTH, H. P., and FLESHLER, B.: Diffuse esophageal spasm, *Ann. Int. Med.* 61:914, 1964.

RYNBERGEN, H. J.: *Teaching Nutrition in Nursing,* ed. 4, Philadelphia, Lippincott, 1959.

SHAFER, K. N., *et al.*: *Medical-Surgical Nursing,* ed. 3, St. Louis, Mosby, 1964.

SHROPSHEAR, G.: Anatomic basis for anorectal disease, *Dis. Colon Rectum* 7:399, 1964.

TRUELOVE, S. C., and REYNELL, P. C.: *Diseases of the Digestive System,* Philadelphia, Davis, 1963.

USHER, F. C., and MATTHEWS, J.: Surgery: treatment of choice for hernia, *Am. J. Nurs.* 64:85, September, 1964.

WILSON, J. P.: Cancer of the colon and rectum, *Nurs. Forum* 4:59, 1965.

WOLFMAN, E. F., JR., and FLOTTE, C. T.: Carcinoma of the colon and rectum, *Am. J. Nurs.* 61:60, March, 1961.

Care of the Patient with Disorder of the Liver, Gallbladder, or Pancreas

39

The Patient with Liver Disease • Specific Liver Disorders
Diseases of the Biliary System • The Pancreas

THE PATIENT WITH LIVER DISEASE

Care of patients with liver disease presents some important challenges in nursing. Two common types of liver disease which are emphasized in this chapter are cirrhosis of the liver and hepatitis. Care of patients with these conditions requires particular concern for nutrition, for health teaching over an extended period, and for meticulous physical care when the patient is acutely ill. Although some work is beginning to be done in relation to liver transplants, it is still in the very early stages. The emphasis in nursing care of patients with liver disease is, therefore, on measures to support the patient physiologically, so that his liver will have the best possible chance to regain adequate function, and to support the patient emotionally during a lengthy and often discouraging period of illness.

Anatomy and Physiology

The liver is the largest glandular organ in the body, weighing between 1.0 and 1.5 Kg. It is located in the right upper abdomen, just under the right diaphragm which separates it from the right lung. The liver has two major lobes, right and left, and two small lobes located on the under surface, the caudate and quadrate lobes. The liver is supported in place by intra-abdominal pressure, as well as by various attachments called ligaments or mesenteries. These attachments connect the liver to adjacent intestines, abdominal wall, and diaphragm. Unless it is abnormally enlarged, the liver is not usually felt by the physician when he palpates the patient's abdomen.

The liver receives arterial blood from the hepatic artery, an indirect branch of the aorta. The portal vein transports blood from the intestinal tract to the liver. After it has traversed vascular pathways inside the liver, the blood is collected by the hepatic veins and transported to the inferior vena cava, and then back to the heart for further circulation.

Microscopically, the internal structure of the liver includes smaller ramifications of the hepatic artery, the hepatic and portal vein, lymphatics, and bile ducts. The cellular constituents of the liver are the hepatic parenchymal cells, which carry out most of the liver's metabolic functions, and the Kupffer or reticuloendothelial cells, which engage in the immunologic, detoxifying, and blood-filtering actions of the liver.

The liver is involved in a multitude of vital, complex metabolic activities. Among the most important functions are the formation and excretion of bile; the utilization, transformation, and distribution of vitamins, proteins, fats, and carbohydrates; the storage of energy-yielding glycogen; the synthesis of factors needed for blood coagulation, including prothrombin and fibrinogen; the detoxification of endogenous and exogenous chemicals, bacteria, and foreign ele-

473

ments which may be harmful; and the formation of antibody and immunizing substances, including gamma globulin.

Diagnosis of Liver Disease and Related Nursing Care

Because different types of liver disease require extremely different kinds of treatment, great care by the physician is required in making the medical diagnosis, and many tests are often necessary. Sometimes the patient becomes weary or frightened by the diagnostic procedures, and it becomes especially important to help him understand the necessity for them. The nurse who understands that jaundice may be due either to liver disease or to obstruction of the biliary tract, and that treatment of the former is medical while surgery is required for the latter, is helped to appreciate the importance to the patient of undergoing diagnostic tests.

Recognition of the importance of accurate diagnosis accents the necessity for nursing intervention which stresses emotional support of the patient during diagnostic tests and explanation to the patient of the procedure for the test. Nursing measures can diminish the patient's discomfort. For example, he is often kept fasting in the morning until blood samples are drawn. Promptly serving his tray as soon as the blood specimens have been taken and making sure that the food served is hot can lessen the patient's discouragement as well as promote adequate nutrition so important in liver disease. Patients with liver disease frequently must have many venipunctures, and sometimes they become very tense about this procedure. While in most hospitals a technician draws the blood, it is essential for the nurse to remain with the patient during the procedure if the patient is frightened. Diverting the patient's attention from the venipuncture by asking him to look at you and to concentrate on squeezing your hand is a useful nursing measure in helping the patient tolerate the venipuncture. Helping the patient tolerate the procedure makes it easier for the technician to draw the blood, lessens the patient's discomfort, and minimizes trauma to the patient's veins.

Liver Function Tests. Most tests of liver function require samples of blood drawn while the patient is fasting. Ordinarily the blood specimens are taken in the morning, and the patient's breakfast is omitted until after the blood has been drawn. A technician from the laboratory usually is assigned the task of seeing that speci-

men bottles are accurately labeled and carefully transported to the chemistry laboratory, and for seeing that tubes containing special additives are used when necessary (for prothrombin determination, for example, to avoid clot formation). Tests which employ dye, such as the BSP test, require calculation of the dose of dye based upon the patient's weight, as well as accurate timing of the period between dye injection and blood collection. Accuracy in carrying out these details is essential and is promoted by careful planning and coordination among all persons involved. In most hospitals the physician injects dye, such as for a BSP test, and collection of specimens is carefully timed after dye is administered. It is important to have an understanding ahead of time about which physician will administer the dye and when the dye will be given. Similar planning should occur with personnel from the laboratory. If telephone reminders are necessary during the test, give the ward secretary a list of persons to be called, indicating the times when the calls should be made.

Total Serum Bilirubin. The level is elevated in jaundice from bile duct obstruction or other causes. (See section on Jaundice.)

Urine bilirubin, urine urobilinogen, fecal urobilinogen are other pigment tests to assist in confirming findings indicated by serum bilirubin testing.

Alkaline phosphatase, serum glutamic oxaloacetic transaminase and glutamic pyruvic transaminase, (SGOT and SGPT), and lactic dehydrogenase (LDH) are liver enzymes whose blood levels help in identification of hepatic neoplasms, obstruction or infection. Liver cells have been found to be rich in enzymes such as transaminase. When the liver cells are damaged by viruses (as in hepatitis) or by alcohol (as in Laennec's cirrhosis), the enzyme is released into the blood stream and is readily measured.

Both albumin and cholesterol are synthesized in the liver. In major liver dysfunction blood levels of both are depressed. Alkaline phosphatase of liver origin is elevated in obstructive jaundice whether of intra- or extrahepatic origin.

Prothrombin time measures the level of a coagulation factor, prothrombin, synthesized by the liver.

Bromsulphalein time (BSP), indocyanine green (ICG) and I^{131} rose bengal are dye-excretion tests which are useful determinants of liver damage. Because BSP is excreted by the liver in the same fashion as bilirubin, the BSP test has been used as a fine measure of excretory function when the level of serum bilirubin is still normal.

SERUM ALBUMIN and GLOBULIN LEVEL, THYMOL TURBIDITY and CEPHALIN FLOCCULATION are tests of liver proteins and may reflect the nature and degree of hepatic disease.

SERUM CHOLESTEROL level is reduced in severe liver damage, but usually elevated with biliary obstruction and liver cancers.

SERUM AMMONIA level may be increased in a failing liver which cannot detoxify this endogenous waste product of intestinal protein metabolism.

More complex tests to define hepatic disorders include LIVER BIOPSY for direct, microscopic analysis of liver tissue. This may be done percutaneously, by passing a special biopsy needle through the skin into the liver, or through a small abdominal incision under general or local anesthesia. Percutaneous needle biopsy is not performed by the physician if there is a bleeding tendency, obstructive jaundice which may result in hidden hemorrhage or bile leakage from the biopsy site.

The patient is asked to sign an operative permit before the biopsy is performed. Preoperative prothrombin time is determined. Sedatives are administered as ordered before the procedure, and the patient is kept fasting. Blood for transfusion will be ordered and kept in readiness in case it is needed. Postoperatively the patient is maintained at rest, and vital signs and the condition of the dressing are observed every hour. Fall in blood pressure, tachycardia, shoulder pain, abdominal pain or distention and staining of dressing with excessive blood or bile are indications of complications, and should be immediately reported to the physician.

ESOPHAGOSCOPY, BARIUM ESOPHAGOGRAM and UPPER GASTROINTESTINAL X-RAYS (GI SERIES) may be ordered to help the physician assess the status of the esophagus and other parts of the upper gastrointestinal tract, because these organs are often affected by liver disease.

PORTAL VENOGRAPHY and HEPATIC ARTERIOGRAPHY are methods by which contrast material is introduced into the hepatic circulation. Appropriate x-ray pictures will then define the character of the blood vessels as well as outline defects within the liver substance. Pressure in the portal venous system can also be determined in patients with portal hypertension and cirrhosis.

LIVER SCAN following intravenous administration of radioactive substances such as Iodine[131],

labeled albumin, or rose bengal, and colloidal Gold[198] can give a picture of liver size, shape and effect due to space-occupying lesions such as tumors (primary or metastatic) or abscess. The pattern of radioisotope uptake may yield information as to the amount of liver damage and help to differentiate various types of disease. No special precautions are required in relation to radioactivity when the patient has received substances such as I[131] intravenously.

SPECIFIC LIVER DISORDERS

Jaundice (Icterus)

Jaundice is a greenish yellow discoloration of tissue due to staining by an abnormally high concentration of the pigment bilirubin in the blood. Normally, total bilirubin concentration is about 1.2 mg. per 100 ml. of blood. If this reaches over 3 mg. per 100 ml. of blood or higher, jaundice is visible. The skin, mucous membrane of mouth and especially the sclerae (white portion of eye) are sites to look for jaundice.

The sign or symptom of jaundice occurs in a multitude of diseases which directly or indirectly affect the liver. It is probably the most common sign of liver disorder. Important to the understanding of jaundice is a knowledge of bile formation and excretion.

When red blood cells are old or injured, they are picked up by the spleen and bone marrow where they are broken down by reticuloendothelial cells. Hemoglobin released from these red blood cells is then reduced to the compound known as "unconjugated" or "indirect" bilirubin. This type of bilirubin then is carried by the blood to the liver where further chemical processes transform it into "conjugated" or "direct" bilirubin. These two forms of bilirubin are distinct, can be differentiated chemically and are important in the clinical discrimination between different diseases producing jaundice.

The "conjugated" bilirubin formed by the liver enters the bile ducts, reaches the intestine and is there transformed into urobilinogen. Urobilinogen is then changed into urobilin, the brown pigment of stool. Urobilinogen enters the blood stream and is carried back to the liver where it is changed into bilirubin for re-excretion in the bile. Another portion of urobilinogen is carried from the intestine to the kidney and is excreted in the urine.

In diseases causing jaundice, the laboratory determination of the type of pigments in blood, urine and stool allows the doctor to arrive at a more accurate diagnosis permitting the most appropriate therapy.

For purposes of discussion, jaundice may be classified in three different forms: (1) hemolytic jaundice (due to the overabundance of breakdown products of blood); (2) hepatocellular jaundice (due to internal liver disease preventing normal transformation of bile by the liver cells); and (3) obstructive jaundice (due to the inability of normally formed liver bile to be passed into the intestine because of duct blockage).

Companion Signs and Symptoms

Jaundice is both a sign and a symptom; it is not a separate disease. The patient's other signs and symptoms are those of the underlying disease.

Pruritus may be an extremely disquieting feature of obstructive jaundice and difficult to control. Soda or starch baths, calamine and other soothing lotions may be helpful. Drugs, including antihistamines, cholestyramine, sedatives, and tranquilizers are sometimes ordered, but are used with extreme care to avoid further possible liver damage.

In addition to the morning bath, sponge bathing with tepid water several times a day may be beneficial in lessening itching. Explain to the patient that scratching can lead to infection of his skin, and help him avoid scratching and skin infections by such measures as:

- Keeping his nails short and clean.
- Avoiding too-warm bed clothes.
- Assisting the patient to find diversion, because concentrating on itching makes it worse.
- Giving the patient a supply of calamine lotion (if ordered) and cotton swabs with instruction to apply it to particularly itchy spots.
- Making special efforts to promote comfort when the patient is prepared for his night's sleep by such methods as soothing backrubs, a starch bath (if ordered), and an evening snack. Itching tends to be worse at night, when the patient's attention is not diverted. If the patient scratches while asleep, have him wear white cotton gloves or mittens while sleeping.

Because of associated blood coagulation defects, jaundiced patients may have bleeding tendencies such as rectal bleeding, tarry stool, blood in urine, bleeding gums, and black and blue marks (ecchymosis) from minor skin trauma. Nursing measures are important in observing for bleeding and in performing procedures in a way which lessens the likelihood of bleeding. For example, intramuscular medicines should be given with small-gauge needles and the injection site should be firmly pressed and observed for hematoma formation. After removing an intravenous catheter, immediate and prolonged pressure should be applied to prevent seepage which allows hematomas to form making the vein unusable. These patients may require frequent blood tests or intravenous therapy so that every effort should be made to preserve integrity of the veins.

Cirrhosis

Pathology. There are several types of hepatic cirrhosis depending on etiology, pathology, and clinical manifestations. Basically it is a disease in which liver damage is followed by scarring with development of excessive fibrous connective tissue. This occurs as the liver attempts to repair itself and leads to considerable anatomical distortion, including partial or complete occlusion of blood channels within the liver.

TYPES OF CIRRHOSIS OF THE LIVER

Laennec's portal cirrhosis (alcoholic; nutritional; toxic)
Postnecrotic cirrhosis (posthepatitis)
Parasitic (following schistosomiasis, malaria, etc.)
Biliary cirrhosis (primary-idiopathic; obstructive)
Congestive (cardiac cirrhosis)

Laennec's portal cirrhosis is most commonly seen in the United States. It is associated with a heavy, chronic alcohol intake, usually coincident with poor nutrition. Laennec's type cirrhosis can also follow chronic poisoning with carbon tetrachloride, a cleaning agent.

Incidence of Laennec's Cirrhosis. This type of cirrhosis is seen most often in males between the ages of 45 and 65 years with a history af alcoholism. Men are affected two or three times more often than women.

Signs and Symptoms. General manifestations of liver damage occur. There are disorders of protein, fat, carbohydrate and vitamin metabolism as well as defects of blood coagulation, fluid and electrolyte balance, and ability to combat infections and toxins.

Clinically, advanced findings include poor nutrition with tissue wasting; poor hemostasis and easy bleeding; vitamin deficiencies; water retention; sodium deficiency; weight loss; weakness, mental dullness; anorexia, nausea, vomiting; intra-abdominal fluid (ascites), low blood sugar (hypoglycemia) and low blood proteins (hypoproteinemia). The skin is thin with dilated veins especially noted over the abdomen. Nose bleeds (epistaxis) jaundice, ecchymosis, scant body hair, palmar erythema (bright pink palms) and cutaneous spider angiomata (tiny pulsatile skin vessels of face and chest) also occur. Testicular atrophy is often seen in men and is probably due to the inability of the damaged liver to metabolize estrogenic factors produced from such organs as the adrenal gland.

A most important factor secondary to hepatic scarring in Laennec's cirrhosis is portal hypertension. The intrahepatic obstruction to the return of portal blood from the intestines leads to backup and diversion of blood through venous pathways in the stomach and esophagus. These engorged collateral vessels are called esophageal or gastric varices. As this obstructed back-flow increases, pressure within the portal system also increases (portal hypertension). The gastric and esophageal veins distend and are then apt to rupture. The subsequent bleeding into stomach and esophagus may be slow, with melena, but is often rapid and may result in massive hematemesis with exsanguination and death. This bleeding is aggravated by clotting disorders common to liver damage.

In addition to hemorrhage, another serious complication of advanced cirrhosis is infection. This is due to lowering of natural resistance as liver function is reduced. Cirrhotic patients are to be protected from other patients with infection and visitors with colds or other contagious diseases.

Hepatic coma may occur in any form of liver failure; it frequently follows a bleeding episode, paracentesis, infection, surgery or other stress. The patient becomes lethargic, drowsy, confused, irritable and eventually stuporous, drifting into coma. Delirium tremens (DT's) may occur early in the development of hepatic coma. The serum ammonia level may be elevated and be a contributing toxic factor.

Care of the Patient with Cirrhosis. There is no specific cure or medicine for hepatic cirrhosis. The aim of therapy is to prevent further deterioration by abolishing underlying causes and to apply supportive measures while the liver attempts to re-establish its functional integrity.

If treatment begins in early phases when signs and symptoms are few and mild, satisfactory recuperation is frequent and long-term prognosis is good. To rescue patients with advanced disease who are jaundiced, hypoproteinemic, have ascites and other manifestations of severe injury is considerably more difficult.

GENERAL SUPPORTIVE MEASURES. Encouraging the patient to eat is a major nursing task. Sustained, adequate nutrition is extremely important in the therapy of cirrhosis. The physician will usually prescribe a diet high in carbohydrates, proteins and vitamins in the form of meat, fish, eggs, milk, fruit and vegetables. Fats are sometimes deleted or included in amounts less than ordinary daily requirements. Tobacco and especially alcohol are prohibited. If a high blood level of ammonia is present and impending liver coma is suspected, proteins (which are ammonia precursors) are omitted from the diet. When improvement occurs, proteins are added to the diet. The anorexia of severe cirrhosis may require frequent, small semisolid or liquid meals rather than three full meals a day. Nausea and vomiting may require parenteral feedings. Vitamin B complex, vitamin K, and vitamin C, liver extract, and iron may be prescribed. Intravenous albumin may be given in severe hypoproteinemia and blood transfusions may be necessary for anemia. Because of the tendency toward salt and water retention (which can lead to edema, circulatory congestion and heart failure) the intake of these substances is carefully regulated and often restricted. Because salt makes food more palatable, its restriction poses a challenge to find other seasonings which the patient enjoys and which he is permitted to have.

Observation of daily weight, intake and output, vital signs, and the color, number, and consistency of bowel movements are important in care of the cirrhotic patient. Changes in any of these indicators of the patient's condition should be reported to the doctor.

Bed rest is ordered if the patient has signs of liver failure such as mental or neurologic disturbance, ascites, jaundice, and weakness. Thoughtful, attentive nursing care can make the difference between a relatively comfortable, really rested patient and an exceedingly uncomfortable, restless one. Helping the patient with bed baths and mouth care, applications of soothing lotions of powders, frequent turning to avoid pressure sores, and easy availability of urinal and bedpan are examples of measures which can increase the patient's comfort during the period of acute illness requiring bed rest.

As the patient's condition improves, helping him to walk and to find quiet diversion are important. Teaching the patient and his family assumes increasing importance as the patient recovers; this teaching requires the collaborative effort of the physician, nurse, and dietitian to help the patient learn how to adapt his way of life to provide the best possible chance of arresting the cirrhotic process. Emotional support is of particular 'importance. Sensitivity to the patient's concerns and willingness to listen can help the patient assess his own motivation and goals, and can assist him in accepting necessary restrictions.

Because immoderate use of alcohol is a significant factor in causing cirrhosis, the assumption is sometimes mistakenly made that cirrhotic patients are necessarily alcoholics. Some cirrhotic patients whose illness is not related to alcohol consumption are burdened by these assumptions of others, and by rejection which, regardless of the etiologic factors in the patient's illness, interferes with treatment and rehabilitation.

THE INCREASED FLUID RETENTION manifested as ascitic intra-abdominal fluid and tissue edema fluid involves several factors and relationships that are not entirely clear. Overproduction of the hormone aldosterone by the adrenal glands probably occurs in cirrhosis. This hormone causes intense sodium and water retention combined with potassium excretion. This, in addition to associated protein deficiency and factors affecting kidney function allows abnormal fluid collections.

Ascites and edema may be partially alleviated by restricting sodium intake to 1.0 Gm. or less per day and giving a diet rich in protein. The drug spironolactone (Aldactone) specifically antagonizes aldosterone, reversing the effects of this hormone so that sodium and water are excreted and potassium is retained. When the abdomen is so tense with fluid that kidney function is impaired, a paracentesis may be required. Even then, only a few liters of fluid are removed, because removal of large quantities of fluid at once can cause drastic shifts between the vascular and extravascular compartments and resultant circulatory collapse.

The rapid removal of abdominal fluid by paracentesis is achieved by carefully introducing a needle through the abdominal wall and allowing the ascites to drain. This may quickly relieve the severe discomfort of distention and difficulty in breathing secondary to a large volume of abdominal fluid pressing upon the diaphragm and lungs. Circulatory collapse (shock) can occur immediately after the tap from acute fluid, mineral and protein shifts acting to replace the lost ascitic fluid. Other complications of paracentesis include perforation of intestine or bladder with peritonitis, and leakage of fluid from the needle site. To avoid perforation of the bladder, it is important to have the patient void before paracentesis. Prior to paracentesis an infusion is usually ordered and plasma is made available for rapid administration if necessary. Pulse, blood pressure and breathing should be carefully observed after this procedure. Any changes in vital signs, abdominal pain or fever should be reported.

Complications. HEPATIC COMA. Coma may occur in any form of hepatic failure. Signs and symptoms have been described. Increased serum ammonia level seems to be related to the development or aggravation of hepatic coma, but is not the absolute cause. Therapy to reduce blood ammonia levels seems to ameliorate the comatose state. Ammonia formed in the intestine by bacterial action on ingested proteins is normally detoxified in the liver by conversion to urea which is then excreted by the kidneys. A failing liver, as in advanced cirrhosis, can no longer break down ammonia and allows it to accumulate in the blood. Also, with portal venous obstruction ammonia-rich intestinal blood may be diverted from the liver, further reducing detoxification.

Therapy of coma includes reducing protein intake to zero; avoiding drugs or stress, and removal of residual protein or blood (if there has been recent hemorrhage) from the intestine by cathartics and enemas. Broad spectrum antibiotics such as neomycin may be ordered in the presence of hepatic encephalopathy. Because it is only poorly absorbed from the gastrointestinal tract, neomycin is used frequently for disinfecting the bowel, thereby lessening the production of ammonia by the intestinal flora. Cleansing enemas are often ordered to reduce the fecal bacterial substrate in the colon. Careful medical support of the comatose patient involves maintenance of fluid and electrolyte balance with parenteral nutrition. Multivitamins are often added to infusions.

Nursing care involves the management of a semicomatose or fully unresponsive patient. Observation of vital signs, frequent turning to avoid pressure sores, mouth care, endotracheal suction to prevent aspiration pneumonia, use of siderails and frequent observation to prevent

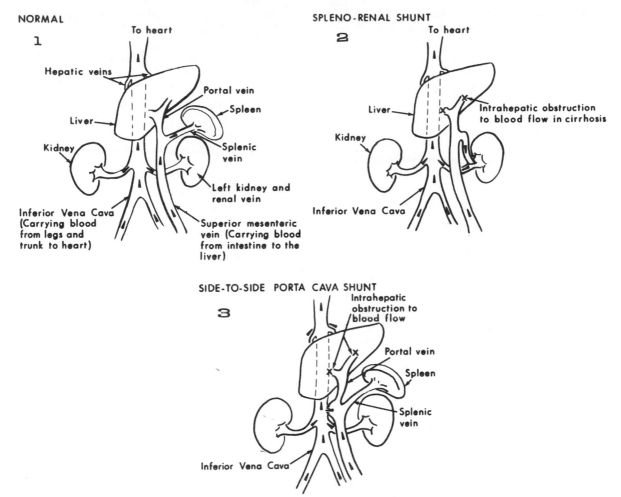

FIG. 39-1. (1) Normal anatomy showing blood flow back to the heart. Note that major veins pass through the liver. (2) Spleno-renal shunt. The spleen has been removed and the splenic vein connected to the left renal vein. Now some portal blood can flow into the inferior vena cava by thus passing the liver. (3) Side-to-side porta caval shunt. The side of the portal vein is anastomosed to the side of the inferior vena cava. Now blood can flow from the portal circulation into the systemic circulation if there is significant intra-hepatic obstruction.

falling, and similar common-sense measures are essential. When it is impossible to reverse the pathologic process, hepatic coma is a terminal state. In other instances, medical and nursing measures succeed and the patient recovers from coma.

PORTAL HYPERTENSION AND BLEEDING ESOPHA-GEAL VARICES. In the scarred cirrhotic liver the intrahepatic veins may be squeezed shut so that blood backs up into the portal vein and on into diverting channels around the esophagus and stomach. If the portal vein itself is obstructed (by tumor, clot, infection or by unknown cause), similar collateral diversion occurs. The buildup of pressure in the portal system (portal hypertension) can be measured by manometry, and an x-ray picture can be taken of the portal vascular system by percutaneous splenoportogram. Before this test is ordered the physician evaluates the patient's bleeding tendency, because a severe bleeding tendency would make the test very hazardous to the patient. It is necessary for the patient to sign an operative permit, and sedation is ordered prior to the test, which is performed in the x-ray department. Under sterile conditions a needle is introduced through the skin into the spleen. Since the venous drainage of the spleen is into the portal vein, the pressure in the spleen will be a good reflection of portal pressure. This is recorded. If it is over 25 cm. of water (18 mm. Hg), it is diagnostic of portal hypertension and indicates the patient is a potential bleeder from esophageal varices. The most life-threatening complication for the cirrhotic patient is hemorrhage from esophageal varices. Patients with cirrhosis of the liver have a high incidence of duodenal ulcers, which may be another cause of gastrointestinal bleeding.

Portal hypertension can be relieved by surgically draining blood from the portal vein into an adjacent systemic vein. As less blood then goes through the portal system, the pressure drops and there is less chance of bursting a collateral vessel with resultant hemorrhage.

The portal vein lies just next to the inferior vena cava. Surgically a connection can be made between these vessels so that portal blood is released into the vena cava, reducing hypertension. This is called a *portacaval shunt* procedure. Sometimes a similar beneficial effect is achieved by connecting the splenic vein (a tributary of the portal vein) to the renal vein (a tributary of the vena cava). This is called a *splenorenal shunt* (see Fig. 39-1).

These are major operations. If done electively or prophylactically to prevent future hemorrhage, the patient should be in the very best possible preoperative condition. The jaundiced, hypoproteinemic patient with electrolyte disorders and ascites is a poor risk and will frequently not tolerate this surgery. Such complications should be rectified before surgery.

Other emergency operations to stop bleeding from varices include direct division and ligation of varices in the stomach and esophagus. Both before and after surgery, the doctors and nurses work as a team to carry out the intensive program of care and observation needed to pull these critically ill people through.

Sengstaken-Blakemore Esophageal-Gastric Balloon Tube. The use of this tube can be hazardous and requires *constant vigil by both doctors and nurses* in order to get the best effect. It has three separate openings. One inflates the esophageal balloon, one inflates the gastric balloon and one aspirates the stomach. The distended, bleeding varices of portal hypertension are in the lower esophagus and upper stomach. As the gastric balloon is inflated to the prescribed pressure, it is gently pulled up. In this way constant application of this balloon to the upper stomach wall squeezes any bleeding vessels shut. Similarly, as the esophageal balloon is inflated, it expands against the esophageal wall and ruptured bleed-

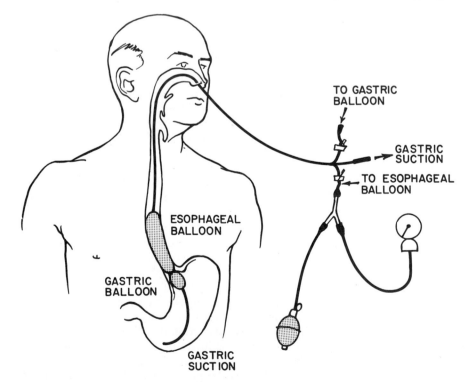

TO GASTRIC
BALLOON

GASTRIC
SUCTION

TO ESOPHAGEAL
BALLOON

ESOPHAGEAL
BALLOON

GASTRIC
BALLOON

GASTRIC
SUCTION

FIG. 39-2. A Sengstaken-Blakemore tube in place. The clamp on the tube that leads to the esophageal balloon is kept tightly closed to maintain the inflated balloon at the prescribed pressure. The clamp is loosened to check the pressure with the manometer. The gastric suction tube is attached to continuous suction to keep the patient's stomach empty and to prevent vomiting, which would dislodge the esophageal balloon. Irrigations of the gastric suction tube may be ordered to prevent clogging with blood.

ing varices are pressed closed. In this way bleeding can be controlled. Through the tube opening into the stomach, clots can be irrigated out (reducing protein by-products of digested blood which lead to ammonia production and possible hepatic coma).

Patients who have this tube in place require continuous nursing care and observation, and for this reason are usually placed in the intensive care unit.

As the patient's condition stabilizes, the tube may be deflated, 24 to 48 hours later. It is hoped that bleeding will not recur. The tube is not removed yet, but kept in place so that rapid reinflation can be carried out if necessary. During this period the patient is observed for melena, further hematemesis, fall in blood pressure, fall in hematocrit and tachycardia, which indicate further bleeding. If bleeding occurs or is uncontrolled, emergency shunt or ligation operations may be necessary.

With this tube in place the patient may be restless, apprehensive and uncomfortable. Simple sedatives, such as antihistamines, may be useful. Barbiturates that are usually metabolized in the liver should not be used.

Viral Hepatitis (Infectious or Serum Hepatitis)

Pathology. Hepatitis is an infectious, contagious disease of the liver caused by a virus. The infection may cause simultaneous damage to the intestine and other organs, but the most significant damage is to liver cells which become necrotic and die. In fatal cases parenchymal damage is severe. Internal damage to the liver may prevent normal bile secretion or excretion causing jaundice in addition to the metabolic dysfunction of parenchymal injury.

Etiology and Incidence. There are two types of hepatitis: both are caused by viruses which, although similar in nature, produce slightly different clinical diseases. Infectious hepatitis is caused by the IH virus, or virus A; serum hepatitis is caused by the SH virus, or virus B.

Both of these viruses resist drying, freezing, heating and other physical and chemical treatment. They can be destroyed by heating at 60° C. for 10 hours. Albumin may be made virus-free whereas whole blood and pooled plasma cannot be decontaminated and are frequent methods of transmission of the virus.

Infectious hepatitis is usually disseminated by contact with contagious virus in the stool of infected people. The virus may be transmitted by close contact with carriers, contaminated food, water or other items apt to be taken orally. Contaminated rectal thermometers, bedpans, and linen harbor the virus, which then reaches the fingers and may be subsequently ingested. Diseased food handlers, cooks or waiters may create an epidemic especially in the army, schools, or similar close community conditions. Virus A also occurs in the blood stream of infected people, so that it can also be transmitted by this route. The virus may be in the blood before, during and after the period of infectivity. Duration of infectivity may be difficult to determine.

Serum hepatitis virus B is found only in blood and is transmitted by transfusions of blood or plasma and inoculation via contaminated syringes, needles, surgical and dental equipment. Carriers are asymptomatic and may be infective for long periods. This condition has risen markedly in incidence in areas of the country where drug abuse is widespread. Drug addicts often use unsterile syringes and contract the disease in this way.

Signs and Symptoms. Serum hepatitis and infectious hepatitis are not clinically distinguishable. The incubation period of infectious hepatitis is from 6 days to 6 weeks whereas serum hepatitis takes 60 to 120 days to develop after infection occurs.

The disease pattern, except for the difference in incubation period, is basically the same. In the preicteric (early or prejaundice) phase, manifestations include fevers, rash, joint pain, lymph-node enlargement, anorexia, nausea, vomiting, weakness, pain over the liver, and diarrhea. The liver may be enlarged and tender to percussion; there is often a distaste for smoking tobacco; fatigue may be profound. The spleen is often palpably enlarged.

All these manifestations may occur with varying speed of onset before jaundice is seen. Icterus may be evident from one to three weeks after onset of symptoms. Occasionally, a patient will die of massive liver failure even before becoming jaundiced. As jaundice appears, patients usually improve clinically with better appetite, less pain, and increased strength. Jaundice usually persists one or two weeks. An important concern of the physician is to differentiate between jaundice due to hepatitis and jaundice due to obstruction.

Prognosis. A small number (less than 1%) of patients will proceed to hepatic coma and death. Most will recover, but they will be forever barred from being blood donors. A few patients will suffer from chronic active hepatitis. These patients usually go on to cirrhosis and death unless corticosteroid treatment slows the active and inflammatory process.

Prevention. Gamma globulin has been used as a preventive against hepatitis with some small success. It may make the attack of hepatitis less severe. It does not give 100 per cent protection; it probably gives no protection against serum hepatitis and it is of no help if the patient already has contracted the disease.

Since at present there is no way for a blood bank to detect the hepatitis virus in the blood of a donor, many hospitals are instituting a policy of preadmission blood donations by the patient himself. Patients scheduled for elective surgery, who may require blood transfusions, are requested to donate their own blood a few weeks in advance of surgery.

With both types of hepatitis, extreme caution is required to avoid direct contact with the patient's blood. The nurse should use great care to see that she is not pricked accidentally by the needle that has been used to withdraw blood from a hepatitis patient. Disposable syringes and needles should be used for these patients. In the unusual situation in which none is available, the needle and the syringe should be rinsed with water and placed in a rack or boat containing solvent or soap solution. If the needles are cared for immediately after use, the chance of anyone's pricking himself with them is lessened.

Needles and syringes should not be used again for a patient until they have been autoclaved at 15 pounds of pressure for a minimum of 20 minutes. If boiling is the only method of sterilization available to the nurse, the equipment should be completely covered by bubbling water for no less than 30 minutes. There is no antiseptic known that kills the viruses, and placing of equipment in alcohol or other antiseptic solutions does not sterilize it against these stubborn organisms. Therefore, this practice is discouraged in any setting, even when there is no known hepatitis patient. Also to be absolutely condemned is the practice of using the same syringe for more than one patient without sterilization of the syringe between uses. When the plunger is pulled back, a small amount of serum enters the syringe. Changing the needle but using the same syringe does not prevent the injection of that serum into the next patient, and hepatitis can be spread from "healthy" carriers in this way.

Treatment. As there is no known drug or medical therapy that directly affects the viruses of hepatitis, the treatment is directed at strengthening the patient's body to withstand the insult of the infection. Rest is a cornerstone of treatment.

Bed rest and a nourishing diet, often one that is higher in protein and carbohydrate, are offered the patient. Although the patient probably will be grateful for the rest, his poor appetite will make it difficult for him to accept the diet.

Nursing Care. Because the treatment is concerned mainly with improving the patient's resistance so that he can fight the virus, nursing care is of paramount importance. Bed rest should not be a mere twisting and turning in an uncomfortable tangle of sheets. Comfortable positioning of the patient, with pillows and changes of bed position, may help him to rest. The nurse also helps to protect her patient from disturbances by maintaining quiet in the halls, explaining the need for rest to visitors, and doing as much as is necessary for the patient at one time so that he need not be bothered at frequent intervals.

His interest in food may be enlivened by an attractively served tray. A small quantity of food does not look as discouraging to the anorectic patient as does a full tray. Hot drinks that are really hot, and cold drinks that are iced are more tempting than those that are lukewarm. Any patient with jaundice (unless the presence of another disease contraindicates the rule) should drink a hearty quantity of fluid each day: 3,000 ml. is a desirable goal. Dehydration can lead to hepatic coma. Color of skin, stool and urine should be observed.

Although the mode of transmission of serum hepatitis and infectious hepatitis is different, the differential diagnosis between the two diseases may be difficult to make. Therefore all patients with hepatitis are usually placed in isolation. Linen is handled separately. Dishes and eating utensils are sterilized. When paper plates are used, they should be heat-retaining and able to contain food without becoming soaked. It is understandable that patients resent being served meals that arrive cold and on soggy plates.

Since the virus of infectious hepatitis lives in the gastrointestinal tract, stool precautions are required. The patient has his own thermometer, and, if it is a rectal thermometer, the nurse is especially careful to scrub her hands after handling it. Since thermometers are known for their poor reaction to autoclaving, it is good economy to throw them away after the patient's discharge from the hospital. This practice is less expensive than trying to sterilize them and possibly infecting another patient with hepatitis. The bedpan is kept for the hepatitis patient's sole use, and it is autoclaved or boiled for an hour when he leaves the hospital. The disposal of feces is carried out according to the hospital rules for stool precautions with strict attention to technic. The nurse is careful to wash her hands well after handling the bedpan. Rubber gloves should be used when she is giving the patient a rectal treatment.

Visitors should be given enough instruction in isolation precautions to enable them to protect themselves. Warn them against close contact with the patient, sharing his food or giving him the bedpan.

Viral hepatitis lowers the patient's resistance to secondary infection. Careful hand washing on entering the patient's unit protects him. No effort should be spared to separate the patient from infective organisms.

Patients generally are kept in isolation until the fever has subsided and the jaundice begins to fade, usually for one or two weeks after the onset of symptoms. As the patient begins to feel well, he may have a tendency to overexert and cause a recurrence of symptoms. The nurse can help to prevent this relapse by encouraging a return to bed if he seems to be a person who drives himself.

Noninfectious Hepatitis (Toxic or Chemical)

Exposure to cleaning solutions with carbon tetrachloride, insecticides, cinchophen (a drug used in arthritis), and a variety of other drugs and chemicals can cause severe liver derangement. Degree of damage, signs and symptoms will vary with the amount of poisoning as well as associated damage to kidneys and other organs. The clinical picture may evolve gradually or abruptly and be indistinguishable from viral hepatitis. History of exposure, high WBC count, acute onset of jaundice and hepatic failure with a rapidly enlarging tender liver usually is more indicative of toxic hepatitis.

Therapy involves removal of the toxic agent, a diet high in carbohydrates, proteins and vitamins, and rest in bed. General supportive and convalescent care is similar to that prescribed for viral hepatitis.

The prophylaxis of this form of disease requires education of children, parents, industrial workers and others by nurses, doctors and public health-minded individuals. Advise the public to read labels carefully and observe precautions in use of cleaning solutions, insecticides and other chemicals; provide adequate ventilation when using volatile chemicals; keep chemicals away from children; take no medicines unless specifically prescribed by the doctor. Often patients will save unused portions of a prescribed medicine, then pass it on to a friend or relative, or even use it for a different condition without medical consultation in order to avoid expense.

DISEASES OF THE BILIARY SYSTEM

Anatomy and Function

The gallbladder is attached to the midportion of the undersurface of the liver. Normally it has a thin wall and a capacity of about 60 ml. of bile. Bile formed in the liver enters the intrahepatic bile ducts and travels to the common hepatic duct. It usually then passes into the cystic duct and is stored in the gallbladder. When required, the gallbladder empties its bile, which now goes out of the cystic duct, into the common bile duct and on into the duodenum. Stones can be found in any portion of this bile system, most frequently in the gallbladder. Arteries, veins and lymphatics are associated with all sections of the biliary tree, and along with the ducts themselves are subject to considerable variation.

The liver forms up to one liter of bile per day. Upon reaching the gallbladder, bile is altered by the absorption of water and minerals to form a more concentrated product. Upon reaching the intestine after gallbladder contraction (stimulated by ingested food, especially fats), this bile functions in the absorption of fats, fat-soluble vitamins, iron and calcium. Bile also activates the pancreas to release its digestive enzymes as well as an alkaline fluid which may neutralize stomach acids reaching the duodenum.

Cholecystitis and Cholelithiasis

These terms signify gallbladder inflammation and stones within the gallbladder. Gallstones represent the most common abnormality of the biliary system occurring in about 20 per cent of people over 40 years. There is progressive increased incidence with aging. They occur in women about four times more often than in men, particularly in women with a history of pregnancies, diabetes and obesity. The etiology of gallbladder stones has not been definitely established. Bile stasis and infection have been generally implicated. Hemolytic anemias associated with excessive bilirubin formations are associated with development of pigment stones; hypercholestolemia is associated with the accumulation of cholesterol type of stones.

Chronic cholecystitis is rarely present without stones. Stones and infections are intimately related. Symptoms in this condition are probably secondary to transient blockage of the outflow of bile due to stones or spasms of the ductal system. Most usually, after a meal containing fried, greasy, spicy or fatty foods the patient experiences belching, nausea, and right upper abdominal discomfort, with pain or cramps. When pain is very severe this is called "biliary colic." Pain may radiate around the right to the back and shoulder. Vomiting may occur.

In simple, uncomplicated colic of chronic cholecystitis with stones, there is no jaundice, fever, chills, liver damage, leukocytosis, or evidence of peritonitis on abdominal examination. Many patients with stones in the gallbladder may never have significant symptomatology.

Diagnosis. In addition to suggestive signs and symptoms, definitive demonstration of cholelithiasis is by the cholecystogram (gallbladder series x-ray). The evening before roentgenography a special dye-containing tablet is given the patient, after which he should fast until the time of testing. The nurse should be sure he gets and takes the tablet and remains fasting during the night. After ingestion, this dye reaches the liver, is excreted into the bile and passes into the gallbladder, making it visible radiographically.

Treatment. Because of the distress associated with this condition, removal of the gallbladder (cholecystectomy) is usually advised. Even in mild cases, because of the possibility of future distress and the complications of acute cholecystitis, cholecystectomy is still advised by many surgeons who prefer to operate electively rather than anticipate a more urgent situation.

Medical Management. Patients known to have gallbladder stones should be advised to avoid fried, greasy, spicy and high cholesterol foods in their diet. These include eggs, pork products, rich dressings, cheese, cream and whole milk. A dietitian should instruct the patient and outline a palatable, wholesome diet also aimed to maintain a reasonable body weight.

During an attack of colic, therapy usually involves rest, a bland liquid diet, and sedation. If vomiting is a feature, hospitalization, nasogastric suction and parenteral fluids may be needed.

Demerol and morphine may be used to reduce severe pain or colic. These drugs should be used sparingly and strictly if necessary because of their known capability to cause spasm of portions of the common duct. Nitroglycerine and aminophylline may be used to attempt relief of spasm; however, many doctors believe these drugs are not often required.

Surgical Management. Patients whose attacks continue or grow worse are usually treated surgically. Cholecystectomy is planned under general anesthesia. The day before surgery a liquid diet helps to keep the bowel clean; after midnight the patient is placed on NPO; the morning of operation a nasogastric tube is usually put in place so that postoperative secretions and swallowed air can be removed from the stomach.

Of particular importance in postoperative care of patients who have had cholecystectomy are:

• Emphasis on deep-breathing and coughing. Because the incision is high on the abdomen, these patients find full expansion of the chest more painful than those with a lower incision.

• Medication for relief of pain must be administered frequently enough so that the patient can rest and carry out his postoperative exercises, but not so frequently that the patient's activity is diminished and his respirations become shallow or even depressed.

• Attention to positioning, privacy, lack of haste, and an attitude of calmness on the part of the nurse can help the patient void before the bladder becomes distressingly distended. Otherwise the patient's tension, physical discomfort, and preoccupation with voiding militate against spontaneous voiding, and catheterization, which might have been avoided, becomes necessary.

For a simple cholecystectomy one or two soft rubber drains are placed in the area of the excised gallbladder to remove blood and bile which may accumulate after surgery. If the dressing is stained excessively with blood or bile, the doctor should be immediately made aware of this.

With a smooth course, the nasogastric tube is usually removed in 24 to 46 hours and liquid feedings are started and gradually progressed to a general low-fat diet. The rubber drain is usually taken out by the third to fifth day. Patients are usually recommended to keep to a low-fat diet indefinitely.

Acute cholecystitis is a progression of chronic cholecystitis in which a stone completely blocks off flow of bile from the gallbladder. If the stone impacted in the cystic duct does not dislodge spontaneously, the walls of the distended gallbladder may become gangrenous causing rupture and subsequent peritonitis. These patients are usually very sick with fever, vomiting, severe abdominal pain and tenderness over the liver. The gallbladder may be so swollen that it becomes palpable; the WBC is high; jaundice may be slightly evident due to associated hepatic inflammation.

Medical management including antibiotics, parenteral fluids and nasogastric suction fails to relieve a significant number of patients. In these cases surgery may be life-saving and consists either of cholecystectomy or cholecystostomy (opening of the gallbladder, removal of stones and placement of a tube for bile drainage to the exterior). If medical therapy is elected and is successful, cholecystectomy is carried out 2 to 3 months after inflammation has subsided.

Choledocholithiasis means the presence of stones anywhere in the ducts of the biliary system. The usual origin is the gallbladder. However, a small number of people form stones within the ductal system even after the gallbladder is removed.

Signs and symptoms are those of cholecystitis and cholelithiasis, but in addition jaundice is typical of this condition. If stones completely block the common duct, the stools will be clay colored because no bilirubin reaches the intestine, and the urine will darken with bilirubin as this pigment backs up into the blood and reaches the kidney.

Treatment of choledocholithiasis is surgical exploration of the common duct, removal of stones and cholecystectomy if the gallbladder is present. At the end of this operation, a small T-shaped tube is placed into the common duct. The small end is placed in the duct lumen aligned lengthwise; the long end comes out through the skin (see Fig. 39-3). If bile flow is temporarily obstructed because of postsurgical spasm of the duct after surgery, this tube will allow decompression by releasing bile externally. Before terminating the operation, dye may be introduced into the T-tube to visualize the ductal tree, insuring that all stones have been removed.

The postoperative care is similar to that following cholecystectomy, except that in this case there is a T-tube to observe. This is connected to straight gravity drainage. The collection bag or bottle is attached to the bed below the level of the operation site. This is to prevent reflux

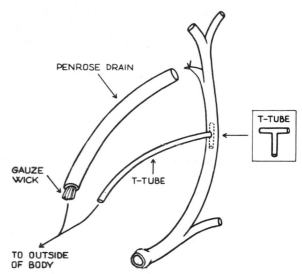

FIG. 39-3. After cholecystectomy the Penrose drain helps to remove exudate from the area formerly occupied by the gallbladder. The T tube diverts bile to the outside.

of bile back into the duct as well as to avoid an excessive height against which bile would have to "climb" in order to drain. Furthermore, the receptacle must have a vent opening to prevent pressure buildup which would hinder bile drainage.

The tube is usually left constantly open. Kinking or allowing the patient to roll over and occlude the lumen must be avoided. It should not be clamped without a doctor's order. Drainage usually amounts to a few hundred milliliters of bile per day since most of the bile is expected to pass on into the intestine. However, if total obstruction is present in the common duct, up to 1 liter of bile may drain and the stool will be light colored.

The T-tube is usually removed after the tenth postoperative day. Frequently a T-tube cholangiogram (in which dye is introduced into the tube and an x-ray picture is taken) is done prior to removal to be sure there is no residual obstruction.

The usual postoperative measures include early ambulation, nasogastric tube aspiration, observation of vital signs and wound drainage for blood or bile.

THE PANCREAS

The pancreas is a gland which has two major functions. As an endocrine organ it produces insulin. This hormone maintains the blood sugar level and is secreted directly into the blood stream. As an exocrine organ it produces a variety of protein, fat and carbohydrate digesting enzymes. These do not enter the blood stream directly, but instead enter the ducts of the pancreas and eventually are released into the lumen of the duodenum, where they act directly on arriving food. By a complex interplay of chemical and nervous stimuli, the pancreas is activated by ingested foods to release its enzymes at the appropriate time for most efficient digestion.

Acute Pancreatitis

The exact etiology of pancreatitis is unknown. In simplest terms pancreatitis may be defined as an inflammatory disease characterized by the destruction of pancreatic tissue as well as functional capability. Pancreatitis may be acute and mild, or may occur abruptly with a fulminant, often quickly fatal course. Later it may occur as a chronic disease, with a long history of relapse and recurrent attacks. Mortality in acute cases may reach as high as 20 per cent.

Pancreatitis is often noted to develop in people with a history of biliary tract disease, high alcohol intake and hyperparathyroidism. However, many persons who develop pancreatitis have no other illness.

Signs and Symptoms. In acute pancreatitis, the most common complaint is severe middle-upper abdominal pain, which may radiate to both sides and straight through to the back. Usually, nausea and vomiting are present. If the pancreatic inflammation is intense, with necrosis and hemorrhage of the gland, peritonitis, severe fluid and electrolyte imbalance and shock may ensue. In fulminant cases the fatty tissue around the pancreas is digested by lipase, a fat-digesting enzyme. Calcium binds with the released fatty acids. In rare cases, this reduces the level of circulating calcium to dangerous levels, resulting in tetany and convulsions. Also, in the more advanced circumstances of hemorrhagic pancreatitis, released blood may discolor the skin of the lateral abdominal wall.

In addition to the various radiologic and blood tests that may be carried out in the diagnosis of pancreatitis, a serum amylase and lipase level are usually ordered. These two enzymes, normal secretions of the pancreas, will appear in elevated quantities in the blood stream of most patients with significant pancreatitis.

Recurrent (Relapsing) and Chronic Pancreatitis

Recurrent pancreatitis is the reappearance of intermittent attacks of pancreatic inflammation after an initial attack earlier in life. With chronicity, there may be partial to ultimate complete loss of function as pancreatic tissue is progressively destroyed.

With the late development of chronic recurrent pancreatitis, stones and strictures may obstruct the pancreatic ducts. Areas of pancreatic breakdown may disrupt to form "pseudocysts" which are fluid-filled pouches budding from the diseased pancreas. These cause symptoms by pressure upon adjacent organs or by rupturing. With the development of chronic pancreatitis, pain, weight loss, digestive disturbances, diabetes, malnutrition and steatorrhea (excessive fat in the stool) occur, in addition to the usual signs and symptoms of acute pancreatitis. These problems are caused by the progressive loss of exocrine and endocrine actions of the gland.

Treatment. In acute pancreatitis measures are taken to relieve pain, reduce pancreatic secretion, restore fluid and electrolyte losses and combat infection. The patient usually receives nothing by mouth and continuous nasogastric aspiration is applied. This will relieve nausea, distention and vomiting as well as reduce stimulation of the pancreas by gastric contents entering the duodenum. Atropine or other anticholinergic drugs may be used to reduce the activity of the vagus nerve, because the vagus nerve stimulates the pancreas. Drugs to decrease the activity of proteolytic enzymes released from the pancreas are used by some physicians to reduce their autodigestive action.

Improvement usually occurs in about a week. The diet initially prescribed is extremely bland with slow progress to a low-fat diet. Alcohol, coffee, tea, and other irritants or rich foods are withheld. Prolonged use of narcotic pain relievers may lead to addiction, a common complication of pancreatitis in its chronic or recurrent stages. Care and thought in the prescription and administration of narcotics is therefore essential.

There is no direct surgical therapy for acute pancreatitis. However, if pancreatic abscess is suspected, this must be drained surgically. Also if acute cholecystitis or obstruction of the common duct are felt to be coincident and/or inciting factors, drainage and simple stone removal may be necessary. Simple bile diversion by cholecystostomy or choledochostomy are felt by some authorities to give relief and hasten healing in acute pancreatitis.

The treatment of chronic, recurrent pancreatitis depends on the etiology and whether or not obstruction of the pancreatic duct is present. If pancreatic duct obstruction is not yet present, abstinence from alcohol, a bland fat-free diet and correction of associated biliary tract disease or hyperparathyroidism may give good results. If there is scarring with stricture and stenosis of portions of the pancreatic duct, a variety of complex surgical measures is available to attempt reconstitution of an unobstructed flow into the intestine.

Pseudocytes of the diseased pancreas can be removed, but often are simply drained directly into the intestinal tract. Chronic pain may be relieved by operative removal of the nerve fibers supplying the pancreas, as well as removal of part or all of the pancreas. The diabetes and digestive enzyme deficiency seen with advanced pancreatic destruction may be treated with insulin and exocrine enzyme replacement.

Nursing Care. Because severe pain is the outstanding symptom of pancreatitis, nursing intervention involves relief of pain by careful administration of prescribed analgesics, and by other measures such as changes of position.

During the acute attack the patient will need mouth care, as does any patient with continuous nasogastric suction. His nasal passage also may feel dry and sore from the tube, and a small amount of glycerine may help. However, be sure that it is only a tiny amount and not enough for him to aspirate into his lungs.

BIBLIOGRAPHY

CHILD, C. G., III: *The Liver and Portal Hypertension,* Philadelphia, Saunders, 1964.

COLCOCK, B. P., and LIDDLE, H. V.: Common bile duct stones, *New Eng. J. Med.* 258:264, 1958.

EKMAN, C. A., and SANDBLOM, P.: Shunt operation in acute bleeding from esophageal varices, *Ann. Surg.* 160:531, 1964.

FLYNN, B.: Esophageal varices: components of nursing care, *Am. J. Nurs.* 64:107, June, 1964.

FOULK, W. (ed.): *Diseases of the Liver,* New York, McGraw-Hill, 1968.

GIVEN, BARBARA and SIMMONS, SANDRA: Acute pancreatitis, *Am. J. Nurs.,* 71:934, May, 1971.

GLENN, F.: Surgical treatment of biliary tract disease, *Am. J. Nurs.* 64:88, May, 1964.

GLENN, F., and THORBJARNSON, B.: The surgical treatment of acute cholecystitis, *Surg. Gynec. Obstet.* 113:265, 1961.

HENDERSON, L. M.: Nursing care in acute cholecystitis, *Am. J. Nurs.* 64:93, May, 1964.

HUYLER, J.: Impaired liver function and related nursing care, *Am. J. Nurs.* 68:2374, November, 1968.

KAPLAN, M., and BERNHEIM, E.: Esophageal varices, *Am. J. Nurs.* 64:104, June, 1964.

LIEBOWITZ, H. R.: *Bleeding Esophageal Varices: Portal Hypertension,* Springfield, Ill., Thomas, 1959.

McINTYRE, N., and SHERLOCK, S.: *Therapeutic Agents and the Liver,* Philadelphia, Davis, 1965.

NACHLAS, M. M., O'NEILL, J. E., and CAMPBELL, A. J. A.: The life history of patients with cirrhosis of the liver and bleeding esophageal varices, *Ann. Surg.* 141:10, 1955.

POPPER, H., and SCHAFFNER, F.: *Liver: Structure and Function,* New York, McGraw-Hill, 1957.

PRESTON, F. W., and KUHRAL, J. C.: Surgical physiology of the pancreas, *Surg. Clin. N. Am.* 48:203, 1962.

ROBINSON, C.: *Proudfit-Robinson's Normal and Therapeutic Nutrition,* ed. 13, New York, Macmillan, 1967.

SALMON, P. A.: Carcinoma of the pancreas and extrahepatic biliary system, *Surgery,* 60:554, 1966.

SCHIFF, L. (ed.): *Diseases of the Liver,* ed. 3, Philadelphia, Lippincott, 1969.

SHERLOCK, S.: *Diseases of the Liver,* ed. 4, Philadelphia, Davis, 1968.

SILEN, W., and GOLDMAN, L.: A clinical analysis of acute pancreatitis, *Arch. Surg.* 86:1032, 1963.

SNELL, A. M.: Liver function tests and their interpretation, *Gastroenterology* 34:675, 1958.

STEWART, R.: Poisoning from chlorinated hydrocarbon solvents, *Am. J. Nurs.* 67:85, January, 1967.

TAYLOR, K., *et al.*: Liver transplant, *Am. J. Nurs.* 68:1895, September, 1968.

The Urologic Patient 40

The Urinary Tract · Diagnostic Procedures · Observations
Care of Patients Who Have Catheters · The Patient with Urinary
Incontinence · Urinary Obstructions · Infection · Nephritis
Nephrosis · Tumors · Other Urinary Tract Conditions

Patients with disorders of the urinary tract not only suffer from the accompanying physical discomfort, but often from embarrassment and anxiety as well. Because disclosure of genitourinary difficulties often involves the sharing of very personal information and the experience of an extensive physical inspection and examination of this part of the body, patients tend to delay seeking medical help. Since the sex organs and urinary tract are in close physical proximity, disturbances of urinary elimination may pose the threat of sexual inadequacy as well. Every effort should be made to protect the patient's modesty and privacy and to deal matter-of-factly with the problem.

Urologic patients, like others, can express their anxiety in a variety of ways. The threatened male patient, for example, may become more immodest and aggressive towards the female nurse than customarily accepted hospital behavior. It is important for the nurse to try to understand the reason for the patient's behavior. However, this does not imply accepting this behavior. Instead, it is necessary to set limits regarding behavior and to listen and talk with the patient regarding his feelings and concerns. Overt sexual behavior of this type may be anxiety producing for the nurse and she may react by withdrawing from the patient. The patient, in turn, becomes more threatened and his self-esteem is lowered even more. Asking the patient to behave more appropriately shows a response to his overt behavior, respect for his capacity to change it, and paves the way for more appropriate anxiety-relief mechanisms such as talking with the nurse or physician about what is bothering him. Not only is it important to understand the patient's emotional response, but also the normal anatomy and physiology of the urinary tract and its alterations during disease.

The urinary tract is one of several waste disposal systems by which the body rids itself of the by-products of metabolism. This system is also essential for the regulation of body fluids and their electrolyte content. When the kidneys are diseased or injured, and their function is impaired, or when there is an obstruction to the free flow of urine to the outside, serious illness is present or imminent. Often, conditions which do develop require long-term care and treatment.

THE URINARY TRACT

The urinary tract consists of the *kidneys,* which manufacture urine, and the various tubes and reservoirs necessary to discharge this fluid from the body. The kidneys have at least three known functions. They excrete excess water and the nitrogenous waste products of protein metabolism; they play a significant role in maintaining the acid-base balance of the body and the equilibrium of plasma electrolytes. Finally, they produce enzymes, such as renin, which acts on certain plasma constituents to form a compound that raises the blood pressure. The kidneys selectively filter over 50 gallons of plasma daily. All but a quart or so of this volume is resorbed back into the circulation every 24 hours.

The formed urine is excreted into the renal *pelves* and carried down the *ureters* to the

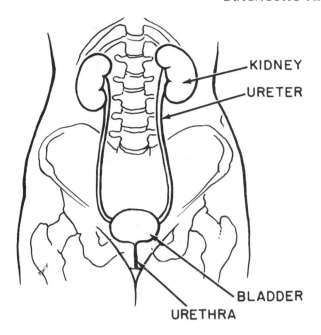

FIG. 40-1. The urinary tract.

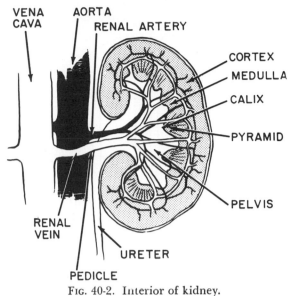

FIG. 40-2. Interior of kidney.

bladder. Here the urine is stored until the capacity of the bladder is reached at which time the patient voids the urine to the outside through the *urethra.* Any disorder which interferes with this process is likely to cause serious repercussions to the patient unless the situation can be corrected. These disorders include interference with the circulation to the kidney, disease of the kidney itself and obstruction to the drainage of the urinary tract.

DIAGNOSTIC PROCEDURES

Urinalysis

A great deal about the condition of the kidneys, the electrolyte balance and the over-all health can be learned by a study of the urine. Urinalysis is the most important diagnostic study of the urinary tract.

The characteristics of normal urine are:

Specific gravity	1.005 to 1.025
Color	Pale yellow to dark amber
Turbidity	Usually clear (cloudiness not always abnormal)
Acidity	pH 4.8 to 7.5
Protein	None to trace
Glucose	None to trace
Red blood cells	0-3 per high power field
White blood cells	0-4 per high power field
Casts	Rare per high power field

A red color to the urine may mean blood, but must be proved by microscopic examination of the sediment. Certain metabolic disturbances, ingested dyes or foodstuffs may impart a red color that is not blood. One-fifth of patients admitted to the hospital with gross blood in the urine (hematuria) have cancer in the urinary tract and this finding requires a complete urologic investigation. Cloudiness of the urine may be due to phosphates (a normal finding) or to white cells, suggesting an infection or irritation of the tract. Proteinuria (usually albumin) may occasionally be normal. More often it implies disease of the system. Little of this material filters through the pores of the normal glomeruli. Casts are molds of the renal tubules and their size will vary with the size of the portion of the nephron from whence they originate. They may be constituted of red cells, white cells, or precipitated protein.

The container in which the urine specimen is collected should be clean and dry; it should be sterile if a culture is to be taken. It is preferable to have the patient void directly into the container that is sent to the laboratory. Taking a urine specimen from a bedpan or a urinal that contains sediment from previous use may result in inaccurate results.

When infection is suspected, a specimen may be taken for culture. In men it is usually sufficient to cleanse the glans penis with an antiseptic and have the patient void about 60 ml., which are discarded, and then void into a sterile specimen

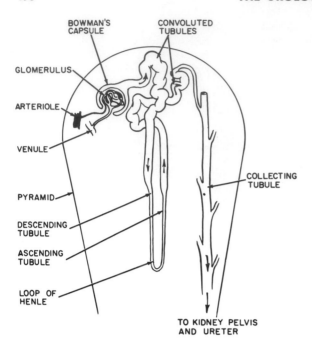

FIG. 40-3. A nephron.

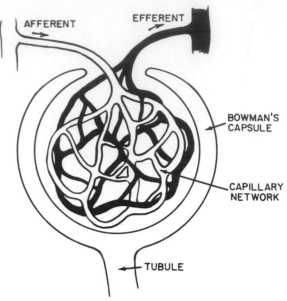

FIG. 40-4. Bowman's capsule.

bottle. Cap the bottle in such a way that it is not contaminated. A male nurse or nursing assistant can help men patients. In women, specimens for culture may be obtained by catheterization. However, because there is always the danger of introducing infection into the urinary tract with a catheter, the "sterile (or clean) catch" procedure is used in many hospitals. The labia are held apart, and the area is cleansed as for catheterization. While the nurse continues to hold the labia open so that the orifice of the urethra is exposed, the patient voids into a sterile container after the initial 60 ml. are discarded.

Since bacteria multiply in urine and to avoid decomposition of its contents, the specimen is delivered immediately to the laboratory or promptly refrigerated on the ward.

Fractionated urine specimens may be obtained in order to identify where a urinary abnormality such as pus is coming from. One method used is the three glass test. The first 60 ml. voided represent urethral washings. A second, similar volume is from the bladder and kidneys. A third specimen, obtained after the doctor performs prostatic massage includes the secretions of that organ. Papanicolaou smears of the urine may identify cancer cells arising from the lining of the kidney, ureter, and bladder. Specimens are

secured in the same manner as described for suspected infection.

Sometimes a specimen of all the urine excreted over a period of time, such as 24 hours, may be needed for examination of such constituents as tubercle bacilli and 17-ketosteroids. The patient empties his bladder immediately prior to the start of the time period and this is discarded. The entire specimen is refrigerated to prevent bacterial growth. To prevent any part of the specimen from being lost or contaminated, the patient is instructed to use separate receptacles for voiding and defecation.

Blood Chemistry

When the nephrons fail to remove waste products efficiently from the body, the blood chemistry is altered. Deterioration in renal function is manifested chemically by rises in the blood urea nitrogen (BUN) and creatinine values, both of which are protein breakdown products. However, there must be a 50 to 75 per cent decrease in function before these values rise. The normal BUN is 8 to 18 mg.%, and creatinine 0.5 to 1.0 mg.%. High blood levels of urea nitrogen can be accompanied by disorientation and convulsions. When you are caring for a patient with kidney disease note any abnormalities in blood chemistry reports. This information can serve as one guide to planning nursing care. For example, if the patient's BUN is high, observe him particularly for disorientation and convulsions and keep necessary protective equipment in readiness, such as side rails and a padded tongue blade.

Other useful determinations are the acid phosphatase, an enzyme produced by the prostate. In 75 per cent of patients with prostatic cancer extending beyond the prostatic capsule, this figure is elevated. Alkaline phosphatase may be elevated with spread of cancer to the bones although other disorders may raise this value.

Blood calcium, phosphorus and uric acid studies may be ordered when the physician is evaluating metabolic causes for certain types of urinary calculi (stones).

Concentration and Dilution Tests. Specific gravity shows the concentration of particles, such as electrolytes, in water. The specific gravity of distilled water is 1.000. Normally, the specific gravity of urine is responsive to the water and electrolyte situation in the body. On a hot day a person who is perspiring profusely and taking little fluid will have urine with a high specific gravity. Conversely, a person who has a high fluid intake and who is not losing excessive water from perspiration, diarrhea or vomiting will have copious urine with a low specific gravity.

When the kidneys are damaged, this ability to concentrate or produce dilute urine is impaired: the specific gravity remains relatively constant, no matter what the water needs of the body are, or how much the patient drinks. It is often fixed low, 1.010 to 1.015. To test for the capacity to adjust the specific gravity of urine, the patient may be dehydrated by restricting fluids, and a specimen taken; then he is well hydrated by giving him a large amount to drink in a short time, and another specimen is taken. The specific gravity of each specimen is tested.

Urea Clearance Test. The ability of the kidneys to remove various substances from the plasma is termed "plasma clearance." The clearance of different substances as a measure of kidney function can be determined by analyzing the concentrations of the substances simultaneously in the plasma and the urine. Normal urea clearance is 60-90 ml. of plasma per minute. A value below 60 ml. indicates decreased renal function. A fasting blood specimen is taken, and the patient voids. The patient drinks several glasses of water and, one hour later, voids again. The exact time between the two urine specimens is recorded on the label of the second specimen. The urea contents of blood and urine are compared. Urine flow per minute is calculated on the basis of the volume of the second specimen and the time between the specimens. In some kidney diseases an elevated urea level in blood and a decreased urea level in urine are expected.

A more accurate glomerular function study is the inulin clearance. Inulin is a polysaccharide which is totally diffusible through the glomerular membrane, but is neither absorbed nor secreted by the tubular walls of the nephron. It continues on into the urine. A carefully monitored intravenous infusion of inulin is required for the test to maintain constant blood levels and the laboratory determinations are more painstaking.

Phenolsulfonphthalein (P.S.P.) Test. Phenolsulfonphthalein (abbreviated P.S.P.) is a red dye that the kidneys excrete after I.V. injection. The amount of dye excreted by the patient is compared with that excreted by a person with normal kidney function. In renal disease, particularly when the tubules are involved, there is a delay in excreting the dye.

The procedure of the test varies slightly from hospital to hospital. It is important that the directions be followed exactly. A few drops of urine lost or a specimen collected four minutes late may mean that test results are inaccurate, and the doctor receives misleading diagnostic data. These are the steps of the test in one hospital:

1. Explain the procedure to the patient.
2. The patient drinks about 400 ml. of water.
3. Twenty minutes later the patient voids. This urine is discarded.
4. The doctor injects exactly 1 ml. (6 mg.) of P.S.P. intravenously. The nurse records the time of the injection.
5. Having the patient void as fully as he can, the nurse collects a series of specimens at these intervals following the injection: 15 minutes; 30 minutes; 1 hour; 2 hours.

The bottles are labeled with the exact time of voiding. The time of the injection is included on the label of the first bottle. Normally 15 to 35 per cent of the dye injected appears in the first specimen, and 80 per cent by the last specimen. If all the urine is not collected, or if the bottles are not labeled accurately, the test results will be inaccurate. If the patient is unable to void at the stated times, catheterization may be ordered by the doctor or a catheter may be inserted for the duration of the study. Patients who are not acutely ill and who are able to assume responsibility for the procedure may be provided with a watch, labeled specimen bottles and written instructions, and instructed to collect their own

FIG. 40-5. (A) A cysto-
scope. (B) A ureteral dilator. Opening and closing
of the dilating end are controlled by the handle.

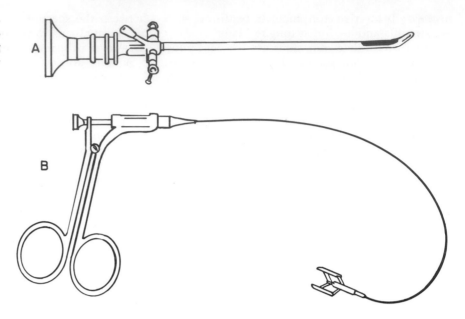

FIG. 40-5. (A) A cysto-
scope. (B) A ureteral dilator. Opening and closing
of the dilating end are controlled by the handle.

specimens. P.S.P. dye becomes colorless in acid urine and red only if the urine is alkaline. The patient should be forewarned that a red color to his urine during the test does not indicate that he is bleeding.

Intravenous Pyelogram (I.V.P.). This x-ray study is based on the ability of the kidneys to excrete radiopaque contrast media in the urine. Injected intravenously, the contrast media shows up the outlines of the kidney pelvis, the ureters and the bladder on x-ray film as the opaque media passes along the urinary tract.

The media contain iodine, to which the patient may be allergic. Reactions of a mild allergic nature such as hives are rather common. If there is a history of allergy, the doctor may inject a very minute amount of media intravenously and observe the patient for five or ten minutes.

Whenever these dyes are used, the nurse carefully observes the response of the patient and promptly reports to the physician any untoward effect such as increasing anxiety, restlessness, wheezing, tachycardia, or signs of cardiovascular collapse. Oxygen, antihistamines, epinephrine (Adrenalin), steroids and vasoconstrictor agents such as metaraminol (Aramine) as well as resuscitation equipment should be readily available in the department where the test is done such as the x-ray or the cystoscopy room, as well as on the ward to which the patient is returned.

If the patient is undergoing an extensive diagnostic work-up, the physician will probably order that barium studies of the gastrointestinal tract be delayed until urologic studies are completed. It may take several days for barium to be removed from the gastrointestinal tract and its presence in the gastrointestinal tract can distort I.V.P. findings. The doctor's orders before the procedure usually include the following:

Nothing by mouth for 12 hours before the pyelogram is scheduled. This fasting dehydrates the patient so that the urine (and therefore the contrast media) will be at maximum concentration.

Cleansing of the bowel, so that its contents do not interfere with visualization of kidneys on the film. Usually, a cathartic is ordered the evening before the test and a rectal suppository or enema may be ordered early on the morning of the pyelogram. Because poor cleansing of the bowels may require that the test be repeated, it is a nursing responsibility to check that the bowel preparation has been effective, even if given by someone else.

Some patients have other conditions that make the usual preparation inadvisable. For example, in peptic ulcer there is the danger of intestinal perforation, and therefore the bowel-cleansing procedure must be modified. After the test, encourage the patient to rest and to take fluids liberally to overcome the dehydration and to flush any remaining dye from the urinary tract. Additional films may be taken as long as 24 hours later, in order to obtain additional information that helps the physician with diagnosis.

Nephrotomogram. This is a variation of intravenous pyelogram. A larger dosage of contrast media is used in combination with body section radiography (laminography). The preparation and observation of the patient is the same as for intravenous pyelography.

Cystourethrography. For this x-ray study, contrast material is instilled into the bladder through a urethral catheter.

Arteriography

Renal arteriograms are used to evaluate the blood vessels to the kidneys and delineate the nature of mass lesions. The surgeon beforehand can obtain accurate information as to the location and number of renal arteries especially since multiple vessels to the kidney are not unusual. The commonly used method is the percutaneous catheter technic. A catheter is passed up the femoral artery into the aorta to the level of the renal vessels. At this point, contrast material is injected directly to produce an aortogram or the catheter may be manipulated into separate arteries individually. After the examination, a pressure dressing is applied to the femoral area for four hours and the pulses in the legs and feet are palpated for signs of interference with the circulation. The femoral area is observed for bleeding. Because of these considerations, arteriography is best done as an in-patient hospital procedure. Preparation is the same as for pyelography.

Cystoscopy and Retrograde Pyelography

Cystoscopy is the visual examination of the inside of the bladder by the doctor using a metal instrument known as a cystoscope (see Fig. 40-5). The cystoscope consists of a sheath with a light bulb for illumination at its tip. A telescope is inserted into the sheath for visualization. The cystoscope enables the doctor to see the interior of the bladder clearly magnified. Inflow and outflow valves allow for irrigation. The size of the cystoscope is graded in the French (F.) scale; usually, 20 to 24 F. is used in adults.

Cystoscopy may be done for the following three purposes:

• Inspection. Prostate, urethra, bladder (dilated with transparent fluid) and ureteral orifices can be seen. Cystoscopy usually is done in instances of bleeding of the urinary tract, since the bleeding may be a symptom of cancer. A catheter may be threaded into each ureter to gather separate specimens of urine from each kidney to indicate which one is affected by pus, cancer cells, tubercle bacilli or other evidence of disease. Contrast media (about 3–5 ml.) can be injected into the catheters to outline the upper urinary tract and a *retrograde pyelogram* is thus obtained. Retrograde pyelograms are usually ordered only when there has been inadequate visualization by intravenous pyelography or when a history of serious allergy to the intravenous media is obtained.

• Biopsy. Specimens of tissue may be taken from bladder or urethra through the cystoscope.

• Treatment. Tumors of urethra or bladder can be treated by electrosurgery (fulguration). Electrodes are passed through the cystoscope tube. Small stones and other foreign bodies can be removed through the cystoscope. Sometimes, larger stones are crushed and then removed. Stenosed ureteral orifices can be incised, ureters dilated, the kidney pelves drained and irrigated, and radon seeds implanted.

Care of the Patient. Cystoscopy can be very frightening to the patient. The more tense he becomes, the more chance there is of increased pain due to spasm of the vesical sphincters. The procedure should be explained, including what the patient will actually feel during it. For example when the cystoscope passes the internal sphincter at the bladder neck and when the bladder is filled, the patient will feel the urge to void.

Additional preparation includes encouraging fluid intake so that adequate urine will be in the ureters for specimens. The patient should drink at least 400 ml. about one hour before the examination, or fluids may be given intravenously, especially if general anesthesia is to be used. Usually, food is withheld because the discomfort of the procedure may cause nausea. If x-ray films are to be taken during cystoscopy, the bowel is cleansed as for an intravenous pyelogram to remove gas and stool, which may throw confusing shadows on the x-ray film. A sedative and a narcotic may be given before cystoscopy. Signed permission must be obtained for this procedure. The examination can be performed without anesthesia or with local, spinal, or general anesthesia. Because the physician must concentrate on the procedure, it is essential that a nurse place her major attention on being with the patient. In some instances one nurse can perform both the functions of assisting the doctor and comforting the patient. If this is not possible, it is desirable to have two nurses present, especially if the patient is awake throughout the examination.

The patient is placed on the examination table in the lithotomy position. A sandbag or firm pillow may be placed under his buttocks to raise them about four inches. The nurse should pad the stirrups for the comfort of the patient and to decrease the pressure on the common peroneal nerves and the blood vessels behind the knees. At best this is an uncomfortable position, and doubly so for an older patient or one with arthritis. When an interval in the examination allows for it, the nurse should remove the patient's feet from the stirrups and flex and extend the legs.

Postcystoscopy Care. When the examination is over, clean the patient's external genitalia and help him to descend from the lithotomy position slowly. Watch for dizziness. Have him rest for a few minutes before proceeding back to his hospital room (via wheelchair or stretcher) or before getting dressed, if he is an outpatient.

The decision whether to perform these examinations on an ambulatory or in-patient basis and the type of anesthesia to be used will depend considerably on the doctor's prior evaluation of the patient, an evaluation that includes emotional as well as physical considerations. Outpatients should rest for a half-hour before going home, and they should not travel unaccompanied. Not only has the patient just been through an uncomfortable procedure, but he may have had sedation. He should not plan to drive a car. Patients who have had spinal anesthesia are hospitalized at least overnight, and they are kept flat in bed for six hours or more after the procedure.

Fluids should be encouraged liberally to dilute the urine and to lessen the irritation of the lining of the urinary tract. The patient should be told that voiding will be painful for about a day. Mild hematuria is not unusual. Discoloration of the urine may be expected if dyes were used. Analgesics, several warm Sitz baths, and explaining beforehand what to expect are ways that the patient's discomfort can be alleviated.

Underlying pathology may be aggravated by the instrumentation. For example, significant prostatic obstruction may culminate in complete urinary retention. If there is precedent urinary infection, instrumentation may be followed by chills, fever and possibly serious septicemia. Observe the patient for these symptoms and promptly report them to the physician. He may

order antibiotics. There may have been damage to the walls of the tract, even perforation (anuria and sharp abdominal pain often accompany perforation).

Ureteral colic occasionally occurs and may be treated with atropine or related drugs. Many patients have a dull ache caused by distention of the renal pelvis with dye. The pain may be relieved by a hot bath or codeine. Out-patients should be instructed to return to the doctor if there is frank bleeding, anuria, pain or fever.

OBSERVATIONS

Because the function of the urinary tract is the elimination of metabolic products and electrolytes, and because it uses water as the vehicle for the movement of these substances, the nurse in observing any patient with a disorder of the urinary tract constantly searches for symptoms of electrolyte and water imbalance. For instance, in greeting the patient in the morning she looks at his lips to see if they are dry. While she bathes him, she inspects his skin. Is it edematous or dehydrated? Does the pressure of a finger leave a mark in the skin, indicating pitting edema? Edema may first become obvious as puffiness around the eyes (periorbital edema). Watch for dependent edema; for example, the patient's hand would swell if it remained over the edge of the bed. Patients who have had swollen ankles when they were ambulatory are delighted to discover that the condition disappears once they are on bed rest, not realizing that now their buttocks are edematous.

Keep track of laboratory reports as they are placed on the patient's chart. They will give you clues to the progress of his illness and the symptoms to watch for.

The physician correlates the laboratory findings with the patient's symptoms. The nurse can help by being especially observant. If calcium is low, you will know to watch for tetany and to keep ampules of calcium gluconate or calcium chloride handy. If the calcium is so low that the patient has had convulsions or is in danger of them, pad the side rails, keep them up, and tape a padded tongue blade to the head of his bed. High potassium will cue you to be especially alert to the rate and the quality of the patient's pulse and to listen to the patient's breathing for moist breath sounds. Whenever there is edema, the patient usually is weighed every day to keep track of possible loss or gain of fluids. Intake and output also are measured. Anemia and other blood changes may lead to a hemorrhagic disorder. Observe for and report to the doctor any bleeding. For example, observe the stool for unusual blackness, which may indicate the presence of old blood from gastrointestinal hemorrhage.

Observation of the urine can reveal a great deal. The daily amount is an important indication of the adequacy of renal function. Less than 500 ml. a day when the intake has been adequate means that there is serious trouble in the urinary tract that should be reported to the doctor. As you record the total intake and output for the 24- or the 8-hour period, see whether the figures are approximately equal. Call any wide discrepancy to the doctor's attention.

Color, consistency and content of the patient's urine should also be observed. Look for sediment, clots and shreds of material; note odor, color and degree of opacity. If the patient has an indwelling catheter, watch the urine as it passes through the glass or plastic connecting tube. This is a better index than the old urine in the drainage receptacle.

Blood pressure is another index of the course of the illness. Note (in the history) the patient's usual blood pressure and what it was on admission. These figures will give you a standard against which to judge your readings. The blood pressure usually is taken every four hours of patients with nephritis, all those with active kidney pathology, and those with uremia. If the blood pressure is not stable, take it more frequently. If the patient seems sluggish or complains of headache, the blood pressure should be taken even more often. A progressive rise should be called to the doctor's attention.

Fluids

Each day, know the specific fluid-intake goal for each patient under your care. Calculate how many glasses he should drink. Plan to give him $\frac{1}{4}$ of the total at night. As a general rule, fluids are encouraged to keep the urine dilute. Dilute urine does not crystallize and form calculi as easily as concentrated urine; in cystitis it burns less on urination; it rids the kidney quickly of noxious substances; and it washes away products of inflammation.

However, fluids may be limited (often to 600–800 ml.) when there is edema, and also when there is kidney failure. If the patient's body is unable to rid itself of water efficiently, damage results from adding more to it.

When fluids are to be encouraged (often to 3,500–4,000 ml.), frequent, small offerings may be more palatable than large quantities presented less often. This is especially true of geriatric patients. Often, the patient himself takes responsibility for his intake. It is better for the patient to help himself as much as he can, because he will feel less helpless. Be sure that the patient understands how much he should drink, how to keep track of the amount, and why the fluids are important.

The fluids available to him may take the form of fresh, iced water in his carafe, certain fruit juices, Jello, Koolade, Seven-up, ginger ale, cola, tea or eggnog served at intervals in the day. When it is important to limit potassium intake, certain fruit juices, tea, coffee and chocolate beverages, all of which have a high potassium content, are limited or omitted. Juices which are high in potassium include grapefruit, orange, prune, tangerine and tomato. Juices which can be included on a 1500 mg. potassium restricted

TABLE 40-1. SERUM VALUES

	NORMAL SERUM VALUE	CHANGES IN PATHOLOGY
Calcium	9–11 mg./100 ml. 4.5–5.5 mEq./L.	Lower in renal failure
Carbon dioxide combining power	50–70 volumes % 21–28 mEq./L.	Lower in acidosis Higher in alkalosis
Potassium	4.0–5.0 mEq./L.	Higher in renal failure

Proteins, total, electrophoretic fractions
    Albumin
    Globulins
	
	58%
	11–14%
		
		Lower in renal failure

Sodium	137–143 mEq./L.	Lower in renal failure
Urea Nitrogen (BUN)	8–18 mg./100 ml.	Higher in renal failure

diet include apple, cranberry, pear, peach, and pineapple (Robinson).

Because of the combination of a large intake of fluids with the symptom of frequency, keep the bedpan or the urinal within easy reach, especially with an older patient for whom climbing in and out of bed may be tiring and dangerous.

When fluids are restricted, the patient should understand the reason. It is unfortunate that a patient may feel psychologically denied when his condition requires that he be restricted in intake; but if he does feel that way, he does. Let him express his hurt or anger.

Of course, thirst is a greater problem in hot than in cool weather. Fluids should be spaced throughout the day, preferably by the patient. Sucking on hard candy or ice may help (however, ice needs to be counted in total fluid intake). Give mouth care with a solution that is pleasant to the patient.

Records of intake and output should be scrupulously accurate; otherwise, the doctor will base his treatment on incorrect information. Every person working with the patient should understand and agree to the method of keeping records and the amount of fluid that the cups and the glasses hold. If the aide believes that the glass holds 240 ml., and the nurse believes it to hold 200 ml., the doctor will read erroneous figures on the chart. Each source of output should be recorded separately and then totaled. For example:

Vomitus	230 ml.
Cystostomy tube	560 ml.
Foley catheter	520 ml.
Total	1,310 ml.

Watch for overhydration (edema, wet breathing sounds) in all patients for whom fluids are encouraged, especially those who are aged and those with a heart ailment or potential renal failure. Patients with edema have severe restriction of their sodium intake. Do not use salt substitutes containing potassium for seasoning without the doctor's approval. Rum, vinegar, mint or cloves probably will be allowed.

Preventing Infection

A rule to remember every time that you approach the patient with a catheter or an irrigating set in hand is that there is danger of introducing microorganisms into the urinary tract with every insertion of something foreign.

Be sure that you proceed with sterile precautions. Did the catheter touch the bedclothes? Discard it and start afresh.

Comfort

Here are some causes of discomfort in the urologic patient and what you can do to relieve them.

• Itching (pruritis). The doctor may order an anesthetic ointment to relieve the itching. Cleanliness helps, too: perhaps this patient can have two baths instead of one a day. Although the skin is not efficient for the disposal of such waste chemicals as uric acid, it is all that the body has available when the kidneys are not functioning, and a clean skin is always more efficient and more comfortable.

• Other skin problems. Use cream or lotion on dry skin instead of alcohol. Keep the sheets under the swollen buttocks taut and free from piercing crumbs. Have the patient change his position frequently. Even lying on the strings of his gown can make a deep crease in the edematous back.

• Odor. Unless urine comes from a necrotic area, as in cancer, or it is infected, it is almost odorless as it leaves the body. The characteristic odor of urine is caused by ammonia, which is formed from urea by bacterial action. The more stale the urine becomes, the more malodorous. It has been said that the quality of the nursing on a urological ward can be judged by sniffing the air. In instances of infection and necrotic tissue, odor can be combated by ventilation, the use of sprays, and, most important, prompt cleaning of the patient as he needs it.

• Dryness of mouth. Mineral oil can be used (a touch of lemon juice with it helps), but be careful to apply only the smallest amount on the applicator, especially in the comatose patient, since aspiration is a danger. Caked blood and crusts can be removed with hydrogen peroxide. However, do not delay mouth care until blood cakes and crusts form. Commercially prepared glycerine-lemon swabs are convenient to use.

• Pain. Sitz baths, when they are allowed, may ease the discomfort of an inflamed urethra. A hot-water bottle (with the doctor's approval) may help the flank ache that sometimes accompanies disease of the kidney parenchyma or pelvis. The burning caused by cystitis is reduced by forcing fluids diluting the urine.

• Long-term bed rest. A consistently quiet position leads to, among other evils, urinary stasis, potassium imbalance, and infection. Without tiring the patient, have him do range-of-motion exercises regularly, and change the gatch level of his bed frequently. Boredom is often a problem for patients on long-term bed rest. Perhaps you can help him to find diversion that will interest but not strain him. The chronicity of his illness may be very discouraging and anger provoking. Irritability may be caused by worries over the hospital bills and his inability to work or over his disease—probably both. The hospital social worker may be able to help to ease his mind about financial troubles.

• Embarrassment and fear. The nurse's matter-of-fact attitude and care in not exposing the urologic patient unduly will help him to accept the necessary treatments. When a man is available on the nursing team, delegate him to perform treatments on the genitalia of the male patient. Catheterization of male patients usually is performed by the doctor.

A man may fear with justification that impotence will follow surgery. Although the patient will probably not discuss this thought with you, suggest that he talk to his doctor, if you detect any hint of such a worry. You can also mention it to the doctor. Also, patients may worry about cancer.

The patient with generalized edema may feel self-conscious about his appearance. The edema of nephrosis gives a bloated look that, in the extreme, is startling.

If a perineal approach is taken to any urologic surgery, the areas around the genitalia and the anus must be shaved. These are difficult areas to shave thoroughly. A good light and a sharp razor are essential.

Preoperative Care

The time that is spent waiting for surgery can be full of anxiety, especially if the operation that is planned is mutilating or changes vital functions. The nurse should follow the surgeon's explanation with opportunities for the patient to ask questions and to talk about his adjustment to the necessary changes in his way of life, such as a different manner of voiding. For instance, other patients who have successfully lived with ureteral transplants might share their experience with the preoperative patient. However, no matter how well-informed the patient is, there will always be a question in his mind as to how he

will be able to get along. The nurse's concern for his welfare may be encouraging to him.

Postoperative Care

The three usual surgical approaches to the urinary tract are: (1) a flank incision just under the diaphragm to reach the ureter and the kidney on that side, (2) an incision in the lower abdomen above the symphysis pubis to reach the bladder (suprapubic), and (3) a perineal incision. Some procedures are done through the urethra. A transthoracic approach may be used for nephrectomy (excision of the kidney).

A flank incision is so close to the thoracic cavity that it is painful for the patient to cough and to breathe deeply. To counter this pain and to help to prevent hypostatic pneumonia, use medications for the pain as they were ordered, and splint the wound site with your hand when the patient coughs. Frequent turning, breathing deeply and early ambulation are indicated.

After kidney surgery, patients may develop gastrointestinal discomfort, such as distention, due to pressure on the abdominal organs during the operation. A nasogastric tube attached to continuous suction may be used, and fluids may be given intravenously until the patient can take them by mouth.

Danger Periods. The two periods when the patient is in the greatest danger from hemorrhage are immediately postoperatively, and the eighth to the tenth days after surgery, when tissue sloughing may occur. Ambulatory patients may be returned to bed rest for these three days. Watch for hemorrhage the eighth to the tenth day after fulguration procedures. With the patient lying on his back or his side, blood may seep under him and not appear on the top of the dressing. Because of its position, this is especially true of a flank incision. During your frequent checks for hemorrhage, feel beneath the patient for dampness, and depress the bed at the point of the bandage, so that you can look for stains.

Detection of Bleeding. When there is a draining catheter left in place postoperatively, it will be easier to detect bleeding if the drainage apparatus is changed every two hours. Use small bottles or large test tubes, which are easier to handle and easier to remember to change, and label each with the time. The bottles can be lined up with a light source such as the window behind them, and their colors can be compared. Normally, you should be able to see a progressive

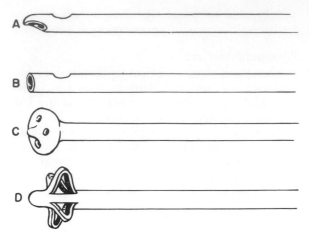

FIG. 40-6. Some catheter tips: (A) whistle-tip, (B) hole-in-tip, (C) de Pezzer mushroom, (D) Malecot 4-wing.

lightening from dark red to pink. If the urine remains the same color, or turns brighter red, call the doctor. After 48 hours the pink should give way to amber or, if the kidneys are working well, and the hydration is good, to yellow.

Protecting the Skin. Some wounds drain urine both through and around a catheter. To prevent skin excoriation and infection, the dressing must be kept dry. Because the dressing may need to be changed every half-hour, nurses often do the dressing changes early in the postoperative course, using aseptic technic. The moisture in the dressing and the frequency of the changes together invite infection, which can be prevented by employing rigid sterile technic and by never allowing the dressing to become saturated.

The skin can be protected in several ways. You can apply zinc oxide, being careful that none enters the wound. Dressings previously soaked in Diaparene (an antiseptic that will prevent the formation of ammonia in urine) and then dried and sterilized can be used. A sheet of rubber may be prepared with a hole in the middle the size of the wound. It then is cemented in place over the operative site. Urine seeping from around the catheter runs over the rubber dam and does not come into contact with skin. However, dressing changes still must be frequent to prevent infection.

Positioning. Patients usually are not restricted in their position postoperatively. Variation of position and frequent change are encouraged to prevent pneumonia. Be sure that no tube is compressed by the patient's lying on it.

CARE OF PATIENTS WHO HAVE CATHETERS

If the patient has one or more catheters in place, it is imperative that the nurses know the function of each tube, and where the inner end of each is placed. Ask if you do not know. Label each catheter (this can be put on the drainage vessel, or on the catheter itself with a tag or a loop of adhesive tape), so that all nursing per-

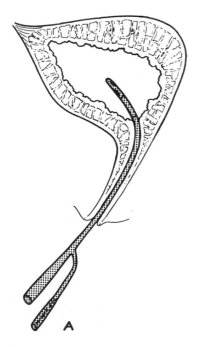

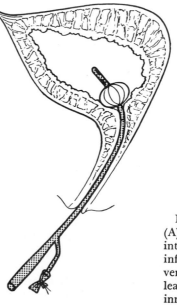

FIG. 40-7. Foley catheter. (A) The catheter is inserted into the bladder. (B) The inflation of the bag prevents the catheter from leaving the bladder. The inner tube that leads to the balloon is tied.

A   B

sonnel can note and chart the material that comes from any drain.

Types of Catheters. There are several types of catheters, suited for different purposes:

• For drainage of urine. This may be a Foley catheter placed in the bladder, a retention catheter in the kidney pelvis, a ureteral catheter, or one for drainage through a suprapubic wound leading to the bladder.

• For external wound drainage. When drainage is expected from a wound, but the surgeon does not wish the dressing to be disturbed frequently, he may incorporate a drain in the dressing. If the wound is infected, this drain may enter the wound superficially. Sometimes it lies near the incision line. The catheter sometimes is used for instillation of antibiotic solution or to keep the dressing wet.

• For splinting. A tube used solely for splinting might be inserted after a plastic repair of the ureter. It is removed two to three weeks postoperatively.

Catheters are measured in the French system. An adult urethra usually takes size 28 to 30 F.; but to avoid pain, size 18 to 20 F. is used for indwelling catheters.

Ureteral catheters are smaller. These catheters are irrigated by using gravity, not plunger-pressure, using a special ureteral syringe and adaptor or with a syringe and blunt needle.

Size of ureteral catheter:	5	6	7	8	9	10
Size of needle:		21	19	18	17	16	15

Ureteral catheters may become obstructed easily if there is purulent or bloody urine. The doctor may order no more than 5 ml. of sterile normal saline to be instilled by gravity and returned by gravity. Notify the doctor if patency of the catheter cannot be established by this type of irrigation.

One way to attach a ureteral catheter to drainage is to punch a small hole with a red-hot needle or pin in the rubber top of a sterile medicine dropper and thread the catheter through it. The medicine dropper is then attached to the glass or plastic connector of the drainage tubing. To prevent dislodgement of the ureteral catheters an indwelling bladder catheter may be attached to them. There may be some leakage of urine around the catheters and the patient's skin care is an important nursing consideration. If there is a ureteral catheter in each ureter, they should be labeled "right" and "left."

Setting up Drainage. When there is a choice, use stiffer rather than softer tubing for drainage, because it will have less tendency to kink. The small-size catheter is connected to the large-size tubing by means of a glass connecting tube.

As soon as the urologic patient with catheters is placed in bed, attach each urinary catheter to the drainage vessel. Label each. Set up the intake and output sheet with a separate column for each source of urine. Pin the drainage tube to the sheet, using an adhesive tab wrapped around the tube. Allow enough tubing between the pin and the patient so that there is no pull on the catheter when the patient turns, but not so much that the tubing will become tangled. Never allow a catheter to be bent at right angles, because this bending clamps it off. Run your eye over the entire length—from insertion into the patient to the drainage vessel—to check for kinks. Coiling excess tubing horizontally so that the urine does not have to flow uphill should keep it free of kinks. The kidney pelvis has a capacity of 5 to 8 ml. If a tube draining it is blocked for a half-hour (clot stuck in the lumen, patient lying on the tube, tube kinked), there will be backup of urine, perhaps strain on the suture line and surely increased pain for the patient.

The end of the tube that drains the kidney pelvis always should be handled with aseptic precautions: use a sterile drainage vessel, and touch the part of the tube near the opening only with sterile forceps or the sterile gloved hand. The tubes that drain the ureter and the bladder are handled sometimes with clean and sometimes with sterile technic, depending on hospital policy.

The drainage end of the tube should be kept above the level of the urine in the vessel.

Observations. When you are caring for urologic patients, the first thing to do is to check all urinary catheters for patency. Fresh catheters draining from the kidney pelvis or the ureter should be rechecked every half-hour, and others at least every two hours. If urine is appearing from a catheter that should not drain, call the doctor at once. If no urine appears from a catheter that should drain, take the following steps:

• Check the length of the tubing from the patient to the vessel for kinks, pressure and other external compression of the tube that may be obstructing the lumen.

• Clamp the tube off near the patient and "milk" the remainder of the tube toward the

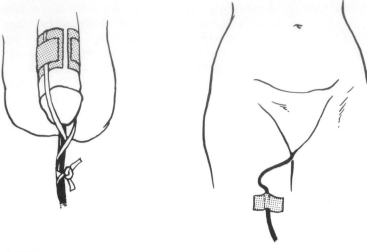

▨ =ADHESIVE TAPE

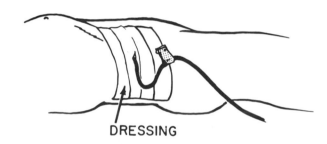

DRESSING

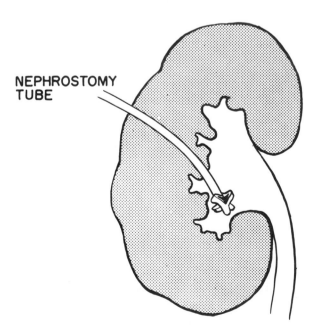

NEPHROSTOMY TUBE

FIG. 40-9. A nephrostomy tube with a Malecot 4-wing tip draining the kidney pelvis.

drainage vessel. Feel for gravel (sediment made of phosphates and other mineral crystals). After milking, release the clamp and watch for urine.

• Disassemble the drainage system (without removing the catheter that goes into the patient) and flush it with sterile saline or water and a sterile syringe. Do not empty the fluid into the drainage vessel if a specimen of that urine is to be sent to the laboratory.

• If urine has not appeared, give the patient water to drink and call for the doctor.

Changing the Catheters. The end of the catheter that goes into the patient should stay in him until the doctor wishes it to come out. Some catheters going into wounds may be sutured in place; others should be firmly taped, except for Foley catheters, which usually maintain their position without outside anchorage. Taping a Foley catheter to the leg is done to prevent pull on the bag, which would cause pressure on the bladder outlet (Fig. 40-8). A catheter that accidentally becomes dislodged from the patient never should be reinserted. A sterile one should replace it, and depending on its location, it may be reinserted by the doctor. Those catheters that are positioned deep into the ureter or the kidney pelvis through a flank incision can, at times, be replaced only by reopening the wound.

Patients who go home with catheters learn to change them while they are still in the hospital. At home they may be helped by a visiting nurse or a family member may be taught. Catheters or tubing for long-term use should be changed also when sand is felt in them. The glass or plastic connectors and tubing are cleaned daily and whenever they become cloudy or plugged. A weak solution of acid such as vinegar will remove the coating.

Drainage and Irrigation. Usually, drainage is accomplished by gravity, though occasionally, weak suction may be used. When the end of the catheter is in the kidney pelvis, only gravity drainage is used.

Catheters are irrigated on occasion with sterile saline or distilled water, but only when there is an order to do so. Generally, irrigation is done to keep the system of tubing open and not to rinse the cavity being drained. Because every irrigation carries with it the danger of infection, sterile technic always is employed. If you put fluid in, and it does not return, you may try very gentle suction *except* in recent postoperative patients and those whose catheters enter the kidney pelvis. If you do not get a return after suctioning once, stop. Reattach the tubing to the drainage system and watch. If nothing has returned after an hour, call the doctor. Keep track of the amount of fluid that was instilled, and subtract that amount from the total output.

The amount of fluid used is ordered by the doctor: a common amount for irrigating urethral tubing is 30 ml. of sterile saline. Never use more than 5 ml. at a time to irrigate tubing that goes into the kidney pelvis. Whenever a patient complains of pain during an irrigation, stop, wait a moment, and then proceed. Irrigations should be done slowly and gently.

If irrigation is required frequently, a closed system may be set up to decrease the chance of infection. Intermittent irrigation can be accomplished by releasing the clamp. When constant irrigation is ordered, a drip device is incorporated into the tubing, and a three-way Foley catheter (one tube admits fluid, one allows for drainage, and the third fills the balloon) may be used. Usually, the fluid is allowed to drip at a rate of 30 to 60 drops a minute. A closed system such as this is not used when the catheter is inserted into the kidney pelvis, because of the danger of admitting too much fluid.

After a catheter is removed from a wound, the closure of the surgical fistula usually is rapid, so rapid that if a catheter should inadvertently slip out of a wound, it may not be possible to replace it after a half-hour has elapsed. If a wound catheter inadvertently slips out, call the doctor immediately. After a catheter is removed by the doctor, observe the site. Urine may drain from it for a short time, but it should gradually stop. When a catheter has been removed from the urethra, observe the patient's voiding pattern, and record the time and the amount. Is he incontinent? If so, is he incontinent in all positions: lying down and standing up? How often does he void? What is the anticipated quantity? Does he void sufficient quantity each time? Sufficient quantity over a 24-hour period?

THE PATIENT WITH URINARY INCONTINENCE

Ordinarily, the excretion of urine is controlled by two sphincters: the internal sphincter, which is close to the most dependent part of the bladder, and the external sphincter, which surrounds the urethra at a lower point. As the bladder fills, nerve endings are stimulated, giving rise to the sensation of needing to void.

The anesthetized, unconscious or senile patient may not receive these stimuli, and in these patients the urinary sphincters relax involuntarily. Also, infection of the urinary system and accidental or surgical damage to either sphincter can cause loss of control. The sphincters may not function adequately when there is local tissue damage, such as in the relaxation of the pelvic floor found in some women. Interference with the spinal nerves, such as that which occurs in tumors of the spinal cord, tabes dorsalis, herniated disk, postoperative edema of the cord and cord injuries, can interfere with the conduction to the brain of the impulse to void, and result in a neurogenic bladder and incontinence. Many paraplegic patients do not know when they void because they have lost all sensation in the lower parts of their bodies. A neurogenic bladder may be spastic, preventing the retention of urine, or it may be flaccid, preventing the complete expulsion of urine. A tidal drainage system, with its periodic filling and emptying simulates normal bladder functioning thus preserving bladder capacity and muscle tone.

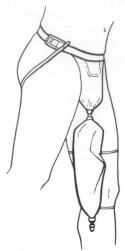

Fig. 40-10. A rubber leg-urinal placed over the penis and held in place with a belt.

Nursing Care

Nursing care is directed at establishing a voiding routine, when that is possible; and when it is not possible, at finding the most convenient way to collect the urine and to keep it off the skin.

Establishing a Schedule. The patient and the nurse together may be able to set up a schedule, so that voiding is regular and predictable. Such a program takes great patience by all concerned. If it is successful, it gives the patient freedom from constant odor, wetness, and the embarrassment of accidents when he may be, for instance, at the movies or with company for dinner. The first step is observation of the patient's pattern of urination. If a pattern is observable, have a bedpan or a commode available (or help the patient to the bathroom if it is possible) just before you both believe that his bladder will empty. As far as possible, avoid any association with childhood experience. This is not the same thing as toilet training in the child, and the patient's dignity should not be affronted.

Fluid intake can be spaced to help to establish a regular time of voiding. Spacing fluids will take experimentation. If the patient limits his fluids before going to bed or going out on a social occasion, be sure that his intake is adequate at other times of the day. A patient with a neurogenic bladder may not void completely. Because of the danger of infection and stone formation, it is doubly important that he drink sufficient fluids—at least 2,000 ml. a day.

Increasing intra-abdominal pressure such as by gentle manual pressure just above the symphysis pubis may aid a patient with a neurogenic bladder to void.

Until a routine is well established, continue to keep a record of the time and the amount voided. Such information can help the doctor to see if there is overflow with retention of residual urine, and it can help the patient to regulate himself.

Rehabilitation. An indwelling catheter may be used to prevent retention of urine and incontinence. Initially, it may be allowed to drain constantly.

Later, if the urologist determines that a reflex is present, a method of bladder training may be instituted. The catheter is clamped and released every one to two hours. In this time the bladder is given a chance to hold urine and then to empty it, thus beginning to re-establish normal function. Gradually, the interval for releasing the catheter is lengthened to three to four hours, giving the bladder a chance to fill more completely. The patient can be taught to release the clamp on his own catheter at scheduled times. The retention-catheter is changed once a week.

The catheter later is removed entirely, and the patient is instructed to void every hour. Usually he is not able to retain the urine longer, and frequent voiding is necessary to prevent incontinence. Gradually the interval is lengthened to two, three or four hours. Since such frequent voiding would disturb the patient during the night, external drainage is used. A rubber sheath is placed over the penis and is connected by rubber tubing to a drainage bottle, or to a disposable urinary drainage bag. Women wear absorbent pads and moistureproof pants. When the patient becomes able to retain the urine longer, the voiding schedule is continued throughout the night.

The process takes a great deal of patience, and accidents do happen during the training period. Be sure that the bed has a full-length waterproof mattress cover. When an accident occurs, promptly change the linen, and assure the patient that this is to be expected during the retraining process. Try to keep him from considering the mishap as evidence that he has failed in his program.

At first many patients void in insufficient quantity, and they must be catheterized after voiding to remove residual urine. Always see that the patient keeps a careful record of his fluid intake and output.

Some incontinent patients never achieve complete freedom from catheters; others do. Success depends not only on the degree of injury but on the motivation of the patient and the amount of skillful help and encouragement that he receives from the staff. Men patients usually do not achieve urinary control as readily as do women, probably because more convenient appliances are available for them than for women. A man can wear a catheter that is connected by means of rubber tubing to a rubber urinal. The urinal is strapped to the patient's lower leg. Each patient should have two urinals, one to wear and the other to wash thoroughly and to hang to dry. The man's trousers cover his urinal; no one need know that he uses it. Women use a less effective device, rubberized pants, plus an absorbent perineal pad. In one way the men are luckier, for there is less likelihood of leakage, and the device is more readily concealed. However, in the long run the convenience of the device often becomes a disadvantage, because the patient becomes dependent on the equipment and is not motivated as strongly to achieve control without it. The presence of the catheter increases the likelihood of urinary-tract infection, an ever-present danger.

Devising a Collection System. When it is important to measure urinary output, and it is expected that the problem will be of a short duration, as in a burned patient, an indwelling catheter may be inserted. When the catheter is in place, be careful that it does not slip out of the bladder. If the patient is irrational, restrain his hands in a way that will not impede movement in bed but will prevent him from pulling the catheter.

The Bed Patient

The male patient who is incontinent, bedridden, and unable to attend to his own needs can have a plastic or a rubber sheath with tubing (condom drainage) placed over the penis and attached to a drainage bottle. Diversion of urine in the female patient is more difficult to accomplish. To protect both the linen and the skin of the patient, arrange the following one above the other, beginning at the mattress and proceeding toward the patient's skin.

> Plastic mattress protector
> Bed sheet
> Waterproof sheet (either rubber or plastic) under the buttocks
> Draw sheet
> Several layers of soft absorbent material. (The bottom layers lie under the patient, and the top layers are folded against the vulva.)
> Liner

The sheet under the buttocks should be large enough so that it does not roll into a wrinkled ball under the patient. The small sheet can be changed without disturbing the basic bed linen. Pads that are placed under and on the patient may be disposable or washable. They should be arranged in proper order before the patient is disturbed. A pile of them ready for use can be kept nearby.

Urea-splitting organisms, among them *Micrococcus ureae,* cause the urea in urine to react with water. An end product of this reaction is ammonia, which causes both the odor of urine and the skin damage. One way to protect skin is to avoid any contact with urine. When this is not possible, an antiseptic, such as methylbenzethonium chloride (Diaparene Chloride), which kills the ammonia-forming organism in urine, may be used. The antiseptic, in ointment or powder, can (with the doctor's approval) be applied to the skin of the incontinent ambulatory or bed patient. Light dusting with an absorbent powder, such as corn starch, also helps to prevent ammonia dermatitis.

If powder, an antiseptic, liners and protective pads are used, there should be no problem with odor or ammonia dermatitis, but these measures should not be a substitute for scrupulous cleanliness and the changing of padding as soon as it becomes wet. The buttocks and the genital area of the incontinent patient should be washed with soap and water several times a day. Unlike feces, urine on the skin is not visible. To prevent skin breakdown, the area actually must be free of urine; it is not sufficient that it appears to be clean. To avoid irritation, be sure to remove all the soap from the skin and to dry it thoroughly. Wash the plastic or rubber sheet with soap and water at least once a day. If an ammonia dermatitis is present, keep the affected area clean, dry and exposed to the air. Exposure to an ordinary light bulb for 20 minutes several times a day, with the doctor's approval, often helps.

The continuous vigilance and the care required by the incontinent patient who is unable to care for himself may seen tiresome. Having the necessary materials right at hand and a planned routine makes quick work of the changes. The reward is a healthy, unbroken skin and a comfortable patient.

The Ambulatory Patient

If it is not possible to establish a voiding routine, the nurse and the patient together should devise some system of collecting the urine. The objective is to provide for the urine an external reservoir that:

- Protects the skin from contact with urine
- Is inexpensive to maintain
- Is convenient for the patient
- Can be worn under clothes
- Does not leak
- Is comfortable to wear

The arrangement should be individualized. For example, if the patient is hemiplegic and cannot use one hand, find or devise a rubber or plastic urinal that he can manage one-handed. If the patient's skin is excoriated, the appliance should not irritate it further. A simple urinal for the ambulatory male patient can be made out of a disposable plastic bag that fits over the penis and is kept in place by taping it to a belt. There are commercially available rubber urinals for men that can be worn under a suit.

Women with incontinence may wear a perineal pad. There are also a number of protective pants on the market that have a rubberized or plastic outside layer and absorbent material inside. These pants can be pinned or snapped in place. (Avoid any reference to these pants as "diapers.") Liners also are available and are worn next to the skin. Because they are nonabsorbent, the urine passes through them; and because they dry

very quickly, they leave the skin dry and free of urine, even though the absorbent material is soaked.

Home Care

Sometimes the decision concerning whether the patient can be cared for at home rests on management of the problem of incontinence—a condition which is embarrassing to the patient, and which the family may find very upsetting. Decisions about whether home care is feasible rest with the family, with the advice and support of the physicians and nurses. Often what appears to doctors and nurses as a family's unwillingness to care for the patient at home actually is fear and uncertainty about the management of such care. A family can be shown that the ambulatory patient usually can care for himself without odor or fuss, or that the bed patient can be changed quickly, easily and inexpensively. The nurse who finds a convenient way to keep the patient clean and dry, and who is able to teach the patient's family how to do this may be able to show the members of the family who wish to care for the patient, but who are uncertain of their skills, how home care can be carried out.

The rehabilitation of the patient with a neurogenic bladder or with urinary incontinence from other causes is often a long-term complex nursing problem. For a more detailed treatment of the

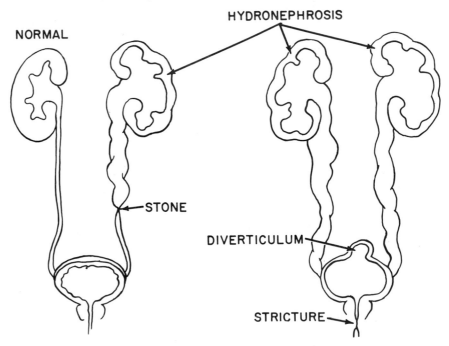

Fig. 40-11. Hydronephrosis caused by blockage of the urinary tract. Note how dilatation occurs above the point of obstruction.

subject, specialized literature is available (see bibliography).

URINARY OBSTRUCTIONS

An obstruction can occur anywhere in the urinary tract—from the kidney pelvis to the tip of the urethra. Obstruction may be caused by a tumor, a stone, a cyst, a kink in the ureter, stenosis or spasm of the ureters, or a diverticulum in the bladder wall that distends and blocks one or more of the three openings (two ureteral, one urethral) into the bladder. In older men an enlargement of the prostate gland is a common obstructing lesion. Congenital strictures are not infrequent, though they may not be discovered until the patient is an adult.

Acquired obstructions include surgical injuries to the ureters and urethral strictures from traumatic instrumentation. Neurogenic dysfunction of the bladder which causes stasis of urine is essentially an obstructive condition.

When urine cannot pass freely by the obstruction, it backs up. For example, if there is closure at the orifice that leads from the right ureter into the bladder, the ureter will become more and more distended as new urine passes into it from above. The back pressure moves into the kidney pelvis, which also becomes distended. Now the parenchyma of the kidney is squeezed between the pressure from the expanding pelvis and the internal pressure of the glomerulus and its continuous formation of urine. Likewise, the tiny blood vessels supplying the kidney tissue are being compressed, a dangerous condition because of the possibility of permanent kidney damage. Waste products accumulate in the bloodstream. When the kidney pelvis is swollen with backflow, the condition is called *hydronephrosis* (see Fig. 40-11).

The lower the level in the tract that the obstruction occurs, the more slowly the kidney pelves become distended with the backflow of urine. When the obstruction is in the urethra, the bladder distends, and finally diverticuli (outpouchings) of the muscular wall can form. Urine becomes trapped in these sacs, stagnates and becomes a culture medium for bacteria. For this reason, infection goes hand in hand with obstruction. The infection may be blood-borne, such as that caused by streptococci, staphylococci, or pneumococci; or it may enter the urethra from the outside, such as that caused by *Escherichia coli*. Control of infection is extremely difficult until the underlying obstruction is corrected.

When the obstruction is minor, and the pressure from backed-up urine develops slowly, there may be no discomfort. However, infection is the rule rather than the exception, and with it come pain and fever. When the kidney pelvis becomes markedly distended, a mass may be palpated through the abdomen. Advanced hydronephrosis causes renal tenderness and pain. If there is a diverticulum of the bladder, the patient may find that he can pass more urine after emptying his bladder and waiting a few minutes. The final quantity of urine comes from the diverticulum sac and may be malodorous.

The aim of treatment is to establish adequate drainage of urine. The first measure that the doctor takes may be temporary, designed to permit free flow of urine, to relieve the retention and to allow the edematous kidney to heal until it is sufficiently healthy to withstand surgery to correct the obstruction. For example, a patient with a ureteral calculus obstructing one kidney accompanied by severe infection may have chills, fever, and hypotension. Under these conditions the patient may be so ill that anesthesia and surgery to remove the calculus may be very risky. Therefore, the doctor, during cystoscopy, may pass a ureteral catheter above the calculus with its tip draining the kidney pelvis. The catheter will not cure the pathology, but it will drain purulent urine from the pelvis and relieve hydronephrosis. When the patient's general condition improves, a more definite procedure can be performed.

As soon as a way for urine to leave the body is established, the patient should be encouraged to drink fluids.

If the obstruction is so complete that a catheter cannot be passed, temporary drainage may be accomplished by inserting a tube into the kidney pelvis through a skin incision (nephrostomy). When the acute process has subsided, surgery can remove the obstruction, repair the stricture, remove the stone, free the ureter from adhesions, or excise the tumor.

Calculi (Stones, Lithiasis)

Etiology. When the salts in urine precipitate instead of remaining in solution, they adhere and form stones. Stones, most of which form in the kidney, can plug the urinary tract, so that obstruction with stasis of urine is frequently found. The exact conditions that cause salts to precipitate are not fully understood. Excessive excretion of calcium, as occurs in patients with hyperparathyroid disease and in some consumers of enormous quantities of milk, tends to encourage stone formation.

Infection (particularly with Proteus species) and stones tend to coexist, but in a particular patient it may not always be clear which came first. Infection can make the urine alkaline, and the result may be the precipitation of calcium. On the other hand, when the pH of the urine becomes excessively acid, cystine and uric acid may precipitate. Patients with gout are likely to form uric acid stones. Osteoporosis (demineralization of bones) may be a contributing factor.

Urinary stones not infrequently occur in patients on long-term bed rest, such as those with fractures or paraplegia. When urine flow is sluggish and there is poor gravity drainage from the kidneys as the patient lies on his back, there may be disuse decalcification of bone, and stones may form. This hazard of immobility may be prevented by nursing action such as active range-of-motion exercises practiced several times a day every day (when they are allowed) and encouraging liberal ingestion of fluids (when they are allowed).

Symptoms. Most small stones pass right through and cause no symptoms at all. However, some are troublesome, because they traumatize the walls of the urinary tract and irritate the lining, or because they clog the ureter or an orifice, preventing urine flow and inviting infection. The symptoms are related to number, size and mobility of the stones.

The following symptoms may occur:

• Hematuria, gross or microscopic, as the stone traumatizes the walls of the urinary tract.

• Pyuria (pus in the urine) due to infection behind the obstruction by the calculus. The patient may experience chills, fever, and can develop serious hypotension and other signs of a gram negative septicemia.

• Retention of urine or dysuria from blockage of the orifice between bladder and urethra. Some patients can void only in unnatural positions; others are unable to void at all.

• Flank pain or ache, related to obstruction.

• Acute renal or ureteral colic, due to violent contractions and spasms as the ureter tries to pass along a stone. The severity of pain is almost inversely proportional to the size of the calculus. Smaller stones frequently travel more rapidly down the ureter causing more forceful ureteral spasm and therefore, greater colic.

The colicky pain is characteristic. It is agonizingly severe, coming in waves that may start in the kidney or the ureter and radiate to the inguinal ring, the inner aspect of the thigh or, in the male patient, to the testicle or the tip of the penis. In a female patient, the pain may go to the urinary meatus or the labia of the affected side. The patient may double up with pain and be unable to lie quietly in bed until it passes. The severity of the pain can cause nausea, vomiting and shock. Often, morphine and antispasmodic drugs are given for relief. Protect the patient from injury as he thrashes about in bed. If he finds it necessary to walk about while in pain protect him from injury brought about by dizziness following narcotic administration. As the pain subsides make him comfortable in bed. Fluids should be encouraged after nausea abates.

Until the kidneys and the ureters are free of stones, the colicky pains tends to recur. The violent spasm that causes the pain may move a stone along, and sometimes after an attack of colic the patient may pass "gravel" or the offending stone itself. On the other hand, a spastic ureter may clamp down on a stone and hold it in place.

In the hospital, the patient who is suspected of having stones should have all of his urine strained through gauze to catch any stones that he may have passed. The stone may be no larger than the head of a pin. At home the patient can void into a clear glass through a small kitchen strainer with cheesecloth lining it. Some stones will be sent to the laboratory for chemical analysis, for the composition of the stones will affect the treatment. Save all the stones (they may be tiny) and show them to the physician.

Treatment. Most ureteral calculi, 1 cm. or less in diameter, will pass into the bladder spontaneously. Unless there is an obstruction at the bladder outlet, such as an enlarged prostate or urethral stricture, they are voided spontaneously as well. The patient newly admitted to the hospital may be observed for several days to see whether the stone will pass from his body. A large fluid intake is encouraged to reduce the concentration of crystalloids in the urine and to foster the passage of stones.

As soon as the acute colic subsides, the patient should be encouraged to walk as well as to drink. An active patient is more likely to pass a stone than a quiet one. Meanwhile, concurrent disorders are treated, and drugs are given to combat infection.

If the stone does not pass spontaneously, and there is continued colic, infection above the stone, or, in the opinion of the doctor, little likelihood of spontaneous passage, surgery is generally performed. Calculi larger than 1 cm. in diameter in the renal pelvis are surgically removed.

For a stone in the renal pelvis, the surgeon may perform one of the following procedures:

• Pyelolithotomy. An incision is made into the renal pelvis, and the stone is removed.

• Nephrolithotomy. An incision is made into the parenchyma of the kidney from the outside to remove a stone in a calyx.

• Calycectomy, heminephrectomy. A proved stone-forming area is excised.

• Complete nephrotomy. The kidney is split from end to end. Each calyx is opened. This operation is most common for a staghorn calculus, a type of stone that tends to fill the kidney pelvis and to take on its shape.

• Nephrectomy. The kidney is removed if the stone has so permanently and severely damaged it that kidney function is no longer possible. This operation is used when there has been unilateral kidney damage, with the other kidney retaining at least some healthy tissue.

Stones in the ureter may be removed surgically (ureterolithotomy). In one method a small incision is made over the stone in the ureter. A drain of the Penrose type is placed at the site of the incision, and the urine is allowed to drain from the wound until the ureter heals. The doctor may attempt extraction of lower ureteral calculi with a variety of stone baskets.

Occasionally, a ureteral stone can be crushed or grasped and pulled out with a special instrument during cystoscopy. Snaring the stone is an extremely delicate procedure because of the constant danger of rupturing the ureter. Usually, this cystoscopic procedure is performed under general anesthesia to avoid any sudden movement of the patient; and if any complications are encountered, open surgery is begun at once. If the procedure is uncomplicated and successful, the patient will have a ureteral catheter attached to straight drainage. The purpose of the catheter is to splint the ureter and to divert the urine past any possible tear in the ureteral wall. It is kept in place for three to four days. At times after a cystoscopy a ureteral catheter will be left in place for 24 hours to dilate the ureter in the hope that stones then will pass through it, or that the stone will be pulled into the bladder when the catheter is removed.

Bladder Stones. Bladder stones may be removed through the transurethral route, using a stone-crushing instrument called a lithotrite. The procedure (called *litholapaxy*) is suitable for small and soft stones. Larger, noncrushable stones must be removed through a suprapubic incision.

The surgery for renal calculi also includes correction of any anatomical obstructions which are thought to contribute to the development of stones. For example, a congenital ureteropelvic junction obstruction may require that the surgeon perform pyeloplasty along with removal of calculi or stones will reform.

Prevention. Patients who have a tendency to form stones should always ingest adequate fluids (minimum 2,500 to 3,000 ml. daily) to help to prevent recurrence. Also, they should be instructed in the methods for straining urine and know that any stone should be brought to the doctor for examination.

The patient should be made aware of the importance of promptly reporting to the doctor any hematuria, burning or other signs of urinary tract infection, and infection anywhere in the body. An infected tooth or an infected cervix may set up a secondary focus of infection in the urinary tract that can help to recreate stones.

Patients with gout must limit their purine intake to prevent uric acid stones. Patients who have had stones of calcium may have to limit their intake of milk and milk products.

When it has been possible to determine the chemical composition of stones that have been passed or removed, dietary treatment then may be attempted to adjust the pH of the urine to keep the urinary salts in solution. However, these diets are not fully effective, and they are not commonly used. Sometimes the desired pH of the urine can be achieved by relatively minor changes in the diet. To acidify the urine, the doctor may suggest that the patient eliminate citrus fruits, fruit juices other than apple and cranberry, and carbonated beverages from his diet. Tomatoes may be eaten for vitamin C. An acidifying agent, such as sodium acid phosphate, may be given. To make the urine more alkaline, the doctor may prescribe sodium bicarbonate or polycitrate solution, and 1 to 3 quarts of orange juice a day. Uric acid stones can be prevented by a low-purine diet and alkalinization of the urine by use of oral sodium bicarbonate. The patient is taught how to check his urinary acidity with litmus or nitrazine paper. A further medical advance is the use of allopurinal, a xanthine oxidase inhibitor. The compound interferes with endogenous production of uric acid by the body. Cystine stones can be prevented in many instances by using a vigorous fluid intake (up to 6 liters a day), stringent alkalinization of the urine, and the oral ingestion of the compound d-penicillamine.

The most effective deterrent to calcium stones, particularly phosphatic ones, is the Shorr regimen. The patient is placed on a low-calcium, low-phosphorus diet to diminish the concentration of these substances in the urine. Basic aluminum hydroxide gel, 30 to 45 ml., is ingested after each meal and at bedtime to precipitate phosphorus as insoluble aluminum phosphates in the gastrointestinal tract, thus further decreasing urinary phosphate output.

Before the patient leaves the hospital, be sure that he understands and can carry out the fluid requirement, any dietary instructions, and his drug or chemotherapy.

Patients who have had recent kidney surgery should avoid heavy lifting.

Urethral Strictures

Since strictures are a form of obstruction, they are a danger to the upper urinary tract. The symptoms may include a slow stream of urine, a forked or spray stream, hesitancy, burning, frequency, nocturia and the retention of residual urine in the bladder, which may lead to distention and infection. A voiding urethrogram helps the doctor to make the diagnosis. If the patient is unable to void, a retrograde urethrogram may be done.

The urologist may treat urethral strictures by:
• Dilatation. This is done with specially designed instruments (bougies, sounds, filiforms and followers) passed very gently into the lumen of the urethra. Although this procedure is done gently, it is still painful. Taking deep breaths may help the patient to relax.

Since forceful stretching of the urethra may cause bleeding and further stricture formation, the doctor gently uses graduated size instruments. He may start with only a 6 or 8 F. Gradually, he increases the size until a 24 or 26 F. can be tolerated. Depending on the cause of the stricture and the patient's response to the therapy, the condition may subside after one or two treatments, but usually periodic dilations are required

indefinitely, or until the condition is corrected surgically. The nurse should help the patient to understand the importance of having these treatments regularly as prescribed and of not waiting until there has been too severe a reduction in the size of the urinary stream or other symptoms of obstruction. After a treatment, the patient may have slight hematuria and he should be told about this in advance so that he will not become frightened. Of course, if a great amount of blood appears, or if bleeding persists, he should notify the doctor immediately. Voiding will be painful for about two days after the procedure. Sitz baths help to relieve the discomfort.

• Internal urethrotomy. The urologist enters the urethra with an instrument called a *urethrotome* and cuts the stricture bands. A large retention catheter then is inserted and maintained in place until the urethra has healed (approximately three weeks).

• Perineal urethrostomy. For very tight, persisting strictures a permanent opening into the urethra through the perineum may be constructed, bypassing the stricture. Following such a diversion of the urinary stream, the male patient must sit to urinate. Providing privacy, emotional support and instruction regarding hygiene after bowel movement to prevent ascending urinary tract infection are part of the nurse's role following this surgery.

• Urethroplasty. The urine is diverted from the urethra by way of a cystostomy tube or perineal urethrostomy tube attached to straight drainage until the urethra has been repaired. In one method of reconstructing the urethra, the constricted area is resected, and a mucosal graft (which may be taken from the bladder) is inserted to restore the continuity of the urethra. Postoperatively, the patient will have a splinting catheter in the urethra that will remain until healing has taken place. This operation may be performed in two stages: urinary diversion at the first operation and plastic repair at the second.

INFECTION

A focus of infection elsewhere in the body—for example, a boil or an inflamed throat—may spread to the urinary tract, particularly the kidney, through the bloodstream or the lymphatics. An infection in the kidney can spread to the tissues of the rest of the urinary tract. An ascending infection (one that starts in the urethra and moves up) is caused commonly by *Escherichia coli*. In men the infection may extend to the tissue of the prostate, the seminal vesicles or the epididymis. The presence of foreign bodies, such as stones and catheters, predisposes to infection. The danger of introducing bacteria with a catheter or with irrigating solution is so great that only the strictest aseptic equipment and technic should be used.

When an indwelling catheter is necessary for a long period, it should be changed periodically, using sterile technic. In some hospitals it is the policy to change indwelling catheters once a week. Patients who have urinary procedures, such as dilations, have samples of their urine tested at intervals for evidence of infection.

The treatment of all urinary-tract infections includes surgical drainage of pus; identification and removal (when this is possible) of contributing factors, such as coexisting stones, obstructions or tumors; increasing the fluid intake, so that there is 1.5 to 2 liters of urine a day; and administering appropriate measures, such as antibiotics, to combat infection.

Tuberculosis

Since the advent of drug therapy, tubercular infections of the urinary tract are less common than they used to be. Tuberculosis of the urinary tract usually occurs secondarily to lesions in the lungs. The upper pole of the kidney is usually first involved and the disease may eventually involve the ureters, bladder, prostate, and scrotal contents. A triple combination of the drugs isoniazid hydrazide (INH), para-aminosalicylic acid (PAS) and streptomycin or cycloserine for at least two years is one mode of treatment.

If the renal tuberculosis does not respond to drug therapy and is unilateral, nephrectomy may be done. Rest in a hospital or at home is part of the treatment. While the pulmonary lesion may be no longer active, in the early stage of treatment the urine will contain the tubercle bacillus. Patients and nurses should wash their hands after contact with the urine, dressings soiled with it should be wrapped in protective coverings and burned, and soiled linen should be treated as contaminated.

Acute Pyelonephritis

Pyelonephritis means infection of the renal parenchyma as well as the lining of the collecting system. In the acute form the patient is clinically quite ill. He experiences pain in the kidney, chills, fever, malaise and nausea. The urinalysis will show pyuria. Frequency and burning on urination may be present if the bladder is also infected. It is often associated with pregnancy and with diabetes.

The patient is placed on bed rest, and liberal fluid intake to keep the urine dilute is urged. These patients are very sick and require attention to skin and mouth care, turning and encouragement to eat. Every effort is expended to prevent both septicemia and the development of chronic pyelonephritis. When there are no complications, the prognosis for complete cure with adequate antibacterial therapy is excellent.

Chronic Pyelonephritis

If the treatment of acute pyelonephritis is not permanently successful (for instance, if the infection is recurrent, or if urinary stasis continues due to an obstruction) the disease may enter a chronic stage. The kidney shows irreversible degenerative changes. It becomes small and atrophic, and the pelvic mucosa becomes pale and fibrotic. Many nephrons are destroyed. If enough nephrons become inoperative, the patient will develop uremia.

Although chronic pyelonephritis may be asymptomatic, the patient can have a low-grade fever, vague gastrointestinal complaints and anemia. There may be acute attacks; some of the patients will develop hypertension due to renal ischemia. Sometimes, stones form in the affected kidney.

Nothing known today can restore scarred kidney tissue. The aim of the treatment is to prevent further damage. Intensive therapy with antibiotics or chemotherapeutic agents is given. Any obstruction is relieved. An effort is made to improve the patient's overall health. A nephrectomy may be done if severe hypertension develops, and if the other kidney can support life. The fight against chronic pyelonephritis is a long one. Prolonged medication and constant attention to general health habits may be a dull and discouraging routine for patients.

In selected patients with chronic pyelonephritis the transplantation of a normal kidney to replace the diseased one offers a new lease on life.

Cystitis

This term means inflammation of the urinary bladder. The contents of the bladder are normally sterile. Bacteria reach the bladder by way of infected kidneys, lymphatics and the urethra. Because the urethra is short in women, ascending infections are more common in women than men. Cystitis is prevented from being even more common than it is by a natural resistance of the bladder lining, which helps to prevent an inflammatory process from taking hold from the occasional invasion of the bladder by bacteria. This resistance cannot be relied on to counter the effects of the introduction of an unsterile catheter into the sterile environment of the bladder.

The symptoms include urgency (feeling a pressing need to void although the bladder is not full), frequency, dysuria (painful urination), perineal and suprapubic pain, and hematuria, especially at the termination of the stream (terminal hematuria). If bacteremia is present, the patient also may have chills and fever. Chronic cystitis causes similar symptoms, but usually they are less severe.

The diagnosis is made by the patient's history, the total physical examination and urinalysis, including culture and sensitivity of the offending organisms to antibiotics or chemotherapeutic agents.

Medical care includes the location and the correction of contributing factors. If there is a partial obstruction, no cure of cystitis will be fully effective until adequate drainage of urine is restored by the removal of the obstruction. Treatment often is prolonged, and it may necessitate many return visits to the doctor after the patient has been discharged from the hospital. For example, dilatation of a contracted bladder with normal saline instillations must be repeated many times.

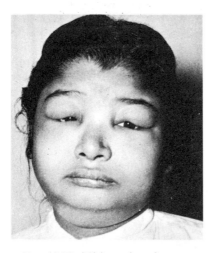

Fig. 40-12. This patient has acute nephritis. (Vakil, R. J., and Golwalla, A.: *Clinical Diagnosis*, Bombay, Asia Pub. House)

If the patient has a fever or other systemic symptoms of infection, he may be put on bed rest. Even though he has urgency and frequency, he needs a great deal of encouragement to take large quantities of fluids. Warm sitz baths may provide some relief. Cranberry juice may be offered to the patient. This acidifies the urine and provides a less favorable climate for bacterial growth. The alert nurse finds out the patient's fluid preferences and provides for these so that the goal of a liberal fluid intake can be more readily met.

Urethritis

Inflammation of the urethra caused by organisms other than gonorrhea is called *nonspecific urethritis*. Gonorrheal urethritis used to be more common than it is now. Urethritis also may be secondary to trichomonal and monilial infections in women.

The distal portion of the normal male urethra is not totally sterile. However, bacteria normally present there cause no difficulty unless these tissues are traumatized, usually following instrumentation such as catheterization or cystoscopic examination. Under such conditions, bacteria may gain a foothold to cause a nonspecific urethritis. The urethral mucosa becomes inflamed and pus forms in the tiny mucus forming glands lining the urethra. Other causes for nonspecific urethritis include irritation during vigorous intercourse.

Gonorrhea, on the other hand, is a specific form of infection which can attack the mucous membrane of a normal urethra. Usually within two or three days after contact, the patient will notice a thick purulent discharge from the meatus.

The symptoms of infection of the urethra are discomfort on urination varying from a slight tickling sensation to burning or severe discomfort, and urinary frequency. Fever is not common and its appearance in the male implies further extension of the infection to such areas as the prostate, testes and epididymi. Treatment includes appropriate antibiotics, a liberal fluid intake, analgesics, warm sitz baths and improvement of the patient's resistance to infection by a good diet and plenty of rest.

The nurse should be gentle when she is catheterizing patients, so that she does not injure the delicate wall of the urethra. The importance of avoiding the introduction of microorganisms with the catheter cannot be overemphasized.

Encourage the patient to drink copiously after all urethral procedures to flush out the lower urinary tract.

The periurethral area of any patient who cannot be placed in a tub should be washed daily with soap, water and a clean washcloth. This should be done by the nurse for the patients who cannot wash themselves well. Urethritis is commonly caused by irritation from indwelling catheters. If a patient has an indwelling catheter the area should be washed more frequently, and especially if the patient is incontinent of feces. It is not sufficient to wash only around anus and buttocks. Avoid wiping toward the urethra. If cotton pledgets are used, wipe from the urethral meatus to the anus in a single stroke and discard the pledget.

NEPHRITIS (BRIGHT'S DISEASE)

The term *nephritis* refers to a group of non-infectious diseases characterized by widespread kidney damage.

Acute Glomerulonephritis

Etiology. Glomerulonephritis is a type of nephritis characterized by inflammation of the glomeruli. It has been repeatedly observed that the symptoms of acute glomerulonephritis appear approximately two weeks after an upper respiratory infection, usually one that has been caused by hemolytic streptococci. Recent influenza, scarlet fever or chickenpox also may be given in the history. The exact relationship between the respiratory infection and the nephritis is not clearly understood. The organisms are not present in the kidney when the symptoms of nephritis appear. The disease may represent an altered tissue reaction to infection, a result of host response rather than damage from infection.

Acute glomerulonephritis occurs most frequently in children and young adults.

Symptoms. Early symptoms may be so slight that the patient does not seek medical attention, though occasionally the onset is sudden, with generalized edema (anasarca), fever, vomiting, anuria, hypertension and dyspnea. There may be cerebral and cardiac involvement. Most patients survive the disease without sequelae, but death from uremia may follow delirium or convulsions, or the patient may die in congestive heart failure.

More often, the patient or his family notices that his face is pale and puffy, and that he has slight ankle edema in the evening. His appetite is poor, and he is up frequently during the night to void (nocturia). He awakens with a headache (due to hypertension). His family and friends find him irritable, and he is out of breath after exertion. The patient may have only one symptom, such as a pitting, dependent edema. Visual disturbances, often due to papilledema or hemorrhage, are common. Nosebleeds may occur. As the condition progresses, he may develop hematuria, anemia, convulsions associated with hypertension, congestive heart failure, oliguria and perhaps anuria.

The laboratory findings may include a slightly elevated blood urea nitrogen and albuminuria. There will be gross or microscopic hematuria, giving the urine a dark, smoky or frankly bloody appearance.

Treatment. There is no specific treatment for acute glomerulonephritis. The therapy is guided by the symptoms and their underlying pathology. The following regimen is usual:

• Bed rest. While the blood pressure is elevated, and edema is present, bed rest may continue for several weeks. When progressive ambulation is slowly started, daily urine specimens are usually collected, and blood pressure is taken daily. Any increase in hematuria, albuminuria or blood pressure is an indication for a return to bed rest.

• Hydration. Fluids should be taken liberally. Since there is damage to the glomeruli, there is a filtration problem. To get rid of waste products the body needs ample fluids. However, fluids are limited to balance output in the presence of marked edema, oliguria or anuria.

• Diet. Sodium is restricted when edema is present. Carbohydrate intake is encouraged, especially when proteins are limited. Vitamins may be added to the diet to improve the patient's general resistance. Iron or liver may be needed to counteract anemia.

• Medication. Antibiotics may be given to prevent a superimposed infection on the already inflamed kidney.

In the seriously ill patient a trial of corticosteroids may be given to attempt to alter the course of the disease. When the blood pressure climbs to high levels, antihypertensive drugs are usually given.

The patient is not considered to be cured until his urine is free of albumin and red blood cells for six months. Return to full activity usually is not permitted until the urine is free of protein for a month.

Prognosis. Most patients with acute glomerulonephritis recover, usually completely. A few develop chronic glomerulonephritis. Subsequent infections with the same strain of hemolytic streptococci usually do not cause a second attack of acute glomerulonephritis. This is in sharp contrast with chronic glomerulonephritis, in which upper respiratory infections must be studiously avoided to prevent exacerbations of the disease.

Chronic Glomerulonephritis

Chronic glomerulonephritis causes irremediable damage to the nephrons. Some disappear entirely. Bands of scar tissue contract the kidney and replace the functioning units. The cortex becomes distorted and shrunken.

Symptoms. A small number of patients with chronic glomerulonephritis are known to have had acute glomerulonephritis. But most give no such history. The symptoms are similar to those of acute glomerulonephritis, but they may be even more individualized. There may be generalized edema, headache and hypertension, visual disturbances, nocturia, dyspnea and albuminuria. Anemia, cardiac failure and cerebral symptoms are not uncommon. The patient who develops anasarca is said to be in the *nephrotic* stage. The generalized edema is due to the depletion of serum proteins, with loss of plasma osmotic pressure. These patients may remain markedly edematous for months or years. Quiescent periods occur between exacerbations. During this *latent stage* the patient is relatively free of symptoms and feels well, although his urine contains protein.

The course of the disease is highly variable. The patient may live for years, with only occasional acute episodes or none at all; or the disease may be rapidly fatal due to uremia.

Complications. Congestive heart failure, pulmonary edema, increased blood pressure that may lead to cerebral hemorrhage, and secondary infection are common and sometimes fatal complications. Blurring of vision and blindness may occur late in the disease. Anemia is usual. Increased capillary fragility causes nosebleeds, purpura and gastrointestinal bleeding in many terminally ill patients. Bronchopneumonia is a serious danger in the nephrotic stage. High blood pressure over a period of months or years may lead to further renal insufficiency. (*Nephrosclerosis* is the term given to kidney disease caused by hypertension in its malignant phase.

The resulting symptoms are those of chronic glomerulonephritis.)

Treatment. No treatment is given during the quiescent stages. Nurses are in a position to assist patients and their families to maintain a healthful regimen for the patient. Everything that can be done should be done to increase his resistance to infection, since a cold may precipitate uremia. He should rest well and eat well and see his doctor regularly. If the patient develops an infection, prompt medical treatment is imperative. Kidney function tests may be done annually. Death from uremia is the usual outcome of chronic glomerulonephritis, but it may be delayed for years with a regimen of healthful living.

When the disease becomes active, often evidenced initially by hematuria and edema, the patient is put to bed. Dietary considerations include low sodium intake and regulation of protein intake. Sedatives, often chloral hydrate, are given for headaches, hypertension, insomnia and irritability. Diuretics containing mercury usually are not given, because they may increase the damage to the kidneys. Intravenous hypertonic solutions may be given to reduce intracranial pressure. If the patient has congestive heart failure, treatment of that condition, with such measures as digitalis, is necessary. Anemia, if it is severe, is treated with transfusions. The symptoms often subside in about three weeks, and very gradually the patient may return to normal activity. Because the restitution of renal function lags behind the patient's clinical improvement, his convalescence should be planned carefully to avoid intercurrent infection, marked exertion and the body stress that may, in turn, affect renal function.

The treatment in the nephrotic stage includes bed rest to decrease the work of the heart, diuretics, and regulation of the diet, including sodium and fluid restriction. During this phase the patient is especially prone to intercurrent infection, and he may die of bronchopneumonia. The patient needs to be protected against infection that is carried to him on the hands or in the throats of hospital personnel and visitors. (See Chapter 56 for Care of the Patient in Renal Failure.)

NEPHROSIS (THE NEPHROTIC SYNDROME)

The term *nephrosis* means a degenerative, noninflammatory disease of the renal tubules. The nephrotic syndrome is characterized by edema, albuminuria, decreased plasma proteins and an increase of blood lipid and cholesterol. There may be degenerative and necrotic lesions of the distal tubules, and renal vasoconstriction. The decrease in blood flow to the kidneys may lead to anuria and uremia. If the damage has not been too severe, and the circulation has not been too greatly impaired, the tubules are capable of regeneration.

The aim of the treatment is to keep the patient alive until his kidneys repair themselves. When the administration of ACTH, or adrenocortical steroids is effective, there is diuresis and lowering or cessation of the loss of protein in the urine. If the patient is not prostrated by the disease he is often treated at home. Bed rest may not be necessary, but he should engage only in moderate activity during the acute phase, and eat a high protein diet to replace the protein lost in the urine. Because of the edema, the diet probably will also be low in sodium content. In the hospital, if intravenous fluids are given (to supply electrolytes), special care must be taken to regulate the rate of the intravenous drip as it was ordered and to watch for signs of pulmonary edema. It is important to keep an account of the patient's weight; he may be retaining fluid.

The disease tends to be even more serious in adults than in children. Death may occur from renal failure, hypertension or intercurrent infection when the patient is on corticosteroid therapy. If the kidneys do not seem to be recovering, and death from uremia is impending, dialysis (see Chap. 56) may be performed to give the kidneys more time to heal.

TUMORS (NEOPLASIA)

Tumors of the Kidney

The malignant hypernephroma (renal adenocarcinoma) is the most common tumor of the parenchyma of the adult kidney. Because the kidneys are deeply protected in the body, tumors can become quite large before they cause symptoms. An abdominal mass found on a routine physical examination or on roentgenograms taken for other purposes may lead to the discovery. These tumors are dangerous, because they usually metastasize early, but may present distressing symptoms only late in the course of the disease. Hematuria may occur if the tumor invades the collecting system. It may be both intermittent and painless. Later, pain may be due to expansion of the kidney or colic-like discomfort from the passage of bloodclots.

The symptoms of a malignant tumor may include weight loss, malaise, unexplained fever, and episodes of hematuria. Sometimes, the first symptom occurs at a secondary, metastatic site. Hypertension is frequent in these patients.

When kidney cancer is diagnosed, a complete removal of the kidney (nephrectomy) and its surrounding perinephric fat may be done. When the tumor arises from the collecting system or in the ureter a complete nephroureterectomy may be done. The kidney and ureter as well as a cuff of bladder tissue is removed because the recurrence rate in any stump of ureter left behind is very high.

Surgery may be followed by x-ray therapy while the patient is still in the hospital or on an outpatient basis. Follow-up cystoscopic examinations are imperative to find any early and newly metastasized areas in the bladder. If the unaffected kidney cannot adequately take over the function of excreting urine, or if extensive metastases are found, only palliative treatment can be given.

Postnephrectomy Care. After a nephrectomy, a Penrose drain is left in place to catch the serous material that collects in the space left by the kidney. Of course, no urine comes from this drain. Note and chart the amount and the characteristics (color, consistency, odor and contents) of this drainage, which may be blood-tinged in the beginning. The drainage should stop after about two days. A sterile safety pin is usually placed on this drain by the doctor so that it cannot disappear into the wound. Because the surgical area is close to the pleural cavity observe the patient for a pneumothorax. In rare instances, the pleura is accidentally nicked during the operation, and air enters the pleural space from the lung and collapses the lung.

Deep breathing is painful because of the proximity of the incision to the diaphragm. Narcotics are given liberally, but the patient must be assisted to deep breathe and cough to avoid atelectasis. Positive pressure breathing treatments may be ordered. Splinting the incision with a binder, or manually, may help the patient to expand his rib cage. The patient may have a gastric tube for several days because paralytic ileus of reflex origin tends to develop. Fluids are encouraged when this tube is removed. Watch for signs of hemorrhage especially during the immediate postoperative period and eight to twelve days postoperatvely when tissue sloughing is apt to occur.

If the hyperextended side-lying position was used for surgery the patient may be troubled by muscular aches and pain. Pillow support and the use of prescribed muscle relaxants may give relief.

Tumors of the Bladder

Bladder tumors may be benign or malignant. In malignant tumors, metastases have usually not occurred so long as the muscle is not penetrated.

The most common first symptom of malignant disease of the bladder is painless hematuria (another instance of the importance of immediately investigating hematuria). Diagnosis is made by cystoscopic examination and biopsy.

Treatment varies according to the type of tumor, and the grade and stage of malignant ones. Small, superficial tumors may be cut out through the transurethral resectoscope by means of an electric cutting instrument. Bleeding can be checked, or tumor tissue may be coagulated in the same manner. Fulguration may be used for small and benign tumors. Patients who have had papillomas removed should return for a cystoscopic examination every three months for the first year, and every six months for the next four years, so that the recurrence of a benign tumor or a new malignant growth can be discovered early.

Radiation therapy for bladder malignancy is presently of debatable merit. Local bladder recurrences of low-grade malignant tumors have been lessened by instillations of the chemotherapeutic agent, thio-tepa.

Some tumors may not be removable by the transurethral method because of their size or their location in the bladder. To remove these tumors a suprapubic incision is made, and the bladder is exposed and thoroughly explored. Part of the bladder may be removed (segmental resection) or all of it (cystectomy).

Bladder Surgery. When a portion of the bladder is removed (segmental resection), its capacity as a reservoir is decreased. Immediately postoperatively, the patient may be able to hold no more than 50 to 60 ml. of urine. This capacity should increase to 200 to 400 ml. within a couple of months (depending on the amount of the bladder that was removed). Fluids should be encouraged during the immediate postoperative period, and the output from both the urethral and the suprapubic catheters should be watched and recorded. The patient becomes aware of being able to hold less urine when his catheters are first removed. Prior discussion of what to expect will help to lessen surprise and anxiety. The patient will need to adjust to the smaller reservoir capacity. For example, he should learn to restrict fluids before retiring or joining a gathering. However, it is important that his total fluid intake for the day be adequate.

After cystectomy, the patient is usually quite ill. The bladder and large amounts of surrounding tissue have been removed. The patient is prone to surgical shock, thrombosis, cardiac decompensation and other circulatory disturbances. Nursing care is similar to that of the patient with major abdominal surgery. In addition, permanent urinary diversion accompanies cystectomy. If the prostatic capsule has been removed, the male patient will be impotent also.

Nursing Care of Patients with Ureteral Transplants

Some operations for urinary diversion are:

• **Ureterosigmoidostomy.** The ureters are attached to the sigmoid colon. The lower colon becomes the reservoir for urine. The patient voids and defecates through the rectum.

The advantage of attaching ureters to the bowel is that the patient is not required to adjust to caring for a continuously draining opening in his abdominal wall. There are no appliances, and there is no need to care for the skin surrounding the orifices. The lower colon acts as a reservoir of sorts (holding about 200 ml.), and the anal sphincter controls the exit from the body of both urine and stool. The amount of urine that can be held is not so great as in the urinary bladder, and the urine liquefies the stool, but some patients learn to regulate themselves so that they can continue with daily activities. This operation is not performed if there is disease of the large bowel such as diverticulitis, or if the anal sphincter is incompetent since the main advantage, voluntary urinary control, is lost.

If the ureters are to be attached to the bowel, microorganisms in the bowel will be minimized preoperatively with the use of a mechanical bowel preparation with cathartics and enemas and a drug such as sulfasuxidine or neomycin. The loss of the usual bacterial flora results in a soft, almost odorless stool. The nurse should observe the stool and chart its characteristics. Patients who have ureteral transplants to the bowel are given a low-residue diet both before and after the surgery, to minimize the formation of fecal material that would contaminate the operative area. The patient is placed on a low-residue diet about three days before surgery, then clear fluids 24 hours prior to operation.

Postoperatively, a sterile rectal tube is left in place for five to ten days to keep the rectosigmoid empty and decrease the chance of urinary leakage through the anastomosis. Ureteral catheters may be brought out through the anus and anchored to the buttocks for about ten days. During the first days after surgery note the hourly or two-hourly drainage. Later the rectal tube may be removed when necessary for defecation and reinserted. The stool at first will be liquid, but as the bowel adjusts to being a reservoir, stools become soft. A low residue diet is usually ordered until the tubes are removed.

Sometimes the patient is taught in the hospital and discharged with instructions to insert a rectal tube each night, anchor it to the skin and attach it to straight drainage if there are problems with the resorption of urinary chloride and resultant hyperchloremic acidosis. The doctor may also prescribe oral sodium bicarbonate. To minimize the absorption of waste products the patient voids (rectally) every two to four hours. He should report symptoms of electrolyte imbalance such as nausea, vomiting, or lethargy.

The major disadvantage of ureterosigmoidostomy is that infection of the ureters and the kidney pelves is very frequent. The urinary tract is unprotected from the organisms that normally inhabit the lower bowel. The patient should be taught to establish a regular routine of drinking 2,500 to 3,000 ml. of fluids daily, and to return to his doctor on the first indication of pain, fever or any other sign of infection. Some patients are placed on a small dose of a sulfonamide or an antibiotic and continue taking the drug for months or years in an attempt to prevent an infection of the urinary tract. Patients should tell hospital personnel on readmission that they void rectally. They do not need laxatives and enemas would force fecal material into the ureters.

• **Cutaneous Ureterostomy.** The ureters are brought to the skin surface. The patient wears one or two rubber collecting cups that drain the urine into a leg bag, an artificial bladder. The patient periodically empties the bag by releasing the stopper at the bottom. This operation is a relatively safe procedure with a low mortality rate, and it is often indicated in debilitated and older patients. Stricture of the ureter at the junc-

tion with skin or fascia is one complication of the procedure. Leakage and odor problems also can occur. After the cutaneous implantation of ureters, the patient returns from the operating room with splinting catheters inserted into the ureters. These catheters remain in place for at least ten days. After that, studies are obtained to determine if the ureters will drain freely to the skin.

During surgery the ends of the ureters are everted and attached to the skin in such a way that a circle of mucosal lining is exposed to the air. It is like rolling the end of a tube back on itself. The purpose is to prevent the ureters from closing. These stoma are called ureteral buds. For about five days postoperatively, sterile wet saline compresses are kept over the exposed urethral mucosa. Saline can be added hourly with an Asepto syringe. Then the entire dressing is covered with several sterile combines to keep the rest of the patient's body from getting wet and to keep the underneath wet dressing sterile. Use zinc oxide, aluminum paste, or petrolatum to protect the skin from maceration. Note the color of the stoma and watch the edema that may occlude the opening.

After the catheters are removed, a collecting appliance is placed over the buds, and urine drains through it to a rubber or a plastic bag that can be attchaed to the leg with straps. Care is taken that the straps are not too tight. The patient visits the bathroom at intervals during the day to release the stopper from the bottom of the bag, emptying it of urine. At night the bag is replaced by a drainage bottle at the side of the bed. The appliance is attached to the skin with bands that go around the patient's body (Whitfield cups), or with adhesive disks, or with cement (Singer cups). The cup is changed every three or four days, and while the patient is still in the hospital, he should learn to care for it himself. Gently wash the skin with warm water and bland soap. Dry it well, for the disk will not stick to wet skin. You can put a sterile cotton ball over the orifices of the ureters while the cup is being changed, so that the urine will not flow over the skin. Look for any signs of irritation of the skin. If it appears to be breaking down, exposure to dry heat and more frequent changing of the cup are indicated. Be sure to check with the doctor if the skin is becoming irritated. Until the skin becomes accustomed to the cups, tincture of benzoin may be ordered. Let it dry on the skin over the area that

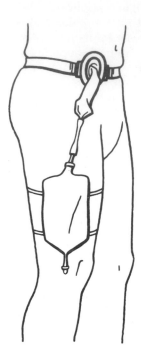

FIG. 40-13. A rubber leg-urinal collecting the urine draining from a ureter implanted into the skin. The end of the bag can be unplugged periodically during the day to empty the bag.

the disk covers. Tincture of benzoin should not be applied directly to the stoma. To function properly, the disk must fit airtight. The patient may take a bath, since the cement is waterproof. The patient may be taught to dilate the stoma with a sterile catheter.

The cup, the tubing and the urinal should be washed with soap and water, rinsed well and allowed to air. Rinsing with a dilute white vinegar solution will help remove encrustations. At home, patients should have two sets, so that one may air while the other is being worn. The urinal should be washed and aired every night while the patient is using a drainage bottle. Referral to a visiting nurse agency is indicated if the patient needs help to care for himself at home.

If urinary drainage stops or if the patient complains of back pain, the doctor should be called immediately since an indwelling ureteral catheter may be necessary. If such catheters are required on a permanent basis (for example, if buds are not formed around the orifices), the patient is taught how to sterilize, irrigate and replace catheters.

● **Ileal Conduit.**

In this operation (the Bricker procedure) a small segment of ileum is resected from the intestines, with its nerve and blood supply kept intact. The proximal end of the segment is closed and the distal end brought out as a stoma in the lower right quadrant. The ureters are anastomosed to the pouch and drain through it. The ileal loop is no longer connected to the gastrointestinal tract. The term "ileal bladder" is a misnomer, since urine is not stored in the pouch; it only passes through it and out of the body via the stoma. The patient wears an ileostomy bag or special ileal conduit bag over the stoma of the pouch. An infrequent complication of this procedure is electrolyte imbalance.

Following construction of an ileal conduit, the patient may have some degree of paralytic ileus for as long as a week. Return of peristaltic activity in the isolated segment of conduit parallels that of the intestinal tract which was re-anastomosed. For this reason, some surgeons will insert a multi-eyed catheter into the stoma at operation and it is not removed for five to seven days. However, the catheter lumen readily becomes obstructed by intestinal mucus and may require frequent irrigations. An alternate approach is the application of a temporary clear plastic ostomy appliance connected to straight drainage. This has the advantage of less likelihood of urinary soilage of the surgical incision and the condition of the stoma can be observed through the plastic. The physician may decide to insert a catheter into the conduit at times to check for residual urine (normally the conduit is nearly empty since it does not have a reservoir function) or to provide for continued drainage should there be a leakage at one of the internal anastomoses.

Because the patient has also had an intestinal anastomosis, he will have a gastric tube in place for several days postoperatively to prevent distention and pressure on the suture line. Observe for and report promptly any symptoms of peritonitis (abdominal tenderness, fever, severe pain, distention) since the intestinal anastomosis can leak fecal material or the ileal conduit may leak urine into the peritoneal cavity. Watch for any signs of distention of the conduit with urine because this puts pressure on the suture line or back pressure on the kidneys. Promptly report pain in the lower abdomen or decreased urinary output.

The mucosa of the ileum produces mucus, which may plug the orifice and prevent the drainage of urine. The mucus may be removed with sterile gauze. The doctor may dilate the stoma daily during the early postoperative period. Until the patient is able to do it for himself, the nurse frequently checks the bag to see that the urine is draining adequately, empties it before it becomes full, and changes the temporary plastic ileostomy bag as needed. Each time his position is changed, at first the nurse, and then the patient, checks to make sure that the drainage system is not impeded in any way.

Additional Nursing Points. Nursing considerations in the care of a patient with ureteral transplants are similar to those in the care of a patient with a colostomy or an ileostomy. For example, in both instances the skin needs protection, the dressings should be changed promptly when they become soiled, the appliances need care and cleanliness, and the patient needs a nurse who can encourage the patient by her matter-of-factness and skill as she changes the dressing. But there are also some differences. The drainage from a ureteral transplant is more liquid; hence it is more difficult to manage. Infection is more prone to occur. This different way of voiding may be difficult for the patient. In the hospital, if he is on a urologic ward, he will see others who use the same method. However, the patient may worry about how he will get along outside the hospital. His own acceptance of the urinary diversion, the equipment and its care can be helped by giving him the responsibility for it in the early postoperative period.

Early ambulation (taking the necessary equipment with him) demonstrates to the patient that he nevertheless can move about, and is not chained to a collecting apparatus at his bedside. If the patient wishes, let him discuss with you his fears and misgivings about the surgery and its effect. By your manner and in your discussion with him, show him that you have confidence in his ability to handle the situation.

Preoperative explanation to the patient, the nurse's familiarity with various collection appliances, and an introduction to other patients who have successfully undergone urinary diversion will do much to allay the patient's fear. During the postoperative period, the patient is measured for his permanent appliance. After this is obtained, the patient is thoroughly instructed, along with another member of his family, in its application, cleaning, and care. Teaching is continued until the patient can leave the hospital confident in his ability to manage his own care alone or with the help of family members or the public health nurse.

A set of written instructions for the patient and family is helpful for home review (Winter). Anxiety in the hospital or on arrival at home may lead to memory gaps or misunderstanding.

OTHER URINARY TRACT CONDITIONS

Trauma

From the back and the sides, the urinary tract is encircled by the ribs, the spinal column and the pelvic girdle. Fracture of any of these bones should alert the nurse to watch for signs of damage to kidneys, ureters or bladder. Any trauma to the lower portion of the body, such as a fall, automobile accident or a gunshot wound, may tear a portion of the urinary tract. The symptoms may not be immediately apparent while the more obvious wounds are being cared for. Watch for anuria in any patient with trauma to the area; perhaps the ureters are cut through, or the bladder may be ruptured. Observe for symptoms of peritonitis: urine is a foreign substance in the abdominal cavity. Check each urine specimen for gross or increasing hematuria. A sample can be left in a test tube for continuing comparison.

Polycystic Disease of the Kidney

This disease is a congenital familial disorder. It is characterized by multiple, bilateral kidney cysts and may not be diagnosed until middle life. As the cysts slowly enlarge, they squeeze the functioning parenchyma between them. The kidneys may become enormous and exert pressure on nearby abdominal and pelvic organs. Nephritis, calculi, infections and hydronephrosis may result from and complicate the condition. The patient may have hematuria, pain, pyuria, anemia, and gastrointestinal symptoms from pressure caused by the expanding kidney. The patient usually is hypertensive. The treatment is the same as that for nephritis. Emergency surgery is required sometimes for hemorrhage. However, there is no cure for polycystic disease, and eventually uremia develops. Because the disease is bilateral, the prognosis is poor. (See Chap. 56 for Care of the Patient in Renal Failure.)

REFERENCES AND BIBLIOGRAPHY
ANSELL, J. S.: Nephrectomy and nephrostomy, *Am. J. Nurs.* 58:1394, 1958.
BECKER, E. L., and THOMPSON, D. D.: Treatment of the nephrotic syndrome in adults, *Mod. Treatm.* 1:78, 1964.
BERGSTROM, N.: Ice application to induce voiding, *Am. J. Nurs.* 69:283, February, 1969.

BERMAN, H.: Urinary diversion in treatment of carcinoma of the bladder, *Surg. Clin. N. Am.* 45:1495, December, 1965.

BLANDY, J.: Urinary bladder substitution and the nursing care involved, *Nurs. Mirror* 122:5, 1966.

BOYARSKY, S.: *Neurogenic Bladder,* Baltimore, Williams & Wilkins, 1967.

CREEVY, C. D.: Ileac diversion of the urine, *Am. J. Nurs.* 59:530, 1959.

DAVIS, J. E.: Drugs for urologic disorders, *Am. J. Nurs.* 65: 107, August, 1965.

DELEHANTY, L., and STRAVINO, V.: Achieving bladder control, *Am. J. Nurs.* 70:312, February, 1970.

DINEEN, P.: The 'sterilization' of endoscopic instruments, *JAMA* 176:772, 1961.

EARLE, D. P.: Management of acute glomerulonephritis, *Mod. Treatm.* 1:49, 1964.

FRENAY, SR. M. A. C.: A dynamic approach to the ileal conduit patient, *Am. J. Nurs.* 64:80, January, 1964.

GIBBS, G.: Perineal care of the incapacitated patient, *Am. J. Nurs.* 69:124, January, 1969.

GLENN, J. F. (ed.): *Diagnostic Urology,* New York, Hoeber, 1964.

GLENN, J. F., and BOYCE, W. H.: *Urologic Surgery,* New York, Hoeber, 1969.

HIGHAM, A. R. C.: Stone in the urinary tract, *Nurs. Mirror* 122:8, 1966.

JACKSON, A. F.: Cancer of the bladder, *Am. J. Nurs.* 58:249, 1958.

KELLY, A. E., and GENSINI, G. G.: Renal arteriography, *Am. J. Nurs.* 64:97, February, 1964.

KEUHNELIAN, J. G., and SANDERS, V. E.: *Urologic Nursing,* New York, Macmillan, 1970.

LITTLEPAGE, S.: Genitourinary injuries—nursing care, *Am. J. Nurs.* 55:973, 1955.

MACKINNON, H.: Urinary drainage: the problem of asepsis, *Am. J. Nurs.* 65:112, August, 1965.

MAINWARING, C.: Clean voided specimens for mass screening, *Am. J. Nurs.* 63:96, October, 1963.

MARSHALL, V. F.: *Textbook of Urology,* ed. 2, New York, Hoeber, 1964.

MOHAMMED, M. R. B.: Urinalysis, *Am. J. Nurs.* 64:87, June, 1964.

MONROE, J., and KOMORIA, N.: Problems with nephrosis in adolescence, *Am. J. Nurs.* 67:336, February, 1967.

MOREL, A.: The urologic nurse specialist, *Nurs. Clin. N. Am.* 4:475, September, 1969.

MULLAN, S.: *Essentials of Neurosurgery,* New York, Springer, 1961.

OBERMEIER, W. B.: Crotch care, *Am. J. Nurs.* 57:618, 1957.

ROBERTSON, C. A.: Manual expression of urine, *Am. J. Nurs.* 59:840, 1959.

ROBINSON, C.: *Basic Nutrition and Diet Therapy,* New York, Macmillan, 1970.

ROBINSON, L.: *Psychological Aspects of the Care of Hospitalized Patients,* Philadelphia, Davis, 1968.

ROSE, J. F.: Management of the patient with trauma of the urinary tract, *Med. Clin. N. Am.* 48:1633, 1964.

SANTORA, D.: Preventing hospital-acquired urinary tract infection, *Am. J. Nurs.* 66:790, April, 1966.

SR. REGINA ELIZABETH: Sensory stimulation techniques, *Am. J. Nurs.* 66:281, February, 1966.

————: The scientific rationale of bowel and bladder training, *Ariz. Med.* p. 13, January, 1966.

SMITH, D. R.: *General Urology,* ed. 6, Los Altos, California, Lange, 1970.

SUTTON, A.: *Bedside Nursing Techniques in Medicine and Surgery,* ed. 2, Philadelphia, Saunders, 1969.

THOMSON, G.: After renal surgery, *Am. J. Nurs.* 61:106, 1961.

TOLLEFSON, D. M.: Nursing care of the patient with an ileac diversion of the urine, *Am. J. Nurs.* 59:534, 1959.

WALSH, M., et al.: Neo-bladder, *Am. J. Nurs.* 63:107, April, 1963.

WHITMORE, W. F., JR., and BONGART, T.: A device for the management of cutaneous ureterostomy, *J. Urol.* 74:603, 1955.

WINTER, C., and ROEHM, M.: *Sawyer's Nursing Care of Patients With Urologic Diseases,* St. Louis, Mosby, 1968.

The Patient with an Endocrine Disorder

41

The Thyroid Gland • The Parathyroid Glands • The Adrenal Glands
The Pituitary Gland

The consequences of diseases of the ductless glands usually are due to overproduction or underproduction of the hormones that the glands secrete, causing a disturbance in the delicate balance that the hormones normally maintain, and often resulting in a widespread chain of pathologic events within the body. Normally, many of the ductless glands respond to stimulation from the pituitary. If the glandular production is increased, the pituitary-stimulating factor is decreased as a counter-regulatory mechanism. This shows down the gland's function. For example, an increase in the production of the thyroid hormones results in a decrease in the amount of the thyroid-stimulating hormone (thyrotropin or TSH) produced by the pituitary gland. Conversely, a decrease in the gland's output is countered by increased pituitary stimulation. In endocrine-disease states this relationship between the pituitary and a target gland may be lost.

THE THYROID GLAND

This gland has the ability to concentrate iodine in the manufacture of thyroid hormones, which help to regulate the production and the use of energy for the body's dynamic processes. The important active hormones that the thyroid gland releases are tetraiodothyronine (thyroxine or T_4) and triiodothyronine (T_3). Iodine is contained in these hormones.

Hyperthyroidism

In hyperthyroidism (also called Graves' disease, thyrotoxicosis and exophthalmic goiter) the patient's metabolic rate is increased, due to an excessive secretion of thyroid hormones.

Etiology. The etiology is unknown. The most acceptable theory is that the abnormality resides within the thyroid gland itself; its normal relationship to the pituitary is lost, and the thyroid becomes autonomously overactive. The consequence is a generalized increase in the body's metabolism. Apparently, any condition which demands that the thyroid produce a large amount of thyroid hormone can precipitate hyperthyroidism: emotional or physical stress, infection, adolescence, pregnancy. Women are afflicted more frequently than men.

Symptoms. Patients with well-developed hyperthyroidism are characteristically restless, highly excitable and constantly agitated. They are emotionally labile, laughing one minute and crying the next. Often, they overreact to situations; they are incapable of resting. The patient may have fine tremors that may necessitate help with eating. Clumsiness, due to tremors, may cause the patient to drop things. Muscular weakness and fatigability are common. The pulse may be as high as 160. Characteristically, there is an increase in the systolic but not in the diastolic blood pressure. The patient may experience palpitations, and, if the condition is untreated, the continued excess activity may lead to cardiac decompensation.

The constant exercise and the high rate of metabolism cause the patient to lose weight, even though his appetite is usually great, and he consumes an extra number of calories. It is important to satisfy the need for food of the patient with a severely overactive thyroid, and even the patient with less severe thyrotoxicosis should eat a high caloric, high carbohydrate diet.

The increased metabolic rate makes the patient intolerant of heat. This symptom can be

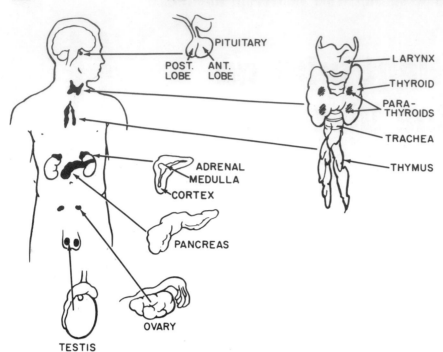

Fig. 41-1. Location of hormone-producing glands in the body.

troublesome on a ward, because ventilation that is comfortable for the patient with Graves' disease; chills the other patients. If possible, the patient should have his own room, in which he can adjust the temperature himself. If this is not possible, at least place the hyperthyroid patient next to the window.

Many patients with hyperthyroidism exhibit bulging eyes (*exophthalmos*) which give them a permanently startled expression. Usually, there is a visible swelling of the neck due to the enlarged thyroid gland.

Other symptoms of thyrotoxicosis include characteristically fine and flushed skin, menstrual abnormalities, changed bowel habits and excessive sweating. There may be hoarseness and difficulty in swallowing, due to the enlargement of the gland.

Diagnostic Tests. The following tests aid in the clinical diagnosis of hyperthyroidism:

Basal Metabolic Rate (B.M.R.). This test determines the rate at which an individual consumes oxygen under standard resting conditions. The patient's temperature must be normal, since each increase in degree of body temperature increases the body's metabolic rate. Digestion and muscular activity also increase the body's consumption of oxygen, and so for this test the patient must have fasted for eight to ten hours, and he must have been lying quietly in bed in as

near a state of complete rest as possible. Minus 11 to plus 11 is within normal limits. The B.M.R. is not as accurate as some other diagnostic tests and is being used less often today.

The nursing care of a patient who is to receive a B.M.R. test is devoted to obtaining and maintaining basal conditions. Explain the need for rest and quiet (even mild excitement or slight muscular exertion can result in large errors in the test results). If the patient knows what to expect, he will be able to help.

The morning of the test, keep the patient's room dark, or the curtains pulled around his bed, until the time of the test. The patient may be allowed to go to the bathroom, but he should return immediately to bed and rest. Or you may bring him a drink of water, a bedpan and the equipment to wash his hands and face and brush his teeth, if these measures will make him feel more comfortable and relaxed. Smoking is not permitted. If the test is not done at the bedside, take the patient to the place of the test in a wheelchair.

Protein-bound Iodine (PBI). Triiodothyronine and tetraiodothyronine are bound to the blood proteins that transport them. Because iodine is contained in the hormones, measurement of the protein-bound iodine in a blood sample reflects the level of circulating thyroid hormone. Although the patient may be active and eat before blood is drawn for these tests, he should not have ingested any unusual amounts of iodine for several weeks before the test. Substances containing iodine, such as some cough medicines and dyes administered for x-ray studies of the gallbladder, for intravenous pyelograms and for bronchograms, will cause errors. Even antiseptic solutions of iodine on the skin should be avoided.

The normal concentration of protein-bound iodine varies with the laboratory method used, but it is usually 4 to 8 μg. per 100 ml. of plasma. Values below and above these figures usually indicate hypothyroidism and hyperthyroidism, respectively.

Butanol-extractable Iodine (BEI). The BEI test measures the protein-bound iodine that is soluble in butanol. This eliminates inorganic iodides (from cough medicine, for example) and inactive iodinated proteins from measurement, since they are not soluble in butanol. Although this test can be more accurate than the PBI test, it is more involved and expensive and therefore is not done routinely.

Radioactive Iodine Uptake Test. The fasting patient is given sodium radio-iodide[131] either as a drink or in capsule form. Diluted in distilled water, the drug is odorless and tasteless. Then, 24 hours later, a *scintillator* (an instrument that measures radioactivity) is held over the thyroid gland to measure the amount of iodine[131] that the thyroid has taken up. The normal thyroid will remove 15 to 50 per cent of the radioactive iodine from the bloodstream. The thyroid gland of a patient with hyperthyroidism may remove as much as 90 per cent.

Thyroid Scanning. The patient ingests sodium radio-iodide[131]. Then a scintillator is passed back and forth across the throat, and a picture of radioactivity is recorded. The pattern of the scan indicates the concentration of the iodine in the thyroid and other tissues and helps the physician to differentiate between the noncancerous and malignant tissue of the thyroid when this test is used with other clinical findings.

I[131] Urine Excretion Test. This test measures the amount of I[131] excreted in 24 or 48 hours. Normally, 40 to 80 per cent is excreted, but a patient with hyperthyroidism excretes less than 40 per cent of the amount ingested. The nurse should be careful to save all the urine specimens during the test period; none should be discarded. The dose is not large enough to warrant isolation precautions for radioactivity. If the patient appears worried, you may tell him that the amount

of radiation in the tracer dose is minute and harmless.

Radioactive T_3 Erythrocyte Uptake Test. In this test the patient's blood is added to triiodothyronine that has been tagged with I[131]. The amount of protein with which the hormone is bound is measured. Generally, high values are correlated with thyrotoxicosis.

Thyroid Suppression Test. When the results of other tests show borderline elevations, the thyroid suppression test may be used. First, a baseline measurement is made of I[131] uptake by the thyroid gland. Then, fast-acting thyroid hormone is given for 7 days, and the I[131] uptake test is repeated. If the patient has hyperthyroidism, the hormone will not suppress the uptake of I[131] by the thyroid, since in hyperthyroidism the gland is autonomous. In persons with a normal thyroid, the administered hormone decreases the amount of thyroid-stimulating hormone produced by the pituitary and, therefore, decreases I[131] uptake, since the pituitary-thyroid relationship is intact.

Because an abnormally high intake of iodine may harm the validity of these tests, foods high in iodine, such as large amounts of iodized table salt, are not eaten for about a week before taking any I[131] tests. Also, medications containing iodine and thyroid extract are avoided.

Blood Cholesterol. In this diagnostic test, 5 cc. of blood are taken from the fasting patient. The normal values are 150 to 250 mg. per 100 cc. of blood. In hyperthyroidism, the patient's blood cholesterol is often lower than normal, but the results of this test vary greatly. The serum cholesterol is elevated in myxedema and can be followed during treatment of this condition.

Treatment and Nursing Care. The treatment for hyperthyroidism may be medical or surgical. The nurse has important responsibilities in both kinds of therapy.

Antithyroid Drugs. These agents block the production of thyroid hormone. Proplythiouracil, methimazole, or another drug of the thiourea group, may be given as medical treatment of hyperthyroidism or as preparation for surgery. The effects of the drug do not become evident until the excess thyroid hormone stored in the thyroid gland has been secreted into the bloodstream. This process may take several weeks. The usual daily dosage of propylthiouracil is 100 to 600 mg., although the dosage has to be individualized for each patient. The drug is excreted rapidly so that the dosage needs to be given at regular intervals during the day whether the patient is hospitalized or not. The nurse should instruct the patient to follow the physician's directions about the number of tablets to take and the intervals at which the drug should be taken. The patient who is treated without surgery usually takes the antithyroid drug for at least a year, and during that time must see his physician frequently.

Toxic effects include agranulocytosis, fever, sore throat, skin rash, enlarged lymph nodes and malaise. If any of these reactions is observed, it should be reported to the doctor, who may discontinue the drug. Periodic hematologic studies should be made to check the white blood-cell count and differential smear.

Radioactive iodine (I^{131}) may be given to a patient with thyrotoxicosis to destroy the hyperplastic thyroid tissue by radiation. Because the thyroid gland is quick to pick up iodine from the bloodstream, the radioactive iodine is taken up and stored in that gland, and for this reason it is currently believed that the usual therapeutic dose does not affect seriously any other tissues of the body. No increase in the incidence of leukemia, cancer of the thyroid or fetal abnormalities has been noted after the use of radioactive iodine in adults. However, as a precautionary measure, young patients and pregnant women usually are treated with surgery or antithyroid drugs. The dosage of radioactive iodine is based on the estimated weight of the thyroid gland, the patient's age, his clinical symptoms, and the emanations from the gland as shown on a scintillator or Geiger counter. The drug is given once, and the patient is watched for several months. If he does not have remission of his symptoms a second dose may be given, and perhaps a third. The internal irradiation allows a dose to be given without endangering the skin. There may be transient symptoms of radiation sickness (nausea, vomiting, malaise, fever), and the gland may feel tender. These reactions are rare. A more common unfortunate sequela of radioactive iodine is hypothyroidism (discussed later in this chapter). It has been reported that as many as 43 per cent of patients treated with I^{131} develop hypothyroidism when they are followed for longer than 10 years. Because this complication may not occur for many years after the administration of I^{131}, patients must remain under medical supervision for many years.

In about six to eight weeks after the initial dose of I^{131} the patient often notices the beginning of remission of his symptoms. The length of time which is required before the patient notices improvement is one of the disadvantages of this treatment. The patient should be instructed to avoid strenuous activity and to eat a nutritious diet.

I^{131} emits gamma and beta rays. Even though gamma rays penetrate tissue (beta rays travel only a few millimeters) the dose administered in the treatment of hyperthyroidism is not large enough to constitute a radiation hazard to others. The patient may be worried about this and also about the effects in his body. The nurse can supplement the physician's teaching and assure the patient that the medication is not a radiation danger.

A third antithyroid drug, Lugol's solution, contains 5 per cent iodine and 10 per cent potassium iodide in water. Iodine causes the gland to involute and become less vascular. For this reason, to decrease bleeding during surgery, patients who are scheduled for a thyroidectomy will often have a short course of iodine treatment preoperatively. For at least two weeks before surgery, 5 to 15 minims, t.i.d., of either Lugol's solution or potassium iodide are given by mouth. Dilute the drug in milk or fruit juice to prevent burning from the iodine and to make it more palatable. Drinking it through a straw will prevent staining of the teeth by the iodine. The maximum effect is expected in 10 to 14 days. Toxic effects may occur if the patient receives iodine for long periods of time, but this is unusual. These effects include symptoms of the common cold, increased salivation, skin rash, fever and, occasionally, a mumps-like syndrome with swollen salivary glands.

Surgery of the Thyroid. Subtotal thyroidectomy is an effective treatment for hyperthyroidism. About seven-eighths of the glandular tissue is removed. Total thyroidectomy may be performed if malignancy is present. Because of the effectiveness of treatment with I^{131}, surgery is more commonly performed when malignancy is suspected, in patients under 35 years of age and in pregnant women for whom the physicians are reluctant to use irradiation.

PREOPERATIVELY, the patient is given a course of antithyroid drugs, a high caloric and high vitamin diet and rest. Usually, surgery is delayed until the patient is euthyroid clinically as well as by laboratory tests. If the hyperthyroidism is not controlled before surgery, there is increased risk of postoperative thyroid crisis. The

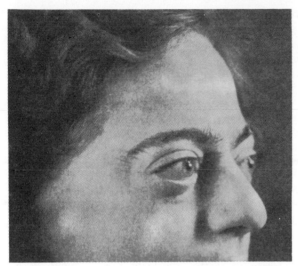

FIG. 41-2. Exophthalmos in Graves' disease. (Cecil, R. L., and Loeb, R. F. (eds.): *A Textbook of Medicine*, ed. 5, Philadelphia, Saunders)

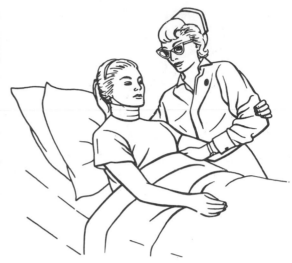

FIG. 41-3. In helping the patient to sit up after a thyroidectomy, the nurse slides one hand under the patient's head to help to support it. The patient's back and neck are supported by the nurse's arm.

patient may be prepared for surgery in his own home or in the hospital; or he may spend several days in the hospital and then go home until he is ready for surgery. The preoperative period may be as long as several months, and the suspense is especially trying for the patient, who usually feels jittery anyway because of the increased metabolic rate.

The patient should be helped by the nurse not to feel ashamed of his restlessness and irritability. The nurse can point out the temporary nature of the highly emotional state, and explain that it is related to the disease. The patient with hyperthyroidism often talks too excitedly and too much, and so the nurse should avoid garrulity. The patient's environment should be as calming as possible. The nurse may help the patient to find diversion that is both restful and enjoyable. Does he like to read? Talking quietly with the nurse may help the patient to relax and rest.

The patient's visitors should help him to rest. Suggest that visitors keep their visits short, calm and pleasant. To help the patient to sleep at night, give him a back rub and straighten the bed just before the lights go out. These measures help to relieve the feeling of warmth and irritability so common among patients with hyperthyroidism.

In preparation for surgery, the patient should be encouraged to eat as much as possible. Keep his glass full of orange juice or eggnog for snacks.

The patient is weighed daily. His blood pressure should be recorded every day. When you are taking the patient's pulse, you should watch for irregularities as well as count the rate. If the patient's heart has been affected by the thyrotoxicosis, he probably will be placed on bed rest. Helping the patient to rest during this period is a great challenge. He will need help in getting comfortable, in settling down to something that interests him and in not feeling lonely. Preoperatively, the patient may be given oxygen to help to meet his increased need for it.

POSTOPERATIVELY, the patient may be placed on his back, with small, firm pillows holding his head still, so that he does not disturb the fresh wound by thrashing. The patient needs constant observation for mucus and frequent, prompt suctioning. When he has reacted, the head of his bed may be moderately elevated. Pillows are positioned under head, neck, and shoulders, with firm support being the objective. The patient should not move his head up and down until the wound has healed considerably. When you are helping the patient to move in bed, support his head, so that it does not fall back or have any strain placed on the neck muscles. When the patient is alone, put his beverage, tissues and whatever else he might need on the overbed table in front of him, so that he does not have to reach over to the stand.

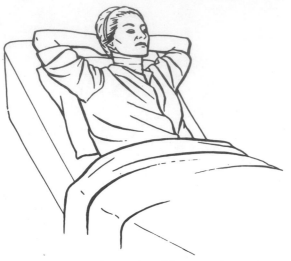

Fig. 41-4. After a thyroidectomy the patient uses her hands to support her head while she raises herself to a sitting position. This support helps to avoid strain on the neck muscles.

The patient usually is allowed out of bed the day after the operation. His head should be well supported while he gets into position to dangle his feet. He should hold his head still with his hands while he walks a step or two, and it should be supported with firm pillows while he sits up in a chair. His attempt to hold his head still may cause a headache that can be relieved by rubbing the back of the neck.

Immediately after surgery watch for symptoms of respiratory obstruction. Edema or bleeding can compress the trachea, causing an inability to breathe. This catastrophe must be treated within minutes by the insertion of an endotracheal tube or by a tracheostomy. A sterile tracheostomy set is kept in the patient's room, ready for immediate use if needed. The patient may be in an oxygen tent during the early postoperative days.

Aspiration is a danger, since there will be depression of laryngeal and tracheal reflexes. Suction as necessary. When swallowing and coughing reflexes have returned, encourage the patent to cough and breathe deeply every two hours the first day. The patient will have pain in the operative site and may be able to cough and to sip fluids better after he has received medication for pain. If he is given morphine, carefully check his respirations, for morphine is a respiratory depressant.

Watch for bleeding. A small amount of blood in the wound can obstruct respirations. Pay attention if the patient complains of a sense of fullness in the wound. Blood may not be evident on the front of the bandage, but it may ooze around to the back of the patient's neck. Periodically during the first postoperative 12 hours, pass your hand behind the patient's neck to see whether it feels damp. When you turn the patient to his side, look for blood on the dressing. If the bandage encircling the neck becomes too tight, loosen but do not remove it, and call the surgeon. Observe for restlessness, apprehension, respiratory distress, an increased pulse or temperature, decreased blood pressure, and cyanosis. Neck swelling may be due to bleeding and accumulation of blood in the wound, distending the tissues.

Infrequently, the recurrent laryngeal nerve is injured during the operation. The patient is hoarse or may be unable to speak due to vocal cord paralysis. Respiratory obstruction may result. Report hoarseness or any voice change to the physician. Encourage the patient not to talk much the first two postoperative days. Steam inhalations may be ordered.

Another infrequent postoperative complication is tetany (muscular hypertonia with spasm and tremor), due to a low concentration of calcium from the inadvertent removal of the parathyroid glands during the thyroidectomy. The patient complains of numbness and tingling of the extremities and muscle cramps. Tetany also can cause laryngeal spasm. The treatment is intravenous or oral calcium.

Thyroid crisis or storm, now a rare complication of thyroid surgery, may occur within the first 12 hours postoperatively. All the symptoms of hyperthyroidism are exaggerated. The patient's temperature may be as high as 106, the pulse becomes very rapid, and cardiac arrhythmias are common. There may be persistent vomiting and extreme restlessness with delirium. The patient becomes exhausted, and not infrequently dies from cardiac failure. The treatment is intravenous sodium iodide, intravenous corticosteroids, oxygen, reserpine to slow the heart rate and cooling by the application of ice, cool enemas or a controlled thermoblanket. Morphine (or other sedation), Lugol's solution, propylthiouracil, and corticosteroids also may be ordered.

Since the incision for a thyroidectomy is made in a crease of the neck, the healed scar is barely visible; it is merely a thin line. If a woman patient seems concerned about it, you may suggest that she wear high-necked dresses and scarves until the scar contracts to its final tiny size. With the surgeon's approval, periodic massage of the operative scar during the first few postoperative weeks may help to obtain a good cosmetic result.

Nontoxic Goiter

The word *goiter* refers to an enlargement of the thyroid gland. Simple goiter is an enlargement without the symptoms of thyrotoxicosis. The enlargement may be caused by a deficiency of iodine in the diet, or by the inability of the thyroid to utilize iodine, or by relative iodine lack owing to increasing body demands for thyroid hormones. Iodine is essential to the production of thyroid hormones. As the gland tries to meet the body's need for thyroid hormones in spite of the relative or absolute deficiency of iodine available to it, it enlarges and becomes more vascular.

The condition occurs in areas where the soil and the drinking water are deficient in iodine, such as portions of the Alps, the Himalayas and other mountain regions. In the United States, endemic goiter areas are the Great Lakes area, Minnesota, Ohio and the Pacific Northwest.

Nontoxic goiter is more frequent in women than in men. It appears (sometimes only temporarily) when there is an increase in the need for thyroid hormone and thus for the iodine to make it—at times of stress, during infection, in adolescence and in pregnancy. In some areas of the world, a large percentage of adolescent girls have nontoxic goiters.

Symptoms. The thyroid gland gradually grows larger. There may be a sense of fullness in the throat. Eventually, the hypertrophy can cause difficulty in swallowing and breathing if the thyroid begins to press on the trachea; otherwise, the general health of the person is usually not affected.

Treatment and Prevention. Oral administration of iodide may reduce the goiter if deficiency is present and treatment is started before irreversible cellular changes have occurred in the thyroid tissue. Many months of treatment may be required. Thyroid hormone may be given instead of iodide. If there is pressure on the trachea or considerable disfigurement, the goiter can be removed surgically.

The body needs very little iodine to satisfy the requirements of the thyroid gland. For the normal adult, 25 to 50 mg. of inorganic iodine a year is sufficient. In this country to prevent iodine-deficient goiters, state boards of health have asked salt manufacturers to add iodine to common table salt—about 0.01 per cent of potassium iodide. Most grocery stores carry iodized table salt, and as a result iodine deficiency goiters are less common than they used to be.

Thyroid Cancer

Thyroid cancer is suspected when there is an enlarged lump which is hard to the touch, invasion of other local structures and when the area of the thyroid containing the lump does not concentrate I^{131} as well as the surrounding normal thyroid tissue. Biopsy may be performed by an incision made in order to obtain the specimen of tissue (open biopsy); or by inserting a needle through which is withdrawn a small amount of tissue (closed biopsy). Most physicians object to the closed procedure, since the needle may miss the cancer; and if it contacts the tumor, it may spread it.

If the tumor is accessible the treatment is surgical and most often radical (total thyroidectomy with removal of the local lymph glands in the neck). However, considerable difference of opinion exists concerning the surgical treatment of carcinoma of the thyroid. Some surgeons advocate total thyroidectomy with radical neck dissection; others advocate the less extensive procedure of thyroid lobectomy.

After the operation thyroid replacement therapy is given in order to replace those hormones that can no longer be produced due to the absence of the thyroid gland, and to suppress pituitary TSH so that it will not stimulate the growth of any residual malignant thyroid tissue.

If there is an inaccessible thyroid cancer, either local or metastatic, which can take up iodine, radioactive iodine may be given. The malignancy will take it up and be destroyed. This effect can be enhanced by administering TSH, because it stimulates increased uptake of the radioactive iodine by the thyroid.

The cure rate of thyroid cancer depends on the type of tumor present. Papillary carcinoma does not grow rapidly, whereas undifferentiated cancer grows more rapidly and is more difficult to control. Since most thyroid cancers are papillary carcinomas, the physician often can convey a certain sense of optimism to the patient.

Hypothyroidism

This disease is due to a deficiency of thyroid hormones, causing a lowered rate of all metabolic processes. It results in a set of symptoms called *myxedema* in the adult. The condition may originate within the thyroid (primary hypothyroidism) or within the pituitary, manifested by TSH lack (secondary hypothyroidism).

Diagnosis. In the TSH-stimulation test there in no increase in I^{131} uptake after the administration of TSH when hypothyroidism is due to primary failure of the gland to function properly. If the hypothyroidism is secondary to pituitary insufficiency and lack of TSH, then administered TSH will increase the I^{131} uptake. An x-ray film of the skull may be taken to examine the pituitary fossa for abnormalities, such as those that may be caused by a tumor. The results of BMR, PBI and I^{131} uptake tests are low, and cholesterol is elevated.

A problem in the early recognition of hypothyroidism is that many of the symptoms are nonspecific, and may not be sufficiently dramatic to bring the patient to the doctor. This condition can go untreated for years. The nurse who notices such symptoms as puffiness of the face, chronic fatigue or intolerance to cold should suggest a visit to the doctor.

Etiology. Atrophy of the thyroid gland may occur after pneumonia, typhoid fever and influenza. Thyroid inflammation and surgery or irradiation for hyperthyroidism also can cause hypothyroidism. Or, the deficiency may be due to an auto-immune process, in which the patient develops antibodies against his own thyroid tissue. Very often the cause is unknown. Women are affected more often than men.

Symptoms. The symptoms of hypothyroidism are opposite in many respects to those of hyperthyroidism. The metabolic rate and both the physical and the mental activity of the patient are slowed. The hypothyroid patient feels lethargic and lacking in energy, dozes frequently during the day, is forgetful and has chronic headaches. The face takes on a masklike, stolid, unemotional expression, yet the patient often is irritable. The tongue may be enlarged, the lips may be swollen, and there is nonpitting edema of the eyelids. The temperature and the pulse are decreased, and there is intolerance to cold. The patient gains weight easily. His skin is dry, and his hair characteristically is coarse and sparse, tending to fall out. A woman patient frequently has a menstrual disorder. Constipation may be severe enough to require daily enemas. The voice of the myxedema patient is low-pitched, slow and hoarse. His hearing may be impaired. There may be numbness or tingling in the arms or legs, unrelieved by change of position. Hypothyroidism may lead to enlargement of the heart due to pericardial effusion and an increased tendency toward atherosclerosis and heart strain. Anemia also may result.

Treatment and Nursing Care. Because his metabolic processes are depressed, the patient may feel chilled in a room that is comfortable for others. In a ward his bed should not be placed next to a window, and he may need extra blankets or a robe while he is in bed. Even though his appetite is poor, he has a tendency to gain weight. The diet is usually low calorie and may be high in roughage and protein. Check daily as to whether or not he has had a bowel movement. Too many days without one may lead to an impaction. Until medication causes the patient's rough skin to soften, apply lotion or cream, especially on the back, the elbows and the feet.

Patients with hypothyroidism are inordinately susceptible to sedative and hypnotic drugs. If any such are ordered (a rare circumstance), watch the patient carefully for narcosis and diminished respirations. The patient may develop respiratory failure. Never ignore the patient just because he is sleeping quietly. Observe him frequently, and count the respirations.

Hypothyroidism is treated by replacement therapy. The patient is supplied with thyroid hormone in the form of desiccated thyroid extract or with synthetic products, such as crystalline thyroxin or triiodothyronine. Thyroid extract is very slow to act; and the dose, given by mouth, can be taken once a day. Patients may be started on 15 mg. of thyroid extract and maintained on the dose found most appropriate. The side-effects of replacement therapy may include dyspnea, rapid pulse, palpitations, precordial pain, hyperactivity, insomnia, dizziness and gastrointestinal disorders. Occasionally, a skin rash may be seen.

Before treatment has become effective, the patient's movement may be so slow that one is reminded of a slow-motion movie. If you ask a patient with severe hypothyroidism to turn over for back care, there may be a considerable interval before he responds. His thought processes are slow. His motion is lethargic. It is important to let these patients do things for themselves and to resist the temptation to do for them, just to get it over with. Do not expect these patients to move quickly, because they are incapable of doing so.

Once the replacement therapy has begun, a dramatic change in the patient's symptoms may be seen in a few weeks. He feels the return of a new interest in life. His hair again becomes soft and attractive, and he can stay awake for 16 hours in one stretch. His mental and physical activities are quickened.

Because these changes in his condition may be rapid and profound, the patient may be hospitalized during the early days of treatment. The nurse has an important responsibility to observe carefully for changes in the symptoms. If the patient's heart or blood vessels have been affected by the hypothyroidism, the sudden improvement in his metabolic rate may impose an additional strain on the cardiovascular system. For instance, if the coronary arteries are sclerotic, they may not be able to supply the heart with sufficient blood for its sudden increase in activity. The nurse should be alert to complaints of precordial pain, dyspnea, and changes in the pulse rate. Report any complaints that may indicate cardiac involvement to the doctor.

These patients usually have to take thyroid extract for the remainder of their lives. A patient who is treated early and is well regulated should continue to feel well. However, periodic visits to the doctor are necessary to ensure continuing the proper dosage. The nurse should emphasize to the patient the importance of keeping his appointments.

THE PARATHYROID GLANDS

The parathyroid glands are tiny bodies, shaped like beans, imbedded on either side of the posterior aspect of the thyroid, or sometimes in the chest. The parathyroid glands are usually four in number, although there may be more. The upper parathyroid is usually found posteriorly, at the junction of the upper and middle third of the thyroid. The lower parathyroids are more variable in location, but usually lie among the branches of the inferior thyroid artery. They may be found in the chest, however. They secrete the parathyroid hormone, which regulates the concentration of calcium and phosphorus in the blood and influences the passage of calcium and phosphorus between bloodstream, bones and urine.

Hyperparathyroidism

Pathology and Symptoms. In hyperparathyroidism, an overproduction of parathyroid hormone results in increased urinary excretion of phosphorus and loss of calcium from the bones. The bones become demineralized as the calcium leaves them and enters the bloodstream. The excess serum calcium that has been taken from the tissues is lost in the urine. The large amounts of calcium and phosphorus passing through the kidneys may lead to stones, pyelonephritis and uremia; thus, renal disease is a serious outcome. The amount of serum phosphorus is decreased. The shift of calcium to the blood from the tissues leads to a chain of events that includes muscle weakness, fatigue, apathy, nausea and vomiting, constipation and cardiac arrhythmias. Excessive blood calcium depresses the responsiveness of the peripheral nerves, accounting for the fatigue and the muscle weakness. The muscles become hypotonic, and this hypotonia is the basis for constipation. Metastatic calcifications can occur, due to the excess of calcium in the bloodstream. Because the bones have lost calcium, there is skeletal tenderness and pain on bearing weight; the bones may become so demineralized that they break with little or no trauma (pathologic fractures).

Diagnosis. The diagnosis is made on the basis of an elevated serum calcium and a low serum phosphorus in the absence of other causes of hypercalcemia. A three-day low calcium diet may be given; and the amount of calcium excreted in the urine may be measured to help to establish the diagnosis and to determine the severity of the disease.

Treatment and Nursing Care. The treatment of hyperparathyroidism is the surgical removal of hypertrophied gland tissue or of an individual tumor. Postoperative nursing care includes observation of the patient for the symptoms of hypoparathyroidism, especially for tetany. Intravenous 10 per cent calcium lactate should be kept at the bedside for the first few postoperative days in case the patient does develop tetany. Usually, it is given in an infusion of normal saline. Until the phosphorus-calcium balance is restored, the patient may be prone to pathologic fractures, and it is important to keep this in mind when administering nursing care.

Hypoparathyroidism

Pathology and Symptoms. The underproduction of parathyroid hormone causes a decrease in calcium and an increase of phosphorus in the blood, with a decrease of both in the urine. The main symptom of hypoparathyroidism is tetany. The patient may feel numbness and tingling in his fingers or his toes or about his lips. A voluntary movement may be followed by an involuntary, jerking spasm. Tonic (continuous contraction) flexion of an arm or a finger may occur. If the facial nerve is tapped lateral to the eye, the patient's mouth twitches. A spasm may occur in the larynx, causing the patient to become dyspneic, with long, crowing respirations as he tries to get air past the constriction. He may become cyanotic and in danger of asphyxia. He may have generalized convulsions or gastric distress. His nails become brittle and break easily. His skin is coarse and dry and his hair is patchy and thin.

Diagnosis. The diagnosis is made on the basis of a low serum calcium and an elevated serum phosphorus in the absence of other causes of hypocalcemia.

Treatment and Nursing Care. The treatment for hypoparathyroidism includes the administration of a vitamin D-like preparation, dihydrotachysterol (also known as A.T. 10 or Hytakerol), or vitamin D_2 (calciferol). These drugs increase the blood level of calcium. The dosage is related to the degree of hypocalcemia, which is determined by frequent measurements of the blood calcium. The urine calcium levels also may be checked.

The treatment of hypoparathyroid tetany also includes the administration of calcium salts, and occasionally parathyroid extract. Calicum gluconate may be given first intravenously, 10 to 50 ml. of a 10 per cent solution in 1,000 ml. of normal saline. Intravenous calcium causes vasodilation; the patient feels hot and nauseated. Calcium is never given intramuscularly, since it causes tissue sloughing. When you are nursing a patient receiving calcium intravenously, be doubly careful that the needle does not slip out of the vein, spilling the solution into the tissues. If the infusion does infiltrate, stop it at once.

Because the correct doses of these drugs may be difficult for the physician to estimate, the nurse should observe the patient frequently for hypercalcemia, which may occur with the administration of any of these preparations. Vomiting, usually one of the earliest symptoms, should be reported immediately to the doctor. It may be followed by high fever, listlessness and coma.

THE ADRENAL GLANDS

Addison's Disease (Adrenal Cortex Hypofunction)

Etiology. Addison's disease can result from destruction of adrenal cortical tissue by tuberculosis or by idiopathic atrophy of the adrenal cortical tissue. It is suspected that excessive stress (overwhelming infection, surgery, or prolonged drain of the body's emergency resources) plays some role in causing insufficient steroids to be secreted. Cancer may invade the adrenal cortex. The disease can result also from the long-term use of large doses of steroids that cause adrenal atrophy by suppressing ACTH. Of course, bilateral adrenalectomy causes a deficiency of the steroids secreted by the adrenal glands. Addison's disease is comparatively rare.

Pathology and Symptoms. Certain corticosteroids regulate absorption, distribution and excretion of body salts and water; a decrease in these hormones leads to increased urinary excretion of sodium and retention of potassium. Dehydration, with reduction of blood plasma volume, results. The patient feels weak and easily tires. His blood pressure, B.M.R. and temperature are low. Because he develops hypotension from sudden changes of position, such as from lying down or sitting up too quickly, he may faint. He is prone to vascular collapse due to poor myocardial tonus, decreased cardiac output and lowered blood pressure. He loses weight, is anemic and may become cachectic. His appetite is poor, and he may suffer from a variety of gastrointestinal symptoms. He feels nervous and has periods of depression. Patients with Addison's disease have an abnormally dark pigmentation, especially of exposed areas of the skin and the mucous membrane, and a decrease in hair growth. Because the patient's body is deficient in those hormones that facilitate the conversion of protein into glucose, he suffers episodes of hypoglycemia. He may develop hypoglycemia five to six hours after eating; the early morning before breakfast is an especially dangerous time. The symptoms of hypoglycemia are hunger, headache, sweating, weakness, trembling, emotional instability, visual disturbances and, finally, disorientation, coma and convulsions.

Acute Adrenocortical Crisis. Because the hormones of the cortex of the adrenal glands are prominent in effecting the body's adaptive reactions to stress, patients with Addison's disease collapse when they are faced with excess stress. Even uncomplicated surgery, such as an appendectomy, requires more physiologic adaptive ability than a patient with Addison's disease usually possesses. Unless he is given steroids, he will experience acute adrenal crisis, which is a severe flare-up of Addison's disease. His blood pressure becomes markedly depressed, perhaps so low as to be unobtainable. The patient is in *adrenal shock,* which is primarily due to lack of hormones.

Addison's crisis is an emergency; death may occur from hypotension and vasomotor collapse. Adrenocortical hormones are given intravenously in solutions of normal saline and glucose. Antibiotics may be ordered because of the patient's extremely low resistance to infection. Vital signs are taken frequently. The patient may have a fever and complain of headache. Morphine and insulin are contraindicated. Keep the patient warm and as quiet as possible. He should not be permitted to do anything for himself until the emergency is over. Corticosteroids and fluids are also important aspects of therapy.

As a precaution in case of acute adrenal crisis, keep two 50 ml. syringes, intravenous hydrocortisone and bottles of 5 per cent dextrose in saline solution at the bedside of all patients with Addison's disease who are not well regulated. If the patient has a weak, rapid pulse, falling blood pressure and cold, cyanotic extremities, lower his head and call the doctor. Salt deprivation, infection, trauma, exposure to cold, overexertion—any abnormal stress—can cause adrenal crisis. The crisis may start with anorexia, nausea, vomiting, diarrhea, abdominal pain, headache, intensification of hypotension, restlessness or a high temperature. Watch for any of these symptoms in all your patients with Addison's disease.

Diagnostic Tests. The pituitary gland secretes ACTH (adrenocorticotropic hormone), which stimulates the adrenal cortex to secrete its own hormones. The most frequently used test for Addison's disease is the determination of the adrenal cortical response to ACTH. The excretion of adrenal cortical hormones is measured after the administration of ACTH in an intravenous solution. Normal persons have an increased excretion of 17-hydroxycorticoids and 17-ketosteroids, whereas patients with Addison's disease show little or no increase. Also, eosinophils in the patient's blood are measured. Normally, a drop of 60 per cent to 90 per cent in the eosinophil count occurs after the ACTH is given, but there is less change in Addison's disease.

Laboratory tests in Addison's disease show a low blood sodium and a high potassium; the B.M.R. is minus 10 to minus 20. A glucose tolerance test (see Chap. 42) may be done. In Addison's disease the glucose in the bloodstream does not rise as high as normal, and it returns to its fasting level more quickly than it would under normal conditions.

Treatment and Nursing Care. Addison's disease is treated by replacement of the missing hormones. Cortisone, 12.5 mg., may be given two or three times a day. Hydrocortisone, 20 to 30 mg. a day, is sometimes prescribed.

Desoxycorticosterone acetate (DCA), 2.5 to 8 mg. by mouth, or 25 mg. every three to four weeks intramuscularly, or fludrocortisone (Florinef), 0.1 mg. daily or every other day, may be given to help to restore normal electrolyte and water balance. The toxic symptoms of an overdose of these drugs include edema, headache, hypertension, and muscle weakness due to potassium depletion. Methyltestosterone, 5 to 10 mg. a day, may be administered orally. The patient may complain of gastric distress, which may be relieved by giving the orally administered hormones during meals. Unless orders to the contrary are given, the last dose of cortisone should be given no later than 4 P.M., since these hormones may make sleep difficult. *Be especially careful that no patient with Addison's disease receives insulin by error; he may die from hypoglycemia.* He is also extremely sensitive to opiates and barbiturates. The dosage of the hormones may be stabilized during the patient's stay in the hospital and continued on a maintenance basis after he is discharged.

It is imperative that the patient take the hormones as prescribed, and that he see his physician regularly. If the patient does not have active tuberculosis, and if he follows his prescribed drug regimen carefully, the outlook for his wellbeing is good (a prognosis that could not have been made before the availability of these hormones as drugs). As in diabetes, the patient's understanding of his condition can mean the difference between disability and an active life. The patient himself must be aware of his body's inability to handle stress of any sort and of the importance of seeking medical attention for the readjustment of dosage whenever he is threatened by stress of any kind: an infection, a car accident (even if he is not noticeably hurt), exposure to cold, an insoluble family crisis or an excessive work load.

Part of the nurse's responsibility to the Addisonian patient is to teach him and his family about the disease, how to protect his health by avoiding stressful situations when it is possible, and to obtain medical adjustment of his drugs when this is indicated. The patient with Addison's disease should not be made to feel that his condition should keep him out of the mainstream of everyday life.

The patient should carry a card stating that he is suffering from adrenal cortical insufficiency. The card should contain such a statement as ". . . Addison's disease. In the event of illness call Dr. (name and telephone number). Give 25 mg. of cortisone every six hours by mouth. If unconscious, give 100 mg. of hydrocortisone intravenously." (Of course, the drugs and the dosages are ordered by the doctor.) Make sure that the patient is given a card to carry before he is discharged from the hospital.

Because of the recurrent hypoglycemia, the patient may do better on five or six small meals than on three big ones. If sodium chloride pills are ordered, they may be tolerated best if they are taken with meals. The salt intake may need to be increased even more during hot weather. Instruct the patient to add extra salt to his food if he has perspired more than usual.

When hypoglycemia occurs, it is treated by giving glucose, orally or intravenously. To prevent recurring episodes of hypoglycemia, between-meal snacks of milk and crackers are preferable to candy and other rapidly absorbed sugars. If the patient's meal is delayed because of diagnostic tests, keep the fasting period to a minimum, and during the fast, limit his activities; keep him in bed and quiet. If he has to leave the ward, have him taken on a stretcher or in a wheelchair.

Because of hypotension and muscle weakness, a patient with this condition is subject to falling. Protect him with side rails unless he is well regulated and well taught. Emphasize the importance of getting out of bed slowly. If he is dizzy on sitting up, he should lie down again. Take his blood pressure if the patient shows any symptoms, such as weakness or faintness, which would lead you to believe that his blood pressure is lower than usual. A change from the previous readings is more important than any one reading.

Cushing's Syndrome
(Adrenal Cortex Hyperfunction)

This condition is the opposite of Addison's disease. An overproduction of adrenal cortical hormones may result (1) from overstimulation by the pituitary gland, with resultant hyperplasia of the adrenal cortex (approximately 70% of patients) (Glenn and Mannix), and (2) from benign or malignant tumors of the adrenal cortex (approximately 30% of patients) (Glenn and Mannix). In a very few patients, Cushing's syndrome is caused by extra-adrenal carcinoma, which produces an ACTH-like substance that causes adrenal hyperfunction and hyperplasia. In Cushing's syndrome, extensive protein depletion occurs, leading to muscle wasting and weakness. Carbohydrate tolerance is lowered, and diabetes may result. There is a redistribution of fat, leading eventually to the typical moonface and buffalo hump that are seen in patients who have had long-term corticosteroid therapy, which can lead to the symptoms of Cushing's syndrome. The skin is thin, and the face is ruddy. The patient becomes progressively weaker, and the symptoms of infection are masked—perhaps most dangerously. Therefore, the nurse should be especially alert for minor signs, a slight sore throat or a small rise in temperature that may indicate the presence of a more severe infectious process. The blood vessels are extremely fragile, the patient bruises easily, and striae may form over extensive skin areas. The bones become so demineralized that the patient may have backache, kyphosis and collapse of the vertebral bodies. Sodium and water are retained; the patient suffers peripheral edema and hypertension. In women, Cushing's syndrome usually produces masculinization with hirsutism and amenorrhea.

Diagnosis. The urine may be examined for 17-hydroxycorticoids (17-OH) and 17-ketosteroids. The former are almost always increased, and the latter are increased or decreased, depending on the nature of the lesion. As is done in the diagnosis of hypofunction, ACTH may be given intravenously and the 17-hydroxycorticoid excretion measured. Patients with bilateral adrenal cortex hyperplasia have a marked urinary increase in both 17-hydroxycorticoids and 17-ketosteroids, while patients with carcinoma of the adrenal cortex may show no such increase. Twenty-four hour urines may be collected for the measurement of urinary hydrocortisone and its major metabolites. Sometimes fractional urines are ordered because normally there is an increase in the excretion of hydrocortisone and its metabolites during the early morning, but this diurnal variation is not seen in Cushing's disease.

Another test is the urinary 17-hydroxycorticoid suppression test, in which a steroid such as dexamethasone is given to suppress ACTH from the pituitary. If, on a low dosage, urinary 17-hydroxycorticoid is not suppressed, the patient probably has hyperplasia of the adrenal cortex. If, on a high dosage of dexamethasone, there is no suppression of urinary 17-hydroxycorticoids, the patient probably has a carcinoma or an adenoma of the adrenal cortex. Hyperplasia and carcinoma may be differentiated also by giving a pituitary stimulant such as Metopirone. Normally and in hyperplasia, 17-hydroxycorticoid in the urine is increased when Metopirone is given, but this is not seen in carcinoma.

Occasionally, an abdominal x-ray film may show an adrenal mass, and an intravenous pyelogram may show changes in the renal shadow caused by an abnormally large adrenal gland.

Treatment and Nursing Care. The treatment depends on whether the disease is due to tumor or to hyperplasia, and on the views of the physician. X-ray therapy to the pituitary may be used if there is hyperplasia. An adrenalectomy may be preferred; the operation may be total or subtotal, unilateral or bilateral. If an adrenalectomy is to be done, adrenal cortical hormone therapy may be started preoperatively in anticipation of the time when the body will be unable to produce its own hormones. However, considerable difference of medical opinion exists concerning the advisability of administering adrenal cortical steroids preoperatively when an adrenalectomy is to be performed. Testosterone propionate, 25 mg. I.M. per day, may be given to help to correct protein depletion; and potassium chloride, 6.0 Gm. by mouth per day, may be given to counteract the effects of decreased blood potassium (hypokalemia).

After the operation the patient is treated as if he had Addison's disease—which, indeed, he now has. A postadrenalectomy syndrome of nausea, vomiting, diarrhea, muscle tenderness and aching should be called to the doctor's attention. Hypotension may be a problem, and the nurse should watch for signs of it. Also, she should observe for such complications as hemorrhage, atelectasis and pneumothorax, since the adrenals are located close to the diaphragm and the in-

ferior vena cava. Patients who have had a unilateral tumor may now have an atrophy of the cortex of the unaffected adrenal gland, and probably they will be given adrenal cortical hormones in slowly decreasing amounts until they produce enough of their own.

Because the adrenal glands and the body water and electrolyte regulation are closely related, both preoperatively and postoperatively, the nurse should keep careful records of fluid intake and urinary output. Preoperatively, the patient is often placed on a low-sodium, high-potassium diet. Because depression is common in Cushing's syndrome, the nurse must be alert for changes in mood and for any suicidal tendencies. The patient needs protection from upsetting situations.

Hyperaldosteronism

Aldosterone is one of the hormones secreted by the adrenal cortex. Primary hyperaldosteronism is a rare disease in which this hormone is produced in excess, resulting in hypertension and renal loss of potassium. The hypokalemia causes muscle weakness, which may progress to paralysis and polyuria. The disease can be caused by carcinoma, adenoma or hyperplasia of the adrenal cortex. Hyperaldosteronism characteristically occurs in early middle life.

The treatment is removal of the adrenal tumor. Preoperative preparation includes potassium replacement for five to seven days and restriction of sodium intake. Postoperatively, intake and output are measured and the patient observed for any signs of urinary dysfunction.

Pheochromocytoma

This term means a tumor, usually of the adrenal medulla, which causes increased secretion of epinephrine and norepinephrine. The symptoms are hypertension (intermittent or, more frequently, persistent), tremor, nervousness, sweating, headache, nausea and vomiting, hyperglycemia, polyuria (increased urination) and vertigo. A diagnostic test for pheochromocytoma is the Regitine (phentolamine) test. Regitine is a drug which neutralizes epinephrine. If the administration of Regitine results in a drop of blood pressure the physician is led to suspect pheochromocytoma. Another diagnostic measure involves measuring the urinary excretion of catecholamines and their breakdown products; this diagnostic measure is both reliable and safe.

The treatment is the surgical removal of the tumor. The operation has been dangerous, especially in the past, because of the wide fluctuation of blood pressure that may occur during and after surgery, due to a sudden liberation or an abrupt stoppage of epinephrine or norepinephrine. Surgery is less dangerous now than in the past, because it is now possible to control the fluctuations of blood pressure preoperatively and during surgery by the use of phenoxybenzamine (Dibenzyline) and phentolamine (Regitine).

THE PITUITARY GLAND (HYPOPHYSIS)

Although the pituitary gland weighs only about 600 mg., it is a key organ. No system or structure of the body is exempt from its influence. There are two secretory parts of the pituitary, the anterior and the posterior lobes. At least nine hormones are secreted by the pituitary gland, only a few of which will be discussed here. Hyperfunction and hypofunction of the gland may be manifested in many ways, depending on which glandular cells of the organ are involved.

The Anterior Lobe

Acromegaly. Hyperplasia or tumors of the anterior pituitary can cause overproduction of the growth hormone (somatropin). When there is excess of this hormone in a youngster before the ends of the long bones are fully united (epiphyseal union), gigantism results. Overproduction of somatropin during adulthood brings about a condition called *acromegaly*, in which the overgrowth of many tissues, including the skeleton, results in a characteristic appearance of coarse features, a huge lower jaw, thick lips, bulging forehead, bulbous nose, and large hands and feet. Headache resulting from pressure on the sella turcica, when the overgrowth is due to a tumor, is common. The patients may become partially blind from pressure on the optic nerve. Women have increased facial hair and deepened voices. Heart, liver and spleen may enlarge. In spite of the patient's enlarged tissues, muscle weakness is a symptom. The joints are hypertrophied and may become painful and stiff. Men often become impotent, and women may have amenorrhea.

Acromegaly is sometimes treated surgically and sometimes by radiation. The tendency now is to treat these patients surgically. Unfortunately, the growth changes due to acromegaly are irreversible, even if the disease is arrested successfully.

Simmonds' Disease. Simmonds' disease or panhypopituitarism, a rare disorder, results from the destruction of the pituitary gland by postpartum emboli, surgery, tumor or tuberculosis. There is a gradual atrophy of the gonads and the genitalia. Because of the impairment of pituitary stimulus, thyroid and adrenals fail to secrete adequate amounts of their hormones. The patient ages prematurely and may become extremely cachectic.

Tumors that threaten pituitary tissue may be irradiated. Surgery is difficult and dangerous because of the location of the gland. Medical treatment includes the administration of substitute hormones of the glands dependent on the pituitary for stimulation.

The Posterior Lobe

Diabetes Insipidus. The hormone vasopressin, also called antidiuretic hormone (ADH), regulates the reabsorption of water in the kidney tubules. In this rare disease there is a reduction in the secretion of ADH, leading to an outpouring of water through the kidneys. The urine is so copious that the patient does not have an unbroken night's sleep. From 15 to 20 liters of urine may be passed in a 24-hour period. The urine is very dilute with a specific gravity of 1.012 or less. The excretion of urine cannot be controlled by limiting the intake of fluids. Thirst is excessive and constant. The need for drinking and emptying the bladder embarrasses the patient and limits his social and work activities; he can never be too far from a bathroom. The patient is weak and anorectic, and he loses weight.

The treatment is the administration of posterior pituitary extract (pituitrin) subcutaneously or by inhalation. The objective is to reduce the patient's urine output to two to three liters during 24 hours.

REFERENCES AND BIBLIOGRAPHY

BEESON, P. B., and McDERMOTT, W. (eds.): *Cecil-Loeb Textbook of Medicine,* ed. 13, Philadelphia, Saunders, 1971.

GREENBLATT, R. B., and METTS, J. C., JR.: Addison's disease, *Am. J. Nurs.* 60:1249–1252, September, 1960.

NORDYKE, R. A.: The overactive and the underactive thyroid, *Am. J. Nurs.* 63:66, May, 1963.

REICH, B. H., and AULT, L. P.: Nursing care of the patient with Addison's disease, *Am. J. Nurs.* 60:1252–1255, September, 1960.

RODMAN, M., and SMITH, D. W.: *Pharmacology and Drug Therapy in Nursing,* Philadelphia, Lippincott, 1968.

WILLIAMS, R. H. (ed.): *Textbook of Endocrinology,* ed. 4, Philadelphia, Saunders, 1968.

The Patient with Diabetes Mellitus

42

Incidence · Etiology · Pathology and Symptoms · Diabetic
Ketosis and Coma · Treatment · Complications · Prognosis
Social Aspects

Diabetes mellitus is a metabolic disease in which there is some degree of insulin insufficiency, resulting in an impairment of the body's ability to metabolize carbohydrate and also fat and protein. Because of the lack of insulin or inadequate insulin action, abnormal amounts of sugar accumulate in the bloodstream and subsequently are excreted in the patient's urine. As the condition worsens, excessive ketone bodies are found in the blood and the urine. Every cell in the body is affected by the metabolic derangement.

INCIDENCE

Almost everyone knows someone with this very common chronic disease. There are approximately 2,000,000 known diabetics in the United States (Public Health Service Publication #1000). No age group is exempt, but diabetes is most frequent between the ages of 40 and 60. The incidence is rising, probably partly because the case-finding methods are better, and because people are living longer and have time to develop diabetes.

The incidence varies among ethnic groups. For example, Jews have a high rate; the incidence curve for Negroes is rising faster than that for whites at the present time; Chinese and Japanese have a lower incidence, and usually they have a milder form of the disease. Among known diabetics, women outnumber men by about one-third. It has been estimated that there are 1,600,000 unknown diabetics in the United States (Public Health Service Publication #1000).

ETIOLOGY

Diabetes is believed to be inherited as a Mendelian recessive characteristic. The disease does not necessarily manifest itself early in life, but (according to this theory) if both parents have diabetes, all of their children will become diabetic if they live long enough. If one parent has diabetes, and the other parent is a carrier of the gene, the chance of their children's developing diabetes is 50 per cent. If both parents are carriers, the chance of their children's developing the disease is 25 per cent. Occasionally, diabetes occurs in persons with no known family history of the disease. The role of genetics in the causation of diabetes is under study and is by no means fully understood (Entmacher and Marks). Obesity may contribute to the development of diabetes in a susceptible person.

PATHOLOGY AND SYMPTOMS

A normal person has a fasting level of 80 to 120 mg. of glucose in each 100 ml. of venous blood analyzed by the Folin-Wu method. Within half an hour after he has eaten, some of the carbohydrate that he has ingested is digested and absorbed into the blood. The blood glucose rises to about 150 mg. per 100 ml. Two hours after eating, the blood glucose has returned to its fasting level. In liver and in muscle, glucose is converted to glycogen and stored. As the body needs fuel, the liver changes glycogen back to glucose and passes it out to the bloodstream, where it becomes available to muscle and other body tissues as fuel for energy. Insulin is an important link in this process; it promotes the storage of glycogen in the liver, it aids in the utilization of glucose by the tissues, and it influences the metabolism of fats and proteins.

Insulin is secreted into the bloodstream by the beta cells of the islets of Langerhans in the pancreas. Diabetics have less insulin available than their metabolic processes require, or, according to some theories, the insulin they produce cannot be utilized effectively. Because they have inadequate insulin activity, the ability of the liver to convert glucose to glycogen is impaired, and the use of glucose by the tissues is impaired.

In diabetes the fasting blood-glucose content may be normal or elevated, but after eating it may rise to high levels (exceeding 150 mg. per 100 ml. of blood or more).

The condition of excess glucose in the blood is called *hyperglycemia*. With so much additional glucose in the blood, some of it is excreted by the kidneys. Glucose usually is found in the urine when it rises over 180 mg. per 100 ml. in the blood. This is called the renal threshold for glucose. The presence of glucose in the urine is called *glycosuria*.

To eliminate glucose, water also must be excreted. Therefore, one of the symptoms of untreated diabetes is *polyuria* (excessive urine). The patient complains of needing to urinate frequently and of passing a large amount each time. Because so much water has been lost in the urine, the patient feels thirsty, and he drinks a great deal (*polydipsia*). Often, the amount that he drinks is not enough to compensate for the loss of the water, and he becomes dehydrated.

While the needed glucose is being wasted, the body's requirement for fuel continues. The patient feels hungry, and he increases his intake of food (*polyphagia*). He becomes hungrier and weaker, and he loses weight, literally starving while he is overeating. To meet the rising need for energy, additional amounts of fats and proteins are metabolized.

DIABETIC KETOSIS AND COMA

Normally, when fat is metabolized, ketone bodies are formed in the liver and transported to muscle and other tissue, where they serve as a source of energy. (Ketone bodies are chemical intermediate products in the metabolism of fat.) In the process of serving as a source of energy, ketone bodies are oxidized to carbon dioxide and water. The more fat is metabolized, the more ketone bodies are formed. The ketone bodies are beta-hydroxybutyric acid, acetoacetic acid and acetone (note that two of them are acids). All three are toxic if they accumulate in the body.

If ketone bodies are produced faster than they can be oxidized in the tissues, they accumulate in tissues and body fluids. Ketone bodies are buf-

fered by the bicarbonate buffer system. Thus, ketonemia causes a decrease of plasma sodium, potassium and alkali reserve. The loss of sodium and potassium salts in the urine further contributes to the development of acidosis. The CO_2 combining power of the blood is reduced, and the alkali reserve of the body is lowered, leading to further electrolyte imbalance. Chloride, particularly, is lost in the vomiting that accompanies acidosis, and sodium, potassium and calcium also are wasted. The increased diuresis causes dehydration, which leads to diminution of the circulating blood volume and fall of the blood pressure. Air hunger (Kussmaul breathing) is common in acidosis. Acetone, being volatile, can be detected on the breath. Finally, if treatment is not given, the outcome is circulatory collapse, renal shutdown and death. This complex is known as *diabetic coma* (though severe ketosis can be present without the patient's being comatose).

Anything that causes glycogen depletion in the liver, and that therefore increases the need for oxidation of fat (for instance, insulin deprivation, infection, surgery, anesthesia, vomiting) may result in an excess of ketone bodies. Infection and surgery invite ketosis and diabetic coma, because they increase the demand for insulin that the diabetic's pancreas cannot deliver.

The metabolic situation is complicated further by overactivity of the anterior pituitary, the thyroid and the adrenal cortex. The secretory activities of these glands may stimulate the formation of glucose, reduce the utilization of glucose, and therefore elevate blood-sugar levels. Although these hormonal interrelations as they affect carbohydrate metabolism are not yet fully understood, there are indications that diabetes is not an uncomplicated disease of merely the islets of Langerhans.

Although diabetes is a highly complex disease, a diagnostic test for its detection is extremely simple. Normally, there is no easily detectable glucose or acetone in urine. In diabetes there may be both. Since glucose is not adequately used, it is excreted in urine. If fats are metabolized faster than the body can utilize the ketone bodies, acetone will appear in the urine. The relative ease of these urinary tests helps to make case-finding programs easier for the early detection of diabetes. However, because sugar in the urine is not always an indication of diabetes, and because not all diabetics excrete sugar in the urine, blood glucose and glucose tolerance tests may be necessary to establish the diagnosis.

Urine Tests

Collection of Urine Specimen. It is important to test the second voided specimen. The first specimen voided may contain urine collected in the bladder for seven to eight hours (as, for example, the first voided specimen in the morning). One wants to evaluate the presence of sugar and acetone *currently*—not for eight hours past. Ask the patient to void, saving the first specimen in case he is unable to give you a second specimen, and then, a half hour later ask him to void again and test the second specimen. This is particularly important if the dosage of insulin is to be based on the results of the test.

When a patient has an indwelling catheter it is essential *not* to take a specimen for testing from the collection bag, as this urine may have been collected over a six- to eight-hour period. Instead, remove the end of the tubing from the collection bag and let some fresh urine run into a clean container for testing.

Both glucose and acetone may be present in the urine at one time of the day and absent at another. For this reason the doctor may order a 24-hour urine specimen or fractional urines. The latter are consecutive specimens collected and analyzed at stated times during the day and the night. The patient saves all his urine in one large bottle. At intervals the nurse takes a specimen from the bottle. She records the volume, empties and cleans the bottle, and returns it to the bedside, so that the patient can start all over again. The usual times for collections are 7 A.M., 11 A.M., 4 P.M., and 9 P.M. Fractional urines give the doctor a picture of the pattern of the excretion of glucose in the urine, and he may judge the timing of insulin injections accordingly.

While the patient is still in the hospital, the nurse teaches him to test his own urine, because once he is at home, he will need to do it himself. By the time of his discharge he should have done it so many times and be so proficient at testing urine for glucose and acetone that he thinks no more of performing the procedure than he does of washing his hands. The patient should be taught not only the technic of urine testing but also the significance of the findings.

Glucose. *Benedict's Test:* Put 5 ml. of Benedict's solution in a test tube. Add 8 drops of urine. Mix. Place in a hot-water bath or, more simply, hold over a direct flame until the mixture has boiled (not so vigorously as to spatter) for 5 minutes. The opening of the test tube should be held away from the face. Allow it to cool, and compare it with the color chart that should be nearby.

COLOR INDICATIONS OF GLUCOSE IN BENEDICT'S TEST

Clear blue	No sugar
Pale green	Trace of glucose
Yellow	Up to 0.5% glucose
Orange	0.5% to 1.5% glucose
Brick red	1.5% and over glucose

This test is the least expensive of the urine tests for sugar. Four ounces of Benedict's solution, a bit less than a month's supply, cost about 65 cents.

Tes-Tape: Dip a strip of Tes-Tape into urine. If sugar is present, the tape will turn green or blue. Only the end of the tape that is not touched by fingers or previously exposed to light or air should be used.

Clinitest: Put 10 drops of water in a test tube. Add 5 drops of urine. Add 1 tablet of Clinitest. Grade the resulting color in accordance with the Clinitest color chart.

Clinistix: Dip the test end in urine and read against the color chart.

An advantage of the last three tests is that the materials are convenient to carry. If need be, a patient can test his urine with these methods in the restroom of an airplane or while he is at a hotel. Because they are quick and easy, these tests are more commonly used than Benedict's test.

Acetone. Although there are several tests for urinary acetone, the most common are the Acetest tablets and acetone test powder. Put 2 drops of urine on the tablet or on a small pile of the powder, and compare with the color chart to show the amount of acetone present. A positive test turns the tablet purple.

Be sure to replace the cap on the bottle, because tablets, powder, and testing strips that have absorbed moisture from the air become useless. These testing materials can be bought in drugstores.

This test becomes especially important when the patient has fever, is vomiting, or consistently has glucose in his urine. These are situations in which the chances for the formation of ketone bodies are the greatest.

Blood Tests

Glucose Tolerance Test. As we have mentioned, normal blood sugar in the fasting person is 80 to 120 mg. per 100 ml. of venous blood by the Folin-Wu method. When the nondiabetic is given glucose orally, his blood-glucose level will return to normal in about two hours (when glucose is given intravenously, the level returns to normal in about an hour). If the patient is diabetic, his fasting blood-glucose level may be high, and it stays even higher for more than two hours after ingesting glucose.

The usual procedure for the standard oral glucose tolerance test is:

The patient receives a high carbohydrate diet for three to five days before the test. The diet contains at least 150 Gm. of carbohydrate per day. This preparation for the test is important, because, without the preliminary diet, blood glucose values may be high as in the so-called hunger or starvation diabetes (Fabrykant, *in* Ellenberg and Rifkin).

Blood and urine samples are taken before breakfast (fasting control).

The patient drinks glucose in water. The dosage is determined by the patient's weight.

Blood and urine specimens are taken at intervals of a half-hour, 1 hour, 2 hours, and 3 hours after the patient has had the glucose. If desired, specimens are also taken at the 4th and 5th hours.

The nurse should put a few drops of lemon juice into the oral glucose solution to help to make it more palatable. Some patients find the drink easier to take if it is well chilled. Note when the patient finishes the glucose, and time the collection of the specimens accordingly. Usually the nurse collects the urine, and a doctor or a laboratory technician takes the blood. Be sure that all specimen bottles are labeled correctly. The patient can have nothing to eat while the test is in progress, but he may drink water.

CO_2 Combining Power. The CO_2 combining power is a general measure of the acidity or alkalinity of the blood. Alkalosis is manifested by an increase above the normal (56 to 70 volumes per 100 ml. of serum), while acidosis is manifested by a decrease in CO_2 combining power.

TREATMENT

Introduction

Treatment of diabetes must be carried out for the rest of the patient's life; therefore the patient (or in some instances, a family member) has the responsibility for carrying out treatment prescribed by the physician, except during periods of illness (such as during complications of diabetes, or some other illness) when physicians and nurses temporarily carry out treatment until the patient can again assume this responsibility. Before the patient can be expected to learn to carry out his treatment, he requires assistance in accepting the fact that he has diabetes, and in dealing with his own feelings about having the disease. The nurse has an important role in helping the patient gradually to accept the condition and begin to understand his feelings about it, and in teaching the patient how to carry out his treatment.

Before beginning to teach the patient it is important to assess how accepting he is of the illness, and how realistically he is viewing it. Does he believe that having diabetes means he will die? Allow opportunity for your patient to talk about his reaction to the diagnosis, and time for him to begin to absorb what it means to him, before starting to teach him to carry out his treatment.

As you explain the necessity for treatment to the patient, try to avoid an unrealistically glib approach. The patient has a potentially serious illness, and most patients know this. An approach which implies, "This is really nothing— all you have to do is spend a few extra moments each morning testing your urine and giving yourself insulin," serves more to relieve staff of their responsibilities to the patient, than to help the patient learn about his illness and deal with his feelings concerning it. Avoid implying a promise that if the patient carries out his treatment faithfully, he will never experience complications. This is not true, and it can form a basis for the patient's later resentment. Explain that treatment will help the patient feel well and avoid complications, but do not say or imply, "If you follow your treatment, you will not have complications."

Coordination between physician and nurse in developing a plan for teaching the patient is essential. However, it is not appropriate for the nurse to wait for a physician's order before considering the patient's need for instruction. Instead, discuss with the physician the ways that both of you can help the patient learn about his condition. Often the nurse assumes that the physician is teaching the patient, and the physician assumes the nurse is teaching him.

Diabetes is especially prevalent among the elderly. Many older diabetics can learn to care for themselves if they are given sufficient time, instruction, and help in overcoming disabilities of age (using a magnifying glass to see the markings on a syringe clearly, or to read the label on a medicine bottle, for example). Although it is useful for a family member also to learn how to care for the elderly person, avoid excluding the patient from instruction and concentrating on teaching a family member, unless it is clear that the patient cannot assume responsibility for his own treatment.

Diet

What the patient eats is one of the most pertinent factors in controlling diabetes. If his intake of carbohydrate is more than he can use or store, eventually he will go into ketosis. If he eats too little food, he ultimately will not only become malnourished but also, if he is taking insulin, be in danger of insulin shock. To prevent both occurrences, he must follow the diet, both in *quantity* and *quality*, that is prescribed for him.

The Prescribed Diet. When a doctor is calculating a diabetic diet, he takes into account the sex, the age, the height and weight, the activity, the state of health, the former dietary habits and the cultural background of the patient. A professional tennis player, like William F. Talbert, diabetic since the age of 10, needs a different diet than would a writer like H. G. Wells, who also was a diabetic. Having diabetes does not obviate the patient's need for a well-balanced diet adapted to his individual life situation.

Although there are some doctors who allow their patients to eat what they like, adjusting the dose of insulin according to the amount of urinary surgar, controlled diet and the goal of sugar-free urine are more common.

Foods. The American Diabetes Association, the American Dietetic Association, and the Public Health Service jointly have prepared exchange lists which assist the patient with meal planning. There are several lists of foods, with each item measured by cup or spoon. On any one list the patient can exchange one item for any other and still obtain approximately the same food value. For example, if the patient's diet allows him one meat exchange for lunch, he can look on a list and see that he can have an ounce of meat or chicken, an egg, a slice of cheese, 1/4 cup of canned fish or a frankfurter. Without deviating from his diet, he can choose

freely from the list of vegetables which are unrestricted.

The following foods are usually excluded from a diabetic diet: sugar, candy, honey, jam, jelly, marmalade, preserves, syrup, molasses, pie, cake, cookies, condensed milk, chewing gum and soft drinks.

The patient should be told that alcohol has a high caloric value. Any alcohol consumed should be counted in his total diet. A large intake of alcohol is not advised, because the high caloric value of alcohol adds greatly to the amount of calories in the prescribed diet, thus reducing the permissible intake of foods necessary for adequate nutrition.

The following foods usually are unrestricted: unsweetened gelatin, clear and fat-free broth, unsweetened pickles, cranberries, rhubarb, coffee and tea, and certain salads.

Dietetic Products. A number of sugarless products are on the market today. Suggest to the patient that he ask his physician about using them. There are two precautions: first, the fats, the proteins and the carbohydrates in such food still have to be counted within the framework of the patient's diet; second, be sure to instruct those diabetic patients who wish to buy these commercially produced foods to *read the label.* The sugar, the fat and the protein contents should be listed. "Low calorie" and "dietetic" are not synonymous with "no sugar."

Teaching the Patient. As is the case with anyone going on a diet, the patient may need help in understanding why it is necessary and in not feeling discouraged. It is important that diabetics eat at prescribed intervals throughout the day to provide a steady supply of carbohydrate in relation to the amount and the kind of insulin that they take. This requirement is especially applicable to patients on insulin. A midafternoon slice of toast and a snack before retiring are often calculated in the diet plan for patients taking insulin.

Before the patient leaves the hospital, be sure that he can realistically plan menus for his meals and snacks from his prescribed diet. Ideally, the patient should be allowed gradually to select and to plan his own diet, with help, before he goes home.

Some diabetics can be controlled on diet alone. These patients have the disease in a mild form; usually, its onset is later in life. The diabetic who is overweight may be placed on a weight-reduction diet by the doctor. It is never healthy for a diabetic (or anyone else, for that matter) to become fat. Diabetes is aggravated by excess weight. If a patient is following his diet and is hungry, he must neither suffer in silence nor adjust his diet or insulin by himself; instead, he should tell his doctor. If he is unable to eat at all, the doctor must be notified immediately. A gastrointestinal upset that is minor for the nondiabetic is a medical emergency for the diabetic if it prevents him from eating the proper foods, or if it causes vomiting or diarrhea.

The better informed the patient is, the more effective will be the control that he will have of his disorder, and, therefore, the healthier he may stay.

Insulin

Insulin is medicine, but it is not a substance foreign to the body. New patients may be relieved to hear that all they are taking is a hormone that is a normal element of the body. Unfortunately, insulin is inactivated by gastrointestinal juices, and therefore it must be injected.

TABLE 42-1. FORMS OF INSULIN

TYPE	EFFECT STARTS WITHIN*	PEAK EFFECTS	EFFECT LASTS FOR
Regular			
Crystalline	½–1 hr.	1– 4 hrs.	6– 8 hrs.
Globin	1–2 hrs.	8–12 hrs.	18–24 hrs.
NPH	1–2 hrs.	8–20 hrs.	20–48 hrs.
Lente	1–2 hrs.	8–20 hrs.	20–28 hrs.
Protamine Zinc	4–8 hrs.	18–24 hrs.	24–36 hrs.

* Effects are greater and last longer with larger doses than with smaller doses.

Forms of Insulin and Action Time. Crystalline insulin is a modification of regular insulin. As you can see in Table 42-1 both of these forms are rapidly absorbed, and usually they are administered 15 to 30 minutes before a meal, so that the insulin reaches the bloodstream at about the same time as does the glucose. Long-acting insulins usually are given 30 minutes before the patient eats. It is the nurse's responsibility to safeguard the hospitalized patient by insuring the correct timing of insulin injection and meals. This is one medication that should always be given on time. If the patient is fasting for a blood-sugar or glucose tolerance test, or for any other reason he does not eat, do not give him his insulin until 15 to 30 minutes before he

takes his regular meal. Exact timing is most important with the quick-acting insulins.

Because regular and crystalline insulins do not last through a whole day (see Table 42-1), a means of prolonging the action was sought. The answer was found in adding certain substances like zinc, globin, and protamine to insulin. Patients can take only one injection a day, instead of two or three, and still not become hyperglycemic at night. However, because of the danger with long-acting insulins of nocturnal hypoglycemia, insulin preparations whose effects are intermediate in time, such as NPH, are used more frequently than protamine zinc insulin.

PZI (protamine zinc insulin) and NPH (neutral protamine Hagedorn) are substances that must be mixed by rotating the container between the palms and gently turning it end over end before withdrawal into the syringe. Do not shake and create a froth, which would make withdrawal of the insulin into the syringe difficult. If the insulin is not mixed well, the dosage received by the patient will vary from injection to injection.

NPH insulin acts more quickly than PZI, and it lasts longer than regular insulin. Lente insulin also acts quickly; the duration of its action is similar to NPH.

Refrigeration prolongs the effective life of a bottle of insulin. Many persons therefore store insulin in the refrigerator. Recently some authorities are recommending that insulin be kept in a cool place, but not in a refrigerator, because storage in the refrigerator can interfere with the even suspension of the insulin solution. When the patient is traveling, he can place the insulin bottle in a thermos or an insulated bag. Note that the bottles are dated. Insulin should not be allowed to freeze, which it does at 32° F.

Injecting Insulin. Insulin comes in units. Units are clearly marked on the bottle and the insulin syringe. U 40 means that 1 ml. contains 40 units; U 80 means that 1 ml. contains 80 units, and so on. The doctor usually specifies both the dose and the unit type of insulin to be used, such as "Regular Insulin, 10 U of U 40." The nurse or the patient would then use the bottle marked U 40 and the syringe marked U 40.

When picking up the syringe, the first thing to do is to match the correct scale to the bottle and the patient's ordered dose. Ten units of U 40 insulin measured on the U 80 scale would give the patient only half of his correct dose.

The U 80 scale is used most frequently for patients who need large amounts of insulin. Since U 80 is twice as concentrated as U 40, larger doses of insulin can be given in smaller amounts of injected fluid.

Teaching the Patient. Teach the patient to vary the site of the injection, so that no two injections are closer than one inch to each other within a two-week period. Repeatedly using the same site might cause tissue damage. Insulin lipo-atrophy, which is atrophy of subcutaneous fat, is an all too common reaction to repeated insulin injections into the same area. It causes deep depressions of the skin and gives an undesirable cosmetic appearance. Lipohypertrophy, which is spongy, painless swelling, also is unsightly. Insulin is poorly absorbed when injected into such damaged tissue.

Patients may use the outer aspects of the thighs, or even the skin of the abdomen, if this is comfortable. It is suggested (Coates and Fabrykant) that insulin be given at a 90° angle with the needle held perpendicular to the skin, instead of the more common 45° to 60° angle. For obese patients a ¾-inch 25-gauge needle may be needed. In thin patients, injecting insulin into a skin fold pinched between the fingers helps to prevent an intramuscular injection. The objective is to place the insulin deep in the subcutaneous tissue, not into the skin, and not intravenously.

Almost all diabetics who need insulin can and should be taught to inject it themselves. Because injection is a daily procedure, it is important that the patient be independent and have control over his own regimen. Teaching can start with the new diabetic in the hospital as soon as he has experienced relief of symptoms and has had a treatment regimen established by his physician. First, he needs to know the essentials of sterile technic; to boil the syringe and the needle for 10 minutes; how to pick up, put down, and hold the syringe without contaminating the needle or the plunger; to wash his hands, and to scrub the vial cap with alcohol. He is shown how to withdraw the insulin; to clean the injection site; to insert the needle, to pull back on the plunger, and to shift his fingers to push the plunger in. Also teach the patient to examine the needle for burrs and dullness before sterilizing it, and how to sharpen it when it is necessary. Of course, all this is too much to learn in one lesson, but the patient should practice every day.

If the nurse is too busy to teach him when he receives his 7 A.M. dose of insulin, perhaps after lunch she can take a pot and a syringe to his bedside and demonstrate sterile technic. The next day, perhaps, the patient can show her how it is done. He can practice manipulating the syringe by himself, acquiring familiarity with it. Disposable syringes and needles are available, and are a particular convenience for diabetics when traveling.

As you well know, it is not easy to learn to insert a needle into the flesh of another person. For many people it is even harder, initially, to give an injection to themselves. It may help some patients to get the feel of the resistance of skin if they first inject solution into an orange or a soft rubber ball. For the first injection into his own skin, the nurse may wish to guide the patient's hands. Remember that although injections have become commonplace in your life, this familiarity is not so for the majority of others. Yet 9-year-olds and 90-year-olds have overcome their distaste for the procedure.

For safety's sake, one other member of the family should learn to give insulin in case the patient cannot do it for himself. The relative can be taught either in the hospital, at home, or in the clinic. The clinic is an ideal place for group teaching. Informal classes in diet, foot care, insulin, and urine testing can lead to group discussions concerning the problems that diabetes causes in the lives and the homes of the patients. The solution that one patient has found may help the others.

The necessity for periodic evaluation of the way the patient is caring for himself cannot be overemphasized. In one study of 162 diabetic patients from three clinics and 22 private practices, it was found that 58 per cent of 115 patients taking insulin made dosage errors (Watkins et al.: Diabetes). The same study showed that, of the 47 patients taking oral drugs, 23 per cent made potentially serious errors. Errors and misunderstanding concerning sterilization of equipment, urine testing, and adherence to prescribed diet were also prevalent (Watkins et al.: Am. J. Pub. Health). Too often a brief program of instruction is given to the newly diagnosed diabetic without necessary follow-up. Often the patient is uncertain about aspects of his self-care, and soon begins to make mistakes.

When evaluating the patient's ability to carry out his own care, it is more effective to ask him to explain what he does and to demonstrate how he does it, than for the nurse merely to repeat to him the instructions which he may have heard many times, but which he may misunderstand or apply incorrectly.

Oral Hypoglycemic Agents

There are two groups of oral hypoglycemic agents: the sulfonylureas, which act by stimulating the beta cells of the pancreas to secrete more insulin; and the biguanides, which act in the cells, promoting the utilization of glucose by muscle and other peripheral tissue.

In the first group are such drugs as tolbutamide (Orinase), chlorpropamide (Diabinese) and acetohexamide (Dymelor). These agents cannot lower blood sugar in a patient who has no pancreas, or in a patient whose pancreas cannot be stimulated to release more insulin. Undesirable side-effects include liver damage (observe the patient for jaundice), especially with chlorpropamide, allergy (skin manifestations seem most common), gastrointestinal disturbances and, rarely, bone-marrow depression. When alcohol is ingested, there may be flushing and headache. Hypoglycemia may occur; this is more frequent with chlorpropamide and acetohexamide than with tolbutamide.

Phenformin is in the biguanide group of oral hypoglycemic agents. There are two types of phenformin (DBI and DBI-TD). Side-effects include gastrointestinal symptoms, a metallic taste and, rarely, ketonuria and lactic-acid acidosis, which may occur with little or no glycosuria. Side-effects are especially likely to be seen in patients with hepatic and renal disease. It is important that patients receiving phenformin routinely test their urine for ketone bodies as well as glucose, and that they have periodic determinations of the plasma bicarbonate level.

A danger of these oral medications is that the patient may underestimate the danger in the progression of his disease; he may fail to remain under medical supervision, or he may neglect his diet, his feet or his urinalysis. He may erroneously reason that his disease can be ignored, because taking a pill is so much simpler than the injections taken by others with the same diagnosis. In talking with the patient the nurse should help him to recognize the need for care, but to lessen anxiety which can interfere with his ability to care for himself. Whether the patient's prescription is for an oral hypoglycemic agent or for insulin, it is usually wise to teach him how to handle a syringe, measure and inject insulin. The patient who takes oral hypoglycemic agents can never be completely certain that he will not require insulin at some future time.

The obese diabetic patient, except in the case of complicating illness, sometimes needs neither insulin nor oral agents, but he does need weight reduction to normal levels. If at normal weight the diabetes is still uncontrolled, then he perhaps will respond to an oral hypoglycemic agent.

Exercise

Exercise is good for diabetes. It improves the circulation, which frequently is rather poor, and it helps to metabolize carbohydrate, thus decreasing the insulin requirement. Of course, if a patient sits at his desk all day Friday and plays touch football Saturday, he will have wide fluctuations in his blood sugar. If his schedule calls for such differences in activity, he should consult his doctor, who may regulate his food and insulin requirements accordingly, and advise him to revise his schedule. During exercise it is especially important for the patient who takes insulin to carry some candy or sugar cubes with him, which he can eat if he feels any of the symptoms of hypoglycemia. (Diabetics should always have some form of easy-to-eat carbohydrate in their pockets or purses, in case of hypoglycemia in such inconvenient places as a subway or a concert hall.)

COMPLICATIONS

Diabetic Ketosis and Coma

The early symptoms of ketosis may be vague, but they become more definite—and serious—as more and more ketone bodies accumulate in the bloodstream unchecked. The patient may have weakness, thirst, anorexia, vomiting, drowsiness and abdominal pain. His cheeks may be flushed, and his skin and his mouth may be dry. There may be an odor of acetone on his breath. Kussmaul breathing, fast, deep and labored, may be evident. His pulse often is rapid and weak, and his blood pressure is low. If he is unconscious, he probably will be restless.

Diabetic coma now occurs less often than formerly, due to more effective regulation of the disease and greater emphasis on teaching patients and families. However, it still occurs. In some instances the patient develops coma in spite of having carefully followed his doctor's recommendations. Such patients may be in the group of severe diabetics whose disease is hard to control. On occasion a patient is admitted to the hospital in diabetic coma who had not known previously that he was a diabetic. Diabetic coma also occurs with greater frequency among persons who have inadequate medical care. One of the most common causes of diabetic coma is infection.

Diagnosis. Only nonspecific treatment (such as intravenous fluids to help to correct the circulatory collapse and the electrolyte imbalance) is instituted when diabetes is known or suspected, until blood and urine samples are taken for the determination of glucose and ketone bodies, electrolytes and CO_2 combining power to confirm the presence and the degree of diabetic coma.

If the patient is comatose, he is catheterized, and a retention urinary catheter may be left in place for future specimens. Some hospitals have a coma cart on which the necessary equipment for diagnosis and treatment of this emergency is collected, so that it is readily available when a patient in coma is admitted. The cart contains urine specimen bottles, test tubes, tubes for blood-sugar and CO_2 combining power tests, intravenous fluids, gastric lavage, and catheterization sets.

Treatment and Nursing Care. Treatment for coma includes the administration of regular insulin. Insulin lessens the production of ketones by making carbohydrate available for oxidation by the tissues and restoring the liver's supply of glycogen. Regular, rather than long-acting, insulin is given for rapid effect.

The nurse observes for a patent airway and suctions mucus away when necessary, keeps the patient flat in bed and notes changes in the patient's condition that indicate deepening of the coma or response to therapy. The nurse keeps the intake and output record, writes down the results of the urine testing each time that a test is performed, charts the insulin given, and her own observations of the patient's symptoms, so that the most current information is immediately and easily available to the doctor at all times.

Insulin may be given every half-hour, and the urine may be tested as often. The nurse should watch for signs of muscular weakness and difficulty in breathing. The patient may be suffering from potassium depletion. Supplementary potassium may be ordered. An edema or gastric aspiration may be necessary, since patients may have gastric dilatation. The gastric contents of a dilated stomach may be vomited and aspirated by the partially comatose patient. In severe cir-

culatory collapse epinephrine or caffeine and a blood transfusion may be needed.

As the patient recovers and is able to take fluids by mouth, the doctor may order milk, salty broth, orange juice, or oatmeal gruel, approximately 120 ml. every hour. Until the patient is well out of danger, the nurse stays with him, observing him, taking vital signs, collecting urine specimens when they are called for, and giving insulin as it is ordered. Specimens of blood and urine continue to be tested for glucose at frequent intervals; and treatment with insulin and carbohydrate feedings (to prevent insulin shock), fluids and electrolytes continues until the diabetes is regulated. Long-term management with diet and insulin resumes.

Hypoglycemic Reaction (Insulin Shock)

When there is too much insulin in the bloodstream in relation to the amount of available glucose—in other words, when blood glucose goes below about 60 mg. per 100 ml. of blood—the condition of hypoglycemia results.

Symptoms. The pattern of symptoms varies somewhat from patient to patient, depending on the degree of hypoglycemia, the patient's individual reaction, and the type of insulin taken. For example, with the long-acting insulins, the symptoms of overdose may be headache, nausea, drowsiness and a feeling of malaise. Many patients who are having an insulin reaction initially experience weakness, nervousness, hunger, tremors and excessive perspiration. Some patients have personality changes that are characteristic for that person. One may become negativistic; another, weepy. Confusion, aphasia, delirium and vertigo may occur. If the hypoglycemia is not relieved, the symptoms may progress to difficulty with coordination, and the patient may see double. If he still is untreated, he may have convulsions and become unconscious; if he is neglected further, he may suffer permanent brain damage, and in very rare cases he may die. The symptoms are variable, but they have a tendency to be repeated in the same person whenever he has too much insulin and too little food. The sequence may be extremely rapid, with the patient convulsing or dropping into unconsciousness before any other symptoms are noticed.

When a diabetic patient is found unconscious, he may be suffering from diabetic coma or insulin reaction. Although it is the doctor who makes the diagnosis and prescribes the treatment, nurses and patients should be familiar with the symp-

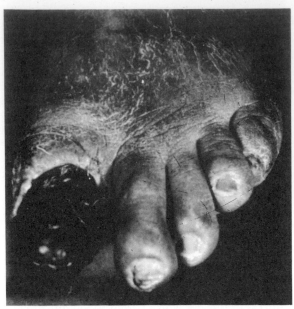

Fig. 42-1. Gangrene of toe. (Dr. W. L. Lowrie, Detroit)

toms of both coma and hypoglycemia, so that these can be noticed in their early stages.

Treatment and Nursing Care. The treatment for insulin reaction is carbohydrate. If the patient is conscious and able to swallow, he is given orange juice, candy, warm tea or coffee with sugar, honey or a dextrose solution. If the patient is unconscious, dextrose will be given intravenously. Whenever there is a diabetic in your care, be sure that there is always some orange juice in the refrigerator, some sugar in the sugar bowl, and some intravenous dextrose in a nearby unlocked cabinet. In a severe reaction the patient may need repeated feedings before the symptoms of insulin reaction are relieved. The doctor may order epinephrine or glucagon to increase the patient's alertness and to stimulate the liver to release some of its store of glycogen.

Patients who develop personality reactions are often not able to treat themselves with sugar, so someone else must do it. While the patient who feels faint and weak often is viewed as sick, the one who becomes obstinate or aggressive may not be treated as promptly. Asking such a patient, "Would you like to have some sugar?" usually evokes the response, "No!" Instead, hand him the sugar or the glass of orange juice, see that he takes it, observe his response and notify the doctor. It is important to teach nursing aides, the family and anyone else who may be with the patient that personality change may represent a hypoglycemic reaction and should be treated as such.

Insulin reaction is as much a medical emergency as is diabetic coma. The nurse stays with the patient, observing him and participating in therapeutic measures. After such an episode the regulation of the patient's metabolism is very difficult for about 24 hours, and he should be under close observation by nurses for further symptoms of imbalance.

Poor regulation of carbohydrate metabolism, with the dangers of diabetic coma, on the one hand, and of insulin shock, on the other, may be brought about by ignorance or carelessness by the patient, by an infection, or by extreme emotional stress. A patient who has been well regulated may become depressed and not care any longer; he may fail to keep his diet, or refuse to test his urine and to take his insulin. A gastrointestinal upset with vomiting may force him to eat less. He may then reason that he needs less insulin, and cut down on his daily dose. This is a dangerous fallacy, and it may lead to ketosis, because illness often increases the need for insulin. Nurses should teach diabetic patients that any slight illness, such as a head cold, is an indication for more frequent testing of the urine, and for particularly careful adherence to the regimen of diet and insulin, or oral hypoglycemic agent. If ketonuria is present, or if the slight illness persists or grows worse, the patient should see his doctor.

Vascular Disturbances

Diabetics are particularly prone to circulatory disturbances. The incidence of arteriosclerosis in diabetics is higher than in nondiabetics. Why this is so is not known. In addition, there are many vascular changes in the diabetic, some of which are not seen in nondiabetics, and some of which become more severe when the metabolic aspects of the disorder are poorly controlled. For example, an almost consistent finding in diabetic patients is thickening of the walls of some capillaries, arterioles and venules (Colwell). It is suspected that these pathologic changes start before there are any symptoms of diabetes, and this is one reason that attention is turned to the identification of prediabetic people.

Any part of the body can be affected by the vascular disturbances, but nerves, eyes, kidneys and legs are particularly likely to be affected. The lower extremities are especially vulnerable

TABLE 42-2. SYMPTOMS OF DIABETIC COMA AND INSULIN SHOCK*

	DIABETIC COMA	INSULIN REACTION
History	Insufficient or omitted insulin	Excessive insulin
	Intercurrent infection	Unusual exercise
	Dietary indiscretion	Too little food
	Gastrointestinal upset	
Onset	Slow, hours to days	Sudden, minutes
Skin	Flushed, dry, hot	Pale, moist, cool
Behavior	Drowsy	Excited
Breath	Acetone	Normal
Respirations	Air hunger	Normal to rapid, shallow
Pulse	Rapid, weak	Normal or slow; full, bounding
Blood pressure	Low	Normal
Vomiting	Present	May be absent
Hunger	Absent	Often present
Thirst	Present	Absent
Urinary sugar	Large amounts	Absent in 2nd specimen
Response to treatment	Slow	Rapid

* Adapted from Lilly Research Laboratories: *Diabetes Mellitus.*

to changes brought about by decreased blood supply to the tissues. In a study of 541 patients, 16 per cent developed foot problems (Whitehouse and Block). Because of lessened blood supply, cramps may occur, infection is not fought effectively and may lead to ulcer formation and eventually to gangrene. Gangrene may necessitate amputation. Surgery is an added strain on the body, and the surgeon and the internist work closely together to regulate the patient's diabetes during the period of extra stress. Uncontrolled diabetes frequently retards wound healing. See Chapter 32 for treatment and nursing care of the patient with an ischemic extremity.

Visual Problems

In diabetics the retinal capillaries tend to develop multiple tiny aneurysms, accompanied by small points of hemorrhage and by exudates. The scarring resulting from repeated hemorrhages eventually may cause blindness.

A blind or a near-blind diabetic has the same need for independence as the sighted diabetic. Perhaps his need is even greater. He should be assisted to rely on himself. He can ask his physician if he can use the Covey technics to test sugar in his urine. A pinch of yeast is placed in a test tube, which then is filled to the brim with urine. A rubber finger cot is stretched over the top, with as little air as possible between the finger cot and the urine. The test tube is left near a 75-watt bulb for 15 minutes. If sugar is present, the heat helps it to ferment, and the finger cot will bulge. The height of the bulge determines the amount

of sugar present. In the beginning this method should be checked by a sighted person who uses one of the conventional technics to help the blind person to correlate the degree of bulge with the amount of sugar shown on a color chart. Insulin can be given with a Tru-Set or a Cornwall syringe. Both can be set so that the plunger cannot be pulled beyond the correct dose. The syringe can be sterilized without interfering with the setting. Aluminum strips on the top of the insulin bottle can be placed so that they point to the center of the rubber stopper and help to guide the needle there.

The partially sighted diabetic may have difficulty seeing the tiny markings on a syringe. A thin strip of tape on the syringe can underline the point at which he should stop the plunger when pulling back.

Neuropathy

Any nervous tissue can be affected. There may be facial paralysis, atony of urinary bladder or stomach, with retention of food, and diarrhea or constipation. However, the legs are the most frequently affected. The patient may experience itching, numbness, tingling, and pain, which often is aggravated at night. There also may be a loss of sensation, so that the patient does not feel intense heat, and he can be burned without realizing it.

Nephropathy

Nodular glomerulosclerosis is frequent among diabetics. The symptoms include albuminuria, edema and hypertension. Renal failure may be the outcome.

Infection

In patients with diabetes, infections heal slowly, and the diabetes itself becomes more severe while the infection persists. Tuberculosis is more frequent in diabetics than in nondiabetics. Carbuncles and furuncles can be a major problem. A cardinal rule for diabetics is: call the doctor at the *first* sign of any illness. The patient with a common cold should go to bed, drink copious fluids, test his urine and call the doctor. Any skin eruption should be brought to the doctor's attention. The patient with an upset stomach should go to bed, take insulin as usual, drink a glass of fluid every hour, test his urine and call the doctor. Anything suspicious or out of the ordinary should be reported to the doctor.

PROGNOSIS

Although diabetics do not have as long a life expectancy as nondiabetics, there has been significant increase in their life expectancy as a result of modern therapy, and, in part, probably as a result of other health measures, such as emphasis among the population as a whole on the hazards of obesity (Entmacher and Marks). Patients whose disease is treated within the first year of its discovery outlive those whose treatment is delayed (McDonald). The patient who understands his disease is better able to keep his diabetes in control than the ignorant patient. The patient whose morale is high is better able to keep his diabetes in control than the depressed patient. The nurse can help by her teaching and her understanding of the discouraging problems of a lifelong disease.

SOCIAL ASPECTS

Prejudice against hiring diabetics is common. Many employers fear that insulin reaction or coma will occur on the job, or that time will be lost due to illness. Therefore, diabetics often have difficulty obtaining employment commensurate with their abilities and their financial needs. The prejudice seems unjustified. Well-regulated diabetics can enter a variety of occupations, such as teaching, nursing, medicine and carpentry. However, employers should know that a person is diabetic, just in case he should need care while he is on the job. The prejudice against employing diabetics leads to concealment of the fact.

Diabetics need not be conspicuous socially. A diabetic can eat in restaurants by developing a keen eye for estimating portions and sticking to foods of known composition. He can pack his own box lunch for picnics.

When the diabetic travels, he can carry his syringe and needle in metal cases that are specially designed to keep the syringe and the needle sterile. Or he can boil the syringe and the needle, using one of the commercial plugs with metal prongs that fits into a cup and boils water in two minutes. Disposable insulin syringes and needles also are available. Insulin can be placed in a cool spot by the hotel window. There is no need for a diabetic to be home-bound.

Helping the patient to acknowledge the condition, and to adapt his way of life accordingly, is a challenge for the nurse. Assisting the patient to recognize the choices open to him (for instance, the choice between learning to follow a diet, and becoming ill from unregulated diabetes) and helping him to learn from his own experiences are measures which can assist the patient to deal effectively with his condition. Too often threats and dire warnings are used in an attempt to frighten the patient into following instructions. Sometimes the nurse adopts a "policeman" role, searching the patient's bedside stand periodically for forbidden food. Such measures are largely ineffective. The decisions about self-care and the will to abide by them must be fostered within the patient since in most instances he carries the responsibility for his own care.

REFERENCES AND BIBLIOGRAPHY

ARNOLD, H. M.: Elderly diabetic amputees, *Am. J. Nurs.* 69:2646, December, 1969.

COATES, F. C., and FABRYKANT, M.: An insulin injection technique for preventing skin reactions, *Am. J. Nurs.* 65:127, February, 1965.

DERR, S. D.: Testing for glycosuria, *Am. J. Nurs.* 70:1513, July, 1970.

JACKSON, H.: Helping a blind diabetic patient become self-dependent, *Am. J. Nurs.* 62:107, November, 1962.

LOCKE, R. K.: Foot care for diabetics, *Am. J. Nurs.* 63:107, November, 1963.

PIRART, J.: Diabetic neuropathy: a metabolic or a vascular disease? *Diabetes* 14:1, 1965.

RODMAN, M., and SMITH, D.: *Pharmacology and Therapeutics in Nursing*, Philadelphia, Lippincott, 1968.

SHAWN, SR. M.: Teaching a patient, *Am. J. Nurs.* 64:126, April, 1964.

WATKINS, J., and MOSS, F.: Confusion in the management of diabetes, *Am. J. Nurs.* 69:521, March, 1969.

WELLER, C.: Oral hypoglycemic agents, *Am. J. Nurs.* 64:90, March, 1964.

ZITNIK, R.: First you take a grapefruit, *Am. J. Nurs.* 68:1285, June, 1968.

Introduction: The Female Reproductive Pattern

43

The Nurse and the Gynecologic Patient • The Menstrual Cycle
Helping the Adolescent to Understand • The Menopause
Disorders of Menstruation • Fertility and Infertility • Religious
Attitudes Toward Birth Control • Summary of Teaching Points

THE NURSE AND THE GYNECOLOGIC PATIENT

Emotional Support

It is sometimes too easy for the nurse to render little or no care to the average gynecologic patient. Such patients usually require short hospitalizations, recuperate quickly from surgery, and assume a large bulk of responsibility for themselves in terms of physical care. The nurse who assumes that her responsibilities for nursing care are limited to the most obvious physical needs of her patients is drastically underestimating the scope of her professional role and depriving her patients of the best possible nursing care.

Besides the basic determination of a patient's physical needs, one of the fundamental requirements of effective nursing care is an ability to hear the patient's requests for reassurance and information and to recognize manifestations of anxiety. The ability to pick up a patient's questions demands sensitive listening because many patients, ashamed of their ignorance, will pose their questions in anecdotal form or attribute them to friends and relatives. A nurse who is listening for such subtleties can often discover the nature of her patient's anxiety and can help by allowing the patient to verbalize her fears and by supplying facts and advice when necessary. It is well for the nurse to remember that a patient whose gynecologic symptoms are sufficient

to require hospitalization is almost certain to be anxious. Many patients fear cancer. This fear is not confined to any one age group, although concern about the possibility of cancer usually increases with age, just as the likelihood of developing cancer becomes greater among women at and after the time of menopause. If the patient actually asks the nurse if she has cancer, the nurse can explain that this is an appropriate question to ask the doctor and encourage the patient to ask it. If the patient is afraid of the possibility of cancer, the nurse cannot take this fear away from her, but by listening supportively the nurse may be able to lessen the patient's anxiety and help her think through just what it is that she fears. In addition to cancer, fear of impairment or loss of reproductive capacity and reproductive organs may cause anxiety in a woman of child bearing age. Many women fear that the capacity to respond sexually may be impaired or lost. Worry how to support another child if the patient is pregnant is another possibility. The possibility of abortion, natural or therapeutic, the relative merits of various birth control methods, ability to carry a fetus to term are some other concerns a patient may wish to discuss with the nurse. It is important to create an atmosphere in which the patient feels free to broach these topics if she wishes. Usually the nurse is not the only source of information and comfort to the patient and recognizing this can

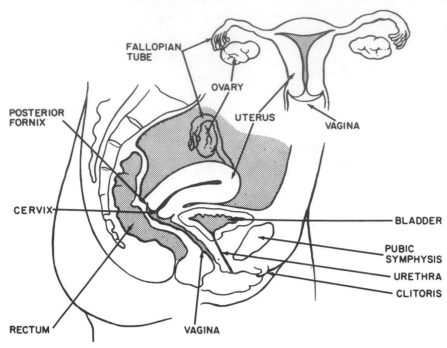

FIG. 43-1. Anatomy of female reproductive organs.

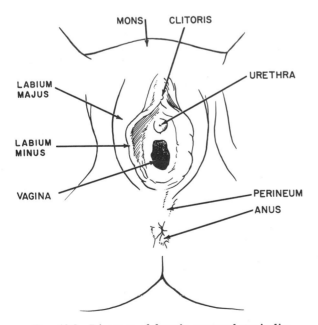

FIG. 43-2. Diagram of female external genitalia.

foster a realistic view of her role. She is one of the persons in whom the patient may confide, and the patient, in confiding, may gain confidence to discuss some of her anxieties with others, such as her physician, her husband, or clergyman. The nurse cannot supply answers to all of the patients' questions. It is often wise to suggest to the patient that she may discuss her fears with the doctor; your listening will have helped her to define her fears. For instance, a seemingly simple operation such as a dilatation and curretage (D and C) may be performed for diagnostic purposes, the outcome of which will most certainly be of concern to the patient. Or, a D and C may be performed on a patient who has aborted to remove products of conception that if left in the uterus would cause vaginal bleeding. Such patients require sensitive emphatic nursing care, and, because their hospitalizations are brief, they need nurses who can quickly "tune in" to them as women undergoing stress.

Teaching the Patient

Public health is the rightful concern of every member of the health team. The nurse in the gynecologic unit has the opportunity to counteract misguided notions about personal hygiene, menstruation, sexual intercourse, birth control and venereal disease. Many women have little understanding of their own body processes. Even among younger women, many have received most of their information about female reproductive functions from mothers and sisters who may themselves be ill-informed and superstitious.

FIG. 43-3. Simplified version of the normal menstrual cycle. (The Upjohn Company, Kalamazoo, Mich.)

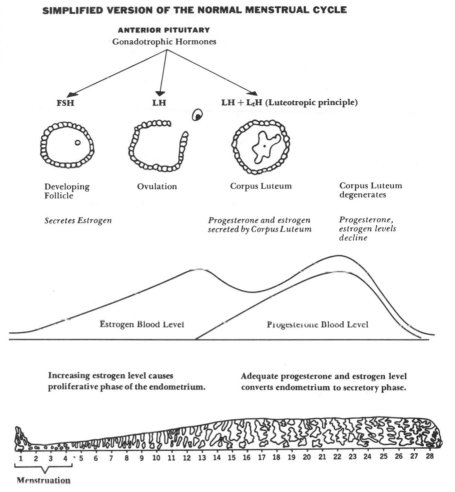

SIMPLIFIED VERSION OF THE NORMAL MENSTRUAL CYCLE

ANTERIOR PITUITARY
Gonadotrophic Hormones

FSH   LH   LH + L$_t$H (Luteotropic principle)

Developing Follicle   Ovulation   Corpus Luteum   Corpus Luteum degenerates

Secretes Estrogen   Progesterone and estrogen secreted by Corpus Luteum   Progesterone, estrogen levels decline

Estrogen Blood Level   Progesterone Blood Level

Increasing estrogen level causes proliferative phase of the endometrium.   Adequate progesterone and estrogen level converts endometrium to secretory phase.

1 2 3 4 5 6 7 8 9 10 11 12 13 14 15 16 17 18 19 20 21 22 23 24 25 26 27 28

Menstruation

How many of your patients believe that bathing is harmful during menstruation? How many take douches daily, using strong and potentially harmful solutions? With the nurse's help, admission to a gynecologic service can provide women an opportunity to learn desirable health practices while they are treated for a particular gynecologic disturbance. Responsible nursing practice means that the nurse takes every opportunity to correct her patient's misunderstandings regarding her own physiology and care.

Anatomy and Physiology Applied

When you are catheterizing female patients, remember that the urethral opening is between the clitoris and the vagina. Have a good light, and look for these landmarks before attempting to insert the tip of the catheter. If you should enter the vagina accidentally, it will be necessary to take a new catheter before proceeding, since the vagina is not sterile. In this event, be sure to discard the used catheter in the area set aside for contaminated supplies. Because the clitoris is a very sensitive organ, poking it with the catheter may cause the patient discomfort. Spread the labia first, placing your fingers carefully so that you do not have to change their position during the procedure, thereby contaminating the area.

Since the vagina is not sterile, and the bladder is sterile, vaginal irrigations are usually done with clean technique, whereas catheterization is always a sterile procedure. Douching usually is contraindicated during late pregnancy and postoperatively. Although the perineal area is not sterile, some situations may require sterile technique in perineal care when clean technique would normally be used. Always wipe anteriorly to posteriorly and use a new cotton ball or sponge for each stroke to avoid bringing any organisms from the anal area to the vagina or the urethra.

Because the urethral opening is so close to the vagina, postoperative care of surgical perineal wounds often is complicated by voiding problems. Dressings should be changed whenever they become wet. After gynecological surgery, patients may have a catheter in place, and catheterization may be ordered preoperatively to empty the bladder fully and to avoid accidental trauma to the bladder during surgery.

THE MENSTRUAL CYCLE

Menarche, the start of menstruation, usually occurs between the ages of 10 and 14. If menses, even if irregular, have not begun by the time that a girl is 15 or 16, the parents should be advised to take her to a gynecologist. He will look for endocrine imbalance, an imperforate hymen, and congenital anomalies. The hymen normally contains an opening adequate to allow the menstrual flow to occur. Occasionally there is no opening in the hymen, and the menstrual flow is held back.

Physiology

Under the influence of the follicle stimulating hormone (FSH) of the anterior pituitary, the ovarian follicle matures along the ovum inside it. With the release of a second pituitary hormone, the luteinizing hormone (LH), the mature follicle ruptures, discharging the ovum, which is drawn into the end of the fallopian tube. This is called *ovulation;* it occurs about every 28 days during the period between menarche and the menopause. After the ovum is shed, the ruptured follicle is transformed into a small body filled with yellow fluid. It is now called a *corpus luteum.*

If the ovum meets a spermatozoon in the fallopian tube and is fertilized, it moves down to the uterus and implants itself in the endometrium, which is prepared to receive it. If fertilization does not occur, the ovum passes through the uterus and vagina and is expelled from the body.

Whether the ovum is fertilized or not, the *endometrium,* a highly vascular glandular tissue lining the inside of the uterus, prepares itself for a possible pregnancy. The development of the uterine endometrium is governed by the hormone estrogen, produced by the maturing ovarian follicle. The follicle is under the influence of FSH. Estrogen production is in turn probably regulated by LH. After the follicle has ruptured, the resultant corpus luteum produces another hormone, progesterone. This stimulates a change in the endometrium, making it richer and thicker in preparation for a possible fertilized ovum. The production of FSH is now inhibited.

If the ovum is not fertilized, the prepared endometrium degenerates and the menstrual flow begins about 2 weeks after ovulation. After menstruation the endometrium again begins to grow thicker and more vascular. Because of these cyclical, hormone-dependent changes, the microscopic picture of the uterus is almost constantly changing. Thus it is important that each gynecologic specimen sent to the laboratory, such as vaginal smears or curettings obtained by scraping the uterus, be marked with the date of the beginning of the patient's last menstrual period.

When conception occurs, the corpus luteum persists during early pregnancy. When conception does not occur, it degenerates and shrinks; and the thickened endometrium, sheds its outer layers with some bleeding. Menstrual flow usually lasts 4 to 5 days, with a loss of 30 to 180 ml. of blood.

HELPING THE ADOLESCENT TO UNDERSTAND

The onset of puberty is characterized by breast development, redistribution of body fat, the growth of pubic and axillary hair and the beginnings of menstruation. The young girl experiencing these changes in herself and in her peers may be very confused and ill prepared to cope with them. The nurse may be called upon to give advice and information.

Since puberty proceeds at different rates for different individuals, many young girls feel embarrassed or ashamed either because they have developed these secondary sex characteristics or because they have not. It helps these young people to know that they will have caught up with one another before they graduate from high school. The nurse can explain this when girls express concern about it. A girl may wonder, but not ask, about the normal vaginal secretion that occurs between menses. If she knows that most women have this discharge, she may be saved some worry.

The amount of discomfort experienced during menses is significantly related to attitudes toward menstruation and toward femininity. This of course does not rule out the possibility of disease or abnormality, and any woman, regardless of age who experiences severe dysmenorrhea should be advised to have a gynecologic examination. Actually, the four or five days of discharge should be accompanied by little or no discomfort. Most doctors believe that there is no reason to curtail activities during menstruation. Many women swim during this period, and some enter athletic contests, apparently without harm. A daily shower or bath should be taken. In contrast to former beliefs, bathing in warm water now is considered not only safe but desirable to lessen odor. There is no reason not to shampoo the hair.

THE MENOPAUSE

The term *menopause* means the cessation of the menstrual cycle. The term *climacteric* is the long period during which ovarian activity gradually ceases. The terms are often used interchangeably, and this period of time is also called the "change of life." The menopause normally occurs between the ages of about 45 and 55.

Physiology

Ovulation gradually ceases and with it the menstrual cycle and the reproductive capacity. The change usually is not sudden; rather, the menses are scanty, or sometimes unusually copious, and irregular for a time before they stop permanently. The uterus, the vagina and the vulva decrease in size. As ovarian function diminishes, so does the production of estrogen and progesterone. The resulting endocrine imbalance may lead to fatigability, nervousness, sweating, palpitation, severe headaches, vasomotor disturbance, and especially, hot flashes which may be so mild and so transitory that they almost escape notice, or which may last as long as two minutes and occur every ten to thirty minutes around the clock. In some instances the hot flashes are disturbing enough to interfere with sleep. Since normal and abnormal changes may readily be confused, it is especially important for women to have regular gynecologic examinations during this period.

Emotional Reactions

To many women the climacteric objectifies the relentlessness of the aging process. The reasons that women often interpret menopause in this way are many, and all centered around the experience of loss. But menopause need not signal the end of useful life to a woman unless she so chooses. Some examples of the fears that have been expressed by women undergoing menopause are:

Loss of role ("My children don't need me any more.") It is clear that this reaction has more to do with the age of the children than the physiological processes of the mother. Nevertheless, many women equate the two phenomena. The woman who has gradually sought experiences and satisfactions in addition to those of caring for her home and family is in a better position to continue this development during the climacteric than is the woman whose interests and satisfactions have been focused almost exclusively on her home and children.

Concern for loss of marital relationship ("Maybe my husband won't want me.") It may be that the woman who voices this fear is actually more afraid of some of the more general concerns of women in that age group; continued sexual satisfaction, wrinkles and grey hair or perhaps her husband's response to his own aging.

Loss of attractiveness and femininity A regular program of enjoyable exercise (not just more housework if the woman is already bored by it), can counteract the tendency to weight gain and muscle flabbiness and provide stimulation and pleasure. Does the woman skate or just take her children to the rink? Does she swim or sit on the beach and watch? Branching out in her tastes, activities, and style of dress can help the woman look and feel more attractive. A new hair style, some new clothes, or learning a new skill can help her feel more confident and energetic.

Fear of physical or mental disability (Getting cancer or having a nervous breakdown.) Instead of just worrying that she might have cancer, the woman can go to the clinic twice yearly for a pap smear and breast examination. Instead of withdrawing from her husband and wondering what his attitudes are about change of life she can talk with him about it, voicing some of her concerns and listening to his. The views of others who are significant to her, such as her husband and children, have important effects upon the woman who is going through the menopause.

Verbalizing such fears does not remove them, but can help the woman to begin to deal with her fears and can help her realize that others have similar concerns. The nurse can help the patient to consider what her own attitudes are toward menopause and aging. Often the woman has not sufficiently delineated her own views on this matter. If her adolescent children think it silly for their mother to return to college or to a job, does she have to agree with them?

Alertness for symptoms of depression among menopausal women is essential for nurses who work with these patients in hospitals or in the community. Depression can be so incapacitating that the patient may be unable to carry on any of her usual activities, or it can lead to suicide. Be especially observant for such communication from the patient as:

- Feelings of worthlessness and uselessness
- Feelings of emptiness and hopelessness
- Lack of interest in others and in usual activities

If you observe such indications of serious depression, report them immediately, so that the patient can be referred promptly for psychiatric treatment. It is difficult to relate to depressed and withdrawn persons. Therefore, make a particular effort to make contact with the depressed patient and to show concern for her while the process of referral is going on and until she is receiving treatment for depression. Such concerned contact by the nurse can help prevent further deepening of depression and can help prevent suicide.

Treatment

There has been considerable discussion and some disagreement still exists among physicians concerning the use of supplementary estrogens for menopausal and postmenopausal women. Some physicians consider the postmenopausal state virtually a deficiency condition and believe that supplementary estrogens should be prescribed. Those who subscribe to this view believe that the woman's overall health will be improved by estrogen administration and that the incidence and severity of some diseases of later life, such as osteoporosis, can be lessened by long term estrogen therapy.

A more widely held view is that decisions concerning estrogen therapy must be individualized. Some of the questions the physician considers are whether by administering estrogens there is a possibility of stimulating the growth of cancer in the uterus or breast. A patient with a history of uterine or breast cancer is not treated with supplementary estrogen, and patients who do receive estrogen supplements are examined regularly for any sign of cancer of the uterus or breast. Some patients experience little discomfort at this period and do not require estrogen therapy. The primary consideration in therapy of menopause, according to physicians who advocate highly individualized treatment, is helping the woman to feel physically and emotionally well and to effectively carry out her roles as wife, mother, and worker. Estrogens, sedatives, tranquilizers or mood elevating drugs may sometimes be prescribed to alleviate symptoms.

The climacteric can be precipitated by the surgical removal of the ovaries or by the radiologic destruction of the ovarian function. Because of the suddeness of the artificially induced menopause, replacement therapy sometimes is given to supply the hormones of which the patient's body has been so abruptly deprived.

DISORDERS OF MENSTRUATION

Dysmenorrhea. Painful menstruation usually is idiopathic (primary dysmenorrhea) and no pathology is found. Mild symptoms are made more severe by fatigue, cold and tension. Premenstrual tension is common. Edema may be present and is sometimes treated by diuretics and a low sodium diet. In some women, discomfort is intensified by an emotional need for more satisfying human contacts. Others fear menstruation or are convinced that they really are sick during this time. Menstruation, by its regular occurrence, calls attention to one's femininity. One way of helping some women who have dysmenorrhea is to help them think through and accept the physiologic phenomena as part of their physical selves, a part that will be with them for more than 20 years. Dysmenorrhea is in some instances related to difficulty in accepting feminine identity and role.

The patient who suffers from dysmenorrhea should visit the doctor to uncover any possible pathology. If none is found, symptomatic relief can be given by the application of heat to the lower abdomen, a hot beverage, rest and, when ordered, aspirin or atropine. Primary dysmenorrhea is generally believed to be peculiar to ovulating women, and therefore appears to be related to progesterone in the second half of the menstrual cycle. Birth control pills, then, are sometimes prescribed to inhibit ovulation, thus relieving dysmenorrhea.

Dysmenorrhea may be secondary to other pathology such as endometriosis, displacement of the uterus, or narrowing of the cervical canal. For some conditions, exercises may be suggested by the doctor. For example, if dysmenorrhea is related to retroversion of the uterus (the uterus tilts backward), the knee chest position may be prescribed. Surgery may sometimes be necessary, as for example in severe endometriosis. However, every effort is made to preserve child-bearing function. The main consideration in therapy of dysmenorrhea is to help the woman feel well throughout her menstrual cycle so that she can continue her accustomed activities. For women in whom emotional difficulties seem to play a prominent part in causing the painful menses, psychotherapy may be helpful.

Amenorrhea, absence of menstrual flow, occurs normally before menarche, during pregnancy, after menopause, and sometimes throughout lactation if the new mother is breast feeding her baby. The term oligomenorrhea refers to infrequent menses. Oligomenorrhea and amenorrhea may be caused by endocrine imbalance, some tumors of the endocrine glands, wasting chronic disease (such as tuberculosis or starvation) and psychogenic factors. There are variations in the extent to which emotional reactions affect the menses. The woman who misses periods should see a gynecologist to determine the cause

Menorrhagia, excessive bleeding at the time of normal menstruation, may be caused by endocrine imbalance, fibroid tumors, emotional upsets, abnormalities of blood coagulation, ovarian cysts, uterine polyps, and a variety of other pelvic abnormalities. Unchecked menorrhagia can lead to anemia. Because the amount of blood loss is difficult to describe, a very rough estimate can be made by asking the patient how many pads or tampons she uses a day. Menorrhagia is a symptom that should bring the patient to a gynecologist.

Metrorrhagia, bleeding at a time other than a menstrual period, may consist of a slight pink or brownish spotting, or it may be frank bleeding. It can be caused by the same abnormalities that cause menorrhagia, or by various abnormalities in the vagina or cervix. Spotting may also occur in early pregnancy, and sometimes it is a warning symptom that abortion is imminent. Some women spot for a day or two midway between menstrual periods. This functional bleeding is thought to be at the time of ovulation and does not indicate pathology. However, metrorrhagia should always be brought to a doctor's attention, because it may be an early indication of cancer. Postcoital bleeding may be an early symptom of cancer of the cervix. It is not the amount of blood that is important; it is the fact that it occurred when no bleeding was expected. Nurses should explain the necessity for a visit to the physician, stressing the importance of an examination but making every effort not to frighten the patient. The nurse who shows concern for the patient and who is supportive in her approach is more likely to persuade the patient to visit the doctor than a nurse who uses scare techniques. Metrorrhagia may be difficult for the menopausal woman to identify if her periods have become irregular. Is the spotting a scanty menstrual flow or an abnormal symptom? When she is in doubt, she should consult a gynecologist, because intermenstrual bleeding is not a normal characteristic of the climacteric.

FERTILITY AND INFERTILITY

Sperm are manufatured in the testes, pass in tubules through the epididymis into the vas deferens and are discharged into the urethra and out of the body by rhythmic contraction of the muscles of the vas deferens and the penis during the sexual climax. The accumulated fluid carrying the spermatozoa is called *semen*. It is alkaline; spermatozoa are rapidly immobilized in an acid environment. In human males spermatozoa are produced continuously, even though they leave the body only periodically.

High in the fundus of the uterus are two openings for the fallopian tubes, along which ova travel from the ovaries to the uterus, and which sperm enter from the uterus. The tubes are about four inches long. After the ovum is shed from the ovary, movement of the cilia at the fimbriated end of the fallopian tube, and muscular contractions of the tube itself draw the ovum down toward the uterus. If the ovum is not fertilized it degenerates and is shed.

The volume of the normal semen ejaculate is 2.5 to 3.5 ml., in which there is an average of 100 million spermatozoa. For conception to occur, it is necessary for a spermatozoon to make its way, by movement of its taillike portion, up the entire length of the uterus and into the fallopian tube, to find an ovum, and to insert its

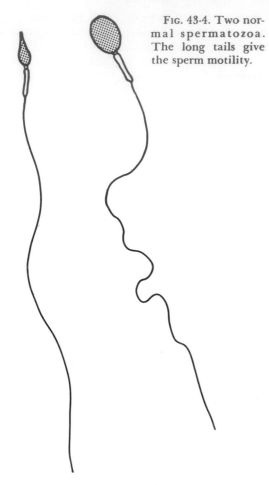

Fig. 43-4. Two normal spermatozoa. The long tails give the sperm motility.

head into the ovum by piercing the outer coat (zona pellucida). Although the actual fertilization is by one spermatozoon, it is probably necessary for more than one sperm to be present in order to dissolve the zona pellucida sufficiently to allow one spermatozoon to enter. Usually, there is only one ovum as a result of ovulation; it is probable that many spermatozoa find their way into the fallopian tubes.

Ovulation apparently occurs midway between menstrual periods, but in individuals there probably is variation in ovulation from month to month. Women are fertile, capable of becoming pregnant, soon after ovulation. A couple wishing to have a baby may be advised by their doctor to have intercourse every other day, from the 10th through the 16th day after the first day of the woman's menstrual period. Alternating days allows for sperm buildup. Couples wanting a baby may not know about ovulation, and they may limit sexual intercourse to the times just before and after menses, when conception is least likely to take place, thus inadvertently practicing rhythm control of conception.

Basal body temperature is useful but a far from infallible indication of when ovulation occurs. To determine it a woman takes her temperature when she first wakes up in the morning, before she drinks anything, smokes or arises. Near ovulation there is a slight drop from normal body temperature, followed by a rise of 0.3 to 0.5 of a degree within the first 24 hours after ovulation.

In about one half of the couples the reproductive difficulty lies with the male. The causes of sterility in men can be general debility, hypopituitarism, hypothyroidism, obesity, infection, absence of a genital organ, undescended testicles (even when they are corrected), orchitis after mumps, irradiation of the testes, and mental stress. Conception can occur when the sperm count is as low as 2,250,000 spermatozoa per milliliter of semen, but the chance of a sperm contacting an ovum is less than when the count is higher. In normal semen, 15 percent or less are nonmotile, and 20 percent or less are formed abnormally. When these percentages rise above 15 and 20 percent respectively, the chance of conception decreases.

Women, like men, may be infertile from systemic causes, or they may have problems interfering with normal ovulation such as a variety of endocrine disorders. Occluded tubes are a significant cause; gonorrheal, streptococcal or other infections can cause tubal strictures that prevent the ova from traveling down and the sperm cells from traveling up the tubes. Endometriosis is a common cause of infertility in women. In both men and women psychological factors sometimes play an important part in causing infertility.

Diagnosis

When a woman is unable to conceive after several years of married life, she and her husband should be examined by the doctor. He probably will give them a complete physical examination to rule out a possible systemic cause. A B.M.R. or PBI (protein-bound iodine) test may be given to determine thyroid function, and the urine may be examined for pituitary gland function. The husband may be examined first, because his examination is made more readily.

INFERTILITY TESTS

TEST	DESCRIPTION	COMMENT
Semen examination	The number, motility and shape of sperm cells from a fresh semen collection is examined under microscope.	1) Absence of sperm cells in *repeated* exams suggests infertility. 2) A low sperm count decreases the possibility of conception.
Testicular biopsy	Tissue is examined to see if sperm cells are being produced.	If sperm are being produced but are not present in the semen, the problem may be an obstructive lesion.
Rubin test	Carbon dioxide is forced through the uterus, the fallopian tubes and into the peritoneal cavity to check for occluded tubes.	In some instances the gas may blow out the obstruction resulting in fertility.
Sims-Huhner (postcoital)	Vaginal and cervical secretions are aspirated 6 to 12 hrs. after intercourse and examined microscopically.	The interreactions of the wife's secretions and the husband's sperm can be observed.
Hysterosalpingography	X-ray study of the uterus and fallopian tubes with radiopaque dye.	Bowel cleansing before the X-ray is usually ordered.
Endometrial biopsy	Microscopic examination of tissue shows whether or not the endometrium has been prepared for surgery.	Frequently done premenstrually or on first day of period. Also used to help diagnose cause of dysmenorrhea and amenorrhea.

Treatment

If a systemic disorder, such as endocrine imbalance or infection, is causing the infertility, the doctor will treat the underlying disorder. Tubal strictures may be treated by surgery, though the operation is rarely successful. Uterine displacement may be treated by the use of a pessary and exercise or by surgery.

In some infertile couples no physiologic defect can be found. There is a psychic factor in fertility that is poorly understood. Sometimes a pregnancy occurs only after the couple have given up hope of conceiving and have adopted a child.

Nurses can help the couple by making sure that they know how and when the ovum is fertilized so that intercourse is not avoided at the midpoint between menses. Does the woman douche immediately after intercourse? The woman whose doctor has advised her to douche, for whatever reason, or who feels that she must douche, should wait until the next morning to do it.

RELIGIOUS ATTITUDES TOWARD BIRTH CONTROL

Those of different religious faith have various beliefs concerning measures used to prevent conception. The doctor advises, the nurse helps, and the couple decide. They make their decision in the light of their own religious beliefs (the pastor helps) and of what they learned from the doctor after requesting information from him. Respect for the patient's convictions is fundamental here as in all relationships in nursing. The teachings of some of the religious groups in America concerning birth control are:

Church of Jesus Christ of Latter-Day Saints (Mormons). "The Church has always advocated the rearing of large families, and birth control, as commonly understood, is contrary to its teachings."[*]

Orthodox Judaism. Some authorities oppose any type of contraception, because it is "wasting of seed." In particular, the man is forbidden to do anything to render the sexual act incapable of producing children. Exceptions to this rule are allowed in times of famine and for some medical reasons.[†]

Reform Judaism. The Talmudic-Rabbinic Law is interpreted to mean that couples, and men in particular, have a duty to propagate

[*] Rosten, L. (ed.): *A Guide to the Religions of America,* New York, Simon and Schuster, 1955; Evans, R. L.: What is a Mormon?, *Look* Magazine 18:67–72, October 5, 1954.

[†] Jakobovits, I.: *Jewish Medical Ethics,* New York, Philosophical Library, 1959; Freehof, S. B.: *Reform Responsa,* Cincinnati, Hebrew Union College Press, 1960; Epstein, L. M.: *Sex Laws and Customs in Judaism,* New York, Block Pub. Co., 1948.

themselves ("Be fruitful and multiply"—Genesis 1:28); and that after a man has had two children there is no immorality in the use of birth control as long as both husband and wife consent. Exceptions to the rule to have children include danger to human life and instances in which the man is fertile, but his wife is sterile, or in which the man is engaged in all-absorbing religious work.‡

Catholicism. Traditional Catholic belief has been that artificial means of contraception are objectively evil. Whenever necessary, and whenever possible, periodic continence (i.e., rhythm) was considered the desirable means of controlling the transmission of life.

While the substance of their teachings has not fundamentally changed, the most recent instructions of the Pope's and national bishops' conferences have been strongly pastoral in content. Much has been written about the concept of "responsible parenthood," the obligation of couples themselves to decide upon the size of their families in terms of many personal and highly variable circumstances, e.g., health, financial conditions, emotional factors, and demographic considerations.

A great deal of recent Catholic literature has also dealt with the conflict of duties and other dilemmas faced by couples who try to limit the size of their families and who at the same time wish to fulfill the demands and rights of conjugal love. This in turn has led the Catholic hierarchy and theologians to give new emphasis to the role of individual conscience. Without diminishing the import of basic religious teachings, couples are expected to exercise their duty to make their own concrete moral decisions in these matters.

Since many aspects of this question are so much in a state of evolution, patients who are in a state of doubt should be referred to a priest for information and counseling.§

---

‡ *Central Conference of American Rabbis at Cape May, N.J.,* vol. 37, p. 369, New York, Central Conference of American Rabbis, 1927.

§ Bird, J., and Bird, L.: The Freedom of Sexual Love. New York, Doubleday, 1967; Curran, C. (ed.): Contraception: Authority and Dissent. New York, Herder and Herder, 1969; Egner, G.: Contraception vs. Tradition: A Catholic Critique. New York, Herder and Herder, 1966; Encyclical of Pope Paul VI: Humanae Vitae. New York, Paulist Press, 1968; McHugh, J. (ed.): Marriage in the Light of Vatican II. Washington, D.C., Family Life Bureau, U.S.C.C., 1968; Valsecchi, A.: Controversy: The Birth Control Debate, 1958-1968. Washington, Corpus Books, 1968.

Protestantism. The various Protestant denominations agree that limitation of conception is acceptable under certain circumstances. There may be differences in interpretation in regard to circumstances and methods. None would probably have argument with this statement: God has laid the responsibility on parents for family planning. The number and the frequency of children should be a responsible choice, with both parents agreeing. Some groups may approve of only abstinence as a method of birth control; most Protestant faiths sanction artificial contraception and rhythm. Motives, more than methods, are important in deciding morality. Responsible parenthood considers the needs and the rights of each child, social and economic situations, and the health and the welfare of the mother and the father.*

SUMMARY OF TEACHING POINTS

Some women may be reluctant to ask questions of a man, even a doctor, whereas they may feel more comfortable approaching a female nurse. Keep yourself approachable, but be gentle and tentative, especially if you meet resistance.

If the doctor has recommended taking a douche, the patient may not know how to do it and may be too shy to ask. The normal processes of menstruation or the menopause may not be understood. A woman may not know how conception takes place, or even how a baby is born. "Where does it come out?" is a question few would ask for fear of being laughed at. A woman who is ignorant may fear to ask questions that are important to her. Be prepared with the correct information. Make it easy for the patient to talk to you in privacy. Encourage her to express her ideas and to voice her questions.

A woman may believe that cleanliness demands that she take a douche after sexual relations and after menstruation. The normal healthy vagina ordinarily requires no vaginal irrigation; unnecessary douching may lead to irritation or infection and it should not be encouraged. A patient should consult her doctor about this. If douching is desirable for her, he

---

* Pike, J. A.: *If You Marry Outside Your Faith.* New York, Harper, 1954; *Responsible Parenthood—A Pronouncement—A Policy Statement of the National Council of the Churches of Christ in the U. S. A.,* Adopted by the General Board, February 23, 1961; Resolution 115, Encyclical Letter of the Lambeth Conference of Anglican Bishops, August 8, 1958.

will tell her so and advise what solution to use. In general douching is being used less and less in the treatment of various gynecologic disorders. In case the physician orders it, here is a review of some significant teaching points to remember:

• Douching at home is done best while the patient is lying down in the bathtub, since sitting on the toilet does not allow the solution to go up in the vagina, and doing it in bed is unnecessarily difficult. Pad the back of the tub with a towel for comfort.

• Teach the patient to insert the nozzle gently upward and backward, and to rotate it when the solution starts to flow.

• The distance should be measured, so that the receptacle of fluid hangs at a height of 12 to 18 inches and not from the top of the door or the shower curtain.

• If the patient has an infectious disease, the nozzle should be boiled between irrigations.

• Teach the patient to regulate the temperature carefully (105° F.) to avoid burning herself and to mix the solution correctly.

• As some solution may drip out after the patient stands up, she may wish to wait a half hour before getting dressed, to wear a pad for a few minutes, or to sit where she is for five or six minutes.

Two other common situations which require teaching among gynecologic patients are perineal care and sitz baths. Patients who have had surgery in the perineal region should have careful demonstrations of how to cleanse the area, particularly in relation to cleansing after a bowel movement. This teaching should begin as soon as the patient becomes ambulatory in the hospital, thus insuring that the patient uses acceptable technique while in the hospital, and later when she goes home. Show the patient how to cleanse from front to back, using disposable cotton pledgets or a disposable wash cloth. Although this technique is especially essential after any perineal surgery, it is an important hygienic measure for all women.

The sitz bath is recommended by the physician as an aid to comfort, healing and cleanliness. A helpful modification of the usual procedure is the use of plastic disposable basins for the sitz bath. The patient can take the basin home with her, making it easier for her to carry out the treatment at home.

The Woman Patient with a Disorder of the Reproductive System

44

Diagnostic Procedures • Dilatation of the Cervix and Curettage of the Uterus (D & C) • Abortion • Ectopic Pregnancy • Infections Endometriosis • Vaginal Fistulas • Relaxed Pelvic Muscles Uterine Displacement

Treatment of the gynecologic patient is undertaken with two objectives: to preserve or restore the woman's health, and to preserve her childbearing capacity, insofar as possible. The first objective is operative throughout the patient's life span; the second, until the woman has passed through the menopause.

Regardless of when pathology occurs, early diagnosis and medical attention are of the utmost value. The nurse familiar with normal function often can help to educate women about the importance of regular gynecologic examinations and the time to seek medical help.

It is very important to recognize that feelings are involved. A permissive atmosphere should be provided for the patient, so that she can come to grips herself with her own emotions. This kind of atmosphere is not achieved by ignoring the patient's feelings. Rather, be sensitive to expressions of anxiety (clear or subtle), and be calm and efficient, so that the patient can feel the security of being among professional people who know what they are doing. If a patient raises a great fuss over some minor procedure, do not cut her off. Perhaps this is her way of communicating the presence of different and more significant fears.

Let the patient know what to expect. A hysterectomy (without oophorectomy) will not cause a sudden menopause, although it is a common belief that it will. Patients may worry about this even though they do not discuss it, and many will

be grateful for an explanation of the terms they hear but cannot interpret.

Common operations for gynecologic disorders include:

Salpingectomy, unilateral, removal of one fallopian tube. It does not cause sterility, but bilateral salpingectomy does. Menses continue.

Hysterectomy, removal of the uterus. Menses stop; but because the ovaries are not removed, hysterectomy does not cause an artificial menopause.

Oophorectomy (ovariectomy), unilateral, removal of one ovary. It does not cause sterility. Bilateral oophorectomy causes sterility and induces an artificial menopause.

In many gynecologic diseases, sexual relations must be suspended; in some conditions, such as very radical surgery for cancer, they must be terminated. This necessity may have a profound effect on the relationship between husband and wife. In either instance, it may help if the doctor discusses this problem with the marital partner as well as with the patient to smooth the way for them to work it out together. Sometimes the nurse can help by suggesting that patient, husband, and physician discuss the matter together.

A youngster in her early adolescent years may be admitted to the gynecologic service of a hospital, perhaps for a dilatation and curettage to diagnose the cause of a delayed menarche. Because she is at an age when she is still forming attitudes about her bodily changes, she may be as embarrassed and upset as an adolescent can be. Spend some time with the young patient, and be sure that she has diversion for the times that she is alone—television, radio, books and some handwork.

Use discretion in choosing a young person's wardmates. Do not place her next to a patient with advanced cancer, or between two women who are likely to elaborate the details of their operations. Make a special effort to help the young patient to understand her condition. If the doctor has hurriedly mentioned to her, "You have an intact hymen," translate this statement, so that she does not imagine some gruesome disease. Be sure to explain procedures to the adolescent patient. It is bad enough to be embarrassed by what the doctor does. To fail to understand the reason for the examination or the procedure adds an unnecessary burden.

DIAGNOSTIC PROCEDURES

The Gynecologic Examination

Most women dread having a gynecologic examination. They are embarrassed about being examined. They fear not only exposure, but also what the doctor may find. The patient usually feels less embarrassed when the nurse moves and acts in a matter-of-fact fashion. It may help to answer an apprehensive patient who has told you that she is frightened or embarrassed by asking what it is which is frightening or embarrassing, and then finding ways, if you can, to lessen fear and embarrassment. For example, suppose the patient says she fears the pain of the examina-

tion. You can explain to her, and have her practice before the doctor arrives, the deep-breathing and muscle-relaxing measures which will lessen discomfort during the examination.

Preparing the Patient. Tell the patient that you will stay with her during the procedure. A nurse *always* remains in the room the *entire* time that a patient is being examined. Be sure that you have all the needed equipment so that you do not have to leave. Make sure to have a

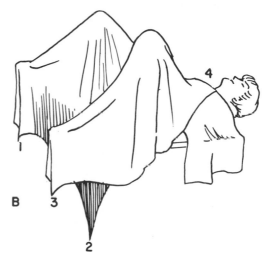

(B) The sheet is turned on the diagonal. One corner (4) is placed under the chin, the opposite corner (2) hangs down between the legs, and the other corners (1 and 3) go over each foot.

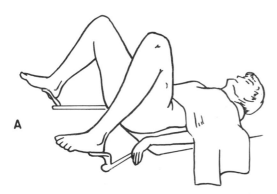

Fig. 44-1. Draping a patient in the lithotomy position.

(A) The patient is placed in this position while she is under a sheet (which was removed for this picture). Note that the patient's hips are right at the edge of the table.

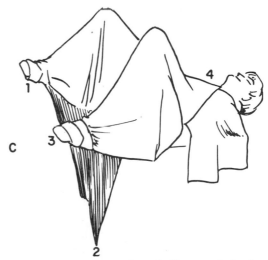

(C) Wrap corners (1) and (3) around the feet. When the physician is ready for the examination, corner (2) is folded up, and only the patient's vulva is exposed.

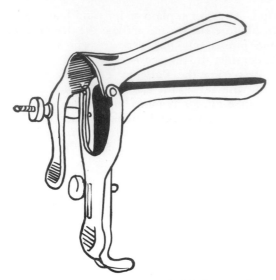

FIG. 44-2. A bivalve speculum. With the mouth of the speculum closed and well lubricated, the speculum is passed into the vagina. Then it is opened to give the doctor a clear view of the cervix. Specula come in various sizes.

speculum of the correct size for the patient. If in doubt, ask the physician before the examination begins. Also, inform the patient that the doctor will ask her questions about her menses: when they started, how frequently they occur, and how heavy the flow is. He will ask her about any pregnancies and perhaps about any vaginal discharge that she may have. Encourage the patient to give a full history.

Instruct the patient to remove her underclothes from her waist down and to loosen anything tight around her waist. Give her a sheet to wrap around her until she is positioned on the examining table. Ask the patient to void, for a full bladder may interfere with the examination. For example, a distended bladder may lead to confusion as to the presence or absence of an ovarian cyst or tumor.

The most common position for the gynecologic examination is the lithotomy position. It is uncomfortable for anyone to maintain. With a sheet around her, the patient sits at the edge of the examining table and lies back. The nurse helps the patient to lift both legs at the same time, and she places the feet in the stirrups. If the stirrups are metal, have the patient wear her shoes for a better grip and more even distribution of pressure on the soles of her feet. Now the nurse places her hands under the patient's buttocks or around the patient's thighs and helps

her slide right to the edge of the table. By draping the patient securely, you do more to reassure her that her modesty will be protected than by anything you say. Sims's and genupectoral (knee-chest) positions are used occasionally for this examination.

Although the vagina is not a sterile cavity, equipment is sterilized each time it is used, to prevent any introduction of pathogens. In addition, it is important, both for preventing infection and for aesthetic considerations, that the patient have a fresh sheet to lie on and that the doctor and the nurse wash their hands after examining a patient and before handling equipment in preparation for the next patient. The necessary equipment is listed in the hospital procedure manual. Have a bright spotlight set up behind the doctor's stool. On occasion, a flashlight held by an assistant will be used.

The Doctor's Examination. The order in which the physician performs various aspects of the pelvic examination varies. It is considered preferable for the physician to begin the examination by observation, first of the external genitalia and adjacent structures, and then of the vaginal walls and the cervix of the uterus through the bivalve speculum.

After examining the external genitalia and performing the visual examination of the vaginal walls and cervix through the speculum, the physician places one or two fingers of his gloved hand into the vagina. By palpation, he examines the structures beyond the orifice. Then, the physician performs the vaginal-abdominal examination. Without removing his gloved fingers from the vagina, he places the fingers of his other hand on the patient's lower abdomen. Between his two hands he can palpate the position, the size, and the contour of the uterus, the ovaries, and other pelvic structures. At the end of the examination the physician may place a gloved and lubricated index finger into the patient's rectum; he can reach as high as the level of the posterior surface of the uterus. The presence of hemorrhoids, fistulas, and fissures can be noted also.

Although the gynecologic examination is uncomfortable, the patient should not feel pain unless disease is present. The more relaxed the patient's lower abdominal muscles are, the better the doctor can palpate the internal organs. Breathing deeply through the mouth may help to relax the abdominal muscles. During the examination the nurse's place is with the pa-

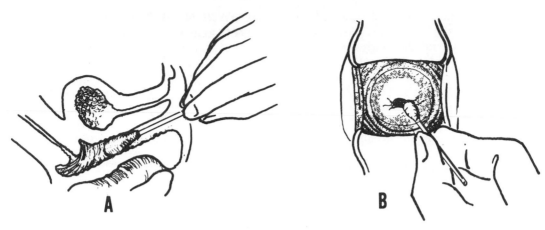

FIG. 44-3. The Papanicolaou test. (A) A vaginal smear can be taken with a cotton-tipped applicator. (B) An endocervical smear can be taken with a cotton-tipped applicator. The smears are spread on a glass slide.

tient—helping her to relax, preventing her from wriggling to the head of the table, talking to her, holding her hand if that seems to give comfort—and not beside the doctor peering through the speculum.

Nursing Care After the Examination. Clean the perineum of any lubricating jelly. Help the patient to slide her hips back from the edge of the table, remove both feet from the stirrups at the same time to prevent strain, and help her off the table. After she has been in the lithotomy position, she may wish to rest for a few moments on the stool or a chair before she gets dressed. Give her a tissue or gauze to wipe off the remaining lubricating jelly, and see that she gets a moment of privacy. Although the nurse wipes the perineum after the examination, the patient may prefer to finish the job. Provide her with a fresh sanitary pad, if she needs one, and the wrappings in which to dispose of the old one. Show her where to dispose of it, and where she may wash her hands. If the doctor used gentian violet, the patient will need a pad to prevent the dye from staining her underclothing. Considerations such as these smooth the way and convey acceptance and caring.

Rinse the used equipment in cold water to prevent secretions from sticking, then scrub it with soap and water, and resterilize it. Wash your hands after cleaning the perineum or touching used equipment. Keep your hands away from your face, especially, to protect your eyes from such infectious organisms as the gonococcus.

If the patient has a discharge, she should not douche before the examination. The doctor may want to see the discharge and to take a specimen for more detailed study.

Cytologic Test for Cancer (Papanicolaou Test)

This test provides a means by which cells that exfoliate may be examined for malignancy. Secretions from various body parts are studied microscopically to determine the presence of malignant cells. In gynecology, the test is used mainly to detect early cancer of the cervix, which is the most common form of malignancy of the reproductive tract in women.

Papanicolaou smears may be taken in the following manner. A small amount of secretion is aspirated from the posterior fornix with a vaginal pipet or an applicator and spread on a glass slide, which is not allowed to dry, but is immediately bathed in a solution of half 95 per cent alcohol and half ether. A solution called Spraycyte may be used instead. It comes in a pressurized bottle and is sprayed directly on the slide.

A cotton-tipped applicator is used to take an endocervical smear. One end of a forked wooden spatula or tongue blade is used to scrape the cervix.

The speculum used to expose the cervix is lubricated only with tap water, because lubricant may interfere with obtaining accurate results of the test.

The diagnosis of endometrial carcinoma is best achieved by dilatation of the cervix and curettage of the uterus (D & C); endometrial smears are another diagnostic measure used to determine the presence of carcinoma. These smears can be taken by use of a malleable cannula that is placed in the uterine cavity and attached to a syringe to aspirate the secretions. As is always the case, the slides are labeled with the source of the smear, the date and the patient's name, and sent to the laboratory. After this test the patient may have a cramped feeling that usually can be relieved by heat over the uterine area or by a mild analgesic. The patient should not bathe for at least two hours, or douche for two or three days before the test, because irrigation may remove the exfoliated cells.

Patients can be taught to obtain their own vaginal smears. Having patients take their own specimens and mail them to a laboratory for examination can increase the number of patients who benefit from this diagnostic test. Some physicians prescribe the test every six months; some, yearly.

Cervical Biopsy

Cervical biopsy is the usual follow-up when a cytologic test is positive or questionable. When the doctor suspects cancer, he may take a tiny piece of the cervix for laboratory examination. This procedure may be conducted in the doctor's office or in the clinic. Thus, preferably, it should be scheduled approximately one week after the cessation of the patient's monthly menstrual flow, when the cervix is least vascular. The patient may have some discomfort, but the procedure is not painful, since the cervix does not have pain receptors. A biopsy forceps is used to obtain the specimen. The specimen, properly labeled, should go to the laboratory in a bottle of 10 per cent formalin or wrapped in a wet saline sponge and waxed paper.

After the biopsy has been taken, bleeding may require additional treatment, such as use of packing. Have the patient rest before she leaves for home. If packing was inserted into the vagina, the patient should be instructed not to remove it until the prescribed number of hours has passed (usually 24). Instruct her to avoid unusual physical strain and heavy lifting for the remainder of the day.

Most patients have slight bleeding for a day. Tell the patient to call the doctor or to return to the clinic if there is serious bleeding. Because of the danger of bleeding and infection, the patient should be instructed not to douche, have sexual intercourse or use tampons until the physician says that she may.

DILATATION OF THE CERVIX AND CURETTAGE OF THE UTERUS (D & C)

Dilatation here refers to expansion of the mouth of the cervix; *curettage* means scraping the lining of a cavity (in this instance the endometrium). This common gynecologic operation often is performed to find the cause of abnormal bleeding and, also, to examine the patient for the presence of malignancy and fibroid tumors. (The scrapings are sent to the laboratory for investigation.)

D & C may be done as part of an investigation of the cause of sterility. In this instance it is performed before menstruation. When the scrapings, which are sent to the laboratory along with the date of the last menstrual period, are examined microscopically, the physician can determine whether ovulation occurred during this menstrual cycle, the adequacy of the endometrial lining, and the state of hormonal balance. Cervical dilatation is performed initially to permit uterine curettage, though it is done also to relieve stricture or stenosis of the cervical orifice, to permit tubal insufflation and, in selected instances, to relieve dysmenorrhea. It is done in the operating room, under a general anesthetic, with the patient in the lithotomy position. Curettage is usually avoided when vagina, cervix or fallopian tubes are infected, because of the danger of spreading the infection.

Preoperative and Postoperative Care (D & C)

Preparation for a dilatation and curettage includes care similar to that of any patient about to receive general anesthesia: food and fluids are withheld for 12 hours prior to surgery; rest, skin cleansing, and safety precautions are important. Opinions concerning whether the patient's vulva and perineum should be shaved prior to D & C vary among different gynecologists.

An enema is usually ordered. Because of their proximity to the operative area, special care is taken to make sure that bladder and lower bowel are empty on the morning of surgery. If the patient has lost a significant amount of blood—for example, during an incomplete abortion—a transfusion will be started. This is unusual, however.

When the patient returns from the operating room or the recovery room, she may be wearing a perineal pad, but probably she will not have a belt to hold it in place. Provide her with a belt or a T-binder to keep the pad in place for comfort and to prevent the sheets from being soiled. She will have a serosanguineous discharge for several days. Packing may be placed within the vagina and the cervical canal. Postoperatively, the nurse should investigate the perineal site and note the drainage on the perineal pad. Immediately after surgery the pad should be observed every 15 or 20 minutes for the first two or three hours. Perineal pads should be used while the packing is in place. Packing is infrequently used now after D & C. When it is used, it is removed after one or two days.

Check for voiding. Chart time and amount of the first voiding. However, voiding problems are usually minimal following D & C. Patients allowed to be out of bed the day of surgery usually void without any difficulty.

Because the cervix is dilated, sexual relations, douching, and tub baths should be avoided until the physician says they may be resumed. The patient should know that her menstrual period may be delayed and that a vaginal discharge may be present during her convalescent period.

Perineal Care. As long as there is sufficient vaginal discharge to warrant a perineal pad, perineal care should be given, whether or not it is ordered by the doctor. The technic will vary from hospital to hospital, but the principles remain the same: keep the area clean and the patient comfortable. A clean rather than a sterile technic is considered adequate in many instances (before going ahead with perineal care or teaching the patient to do it, you would find out which technic is required). Many hospitals use a disposable washcloth, especially for ambulatory patients.

In some hospitals perineal care is given as a warm sitz or tub bath. The tub bath, relaxing in itself, is often preferred by the patients. Of course, the tub is scrupulously cleaned between patients. In some hospitals individual disposable basins are used for sitz baths. To many patients, perineal irrigation is particularly comfortable. Sterile or clean water, 100° to 105° F., is poured over the vulva from a pitcher no higher than six inches over the patient. The perineum can be dried with sterile cotton balls or a clean washcloth, depending on the technic used.

The nurse should give perineal care during at least the first 48 postoperative hours. Giving perineal care affords the nurse an excellent opportunity to observe the surgical area. Perineal care always should be done after a bowel movement and after voiding. No patient with sutures should give herself perineal care. She cannot see the area, and a piece of cotton or washcloth might catch on a suture and pull it, or stay there and induce infection. Also, the perineal area with sutures deserves the nurse's direct observation several times a day. Likewise, when packing is in the vagina the nurse should give the perineal care, being especially careful not to dislodge the packing. Embarrassment of the patient can often be minimized by draping, ensuring privacy, and by sure movements.

ABORTION

Abortion is the termination of a pregnancy before the fetus is viable. The term *abortion* is used to designate interruption of pregnancy before the fetus weighs more than 500 Gm. (about 20 weeks of gestation). Between this time and a full-term delivery, the expulsion of the fetus is referred to as a *premature birth*.

Types of Abortion

Spontaneous Abortion. About 10 per cent of all pregnancies result in spontaneous abortion ("miscarriage" is the layman's term), usually before the 12th week. (The nurse might keep in mind when talking to patients that some people associate the word *abortion* only with criminal abortion, and for them "miscarriage" may be more acceptable.) Abnormalities of the fertilized ovum or the placenta, inconsistent with life, are believed to be the most frequent cause. Maternal disease, such as a severe acute infection, endocrine imbalance or a chronic wasting disease, may be a cause. Physical trauma rarely causes abortion; emotional trauma may cause it.

Abnormal uterine bleeding in any woman during her childbearing years may indicate an abortion in the early weeks of gestation—so early in her pregnancy that she is unaware that she was pregnant. Pain and bleeding are common symptoms. The pain may be so mild that it is disregarded or as severe as labor pains. Bleeding may range from spotting to hemorrhage. Generally, spontaneous abortion occurs six weeks or so after the fetus has died.

Threatened Abortion. Bleeding or spotting may indicate that abortion is threatened. Other signs may be cramps or backache. Only about half the women who have these symptoms lose their babies; in the others the pregnancy may proceed entirely normally.

Incomplete Abortion. Some of the products of the pregnancy are expelled, and some (usually a portion of the placenta) are retained. Incomplete separation of the placenta from the uterine wall causes hemorrhage. In a *complete abortion* all of the products of conception are expelled.

Missed Abortion. The fetus dies, but is not expelled. It may be retained two months or longer.

Therapeutic Abortion. Such an abortion is induced by a physician for medical reasons. The decision to terminate a pregnancy usually is made by more than one physician, and the husband is consulted as well as the patient. Some religions, such as the Roman Catholic, forbid therapeutic abortion despite the relaxation or absence of legal restrictions. State laws are changing, and it is essential for the nurse to keep abreast of the laws in her state which pertain to therapeutic abortion. In some states therapeutic abortion is permitted only when the life of the mother is at stake. In some states newer laws include the following as a basis for therapeutic abortion: threats to the mother's health, pregnancy resulting from rape or incest, severe psychiatric disturbance of the mother, and the likelihood of the child being born with serious abnormalities (as may occur, for example, if the mother had German measles during the first trimester).

Criminal Abortion. This is the illegal termination of pregnancy. Women who seek this procedure usually either attempt it themselves by taking large amounts of drugs, and thus run the risk of poisoning themselves (this approach almost always fails to empty the uterus), or put themselves in unskilled hands for a crude curettage. There are three outstanding dangers to the latter procedure: rupture of the uterus, infection and hemorrhage. Women who consider criminal abortion may be helped by counseling and by referral to a social service agency such as the Florence Crittenton League and the Salvation Army. These are examples of agencies to which an unmarried pregnant woman can turn with the assurance of anonymity. These agencies offer social case workers, shelter during the last months of pregnancy, obstetrical service and, when desired, adoption facilities.

When you are caring for a patient who has entered the hospital for the treatment of a complication of criminal abortion, it is helpful to recognize your own feelings about the situation. It is all right to feel however you do, but the patient needs to be treated only as a patient (and she may be very ill). This patient probably will be in extreme need of an emotionally low-pitched, non-judging environment, and of nurses who are concerned for her welfare and who convey to the patient a feeling of being accepted and cared for.

Habitual Abortions. Such abortions occur repeatedly without apparent cause. Bed rest and hormonal therapy have helped some women who habitually abort to carry a fetus to term. Emotional support can be an important factor in helping the patient carry the baby to term. If abortion does occur, support from the physician and nurse can assist the patient to deal with the loss of her baby. The fear of being unable to carry a baby to term is very common among women who have once suffered a spontaneous abortion.

Treatment

A pregnant woman should report the first signs of a vaginal discharge, bleeding or cramps to her doctor. He probably will advise bed rest and a light diet, and warn her against any straining, such as when she moves her bowels. She should save all formed vaginal discharges for the doctor to examine. The doctor may order a sedative or a tranquilizer to help her rest quietly. If the bleeding stops, he may allow her out of bed in several days, but only for quiet activity. If abdominal pain becomes severe or uterine bleeding increases, abortion may be imminent, and the doctor probably will hospitalize the patient. An incomplete abortion is treated by curettage. The patient may enter the hospital bleeding profusely. Typing and cross matching are done, and an infusion is started. Sometimes a transfusion is necessary. In missed abortion the uterus usually is allowed to empty itself. Occasionally it is necessary to remove the dead fetus. In incomplete abortion, drugs such as oxytocin and ergonovine are frequently used to make the uterus contract and to control bleeding.

Nursing Care

The nursing care after an abortion is similar to that given after a D & C or that given any time after the cervix has been dilated. Perineal care is given as long as there is a discharge; because the cervix is dilated, the patient should not have douches or sexual intercourse.

If the abortion is threatening, there is the possibility that a quiet stay in bed will save the baby. If the abortion is imminent, or incomplete, bed rest will prevent the increase of bleeding by activity. The patient should be observed carefully and repeatedly for hemorrhage. Save all large clots and tissue for the doctor to examine. The patient should not use the toilet; instead, she should use the bedpan to avoid passing the fetus or the placenta unnoticed. If the patient begins to have cramps, inform the doctor immediately.

A patient with a threatened abortion may remain on bed rest for a long period of time. A few women spend the major part of the nine months in bed, although they may not be in the hospital for the entire time. Many of these women carry the infant to term, but the husband or a relative has to take care of the household. For a woman who wants a baby, the suspense of a threatened abortion is very difficult, but she is usually motivated to follow the prescribed treatment, including bed rest, if necessary. She may be resentful that other women are able to carry a baby without having to stay in bed. She may feel guilty because she has to be waited on and cannot contribute to the work of the household. Because she has little exercise in bed, her diet should be light but nutritionally sound.

A woman who has aborted may grieve over the lost baby. Her emotional reaction will be governed by many factors; for example, it will make a great difference whether the patient is 20 years old or nearing the end of her childbearing period. If she seems bitter over losing the baby, encourage her to recognize this emotion. She will still be angry, but being listened to will give her some relief. If there is likelihood that the patient can again become pregnant, the physician explains this to her. Although knowledge that she is likely to conceive again does not take away the loss of the fetus, it can help the patient deal with her grief and begin to look forward to becoming pregnant again.

ECTOPIC PREGNANCY

This term refers to the implantation of the fertilized ovum outside the uterus. The fallopian tubes are the most common ectopic site, but implantation may occur elsewhere, such as in the abdominal cavity. The fetus starts to develop just as it would in the uterus. In most cases the patient has all the classic signs of pregnancy. In addition, she may complain of spotting and pain in the lower abdomen.

Because there is so little room for expansion in the tube, the enlarging fetus and the placenta will rupture it. The diagnosis of a tubal pregnancy is rare until rupture occurs. The patient has a sudden, sharp pain, and often she is admitted to the hospital in severe shock from hemorrhage. Profuse bleeding occurs both vaginally and into the abdominal cavity. The patient is taken immediately to the operating room, and a salpingectomy is usually performed. Preparing the patient for the operating room has to be accomplished with speed. Treatment for shock and hemorrhage is instigated immediately. Blood transfusions are given as soon as blood typing and cross matching are done.

After the operation, careful and frequent observation of vital signs is imperative, until they are well stabilized. The nature and the quantity of the vaginal discharge should be noted and perineal care given as long as there is any vaginal discharge. Preoperative bleeding into the abdominal cavity may cause peritonitis postoperatively; therefore, abdominal pain, nausea and vomiting should be reported to the physician. The rupture of a tubal pregnancy is a sudden and shocking event not only for the patient, but also for the family. The patient probably will need some time postoperatively to assimilate the experience and to accept the fact that she has lost the baby.

INFECTIONS

Vaginitis

The normal acidity of the vaginal secretion at maturity (pH 3.5 to 4.5) is a natural defense against infection. Nevertheless, a variety of pathogenic organisms can invade and infect the vagina—most commonly the protozoon *Trichomonas vaginalis* and the fungus *Candida albicans*, and certain bacterial species.

An abnormal vaginal discharge is a prominent symptom of vaginal infection. It may be copious and malodorous, and often it is irritating, causing itching and redness of the perineum and the anus. If the mouth of the urethra is affected, the patient may have urinary symptoms, such as burning on urination and the feeling that she has to void frequently. Also, there may be some discomfort in the lower abdominal region. In contrast with an abnormal discharge, a normal vaginal discharge has little odor and is colorless.

Normal vaginal discharge changes in character and amount during the menstrual cycle, usually becoming more noticeable at ovulation and before menses. It varies from clear to cloudy.

Trichomonas vaginitis can cause a white, frothy, highly irritating leukorrhea, and candida infection can cause a leukorrhea that has the consistency of cottage cheese and itches intensely.

The patient often is treated as an outpatient. Diagnosis of trichomonas vaginitis is made upon microscopic examination of the vaginal secretions. The patient should not douche before the examination, since washing away the secretions will prevent the doctor from noting their characteristics and from taking an adequate smear. After determining the cause of the infection the doctor may swab the infected area with a cleansing solution, using cotton balls on a Kelly clamp. A vaginal jelly or suppository may then be inserted, or tampons may be prescribed to absorb the discharge. A sulfonamide cream may be given intravaginally to combat streptococcal or staphylococcal infection. Douches are sometimes ordered for cleansing and esthetic reasons. Döderlein's bacillus, by favoring the production of lactic acid, serves to maintain an acid medium as a natural defense mechanism. Trichomonas prefers an alkaline climate. Oral beta-lactose may be ordered. Flagyl, a specific drug for the treatment of trichomonas vaginitis, is taken orally. A treatment course may be ordered for ten days. Mycostatin is another drug frequently prescribed. Intravaginal creams also may be employed. When a vaginal cream is prescribed its use is continued through the menstrual period, because this is a time when the secretions become more alkaline.

Monilial vaginitis, caused by the fungus *Candida albicans,* is a common infection during pregnancy and after antibiotic treatment for other reasons (the antibiotics destroy the normal vaginal flora). It also is frequent in diabetics whose urine contains sugar (the monilial fungus is supported by carbohydrates), and occasionally this infection is seen after long-term corticosteroid therapy. A marked increase in the incidence of monilial vaginitis has accompanied the use of oral contraceptives.

Nystatnin (Mycostatin), an antibiotic fungicide, may be given orally and in suppositories, one at bedtime for 15 nights. When the perineum is badly irritated, Mycostatin ointment may be prescribed to be applied locally t.i.d. If the patient has diabetes, the elimination of glycosuria through the control of the diabetes is an aspect of the treatment. Gentian violet may be painted onto the vaginal mucosa several times a week. After the medication is applied, the doctor may insufflate the vagina with cornstarch or other drying powders, since the infecting organisms thrive better in a moist environment than a dry one.

Teaching a Patient the Aspects of Treatment and Self-Care. Before the patient leaves for home, be sure that she understands every detail of what she needs to do. In most instances, the treatment will be performed by the patient at home. Can she obtain the vaginal suppository if one is ordered? Does she know that she should wash her hands before inserting a vaginal suppository? Does she know that she should be in the dorsal recumbent position, use her longest finger and aim up and back, toward the posterior fornix? Some suppositories and creams come with long applicators that the patient may not know how to insert. She needs to learn how to hold the applicator, to lie down on a bed with her hips elevated on a pillow, how to insert the applicator and to stay in this position for 10 to 15 minutes when cream or suppository is used so that it will melt and the dissolving medication will cover the vaginal vault. A good way to use a vaginal suppository is to insert it in bed upon retiring. It probably will not dislodge and will melt during the night. The next morning a perineal pad may be worn, or a tampon inserted instead if the pad is irritating to the already infected perineum. When douches form a part of the treatment they should be used before insertion of the suppository.

Vaginitis can be stubborn and discouraging. Vigorous early treatment may overcome its tendency to become chronic. At best, the patient can expect at least six weeks of treatment before she is cured. At worst, vaginitis persists for years, recurring at the very moment when it appears to be cured. Patients with long-term vaginitis are understandably discouraged. They are tired of the malodorous discharge, of wearing perineal pads every day of the month, of going to the doctor for treatment.

Be available if the patient needs someone to talk to about her vaginitis, or if she needs to talk with someone who is not involved in her family life about how to set up a more healthful regimen for herself. The fact of having a discharge is in itself upsetting, and to many it suggests uncleanliness. An infection of the genital area is often linked with venereal disease, even if it is not venereal. The patient may ask whether or not it is infectious and a hazard to her family; and if it is not a venereal disease, what is it? The patient may ask whether she should use the same toilet seat as the rest of the family. Most infections are not transmitted this way. Of course, if some discharge drops on the seat, she would wash it off with soap, water and some antiseptic cleansing agent.

Perineal Pruritus

For obvious reasons, there is no worse place to itch than the perineum. Itching of the perineum can be caused by a deficiency of vitamin A (especially in older women who do not eat enough butter, milk and yellow vegetables); an irritating vaginal discharge; sugar in the urine of those with uncontrolled diabetes mellitus (diabetic vulvovaginitis); uncleanliness; leukoplakia; urinary incontinence; an inflammatory skin disease or local skin infection such as moniliasis, scabies and pediculosis pubis. Allergic reactions to fabric or dye can produce or contribute to the pruritus, which is a symptom, not a specific disease. It is seen in many genital conditions, both in the presence and in the absence of a vaginal discharge.

The treatment is directed at the underlying cause. Obese patients are especially prone to suffer pruritus, because as they walk the skin surfaces rub against each other. In such cases a light dusting with cornstarch may help to decrease the friction. Itching may be severe. If the patient must scratch, the chance of infection can be minimized by keeping the hands clean and not using the nails. The doctor may approve of cold or hot compresses or applications of calamine lotion to help to relieve the itching. Clothing should be light and nonrestrictive. Girdles or pants with long legs keep the skin surfaces separated and are a great comfort, especially in hot weather.

Cervicitis

Cervicitis (inflammation of the cervix) may be caused by a number of infectious organisms. Streptococcal and staphylococcal infections are common, especially after childbirth, when the organisms are able to enter the cervical tissue through small lacerations. Gonorrhea is a frequent cause of cervicitis, and cases from this cause have increased alarmingly in recent years. Cervicitis also may be caused by a change in the pH of the cervical secretions (which are normally alkaline pH 7.5 to 8). Cervicitis also may be due to cancer, and it is thought that the constant irritation of chronic cervicitis from any cause can lead to cancer.

Inflammation can cause erosion of cervical tissue, which may cause spotting or bleeding. Leukorrhea is the prominent symptom. There may be *dyspareunia* (painful sexual intercourse) or slight staining after sexual intercourse. Early cervicitis may fail to show any symptoms at all. A severe cervicitis may cause a sensation of weight in the pelvis. Unless acute cervicitis is treated promptly, it has a tendency to become chronic and difficult to cure. Examination of the cervix six weeks after giving birth, in addition to regular gynecologic examination for all women, is important in discovering the condition before it becomes chronic.

Treatment and Nursing Care. Acute cervicitis may be treated with douches and antibiotics locally and systemically. Chronic cervicitis may be treated with electrocautery. The procedure is usually done in the doctor's office or the clinic five to eight days after the end of the menstrual period. The patient is put in lithotomy position, a vaginal speculum inserted, and the cervix painted with an antiseptic. The nurse should be sure that the doctor has a good light. He may first take a biopsy for a microscopic examination for cancer cells. The eroded tissue is touched with a thin electrical rod, burning strips around the mouth of the cervix, destroying any cysts present. Usually no anesthesia is used, since there is no pain. If the cautery blade is inserted into the cervical canal, there may be a momentary cramping sensation.

For a day or two after electrocautery the patient should rest more than usual. No straining or heavy lifting should be undertaken. If slight bleeding occurs, the doctor may advise bed rest. Frank bleeding should bring the patient back to the doctor. Cervical or vaginal packing, or electric coagulation of the bleeding vessel, may be necessary. Be sure that the patient knows to expect a gray-green slough (discharge) for about three weeks after cautery. The discharge is watery at first, and then as the burned tissues become necrotic, the discharge becomes malodorous. Slight bleeding may occur about the 11th day. The doctor will wish to re-examine the cervix two to four weeks later. Dilatation is done if there is cervical stenosis. Sexual relations should not be resumed until the doctor gives his approval. Healing takes six to eight weeks.

Severe chronic cervicitis may be treated by *conization* (removal of the diseased portion of the cervical mucosa). The procedure is done with an electric instrument that simultaneously cuts tissue and coagulates the bleeding area. The patient usually is hospitalized, but not always, and anesthesia may or may not be given.

As with cautery, approximately six to eight weeks are required for healing. The follow-up visits (usually about every two weeks) to the doctor are most important, so that he may observe the patency of the cervix. Successful treatment eliminates the distressing leukorrhea, may aid fertility and eliminates the constant irritation.

Pelvic Inflammatory Disease (P.I.D.)

This is a term used to describe an inflammatory disorder of the plevic organs (except the uterus). There may be inflammation of the ovaries (oophoritis) or of the fallopian tubes (salpingitis); pus in the fallopian tubes (pyosalpinx); inflammation of the pelvic vascular system or of any of the pelvic supporting structures.

Infection may enter these structures through the vagina, the peritoneum, the small gap between the tubes and the ovaries, the lymphatics, or the bloodstream. The most frequent cause is the gonococcus, although other organisms, such as streptococci and staphylococci, may also cause it.

P.I.D. caused by the tubercle bacillus spreads most frequently by the bloodstream, and it may occur years after the primary lesion in the lungs has become inactive. The patient with tuberculous P.I.D. may have night sweats, weight loss and an afternoon rise in temperature. Antituberculosis drugs are usually ordered. Tuberculosis is not often found now in these organs, since chemotherapy helps to control the primary pulmonary infection.

Symptoms of P.I.D. may include a malodorous discharge that is infectious and should be handled with care by both patient and nurse to prevent spread of the disease. There may be backache, severe or aching abdominal and pelvic pain, a bearing-down feeling, fever, nausea and vomiting, menorrhagia, and dysmenorrhea. Pain may be felt during sexual intercourse or a pelvic examination. Severe infection may cause urinary symptoms or constipation.

The patient with acute pelvic inflammatory disease usually is hospitalized and kept in bed. Often the bed is adjusted to a semisitting position to facilitate pelvic drainage and to help prevent the extension of the infection upward. Antibiotics usually are administered, and warm lower abdominal applications may be ordered. Heat improves the circulation to the area. Warm sitz baths may be given. The tub should be well scrubbed afterward to prevent the spread of infectious organisms. Douching is usually avoided because there is danger that the infection will be spread by it.

If there is leukorrhea, the perineal pad should be changed frequently. Wrap it in paper before discarding it, or provide the patient with bags in which to deposit it. Be sure that the patient, and any auxiliary personnel who care for her, wash their hands well after changing the perineal pad. When there is copious discharge, perineal care should be given each time that the pad is changed, and after the patient uses the bedpan. When the causative organism is particularly infectious, as in gonorrhea, the patient is placed on isolation precautions, and whoever gives the patient perineal care should wear gloves. Amount, color, odor and appearance of the discharge should be recorded daily on the nurse's notes. Tampons should not be used, because they may obstruct the flow of discharge. If the infectious process of P.I.D. is not treated early, it may localize and form an abscess.

One way of preventing pelvic inflammatory disease is early medical attention to such symptoms of infection in the genital or urinary tracts as a feeling of pressure in the pelvic area, burning on urination and leukorrhea. Early treatment may prevent the infection from moving up the genital tract. When early treatment of acute pelvic inflammatory disease is delayed or inadequate, the infection may become chronic.

After discharge from the hospital the patient should refrain from sexual intercourse as long as leukorrhea or any other abnormality exists, since intercourse tends to extend the infection and may also infect the husband's genitourinary tract.

Puerperal Infection

Puerperal infection is the term given to an infection, usually streptococcal or staphylococcal, which follows childbirth. The infection often centers in the endometrium, but it may spread anywhere in the pelvic and peritoneal cavities. It can cause generalized sepsis after entry of the organisms into the bloodstream. Puerperal infection is a grave danger of criminal abortion during which unsterile instruments are used. The retention of bits of the placenta after a normal delivery provides a good culture medium for pathogenic organisms. Also, rupture of the membranes several days before delivery, postpartum thrombophlebitis, and delivery of a baby under unsterile conditions may lead to puerperal infection. Careful technic to prevent infection is extremely important once the patient's membranes have ruptured.

The patient with a puerperal infection is febrile and, if the endometrium is involved, she will have tenderness in the area and a vaginal discharge. Antibiotics or sulfonamides are given to combat the infection. If there is retention of placental fragments, D & C is performed. In bed the patient is placed in a semisitting position. Change of position is encouraged to facilitate pelvic drainage and to help to prevent thrombophlebitis in the legs. The patient is usually given a supportive, high vitamin diet. Thorough handwashing by the personnel caring for the patient is necessary before and after any procedure in which the genital area is touched. Frequent perineal care and change of the vaginal pad provide some comfort to the patient and help to prevent extension of the infection.

ENDOMETRIOSIS

This is a condition in which tissue that histologically and functionally resembles that of the endometrium is found outside of the uterus—most frequently on the ovaries, commonly elsewhere in the pelvic cavity, and occasionally in the abdominal cavity. Endometrial tissue has been reported even in the thigh and the forearm. The ectopic tissue apparently responds to estrogen, and perhaps also to progesterone, stimulation. It menstruates when the uterus does, and it shrivels after menopause and may regress during pregnancy. Endometriosis is serious, since the tissue bleeds into spaces that have no outlets. The free blood causes pain and adhesions. During menstruation, dysmenorrhea may be severe and bleeding copious. The fallopian tubes may be occluded, causing sterility. If the endometrial tissue is enclosed in an ovarian cyst (chocolate cyst) there is no outlet for the monthly bleeding. Occasionally the cyst ruptures, spilling its old blood and endometrial cells into the pelvic or the abdominal cavity. There may be menorrhagia, metrorrhagia, dyspareunia and pain on defecation.

This condition is relieved by menopause: natural, surgical, or radiologic. However, because it is a disease of women in their childbearing years, an artificially induced menopause raises many problems. Surgical treatment often is designed to remove the cysts and as much of the ectopic tissue as possible, and to free the adhesions caused by bleeding, without destroying the childbearing function. Endometriosis that is widespread throughout the pelvic organs may necessitate extensive surgery, such as panhysterectomy (removal of the uterus, both fallopian tubes and ovaries). Sterility of course results. One aspect of medical management is to give the patient hormones to keep her in a nonbleeding phase of her menstrual cycle for a prolonged time, such as nine months. Sometimes this therapy controls the ectopic tissue, so that the patient is symptom-free for several years. Small doses of testosterone (5 mg. a day) may relieve the symptoms without making the patient infertile. Synthetic oral progestins prevent ovulation while the patient is taking the hormone, but pregnancy can occur when the drug is discontinued. Large doses are required to prevent break-through bleeding. Norethynordrel (Enovid) and norethindrone (Ortho-Novum) are two such synthetic hormones. Patients taking these drugs may experience nausea, vomiting and diarrhea. Taking the tablets with food may reduce the nausea. Breasts may become tender, and there may be dizziness, weight gain and stomach cramps. Patients should be taught good leg care (such as not using round garters, not sitting for long periods with legs crossed, and using supportive stockings if there are varicosities), because these synthetic hormones may cause thrombo-embolic phenomena. If the patient notices vaginal bleeding during hormonal therapy, she should notify the doctor. The dosage may need to be increased.

Benign Tumors of the Uterus

Myomas (fibroids) growing in the uterine wall are the most common tumor of the female pelvis. The development of these tumors is believed to be stimulated by estrogen. They may be small or large, single or multiple. Growth is usually slow except during pregnancy. Fibroid tumors can occur in various locations in the uterus: subserous, intramural, and submucous. The latter are most frequently associated with excessive menstrual bleeding.

Sometimes, this benign tumor causes no symptoms, and the woman is unaware of its existence. When there are symptoms, menorrhagia is the most common. Also, the patient may have a feeling of pressure in the pelvic region, dysmenorrhea, anemia (from loss of blood), and malaise.

The treatment of benign uterine tumors is governed by a number of factors. An asympto-

Ovarian Cysts and Tumors

Ovarian Cysts	Comments	Treatment
Follicular cysts	Caused by retention of fluid, they are often symptomless and may disappear.	Usually no treatment is required; needle aspiration or surgical excision may be required.
Corpus luteum cysts	These cysts form when the corpus luteum fails to regress after the discharge of the ovum.	Surgical excision of the corpus luteum may be necessary; the rest of the ovary can usually be saved.

Ovarian Tumors	Comments	Treatment

Benign:
  Serous
  pseudomucinous
  Fibroma
  Cystic teratoma
  (dermoid)
	May cause cessation of menstruation, hirsutism, atrophy of the breasts, sterility.	Surgical removal of tumor, occasionally oophorectomy; reversal of sexual changes follows.

Malignant	May cause (1) pressure on the bladder leading to frequency and urgency or (2) pressure on the portal blood vessel leading to ascites. In the late stages there is weight loss, severe pain and G.I. symptoms.	Panhysterectomy Deep X-ray therapy Chemotherapy

matic tumor in a woman who wishes to have children usually is watched closely by her gynecologist, but it is not treated. The patient is reexamined every three to six months. A Papanicolaou smear is taken at least once a year.

When the patient has had abnormal bleeding, she may be admitted to the hospital, and a D & C may be performed to determine the cause of the bleeding, which may be a coexisting condition, unrelated to the fibroid. Sometimes, a curettage is performed to control the bleeding. Although it does not remove the tumor, it preserves the uterus, and it may make immediate, more extensive surgery unnecessary. Surgical removal of the tumor (myomectomy), which also preserves the uterus, may be performed. These operations are done only when the doctor feels sure that the tumor is benign. Further surgery in the future often is required—if possible, after the patient's family is complete. A hysterectomy is performed when the symptoms are severe and incapacitating. Myomectomy or hysterectomy may be done through a vaginal or an abdominal approach. If the patient is a poor operative risk, and the symptoms are extreme, the tumor may be treated by radiation. The disadvantage of irradiation is that it brings about an artificial menopause, which surgery does not cause, since it does not affect the ovaries.

Cancer of the Uterus

Cervical Cancer. The most common malignancy of the female reproductive tract is cancer of the cervix. Only cancer of the breast exceeds it in frequency. Routine inspection of the cervix, with Papanicolaou smears and biopsy of suspicious tissue, is imperative for early diagnosis. When cancer is suspected or diagnosed, the physician may do a Schiller's test. The cervix is painted with an iodine preparation. Biopsies are taken of all unstained tissues, since cancerous tissues are among those that remain unstained.

Cure is possible if the disease is discovered before it has spread. When the cellular change is still confined to the mucosal layer of the cervix, it is called *carcinoma in situ*. Invasion of surrounding tissue may not occur for five or more years after the pre-invasion period. In this early stage there are no symptoms. Even when the cancer has begun to invade the cervix, there still may be no symptoms. Bleeding is the most prominent symptom.

At first, there is spotting, especially after slight trauma, such as douching or intercourse. Later, if the condition is still untreated, the discharge continues, growing bloody and malodorous as the cancerous tissue becomes necrotic. There may be pain, symptoms of pressure on bladder or bowel, and the generalized wasting of advanced cancer.

If the patient wants children, and the disease is still *in situ,* it may be treated by a cone-shaped amputation of the cervix, leaving the fundus in place for childbearing. Postoperatively the patient is monitored with frequent Papanicolaou smears. Usually, however, a hysterectomy is performed if the cancer has not spread. If the cancer is invasive, it is treated by radical surgery, such as hysterectomy with pelvic node dissection and radium inserts, x-ray or radioactive cobalt therapy, or drug perfusion.

Theoretically, all cancer of the cervix begins in situ. It may take 10 to 15 years to become invasive. Therefore, regular Papanicolaou smears are very important for women in their 20's. The means are theoretically available for completely eliminating cancer of the cervix as a cause of death.

Cancer of the Fundus. Carcinoma of the fundus occurs most frequently, and yet not exclusively, in menopausal and postmenopausal women. Bleeding is the earliest and commonest symptom. Before the menopause it may appear as menorrhagia. All vaginal bleeding after the menopause must be investigated.

When cancer is suspected after a gynecologic examination and a Papanicolaou smear, the patient may be admitted to the hospital for a diagnostic curettage. This procedure is not without danger, because the scraping may spread the cancer cells.

If malignancy is revealed, the treatment is directed at removing the tumor. A hysterectomy may be done; radium, in a rigid applicator or interstitial needles, may be inserted into the uterine cavity, or deep x-ray therapy may be given to the pelvis. If the tumor is large, it may be irradiated before surgery to reduce its size. Radiation may follow surgery if metastases are suspected.

Cancer of the Vulva

This is a relatively rare malignancy usually occurring in women past their 60's. Pruritis is the most frequent early symptom. Later, there may be a bloody discharge, enlarged nodules (as the adjacent lymph nodes become involved), ulceration, edema and a visible mass; finally, there is severe pain. As the cancer ulcerates, there may be a bloody, perhaps a purulent, discharge from the vulva.

Diagnosis is confirmed by biopsy. Vulvectomy with removal of the inguinal lymph nodes (radical vulvectomy) is the treatment of choice. After five years 60 to 75 per cent of the patients are alive and considered to be cured. When the disease has spread to an inoperable stage, radiation therapy may be used. There then may be exaggerated tissue reaction, causing the patient to have considerable discomfort.

In view of the patients' average age, the operation may be done in two stages: first the vulvectomy and later the groin dissection. The patient usually is very uncomfortable after vulvectomy, and she probably will need frequent administration of analgesics for at least two weeks. Because the urethra is involved in the operation, the patient will return from surgery with a Foley catheter inserted into her bladder. A record should be kept of urinary output. Placing the patient in a semirecumbent position may relieve some of the pressure on the sutures, which will probably be taut. However, she should not remain in one position, even if a comfortable one is found. When she is on her side, the upper leg should be bent and supported with pillows to prevent pull on the operative area. She should do leg exercises frequently—at least once an hour during the early postoperative period. She should be assisted with passive movements until she can move her legs herself. Straining at stool should be avoided. The patient will be given enemas preoperatively and a low-residue diet postoperatively. After she does have a bowel movement, the nurse should avoid contaminating the wound when cleaning the anal region.

The initial pressure dressing is held in place with a T-binder. After this dressing is removed, give frequent perineal care (sterile technic, usually). Sterile saline, peroxide, or an antiseptic solution may be ordered for cleaning the surgical area. If drains are inserted, be careful that they are not disturbed; note and record drainage from them. Heat-lamp treatments are used to dry the area after perineal care and also to improve the circulation, thus promoting healing. After the sutures have been removed, warm sitz baths may be given. Also, these may help the patient to urinate after the Foley catheter has been removed. Assure her of privacy during perineal care, the heat-lamp treatments, and the sitz baths.

When cancer of the vulva is inoperable, wet dressings and perineal irrigations with a deodorizing solution may help to control the odor and the infection that so often occurs in the ulcerating neoplasm.

General Nursing Care of Patients with Gynecologic Tumors

Because gynecologic tumors can be a threat both to life and reproductive power, the patient should receive as much emotional support as possible from the nurse. It is helpful to the patient for the same nurse to care for her consistently, so that there is time for rapport to be established and for the patient to feel free to discuss her thoughts. The desire for children, the fear of returning to the doctor for observation of a fibroid, the fear of cancer, the dread of mutilation and of the loss of femininity are emotions that lie deep. Sterility, resulting from some gynecologic surgery and usually from gynecologic irradiation, often requires severe adjustments by the patient. Postoperative tearfulness, which is fairly predictable, may be based on hormonal changes as well as a feeling of depression. If it seems helpful, discuss the patient's reactions with the family, so that they, too, can support her while she makes her difficult adjustment. Lend an emphatic ear to the husband, since his wife's condition has a special meaning to him as well. Perhaps you can help him to help her.

Preoperative preparation may include vaginal suppositories and catheterization to minimize the chance of damaging the bladder (or, perhaps the order will read to make sure that the patient voids). She is usually given an enema. The perineal preparation of the skin usually is done with the patient first in the lithotomy position and then in Sim's position to shave the anal region.

A hysterectomy or the removal of a large tumor causes sudden shifts in the body spaces, and distention is a frequent and uncomfortable complication. A heating pad and a rectal tube may be ordered, and the patient usually is kept on a light diet until peristalsis is re-established. A carminative enema may be ordered about the third postoperative day.

A patient with a vaginal hysterectomy will wear perineal pads. In some hospitals, sterile pads are used. Change the pads frequently, and be sure that the patient has a T-binder or sanitary belt to hold them in place. There will be some serosanguinous drainage, particularly if a radical operation was done. The patient should have frequent perineal care, including after each use of the bedpan. The ambulatory patient who gives herself perineal care still needs the nurse to observe the operative area at least once every eight hours. Watch for hemorrhage. With both a vaginal and an abdominal hysterectomy, there should be no more bleeding than is seen in a normal menstrual period. Check the perineal pad every 10 to 15 minutes during the first few postoperative hours, and then every hour for the rest of the day. There will be a moderate to a slight amount of drainage for the first one or two days, and some spotting for about two weeks. Frank bleeding is not expected. Bleeding may, of course, be internal.

Patients who have had perineal surgery may have discomfort from perineal stitches. Heat in the form of a lamp, sitz baths or warm perineal irrigations may be ordered.

Inability to void is a frequent postoperative complaint because the urinary tract is in the operative vicinity. There may be edema, inflammation and loss of muscle tone of bladder and urethra. A Foley catheter usually is inserted preoperatively, and removed on about the fourth postoperative day. After removal, the patient often is catheterized immediately after each spontaneous voiding to note the amount of residual urine, until there is no more residual than 50 to 80 ml. Note and record the first few times that the patient voids spontaneously. Is the amount adequate? Is it bloody? (Occasionally, surgical injury to the ureter or the bladder occurs during gynecologic surgery.) Decreased urinary output and a low backache may indicate that a ureter has been ligated.

Thrombophlebitis is a common complication of hysterectomy. The surgery itself, or the position of the patient during surgery (the lithotomy position is used for vaginal hysterectomy) may interfere with circulation. Frequent turning and active exercises of the legs are in order. To avoid the pooling of blood in the pelvis and pressure on leg veins, help the patient to exercise, and do not put the knee gatch up or raise the head of the bed higher than midsitting position. The patient should lie flat for short periods during the day. She probably will be out of bed, with help, the day after surgery.

Occasionally, a patient will have the entire contents of her pelvis removed (*pelvic exenteration*). This operation includes a panhysterectomy, a cystectomy, removal of the rectum and an abdominal-perineal resection. A colostomy is done and the ureters are transplanted into the skin or into the ileum. Both the physical and the emotional trauma resulting from this extensive surgery can well be imagined, considering the radical alterations in physiology and the extensive adjustments in activities of everyday living. If the patient is not already past the menopause, she will have a surgical menopause. Because of the severity of the operation, the water and electrolyte regulation will be upset. After vaginectomy the patient will be unable to have sexual intercourse, unless there is sufficient remaining vagina to permit it. Weakness and fatigue will be all-consuming for some time after surgery. In addition, the patient has to adjust physically and emotionally to both a colostomy and a ureterostomy.

On returning home after any kind of gynecologic surgery, the patient should know that heavy lifting, straining, or active sport should not be undertaken for several months. Swimming is usually permitted, but horseback riding is not. Any constrictive clothing, such as a panty girdle, which binds in the area of the groin, should not be worn.

Care of the Patient with Inoperable Malignancy. Death from cancer of the reproductive tract is often prolonged. It may be caused by uremia, as the ureters slowly are shut off by the growth. The patient frequently has severe pain and is emaciated. In addition, there is a thick, foul-smelling vaginal discharge, which is extremely distressing to the patient. She needs frequent perineal care and cleansing douches. Chlorine solutions may help to control the odor. If ascites is present, a sitting position will aid respiration. Sensory nerve connections may be severed to relieve intractable pain. A chordotomy destroys the pain tract at a specific level in the spinal cord.

VAGINAL FISTULAS

Fistulas may be congenital or a result of obstetric or surgical injury, but the most frequent cause in adults is a breakdown of tissue due to cancer or irradiation. The opening may be between a ureter and the vagina (*ureterovaginal* fistula); between the bladder and the vagina (*vesicovaginal* fistula); or between the rectum and the vagina (*rectovaginal* fistula).

A large fistula causes the patient endless distress. An opening between the urinary tract and the vagina means that there is continuous leakage of urine from the vagina. The vaginal wall and the external genitalia become excoriated, and often they become infected. The patient may not void at all through the urethra, since

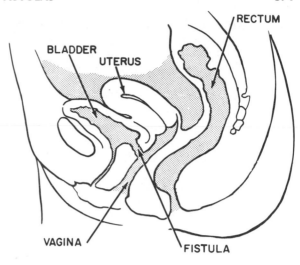

FIG. 44-4. A fistula between bladder and vagina (vesicovaginal fistula).

there may be no accumulation of urine in the bladder. Rectovaginal fistulas cause fecal incontinence and discharge of flatus through the vagina. The feces added to the leukorrhea that is already present, or that is initiated by the passage of stool over the vaginal mucosa, are so distressingly odorous that the patient easily withdraws from social contacts. Frequently, the tissues are in such poor condition that surgical repair is not possible.

Treatment and Nursing Care

Surgery is only performed under as close to optimum conditions as possible: when inflammation and edema have disappeared, and this may mean months of waiting. Unfortunately, surgery for a rectovaginal fistula is frequently unsuccessful.

When operation is done for a rectovaginal fistula, both preoperatively and postoperatively the patient is placed on sulfasuxidine or sulfaguanidine to clean the bowel of colon bacilli. She is given a light, low-residue diet preoperatively, to keep the stool soft, and an enema and a cleansing vaginal irrigation the morning of surgery. Postoperatively, the patient may be kept on clear fluids for several days to inhibit bowel activity, and then she may be graduated first to a light, low-residue diet and then to a general diet. Paregoric may be given to constipate the patient in the early postoperative period. The genitalia may be kept clean and warm perineal irrigations, and perineal heat-lamp treatments may be ordered to promote healing and to lessen discomfort. Because patients with vaginal fistulas often are debilitated, they need attention to overall health measures, such as an adequate diet, fluids and rest.

After repair of a vesicovaginal fistula, a Foley catheter will be inserted. Note its drainage carefully. If the tube becomes blocked, and the bladder is allowed to fill, the pressure may break down the surgical repair and cause the fistula to reappear. If irrigations are ordered, do them very gently, so that no pressure is applied to the suture line. Vaginal serosanguinous drainage is expected. The absence of urine in the vagina indicates healing of the fistula. If douches are ordered, the pressure should be kept to a minimum.

When the fistula cannot be repaired, as in advanced cancer, frequent sitz baths and deodorizing douches help to control infection and odor and to make the patient feel cleaner. A perineal pad or rubber pants will be needed. Before she joins a social gathering, a woman with a rectovaginal fistula may give herself a low, gentle cleansing enema. If the enema is to be effective, the tube must be inserted above the point of the fistula, and directed away from the opening.

The patient with a fistula usually is discouraged and uncomfortable. It is difficult for her to feel clean. She is always wet with urine, which perhaps is mixed with feces. Not only does she feel the opposite of fastidious, but her skin becomes raw and irritated.

Although the problems remain serious as long as the patient has the fistula, certain measures may help to make her more comfortable. She may wear an absorbent material, such as a perineal pad. Frequent changes of the pad and sitz baths help to reduce odors and lessen the irritation of the skin. Wearing a liner next to her skin helps to keep the urine off the skin. Some patients are soothed by a light dusting of cornstarch. Waterproof underpants are sometimes worn to protect clothing and furniture.

RELAXED PELVIC MUSCLES

When the muscles and the fascia that support a structure relax, the structure sags. After unrepaired postpartum tears, childbirth, multiple births, or sometimes without apparent cause (perhaps from a slight congenital weakness), the floor of the pelvis relaxes, and uterus, rectum or bladder may herniate downward. The bulging of the bladder into the vagina is called a *cystocele,* the most common type of poor pelvic support. Herniation of the rectum into the vagina is called a *rectocele.* Downward displacement of the uterus is called *prolapse.* A cystocele and a rectocele usually accompany uterine prolapse. The presence of the uterus low in the vaginal vault is spoken of as a *first degree prolapse;* a *second degree prolapse* is the extension of the cervix beyond the vaginal os; and when the entire uterus hangs outside the body, a *third degree* or *complete prolapse* (procidentia uteri) is present. The improved obstetrical care now available to many women before, during and after delivery has greatly reduced the incidence of postpartum pelvic relaxation as a result of childbirth.

Symptoms may include backache, pelvic pain, fatigue, and a feeling that "something is dropping out," especially when lifting a heavy object, coughing, or with prolonged standing. A cystocele may cause difficulty in emptying the bladder, resulting in stagnation of the urine and possible cystitis. There may be stress incontinence: a little urine seeps out every time that the woman coughs, bears down or strains. A rectocele can cause difficulty in evacuation; constipation can result. In some instances, the patient may need to put her finger into her vagina and apply pressure to the posterior vaginal wall to reduce the herniation before she is able to evacuate the stool collected in the pocket.

Any tissue that protrudes below the vaginal orifice is subject to irritation from clothing or rubbing against the thighs in walking. This is especially seen in second and third degree prolapse. Ulceration and infection frequently follow. These symptoms are annoying and they may be incapacitating. They may forbid standing for a long time, walking with ease, or lifting and other activities that are difficult to avoid.

Treatment and Nursing Care

The surgical repair of a cystocele is called *anterior colporrhaphy.* Repair of a rectocele is called *posterior colporrhaphy.* Repair of the tears (usually old obstetric tears) of the perineal floor is called *perineorrhaphy.* The operations are done by the vaginal route and occasionally under local anesthesia. A vaginal hysterectomy may be done to remove a completely prolapsed uterus.

The patient may be kept on bed rest for one or two days before surgery to decrease any edema of the area. The bed should not be placed in a high sitting position, which would increase congestion to the pelvic region. Before posterior colporrhaphy an enema is given to empty the bowel.

Postoperatively, perineal dressings are not commonly used; rather, perineal care is given several times a day, and always after the patient has urinated or defecated. A heat lamp is sometimes ordered to dry the area and to promote healing. Every effort is made to prevent pelvic pressure and stress on the suture line. An ice pack may be ordered to relieve edema and pain, and this should be placed so that the weight of the pack lies on the bed and not on the patient. If sitz baths are given, a rubber ring should be placed in the bathtub. Until healing has taken place, the patient may be more comfortable sitting on a pillow placed over a rubber ring. About the third or fourth postoperative day, the patient may be given a suppository or a cathartic by mouth. The patient is instructed not to strain when having a bowel movement.

After an anterior colporrhaphy, a Foley catheter usually is inserted to keep the bladder empty, since overdistention of the bladder could weaken the repair. The Foley catheter often is attached to straight drainage while the patient is in bed. When she is ambulatory, find out whether the catheter is to be clamped, or whether straight drainage is to be continued. Clamping may be ordered to allow the bladder to fill to increase its muscle tone. However, it should be released every four hours to prevent overdistention. If the patient does this herself, check it. No more than 150 ml. should accumulate in the bladder.

After the catheter is removed (two to seven days postoperatively), observe for adequate voiding. The patient should urinate every four hours, but she may have frequency without adequately emptying the bladder. Catheterization for residual urine may be ordered. Urinary output should be measured for the first day or two.

Because these conditions are most frequently found in older women, sometimes there are complicating diseases that make surgery too great a risk to be undertaken. Under such circumstances the displacement may be reduced by inserting a pessary, which repositions the uterus. The pessary should be kept as clean as possible to avoid infection. A sterile lubricant should be applied to it before it is inserted. Once the pessary is in place, the patient should feel nothing. Discomfort may indicate that it is placed incorrectly, or

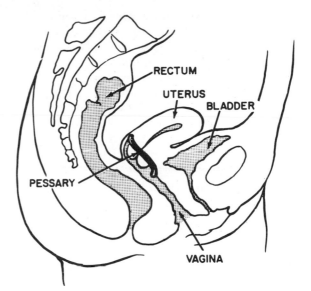

FIG. 44-5. Ring pessary in place.

that it is causing irritation. The appearance of leukorrhea may indicate an infection, in which case the patient should see the doctor immediately. The pessary usually is kept in place for six weeks at a time. The patient should return to the doctor one week after its insertion and then about every two months. If the pelvic floor is very relaxed, and there is danger of the pessary's falling out, a string may be attached to it and pinned to the clothing. Hard rubber or plastic pessaries have less tendency to become soggy than soft rubber ones. Assuming the knee-chest position for a few minutes once or twice a day helps to keep the genital organs and the pessary in good position. Modern surgical technics, and concern over the possible harmful effects of chronic irritation from the pessary, have made the use of pessaries infrequent.

Pelvic relaxation happens over the years. It is not uncommon for a woman to tolerate the increasing discomfort until a more "convenient" time for surgery. She may wait until cystitis is well developed. All nurses, and particularly those in public health and industry, are in a position to urge early medical attention before complications become severe, and the condition is incapacitating.

UTERINE DISPLACEMENT

In some women the position of the uterus is abnormal. Displacement usually is congenital; sometimes backward displacement is due to childbearing. *Anteflexion* is the term given to a uterus that is bent forward at an acute angle. In *retroversion* the uterus tilts backward. In *retroflexion* the fundus is bent backward on the cervix (the opposite of anteflexion).

Displacement may be asymptomatic, or it may cause backache, dysmenorrhea or sterility. The condition may be treated by the insertion of a pessary and the assumption of the knee-chest position several times a day. If the displacement causes severe discomfort, or if there is a chance for sterility to be corrected, surgery may be attempted, during which the uterus is moved to a more natural position.

REFERENCES AND BIBLIOGRAPHY

ALPENFELS, E. J.: Cancer in situ of the cervix; cultural clues to reactions, *Am. J. Nurs.* 64:83, April, 1964.

BREWER, J., MOLBO, D., and GERBIE, A.: *Gynecologic Nursing*, St. Louis, Mosby, 1966.

CIANFRANI, T., and CONWAY, M. K.: Ectopic pregnancy, *Am. J. Nurs.* 63:93, April, 1963.

DEUTSCH, M.: *The Psychology of Women*, 2 vols., New York, Grune, 1944.

DONALDSON, S. S., and FLETCHER, W. S.: The treatment of cancer by isolation perfusion, *Am. J. Nurs.* 64:81, August, 1964.

FITZPATRICK, G.: *Gynecologic Nursing*, New York, Macmillan, 1965.

FRANCIS, G. M.: Cancer: the emotional component, *Am. J. Nurs.* 69:1677, August, 1969.

FUNNELL, J. W., and ROOF, B.: Before and after hysterectomy, *Am. J. Nurs.* 64:120, October, 1964.

GELBER, I.: Family planning in a growing world, *Am. J. Nurs.* 64:98, August, 1964.

GUSBERG, S. B.: Cancer in situ of the cervix, treatment as preventive medicine, *Am. J. Nurs.* 64:76, April, 1964.

GUTTMACHER, A. F.: Family planning: the needs and the methods, *Am. J. Nurs.* 69:1229, June, 1969.

IORIO, J.: *Principles of Obstetrics and Gynecology for Nurses*, St. Louis, Mosby, 1967.

KLEEGMAN, S., and KAUFMAN, A.: *Infertility in Women: Diagnosis and Treatment*, Philadelphia, Davis, 1966.

LAMMERT, A. C.: The menopause—a physiologic process, *Am. J. Nurs.* 62:56, February, 1962.

LEWIS, G. C.: Cancer in situ of the cervix, screening and diagnosis, *Am. J. Nurs.* 64:72, April, 1964.

LEWIS, G., WENTZ, W., and JAFFE, R.: *New Concepts in Gynecological Oncology*, Philadelphia, Davis, 1966.

MALONE, A.: The nurse in a fertility clinic, *Am. J. Nurs.* 57:348, 1957.

MATHIS, J. L.: The emotional impact of surgical sterilization on the female, *J. Oklahoma State Med. Assoc.* 62:141-145, 1969.

McGOWAN, L.: New ideas about patient care before and after vaginal surgery, *Am. J. Nurs.* 64:73, February, 1964.

MEAD, M.: *From the South Seas—Studies of Adolescence and Sex in Primitive Societies*, New York, Morrow, 1939.

MENAKER, J. S.: When menstruation is painful, *Am. J. Nurs.* 62:94, September, 1962.

MILLER, N., and AVERY, H.: *Gynecology and Gynecologic Nursing*, ed. 5, Philadelphia, Saunders, 1965.

MILLER, O.: Nursing care after pelvic exenteration, *Am. J. Nurs.* 62:106, May, 1962.

NEWTON, M., and ODOM, P. L.: The menopause and its symptoms, *Southern Med. J.* 57:1309, 1964.

NOVAK, E. R.: Benign ovarian tumors, *Am. J. Nurs.* 64:104, November, 1964.

NOWAK, P. A.: Nursing care in isolation perfusion, *Am. J. Nurs.* 64:85, August, 1964.

PARKER, E.: *The Seven Ages of Woman*, Baltimore, Hopkins, 1960.

ROBBINS, L. C., and WALKER, E.: Cancer in situ of the cervix; problems of control, *Am. J. Nurs.* 64:80, April, 1964.

STEPHENS, G.: Mind-body continuum in human sexuality, *Am. J. Nurs.* 70:1468, July, 1970.

STURGIS, S. H.: Treatment of ovarian insufficiency, *Am. J. Nurs.* 64:113, January, 1964.

WATKINS, E. W., and SULLIVAN, R. D.: Cancer chemotherapy by prolonged arterial infusion, *Surg. Gynec. Obstet.* 118:3, 1964.

WEISS, S. M.: Psychosomatic aspects of symptom patterns among major surgery patients, *J. Psychosom. Res.* 13:109-112, 1969.

WILSON, R. A., and WILSON, T. A.: The fate of the non-treated post-menopausal woman: a plea for the maintenance of adequate estrogen from puberty to the grave, *J. Am. Geriat. Soc.* 11:347, 1963.

The Male Patient with a Disorder of the Reproductive System

45

Benign Prostatic Hypertrophy • Cancer of the Prostate
Disorders of the Testes and Their Adjacent Structures

Embarrassment, fears of impotence and the feeling of loss of manly self-esteem frequently make a disorder of a reproductive organ hard for the patient to bear. It is important for the nurse to realize that although the patient may more readily discuss his concerns with a knowledgeable man, for example the physician, the nurse should show a willingness to listen to the patient. (Sometimes the firm belief that the patient does not wish to discuss these concerns with the nurse has more to do with the nurse's discomfort over the topic rather than with the patient's reluctance to discuss it.) If the patient appears worried about his illness or an impending operation, a knowledgeable nurse can let him know that his fears are neither strange nor unexpected, and that he may discuss any matters that he wishes. If the patient seems unduly shy or hesitant, the nurse might mention her observations to the physician so he may open the subject with the patient, in addition to herself spending time and showing concern for the patient. The patient himself decides how he wishes to proceed.

The male lower urinary tract and reproductive system are so closely associated that disorders in this area frequently affect both systems. This is in contrast to the female where, although close together, these systems are somewhat more separate. The male genital system consists of the testes which produce sperm and the epididymides and vas deferens which deliver the sperm to the prostate and seminal vesicles. The bladder urine and seminal fluid are both discharged, although separately, to the outside through the urethra, which traverses the penis.

BENIGN PROSTATIC HYPERTROPHY

The prostate gland is an accessory sex organ which produces the majority of the seminal fluid. This fluid contains zinc, invert sugars and other substances necessary for nutrition of the sperm. The prostate is located just below the urinary bladder. The urinary stream travels through the center of the gland in the prostatic urethra. With advancing age and seemingly under the influence of male sex hormones, the peri-urethral glandular tissue undergoes hyperplasia, with gradual enlargement of the gland. This outward expansion is not of any clinical importance. However, inward encroachment of this tissue which diminishes the diameter of the prostatic urethra certainly is.

The symptoms of "prostate trouble" are all secondary to an increasing impediment to urinary flow. Symptoms appear gradually. At first the patient may notice that it takes more effort to void and there is decreasing force and narrowing of the urinary stream. As the residual urine remaining in his bladder accumulates, the bladder fills more quickly, and the patient finds that he has the urge to void more and more frequently. Urgency, to the point of incontinence, is common. At night he awakens for trips to the bathroom. There may be difficulty in starting the stream, and hematuria when it does start. Residual urine is a good culture medium for bacteria, and if infection results, symptoms of cystitis also will be present. The combination of hesitancy, narrowed stream, straining to void, frequency, urgency and nocturia is known as prostatism. Any obstruction in the lower urinary tract can cause these symptoms, but the most common is prostatic enlargement.

Diagnosis

If the patient has prostatic hypertrophy, the doctor will feel the gland to be enlarged and elastic. Cystoscopy will reveal the extent of the infringement on the urethra and the effects on the bladder. Pyelography will give information about the possible damage to the upper urinary tract due to the backup of urine. Blood chemistry tests are done to reveal kidney malfunction. Measurement of significant quantities of residual urine (usually at least 60 ml.) adds to the data confirming the diagnosis.

Treatment and Nursing Care

Symptomatic benign prostatic hypertrophy is treated by surgically removing part of the prostate gland. Unless the patient has marked symptoms or is totally unable to void, a urethral catheter is not inserted preoperatively. The history will tell the doctor whether the patient has had an acute episode of retaining his urine, or whether he has been building up larger and larger residual amounts over a long period of time. If the patient has gone into sudden acute retention, a urethral catheter is inserted and connected to straight drainage. If, on the other hand, the history suggests a gradual worsening of chronic retention, a rapid complete emptying of the bladder may have dire consequences. These include a profound hematuria due to rupture of the numerous stretched mucosal blood vessels and postobstructive diuresis. In a chronically obstructed patient, the sudden, complete relief of obstruction by means of a catheter may be followed by a marked diuresis with loss of large amounts of sodium in the urine. If unnoticed and unreplaced, the salt and water loss may be serious enough to cause the patient to go into shock.

Consequently, if the retention is chronic, the physician will want to decompress the patient's bladder slowly (over a period of hours) to avoid the bleeding that sometimes accompanies a rapid withdrawal of urine from a bladder that has been chronically distended. Decompression drainage effects a gradual emptying of the bladder and also helps to maintain bladder tone, because the urine, with free flow maintained through the catheter, must be pushed uphill. Note that the top end of the Y-tube is left open to the air as a safety vent should the intravesical pressure (pressure in the bladder) become too high. The apex of the Y-tube is placed six to eight inches above the level of the pubis. The Y is gradually lowered one inch an hour until it is at bladder level and eventually is replaced by straight drainage. The two most important precautions are: be sure that the entire tubular passageway from the patient to the bottle is patent, and that the level of the Y-tube is as it was ordered.

Preoperative Regimen. During the preoperative period, the patient is put on a healthful regimen, with emphasis on copious fluids, a good diet and rest periods. Other illnesses are treated,

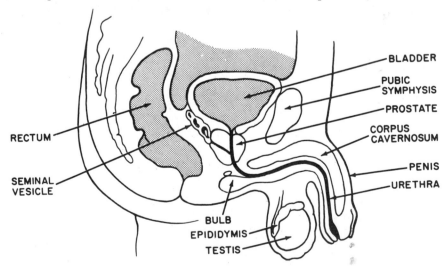

Fig. 45-1. Male genitourinary tract.

such as regulation of diabetes and digitalization for heart failure.

If catheter drainage is not provided, the patient is taught to measure his urine and keep a record of the time and the amount that he voids each 24 hours. When you look at the chart you may see an abnormal pattern that will be fairly consistent from day to day for this patient.

If during the preoperative evaluation period the physician finds significant damage to the upper urinary tract, he may elect to perform a suprapubic cystostomy (a small suprapubic incision into the bladder through which a catheter is inserted). This type of urinary drainage bypasses the prostate until there is adequate recovery of renal function so that a definitive operation on the prostate can be performed safely. The use of the suprapubic catheter for long-term drainage prevents epididymitis and other serious infections associated with prolonged use of a urethral catheter. The patient may be sent home with this drainage for several months. He and a family member need instruction in the care of the catheter and skin before discharge from the hospital.

Types of Surgery

(See following section for nursing care of the prostatectomy patient.)

As benign prostatic hypertrophy develops, the hyperplasia of the periurethral glands forms an adenoma which comprises the bulk of the prostate. The adenoma thins and compresses the surrounding true capsule of the gland. Between the adenoma and capsule there is a plane of cleavage which can be developed easily by the surgeon. The aim of all surgical procedures for benign prostatic hypertrophy is removal of the adenoma leaving the true capsule behind. Subsequently, the patient urinates through this fossa. Healing, by re-epithelialization, occurs over a two- to three-month period. At open operations (retropubic, perineal, or suprapubic prostatectomy), the surgeon develops the cleavage plane between the adenoma and capsule by either finger or sharp dissection. The adenoma is removed along with the mucosa of the prostatic urethra. The transurethral method accomplishes the same objective except that the adenoma is removed piece by piece through an instrument inserted through the urethra.

Transurethral prostatectomy is the easiest of the four operations for the patient, since there is no external wound. It is performed most frequently on patients with complicating conditions, such as heart disease and advanced age, and those with a small amount of prostatic hypertrophy. Hemorrhage can result around the eighth to tenth day when tissue sloughing may occur.

The surgeon's preference, his experience with various technics, the size of the adenoma, and the general condition of the patient play a part in the type of operation performed. If the patient is very obese, the doctor may prefer the transurethral or perineal approach rather than an abdominal one.

Patients may become discouraged if they observe another patient who entered at the same time with the same complaints going home one week after a transurethral resection. Help such a patient to understand that the transurethral approach would not have been the best procedure for him, and that results, even with the same operation, differ from patient to patient.

Although the majority of patients retain potency following operations for benign prostatic hypertrophy, there is a significant percentage in whom it is impaired following perineal surgery. Consequently, the perineal approach is reserved either for the elderly or in patients in whom there is a strong suspicion of cancer and a radical prostatectomy may be planned. There is also some danger of injury to the rectum resulting in incontinence and possible fistula formation. Following simple perineal prostatectomy patients generally do not require catheter drainage for longer than one week.

Preoperatively, many surgeons will order a bowel prep to decrease postoperative fecal wound contamination.

Nursing Care After Prostatectomy

No matter which surgical approach is used, there are general principles of care applicable to postprostatectomy patients.

When the patient returns to the ward, his catheter or catheters are attached to the prescribed type of drainage. Output of each is separately recorded.

The patient may also return to his bed with a Penrose drain inserted into the tissues of the operative site. This drain does not enter the urinary tract. The drain removes blood and urine that have leaked into the area. The Penrose drain is removed when all drainage has ceased.

The following are matters of considerable import following prostatectomy:

Bleeding. Clear urinary drainage following any type of prostatectomy is rare. Hematuria is generally present. However, frank bleeding is a serious emergency and a potential complication for several days after surgery. Note the color of the urine and the presence of any clots. Bright red blood indicates an arterial bleeding source while a deep black red suggests venous oozing. Clots can obstruct the catheter causing spasm, pain and further bleeding. Therefore, the catheter must remain patent at all times. Check the bladder for fullness and tenderness. If these are present, the bladder could be distended with clots and the physician should be promptly notified.

To control arterial bleeding, the surgeon may put traction on the urethral catheter. One method used is that of taping the inflated catheter to the thigh. The traction may be maintained for six hours, but after this there is danger of damage to the bladder sphincter causing temporary incontinence. The physician may order the tension to be decreased gradually or may reapply more gentle traction overnight. The patient has a sensation of having a full bladder even though the bladder is empty. If he tries to void around the catheter the bladder muscles contract causing a painful spasm. The nurse can explain to the patient that the bladder is kept empty by the catheter and that trying to void causes irritation to the bladder mucosa. Encouraging fluid intake (if permitted) helps to decrease bladder mucosal irritation because there is a constant passage of fluid over the irritation. Explaining to the patient why he feels this need to urinate may help him not to worry about it.

Drainage and Irrigation. The doctor usually orders straight drainage without irrigation. Overzealous irrigation may induce further bleeding and cause frequent and uncomfortable bladder spasms. The nurse follows the doctor's orders regarding when to irrigate, how much solution and what kind of solution to use.

In selected patients, continuous irrigation, regulated by a drip mechanism, is ordered. The continuous gentle flow of fluid helps to prevent clots from forming in the bladder and plugging the catheters. The drip is regulated to maintain the drainage at a light pink. When this through-and-through irrigation is ordered, the urethral catheter is usually used for inflow and the cystostomy tube for outflow. The danger of bleeding is increased if the irrigating fluid is continued when the outflow is obstructed by clots.

Normal saline is preferred for irrigation, especially if large volumes are necessary, to prevent dilution of blood as a result of absorption of the irrigating solution.

When the urethral catheter is removed, the time and amount of each voiding should be recorded for several days. The patient may be instructed to do this. Occasionally, if urinary function does not progress satisfactorily, the catheter may have to be reinserted.

Bladder Spasms. It is important that the nurse distinguish between catheter obstruction and bladder spasm. Usually with catheter and, consequently, bladder obstruction there is gradual and increasing discomfort with absence of urinary output. The bladder becomes distended and is tender on palpation. Relief of the obstruction is urgent. If there is an order for catheter irrigation by the nurse she should do this gently. If patency is not achieved, or there is no order for irrigation, the urologist should be notified.

When bladder spasm without catheter obstruction is present, the patient will have a urinary output, but pain may be constantly present or intermittent. Some bladder spasms are extremely painful, but fortunately each spasm lasts only a few seconds. Narcotics do not seem to lessen the spasms, but they will help to decrease pain from the operative area. An antispasmodic drug such as Pro-Banthine (propantheline) may be ordered. Bladder spasms generally lessen in severity after 48 hours.

Dressings and Wounds. The nurse changes cystostomy and perineal dressings as frequently as necessary to keep the patient clean and dry. Care must be taken not to disturb any tissue drains placed by the surgeon. Montgomery straps simplify frequent dressing changes. Strict aseptic technic is essential to prevent wound infection.

After a cystostomy tube is removed, the suprapubic wound frequently leaks urine for a few days. A saturated, wet dressing, smelling of urine, and wet bed clothes can be very uncomfortable and embarrassing to the patient. If his dressings are not changed promptly when necessary, he may attempt to keep dry by restricting his fluid intake. The nurse encourages liberal fluid intake (when the patient's medical status permits) by demonstrating to the patient that he will have his dressings changed promptly and by attempting to provide the type of liquid which is most appealing to him.

Observe and chart the amount of urine that comes from the wound and the condition of the skin surrounding it. To prevent irritation, the skin should be washed frequently. A medicated powder or ointment may be prescribed if irritation develops. The wound heals slowly, depending to a great extent on the general health of the patient. If it becomes infected, the healing is even slower.

Although a perineal wound may not be as painful as an abdominal incision, the patient may experience some discomfort sitting for the first week or two. A male T-binder is used to support the dressing. In some instances, beginning on the second or third postoperative day, special wound care consisting of cleansing the incision with surgical soap and water followed by exposure to a heat lamp is performed three times daily. The procedure is completed by applying an antiseptic and a dry sterile dressing. Sitz baths may be ordered after removal of the drains. By ten days after operation, perineal wounds are well on their way to healing in most instances. Early postoperative patients should have help (given preferably by a male nurse) in cleansing after a bowel movement to avoid contaminating the wound. Much of the nursing care following a perineal prostatectomy is the same as that for any perineal or rectal procedure: for example, sitz baths, and the maintenance of extreme cleanliness.

Rectal Precautions. Generally, the use of rectal tubes, rectal thermometers, and enemas is not resumed until at least a week following prostatectomy to avoid perforation or hemorrhage. This precaution is observed especially for patients having perineal surgery.

Bowel Hygiene. After prostate surgery the patient should be cautioned to avoid straining to have a bowel movement because this can cause prostatic hemorrhage. Stool softeners may be ordered daily, or a mild cathartic may be ordered after the third day. Copious fluids and dietary roughage, as permitted, help to prevent constipation.

Convalescence. Since most patients having prostatic surgery are in the older age group, surgery can be a severe strain and one more contributory factor to pre-existing depression. Personality change as a result of the increased emotional and metabolic stress should be antici-

pated after surgery. As the patient gropes for a return of emotional balance, the nurse, rather than avoiding him, makes an effort to make him feel wanted and valued. An aspect of her relationship with the patient is established by nonverbal communication: her frequent appearance at his side when he feels most desperate, the good physical care she gives, the expression on her face and the way she moves, all convey to the patient that she wants to care for him, no matter what his mood.

After discharge from the hospital, the patient should continue to follow established fluid and bowel routines and follow his doctor's orders for physical activity. Generally, no lifting or straining is permitted for several weeks.

Many patients having prostatectomy will be single, retired, living alone, and confronting the myriad problems of the elderly in our society. A referral to a visiting nurse agency and other community resources may be indicated.

CANCER OF THE PROSTATE

Prostatic carcinoma is most common in men over the age of 50. As life expectancy increases, more and more men live to the age group of highest incidence of this disease. Along with cancer of the lung and gastrointestinal tract, it is among the more common malignancies of older men.

Symptoms. At first there are no symptoms, and none may occur for years. The disease usually starts as a nodule in the posterior lobe of the gland which is farthest away from the urethra. If the tumor grows large enough, it will obstruct urinary flow and cause frequency, nocturia and dysuria. Thus, a patient with cancer of the prostate who has urinary symptoms usually has more advanced stage of the disease. Many patients who have prostatic cancer also have benign prostatic hypertrophy, and the symptoms of urinary obstruction may be due to the latter condition. Spread of the cancer is by way of the blood stream and lymphatics to the pelvic lymph glands and skeleton, particularly the lumbar vertebrae, pelvis, and hips. The first symptoms may be back pain or sciatica due to metastases to the nerve sheaths. In 75 per cent of patients with prostatic cancer extending beyond the prostatic capsule, the acid phosphatase, an enzyme produced by the prostate, is elevated in the blood. Because early cancer of the prostate is asymptomatic, and because cure is possible only when the disease is discovered early, regular annual or biannual rectal examinations of all men over 50 are as important as are regular gynecologic and breast examinations for women.

Treatment and Nursing Care. In the presence of a solitary nodule in a younger patient (usually under 70 years), an open perineal biopsy with frozen section may be suggested. The surgical approach is as for simple perineal prostatectomy. If the nodule is benign and the patient has symptoms of prostatic obstruction, a simple prostatectomy can be performed at that time. If the nodule is seemingly localized cancer, a radical perineal prostatectomy can be performed. In contrast to prostatectomy for benign disease, the so-called radical operation involves en bloc removal of the entire prostate with its capsule and the seminal vesicles. The bladder neck is sutured to the membranous urethra over a Foley catheter which is left indwelling for 10 to 14 days. Disadvantages of the operation include virtually guaranteed impotence (versus a chance to be cured of cancer) and some serious difficulty with urinary control in 5 to 10 per cent of patients.

Preoperative Care. If the patient is to have radical surgery through a perineal approach, bowel preparation usually includes enemas, a liquid diet the day before the operation, and a drug such as Neothalidine. After surgery the patient is kept on a low-residue diet until healing occurs, so that he does not strain at stool. He may be given camphorated tincture of opium to constipate him for several days immediately postoperatively.

Postoperative Care. The patient returns to his unit with a Foley catheter placed so that the balloon supports the urethral anastomosis to the bladder neck. Care must be taken that the tube is not displaced from this position. The nurse remains watchful for hemorrhage. She notes and records the color of the urine. The Foley catheter is removed in 10 to 14 days. The patient will have a tissue drain. Initially, there may be seepage of urine through the wound, but this should stop in about two days.

Perineal irrigations may be ordered to help to keep the wound clean and to decrease pain and inflammation. After the sterile dressing is removed, the nurse irrigates very gently with the solution that is ordered, often a mild antiseptic, such as hydrogen peroxide. This treatment gives the nurse an excellent opportunity to observe the wound's progress in healing and to observe for signs of disturbance in the healing process.

Additional wound care and nursing measures are similar to those carried out for the patient following rectal or perineal surgery.

The perineal dressing is very close to the rectum. Do not allow it to remain soiled with fecal matter. Since a fistula easily develops in the fragile tissue of the operative site, do not insert anything into the rectum—no rectal thermometers, no rectal tubes, no enemas—nothing unless specifically ordered by the surgeon. Fluids should be encouraged to 3,000 ml. a day, unless there are orders to the contrary.

Often, patients are assisted out of bed the second postoperative day. They should sit on a firm, even surface. They should never sit on a rubber ring or an air mattress, either of which could cause compression of or congestion in a portion of the operative site.

If urinary or fecal incontinence results, some patients may be helped to regain fecal control by doing perineal exercises to improve muscle tone and by regulating their diet. Perineal exercises may be done by contracting and relaxing the gluteal muscles. Teach the patient to observe the effects of various foods, and instruct him in an adequate diet. He should avoid only particular foods that cause diarrhea, and not any important food groups. Dietitian, doctor and nurse work with the patient to help him to establish a dietary regimen that results in good nutrition and regular, formed bowel movements.

The thought of incontinence for the rest of his life may be very depressing to the patient. Teach him how to keep himself dry and odor-free, so that he will not feel shy about mixing with other people. Teaching the patient to care for himself should start while he is in the hospital and has the support of the staff. One object of this teaching is to make self-care as simple and routine as possible, so that the patient will be relatively free to concentrate on matters other than his condition.

Prognosis. The outlook for most patients with prostate cancer is relatively good in that many men who are obviously incurable may experience prolonged palliation on conservative therapy. Manipulation of the patient's hormones may give surprising, if temporary, relief of symptoms. Where there had been severe pain, there may be none; where there was bladder neck obstruction, urine may flow freely. Many tumors will progress under the influence of androgens and regress on estrogens. Following the decrease in androgens by castration (bilateral orchiectomy) and treatment with estrogens, 50 per cent of men with "incurable prostate cancer" will be reasonably comfortable and well five years later. Because of fluid retention problems associated with estrogen therapy, the patient with congestive heart failure must be very carefully observed. A low salt intake is recommended.

As androgens are decreased, and estrogens are given, the patient's voice may become higher, his hair and fat distribution may change, and his breasts may become tender and enlarged. Also, gastrointestinal disturbances may occur. Because the doctor regulates the dosage according to the response of the patient, it is important that the nurse's observations be especially accurate and her charting up-to-date.

If, even after drug therapy, the tumor obstructs the bladder neck, a transurethral prostatectomy may be necessary to establish urinary drainage. Occasionally, permanent suprapubic drainage will have to be established.

Once the suppressive effects of the estrogen treatment wear off (a period which may be quite a few years), the disease progresses more rapidly. For some patients, a second remission, although not as pronounced, may be obtained by hypophysectomy (removal of the pituitary).

In the late stage of the disease, there may be severe pain which may be treated by chordotomy. Radiation therapy may give some relief from painful metastases.

DISORDERS OF THE TESTES AND THEIR ADJACENT STRUCTURES

Cryptorchidism (Hidden Testicle)

Failure of the testicle to lie in the scrotum is known as cryptorchidism (or undescended testicle). At least one testis must be in its normal position in the scrotum for the patient to have reproductive function. The undescended testis may lie in the inguinal canal, abdominal cavity, or rarely in the perineum or femoral canal. If undescended testes are not placed in the scrotum by age five or six, the likelihood of their being good sperm producers diminishes markedly. Undescended testes have a significantly higher incidence of malignant degeneration whether or not they are placed in the scrotum, but the overall incidence of tumors of undescended testes is low. In some individuals, undescended testicles find their way into the scrotum without treatment during childhood or at puberty.

The treatment may consist of a short (one week) trial of hormone (gonadotrophin) therapy. If there is no response within three weeks, surgery may be performed (orchiopexy). After orchiopexy the patient may have three wounds: inner thigh, scrotal and inguinal. The surgeon makes an inguinal incision and locates the testis. It is held in the scrotum on tension to a taped rubber band attached to a suture through the lower pole of the testis and to the skin of the upper thigh. The suture is usually removed in five to seven days. Often there is an associated congenital hernia which is repaired at the time of orchiopexy. The patient can move his leg, but, of course, undue pressure should not be placed on this traction. The nurse should inspect the traction, which will be outside the dressings, several times a day to make sure that it is functioning well.

Adolescent boys who have this operation may be particularly embarrassed to have a female nurse present during dressing changes or to have her inspect the dressings. If there is a male on the nursing team, the patient may feel more comfortable in his care. Some young people in their embarrassment will joke excessively. A matter-of-fact but friendly and accepting manner on the nurse's part may help them to re-establish poise.

Epididymo-orchitis

Infection and inflammations of the testis and epididymis usually occur simultaneously. The most common cause is infection ascending via the vas deferens and its surrounding lymphatics from a prostatitis. A less common cause of acute epididymitis is untreated gonorrhea.

The symptoms are chills, fever, scrotal pain and tenderness. The scrotal skin may be erythematous and tense. The doctor can palpate a markedly swollen testis and epididymis. Elevation of the scrotum with a 4-tail bandage or adhesive taped across the upper thighs (Bellevue Bridge) relieves the pain considerably by lessening the weight of the testes.

Strict bed rest usually is ordered during the early stage. An ice bag may be ordered to help to relieve the pain. Place it under the tender scrotum; not on top of it or leaning against it. Do not keep the cold bag constantly next to the skin, because it may damage tissue. On an hour, off a half-hour is one routine that may be followed. Heat is not applied to the scrotal area, because spermatozoa are damaged by heat that is even a few degrees above body temperature. (The normal temperature of the scrotum is lower than that of the rest of the body.) As with any infection, copious fluid intake is encouraged. Antibiotics may be ordered.

Orchitis without epididymal involvement is most often caused by mumps occurring after puberty. This viral orchitis may result in testicular atrophy and sterility. For this reason men who have not had mumps as children and who are exposed to it are advised to receive immediate medical attention. The administration of gamma globulin may have the effect of lessening the severity of mumps if it develops. Commonly, there will be a sudden onset of chills, fever and testicular swelling one or two weeks after the parotid swelling. Urethritis may also be present. Besides local treatment, the doctor may prescribe corticosteroids.

Bilateral epididymitis frequently leads to permanent azoospermia (absence of sperm), especially when the infection recurs frequently, or when it becomes chronic. Vasectomy (removal of the vas deferens) prevents recurrent attacks, but it causes sterility if it is performed bilaterally.

Torsion (Twisting of the Spermatic Cord)

This condition occurs in prepubescent boys and men whose spermatic cords are (congenitally) unusually unsupported in the vaginal sac and are freely movable. Torsion may follow severe exercise, but it also may occur during sleep or following such a simple maneuver as crossing the legs. There is a sudden, sharp testicular pain and local swelling. The pain may be so severe that nausea, vomiting, chills and fever occur. The testis is extremely tender and the usually posterior epididymis may be located anteriorly. In contrast to inflammatory conditions, elevation of the scrotum will increase the pain by increasing the degree of twist.

Treatment consists of immediate surgery to prevent atrophy of the spermatic cord and to preserve fertility. The torsion is reduced, excess *tunica vaginalis* (the membrane surrounding the testis) excised and the testis is anchored with sutures in the scrotum. A similar prophylactic procedure may be performed on the opposite side.

Hydrocele

The testis is surrounded by a membrane called *tunica vaginalis*. Normally, there is a small amount of fluid in the space between the testis and this membrane. A large accumulation of fluid in that space is known as *hydrocele*. This common cause of scrotal enlargement may be due to an infection, commonly epididymitis or orchitis, or trauma; the majority occur without known cause. When the accumulation of fluid is slow (chronic hydrocele), there is usually no pain, even when the scrotum becomes as large as a grapefruit. A hydrocele causes few symptoms in most instances except for its weight and unsightly bulk. Acute hydrocele is accompanied by both pain and swelling and may follow trauma or local infection.

Treatment, if indicated, consists of surgical excision of the sac. Aspiration is rarely done, particularly since the fluid will reaccumulate and there is a real danger of introducing infection. Postoperatively, the patient has a drain and a pressure dressing. A snug support is required for some weeks afterward.

Varicocoele

This condition usually occurs on the left side of the scrotum and consists of dilation and tortuous clumping of tributaries of the spermatic vein. Swelling and a dragging pain are the major symptoms. Very rarely does a varicocoele per se cause enough symptoms to warrant surgery. In certain instances of infertility, correction of a varicocoele has resulted in significant improvement in the semen specimens, for unknown reasons. The surgery involves an inguinal exploration of the spermatic cord with ligature and division of the major spermatic vein tributaries in this region.

Cancer

Malignancy can occur anywhere in the male reproductive system but is not common in the testes. Testicular tumors tend to metastasize early, and the first symptoms may be related to the secondary site of growth. The symptoms may be abdominal pain, general weakness and aching in the testes. Gradual or sudden swelling of the scrotum always should receive medical attention.

The diagnosis is most often made when the doctor discovers a hard, nontender scrotal swelling. If testis cancer is suspected, the operation suggested is an orchiectomy performed through an inguinal incision. Biopsy risks spilling tumor cells and these tumors are highly malignant.

Depending on the pathology, further treatment may be radiotherapy to the lymph glands (paraaortic nodes), surgical removal of these glands followed by radiotherapy or chemotherapy with actinomycin-D. When radical lymph node dissection through a thoraco-abdominal incision is done bilaterally, the procedure involves extensive surgery, and the patient is very uncomfortable postoperatively. Because the tissue supporting the kidneys may have been removed, he may be kept in a Trendelenburg position for a week or two to help to maintain the kidneys in good position. In this position it is difficult to eat, to read, to urinate and to defecate. X-ray therapy is begun usually immediately after surgery.

Infertility

See Chapter 44 for discussion of infertility.

REFERENCES AND BIBLIOGRAPHY

DICK, V.: Carcinoma of the prostate gland with metastases, Surg. Clin. N. Am. 42:771, 1962.

FLINT, L., and HSIAO, J. H.: Radical prostatectomy for carcinoma: a review and perspective, Surg. Clin. N. Am. 47:695, June, 1967.

KASSELMAN, M. J.: Nursing care of the patient with benign prostatic hypertrophy, Am. J. Nurs. 66:1026, May, 1966.

KEUHNELIAN, J., and SANDERS, V.: Urologic Nursing, New York, Macmillan, 1970.

MARSHALL, V.: Textbook of Urology, ed. 2, New York, Hoeber, 1964.

MOREL, A.: The urologic nurse specialist, Nurs. Clin. N. Am. 4:475, 1969.

MOSSHOLDER, I.: When the patient has a radical retropubic prostatectomy, Am. J. Nurs. 62:101, July, 1962.

PATRICIA, SR. M., and FLOYD, L. C.: Nursing care in prostatectomy, Canad. Nurse 59:833, 1963.

PATTON, J., and ROSS, G.: The painful testicle, Hosp. Med. 3:24, June, 1967.

PURDEY, A.: Prostatic tumors: (2) nursing care, Am. J. Nurs. 56:986, 1956.

ROBINSON, L.: Psychological Aspects of the Care of Hospitalized Patients, Philadelphia, Davis, 1968.

WINTER, C., and ROEHM, M.: Sawyer's Nursing Care of Patients With Urologic Diseases, St. Louis, Mosby, 1968.

The Patient with Breast Disease

46

Physiology of the Breast · Incidence of Breast Disease · Diagnosis
Cystic Disease · Breast Surgery · Treatment of Metastatic Cancer
Breast Abscess

PHYSIOLOGY OF THE BREAST

The breast is a complicated glandular organ that produces milk after pregnancy. Considerable space in the breast is devoted to a network of ducts that carry milk to the nipple. The lymphatic and the blood supplies are rich.

The breast manufactures milk from elements in the blood. The transformation of amino acids and glucose in the blood to the proteins and the lactose in milk is a chemical process not yet fully understood. To make 30 ml. of milk, it has been estimated that the breast must process 12,000 ml. of blood.

Although the most dramatic changes occur in the breast during its preparation for its primary function—lactation—the mammary glands are a part of the female reproductive system, and thus they respond to the hormonal cycle associated with menstruation. Estrogen, secreted by the ovaries, brings about the growth and the development of the duct systems and suppresses lactation. Progesterone, secreted by the corpus luteum of the ovary, stimulates lactation, as does prolactin, an anterior pituitary hormone.

INCIDENCE OF BREAST DISEASE

The most common breast disorder is cystic disease, occurring at a rate of approximately 125 cases per 100,000 women (Davis). Benign tumors, such as fibroadenoma, are less common than cystic disease, but they are common enough so that you probably will care for many patients with this diagnosis.

In American women the breast is the most common site of cancer. In 1968 cancer of the breast was responsible for more deaths among women (about 28,000) than malignant neoplasms of any other site (Metropolitan Life Insurance Co.). It is estimated that 1 of every 25 women in the United States today will develop breast cancer (Haagensen). When the disease is discovered and treated early, the five-year level of cure for small lesions is about 80 per cent. After 20 years it drops to 60 per cent (Robbins). More than half survive at least five years after diagnosis.

This disease can occur at any age, but it is most common during and after the menopause. The longer a woman lives, the greater is her chance of developing breast cancer. The disease is more common in women who have a relative who has had the disease, and it is less common in those who have nursed babies. Each year more than 50,000 women in the United States have a *mastectomy* (removal of a breast). Your patient may be helped by knowing that it is not she alone who has lost a breast. Though it primarily affects women, men, too, can develop breast cancer.

DIAGNOSIS

Although cysts and tumors start microscopically, when they grow larger, they sometimes cause physical changes in the breast that may occur before there is any discomfort or pain. Because women have a better chance for cure when cancer is detected early, every lump and every change in the appearance of the breast should be brought immediately to medical attention. The earlier cancer is diagnosed, the less chance that it has spread. Axillary lymph nodes and the internal mammary lymph nodes drain the breasts. Enlarged nodes occur in breast abscess and cancer. The rate of survival is not as great if the lymph nodes are involved. The five-year 80 per cent survival figure applies to small lesions—less than 3 cm. in diameter and with negative nodes (Robbins).

Signs and Symptoms of Breast Disease

Pain. At times breast pain may be normal. It is not uncommon for the breasts to become enlarged, lumpy and tender during the period immediately before menstruation. These physical changes probably are associated with the hormonal changes of the reproductive cycle, and they may be due to an increase in extracellular fluid tension, but the mechanism is not fully understood. Women with cystic disease also frequently experience fullness, tenderness to the touch, and some pain in the breast immediately before they menstruate.

Lumps. This is one of the prime symptoms of breast disorder. The chief importance of self-examination lies in the discovery of lumps. A lump may be a cyst, a benign tumor or a malignancy. Many lumps disappear at the time of menses and only those present postmenstrually are significant. Characteristically, malignant lumps are painless in their early stages. The differential diagnosis can be made by a physician, but only if it is brought to his attention. Rarely in malignancy, a lump in the axilla is the first sign that is noticed. In those women who do not regularly have breast examinations—most lumps are discovered by accident. For example, a woman receives a sharp blow to her breast. That night the area is still tender, and she puts a hand up to it. She discovers a lump. The lump was not caused by the blow, but its discovery was.

Nipple Discharge. A discharge that spots the brassiere or drips out without being elicited requires medical attention immediately. Cheesy and milky discharges are usually of no significance. Bloody, brown or clear fluid discharges should be checked immediately.

Change in Appearance. A breast with an adhering lump near the surface may *dimple* the skin outside, or it may cause the nipple *to retract*.

A deep-adhering cancer may fix the breast tissue to the underlying pectoral muscle. There may be a change in *firmness, redness, chapping* of the areolar area, *erosion* or *edema*.

Examination

Self-Examination. In order to discover carcinoma of the breast early enough so that its excision will be life-saving, regular examination of their breasts by all women is advocated. The best protection against cancer is effective early action. If every woman in the United States visited her physician every three months for an examination of her breasts, the death rate from this disease would drop. But such frequency of medical visits is not practical.

The following technic is suggested for self-examination of the breasts:

• Sit or stand in front of your mirror, with your arms relaxed at your sides, and examine your breasts carefully for any changes in size and shape. Look for any puckering or dimpling of the skin, and for any discharge or change in the nipples.

• Raise both your arms over your head, and look for exactly the same things. See if there's been any change since you last examined your breasts.

• Lie down on your bed, put a pillow or a bath towel under your left shoulder, and your left hand under your head. (From here on, you should feel for a lump or a thickening.) With the fingers of your right hand held together flat, press gently to feel the inner, upper quarter of your left breast, starting at your breast bone and going outward toward the nipple line. Also feel the area around the nipple.

• With the same gentle pressure feel the lower inner part of your breast. Incidentally, in this area you will feel a ridge of firm tissue or flesh. Do not be alarmed. This is perfectly normal.

• Now bring your left arm down to your side, and still using the flat part of your fingers, feel under your armpit.

• Use the same gentle pressure to feel the upper, outer quarter of your breast from the nipple line to where your arm is resting.

• And, finally, feel the lower outer section of your breast, going from the outer part to the nipple.

• Repeat the entire procedure as that described above on the right breast.

• Examine your breasts every month right after your period. Be sure to continue these checkups after your menopause.

• If you find a lump or a thickening, leave it alone until you see your doctor. Most breast lumps or changes are not cancer, but only your doctor can tell.

In spite of the excellent educational program of the American Cancer Society, there has not been a significant drop in the death rate due to cancer of the breast. Many women are not aware of what they themselves can do to discover early disease. Some women have not been exposed to the idea of self-examination. Others have, but fail to attend to it. Small early cancers can only be found by regular examinations.

Helping with Emotional Factors. In the education of women for protecting themselves from death from cancer of the breast, the imparting of knowledge is not enough. The educator also must understand why there is resistance to action, and how people may be helped to overcome their apparent indifference. Apathy, fear and the magical belief that cancer will happen to the other person and not to oneself leads to resistance to regular examinations of the breasts in the search for lumps. Fear may lead to "forgetting" or refusing to do the monthly examination; or, on the other hand, it may induce such concentration on the breasts as to lead to daily examinations. One woman said, "I'd hate to examine my breasts. I couldn't do it! Both my mother and my father died from cancer. Last night I dreamed about it and woke up in a cold sweat from the nightmare. I have a terrible phobia about it. I'm so frightened that I hate to wash under my arms, I'm so afraid that I'm going to feel something there. Of course, I do wash, but never without thinking about cancer." Instead of examining herself, this woman visits her doctor regularly every six months. A wise nurse would encourage this woman to continue the regularity of the visits, without pushing her on the point of self-examination. The nurse should be flexible, accepting the compromise, lest her patient's fear take the form of resistance to any type of examination.

The knowledge that two-thirds of all breast operations are for benign lesions (Lewison and Taras) is not necessarily reassuring. The patient knows that she may be in the other third. Those who have seen a close relative die of cancer of the breast may find self-examination especially difficult.

Some women fear the cure as much as the disease. Breast amputation is mutilating; irrevocably it alters a woman's body, and particularly significant is the fact that it affects a part of her body intimately associated with sexual fulfill-

ment and childbearing. Concern with appearance after surgery may be mitigated only partly by the use of prosthetic devices. The change in her body is one that the woman herself must learn to accept and cope with, regardless of what measures she may use to conceal the disfigurement from others.

These are deep and significant feelings, not to be ignored. Nurses should help women to come to grips with these feelings by listening to them. Without prying, help the woman to identify exactly what it is that troubles her. Help her to talk to you and her physician without feeling ashamed. Provide her with the factual information that she needs. The patient needs a great deal of support from the physician, nurse, office secretary, friends, and family.

Fear of cancer is not limited to those outside the medical and the nursing professions. The United States culture is one which places high value on the female breast as a primary source of identification with the feminine role. Since most nurses are women, some may find the care of patients with breast cancer threatening and anxiety producing because of their vulnerability to this disease. Unwittingly, they may avoid the patient except for highly structured activities such as teaching exercises. If the nurse is to be supportive of patients she must have the opportunity to become aware of her own feelings and reactions.

Some women seem to survive the surgery without damage to their self-concepts. One woman who had had a bilateral mastectomy said, "My breasts weren't *me*. The *me* is still there." This woman suffered no depression postoperatively and says that when she is dressed she does not feel that her appearance is markedly altered.

Examination by a Physician. All women should have their breasts examined by a physician at least once a year. Those over 30, those with cysts, and those who have a relative who has had cancer should be examined every six months. Women should go immediately to a doctor when a lump in the breast is discovered.

To investigate a breast lump the doctor completely palpates the breasts and nodes. Palpation of adjacent (such as axillary) lymph nodes helps the doctor to determine evidence of cancer that has spread. The spread to lymph nodes sometimes is diagnosed by biopsy. He inspects the breasts from every angle with the patient sitting, standing, and bending. *Mammography,* or soft tissue roentgenography of the breast without the injection of a contrast medium may be ordered. On these films it is possible for the radiologist and the surgeon to distinguish with considerable accuracy a benign from a malignant lump, and also to discover lesions that are still too small to palpate.

When a malignancy is suspected, the surgeon usually takes a biopsy to confirm the diagnosis. *Aspiration biopsy* can be done in the doctor's office under local anesthesia. A large-core needle attached to a syringe is inserted into the tumor. Applying suction, a core of tissue is withdrawn into the bore of the needle by the physician. The material is smeared on a glass slide, fixed and stained, and sent to the pathologist.

Recurrent cysts may be aspirated periodically to facilitate examination of the breasts in the search for a new lump that may be cancer. Malignancy in the breast seems to be somewhat more common in patients with cystic disease than in women with normal breasts (Davis). The most important point in the nursing care of these patients is to encourage them to have regular examinations. The search for new lumps is complicated by the already existing ones caused by the cysts, but the woman who becomes familiar with her own breasts by periodic examination often can identify new growths.

Incisional biopsy is performed in the operating room. The microscopic frozen section is performed by the pathologist while the patient is anesthetized. The doctor is guided in his treatment by the pathologist's report.

Thermography, an additional diagnostic method under investigation, is based on the principle that neoplastic tissues produce more heat than surrounding tissues due to their high metabolism. The heat is transmitted to overlying skin and the infrared radiation can be detected and a heat "image" produced by scanning devices. Temperature difference between normal and malignant tissue is in the range of 2° F. (Spratt and Donegan).

Roentgenograms may be taken to determine whether or not there are metastases to bone.

CYSTIC DISEASE

Chronic cystic mastitis is not inflammatory (as the word *mastitis* would imply). In this disorder normal breast tissue proliferates and forms many masses throughout the breasts. The masses become fibrotic and block the ducts, causing cysts to form.

Cystic disease of the breast may cause no symptoms other than lumps, or the breast may be tender, especially premenstrually. There may be shooting pains one or two days before menstruation. A well-fitted brassiere may be advised by the physician. During periods when the breasts are tender, the patient may feel more comfortable if she wears a brassiere during the night as well as the day. Multiple cystic disease sometimes is treated by simple mastectomy. The areola may be saved, and reconstruction surgery may be done with fat and fascia or a plastic insert to preserve the appearance of the breast (augmentation mammoplasty).

A single breast cyst may develop, frequently with a bluish color, which has prompted the name *blue-domed.* Cysts usually are movable in the surrounding breast tissue. They have far less tendency to adhere and to cause retraction than does cancer.

BREAST SURGERY

Preoperative Care

A benign tumor usually is excised. When there is malignancy, the surgeon usually removes the pectoralis major, the pectoralis minor, and the entire breast along with the adjacent lymph nodes in an attempt to remove all of the cancer cells from the patient's body: this is a *radical mastectomy.* A *simple mastectomy* is removal of a breast without lymph node dissection.

Other procedures for malignancy include simple mastectomy with axillary dissection, extended radical mastectomy with chest wall resection, and superradical mastectomy in which the sternum is split and the lymph nodes are dissected from the mediastinum. Since the latter two procedures involve opening the thoracic cavity, additional postoperative care is required.

In surgery for a lump in the breast, the preparation of the patient for operation is for the more extensive operation, because until the doctor sees the pathology report he does not know whether the lesion is benign or malignant.

The spread of cancer is capricious and inconstant. It may begin early or late. At first it is microscopic, and is not detectable grossly. A very small lump in the breast may have sent some cells along the lymphatics to the axillary nodes. Cancer spreads through the lymphatics and blood vessels.

Before surgery the patient should be told by the surgeon that a radical mastectomy may be necessary. Skin preparation includes the axilla. Blood typing and cross matching are done. The operative permission includes radical mastectomy.

This is a time of tension and suspense for the patient. She does not know whether she will awaken from the anesthesia with only a lump removed or an entire breast removed and a diagnosis of cancer. Help her in every way possible to face the impending operation.

It may be easier for her to talk to a woman about her fears than to a man. Be sure that you know what the surgeon has told her. She may not know that cancer is the disease in question (although that would be rare today), and the word should not be used first by you. Let the patient talk without adding to her anxiety. Some prefer not to mention the word "cancer," even though they are aware that it is a possible diagnosis. Assure her that her breast will not be removed unless the doctors know that this operation will be necessary for her health. If she has doubts about this subject, either preoperatively or postoperatively, let her express them, but continue to convey the idea that the operation is necessary. When the patient seems unable to accept the surgery, this should be discussed with the surgeon before the operation is performed. This is essential in order to help to lessen serious postoperative sequelae, such as severe depression or the patient's inability to recognize and to acknowledge that a breast has been removed.

When there is no doubt that a radical mastectomy must be done, a short visit from a recovered patient may assist the patient to accept the surgery more readily.

The Operation

The patient is prepared for a radical mastectomy and is kept under general anesthesia while the biopsy specimen is being examined. The pathologist requires about 15 minutes to make his diagnosis of the tiny piece of tissue. If the diagnosis is of a benign tumor, the surgeon may simply excise it and close the wound.

The excision of a benign breast tumor is minor surgery. If it were not for the possibility of performing a radical mastectomy, many benign tumors could be removed under local rather than general anesthesia. The surgery is over quickly, and the incision is small; the patient usually goes home after two or three days in the hospital.

If at operation the pathologist's report shows that the lesion is malignant, the surgical drapes are changed, and the operating team rescrubs and proceeds with a radical mastectomy.

A drain often is inserted to prevent the accumulation of fluid in the wound. A skin graft (often from the anterior thigh) may be required to close the resulting wound. When there is a graft, a drain may be left in the axilla to drain fluid that may form under the graft and prevent its "take." If a graft has been done, pressure dressings are applied on both the donor and the recipient sites.

If the cancer is so far advanced that there are metastases to other portions of the body, the removal of the breast will not cure the disease, and a mastectomy may not be done. A simple mastectomy may be performed to remove a grossly enlarged, draining breast to make the patient more comfortable.

The combined operations—breast amputation and bilateral oophorectomy for node metastases from breast cancer—are performed in premenopausal women by a significant number of surgeons. Because the ovaries are removed to eliminate the source of estrogen from the body, no replacement estrogens are given to help to relieve the distressing symptoms of the surgical menopause. The suddenness of the lack of estrogen supply frequently causes these patients more severe menopausal symptoms than those associated with natural menopause.

The two operations, singly or in combination, are threatening to a woman's image of herself, especially for women of childbearing age. The one operation prevents a woman from having children, and the other mutilates her appearance.

Because some surgeons believe the risk is high for the development of another primary cancer in the remaining breast, the surgeon may recommend that the remaining breast be removed.

Postoperative Care

Patients who have had a radical mastectomy frequently discover their diagnosis for themselves when they are beginning to recover from anesthesia. Unlike many other types of surgery, this operation makes the diagnosis evident to the patient. The doctor and the family have no time to talk over how, if, and when to break the news to the patient. The patient, whose emotional and physical resources have been lowered by anesthesia, surgery, drugs, and suspense, needs a nurse to be there to help her at the time of the anguish of discovery.

Arm Position. Because in radical surgery the incision is extensive, disturbing the integrity of a large area of skin and muscle, immediately after the surgery the upper arm on the affected side is prevented from excessive motion, especially abduction. That arm may be bandaged to the body, with the elbow bent at a right angle, especially if grafting has been done. Motion might pull the graft free of its attachments. Whether the arm is bandaged or not, do not allow abduction of the arm on the affected side. The arm must be kept especially still when grafting has been done. A pillow may be placed under the arm to help to support it and to elevate it above breast level at least for the first day. This aids in preventing lymphedema that commonly develops postoperatively from interference with the circulatory and lymphatic systems. If the arm is bound to the body, watch the hands for signs of impaired circulation (swelling, cyanosis, coldness, tingling). If you note such signs, call the surgeon.

The Dressing. Drains may be inserted at the time of surgery to remove the serous fluid that collects under the skin, thereby delaying healing and predisposing to infection. A drainage tube may be attached to low-pressure suction such as the Hemo-Vac which enables the patient to be easily up and about and eliminates the need for constantly reinforcing dressings. Drainage tubes are irrigated daily by the physician in order to free any clots.

Some wounds drain copiously. Note and chart color, amount, odor, and consistency of any drainage, whether from a drain or on the dressing. Watch the dressing for drainage and oozing, and report any evidence of these to the doctor. Feel with your hand under the patient's side, since fluid seeping from the wound may not be visible on the front of the bandage, but it may flow underneath the patient. Immediately after the operation, check the dressing at least every 15 minutes. On the second and the third postoperative days check it at least three times a day, but do not disturb it. The dressing, which is bulky to hold the skin flaps down, usually is left in place until the fifth to the ninth day after the operation, depending on whether a graft was used and the preference of the surgeon. At that time the dressing is changed.

Every effort should be made to assist the patient to look at the incision before going home but she should not be pushed into this at the time of the first dressing change. In addition to the incisions, stab wounds for drains are also present and the over-all appearance can greatly upset the patient who may react with hysteria, anger, crying, depression, or withdrawal. Helping the patient involves anticipation of and sensitivity to her reaction. Timing the encouragement for the patient to look requires an assessment of the patient's state of readiness. When the patient's refusal continues, a lead such as "You seem not to be able to look at the incision," can be helpful in initiating discussion. Chiding the patient that she'd best be prepared before she goes home is not helpful. Sometimes, having the husband, daughter, or other person who will help the patient at home come to the hospital for the dressing change is beneficial. The nurse can offer support and answer questions.

The patient needs to know that in time, redness, swelling, and irregularity disappear, the scar becomes less prominent, and the tissues more normal in color. The healing period for the wound is four to eight weeks for most patients. Pressure dressings may be continued after the initial dressing change and dressings are changed daily until healing occurs.

Helping the Patient Toward Self-Sufficiency. Since dressings tend to constrict the chest, the patient needs to be assisted to cough deeply and take deep breaths. Pain is considerable and narcotics are given liberally as ordered by the physician. Because the movement of the chest is painful and opiates depress respirations, help the patient to take full breaths after medication for pain has had its effect.

The patient may be helped out of bed for the first time on the operative night or the next day. Patients who have had radical surgery, with or without drainage, are helped to walk as soon after surgery as patients who have had a simple mastectomy. If the patient needs assistance as she walks, support her on the *unaffected* side. She will have a tendency to splint the operative site and to balance herself by hunching that shoulder. Encourage her to keep the shoulder level and the muscles relaxed. For approximately two weeks (the length of time varies with the surgeon's preference) the arm on the affected side usually is supported in a sling whenever the patient is out of bed.

Immediately postoperatively, help the patient with those activities that she cannot do for herself. For example, cut her meat for her. To avoid placing her in the dependent and the embarrassing position of having to ask for this service, perform it before she asks. However, as soon as it is possible, help her to be independent and to do everything for herself that she can. Try to encourage her to be self-sufficient in a way that minimizes the chances for her to misinterpret your intentions to mean that you do not want to be bothered with her.

Exercises of the affected arm will be ordered by the physician and in some institutions begin about the third or fourth postoperative day. With grafting, no exercise is used without definite written orders from the surgeon. In patients who do not have grafts, exercises are frequently preceded from the first postoperative day by such activities of daily living as brushing the teeth, washing the face, and combing the hair with the affected hand. Squeezing a rubber ball stimulates circulation and helps restore function. Exercises prevent shortening of muscles, contractures of joints, and loss of muscle tone.

Active exercises are always more effective than passive ones. As soon as the doctor has given his permission, the patient starts on a regular program that can enable her to perform all the activities in which she used her arm preoperatively. The first exercises may be opening and closing the hand, flexing and extending the fingers, and bending the wrist forward and backward. In some hospitals no order is needed to commence these exercises, and they are started on the first postoperative day. There is a psychological as well as a physiologic point to starting active exercises soon after surgery. This is something that the patient herself can do to aid in her recovery. When the drains are removed, and the first dressing is changed, the surgeon may consider that the wound has healed sufficiently so that the patient can abduct her arm. Raising the elbow away from the body may be started. If fluid collects in the wound, exercises are delayed.

Whenever the exercises start, it is important for the return of full function that they be practiced regularly. The removal of the pectoral muscle causes some temporary loss of strength, but no loss of arm function. Though the arm on the affected side will present the most difficulty, exercises should be bilateral to avoid pain and postural change resulting from inconsistent development and consequent structural change.

Some hospitals have group classes for postmastectomy patients. Doing exercises with other women who have the same difficulties can help a patient to feel that she is not odd or clumsy, and that she is one among others who share a common problem and have common goals. A mimeographed pamphlet that can be given to the patient, illustrating the exercises, may help her to practice those ordered for her. *Help Yourself to Recovery*, a pamphlet written for patients, describes postmastectomy exercises. Published by the American Cancer Society, it is available from your local Cancer Society chapter.

The teaching of exercises is important but it should not be the focus of the nurse-patient relationship. The feelings and reaction of the patient afford the framework in which the nurse teaches. A perfect teaching plan can be a failure if the patient is not ready to learn or is so anxious that her perception is distorted. Because patients vary in their grief reactions, some may be too depressed to be able to meet the nurse's expectations for participation in self-care activities. The normal healing processes of grieving cannot be accelerated and some patients need more time, artful listening, gentle suggestion, and passive performance by the nurse before they are able to accept the changes in themselves and be ready to learn. As the patient's mourning and depression lessen, she will be able to be more aware of how the exercises are helping her and become a more active participant in the learning process.

Skin Care. After the bandage has been removed, help the patient to care for the skin area herself. She should wash it gently with a soft washcloth and soap. Complete healing of the wound takes considerable time and varies with the patient's state of health and complicating factors, such as wound infection. Whereas some patients have healing in two months, others may require six to eight months for complete healing. It is not unusual for patients to have some discomfort in the operative site for several months. One described the discomfort thus: "It pinches and pulls and feels as if it is bandaged with sandpaper." Cold cream, pure lanolin or any emollient may be applied to the scar. Talcum powder may relieve itching.

Attitudes. The emotional significance of a mastectomy varies from patient to patient. To some it is but a surgical experience, and life continues as before. To others it means the first signal of the death process. Many of the women

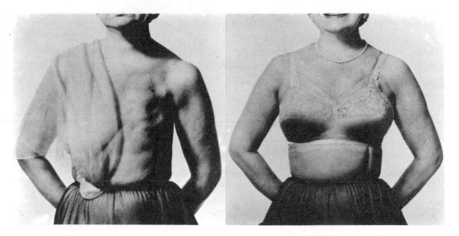

FIG. 46-1. (*Left*) Radical mastectomy scar. The slight irregularity is typical. (*Right*) Same patient fitted with a prosthesis. (Identical Form, Inc., New York, N.Y.)

are occupied with thoughts of death, but find no one with whom to discuss it freely. One study shows that the impact of the significance of surgery is more likely to be felt fully once the patient has returned home than in the hospital (Quint). Yet family and friends understandably tend to avoid conversations about death, and the patient is expected to carry on as before. Not only are family and friends emotionally involved with the patient, but a conversation about another's impending death is a reminder that one, too, will die.

The postmastectomy patient often feels isolated, with no one to help her face the annoying problem of the healing incision and the larger problems of social acceptance and worry about death. How effectively the patient maintains her contacts with family and friends when she returns home is determined by her prior relationship with them and by her attitude, and theirs, to the surgery. The nurse can encourage the patient to maintain her ties with friends and family during hospitalization by showing courtesy to the patient's visitors and by assisting the patient, if she needs help, when she wishes to write letters or to make telephone calls. Perhaps the greatest help that the nurse can render in aiding the patient to maintain her ties with others after discharge lies in showing acceptance of the patient and willingness to help her come to grips with the impact of the surgery. The skillful nurse allows her patient to express what she wishes concerning the meaning of the operation to her, without suggesting what it should mean, might mean, or has seemed to mean to other patients.

If the patient learns to care for her skin while she is still in the hospital and has your support

and interest, she may have less tendency to shun the scar once she gets home. If she is repelled by the sight of it, allow her to tell you. Show interest in its progress of healing, and help her to become used to it. You can tell her that the scar will become less noticeable in time. For example, the married patient who can begin to accept her scar before she leaves the hospital can help her husband to feel less shy or embarrassed about it, and then in turn he can help her to feel more comfortable about it.

A Prosthesis. On discharge from the hospital the patient is seldom ready to wear a commercial prosthesis because the wound is not healed. Helping the patient to make a prosthesis while she is still in the hospital shows her that she can present a natural appearance when dressed. After the physician has given permission, the patient can be fitted for a prosthesis. (Perhaps the more acceptable word to the patient will be "falsie.") Until a prosthesis is obtained, and when the doctor approves, a makeshift one to be worn over the dressing can be fashioned, using the patient's brassiere. For example, suggest that the patient tack a sanitary pad into the cup that fits over the affected side (providing her, of course, with the pad and the sewing implements). Sew one end to the middle section of the brassiere and the other end to the back, so that the pad extends under the arm and fills in the space left by the loss of the muscle and the glandular tissue. Then fluff some absorbent cotton and stuff the area between the brassiere and the pad until the contour of that side is similar to that of the breast on the other side. Change the pad and the cotton daily to keep them clean and to avoid matting. Be sure that this improvised "falsie" does not exert pressure on the shoulder. If it does, the patient can insert a small strip of elastic tape in the shoulder strap. When the patient gets dressed in her own clothes, and before she is allowed to wear a commercial prosthesis, a V-shaped elastic insert from her brassiere to her girdle will prevent that side of the brassiere from riding up. This is a very important point, because if the patient feels that the cotton is about to pop out from the neck of her dress, she will be unnecessarily self-conscious, have a tendency to keep pulling at her brassiere, and refrain from using her arm on that side freely and naturally.

When the surgeon tells the patient that she may wear a commercial prosthesis, she has her choice of several different types. Some are made of foam rubber; others are inflated with air or filled with fluid. Sponge rubber is light and easily washable. Excessive heat and of course, careless handling should be avoided. If a rubber prosthesis is worn under a bathing suit, it can be squeezed dry unobtrusively with the forearm while the woman dries her face with a towel. Any prosthesis in a bathing suit should be tacked in. The prostheses that are filled with water assume natural contours in keeping with those of the other breast as the woman changes position. These prostheses feel more like a normal breast and even assume body warmth.

It is especially important for nurses to know where to refer their postmastectomy patients, since it is frequently the nurse to whom the patient will turn for help.

Some surgical supply houses and corsetiers who sell breast prostheses have an experienced female prosthetist who can give the patient a correct fit and instruct her in the care of the prosthesis. Such stores may be found in the yellow pages of the local telephone directory. Many large department stores carry prostheses, at a cost of about $18.00. Some companies have excellent pamphlets prepared for postmastectomy patients. Be sure that the doctor approves of the literature, the prosthesis and the store before suggesting any of these resources to the patient. The addresses of several stores can be given to the patient. Some hospitals keep samples of different types of breast forms to show to the patients.

Complications of Breast Surgery

Some postmastectomy patients develop sympathetic pain in the other breast. Encourage such a patient to call this symptom to the atten-tion of her doctor. It usually does not represent organic disease. At times the remaining breast becomes larger postoperatively.

The amputation site may become infected, or serous fluid may collect beneath it. When you are changing the dressing, and after the dressing is no longer necessary, inspect the wound daily. Look for pockets of swelling, redness, discharge, odor, and breaks in the suture line.

Slight and transistory swelling of the arm is relieved usually as soon as the arm regains function. However, in some postmastecomy patients lymphedema is disabling. It may develop shortly after the operation or years later. The cause is unknown, but it is believed that an infection that obstructs lymphatic flow can cause this distressing complication. Radiation may aggravate it. Because infection may play a role in its etiology, and because the complication may occur years later, women who have had a mastectomy should be told to treat as serious even slight infections of that arm and that hand. Any symptoms of infection of the hand or cellulitis of the arm (fever, pain, red streaks on the arm) should bring the patient immediately to her doctor. Cutting the cuticles should be avoided, because it may lead to infection. The patient should exercise care not to break the skin when she cuts her nails, and hangnails should be cut, if at all, by a physician. Most women are understandably reluctant to go to a doctor to have a hangnail cut, but they must be warned not to pull at it or to bite it, to keep it very clean, and to report to the doctor at the slightest sign of soreness or infection. The healthy, unbroken skin is the best protection against a minor infection that may lead to the major complication of edema of the arm. Night creams may help to keep the skin soft. Patients with lymphedema should not be given any form of injections or vaccinations in the affected arm.

Edema of the arm is treated by antibiotics to abolish the underlying infection; however, this treatment is effective only if it is applied before fibrosis has blocked lymphatic outflow. Often the patient is hospitalized, and her arm is kept elevated on a pillow. An air pressure machine may be used. It automatically fills the segments of the sleeve with air, exerting progressive cumulative pressure on the arm. The most distal portion of the sleeve fills first, then the next, and so on, forcing fluid past incompetent lymphatic valves toward the heart. After all the segments are filled, the air is released, and the cycle starts over again. The machine is set approximately 5 mm. below the diastolic blood pressure. This treatment must be used several times a day to be effective. Significant arm edema can be controlled in some cases with the use of an elastic sleeve or Ace bandage. Patients who are obese will need help in losing weight, as obesity complicates the reduction of the edema. Low sodium diets and diuretics are sometimes prescribed.

TREATMENT OF METASTATIC CANCER

It is estimated that slightly over two-thirds of the individuals affected with mammary cancer will sometime during their lifetime have disseminated mammary cancer. Metastases often cause pain in the new site. Lymph nodes are most commonly involved in metastasis with bone and pulmonary involvement following in order. Many organs and systems can be affected before death. When bone becomes involved, there is danger of pathologic fracture (fracture after slight or no trauma). The patient is taught to take precautions against falling and to avoid bumps. Without frightening her, encourage her to keep regular appointments with her physician.

Treatment varies with the physician and specific type of metastasis and is aimed at providing the greatest period of palliation for the patient. All forms of treatment carry the possibility of unpleasant side-effects and complications.

Hormonal Therapy. Normal function of the mammary gland is dependent on the action of several stimulating hormones. Changing the hormonal environment of the body should inhibit the growth of the primary tumor or metastatic tissue elsewhere in the body derived from the primary tumor. The hormonal environment of the body can be changed by *ablation* (removal) of an endocrine organ or by *addition* of exogenous sex hormones.

Endocrine ablative procedures include prophylactic or therapeutic destruction of the ovaries or testes (castration) by surgery or radiotherapy. Also, the adrenal gland is capable of producing estrogen. Bilateral adrenalectomy sometimes is performed in women who have estrogen-dependent metastatic cancer, and whose vaginal smears continue to demonstrate a high level of estrogen activity. This operation may cause the cancer to regress and the patient to feel less distress. Lifetime replacement of cortisone with adjustment of dosage in times of stress is necessary after adrenalectomy.

The removal of the pituitary gland (hypophysectomy) may be done in the treatment of estrogen-dependent tumors to suppress both the adrenal glands and the ovaries. Other endocrine glands will be suppressed as well, and the patient may require adrenal and thyroid replacement therapy. After both adrenalectomy and hypophysectomy the nurse should watch the patient for polyuria and other water and electrolyte balance disturbances. Stress may bring about symptoms of adrenal or pituitary insufficiency. (See Chap. 41 for a more detailed discussion of observations to be made and nursing care in these conditions of endocrine imbalance.)

Additive hormonal therapy to change the internal environment includes the use of androgens, estrogens, progesterone, and cortisone.

Large doses of estrogen and testosterone are used sometimes to help to alleviate the pain, the weight loss and the malaise of metastatic cancer in postmenopausal women. Estrogen is contraindicated in premenopausal women, for whom large doses of testosterone propionate may be ordered for its antagonistic effect. Hormonal treatment does not cure cancer that has spread, but it may increase the life span by months or even years, and it makes some patients more comfortable during much of this time. Why the hormones have this effect is unexplained.

Estrogen therapy can cause nausea and vomiting, pigmentation of the nipple and the areola, and uterine bleeding. Stress incontinence is frequent. Sodium may be retained, leading to excessive storage of intercellular fluid and edema. To help to relieve this situation, diuretics and a low-sodium diet may be ordered. Large doses of estrogen sometimes cause the mobilization of calcium into the bloodstream. When this happens, the kidney may be damaged in excreting the excess calcium.

Intramuscular androgen (testosterone) therapy is used especially when there are metastases to bone. Patients may have increased bone pain after the first few injections, but as therapy continues, pain frequently is lessened, there is some recalcification of bone, and the patient gains appetite and weight. Androgen therapy may cause fluid retention and distressing symptoms of virilization, such as a deeper voice, hirsutism, and increased libido.

The results of therapy aimed at decreasing the amount of estrogen in the patient's body may be observed by vaginal smears and studies of the urinary excretion of estrogen and calcium.

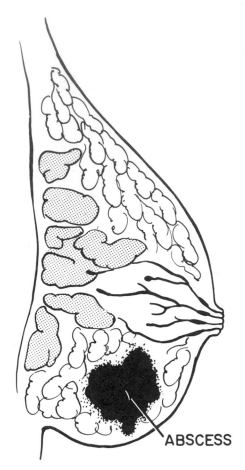

ABSCESS

Fig. 46-2. A breast abscess.

Radiotherapy may be given preoperatively or postoperatively. If the surgeon finds that the axillary nodes contain cancer cells, a series of x-ray treatments may be ordered prophylactically, even though the nodes have been removed. Postmastectomy exercises should continue during the x-ray treatments. For palliation purposes, radiotherapy may be directed to treatment of primary tumors, regional or distant metastases especially to bone, or local recurrence to the chest wall.

Chemotherapy. Metastases to soft tissue and bone are most responsive to chemotherapeutic agents. The purine antagonist 5-fluorouracil (5-FU) and the alkylating agent thio-TEPA (N, N', N"—triethylenethiophosphoramide) are the most useful chemotherapeutic agents for the treatment of mammary carcinoma. These drugs may cause bone marrow depression, granulocytopenia, anemia, nausca and vomiting, hypotension, dermatitis and malaise, diarrhea and stomatitis.

The use of any of the above measures may prolong the patient's life and make her more comfortable. Many eventually will succumb to the disease, but some will die from other causes. Some patients are symptom-free for long periods and lead relatively comfortable and fruitful lives. Unfortunately, others, like the young woman with galloping metastases, may die quickly. Still more might have to endure long periods of suffering before they succumb. The victims of breast cancer offer to nursing unlimited challenge.

BREAST ABSCESS

Abscesses occur most frequently as a postpartum complication. Fissures and cracks in the nipple provide an entry for organisms, especially staphylococci, which thrive in milk. The patient usually is hospitalized, placed on isolation precautions, and treated with antibiotics. A localized lesion may be incised, drained and packed. Because the soiled dressings are highly infectious, the nurse should keep a separate dressing tray at the patient's bedside.

Apply Montgomery straps, so that the frequent removal of adhesive tape will not irritate the skin. If warm soaks are ordered, apply zinc oxide to the surrounding skin to avoid maceration. A massage of the neck and the shoulder muscles on the affected side may help to decrease the pain by relaxing those muscles. Support the arm and the shoulder with pillows. Instruct the patient not to shave axillary hair on that side until the healing is complete. A postpartum patient admitted to the hospital with a breast abscess often is worried about the new baby she had to leave in someone else's care at home, and about the added expense of a second and an unexpected hospitalization.

REFERENCES AND BIBLIOGRAPHY

ALEXANDER, S. E.: Nursing care of a patient after breast surgery, Am. J. Nurs. 57:1571, 1957.

AMERICAN CANCER SOCIETY: Help Yourself to Recovery (pamphlet), New York, American Cancer Society, 1957.

————: Personal Memo for Today; BSE [Breast Self-examination] (pamphlet), New York, American Cancer Society, 1958.

BARD, M., and SUTHERLAND, H.: Psychological impact of cancer and its treatment. IV. Adaptation to radical mastectomy, Cancer 8:656, July-August, 1955.

BONSER, G. M., et al.: Human Breast Cancer, Springfield, Ill., Thomas, 1961.

BOUCHARD, R.: Nursing Care of the Cancer Patient, St. Louis, Mosby, 1967.

CARRINGTON, E. R.: Epidemic puerperal breast abscess, *Am. J. Nurs.* 58:1683, 1958.

CURRENT CONCEPTS IN CANCER: Carcinoma of the Breast, Stage I—Surgical Spectrum, *JAMA* 199:132, March, 1967.

DAVIS, H. H., *et al.*: Cystic disease of the breast: relationship to cancer, *Cancer* 17:957, 1964.

DIETZ, J. H., JR.: Rehabilitation of the cancer patient, *Med. Clin. N. Am.* 53:607, May, 1969.

EDWARDS, B. F.: Endoprostheses in plastic surgery, *Am. J. Nurs.* 64:123, May, 1964.

EGAN, R.: Mammography, *Am. J. Nurs.* 66:108, January, 1966.

FARROW, J.: Rehabilitation following radical breast surgery, *CA* 16:222, November-December, 1966.

HAAGENSEN, C. D.: *Diseases of the Breast,* Philadelphia, Saunders, 1956.

HARRIS, H., and SPRATT, J. S., JR.: Bilateral adrenalectomy in metastatic mammary cancer, *Cancer* 23:145, January, 1969.

HARTLEY, L., and BRANDT, E.: Control and prevention of lymphedema following radical mastectomy, *Nurs. Res.* 16:333, Fall, 1967.

HIGGINBOTTOM, S.: Arm exercises after mastectomy, *Am. J. Nurs.* 57:1573, 1957.

HUBBARD, T. B., JR.: Prophylactic mastectomy for the prevention of the second primary, *JAMA* 201:530, August, 1967.

JORSTAD, L. H.: *Surgery of the Breast,* St. Louis, Mosby, 1964.

LEWISON, E. F.: The treatment of advanced breast cancer, *Am. J. Nurs.* 62:107, October, 1962.

LEWISON, E. F., and TARAS, O. O.: Chronic cystic mastitis, *Am. J. Nurs.* 59:690, 1959.

MAYO, P., and WILKEY, N.: Prevention of cancer of the breast and cervix, *Nurs. Clin. N. Am.* 3:229, June, 1968.

MERCADO, R.: Radiotherapy, *in* SPRATT, J., and DONEGAN, W.: *Cancer of the Breast,* Philadelphia, Saunders, 1967.

METROPOLITAN LIFE INSURANCE CO.: *Statistical Bulletin,* vol. 50, March, 1969.

NEW YORK CITY CANCER COMMITTEE OF THE AMERICAN CANCER SOCIETY: *Dial for Life* (pamphlet), New York, The Committee, 1960.

PEREZ, M. C.: Pathology of mammary carcinoma, *in* SPRATT, J., and DONEGAN, W.: *Cancer of the Breast,* Philadelphia, Saunders, 1967.

QUINT, J. C.: The impact of mastectomy, *Am. J. Nurs.* 63:88, November, 1963.

ROBBINS, G.: Personal Communication.

RODMAN, M., and SMITH, D.: *Pharmacology and Drug Therapy in Nursing,* Philadelphia, Lippincott, 1968.

SPRATT, J., and DONEGAN, W.: *Cancer of the Breast,* Philadelphia, Saunders, 1967.

THORNBLAD, I.: Hormonal ablative therapy for the premenopausal patient with advanced cancer, *Nurs. Clin. N. Am.* 2:659, December, 1967.

WOLF, E.: Nursing care of patients with breast cancer, *Nurs. Clin. N. Am.* 2:587, December, 1967.

The Patient with Venereal Infection

47

Gonorrhea • Syphilis • Lymphogranuloma Inguinale • Chancroid
Granuloma Inguinale • Nursing Care of Patients with
Venereal Diseases

A venereal disease can be described as one that is communicated through sexual intercourse with an infected person. The major part of this chapter deals with syphilis and gonorrhea, the two most common venereal diseases.

GONORRHEA

Gonorrhea is a bacterial infection. The primary site of infection is the genital tract, from which the disease can spread to other parts of the body.

Incidence. Gonorrhea is the most common of the venereal diseases. The disease is worldwide, but there is no country that has accurate statistics of its incidence. The reluctance of physicians to report the disease in their patients, due to the social stigma associated with it, interferes with accurate reporting of cases. The number of reported cases of gonorrhea in the United States has risen from 142 per 100,000 in 1962 to 263 per 100,000 in 1969 (U.S. Center for Disease Control, Atlanta). Some of this increase is believed to be due to an increase in the proportion of cases that are reported. However, in the United States, as well as in many other countries, there has been a real increase in the number of cases of gonorrhea over recent years. Gonorrhea is now one of our foremost health problems. The problem of spread of the disease is intensified by the fact that infected persons may be asymptomatic. The person who has no symptoms but who harbors the infection may unknowingly spread the disease.

Etiology. The organism responsible for gonorrhea is the *Neisseria gonorrhoeae* (also called the *gonococcus*), named for Neisser, who first described it in 1897. The bacterium is gram-negative, and it resembles a pair of tiny kidneys. The gonococcus does not live long on a dry surface, and the likelihood of adults contracting the disease by ways other than sexual intercourse is minimal, and perhaps not possible. However, newborn infants may contract the infection from the mother's birth canal, and infants and young children may contract the infection from contamination by fingers or articles, on rare occasions. Natural immunity is not acquired after having an infection.

Symptoms. The usual incubation period is three days to two weeks after intercourse with an infected person. In men, the infection first settles around the mouth of the urethra, so that the first symptom usually is burning and pain on urination, followed by a yellowish discharge containing pus. In women the organisms frequently invade Skene's or Bartholin's glands, sometimes causing abscesses at these sites. However, many infections in women are asymptomatic for long periods of time.

If the disease is not treated, the infection may move up into the uterus and the fallopian tubes in women, and into the epididymis in men. The thick pus can clog completely both fallopian tubes, bind them with strictures and render a woman sterile. The adhesions may cause pain, disturb menstruation, or cause ectopic pregnancy. If the infection spreads still further it can cause a generalized infection of the abdominal cavity (peritonitis). Intercourse, douches and menstruation may spread the infection upward. Men may develop prostatitis, epididymitis, and infection of the seminal vessels. Adhesions of the urethra can result in urinary symptoms, and adhesions of the tract along which spermatozoa travel can result in sterility.

The infection, if it still is untreated, may enter the bloodstream, causing the patient to have typical symptoms of septicemia: fever, chills and malaise. Once the organisms are in the bloodstream, they have access to every part of the body. They may cause arthritis, or more rarely meningitis or endocarditis. All these complications are quite rare, considering the tremendous number of cases of gonorrhea.

Laboratory Diagnosis. In men a stained smear of the urethral discharge demonstrates the gonococcus. In women, however, smears are not reliable, and cultures should be obtained using special medium and growing conditions which promote the growth of the delicate gonococcus.

Treatment. The recommended therapy for men is intramuscular penicillin, 2.4 million units. For women, 4.8 million units of intramuscular penicillin given at one session in two or more sites is recommended. Many penicillin resistant strains of gonococci are emerging. If the patient is allergic to penicillin, or if the organism is resistant, another antibiotic, such as one in the tetracycline family, can be equally effective.

SYPHILIS

Syphilis (lues) is a venereal disease that can result in widespread destructive lesions in the body. Syphilis exists throughout the world, and it is the second most prevalent venereal disease in the United States. As is the case with gonorrhea, the hope that availability of antibiotics would markedly decrease the incidence of syphilis has proven unfounded.

Etiology

The cause of syphilis is a thin spirochete known as *Treponema pallidum*. A most significant fact about this spirochete is that it must stay wet to live. It is also sensitive to cold, and soap kills it. The transmission of syphilis is by sexual intercourse, although theoretically other types of intimate contact might also transmit syphilis. (Syphilis can also be transmitted via the placenta from the mother to her infant. Congenital syphilis will be discussed later.) Persons with untreated syphilis are infectious for about one year, and rarely are they infectious during the later latent period. Persons with primary syphilis who are successfully treated rapidly become noninfectious: the organisms usually dis-

appear from the lesions within 24 hours of the start of therapy.

Laboratory Diagnosis

A definite diagnosis of syphilis is made when the spirochetes are identified microscopically by dark-field examination of a smear taken from a lesion. This is the only way to make a definite diagnosis in the early stage of the disease. After the disease is well established in the body (about three weeks after infection), a positive blood test can help to establish the diagnosis. Many serologic tests for syphilis have been devised since the original Wassermann test. These tests frequently have been named after their inventor and fall into two general classes: the nontreponemal tests and the treponemal tests. The VDRL (Venereal Disease Research Laboratory) and the RPR (Reiter Protein Reagin) are the most common of the nontreponemal tests. The FTA-ABS (Fluorescent Treponemal Antibody-Absorption) is the most common of the treponemal tests.

Treponemal tests are more specific than nontreponemal tests. However, because the VDRL and the RPR are relatively simple and inexpensive, they have become the standard screening tests. Treponemal tests are reserved for special cases, to rule out false positive reactions. False positive results sometimes are seen in patients who have collagen diseases, or who recently have been inoculated. A positive serologic test, like a positive tuberculin, may remain so throughout the patient's life and does not necessarily indicate active disease. The presence of lesions and the adequacy of any past therapy are the usual criteria determining the need for treatment.

A majority of the states require a serology test for syphilis before a marriage license is issued. In the Armed Forces and some industries, blood tests for syphilis are done for routine screening. In many hospitals a serology test for syphilis is routine for all newly admitted patients.

Symptoms

After direct contact with a syphilitic lesion, as in kissing or sexual intercourse, the spirochetes enter the mucous membrane through tiny cracks and immediately establish a colony there. They also spread through the circulation almost immediately, and in about three weeks the patient may notice a chancre, the first lesion of syphilis. This is the *primary stage*. A chancre is a painless, round lesion on the genitalia, inside the wall

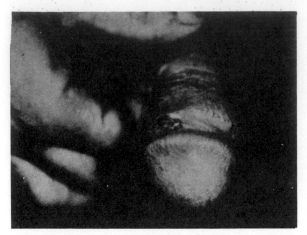

Fig. 47-1. Chancre, the primary lesion of syphilis. (Medichrome—Clay-Adams, Inc., New York, N.Y.)

of the vagina, on the nipple, or perhaps in a crack in the side of the mouth. The untreated chancre is alive with millions of spirochetes. It disappears entirely within two to five weeks. During this period some people have headaches, and most have enlarged lymph nodes near the chancre, but in general the patient feels well. A person who is ignorant of the disease is given little hint of the dangers that lie ahead if he fails to obtain treatment.

The *secondary* stage of the disease starts about six weeks after the initial infection. Many persons (but not all) with untreated syphilis show a skin rash during this period. The rash can take any form; frequently, it is diffuse, and it leaves as suddenly as it appeared. On mucous membrane surfaces, such as about the anus or in the mouth, luetic plaques (condylomas) may develop. These tend to crack and to ulcerate, and they are highly infectious. Sometimes the patient loses hair in patches, giving the head a characteristic moth-eaten appearance. The patient may have fever, headache, malaise and a sore throat; or, on the other hand, he may still feel well.

By now the serology test will be positive. During this stage there is generalized enlargement of the lymph nodes. Cutaneous and lymph node changes are the most prominent features of secondary syphilis. Other manifestations, such as iritis, arthritis, or even meningitis may occur, but are rare. After a few weeks it is usual for the symptoms to disappear. Although they come back, to disappear again, the untreated and unsuspecting patient may still be unaware of the seriousness of his illness.

The disease now enters a latent period. The patient feels well, and he has no symptoms related to syphilis. Some of the untreated infected persons will be troubled by the disease no longer. The others are not so fortunate. This disease is quiescent, perhaps for a year, often four or five years, and perhaps for 20 or 30 years.

Complications

At the tertiary stage, symptoms of the serious, damaging late complications begin to appear. Because the spirochete has had access through the bloodstream to all the tissues of the body, any organ now can be stricken with syphilis. Most commonly affected are the aorta, the eye and the central nervous system. Spirochetes may cause either widespread disease or local disease with a fibrous reaction. These well-defined local lesions are called *gummas*. They have fewer syphilis organisms than the earlier chancre, but they do contain a certain number. Gummas may develop anywhere in any tissue, but they appear most frequently in skin, bones, liver, larynx, and (in men) testes. Wherever these lesions occur, they may give rise to symptoms of dysfunction of the infected organ.

Even though the effects of the organisms on the internal organs may be devastating, the patient with tertiary syphilis generally is not a hazard to others. The elderly patient, for example, who is admitted to the hospital with a late cardiovascular disease due to lues has no discharging lesion and there is no reason to use special precautions for preventing spread of disease.

Complications to Pregnancy. Pregnant women with untreated syphilis commonly have a miscarriage; if the baby is carried to term, it may be stillborn, or it may be viable with congenital syphilis. In congenital syphilis, the fetus contracts the infection from the mother, through the placenta. Congenital syphilis may cause severe damage to practically any organ, including the central nervous system.

Cardiovascular Complications. A manifestation of late syphilis that is dangerous to life is the involvement of the cardiovascular system. The patches of necrosis produced by the disease in the walls of blood vessels weaken that area of the wall, leading to aneurysms. The development of aneurysms commonly occurs in the aortic arch. The pulsing aneurysm can balloon out, pushing all other structures—lungs, nerves, even vertebrae—out of its way. It can grow larger and larger, with its wall becoming thinner and thinner, until it bursts, and the patient bleeds to death.

In the heart the spirochetes may invade the aortic ring or the aortic valves, causing narrowing of the coronary vessels and coronary insufficiency, or valvular damage and aortic insufficiency.

Neural Complications. Syphilitic lesions of the nervous system occasionally cause meningitis, which responds to antiluetic treatment. Another manifestation of central nervous system involvement is general paresis, a chronic syphilitic meningoencephalitis. At first the patient exhibits slight changes in personality, which may start 10 or 20 years after his original infection. Memory and judgment become impaired. The mental state varies from euphoria to depression to paranoia. Optic atrophy with blindness may occur. If the disease progresses, the patient becomes totally helpless, both physically and mentally, and eventually expires.

In tabes dorsalis (also called *locomotor ataxia* or *syphilitic posterior spinal sclerosis*), the posterior spinal nerve roots, the posterior columns of the spinal cord and the posterior root ganglia become infected and degenerate. The syndrome may appear 5 to 20 years after the original infection. Because the kinesthetic fibers are the first ones to be affected, the first symptoms are pain and a loss of position sense. Pain, frequently in the legs (although it also may occur in the arms or the trunk) is severe, knifelike and burning. Tabetic crisis is an acute attack of severe abdominal pain with vomiting.

The patient with tabes dorsalis has eye involvement. For example, his eyes accommodate to near and far vision, but his pupils do not react to light (Argyll Robertson sign). Optic atrophy with blindness may occur.

Charcot Joint. A further complication that is found most often in patients with tabes dorsalis is the Charcot joint. The joint atrophies due to syphilitic involvement of its innervation. It becomes hypermotile, and it will not support weight. The knee and the spine are most frequently involved.

Treatment

Early. A single injection of 2.4 million units of long lasting penicillin, or daily injections of procaine penicillin (600,000 units for 10 days) cures early syphilis. Unlike *Neisseria gonorrhoeae*, there is no evidence that Treponema pallidum becomes penicillin resistant. Periodic follow-up is indicated, and serologic tests should be repeated every three months for one or two years. Infection does not give natural immunity. Reinfections do occur, but not so commonly as with gonorrhea.

If the patient cannot tolerate penicillin, he may be treated with tetracycline or erythromycin.

Late. In the later stages of syphilis, penicillin or another antibiotic is given but the spirochetes may be less susceptible to the drugs than they are in early syphilis. Damaged organs cannot be restored to complete function. Therapy is also directed at the treatment of any damaged structures of the body, with specific measures dictated by the pathology and the symptoms. For example, the treatment and nursing care of the patient with cardiac symptoms caused by syphilis is similar to that given any patient with heart disease, and the patient with an aortic aneurysm due to syphilis may undergo surgical treatment.

LYMPHOGRANULOMA INGUINALE (LYMPHOPATHIA VENEREUM)

This disease is caused by one of the large viruses. It starts with a fleeting, asymptomatic ulcer. The disappearance of this lesion is followed by an enlargement of the inguinal lymph nodes. Abscesses form, which become necrotic and may suppurate through the skin. These lesions are called *buboes*. The patient feels weak and has fever, chills and anorexia. If untreated, late persistent edema (elephantiasis) of the genitals, and rectal stricture may result.

Diagnosis is made by the Frei test, in which antigen is injected intradermally. The test is read in 48 to 72 hours. Broad spectrum antibiotics such as tetracycline are the treatment of choice. Lymph nodes may be aspirated, but should not be incised.

CHANCROID

Chancroid is an acute disease characterized by large multiple ulcerations of the genitals. Regional lymph nodes are also involved with abscess formation. The causative organism is *Hemophilus ducreyi*. This bacterium is difficult to isolate, and diagnosis is made on the basis of the clinical findings, and exclusion of other venereal diseases, such as syphilis. Of course, the two diseases may occur concurrently in the same patient. Sulfonamides and tetracyclines are effective therapy for chancroid.

GRANULOMA INGUINALE

Granuloma inguinale is a slowly progressive disease of the skin and mucous membranes, with some involvement of the lymph nodes. Ulcerative, nodular, and scarring forms occur, with gradual extension over the genital and inguinal areas. Severe, mutilating effects occur in untreated patients, who have an increased likelihood of developing carcinoma in the involved areas. The causative organism is *Donovania granulomatosis,* a bacterium which can be demonstrated by biopsy. Antibiotics of the tetracycline type are effective therapy.

NURSING CARE OF PATIENTS WITH VENEREAL DISEASES

Physical Measures

Venereal disease is usually treated on an outpatient basis. "Routine" isolation precautions are unnecessary for patients with syphilis or gonorrhea. The unnecessary use of such precautions as gowns and masks can lead the patient to feel rejected. Because of the stigma associated with venereal disease, it is especially important to convey acceptance to the patient, and to avoid measures which are likely to cause him to feel isolated.

While this patient has a discharge, contact with the discharge while it is still wet is avoided. For example, the nurse would wear gloves if she gives an enema, the patient should wash his hands after going to the bathroom, and the female patient should wash her hands after changing the perineal pad she wears while she has a discharge. Because the gonococcus has special predilection for the eye (gonorrhea used to cause a large percentage of the world's blindness, infecting newborn babies when they passed through the vagina), both the nurse and the patient should be especially careful to wash their hands before touching the face, after coming in contact with the discharge. In some hospitals the linen is considered contaminated for the first one or two days after treatment for gonorrhea is started. However, this organism dies so quickly on drying that the danger of spread of the disease by any means except direct contact with the still-wet discharge on mucous membrane or an open cut is practically non-existent.

If a patient known to have untreated primary syphilis is admitted to the hospital, precautionary measures are applied to avoid direct contact with the lesion during the brief period that the spirochetes are still alive in it after treatment has been instituted. For example, the nurse would wear gloves if she were giving care which required touching the chancre.

Attitudes

The nurse who is aware of her own feelings will have less tendency to shun or belittle the patient, or subtly to punish him by what she says or does. The patient's disease will be reported to the Board of Health, but no punitive action is involved. The records are confidential; the name of the informant never is revealed.

Attitudes of patients toward their illness are especially important in control of venereal disease. Some patients report to a venereal disease clinic with trivial symptoms, while others whose symptoms are acute require all the persuasion of a skilled nurse or other public health worker to convince them that they need medical attention. Between these two extremes are patients who come to the clinic with a realistic appreciation of their need for treatment, either because a sexual partner has named them as contacts, or because of the symptoms they are experiencing.

One of the major problems in venereal disease control is its prevalence among young people.

The nurse in her own community can do a great deal to bring young people with venereal disease to treatment, by being approachable and nonjudgmental, and by participating in programs which educate young people about various health problems, including venereal disease.

The problems created by venereal disease are added to those already faced by adolescents and young adults. For older patients, the problems may be slightly different, but they are no less severe. A man has to tell his wife that he has been unfaithful to her, because the wife must be examined to determine if she is infected; or a woman becomes terrified of infecting her children.

Venereal disease is not limited to any socioeconomic group, although the patient in a high socioeconomic class will probably be treated by his own physician, rather than in the clinic. The patient who comes from a high socioeconomic class and who secures private treatment is probably less likely to have his disease reported to health authorities than is a lower class patient who seeks care at a clinic. Attitudes toward the diseases may vary according to the socioeconomic level. In some groups the acquisition of gonorrhea is considered halfway between a joke and

REPORTED SYPHILIS AND GONORRHEA CASES
PER 100,000 POPULATION

All Areas Reporting in the Continental United States*

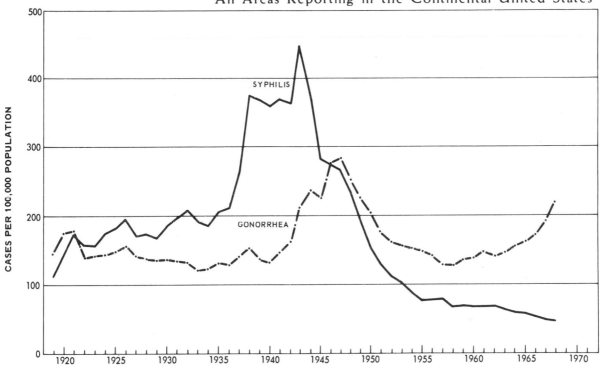

FIG. 47-2. Note that the incidence of gonorrhea is considered higher than that of syphilis and that both diseases have their highest incidence among young people. (United States Department of Health, Education, and Welfare, Public Health Service, October, 1967)

a sign of virility. This attitude may not be so acceptable to the nurse with a middle-class background, yet this patient also will need her teaching and understanding. This patient will also require help in realizing that gonorrhea is a serious disease which can cause severe illness and disability.

The increasing transmission of venereal disease, both syphilis and gonorrhea, through homosexual intercourse poses a difficult problem. Contact-tracing is especially difficult and is often impossible under these circumstances, because of the social stigma of homosexuality. Another difficult problem is posed by transmission of venereal disease from infected adults to children. Because of the stigma involved, treatment may not be sought. It is especially important for all who work in the field of venereal disease—pre-vention, detection, and treatment—to deal with their own feelings about sexual practices in a way which does not impede the reporting and treatment of venereal disease.

In working with patients who have venereal disease the nurse is especially careful always to respect the patient's privacy, and to avoid condescension.

It is not safe to have the attitude that a "single injection of penicillin cures venereal disease, so why be afraid of it?" The security given by the knowledge that venereal disease is cleared up by a single injection leads some people to be careless in attending to the early symptoms. Because they are sure of a cure, they may delay seeking it until the disease has spread. A careless attitude about reinfecting oneself or others may develop.

The entire disappearance of venereal disease was optimistically predicted after the discovery of the effectiveness of antibiotics. Less money was appropriated for case finding, and less attention paid to public education. It has now become clear that efforts to control venereal disease must be intensified. The development of penicillin-resistant strains of the gonococcus has intensified the urgency of the problem by contributing to more frequent treatment failures. It remains to be seen whether a program of medical and epidemiologic measures can effectively check the spread of venereal disease in this country.

REFERENCES AND BIBLIOGRAPHY

BEESON, P. B., and McDERMOTT, W. (eds.): *Cecil-Loeb Textbook of Medicine,* ed. 12, Philadelphia, Saunders, 1967.

BROWN, W. J., and LUCAS, J. B.: *Tice's Practice of Medicine,* Vol. III, Ch. 19, New York, Harper, 1962.

BROWN, W. J.: Acquired syphilis—drugs and blood tests, *Am. J. Nurs.* 71:713, April, 1971.

CALABRO, J. J.: Gonococcal arthritis in the young, *New Eng. J. Med.* 279:1002, October, 1968.

CALDWELL, J. G.: Congenital syphilis: a non-venereal disease, *Am. J. Nurs.* 71:1768, September, 1971.

CATTERALL, R. D.: *A Short Textbook of Venereology,* London, English University Press, 1965.

DESCHIN, C. S.: VD and the adolescent personality, *Am. J. Nurs.* 63:58, November, 1963.

DUBOS, R. J., and HIRSCH, J. G.: *Bacterial and Mycotic Infections of Man,* ed. 4, Philadelphia, Lippincott, 1965.

EDITORIAL: Excelsior, *JAMA* 203:592, February, 1968.

———: Gonorrhea, *Lancet* 1:675, March, 1968.

GOLDSBOROUGH, J. D.: On becoming nonjudgmental, *Am. J. Nurs.* 70:2340, November, 1970.

KING, A.: *Recent Advances in Venereology,* Boston, Little, Brown, 1964.

LENZ, P. E.: Women, the unwitting carriers of gonorrhea, *Am. J. Nurs.* 71:716, April, 1971.

MATHEWS, ROSEMARY: TLC with the penicillin, *Am. J. Nurs.* 71:720, April, 1971.

MOYER, P. J., and CONOVER, B. J.: The now style of campus nursing, *Am. J. Nurs.* 70:1901, September, 1970.

PODAIR, S.: *Venereal Disease,* Palo Alto, Fearon, 1966.

RUSSELL, B., and LOFSTROM, L.: Health clinic for the alienated, *Am. J. Nurs.* 71:80, January, 1971.

SCHWARTZ, W. F.: Communities strike back, *Am. J. Nurs.* 71:724, April, 1971.

STATISTICAL BULLETIN, vol. 50, New York, The Metropolitan Life Insurance Company, April, 1969.

TOP, F. H., SR.: *Communicable and Infectious Diseases,* ed. 6, St. Louis, Mosby, 1968.

U.S. DEPARTMENT OF HEALTH, EDUCATION, AND WELFARE, PUBLIC HEALTH SERVICE: *Syphilis: a Synopsis,* Washington, D.C., U.S. Government Printing Office, 1968.

VANDERMEER, DANIEL: Meet the V.D. epidemiologist, *Am. J. Nurs.* 71:722, April, 1971.

The Patient with a Dermatologic Condition 48

Injury and Disease of the Skin • The Problem of Disfigurement
Nursing Care of Patients with Skin Disease • Common
Dermatologic Conditions • Premalignant and Malignant Skin Lesions

Since the skin is in constant contact with the environment, it is unusually subject to injury and irritation. Nurses are in a strategic position to help others to maintain a normal, healthy skin. In bathing a hospitalized patient or in teaching patients in outpatient departments, industry, or their homes about sound practices in skin care, the nurse can help others to avoid abusing the skin and subjecting it to disease or injury.

Probably no other organ in the body is so subject to the application of remedies without medical advice. The accessibility of the skin makes such self-treatment commonplace. Although most people recognize the importance of healthy skin as an asset to personal appearance, those who unhesitatingly seek medical advice for other symptoms try a variety of nostrums on skin lesions, often making the condition worse. The idea that skin disease is never serious and therefore can be trifled with is far from the truth.

Cleanliness. Our culture values cleanliness, beauty and the avoidance of body odors. Skin diseases of all sorts are often attributed to poor personal hygiene, and a vigorous program of scrubbing and cleansing is undertaken sometimes to "clear the condition up." Popular advertising reinforces these ideas, and it emphasizes the wonderful properties of various soaps and cleansers. How clean does skin have to be to be healthy? If one bath is good, are two better?

Thorough scrubbing with soap and water or a detergent does temporarily reduce the number of bacteria, but the number rapidly returns to previous levels. Countless bacteria, most of them nonpathogenic, normally exist on the skin. Be-

cause most skin disorders of adults in this country are not related to germs and dirt, vigorous cleansing is not a cure-all. In fact, many conditions, such as those related to excessive dryness or to allergy, are made worse by preparations that increase skin dryness by removing natural oils, or that further irritate a sensitive skin with a variety of perfumes and colorings. People with an oily skin need to bathe more frequently than those with a dry skin. Older people, especially women, tend to have dry skin. Often, they cannot tolerate the drying effect of a hot tub bath daily. Instead, they may sponge-bathe the hands and the face, the axillae, the genital region, and the feet daily and take a tub bath or a shower two or three times a week. Lukewarm water is less drying than hot water. Bathing quickly rather than luxuriating in a leisurely bath is also less drying, because it avoids prolonged contact with soapy water. Adding a little oil to the bath water also lessens the drying effect.

Sweat glands are present over the entire body, but they are especially abundant in axillae, forehead, palms, and soles. In adults perspiration in the axillary region has an odor that is considered unpleasant. Deodorants are commonly used by both men and women to banish it. When bathing a patient, the nurse should apply the patient's deodorant if he is unable to do so or, if he wishes to purchase some, help him to obtain information about whether and where it is sold in the hospital.

Preventing Dryness. The sebaceous glands, which surround the hair follicles, secrete sebum, an oily substance that protects the hair and skin from becoming excessively dry. However, some persons produce less sebum than desirable for keeping the skin soft. This is particularly common during later life.

Heredity is important in determining the type of skin that a person will have. It is often noted that very dry or oily skins are most common among persons who have a family history of these conditions.

Creams help to keep the skin soft and smooth by reducing the loss of moisture from the skin. Creams and creamy lotions help to prevent dryness and chapping, particularly during cold weather, when moisture is lost more quickly. But regardless of additions of estrogenic hormones, creams cannot "restore youthful beauty." Their value lies primarily in the cream, rather than in the hormones. Most people, as they grow older, find that creams and lotions applied to face, hands, elbows and feet help to keep the skin smooth and soft. Wearing rubber gloves during the use of soaps and detergents for laundry and dishwashing also is helpful in preventing dryness. Such simple measures can reduce greatly chapping and cracking, which make the skin not only unattractive and uncomfortable but also vulnerable to infection and rashes.

Dandruff. People who have oily scalps need to shampoo the hair more frequently than do those with dry scalps. Pronounced oiliness and the shedding of greasy scales (commonly described as dandruff) require advice and treatment by a dermatologist. This condition is quite common, and many people either neglect it entirely or indulge in self-medication. If neglected, dandruff can be a factor in the thinning and the loss of hair. Regular brushing and shampooing and the avoidance of such constricting apparel as tight hat bands are important in preserving a healthy scalp.

Sunlight. Skin tanning in response to exposure to sunlight helps to protect it against the damaging effects of excessive ultraviolet light. But exposure to sunlight can be either a bane or a blessing, depending on the condition of the patient's skin and on the length of the exposure. For example, acne usually is improved by exposure to sunlight. But a prolonged exposure, particularly of fair-skinned persons whose skins tend not to tan effectively, can cause a painful sunburn. Adolescents and young adults tolerate exposure to sunlight better than older persons do, because the skin becomes thinner, drier and less protective with increasing age. Prolonged exposure to sun eventually causes the skin of farmers, sailors and other outdoor workers to become coarse and leathery. Skin cancer is more common among those whose skins have had excessive exposure to sun and wind. People who work outdoors can avoid unnecessary exposure by wearing wide-brimmed hats and by covering the skin (wearing a T-shirt as well as trunks or slacks).

The condition of the skin is indicative of one's general health. Good health habits help to keep the skin, as well as the rest of the body, in good condition. Plenty of sleep, relief of worry and tension, regular exercise and an optimum diet are important.

Nursing Considerations

What particular dermatologic problems are often encountered by the hospitalized patient, and how can the nurse help to prevent them? Here are some ways:

• Remember that the alkalinity of ordinary soaps sometimes causes irritation, especially in older, bedridden patients. The doctor may suggest a soap substitute of neutral pH, such as pHisoderm, Dermolate, or Lowila.

• When you are giving a bed bath, rinse the soap off with clear water. Never leave the cake of soap in the bath water, because it makes the water soapy and also wastes soap. Use a soap dish. If one is not available, a folded paper towel will do. Change the water in the basin frequently, so that the process of rinsing is not actually a reapplication of soap.

• Use the method that provides the best possible rinsing compatible with the degree of activity permitted the patient. A patient who can have a tub or a shower with assistance should have this rather than a bed bath.

• Instead of giving "routine baths," especially for long-term patients, plan ahead and allow time for shampoos and care of the nails. To give a complete bath daily, but to allow no time to give a shampoo for two months reflects lack of planning.

• Keep the patient's elbows covered by seeing that the sleeves of his gown or pajama top stay down over them. Creams and lotions applied to the elbows and the knees help relieve dryness.

• If you notice skin lesions, avoid washing them with soap and water. Do not try to clean off any scales or exudate, since the appearance of the lesions is important to the doctor in making a diagnosis. Report the symptom to the doctor promptly, and be ready to answer questions concerning the medicines that the patient is receiving. Drugs are a frequent cause of skin lesions in hospitalized patients.

Nurses can apply these measures to safeguard the health of their own skin, and, in addition, they can take the following special precautions against specific occupational hazards:

● Avoid unnecessary contact with medications; many of them can cause allergic skin reactions. Careful handling of syringes, needles and of the medicines themselves can greatly reduce physical contact. If a medicine spills on your hands, wash it off promptly. Never indulge your curiosity by tasting medicines!

● Thorough hand washing is important in preventing the spread of infection. Because you must wash your hands so often, use hand cream or lotion liberally, and be sure to dry your hands well after washing. These precautions will help to prevent chapping and cracking of the skin.

● If a patient has a skin disease, ascertain whether or not it is contagious. If it is, follow the necessary medical aseptic technic. (This rule applies, of course, to any contagious condition, dermatologic or otherwise.)

INJURY AND DISEASE OF THE SKIN

By the time that he has reached adulthood, almost everyone has had some kind of contact with some of the common disorders of the skin. For example, allergy is an important cause of skin disease. And because of its constant contact with the environment, the skin frequently is injured. The skin has been described as a "mirror of the emotions", emotional stress is a frequent cause and a complicating factor in many dermatologic conditions. Congenital abnormalities may occur. Hormone imbalance during adolescence is believed to be responsible for acne. Infections and malignant changes also may involve the skin.

The following are some common causes of skin diseases with examples of the resulting conditions.

● Allergy—urticaria (hives)
● Congenital lesions—nevus (mole)
● Emotional disturbances—neurodermatitis (a form of eczema)
● Hormonal imbalance—acne
● Infection—furuncle (boil)
● Malignant growth—malignant melanoma
● Trauma—accidents: burns, lacerations; radical surgery, such as that for cancer of the head and neck.

Disorders of the skin may be classified also according to the degree of the involvement of the entire body. For example, a burn may be small and produce only local symptoms; or it may cover a large area of the body and produce systemic as well as local symptoms, because of the marked physiologic disturbance accompanying it (see Chap. 57). Some diseases of the skin produce only local manifestations—acne, for example. On the other hand, many systemic diseases produce dermatologic symptoms; measles and syphilis are examples. Systemic lupus erythematosus and scleroderma are diseases that affect many systems of the body, including the skin. Both of these diseases affect collagen, a connective tissue widely distributed in the body.

THE PROBLEM OF DISFIGUREMENT

The condition of the skin determines to a great extent the appearance that an individual presents to others. A clear, radiant skin is always pleasant to behold. Our society places a high premium on youthful beauty, and advertising continues to hammer home an ideal which, though patently unrealistic, is nonetheless highly persuasive. What effect has this on the person whose skin is disfigured from disease or trauma? Skin diseases have long been associated with immorality, uncleanliness and contagion. Despite the fact that these associations are usually unjustified, an inflamed and pimply skin just does not convey the look of fresh cleanliness that a clear skin does. Some skin lesions exude serum that has an unpleasant odor, further adding to the impression of uncleanliness. Only a very few skin diseases are contagious; nevertheless, many persons have a fear of touching the person with skin disease, or even of being near him. People whose faces have been scarred by burns or cuts may be severely disfigured, and may have even their facial expressions changed for the worse.

It is not difficult to understand why people who suffer severe facial disfigurement often undergo personality changes. They become acutely and painfully aware of the stares, the avoidance, and even the revulsion of other people, and they tend to withdraw from social and business contacts. Many occupations are closed to those who are disfigured, particularly jobs that place heavy emphasis on personal attractiveness, such as those of a receptionist, an airline stewardess, or a salesman.

More instances of disfigurement are seen nowadays. Cancer of the head and neck is treated more often by radical surgery, as new advances in surgical technics are developed. Although the malignant cells may be removed successfully, the problem of disfigurement remains. People with severe injuries of the face and the neck have a better chance of survival, because of such treatments as antibiotics and parenteral fluids. Plastic surgery has worked wonders for many of these patients—by such methods as reconstructing an ear so skillfully that it scarcely can be distinguished from the normal ear. Nevertheless, some patients are so severely mutilated that they remain disfigured despite all that plastic surgeons can do for them. Rehabilitation must emphasize function, but we must not forget that appearance is important, too.

Learning to accept those who are disfigured is a big challenge. Often, the nurse is the one who is with the patient when he becomes aware of the change in his appearance. It is easy to preach acceptance, but it is not always easy to act on it, because we nurses, too, are not immune to prejudice. The points listed below may seem so commonplace as not to deserve mention; but perhaps because the care of disfigured patients is often difficult, the list will help to spell out some of the ordinary little things that we can do to help the patient to feel accepted. The patient will notice; he will be an amazingly sensitive observer of our reactions, because they serve as a foretaste of what is to come.

• When dressings or treatments are required, do not hesitate to touch the part as you minister to the patient. Use only the logical and the necessary protective technics. For example, gloves should be worn only if the skin disease is contagious, and their purpose should be explained to the patient. Even if the patient is physically able to carry out his own treatments, arrange to do some part of the care of the lesions yourself as a way of demonstrating acceptance of the patient and his condition. Understanding the disease will help you to feel sure of yourself, so that you can use a firm rather than a gingerly touch.

• Neither stare at the patient's disfigurement nor avoid the sight of it. Try to look at the patient—at all of him, including his rash or his scar—in the same way that you would look at any other patient.

First experiences with severely disfigured persons can be trying. You may feel shock at first, or pity, or revulsion. Recognizing how you feel will help you to control the expression of your feelings to the patient. Gradually, in working repeatedly with the same patient, or with others who have a similar disability, you will find that the changed appearance can be accepted more easily as a temporary, or even a permanent, part of your patient.

Having begun to recognize and to cope with your own feelings, you can understand more readily the reactions of the patient's family, friends and co-workers to his condition. Part of your task lies in helping them. You can:

• Demonstrate by your behavior that you accept the patient, with his changed appearance. Your assurance as you approach and minister to him can convey this.

• Give the family members an opportunity to talk with you away from the patient, as well as in his presence. They may fear that others will stigmatize the patient, and this dread can be a powerful threat.

Treatment of Skin Disease

Both local and systemic treatment may be used in skin disease. Lotions, powders and ointments may be applied to soothe and to soften the skin (*emollients*), to relieve itching (*antipruritics*), to protect the lesions, to provide a vehicle for other medications, and to stimulate the healing of chronic lesions. In addition, local preparations may be keratolytic (dissolving thickened or horny skin), antiseptic or antiparasitic. Here is an example of each of these types of preparation:

• Emollient—lanolin
• Antipruritic—calamine lotion
• Protection—zinc oxide ointment
• Vehicle for other medication—bacitracin ointment
• Stimulation of the healing of lesions—coal tar ointment
• Keratolytic—salicylic acid plaster (contained in many corn plasters)
• Antiseptic—potassium permanganate solution
• Antiparasitic—Desenex powder

Local preparations for the skin often are combinations of several ingredients carefully chosen by the dermatologist for their specific effect. Even patients who have similar skin disorders may respond very differently to a particular preparation. It is always unwise to recommend any local preparation for the treatment of a disease of the skin, even though you have observed that it has helped patients with apparently similar conditions.

Systemic treatment usually forms part of the patient's management. Most skin disorders grow worse when the patient is tired or under emotional stress. Therefore, rest and sleep are an important part of treatment.

Diet also may be an important part of treatment. For instance, most patients with acne find that the condition grows worse after eating chocolate. A patient may develop hives (*urticaria*) from eating fish, and therefore he may have to eliminate it from his diet.

Since some skin diseases are manifestations of systemic disorders, the variety of drugs given is as broad as the study of pharmacology itself. These are some commonly used preparations:

• Corticosteroids help to relieve many severe skin diseases. They do not cure the disease, but they often relieve the symptoms, sometimes with dramatic speed. As is true of their use in other diseases, these drugs can have serious toxic effects. Therefore, they are used primarily to relieve acute attacks. Continued use in long-term conditions brings greater risk, and it is justified only when the disease itself is very serious and cannot be relieved by other treatments.

• Antihistamines frequently are prescribed when allergy is a factor in causing the disease, and for the relief of itching.

• Sedatives and tranquilizers are used to help the patient to relax and rest.

• Antibiotics are used to treat infection.

Sunlight is important in the treatment of some dermatologic problems. For example, its effects —bacteriostasis, drying and mild peeling of the skin—are helpful in acne. Exposure to ultraviolet light can produce a similar effect in much less time, and ultraviolet treatments often are given by dermatologists. Usually, only the part being treated is exposed to the light. Any type of heavy cloth or opaque paper can be used to protect the other parts of the body from exposure.

X-ray therapy provides relief from the symptoms of a variety of skin diseases. The dosage is measured carefully, and the number of treatments that can be given safely to any one area of the body is limited. Excessive use can cause loss of hair or thinning, dryness and wrinkling of the skin; and it may even predispose to malignant changes in the skin. When very large doses are given, deep burns may result. Sometimes, when a dose of radiation is given to treat cancer of other organs, the skin becomes pink and dry as an unavoidable consequence. However, because of mounting concern over the hazards of radiation therapy, this form of treatment is now used less commonly for benign conditions. (See Chap. 14 for further discussion of radiotherapy.)

NURSING CARE OF PATIENTS WITH SKIN DISEASE

Often the doctor wants to examine the skin of the patient's entire body, including the scalp and the perineal region, even though the patient may state that the condition is limited to only one part. Remember to adjust the light to facilitate the examination and to drape the patient carefully. Expose only those areas being examined at that time. Patients with skin disease are particularly sensitive to being examined, even by doctors and nurses. The examination may not be limited to the skin. Some skin diseases are related to systemic illness, and the doctor examines blood and urine, he notes temperature, pulse and respiration, or he takes a biopsy. Any aspect of physical examination may be required. The necessity for the tests must be carefully explained to the patient, who may see no connection between them and the lesions on his skin.

Itching

Although itching (*pruritus*) is a common and very distressing symptom of many skin diseases, the mechanism of itching is still somewhat obscure. The itch impulse probably has a lower frequency and intensity than the pain impulse, thus differentiating the feeling of pain from the sensation of itching. Certain factors tend to make itching worse: excessive warmth (as from too many blankets); rough, prickly fabrics; emotional stress; and idleness. Itching usually is worse at night, probably because the patient's attention is not occupied, and he is therefore more aware of the sensation.

Severe itching is agony. Scratching leads to trauma and excoriation, and often it leads to infection. Helping the patient with severe pruritus to obtain some degree of comfort and to avoid catching is a challenge to all who care for him. Reminders not to scratch are little help; usually, all that is accomplished is that the patient grows tired of being scolded, and the nurse is irked, because he does not stop scratching. Instead of scolding the patient, try the following:

• Divert his attention from the itching. A game of cards with another patient or painting a picture can work wonders. Here is a word of caution: the materials that the patient uses should not irritate his condition. A patient who is allergic to wool obviously should not knit a woolen sweater.

• Provide enough clothing and bedding for comfortable warmth, but avoid overheating. Carefully check the temperature of the room to avoid chilling or excessive warmth.

• Encourage your patient to keep his nails short and very clean. This will minimize trauma and infection from scratching.

• If the patient scratches while he is asleep, have him wear white cotton gloves at night.

• Help the patient to avoid emotional upsets. If he does not get along with his roommate, perhaps he could be moved to another room.

• When the sensation of itching is acute, and the patient cannot resist the impulse to touch his skin, have him press his finger or hand against it, without scratching.

• Help the patient to sleep. A back rub, a snack or a chance for some quiet reading may help him to relax and go to sleep. Note carefully any bedtime treatment or medications ordered to relieve the itching or to promote sleep.

A variety of treatments may be ordered by the doctor to alleviate itching. The treatment of the disease itself, thus eliminating the cause of the symptom, is, of course, the most effective. However, in waiting for curative treatment to take effect, or in treating conditions in which complete cure is unlikely, much relief of itching can be achieved by symptomatic treatment. Wet dressings or starch baths often help. The relief of emotional tension helps to reduce itching; sedatives and tranquilizers often are ordered for this purpose. Soothing lotions, such as calamine, often give temporary relief. When allergy is a factor, antihistamines may provide considerable relief.

Dressings

If dressings are needed, apply them so that they fit snugly and yet do not bind. Dressings applied to open, denuded areas should be sterile. Cotton should not be placed next to the skin, because of its tendency to stick to moist surfaces. Gauze or cotton cloth may be used. Tubular cotton gauze, which is thinner but similar to the stockinette used under casts, is easy to apply, and it stays smoother than roller gauze. If this material is not available, a long, white cotton stocking or a sock will serve. Cut the foot out of the stocking, and you have a tubular dressing that can be applied over an arm or leg. Avoid applying adhesive tape directly to the skin, because it can cause trauma and irritation.

Wet Dressings. When applying a wet dressing, find out first whether the procedure is to be clean or sterile. The nature of the lesion (acute or chronic; open, weeping, or dry) helps to determine whether sterile technics must be used. In either case, scrupulous cleanliness is important. Here are some points to remember in contrasting clean and sterile technic for a wet dressing:

Clean	*Sterile*
1. Clean bowl, washed, dried and reused by the same patient; sterilized before it is used by another patient.	1. Sterile bowl, used only once and then resterilized.
2. Gauze, or cotton cloths. Gauze may be remoistened and reused by the same patient. Discard when it is soiled.	2. Gauze or cotton cloths that have been autoclaved. Use during one treatment only.
3. Dressing may be handled by patient or nurse after washing hands thoroughly.	3. Two sterile forceps, to use when placing compresses in solution, wringing them out, and applying them. Depending on the size and the location of the area to be covered, and the amount of handling of the dressing that is necessary, sterile gloves may be needed, so that dressings can be handled directly with the gloves.

Wet dressings have a cooling and a soothing effect, produced by the evaporation of the moisture from the dressing. To avoid chilling, make certain that the rest of the patient's body is kept warm.

Wet dressings may be applied by either the open or the closed method:

Closed	*Open*
Moist compresses are applied and then covered with waterproof material, such as plastic sheeting or waxed paper.	Moist compresses are applied and left open to air. Do not cover the part with bedclothes. The foundation of the bed is protected by laying a rubber or a plastic sheet, covered by a cotton draw sheet or treatment towel, under the part.

Several points must be considered in keeping the dressing wet:

• A dressing that is completely dry (it should not be, but you may be the first to discover a dressing that needs attention) should never be moistened by pouring solution over the dry, outer layers of the gauze. The solution may not even penetrate to the gauze next to the patient's skin, and the solution can carry dirt inward from the surface of the dressings. Remove the dressings completely, and resume the treatment by immersing fresh dressings in a bowl of solution and applying them as ordered.

• An open dressing that is changed frequently enough to prevent soiling and is not allowed to dry out usually may be remoistened at intervals, using an Asepto syringe.

• If the dressing is not only dry but also stuck to the skin, first remove the outer layers of gauze, then moisten the inner layer with solution, using an Asepto syringe. Never pull roughly at a dressing that is stuck, because this action will cause pain and trauma.

• A closed dressing that is protected by outer wrappings may usually be remoistened by squirting solution on it with an Asepto syringe, provided that the dressing has not dried out.

Often, the patient can assist in keeping the dressing moist, provided that sterile technic is not necessary; the area is one that he can reach; his physical condition permits; he is shown how to do it; and the necessary supplies are provided for him. The nurse is always responsible for seeing that the treatment is carried out, whether or not she performs every aspect of it herself.

Starch Baths. Starch baths (colloid baths) are useful in relieving itching. Usually, they are ordered at bedtime to help the patient to sleep. The patient may be able to carry out the treatment with only a little help, as long as he is physically able. He should be carefully instructed, and there must be an effective call system in the bathroom, so that he may signal for help if he needs it.

Fill the bathtub with lukewarm water. Add one pound of cornstarch or laundry starch, and stir the water so that the starch is mixed through it. Have the patient immerse his whole body by stretching out full length in the tub. A washcloth or a compress may be used to apply the solution to the face and any other parts not covered by the solution. The cloth or compress should be applied gently, without rubbing

the skin. Soap is not used with the starch bath. Although the primary purpose of the bath is soothing, it also helps to cleanse the skin. Unless this fact is explained to the patient, he may reach for the soap, and its use could irritate his skin. The bath often is ordered for 20 to 30 minutes at a time. The bathroom should be comfortably warm, and more hot water should be added occasionally to prevent the patient from becoming chilled. When the treatment is over, the skin should be patted dry. Never rub it, since rubbing would cause irritation.

At his point the patient needs the nurse's assistance most. Whatever local medication is ordered should be taken to the bathroom and applied immediately after the patient's skin has been dried. Irritation and increased itching may result if the application of the local medication is delayed after the bath. The patient should not putter around cleaning up the bathroom, but he should go right to bed; otherwise, the soothing effect of the treatment will be lost. Often, patients with a skin disease are susceptible to chilling, particularly after a bath. Therefore, make sure that the patient wears his bathrobe and his slippers to and from the bathroom.

COMMON DERMATOLOGIC CONDITIONS

Acne

Acne is one of the most widespread skin conditions. The cause is not fully understood, but acne characterisically occurs during adolescence, and it is believed to be related to the hormone changes during that period of life when the secondary sex characteristics are developing. Other factors can aggravate the condition, although they alone do not cause it. Fatigue, emotional stress and eating too many rich foods, such as chocolate and ice cream, are examples.

The skin of the affected areas (usually face, chest and back) is excessively oily. The lesions consist of comedones (blackheads), papules (pimples), and pustules (pimples filled with pus). In severe cases, cysts sometimes occur, appearing as large, reddish swellings. The severity of the condition ranges all the way from an occasional pimple, which during adolescence is so common that it is considered to be almost normal at this age, to a face that is covered with bright-red pimples and peppered with blackheads. Severe acne, if neglected, can lead to the formation of deep, pitted scars that leave the skin permanently pock-marked. Oiliness of the scalp and the shedding of greasy scales (seborrhea) often accompany acne. Infection and the formation of pustules are fostered by picking and squeezing the lesions.

The possibility of scarring from severe acne is too often overlooked. These scars are *not* outgrown, and they can spoil a complexion for life. But probably the emotional scars are just as important. For some young people these matters mean just temporary distress, but for others who feel less secure, who already have difficulty in making friends, severe or unusually prolonged acne can interfere seriously with their developing into poised, confident adults. Acne that is in any way pronounced or unsightly should be treated—the more prompt the treatment, the less likelihood of scars, physical or emotional.

Treatment. Despite the fact that there is as yet no swift and certain cure, a great deal can be done to relieve the symptoms and, in time, to help them to disappear. Instruction in personal hygiene from a person whom the patient considers to be an authority on health matters is heeded more often than the advice, however kindly, of parents and neighbors.

The doctor can remove the blackheads and drain the pustules with special instruments. This process never should be attempted by the patient or by family and friends, because infection and scarring can be caused by unskilled manipulation. "Hands off" is an ironclad but difficult rule that the patient must learn to follow. The patient is instructed to keep his fingernails short and clean, since this helps to prevent infection of the skin lesions. He should wash his hands thoroughly before applying medication or carrying out any other treatment of the lesions. Mild soaps that do not irritate are preferable to hard or highly perfumed varieties. Medicated preparations should be used only with the doctor's advice. Some physicians recommend washing the skin with an antibacterial soap to keep the number of staphylococci on the skin to a minimum. Sometimes, an abrasive soap, rubbed in gently, helps in peeling the skin. The diet should exclude any foods that the patient has found make the condition worse. Chocolate and nuts are common offenders, as are other fatty foods, such as salad dressing, fried foods and bacon.

Healthful living can help to relieve acne. The skin often improves after such everyday treatment as plenty of fresh air and exercise, improved diet and more sleep.

Exposure to sunlight is beneficial, because it lessens oiliness, reduces the number of infection-causing bacteria and causes peeling of affected skin. The combination of increased exercise, relaxation and sunlight often makes acne improve during the summer. But the exposure to the sun should do no more than produce slight pinkness and peeling; a painful sunburn is not beneficial. Short treatments with ultraviolet light, administered by the doctor, provide benefits similar to exposure to direct sunlight, and they have the added advantage of year-around application and controlled dosage to prevent burning.

White lotion (lotio alba) is useful in drying the skin and decreasing the severity of the lesions. Other treatments sometimes used for acne include antibiotics and vitamin A. Hormones (contraceptive pills) are sometimes given to prevent ovulation and the formation of progesterone, since progesterone aggravates acne. Patients who do not respond to other treatment may occasionally be treated by x-ray therapy. Because of the increasing concern over the hazards of x-ray therapy, and the advent of other treatment measures such as corticosteroids, x-ray therapy is less commonly used now in the treatment of acne. Nevertheless, this treatment relieves the acne by decreasing the activity of the sebaceous glands, thus reducing the oiliness of the skin. The scarring that has already occurred from acne lesions can be made less conspicuous by *dermabrasion*. Lotions containing corticosteroids have been effective in treatment of severe acne. Corticosteroids are sometimes administered orally for this purpose. In general, face creams are to be avoided.

Seborrheic Dermatitis

The common term for mild seborrheic dermatitis is *dandruff*. The symptoms are familiar: oily scalp, formation of greasy scales, itching and irritation. Severe cases have inflammation with redness, swelling and, sometimes, exudation and pyogenic infection. Seborrheic dermatitis frequently accompanies acne, but unlike acne it is not limited typically to adolescence. Often, it persists throughout adulthood. It affects the scalp primarily, but it may spread to the eyebrows, the skin around the ears, the sides of the nose, and the forehead near the hairline, causing the skin in these areas, as well as the scalp, to be red, oily and scaly.

Normally, new cells are constantly being formed and pushed to the outside of the skin, where they die and are gradually and imperceptibly shed (*keratinization*). In the presence of certain diseases, such as seborrheic dermatitis, keratinization is speeded up, and scaling becomes visible.

Why so many people suffer from oily scalps and dandruff is not understood clearly. Sometimes, the condition makes its appearance, together with acne, during adolescence. Prompt and persistent treatment often results in great improvement, to the degree that only good scalp hygiene is required to avoid a return of the condition. However, many people are not so fortunate and continue to require regular medical treatment to control the symptoms. These individuals have chronically overactive sebaceous glands; the condition may be related to heredity, emotional tension, a diet too high in fat, or endocrine imbalance.

Treatment. The treatment includes regular cleansing, application of local medication between shampoos, and a regimen of healthful living. When the oiliness is severe, shampoos may be needed as often as daily. Although the scales are removed by washing, they promptly accumulate again until the condition is controlled. The doctor rather than the hairdresser should be consulted about the selection of a shampoo. The doctor will advise the use of an antiseborrheic shampoo such as Selsun, or Fostex cream. When the condition is unresponsive, mildly antiseptic lotions or medicated ointments may be prescribed for use between shampoos. The lotions should be applied directly to the scalp rather than to the hair. Explain the importance of systematically applying medication to his entire scalp by parting the hair frequently and reaching all areas of the scalp. Regular exercise, sufficient rest, and relief of emotional tension are important aspects of therapy.

Allergic Reactions of the Skin

The skin is one of the organs most frequently affected by allergy. (The phenomenon of allergy is discussed in Chap. 6.) The allergic response of the skin is characterized by dilation of the blood vessels, causing redness and swelling, and sometimes by vesiculation (blister formation) and oozing. Itching is a prominent symptom.

Allergic reactions of the skin commonly are caused by substances with which the skin has contact, such as cosmetics, fabrics or chemicals. The resulting disorder is called *contact dermatitis*. The condition also may be caused by drugs (dermatitis medicamentosa) and foods. Penicillin frequently causes urticaria.

Irritants are differentiated from contact allergens in that an irritant, if it is used in sufficient quantity, causes skin inflammation in almost everyone, whereas an allergen provokes a reaction only in the small proportion of people who are hypersensitive to that particular substance.

Patch tests, which place small amounts of various substances in direct contact with the skin, may be helpful in identifying the causes of the reaction. A wide variety of substances may be used, such as a sample of the patient's lipstick or nail polish. A careful history is very important in any allergic condition. For example, it may be discovered that the patient has taken some new drug or has tried a new cosmetic.

Urticaria (Hives); Angioneurotic Edema

The most familiar example of urticaria is a mosquito bite. The skin reacts to the insect's bite with a *wheal* (a roundish, white elevation) that is surrounded by an area of redness and itches furiously. Imagine being covered with mosquito bites, and you will have some idea of the misery of a severe case of urticaria. The wheals are a result of localized edema, due to increased capillary permeability. Urticaria is usually an allergic response, although sometimes emotional stress seems to cause the condition.

In *angioneurotic edema* that part shows an all-over swelling rather than the patchy swellings of hives. The lips may be swollen to three times their normal size, or the tissues around the eyes may be so edematous that the patient cannot open them. Patients with allergic reactions must be observed for the symptoms of respiratory obstruction, because edema of the larynx may interfere with respiration.

The treatment of urticaria and of angioneurotic edema includes avoidance of the allergen and the use of antihistamines and epinephrine and, in severe cases, corticosteroids. Cold compresses applied to the affected areas help provide relief. When angioneurotic edema and urticaria are associated with emotional tension, counseling, tranquilizers and sedatives are useful.

Eczema

The term *eczema* refers to a group of skin diseases that tend to be chronic and are related to heredity, allergy, emotional stress and, possibly, endocrine disorder. The lesions consist of tiny vesicles (blisters) on reddened, itchy skin.

The vesicles sometimes burst, causing the area to weep and later to form crusts from the dried fluid. The skin of the affected area is red, dry and scaly. Leathery thickening (lichenification) and darkening of the skin result from continued irritation and scratching. A form of eczema called *infantile eczema* occurs in children under the age of two. Our discussion will be confined to the chronic type of eczema frequently seen in adults. It is called *atopic eczema* or *neurodermatitis*.

Eczema typically occurs in the folds of the elbows and the knees and on the neck and the face. During acute attacks it may spread widely to other parts of the body. The symptoms tend to come and to go. The patient may have a severe flare-up that necessitates absence from work or school. Several months later he may have no symptoms of the disease, and he may remain symptom-free for months or even years. However, the condition tends to recur. Frequently, an exacerbation of eczema can be traced to an emotional upset. At other times the immediate cause of the attack is obscure. People with chronic eczema frequently have patches of thickened, dark skin in the bends of their elbows and knees or on their necks. These patches persist long after the acute attack subsides. During an acute attack these areas become red, scaly, oozing and crusted, and later they revert to their darkened leathery appearance. A form of eczema occurs in the perineal region, causing itching and inflammation. Sometimes, the condition is referred to as *pruritus ani* (itching of the anus) or *pruritus vulvae* (itching of the vulva).

Treatment. Caring for the patient with eczema demands the utmost in skill and understanding. Medical treatment includes local creams and ointments that are soothing and antipruritic, such as hydrocortisone cream. If the skin is very inflamed, wet dressings or starch baths may be ordered. Antihistamines often help to relieve the symptoms. Sedatives and tranquilizers may be necessary to calm a tense, restless patient. Corticosteroids are sometimes administered orally when the symptoms are very severe. Rest and sleep are essential treatments, and yet difficult to provide because of severe itching and discomfort. Sedation can help to break the cycle of insomnia, tension, itching and scratching. X-ray therapy is occasionally used in controlling acute attacks.

The patient should understand the importance of giving a complete account of his previous treatment if he consults a new doctor. This directive is especially important in relation to x-ray therapy, because there is a limit to the number of treatments that may safely be administered to any one part of the patient's body.

The nurse can play an important role in helping the patient to learn to manage his condition. Here are some suggestions:

• Avoid talking down to the patient. Many observers have commented that patients with eczema tend to be high-strung, intelligent, ambitious people. No such generalization can be applied to each individual patient; nevertheless, it is worth keeping in mind as you care for your patient, if only as a stimulus to your observation of whether it may be relevant.

• Try to understand some of the social and the emotional pressures that may affect the patient besides his physical discomforts.

• Help your patient to feel less tense. Give him a chance to talk; help him to find diversion and to obtain adequate sleep.

• If emotional tension seems to play a large part in causing the condition, avoid giving the patient the impression that you think he could snap out of it, or that he has purposely brought it on himself.

• Remember that eczema is not contagious. Do not be afraid to go near the patient.

• If allergy plays a major role in causing the attacks, learn specifically what allergens the patient must avoid, keep them away from him when he is in the hospital, and teach him to recognize and avoid them when he goes home.

• Ointments should be applied sparingly; otherwise, they will be wasted and cause clothing to become unnecessarily soiled.

• Some soiling of underwear is inevitable while the condition is acute. Wearing white cotton panties help to protect clothes. (Cotton is more absorbent than nylon or an elasticized fabric.) If the weeping of the lesions is severe, a perineal pad may be necessary until the condition improves.

• Toilet tissue, especially if it is rough or highly colored, may be irritating to an already inflamed skin. After a bowel movement, soft cotton pledgets and plain water may be used for cleaning. The small pieces of cotton can be flushed down the toilet after use.

• Soap should not be used, because it irritates the lesions.

• For aesthetic reasons, cleaning and drying should be carried out with some soft disposable material like cotton. All that is necessary is the observance of good practices of personal hygiene, such as not sharing towels and careful hand washing, since the condition is not contagious.

Other Common Dermatologic Conditions

Psoriasis. Both men and women are affected by psoriasis, usually during young adulthood and middle life; men are affected more often than women. The cause is unknown. It may be related to metabolic disorder, heredity or emotional conflict.

The disease is characterized by patches of erythema (redness), covered with silvery scales, usually on the extensor surfaces of the elbows and the knees, the lower back and the scalp. Itching is usually absent or slight, but occasionally it is severe. The lesions are obvious and unsightly; the scales tend to shed.

The following measures are used to treat psoriasis:

• Local medication. A variety of ointments, such as those containing ammoniated mercury, salicylic acid and coal tar are used.

• Diet. Avoidance of alcohol is recommended.

• Actinotherapy. Exposure to sunlight or to ultraviolet light helps; x-ray therapy is occasionally used.

• Systemic medication. Vitamin A, sedatives, tranquilizers, antihistamines and corticosteroids sometimes are administered. Folic acid antagonists such as methotrexate are sometimes given.

The prognosis is guarded. Some patients respond very well to treatment. However, the condition tends to recur. Some patients obtain little relief from therapy and are easy prey for a variety of widely advertised remedies promising quick relief.

Rosacea. More common in women than in men, rosacea typically occurs during middle life. Emotional stress, anxiety, tension, endocrine disturbance, hypochlorhydria and coexisting seborrheic dermatitis may all play a part in causing rosacea.

The symptoms include flushing of the face, particularly of the cheeks and the nose. Papules and pustules form on the flushed skin.

The treatment includes:

• Local medication. Sometimes, white lotion (lotio alba) is prescribed.

• Diet. Coffee, tea, chocolate, nuts, and alcoholic beverages are restricted, as are highly seasoned foods.

• Exposure to sunlight or ultraviolet light may be helpful.

The administration of hydrochloric acid is often helpful. Estrogenic hormones and corticosteroids are sometimes employed. Antibiotic therapy may be given on a long-term basis.

Patients who are willing and able to accept counseling and to take the prescribed medication often obtain relief of the symptoms.

Dermatitis Venenata. This condition is caused by contact with a substance that produces inflammation of skin; the oleoresins (plant oils and juices) of poison ivy, poison oak and poison sumac are common offenders in this country.

Dermatitis venenata can be prevented by:

• Learning to recognize the plants and to avoid them.

• Wearing clothing that protects the skin from contact when a person is obliged to walk through areas where the plants exist (slacks, closed shoes, and socks rather than open sandals, no hose, and shorts or a skirt).

• Prompt and thorough cleaning of the exposed skin with soap, followed by application of alcohol, helps to remove the oleoresin from the skin after exposure. The cleaning should be done preferably within the first few minutes after contact, as the oleoresin later becomes fixed in the skin, and can no longer be removed.

• Desensitization by repeated administration of minute quantities of an extract of the oleoresin; this method of prevention is reserved for persons who are extremely sensitive to a particular plant.

The symptoms of dermatitis venenata include redness, itching, formation of blisters, and edema. Usually, the symptoms are limited to the point of contact—for example, legs or hands. In unusually severe cases the eruption may involve large areas of the body, and the edema may be severe. The symptoms usually subside in about seven days, although in severe cases they may last longer.

Wet compresses of potassium permanganate solution or Burow's solution may be ordered to soothe and to lessen itching. Lotions also may be ordered, such as calamine. Injections of the plant extract are not given during an acute attack, because they may cause exacerbation of the symptoms.

Impetigo Contagiosa. More common in children than adults, impetigo is caused by a streptococcal or a staphylococcal infection of the skin. The symptoms include erythema and vesicles that rupture and are covered with a sticky yellow crust. Face and hands are common sites.

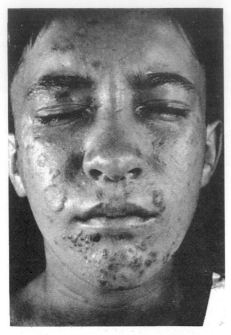

FIG. 48-1. Impetigo. Note crusts that form over lesions. (Medichrome—Clay-Adams, Inc., New York, N.Y.)

Impetigo is highly contagious, and contact by other persons with the lesions or the exudate should be avoided carefully. The patient should never share his towel or bed linen. Meticulous hand washing after applying any medication is important. The patient himself should avoid touching the lesions unnecessarily. Because the condition can be spread from one part of his body to another, as well as to other people, he should wash his hands immediately after touching the lesions.

The crusts should be removed with soap and water, or with mineral oil, before any local medications are applied. Remember that applicators or gauze used for this purpose must be wrapped carefully and immediately discarded. Various preparations may be ordered, such as neomycin-bacitracin ointment, ammoniated mercury ointment, or gentian violet.

Usually, the condition is cured in a week. However, it can be especially severe in the newborn, and it can even cause death.

Herpes Simplex (Cold Sore). Herpes simplex is caused by a virus. It is believed that many people harbor the virus, and that a variety of factors, including colds, fever, emotional upsets and menses may precipitate the appearance of herpes simplex.

A group of blisters occurs on reddened, inflamed skin, usually near the mouth, or on the genitals. Usually, pain and burning accompany the lesion. Herpes simplex often is called a cold sore or a fever blister. The lesions subside in about a week. Some people are especially susceptible to herpes simplex, and they have frequent recurrence of the lesions.

Usually, the symptoms are mild, and the condition subsides without treatment. No specific treatment is available that can shorten the duration of the lesion. Sometimes smallpox vaccine is administered in an effort to control recurrent eruptions of herpes simplex.

Herpes Zoster (Shingles). Herpes zoster is caused by a virus. The virus is the same one that causes chickenpox. The cutaneous lesions usually follow the course of a sensory nerve.

Before skin lesions appear, the patient usually experiences fever and malaise. Erythema and vesicles then appear, usually on the trunk or the face, along the course of a sensory nerve. Neurologic pains occur, and they may be severe, particularly in elderly persons. The condition subsides in about three weeks; however, the neuralgia may persist for months or even longer.

No specific treatment is available. Analgesics are ordered for the relief of the pain. Local applications like calamine lotion are used to soothe the lesions. In older people systemic corticosteroids may be given. Clothing should be loose and non-irritating.

Furuncle, Carbuncle, Furunculosis. Streptococci, staphylococci and other pathogenic organisms sometimes exist harmlessly on the surface of the skin, but when the normal protective functions of the skin are impaired these pathogens may cause infection. For example, dryness and chapping of the skin may result in cracking, which allows microorganisms to enter and to cause infection. These lesions usually are caused by staphylococcal infection. Often, an injury, such as that caused by squeezing a pimple is the immediate cause, since it allows infection to enter through a break in the skin. Furunculosis is frequently due to lowered resistance, poor general health, and poor diet. Sometimes virulent strains of hospital-type staphylococci are the cause.

The descriptive symptoms of these conditions are:

• Furuncle: A whitish, raised, painful lesion, surrounded by erythema. The area feels hard to the touch. After a few days the lesion exudes pus, and later a core. It heals, leaving a tiny scar. Neglect or mismanagement can cause a larger, obvious scar.

• Carbuncle: A large swollen lesion, often on the back of the neck, surrounded by erythema. It is acutely painful; it has several openings through which pus drains.

• Furunculosis. In addition to multiple boils, the patient may have fever, anorexia, weakness and malaise.

Hot wet soaks are used to localize the infection. Often, for a single boil, this is the only treatment necessary. Antibiotics, such as penicillin or erythromycin, may be ordered to control the infection. Often, large doses are prescribed when fever is present, or if the lesion is a carbuncle. Incision and drainage may be necessary sometimes. When boils recur frequently, staphylococcus toxoid and autogenous vaccine (vaccine derived from the organism infecting the patient) may be given. Measures to improve general health are important in treating furunculosis.

The patient never should pick or squeeze a boil, as this practice favors spread of the infection to surrounding tissues or even to the bloodstream, causing septicemia. The exudate should be allowed to escape through the opening without the patient's squeezing the lesion or picking the top off. Drainage from a boil is infectious; strict medical aseptic technic is essential to prevent the spread of the infection to other parts of the patient's body or to other persons.

Sebaceous Cysts. Sebaceous cysts are caused by obstruction of the duct of a sebaceous gland. The gland continues to secrete sebum despite the obstruction, thus causing accumulation of an oily secretion in the blocked duct. A swelling appears which at first is small, but which can grow to be large and unsightly. Treatment of the condition is surgical excision of the cyst, or cysts. If the lesion is small it may be removed outside the hospital; larger cysts must be dealt with in a hospital operating room.

Dermatophytosis (Athlete's Foot). Dermatophytosis is a fungus infection most common in young adults. Usually, dermatophytosis first affects the toes, and particularly the skin between them. The affected skin becomes red, scaly, cracked and sore. Sometimes, the condition also affects the sides of the toes and the soles of the feet. Sometimes it spreads to hands, axillae and groin. The nails may become involved also and are characteristically yellow, friable and opaque. The treatment includes benzoic and salicylic acid ointment (Whitfield's ointment) and undecylenic acid (Desenex powder and ointment). Many other remedies are available. (Before local medication is applied, scales and dead skin should be gently removed.) An antibiotic, griseofulvin, is useful in treatment. Griseofulvin is given orally in doses of 125 mg., four times daily. The drug may be required for many weeks in order to eradicate the infection. Side-effects include urticaria, headache, nausea and diarrhea. In severe cases corticosteroids may be administered for a limit time (such as one week) to lessen the inflammation.

The disease may be transmitted from person to person through towels, locker room and bathroom floors. Towels and slippers should not be shared, and those using locker rooms or "community" bathrooms in dormitories should avoid going barefoot. Early diagnosis and treatment are important in preventing spread. Keeping the feet (particularly the area between the toes) dry increases resistance to the infection. People whose feet perspire freely often find that powdering between the toes helps to keep the area dry. Washing and drying the feet, putting on clean, dry socks and a different pair of shoes after coming home from work is another aspect of personal hygiene that helps to keep the skin of the feet healthy.

Because the fungus can survive in shoes, slippers and socks and these can constitute a source of reinfection, socks should be boiled after each use; slippers and shoes may have to be discarded. The fewer articles that the patient touches with his feet, the less is the problem of disinfection, and the fewer are the chances of reinfection. For example, it is preferable for the patient to wear clean socks at all times, even at night, rather than to place his bare feet in contact with slippers and bedding. Shared bath mats can be a source of infection for others. If the patient uses a separate towel as his bath mat, it can be more easily boiled and laundered than a heavy bath mat or a rug— and is therefore less likely to spread infection. The patient should clean the tub or the shower floor with a disinfectant, such as creosol (Lysol), after each use.

Infestation and Bites. An infestation with pediculi (lice) results in *pediculosis*. The following terms are used to describe pediculosis:

• Pediculous capitis—infestation of the hair or the scalp.

• Pediculous corporis—infestation of the body surfaces with a louse larger than the one that affects the scalp and the hair. This parasite and its eggs may be found also in the patient's clothing—particularly within cuffs and seams.

• Pediculous pubis—infestation of the pubic area with a very tiny louse shaped like a crab—hence the lay term, *crabs.* Although this condition occurs primarily in the pubic area, it may occur also in the hairy areas of the axilla.

The symptoms of pediculosis include itching, scratching and irritation of the skin. Scratching denudes the skin, making is susceptible to infection. Eggs are deposited on the hair near the scalp, and they may be confused with dandruff. These eggs, often called *nits,* cannot be brushed out as dandruff can, but they are attached firmly to the hair. The lice are tiny, grayish-brown creatures that may be seen when they move on the scalp.

Benzyl benzoate and benzine hexachloride are contained in a variety of ointments, powders and lotions that are effective in killing pediculi. Kwell lotion and shampoo are commonly used preparations. Although the pediculi can be promptly killed by these modern remedies, repeated infestations are likely if the individual continues to have close contact with others who harbor the parasites, and if personal hygiene is poor. Pediculosis capitis can be spread by shared toilet articles, like combs, and by close personal contact, such as that occurring in crowded places. Pediculosis pubis can be transmitted by toilet seats and by sexual intercourse.

Scabies is caused by infestation with the itch mite (*Sarcoptes scabiei*). The symptoms include intense itching, which usually is worse at night, accompanied by excoriation and burrows (the lesion caused when the female itch mite invades the skin, burrowing underneath, leaving a dark line). The lesions occur most often between the fingers and on the forearms, the axilla, the waistline, women's nipples, men's genitals, the umbilicus, and the lower back.

Kwell or benyl benzoate in lotions and ointments are highly effective in treating scabies. Thorough bathing, clean clothing, and the avoidance of contact with others who have scabies are essential in preventing recurrence. Before any treatment is started, the patient should have a thorough bath. After medication has been applied, he should have a complete change of clothing.

The itch mite can be transmitted readily from one person to another by close personal contact and by sharing towels and clothing.

Bedbug bites are caused by tiny, dark-brown insects that infest mattresses and wooden bed frames. In heavily infested dwellings, bedbugs may live in crevices of the woodwork or in upholstered furniture. Although they are more common in crowded, unsanitary homes, bedbugs may be brought into any home on clothing or even on newspapers. The symptoms of bedbug bites include the appearance of wheals (hives) with central points or dots. These lesions may appear on any part of the body, but they are most commonly found on the wrists, the ankles and the buttocks. Usually, the bites require little local treatment. Sometimes, calamine lotion or witch hazel is applied to soothe the lesions. The services of an exterminator are frequently required to get rid of the bugs.

SOCIAL AND EMOTIONAL IMPLICATIONS. The diagnosis of pediculosis or scabies or bedbug bites often causes embarrassment and is difficult for many people to accept. This is true whether the patient comes from a clean home in a good neighborhood, or whether he lives in a slum. To the poor person who lives in a crowded, dirty environment the condition may be viewed as further evidence of economic and social disadvantages. Whether or not it is common in his neighborhood, he will be sensitive to the attitudes of those who care for him. Indications of disgust and distaste will serve to make the patient less willing to seek treatment the next time that he needs health care. If the nurse herself sees the condition as a willful neglect of personal hygiene, or as a result of laziness and irresponsibility, her attitude of condemnation will show through—despite even a smile or a greeting.

However, if the nurse recognizes the interdependence of social, economic and health factors, she will be better able to understand the degree to which people can be the victims of poverty and lack of opportunity. The nurse who can accept the patient—even the one with pediculosis —has taken the biggest and most important step in helping that patient to recover from the condition and to learn to prevent its recurrence. Instruction must be handled with great tact.

PREMALIGNANT AND MALIGNANT SKIN LESIONS

Skin lesions usually are readily observable, thus facilitating prompt diagnosis and treatment. Nurses have a responsibility to teach people to seek medical advice for any lesion that persists.

SYSTEMIC CONDITIONS WITH DERMATOLOGIC SYMPTOMS

Conditions with grave prognoses

CONDITION	CAUSE	DESCRIPTION	TREATMENT	NURSING CONSIDERATIONS
Pemphigus	Unknown; may be hereditary	Bullae (large blisters) appear and rupture, leaving a raw lesion with an offensive odor and intense itching.	Baths or wet dressings with mild antiseptic solutions. Neo-calamine lotion to relieve itching. High protein diet to compensate for protein lost through weeping lesions. Chemotherapy.	1. Observe for toxicity to drug therapy which may be prolonged
Systemic lupus erythematosus	Believed to be auto-immune disorder; affects collagen	Red butterfly pattern over the cheeks and bridge of the nose; painful joints; edema; fever and anemia. Kidneys, heart and lungs may be affected.	Steroids plus local symptomatic therapy.	2. Foster independence for as long as possible
Scleroderma (Progressive systemic sclerosis)	Unknown; some evidence suggests an auto-immune cause	Hardening of collagen in many organs. Skin becomes tight and smooth; movement becomes difficult. The heart and lungs may be affected causing dyspnea, cyanosis and edema. The esophagus and intestines are often involved.	Symptomatic treatment including ointments, massage, heat, physiotherapy and hydrotherapy. Cortisone may be used.	3. Meticulous care improves patient's comfort 4. Be available to lend emotional and physical support when necessary

OTHER SYSTEMIC CONDITIONS WITH DERMATOLOGIC SYMPTOMS

CONDITION	CAUSE	DESCRIPTION AND COURSE	TREATMENT
Erysipelas	Hemolytic streptococcus	Chills, fever, headache and a raised, reddened area of the skin which spreads rapidly and is sometimes accompanied by blistering.	Antibiotic therapy.
Erythema nodosa	Believed to be an allergic reaction to drugs or to viral or bacterial infections.	Red, tender nodules in cutaneous and subcutaneous tissues. Shins, thighs and forearms are commonly involved. Possibly fever and malaise.	Identify and, if possible, remove the cause. Salicylates, bed rest and corticosteroids for symptomatic relief.
Polyarteritis (Periarteritis nodosa)	Unknown	Nodules appear along the course of arteries. There may be muscle and joint pain, nausea, vomiting, diarrhea, abdominal pain, fever and weight loss.	Symptomatic; includes analgesics, rest and corticosteroids.
Erythema multiforme	Undetermined; may be secondary to drug reaction or infection.	Eruption of red macules, papules, vesicles and bullae affecting the wrists, hands, elbows, knees, feet and face. Systemic symptoms may involve muscles, GI, urinary, respiratory and nervous systems.	Treatment of any underlying conditions. Soothing lotions Antihistamines Symptomatic therapy

If it is malignant, prompt treatment often can prevent spread and cure the condition.

Several factors predispose to malignant changes in the skin:

• Prolonged, repeated exposure to ultraviolet rays. Sailors, farmers, overzealous sun bathers and others who are exposed to a great deal of sunlight are particularly vulnerable.

• Exposure to radiation.

• Ulcerations of long duration and scar tissue.

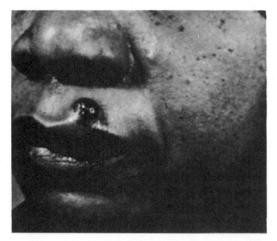

FIG. 48-2. Melanoma. (Medichrome—Clay-Adams, Inc., New York, N.Y.)

Both are prone to malignant changes.

Precancerous Lesions. Some lesions are considered precancerous. *Leukoplakia* is characterized by shiny white patches that usually occur on the mucous membrane of the mouth or the female genitalia. If leukoplakia occurs in the mouth, smoking is definitely contraindicated, because it makes the condition worse. Rough, jagged teeth should be replaced, so that they do not irritate the lesion. Surgical excision of the lesions often is recommended because of the danger of cancer. The lesions also may be removed by electrodesiccation.

Birthmarks (nevi) are of various kinds, including vascular nevi (*angiomas*), brown moles and black moles. The lesion may not be visible at birth; however, the beginnings of the lesion are present at birth and may appear later. Black, smooth moles are the most likely to become cancerous. However, any mole that becomes irritated, bleeds or begins to grow larger should have prompt medical attention. Surgical removal usually is recommended. Light brown moles that are not located where irritation from clothing is a problem usually do not have to be removed unless it is desirable for cosmetic reasons.

Senile keratoses are brownish, scaly spots appearing on the skin of older persons. They are most likely to occur on exposed portions of the skin, such as the face, the ears or the hands. Patients who develop senile keratoses should be advised to seek medical attention. Because the lesions are common and seem to be insignificant, they often are disregarded. But they may become malignant, and their removal usually is recommended.

Malignant Lesions. Malignant growths of the skin usually are primary lesions. The spread to other parts of the body may be prevented by prompt removal of the malignant tissue. *Epithelioma* is a common type of skin cancer. It arises from the surface layers of the skin. If promptly treated by surgical excision, electrodesiccation, or x-ray therapy, these lesions usually are controlled promptly. On the other hand, *malignant melanoma* is a highly malignant, rapidly spreading lesion. Usually it is coal-black. Wide surgical excision may be attempted to save the patient's life; however, because of the rapid spread, the prognosis is poor. *Squamous-cell carcinoma* is another dangerous type of lesion, because it tends to metastasize to internal organs. This type of cancer often occurs on the tongue or the lower lip. (Chronic irritation from pipe smoking is a common causative factor in lesions involving the lower lip.) Depending on the size and the location of the lesion, the treatment may involve electrodesiccation, surgical excision, or x-ray therapy.

REFERENCES AND BIBLIOGRAPHY

ABEL, T. M.: Facial Disfigurement, *in* GARRETT, J. F. (ed.): *Psychological Aspects of Physical Disability,* Washington, D.C., U.S. Government Printing Office, (n.d.).

ALLEN, L. G.: Facts and fancies about cosmetics and aging skin, *Nurs. Clin. N. Am.* Vol. 2, No. 2, Philadelphia, Saunders, 1967.

BAER, R., *et al.*: Changing patterns of sensitivity to common contact allergens, *Arch. Derm.* 89:3, 1964.

BEHRMAN, H. T.: Hormone creams and facial skin, *JAMA* 155:119, May, 1954.

BUTTERWORTH, T., and STREAN, L.: *Manual of Dermatologic Syndromes,* New York, McGraw-Hill, 1964.

CAHN, M. M.: The skin from infancy to old age, *Am. J. Nurs.* 6:993, July, 1960.

DuBois, E. (ed.): *Lupus Erythematous,* New York, McGraw-Hill, 1966.

GOLDMAN, L.: Prevention and treatment of eczema, *Am. J. Nurs.* 64:114, March, 1964.

JOHNSON, S. (ed.): *The Skin and Internal Disease,* New York, McGraw-Hill, 1967.

LEIDER, M., and ROSENBLUM, M.: *A Dictionary of Dermatological Words, Terms, and Phrases,* New York, McGraw-Hill, 1968.

LEWIS, G. M., and WHEELER, C. E.: *Practical Dermatology,* ed. 3, Philadelphia, Saunders, 1967.

MACKENNA, R. (ed.): *Modern Trends in Dermatology,* Washington, D.C., Butterworth, 1966.

MACKENNA, R., and COHEN, E.: *Dermatology,* London, Bailliere, 1964.

MUSAPH, H.: *Itching and Scratching,* Philadelphia, Davis, 1964.

SAUER, G. C.: *Manual of Skin Diseases,* ed. 2, Philadelphia, Lippincott, 1966.

SHAW, BERNICE L.: Current therapy for burns, *RN,* 34:33, March, 1971.

The Patient Undergoing Plastic Surgery

49

Cosmetic Surgery and Functional Improvement • Skin Grafts
Nursing Care of Patients Who Have Plastic Surgery

The terms *plastic surgery* and *reconstructive surgery* often are used interchangeably to refer to the repair of defects that may be congenital or acquired through injury or radical surgery. The repair surgery may have been performed for cosmetic purposes or to improve function. For example, a crooked nose may be straightened, or contracted scar tissue in the axilla may be freed to restore normal motion to the arm. A deformed hand may be totally reconstructed by repair of tendon, bone, nerve or skin. An eyelid that has been damaged by trauma or by surgery for cancer may be repaired by means of a pedicle graft or advancement flaps. The four main kinds of conditions treated by plastic surgery are:

1. Congenital deformities, such as harelip and protruding ears
2. Deformities resulting from trauma, such as burns and automobile accidents
3. Conditions for which the patient seeks cosmetic surgery, such as face-lifting
4. Disfigurement resulting from malignant disease, such as cancer of the mouth

This highly specialized treatment combines art and medicine. In cosmetic surgery the aim is not to produce beauty as such, but beauty in the sense that the changed appearance is appropriate for the particular patient and blends unnoticeably into his features, producing a natural appearance.

COSMETIC SURGERY AND FUNCTIONAL IMPROVEMENT

Plastic surgery holds the promise of a more normal appearance and improved function for many patients. Both appearance and function are important considerations; however, their relative importance varies with the part of the body involved. For instance, function is a prime consideration in reconstructive surgery on the hand, and appearance is of particular significance in surgery involving the face. Surgical treatment that produces the greatest functional improvement may not be the same as that which leads to the most satisfactory cosmetic result.

When we think of cosmetic surgery, we usually think only of the face and the neck. Although these areas are involved frequently in plastic surgery, it is by no means limited to them. The degree of disfigurement can range from slight to marked; however, it may not be a reliable indicator of the patient's reaction to his condition. A very tiny flaw may seem like a huge blemish to a person who is very sensitive about his appearance. Cosmetic surgery may bring great relief to patients who are very conscious of, for example, a hooked nose; straightening the nose may bring the person a new feeling of poise and assurance.

However, people who tend to blame all their failures and disappointments on what may seem to others a barely noticeable blemish have unrealistic expectations of what plastic surgery can accomplish. Sometimes, plastic surgery is contraindicated if the patient's dissatisfaction with his appearance seems to be an expression of a deeper emotional problem.

Here are a few example of plastic surgery performed for cosmetic purposes:

• *"Face lifting"* and *blepharoplasty.* Most of the incision for face lifting is made in the hairline. Wrinkles are removed by the tightening of fascia and skin and the removing of excess skin.

Most of the fine scar, resulting from surgery, is concealed by the hair. Modern face-lifting technics produce results that are longer lasting than was the case with formerly used technics. Although more time is necessary to evaluate how long the results of these newer procedures last, it is believed that one face-lifting procedure will suffice for many years.

Frequently blepharoplasty (eyelid reconstruction) is carried out as part of the surgical procedure, in an effort to remove the aged appearance which frequently sets in at about the age of 50. At about this time of life the elastic fibers of the dermis relax, and some of the subcutaneous fat that produces a youthful look becomes absorbed. In eyelid reconstruction, incisions are made which are hidden in normal crease-lines. The excessive eyelid skin and orbital fat (if necessary) are removed.

• *Rhinoplasty*. Since the nose is the most exposed part of the face, it is frequently injured, often without the individual's remembering the accident. Reconstruction of the tissues has developed to a fine art. Usually within two to three weeks after the surgery the patient's improvement in appearance, breathing, and senses of smell and taste are apparent. With these improvements come greater poise, assurance, and improved morale.

• *Dermabrasion* is a technic for removing surface layers of scarred skin. It is useful in lessening such scars as the pitting from severe acne. The outermost layers of the skin are removed by sandpaper, a rotating wire brush or a diamond wheel. A local anesthetic, such as ethyl chloride-freon mixture may be used during the procedure. Afterward, the skin feels raw and sore, and some crusting from serous exudate occurs. Patients frequently say that the discomfort is much like that from a burn. The patient is instructed not to wash the area for five or six days, until sufficient healing has occurred. He should avoid picking or touching it, since this contact might cause infection, or produce marking of the tissues.

• *Tattooing* is used to change the color of the skin. Pigments are blended to just the right shade for the patient's skin and then are implanted into it. The treatment is useful in covering up dark red birthmarks (port wine stains), and in matching the color of grafted skin to its surrounding skin more exactly. However, the pigments may shift position beneath the skin so that they are no longer effective in covering up the blemish. Also, the pigments sometimes look

different in environments of various temperatures. For example, a tattoo that is not noticeable at room temperature may become noticeable, due to color change, when the patient goes out into the cold.

Tattooing and dermabrasion usually are carried out in the doctor's office or in a clinic.

• *Artificial parts* may be used to camouflage defects. For instance, part of a nose or an ear may be made of plastic to match the patient's features so exactly that it is hard to tell which is the prosthetic part, and which is the natural. Plastic materials are also used as framework or supporting structures over which the patient's tissues grow. For instance, a plastic material, such as silicone rubber, may be used beneath the skin to correct an underdeveloped chin.

• *Mammoplasty* may be performed to change the size and the shape of the breasts. Very large breasts may make a woman self-conscious, contribute to poor posture, and interfere with breathing. Excess tissue is removed surgically under general anesthesia. Afterward, the patient must wear a firm supporting brassiere for several months until healing is complete, and the tissues are firm. Surgery is sometimes undertaken to enlarge small breasts (augmentation mammoplasty). Tissues from the patient's own body, such as a buttock, or plastic materials, such as silicone gel within a silastic bag, are used as an implant between the chest wall and the breast. Placing the material between the chest wall and the breast, rather than inside the breast, has two advantages: (1) the function of the breast is unimpaired: the woman can lactate normally; and (2) the possibility of carcinogenesis from introduction of foreign materials in breast tissue is obviated.

SKIN GRAFTS

Skin grafts may consist of *autografts* (skin transplanted from one part of the patient's body to another) or of *homografts* (skin transplanted from one person to another). Only autografts or skin transplanted from one identical twin to another can become a permanent part of the patient's own skin. However, homografts are useful in temporarily closing large defects, thus preventing further loss of tissue fluid. Although the homografts slough away after one or more weeks and must be replaced by autografts, they tide the patient over the critical period of his illness and help him to recover enough to permit the use of

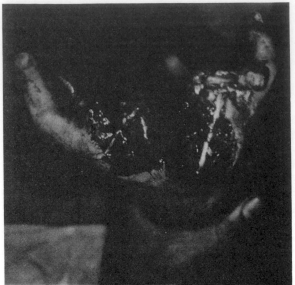

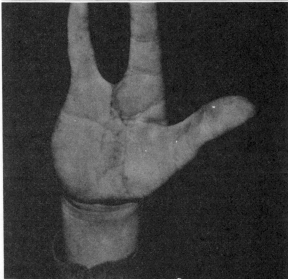

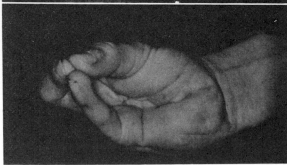

Fig. 49-1. (*Top*) Hand mangled in an accident. (*Center*) After plastic reconstruction. (*Bottom*) There is good function in this hand. (Dr. Alvin Mancusi-Ungaro, Montclair, N.J.)

autografts. Other body tissues, such as bone and cartilage, also may be used as grafts.

In order for grafts to "take," there must be a sufficient blood supply to the part and an absence of infection. The graft must stick close to the tissues on which it is to grow; excess blood or serous fluid can cause the graft to become separated from the tissues and to fail to grow. Sometimes warm, moist saline compresses are placed on pedicle grafts. The skin being transplanted by a pedicle has blood supplied from the donor site. The warmth transmitted to the recipient bed through the graft is believed to favor the development of blood circulation in the graft. Such drugs as tolazoline (Priscoline) and alcohol are sometimes administered because they, too, cause vasodilation, thus increasing the blood supply in the recipient bed.

Several different types of skin grafts are in use. The doctor selects the kind best suited to the needs of each patient. *Free grafts* are those that are completely severed from the donor site and transferred to the recipient site. In *pedicle* or *tube grafts* two or three sites may be involved. A piece of skin is freed at one end, and the free end is allowed to grow onto the recipient site, while the other end is still attached at the original site. The flap of skin receives its blood supply from the original site until the blood supply is sufficiently well established for it to be transferred to the recipient site.

Pedicle grafts are used when thick pieces of skin that could not survive an interruption of blood supply are transplanted. Pedicle grafts can carry tissues other than skin with them, such as bone and fat.

Usually, it takes about three or four weeks for sufficient blood supply to be established to permit severing the skin completely from the donor site. Meanwhile, depending on the location of the parts involved, the patient may have to be in a very awkward position. Sometimes, a cast is used to fix the parts in the proper position and to prevent movement until the flap can be freed from its original site.

Skin grafts vary in thickness. The Ollier-Thiersch graft consists of large pieces of skin varying in width from one-half to nearly the full thickness of the skin. This type of graft, also called a *thick split skin graft,* is widely used. Large slices of skin may be removed by a *dermatome,* a mechanical cutting device that can be adjusted so that precisely the desired thickness of skin will be evenly removed.

Pinch grafts consist of small cones of skin that are lifted, cut off and transplanted to the graft area. They look like little islands, or dots of skin, set on the recipient site. The pieces of skin grow together, so that when healing has occurred, the entire area is completely covered. Pinch grafts do not give as smooth an appearance as other grafts; the skin appears rough and pebbly. Therefore, such grafts are used on areas of skin that will be covered by clothing.

Full-thickness grafts (Wolfe-Krause grafts) are composed of a full depth of skin. They give the best cosmetic appearance, and therefore they are used for face, neck and hands when feasible. The supply of skin from the patient's own body that is suitable for use as full-thickness grafts is limited. Sufficient skin for this purpose may be procured when the defect is small, but it may be difficult to obtain enough suitable full-thickness skin to repair a large defect. The surgeon must consider also matching the skin for color and texture. For example, color and texture of skin from the abdomen are quite different from those of the skin of the face.

NURSING CARE OF PATIENTS WHO HAVE PLASTIC SURGERY

Classifying surgery as *minor* or *major* has many pitfalls. Much of plastic surgery is referred to as minor, because the areas involved usually are superficial and readily accessible. Nevertheless, the success or the failure of the surgery has grave consequences *for the patient*. Permanent grafts must be obtained from the patient's own skin; yet, when large areas of a patient's skin have been destroyed by trauma, such as a severe burn, the amount of healthy skin available for grafting is limited. The failure of the graft to grow can mean that another operation is necessary, or that the procedure cannot be repeated because of the scarcity of healthy skin. Most patients who undergo plastic surgery already have suffered a great deal.

The nurse has an important part to play in insuring the success of a plastic-surgery procedure. For instance, care must be taken to avoid excessive pressure that might impair circulation. (A bandage that is too tight can interfere with circulation.) The part must be protected from injury. Do not let the patient lie on or bump the area. The most meticulous aseptic technic is necessary to prevent infection. If a warm, moist dressing is ordered, make sure that the solution is sterile, that it is poured into a sterile basin, and that it is wrung out and applied with sterile forceps. It should be about 105° F. A dressing that is too hot could damage the tissues rather than help them to grow. Never change a dressing unless the doctor specifically requests it; removing the dressing may take the graft with it. Report to the doctor any evidence of bleeding or of pus on the dressing.

Patients with skin grafts have two sites to be cared for before and after the surgery—the donor site and the recipient site. Usually, the skin of the donor site is shaved before the patient goes to the operating room. The surgeon will specify which area (often the upper thigh) is to be prepared. The recipient site is the wound or the defect to which the grafts will be applied. The surgeon will specify the particular care needed for this area, too. Postoperatively, the nurse must observe both the donor area and the recipient area. For instance, a sheet or a slice of skin may have been removed from the anterior thigh by a dermatome, leaving a raw, weeping surface. Often, petrolatum gauze is placed over the wound and covered by a dry dressing. The nurse must observe this area for any sign of infection or bleeding, and she must protect it from injury until it has healed.

Whether the patient has skin grafting or reconstructive surgery of some feature, such as his nose, it is important for him to understand what to expect from the surgery. The surgeon will discuss the operation with the patient in advance, but there may be many times during his recovery when the patient will turn to the nurse for repeated explanation and reassurance. For instance, immediately after plastic repair of the nose (rhinoplasty), the patient's nose may be swollen and bruised. His first thought may be that he looks worse than ever. Help him to understand that he cannot evaluate the results of the surgery until the healing has taken place.

Be especially careful not to respond to the patient's apprehension concerning the outcome of surgery with promises of favorable results. Because most patients feel considerable tension about the outcome of plastic surgery, they may question you repeatedly about matters that should be discussed with the surgeon. Allow the patient to express his concerns and explain that he will have the opportunity to discuss the matter further with his physician. Because some patients are hesitant to voice some of their worries to the doctor, it is important for the nurse to mention to the physician the questions which the patient has raised, so that he can talk further with the patient about them.

The patient's reaction to the change in his appearance may sometimes seem baffling—particularly when the surgery results in a considerably improved appearance. Instead of immediately showing pleasure and gratitude, the patient may cry. (Even when a change in his body is a cosmetic improvement, some loss of the patient's "old self" is inevitable, and grief can occur over the loss, even of a deformity.) Ordinarily, grieving is short-lived when the surgery results in improved appearance. It is important during this period to help the patient to realize that his reactions are acceptable and not unusual. Give your patient opportunity to talk about his feelings concerning his changed appearance. Another possible reaction after plastic surgery is hostility, which the child may show by tantrums and fighting with neighborhood children, but which in an adult is more likely to be expressed as crankiness, impatience, and general dissatisfaction. Reasons for such behavior are individual, and each patient must discover these and deal with them himself. An accepting, concerned listener can help him to do so. Possibly he has stored up anger as a result of many years of humiliation over a deformity, and once it is removed, so too is the muzzle he has placed on the expression of his anger.

Sensitivity is required in helping the patient to resume his contacts with others after surgery. This is especially problematic if the patient's appearance has been altered for the worse. For example, a patient who has been badly burned may have his disfigurement only partially alleviated by plastic surgery, and this improvement may be the result of numerous operations over a period of many months. The patient may dread being seen by family and friends but be badly in need of the encouragement and support their visits can bring. Often the nurse can help in such situations, by gently preparing visitors before they enter the room for the first time.

Tactfully encouraging the patient's contact with other patients on the unit can also help lessen his isolation. Careful assessment of the patient's readiness, and that of other patients, is important. For example, a patient who is painfully selfconscious about his appearance may tolerate and then begin to enjoy the visits of a quiet person who comes to offer some brief service, such as sharing a newspaper, but be overwhelmed by being wheeled to a solarium where a group of patients is gathered.

REFERENCES AND BIBLIOGRAPHY

ABEL, T. M., Facial disfigurement, *in* GARRETT, J. F. (ed.): *Psychological Aspects of Physical Disability,* Washington, D.C., U.S. Government Printing Office, (n.d.).

BARSKY, A.: *Principles and Practice of Plastic Surgery,* ed. 2, New York, McGraw-Hill, 1964.

CONWAY, H., and NAYER, D.: Skin grafts, *Am. J. Nurs.* 64:94, November, 1964.

DE RAMOS, LOUISE M.: Total scalp loss, *Am. J. Nurs.* 71:1404, July, 1971.

EDWARDS, B. F.: Endoprostheses in plastic surgery, *Am. J. Nurs.* 64:123, May, 1964.

GIBSON, T. (ed.): *Modern Trends in Plastic Surgery,* Washington, D.C., Butterworth, 1966.

MacGREGOR, F. C., *et al.*: *Facial Deformities and Plastic Surgery,* Springfield, Ill., Thomas, 1953.

McGREGOR, I., and REID, W. H.: *Plastic Surgery for Nurses,* Baltimore, Williams & Wilkins, 1966.

PEET, E., and PATTERSON, T.: *The Essentials of Plastic Surgery,* Philadelphia, Davis, 1963.

WOOD-SMITH, D., and POROWSKI, P. (eds.): *Nursing Care of the Plastic Surgery Patient,* St. Louis, Mosby, 1967.

ZAYDON, T. J., and BROWN, J. B.: *Early Treatment of Facial Injuries,* Philadelphia, Lea, 1964.

Intensive Care Nursing 50

The concept of intensive care involves a concentration of medical and nursing staff and allied health personnel specially prepared to observe, assess, and treat critically ill patients with the assistance of various kinds of technology. The patients may have the same diagnosis, such as acute myocardial infarction. Or, in a mixed intensive care unit there can be patients in acute renal or respiratory failure, patients after cardiac surgery or severe trauma, patients with third-degree burns, septicemia, postsurgical complications, or metabolic crises such as diabetic keto-acidosis, among other diagnoses.

Because of the need for close and constant observation and the potential for deterioration of the patient's condition, the ratio of nurses to patients is high. But a high nurse-patient ratio is not the essence of intensive care nursing. Skilled intensive nursing care is a blend of expertise in the technical-judgmental skills and the interpersonal skills exercised in behalf of the patient and family caught in a life-death crisis, many for the first time.

The importance of performing technical tasks in a knowledgeable, precise, and manually dexterous manner with necessary adjustments to the individual patient cannot be overestimated. The nurse who traumatizes a patient because of an unskilled attempt at nasal or oropharyngeal suctioning can cause the patient to resist or refuse to be suctioned again despite his need.

The patient admitted to an intensive care unit has special problems different from the patient admitted electively. His illness is most often acutely disruptive of his work or home life. The nature of his admission by ambulance with siren screeching, the rush of personnel, and the emergency therapies, serve to reinforce the message which his pain, or dyspnea, or bleeding, or vomiting has already conveyed to him—that he is gravely ill and can even die. The sights and sounds and smells which surround his small living space in the intensive care unit are foreign and threatening to him. It is hard to distinguish night from day when lights are on all the time and activity is constant. Restrained from moving by intravenous lines, monitoring electrodes and various kinds of other devices, and separated from family and friends, the acutely ill patient faces a fearsome burden. Nursing assists the patient to cope with all of these strange and threatening conditions so that his major efforts can be directed toward the work of healing.

Providing emotional support for the ICU patient is as much a part of sound physiologic care as is the overtly technical procedure. The patient's psychological response to an acute physical problem stresses his cardiovascular, respiratory, and endocrine systems. Increase or decrease in heart rate, cardiac arrhythmias, hyperventilation with subsequent shift in pH, and the outpouring of catecholamines from the adrenal gland are examples of physiologic responses to stress. These responses are also experienced at times of crisis by members of the staff, as well as by the patient's family or associates in the waiting room. Just as one needs specialized education to deal with newer technical aspects of care, so do the members of the intensive care staff need continuing assistance to deal with their own emotional responses so that they can be more supportive of patients and visitors.

If the nurse does not recognize or understand her own feelings and receive help to deal with them, she may protect herself by preoccupation with the technical aspects of care and unwittingly ignore the persons to whom the care is given.

There is considerable challenge and satisfaction in intensive care nursing. Many lives are saved by a caring, competent team. Newer treatment modalities offer new opportunities for sharing and collaboration between physicians and nurses in the interest of quality patient care.

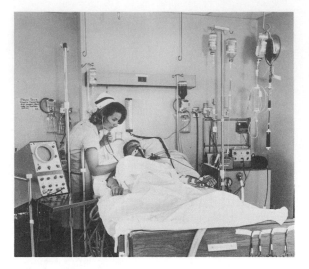

Fig. 50-1. Nursing the patient in a modern intensive care unit. (Winter, P., and Lowenstein, E.: Acute respiratory failure, *Sci. Am.* 221:23, November, 1969; courtesy of Edward Lowenstein, M.D., Massachusetts General Hospital)

Inevitably, some patients will die. They and their families need as much support and dignity as the situation permits. The other patients need an honest answer to their question, "Where is Mr. Jones?" Such an answer is, "Despite all we could do for him, Mr. Jones died this morning." To attempt to give a false answer such as "The patient was transferred" destroys the patient's confidence when the truth is inevitably found out.

Sudden death means that the patient and his family have had no time to prepare for it; the news may overwhelm them. In their shock and sorrow they may feel aggressive against the hospital staff. The nurse should understand their reaction, even though it may be difficult for her to listen to them, and explain that everything possible was done for the patient.

The surviving patient's stay in the ICU is generally a short one and he is transferred out as soon as possible to a general hospital area. A study has shown that patients who are not prepared for this transfer through early anticipation of the time of transfer, discussion of the meaning of the move, weaning the patient from equipment such as a cardiac monitor on which he may have developed a degree of dependence, and acceptance by a knowledgeable new nursing staff, may experience sufficient stress to cause a major setback (Klein). In addition to patient preparation, the staff on the general nursing unit needs a full nursing history and well-developed written nursing care plan so that the nursing care can continue without disruption.

The nurse with sound academic and clinical preparation, knowledge of scientific principles, and ability to combine intellectual alertness with humane understanding is prepared to work in an intensive care setting. Taking the leadership role in planning and giving nursing care to the seriously ill patient requires much more instruction than this book can give.

This section is intended to assist the reader:

- To recognize and evaluate the nursing needs of patients who become critically ill unexpectedly on a medical or surgical unit;
- To recognize the early warning signs of life threatening conditions and the appropriate nursing intervention;
- To learn about the nursing problems involved in care of critically ill patients so that the nurse can prepare the patient when possible for transfer to a specialty unit, can participate with the other team members in the nursing care of seriously ill patients, and can assist in formulating and carrying out an effective plan of nursing care for the patient who survives the period of critical illness.

REFERENCES AND BIBLIOGRAPHY

DeMeyer, J.: The environment of the intensive care unit, *Nurs. Forum* 6:262, 1967.

Klein, R., *et al.*: Transfer from a coronary unit: some adverse responses, *Arch. Intern. Med.* 122:104, 1968.

Kornfeld, D., *et al.*: Psychological hazards of the intensive care unit: nursing care aspects, *Nurs. Clin. N. Am.* 3:41, March, 1968.

Lambertsen, E.: The nature and objectives of intensive care nursing, *Nurs. Clin. N. Am.* 3:3, March, 1968.

Michaels, D.: Too much in need of support to give any?, *Am. J. Nurs.* 71:1932, October, 1971.

Strauss, A.: The intensive care unit: its characteristics and social relationships, *Nurs. Clin. N. Am.* 3:7, March, 1968.

VerSteeg, D.: If I could hold your hand, *Am. J. Nurs.* 68:2554, December, 1968.

The Patient in Shock 51

Prevention • Signs, Symptoms and Observations • Treatment and
Nursing Care Implications • Prognosis and Complications

Why blood vessels occasionally fail to maintain the balanced constriction that maintains normal pressure is not completely understood. It is known that master adjustment centers in the brain can be impaired by drugs, by hypoxia, by anesthesia and by trauma, among many examples, and that poor vascular tone can result. Despite much investigation, agreement on the exact pathophysiologic disturbances involved in shock or on modes of treatment has not been reached. It is agreed that shock is a complicated series of interwoven events—vascular, hormonal, neural, metabolic, and hemodynamic.

Shock is a clinical syndrome indicating inadequate circulation that results from a variety of causes. Inadequate circulation leads to tissue hypoxia. Regardless of the cause, prolonged shock is incompatible with life. The faster the shock state can be reversed, the greater the chance of uncomplicated recovery for the patient. There are few instances in the care of patients where careful attention to nursing practices and principles are as important to recovery as in the management of the patient in impending or actual shock.

Shock can be classified according to etiology:

Hematogenic shock, in which there is a reduction in the volume of circulating blood (hypovolemic shock). This type of shock may be caused by hemorrhage, in which blood is spilled from the usually closed system of arteries and veins. Other causes include severe burns, in which a large amount of fluid seeps from the circulatory system into the injured area; and the loss of large amounts of fluid in vomitus and diarrhea. Hemorrhage into a cavity, such as thoracic or abdominal, may be hidden from sight, but it is just as deadly as the hemorrhage one can see from an external wound.

Cardiogenic shock, in which the circulatory failure involves faulty pumping of the heart. A common cause of cardiogenic shock is acute myocardial infarction.

Vasogenic shock, in which there is diffuse vasodilation, resulting in an increase in the size of the vascular bed. When blood becomes trapped in small vessels and in the viscera, it is lost temporarily to the mainstream of circulating fluid. The skeletal muscles and the viscera may become engorged with blood, while the volume of circulating blood is reduced dangerously. This type of shock is *normovolemic.* That is, the amount of fluid in the tubes of the circulatory system is not reduced, but it is not circulating in such a way that permits effective perfusion of the tissues. Anaphylaxis is an example of vasogenic shock. (See p. 75 for a discussion of anaphylactic shock.)

Neurogenic shock, which results from an insult to the nervous system. Intracranial damage and certain drugs can cause neurogenic shock. Vasodilation is a prominent feature.

Psychic shock, in which pain, severe fright or other strong emotion interferes with normal vascular control. A frightened patient makes a poor surgical risk.

Bacteremic shock, which may be seen in any overwhelming bacterial infection, usually occurs in the patient who is succumbing to his infection. Bacteremic shock is more common in patients whose bacteremia is caused by gram-negative organisms. Endotoxins released by the organisms probably are a major cause.

PREVENTION

The ability of an individual to avoid shock cannot be predicted. The patient who has undergone a known cause of shock is safer when cared for as if shock might develop. All accident victims and patients with acute myocardial infarction, for example, should be treated as if shock were imminent. Frequent observations of the patient and his vital signs to maintain an appraisal of the circulatory state are ordered until the occurrence of shock is no longer considered probable. All postoperative patients belong in this category. Even if the surgical procedure involves practically no blood loss, the stress of going to surgery, the anesthetic and the necessary trauma of the surgical incision are influences that can contribute to shock.

Careful preoperative preparation, both physical and psychological, is important in preventing shock. However, hypovolemia is more significant as a cause of shock than such factors as anesthetic agents and psychic stress.

Nurses should become expert at estimating fluid loss. How many ml. are in a puddle of vomitus on the floor? How many ml. are soaked into the bed linen after a severe nose bleed? How much fluid can a saturated 4-inch square sponge hold? One way to train the eye is to take a known amount of fluid and pour it on the floor, in a sheet, on a sponge and see what it looks like. Another way to estimate fluid loss is by weight. For example, in the operating room weigh a dry sponge. Then weigh a blood-soaked one and subtract. A healthy adult can lose up to about 500 ml. of blood without need for replacement. The ill, the elderly, the poorly nourished need replacement therapy for less blood loss. Central venous pressure monitoring is being used more frequently prophylactically in the elderly patient undergoing surgery in order to better evaluate volume replacement needs.

The nurse must watch for signs that the body is being forced to call on major defenses to maintain blood pressure. Although deep shock can develop in minutes, more often there is a warning period. In hypovolemic shock the rate of volume loss is most directly related to the speed with which the symptoms of shock appear. For example, the patient whose aorta ruptures, progresses almost instantaneously to profound circulatory collapse, whereas the patient sustaining a venous hemorrhage will go into shock in a more orderly, step-by-step fashion through the sequence of symptoms indicating impending circulatory collapse.

SIGNS, SYMPTOMS AND OBSERVATIONS

Every nurse should be thoroughly familiar with the signs and the symptoms of shock, so that when they occur, she will know what to do and, just as important, what not to do. The signs and symptoms are not difficult to remember once they are correlated with the pathologic changes that cause them.

Skin

Peripheral blood vessels constrict to direct blood from the skin to more vital organs. Ischemia renders the skin pale and cold. It is clammy due to activation of the sweat glands. There may be cyanosis especially of the fingernail beds, lips and ear lobes. Cyanosis means severe tissue hypoxia. Its absence, however, does not mean the absence of hypoxia. Recognition of cyanosis may be obscured by deep skin pigmentation, anemia, and poor lighting conditions.

Arterial Blood Pressure

Blood pressure is a valuable but not an infallible index of shock. Organ blood flow, not blood pressure, is the critical determinant.

Systolic blood pressure falls due to reduced cardiac output. For some adult patients, the situation is:

	SYSTOLIC BLOOD PRESSURE
Average, normal	100—130 mm. Hg
Impending shock	90—100 mm. Hg
Shock	Below 80 mm. Hg

The usual pressure of the patient should be known. Regardless of the numerical figure, the consistent progressive fall of blood pressure with a rapid, thready pulse is a serious sign. In the early stages of shock the blood pressure may not yet have fallen. A rapid pulse, apprehension, or air hunger may be the only indication of impending shock. The physician should be made aware of any fall in systolic blood pressure below 100 mm. Hg or any fall of 20 mm. Hg below the patient's usual blood pressure when this is an unexpected occurrence.

Blood pressure measurement may be difficult or even impossible to obtain or may give falsely low readings. This is particularly true of those patients with peripheral vessel arteriosclerosis compounded by the effects of vasopressor drugs. Intra-arterial blood pressure monitoring is becoming more commonplace because it is more accurate than the usual indirect auscultatory method.

The systolic blood pressure level may be ascertained by palpation, using a sphygmomanometer with the fingertips on the radial pulse. After the cuff has been inflated sufficiently to obliterate the pulse, the column of mercury is reduced sufficiently for blood to begin flowing through the radial artery. The systolic blood pressure is recorded as the point at which the radial artery is palpable. When peripheral arterioles are constricted in shock, diastolic pressure rises initially because blood has to be at an increased pressure to flow through the constricted vessels.

Pulse

Cardiac output is depressed in shock. A compensatory tachycardia occurs in an attempt to raise the output.

Pulse pressure is the difference between the systolic and diastolic blood pressures. In shock, a fall in systolic blood pressure with a rise in diastolic pressure results in a narrowed pulse pressure. The small spurts of blood passing in the artery feel more like a quiver than the thump of a full pulse. It is often described as a "rapid, thready pulse."

Tachycardia associated with easy compression of the radial pulse is an early sign of shock. It precedes the thready nature of the pulse in established shock. In the later stages of shock, the pulse is imperceptible.

Respiration

In shock, the tissues are receiving less oxygen. In response, the patient tries to gain more oxygen by breathing faster (tachypnea). Rapid respirations are helpful in moving blood along in the large veins toward the heart. The respirations are shallow and there may be grunting. In earlier stages the patient is hungry for air, but in profound shock the respiratory rate decreases to two or three a minute. To treat hypoxia, humidified oxygen is given.

Temperature

Heat regulating mechanisms are depressed in shock and heat loss is increased by added diaphoresis. With the possible exception of bacteremic shock, subnormal temperature is characteristic. Since there is a definite temperature range for cellular function and enzyme activity, the patient should be kept comfortably warm through control of environmental temperature and light blankets. Direct heat to the skin should not be used since it causes vasodilatation, further increasing heat loss and reducing the flow to critical organs. Heat also raises the metabolic rate, which raises the tissue requirement for oxygen.

Restlessness and Pain

Restlessness in shock is caused more often by hypoxia than by pain and may be relieved by oxygen administration. Pain can cause or enhance shock and it lessens the patient's adaptive response.

Narcotics cause further respiratory and circulatory depression. Opiates administered subcutaneously or intramuscularly to patients already in shock often are not absorbed effectively from the tissues because of the diminished circulation. If several injections of narcotics are given during shock, a double or triple dose may be absorbed when the patient's circulation improves, causing serious toxic effects. This result can happen with any drug given by an intramuscular or subcutaneous route. When symptoms of shock are present, the nurse should call the doctor and in the meantime withhold all previously ordered drugs. Narcotics should be given very judiciously to a postoperative patient whose blood pressure is falling, or to a patient who shows other symptoms that may indicate the approach of shock. The doctor may give the drug in such situations intravenously in a diluted bolus dose administered slowly and titrated to the patient's response.

pH and Blood Gases

The measurement of hydrogen ion concentration (pH), oxygen tension (Po_2) and carbon dioxide tension (Pco_2) in arterial blood is an effective way to evaluate lung function, lung adequacy, and tissue perfusion.

Arterial blood gas specimens may be drawn from a direct arterial puncture and may be serially or continually monitored with an indwelling arterial catheter. Venous samples are taken through a central venous catheter, not from a peripheral vein.

Central Venous Pressure

Central venous pressure (CVP) is the pressure of the blood in the right atrium or venae cavae. It serves to distinguish relationships among the hemodynamic variables in shock—the venous return, the quality of the pump, and vascular tone. Thus it is a critical guide in the management of the patient in shock. Normal central venous pressure is 0 to 4 cm. of water in the right atrium and 6 to 12 cm. of water in the venae cavae with a reference point at the midaxillary line.

An isolated CVP reading is of little value unless it is unusually high or low. Central venous pressure is best used by obtaining a baseline value and then taking frequent readings. The response of the patient to drug therapy or to volume expansion or contraction can then be evaluated. To be accurate, the zero level on the manometer must always be at the same height in relation to the patient's right atrium.

Effects on Vital Organs

Kidney. Vasoconstriction in shock contributes to a marked reduction in renal blood flow. Many physicians believe that the rate of urine formation is the most important indicator of the status of the shock patient. The patient in shock or impending shock needs an indwelling urethral catheter and hourly measurement of urine output. The physician should be notified of urinary output below 30 ml. per hour so that therapy may be initiated promptly to promote adequate renal perfusion.

With rapid reversal of the shock, urine output usually returns promptly. Continued oliguria after reversal of shock indicates renal damage secondary to ischemia.

Brain. Alteration in cerebral function is often the first sign of impaired oxygen delivery to the tissues. Mild anxiety, increasing restlessness, agitation or other change in behavior can be clues in advance of the more obvious signs of shock. As the condition deteriorates, the patient becomes listless, stuporous and finally unconscious.

Heart. Minimal essential myocardial perfusion pressure to maintain coronary artery blood flow is considered to correspond to a systolic pressure of about 80 mm. Hg. Below this the myocardium becomes increasingly hypoxic. The force of myocardial contraction decreases and the potential for dangerous cardiac arrhythmias, including ventricular fibrillation, increases.

TREATMENT AND NURSING CARE IMPLICATIONS

The nurse who is alert and has recognized the early warnings can bring help to the situation while the body's defenses are still in control. If a patient shows early warning signs of shock,

the physician should be notified. While waiting for him, the vital signs should be monitored and oxygen administered. An intravenous line should be opened for drug therapy. Obvious causes, such as external hemorrhage, should be controlled. A nurse should remain with the patient to observe him and to reassure him.

The treatment of shock depends on the clinical assessment of the patient and the complex hemodynamic variables involved. Treatment of hypoxia, pain, and cardiac arrhythmias proceeds concurrently with treatment of the shock state.

Replacement Therapy

Hypovolemic shock is best treated with the type of fluid that is being lost. In hemorrhage, this is whole blood; in burn shock, plasma; in extreme vomiting and diarrhea, solutions containing electrolytes. When blood is given, the doctor usually orders that the transfusion run rapidly while the blood pressure is low, and that the rate of administration be slowed to the usual 40 drops a minute when the blood pressure rises. At times, in order to keep pace with blood loss, several simultaneous transfusions are given. Blood may be forced by pressure into a vein to achieve more rapid introduction into the circulation than could be accomplished by free flow of the blood. When whole blood is desired but not available, the intravenous infusion may be started with plasma, concentrated albumin, low molecular weight dextran or saline, until blood can be obtained.

Volume loading, or infusing measured increments of fluid while observing CVP response, serves two purposes:

1. It establishes a true CVP. Initial low or normal levels are meaningless unless the response to an additional fluid load is observed.

2. As a therapeutic measure it serves to increase the effective circulating blood volume and increase cardiac output.

When the CVP is initially elevated or rapidly rises to high levels with volume increments of fluid, intravenous fluids are deferred. Efforts to improve the pumping effectiveness of the heart are then made with drug therapy.

Pulmonary Edema. The nurse remains alert for symptoms of overdose of fluids into the vascular system. CVP rise above 15 cm. H_2O indicates the inability of the right heart to accept a further fluid load. If more fluid arrives at the heart than the left side of the heart can hold and move forward, blood accumulates in the lungs. Its rising pressure in the pulmonary vessels squeezes some fluid from the vessels into alveoli. This fluid (pulmonary edema) can drown the patient. During hypovolemic shock, when an inadequate volume of blood is reaching the heart, the infusions of blood or other replacement therapy are providing the heart with something to pump. As the blood pressure improves, and as the fluid of the infusions, plus the body's own blood supply, reach the heart effectively, an overload may develop. The nurse will notice that the patient feels as if he cannot breathe well, and his respiration will be rapid and may sound moist. Frothy pink sputum may be coughed up. All these signs point to the complication, pulmonary edema, and without immediate help this can be as serious as the shock state. The infusion should be stopped and the physician notified.

Drugs

It is postulated that the effects of the sympathetic nervous system are mediated by receptors located throughout the body called adrenergic receptors. Adrenergic receptors are classified as alpha and beta on the basis of their characteristic responses.

When stimulated, alpha receptors cause constriction of the smooth muscle of blood vessels supplying skeletal muscle, the splanchnic vascular bed, skin and mucosa.

Beta adrenergic stimulation results in excitation of the S-A node resulting in increased heart rate, increased cardiac conduction (positive chronotropic effect) and increased myocardial contractility (positive inotropic effect). Also, the smooth muscles of the arteries, veins, and bronchi are relaxed, resulting in dilation.

Alpha and beta adrenergic blockers prevent the effects of alpha and beta stimulators, respectively.

Alpha and beta adrenergic stimulating drugs as well as alpha adrenergic blocking agents can be used in the treatment of shock.

ACTION	DRUG
Alpha stimulator causing vasoconstriction	Vasoxyl Neosynephrine
Beta stimulator causing vasodilatation and positive inotropic effects	Isuprel
Alpha and beta stimulator causing vasoconstriction and positive inotropic and chronotropic effects	Levophed Aramine Wyamine Epinephrine
Alpha adrenergic blocker causing vasodilatation	Dibenzyline Regitine Thorazine

Alpha and Beta Adrenergic Stimulators

Levophed (levarterenol bitartrate). Using the 0.2 per cent commercially prepared levarterenol bitartrate solution, 4 ml. may be added to 1,000 ml. of glucose in distilled water. The solution is titrated intravenously using a pediatric drip and the blood pressure is checked every five minutes to prevent wide swings. The rate of administration depends on the patient's blood pressure, the desired blood pressure ordered by the physician, and the concentration of the solution.

For example, the doctor may request that the patient's blood pressure be kept as close to 100/70 as possible. If the systolic pressure falls below 100, the nurse speeds up the flow of levarterenol; if it rises above this figure, she slows it down. A patient receiving this drug needs the constant attention of the nurse. If his blood pressure suddenly shoots up, he is in danger of a cerebral hemorrhage.

If a solution containing levarterenol infiltrates the tissues, the infusion should be discontinued immediately. The drug causes such profound vasoconstriction that the tissues it contacts directly become severely ischemic. The tissues can become necrotic and slough away, leaving a serious wound to be treated. For the moment, treatment of shock takes precedence over all other problems. However, if the patient's condition allows attention to the injury produced by the infiltration, the doctor may inject a vasodilating drug, Regitine, into the area, or he may ask the nurse to keep the wound covered with ice-water dressings or an icebag. Another venipuncture site must be selected.

Aramine (metaraminol bitartrate). Aramine may be given by any parenteral route:

ROUTE	EXPECT PRESSOR EFFECT WITHIN	AVERAGE DOSE
I.V.	1 to 2 minutes	15 to 100 mg.*
I.M.	10 minutes	2 to 10 mg.
Subcutaneous	5 to 20 minutes	2 to 10 mg.

* Doses as large as 50 to 100 mg. are given in infusions.

The dosage is regulated by the patient's response, especially his blood pressure. Sloughing of tissue due to infiltration of the solution is less likely than with levarterenol, but it may occur. Administration of Aramine has to be regulated very carefully, as the effects can accumulate. The maximum effect may not be in evidence until ten minutes after the drug is given. Overdose can lead to hypertension and cerebral hemorrhage. Aramine is given subcutaneously or intramuscularly only when shock is mild, and there is sufficient circulation to absorb it; if it is given in profound shock, not only will the patient fail to achieve the intended effect, but the drug will remain in the tissues to be picked up by the bloodstream when the patient's circulatory state improves, at which time an overdose might be received.

Some practical points about vasopressor therapy used as guides by the physician are:

• Blood pressure should be raised no more than 20 to 30 mm. Hg below the preshock normal level. If this is not known, systolic blood pressure should be kept between 90 to 100 mm. Hg. Excessive elevation of blood pressure produces marked vasoconstriction, reduces cardiac output and increases cardiac work and irritability.

• Prolonged use of vasopressors is not recommended and the dosage should be reduced or the patient weaned from them as soon as possible. They should be used as emergency drugs only.

Epinephrine (Adrenalin) may be given in anaphylactic shock. It increases the output of the heart and the force of the cardiac contraction; it constricts the blood vessels of the skin and increases blood pressure. It may be given intravenously in the dose of 0.5 ml. of a 1:1,000 solution. Tremors, dyspnea, chills, increased apprehension, nausea, vomiting, cyanosis, perspiration and headache may follow the administration of epinephrine. Adrenalin is a dangerous drug in hypovolemic shock or any other physiologic state in which the cardiac muscle is ischemic because the drug may cause death by ventricular fibrillation. One of the actions of Adrenalin is to increase cardiac irritability, and this action is enhanced whenever myocardial oxygenation is compromised. Its use in shock usually is limited to anaphylactic shock.

Beta Adrenergic Stimulator: Isuprel (Isoproterenol). The vasodilating effect of Isuprel promotes increased skin, renal, coronary, and cerebral blood flow. Because it increases heart rate and speed of conduction and is a myocardial irritant, patients receiving Isuprel require careful monitoring for increased heart rate above that ordered by the physician, and for signs of ventricular irritability manifested by dangerous forms of ventricular premature beats. Since vasodilation can lead to further hypotension, Isuprel is used in conjunction with volume replacement and central venous pressure monitoring. The drug is titrated intravenously in a concentration of 1 to 4 mg. per liter using a pediatric drip. The patient receiving Isuprel should not be left

alone. The drug is ordered to be discontinued if tachycardia at a specified rate, ventricular irritability, or further hypotension develop. The response of the patient receiving Isuprel is not evaluated strictly in terms of blood pressure, but rather in regard to evidence of improved perfusion. Increase in urinary output and "pinking" of the skin are positive signs.

Alpha Adrenergic Blocking Agents. These drugs are not vasodilators, but act as such by reversing norepinephrine-induced vasoconstriction. They may increase organ blood flow. Dibenzyline (phenoxybenzamine), Regitine (phentolamine) and Thorazine (chlorpromazine) are useful as alpha blocking agents. Because they produce marked venodilatation and increase the volume of the venous reservoir, central venous pressure has to be monitored carefully when they are used. Adequate quantities of a plasma expander should be available at the bedside.

Steroids

Even though there is no deficiency of steroids in the body during shock, corticosteroid therapy seems to help to maintain blood pressure. Particularly in bacteremic shock, which has not responded to the usual supportive measures, intravenous hydrocortisone may be given. Dosage may be as high as 2.0 gm. a day.

Pharmacologic agents used for the shock patient are potentially hazardous. Regardless of the physician's choice of drug or combination of drugs, the nurse must realize their benefits as well as their hazards, meticulously administer them, and intelligently observe the patient's response.

Position

In the *Trendelenburg* position the legs and the feet are raised, and the head is lower than the rest of the body. Usually the position is accomplished by elevating the foot of the bed on shock blocks, or by turning a crank that raises the foot of the bed (not the knee gatch, but the whole bottom of the bed). The slope should be gentle, because too great a tilt will throw the patient's abdominal viscera up against his diaphragm and impede breathing. The simple maneuver of elevating the patient's legs might return as much as 500 ml. of blood to the general circulation. Therefore, in impending shock, if the patient's legs have been up, as in a lithotomy position, do not put them down without a doctor's order or presence.

Because in shock position the head is lower than the rest of the body, blood flow to (but not from) the brain is facilitated, and this affords the brain some protection.

Patients in shock from conditions resulting in increased intracranial pressure (after brain surgery, for example) are positioned flat in bed, or even in a low sitting position, because lowering the head could result in further increase in intracranial pressure.

Patients in cardiogenic shock may benefit from a low Fowler's position. Respiratory excursion and pulmonary expansion are enhanced when the diaphragm is lower.

Activity

The patient in shock needs to have his metabolic activity kept to a minimum without introducing further hazards of immobility. Physical and emotional activity increase cellular needs for oxygen and nutrients and increase the formation of metabolites. Positioning, lifting, and turning are done gently by the nurse. Care should be planned so that the patient has some periods of uninterrupted rest. He needs to be protected from unnecessary and controllable stimulation. Visitors are limited. Understandably, they are distressed and need to be approached humanely and counseled regarding the rationale for rest.

PROGNOSIS AND COMPLICATIONS

When shock has progressed too far before treatment is started, or when, despite prompt treatment, the patient fails to respond, or when the underlying condition, such as a huge infarction of the myocardium, cannot be effectively treated, death follows.

Fortunately, when shock is treated adequately and promptly, the patient usually recovers. As vital signs return to normal, careful withdrawal of therapeutic measures can be made gradually.

A grave complication is failure of the kidneys to resume work after blood pressure improves. The nurse records both the amount of urine and the time of voiding. She should inform the doctor if no urine is excreted and blood pressure has been satisfactory for two hours, or if less than 25 ml. per hour is being put out.

Other complications may occur that are not always observable until the patient has recovered from shock. There may be a clot that formed in the slow-moving blood. Even in uncomplicated recovery the patient requires a period of convalescence to end the effects of the changes the body commanded when it called out its defensive reactions to fight shock.

REFERENCES AND BIBLIOGRAPHY

Ayres, S., and Giannelli, S., Jr.: *Care of the Critically Ill,* New York, Appleton-Century-Crofts, 1967.

Beland, I.: *Clinical Nursing: Pathophysiological and Psychosocial Approaches,* ed. 2, New York, Macmillan, 1970.

Betson, C.: The nurses' role in blood gas monitoring, *Cardiovasc. Nurs.* 7:83, November-December, 1971.

Betson, C., and Ude, L.: Central venous pressure, *Am. J. Nurs.* 69:1466, July, 1969.

Davis, L. (ed.): *Christopher's Textbook of Surgery,* ed. 9, Philadelphia, Saunders, 1968.

Guyton, A.: *Textbook of Medical Physiology,* ed. 3, Philadelphia, Saunders, 1966.

Morris, D.: The patient in cardiogenic shock, *Cardiovasc. Nurs.* 5:15, July-August, 1969.

Rodman, M., and Smith, D.: *Pharmacology and Drug Therapy in Nursing,* Philadelphia, Lippincott, 1968.

Simenone, F.: Part I. The nature of shock, Part II. The treatment of shock, *Am. J. Nurs.* 66:1286, June, 1966.

Sun, R. L.: Trendelenburg's position in hypovolemic shock, *Am. J. Nurs.* 71:1758, September, 1971.

Respiratory Insufficiency and Failure

52

Lung Function • Results of Lung Dysfunction • Acidosis and Alkalosis • Acute Respiratory Failure

The acute disruption of breathing and increasing anxiety go hand in hand. Only when normal breathing is compromised does the realization that disruption of breathing leads quickly to death enter awareness. Regardless of the cause, survival is threatened and the human organism reacts swiftly and strongly to respiratory failure with emergency neural adaptive mechanisms. As breathing is facilitated, anxiety is reduced, and as anxiety lessens, breathing improves. The patient with continued respiratory distress has the double task of dealing with the underlying disease process and the anxiety generated by it. The major objectives of nursing care for the patient in respiratory distress are to facilitate ventilation (O_2 intake and CO_2 removal) and to reduce the work of breathing. Competent observation, judgment, technical ministration, and emotional support of the patient are the ingredients of nursing care of the patient in respiratory distress. The nurse's supportive presence is a powerful factor in relieving apprehension.

Because life processes depend on the continuing availability of oxygen to the mitochondria of each body cell, all intensive care patients can be considered to be respiratory patients as well. Some will have respiratory disease as their major problem; all require nursing action which prevents respiratory complications. The encouragement of periodic sighing and coughing, deep breathing exercises, correct positioning with a regular routine of turning, and chest physiotherapy (see Chap. 24) within the limitations of the individual patient become part of the care plan for each patient in the intensive care unit.

LUNG FUNCTION

The main function of the respiratory system is to exchange oxygen and carbon dioxide between ambient (atmospheric) air and the blood. Usually it has sufficient reserves to maintain normal partial pressures or tension of these gases in the blood during times of stress. If, however, there is too much interference with the following aspects of lung function, respiratory insufficiency develops.

Ventilation is the movement of air in and out of the lungs in volumes sufficient to maintain normal *arterial* oxygen and carbon dioxide tensions.

Perfusion of the lungs is the filling of the pulmonary capillaries with venous blood returning from the systemic circulation via the right ventricle.

Diffusion is the process whereby oxygen and carbon dioxide are exchanged across the alveolar-capillary membrane.

Distribution is the delivery of ambient (atmospheric) air to the separate gas exchange units in the lung.

Surfactant, a lipoprotein substance secreted by the alveolar cells prevents alveoli from collapsing as they get smaller and from rupturing as they expand. Sighing or other mechanisms which increase alveolar inflation stimulate alveolar cells to produce surfactant.

RESULTS OF LUNG DYSFUNCTION

Abnormalities in ventilation, perfusion, diffusion, or distribution lead to the following conditions:

Hypoxia, or the diminished availability of oxygen to the cells of the body

Hypoxemia, or reduced oxygen in the body fluids (refers particularly to oxygen in arterial blood)

Hypercapnia, or excess carbon dioxide in the body fluids

Hypocapnia, or lessened carbon dioxide in body fluids

The patient who is hypoxemic but normocapnic (without hypocapnia) would have a low arterial oxygen tension. He is not receiving sufficient oxygen into the pulmonary capillaries. A frequent cause of this is atelectasis and veno-arterial shunting. We would expect the patient to be restless, anxious, and to have tachypnea (rapid respirations) and tachycardia. As the condition progresses, the patient would show other signs, such as duskiness, cyanosis, sweating, cardiac arrhythmias, and he might be combative or confused. The doctor would direct therapy toward improving oxygenation by such means as vigorous suctioning, supplemental oxygen, chest physiotherapy, humidification, or bronchoscopy to remove mucus plugs.

The patient who is hypoxemic and hypercapnic has a low arterial oxygen tension and elevated carbon dioxide tension. This is a result of alveolar hypoventilation. As carbon dioxide accumulates in the blood, the patient develops headache and becomes successively drowsy and then comatose. The hypoxia is the last remaining stimulus to respiration since the respiratory center becomes narcotized or "anesthetized" from excessive carbon dioxide. The patient is in a state of respiratory acidosis. To give the patient oxygen only, despite his bluish appearance, would take away his last stimulus to respiration and, though his color might improve temporarily, he could die from respiratory arrest. The physician would order assisted or controlled ventilation with intubation and a mechanical respirator. Evacuating carbon dioxide allows adequate oxygenation to take place. Because mechanical ventilators are very powerful, the doctor will want the reduction of carbon dioxide to take place slowly over several hours rather than sev-

eral minutes. If there is a precipitous rise in pH by ventilatory removal of CO_2, there can be dangerous fluctuations in myocardial potassium with serious cardiac arrhythmias. What had been the state of respiratory acidosis could swiftly become metabolic alkalosis.

The patient who is both hypoxemic and hypocapnic would be one, for example, in serious shock where all body processes are depressed. The physician would attempt to control the patient's respiration and maintain alveolar ventilation with a volume-limited respirator.

ACIDOSIS AND ALKALOSIS

(Acidemia and Alkalemia)

The kidney, as well as the lung, together with the body fluids and electrolytes and several buffer systems, acts and reacts to keep the arterial pH (hydrogen ion concentration) within the normal limits of 7.39 to 7.45. Since normal pH is essential for correct enzyme action and cellular metabolism, the body's ability to make adjustments is of critical importance. Life cannot be maintained for more than a few moments when pH falls to 7.0 or rises to 7.8.

Alveolar ventilation determines the amount of carbon dioxide in the body. An increase in carbon dioxide, present in body fluids primarily as carbonic acid, decreases the pH below the normal of 7.4 (acidemic). A decrease in carbon dioxide increases the pH above 7.4 (alkalemic). The hydrogen ion concentration, or pH, affects the rate of alveolar ventilation by a direct action of hydrogen ions on the respiratory center in the medulla oblongata.

The kidney contributes to the normal pH by maintaining serum bicarbonate between 26 to 28 mEq. per liter and excreting excess hydrogen ions.

The lung and kidneys combine to maintain the carbonic acid to bicarbonate ratio at 1:20, fixing the pH at about 7.4.

In the critically ill patient, various homeostatic mechanisms operate to compensate for altered physiology. Buffer ratios shift, the lung can "blow off" carbonic acid as carbon dioxide, or the kidney can excrete more bicarbonate in an attempt to maintain normal pH. Compensatory mechanisms, however, can become overstressed and fail, and dangerous clinical conditions develop which in the intensive care patient are generally superimposed on an already serious underlying condition. The patient's condition is said to be compensated as long as the ratio of carbonic acid to bicarbonate remains 1:20.

By convention, disturbances in pH which involve the lung and carbonic acid levels which result from dissolved carbon dioxide are termed respiratory; the other disturbances are termed metabolic. At times, metabolic and respiratory derangements coexist. Blood gas studies done on a sample of arterial blood enable the physician to assess the acid-base balance dependably and rapidly. The blood may be withdrawn by single arterial puncture or repeated samples may be drawn from an indwelling arterial catheter. A heparinized syringe is used and, after careful filling to avoid bubbles, it is capped with a syringe cap or a round toothpick. If delay in analysis is anticipated the syringe is immediately immersed in ice. This decreases the metabolic activity of the blood cells and prevents oxygen consumption in the syringe.

Some laboratory values of importance in the care of the respiratory patient or other patients requiring assessment of acid-base balance are:

ARTERIAL BLOOD

pH	7.39-7.45
Pa_{O_2}	100 mm. Hg breathing room air 300-600 mm. Hg breathing 100% oxygen
Pa_{CO_2}	35-45 mm. Hg
O_2 saturation	96-100% (per cent oxygen attached to hemoglobin compared to how much could be attached)
Bicarbonate	20.0-29.0 mEq./L.

Because of the numerous ways in which individuals can vary in their response to illness, laboratory tests serve as guides, but are not black and white indicators of the overall clinical condition of the patient.

Laboratory reports of blood gases require prompt decision making; they cannot be relegated to a spindle for the physician to look at the following morning. In many hospitals an intern or resident maintains a close check on the patient's condition. In some hospitals specially prepared nurses review the laboratory and clinical data and make adjustments in therapy according to previously written physician's orders or following telephone communication with him. Close observation of the patient, including his general behavior, state of consciousness, skin turgor, urinary output, rate and depth of respiration, muscle function, intestinal function, and abdominal distention, is an essential nursing activity.

ACUTE RESPIRATORY FAILURE

Acute respiratory failure, or acute ventilatory failure, is a life-threatening complication in which alveolar ventilation becomes inadequate to maintain the body's vital need for oxygen supply and carbon dioxide removal. Though the signs are not specific, the patient initially may be restless, agitated, confused, and diaphoretic.

Tachycardia or other cardiac arrhythmias and signs such as flapping tremor (asterixis) are prone to develop. Though laboratory confirmation of acute respiratory failure will show different correlations with each patient's clinical condition, one general guideline is that acute respiratory failure will reveal a Pa_{O_2} of less than 50 mm. Hg, a Pa_{CO_2} of more than 50 mm. Hg, and a pH of less than 7.30 (Nett and Petty).

The most frequent circumstance of acute respiratory failure is when a patient with moderate to severe chronic obstructive lung disease (see Chap. 24) develops an acute bronchopulmonary infection, is over-sedated, undergoes general anesthesia, has chest trauma or incurs some other type of insult to his already embarrasssed pulmonary reserve. Other patients with neurological disorders, acute poisoning, or surgical intervention (especially abdominal operations) are susceptible to respiratory failure.

At first the patient may be alert but he is apprehensive, dyspneic, wheezing, and perhaps cyanotic. There is marked use of the accessory muscles of respiration. Though the patient often looks as if he would benefit from sedation because of his apprehension, the doctor prescribes therapy aimed at relieving the patient's symptoms by improving ventilation. Sedation, alone, can further depress respiratory effort. In the presence of continued hypoventilation, cardiac arrhythmias, hypotension and congestive heart failure can develop.

If CO_2 retention develops slowly, there is time for the kidneys to excrete chlorides and reabsorb bicarbonate and sodium ions, thus maintaining the pH within normal limits. If the renal mechanisms fail to compensate for rapidly accumulating CO_2, the pH falls below the normal 7.39 and respiratory acidosis develops.

Treatment Modalities

The physician plans a program of care for the patient which encompasses the following aspects of management:

- Clearing the airways
- Combating bronchospasm
- Giving oxygen for hypoxemia while assisting or controlling ventilation
- Humidification
- Combating infection
- Monitoring clinical and laboratory values
- Treating cardiac and circulatory status
- Maintaining fluid and electrolyte balance

Essential to nursing management of the patient is understanding the aims of therapy, explaining these to the patient as they are about to involve him, skilled observation and judgment, technical expertise with various forms of equipment utilized by the respiratory care team and establishing effective communication with the patient so that he knows what is expected of him and knows what he can expect of others. The patient's fear is lessened when he is assisted to remain in control of his situation for as long as possible. When he can no longer do so, he must have the confidence that he can temporarily relinquish the control to others who are concerned and competent to do the job for him.

Airway Maintenance

Cough is the major mechanism for clearing the tracheobronchial tree of abundant, tenacious mucus. Effective coughing requires that the patient be assisted to a sitting position, that he take a deep breath prior to coughing, and that he use his abdominal and accessory respiratory muscles to forcefully exhale and cough. In the event that the patient's cough is ineffective but he is conscious and cooperative, the physician may wish to stimulate coughing by tracheal irritation with a catheter. The use of the intermittent positive pressure respirator serves to inflate the lungs and enhance the ejecting mechanism of the cough by driving air past mucus secretions.

Simply giving the patient an IPPB treatment is not enough. After the treatment, the patient must be assisted to cough or the treatment will be ineffective. Thus, he requires nursing attention even if another member of the respiratory care team, such as the inhalation therapist, actually turns on his machine.

Encouraging fluid intake within the maximum limits of the patient's treatment regimen aids in preventing the drying of secretions. Turning and positioning the patient every hour and performing chest physiotherapy aid in directing mucus to the main airway from whence it can be expelled.

Secretions often must be thinned to be expectorated. To be most effective, sterile solutions or medications must be delivered to the mucus-covered surface. Nebulization therapy is the least traumatic and most effective method of accomplishing this.

When the patient cannot cough effectively despite therapy, the physician may utilize nasal-tracheal suction. Passage of the suction catheter is facilitated if the patient is sitting upright and leaning slightly forward with his jaw extended. An assistant can grasp the patient's tongue. A 16-inch, size 1824 F. catheter, lubricated with a water-soluble substance, is inserted gently, without suction, into the nostril. As the patient coughs or pants repeatedly, the glottis opens and permits the catheter to be passed between the vocal cords and into the trachea. The catheter is attached to a suction apparatus with a "Y" connection. As the opening of the "Y" is occluded, gentle suction (40 cm. of water) is applied. The catheter is rotated between the left thumb and forefinger to sweep the walls. Suction is applied for no longer than 15 seconds at a time. The catheter can be guided into either main bronchus by turning the patient's head to the side opposite that to be catheterized. Sterile normal saline, 5 to 10 ml., can be inserted into the trachea through the catheter once it is in place. The catheter can be left in place between periods of suctioning, but oxygen is given during these intervals. As the catheter is withdrawn, suction is applied to clear the oropharynx of secretions.

Endotracheal Intubation

Suctioning can be accomplished also through an endotracheal tube which the physician inserts through the nose or mouth. It can remain in place for several days, and when its cuff is inflated to provide a tight connection, it can be attached to a respirator for controlled ventilation. The patient, however, cannot speak and may have difficulty swallowing. Sedation may be ordered for him as long as respiration is controlled. Suctioning is not as effective as when tracheostomy is done, but the time delay, surgical trauma, and complications of tracheostomy are avoided. Once the patient is intubated with

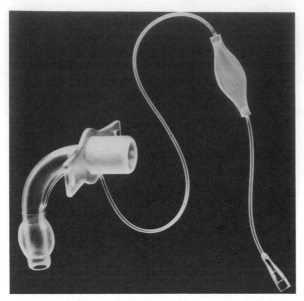

Fig. 52-1. Bassett cuffed tracheostomy tube. (Portex, Ltd., Hythe, Kent, England)

an endotracheal tube, the following points are important considerations:

Placement of the Tube. If the tube is not anchored securely to the exterior, it can slip into the right main stem bronchus. Then the left lung would not be ventilated and is actually completely obstructed from the flow of air. When the patient is intubated, both sides of the thorax should rise evenly during inspiration. Because this is not always a reliable sign, both sides of the lung should be auscultated with a stethoscope to hear the flow of air. The physician or nurse can do this.

The tube can also be misplaced and pass into the esophagus. If the patient is still breathing spontaneously, breath sounds will still be heard in both lung fields. The physician can check correct placement of the tube by attaching it to an "Ambu" bag or other type of anesthesia bag and, while squeezing the bag, simultaneously auscultate the thorax.

Because of dangers of tube displacement it is not generally considered advisable to turn this patient from side to side. Suctioning is used to prevent airway obstruction.

Obstruction of the Tube. Absence of breath sounds in either or both lungs can indicate obstruction of the tube. The tube can become obstructed by: (1) secretions; suctioning and liquefying secretions is required; (2) kinking of the tube; (3) biting down on the tube by the

patient; this can be prevented by the use of a bite block or an oral-pharyngeal airway; (4) the cuff, which, when inflated, provides a tight seal between the tube and the trachea can slip down and occlude the orifice; and (5) the distal end of the tube, which may press on the wall of the trachea. All of the above situations demand emergency action because of the immediate danger of asphyxiation.

Removal of the Tube
• Accidental removal by the patient must be guarded against as this can result in laryngeal edema or spasm and predispose to respiratory arrest.
• The physician makes the decision to remove the tube when the patient's vital capacity, measured with a ventilometer, is adequate. Blood gas values are also used as a guideline for tube removal.
• The endotracheal tube should be removed only by a person who can replace it if necessary. The necessary emergency equipment should remain at the bedside.
• Before the cuff is deflated, the pharynx is aspirated so that secretions do not gravitate downward. The tube is usually removed with the patient in semi-Fowler's position. Laryngospasm can occur. If so, the physician gives air by positive pressure with an "Ambu" bag; he may re-intubate the patient, and may order muscle relaxants.

Postextubation Care
• High or semi-Fowler's position promotes chest expansion and optimal alveolar ventilation.
• The patient's posterior pharynx may be dry and he may be hoarse. Humidification aids in preventing further complications. Hard candy may be comforting.
• The patient should be observed carefully for signs of laryngeal edema or increased respiratory distress.

Tracheostomy

An opening into the trachea with insertion of a cuffed tracheostomy tube provides a portal for suctioning and the tube can serve as a connection for a respirator. Complications of tracheostomy include infection, bleeding, tracheal trauma, and pneumothorax. Humidification is necessary to prevent drying and incrustation of the mucous membrane in the trachea and the main stem bronchus. Crusts can break off, obstruct the lower airway, and cause asphyxiation.

Ideally, a new disposable suction catheter and disposable sterile glove should be used each time the patient is suctioned, and these are then discarded. The frequency of suctioning depends on the amount of secretions present.

Because of the danger of necrosis of the tracheal wall, the cuff of the tracheostomy tube should be deflated on a regular basis. Physicians have their own preferences regarding deflation routine. These vary, for example, from 15 minutes of deflation every two hours to five minutes of deflation every hour. The amount of air injected into the cuff should be just enough to prevent an air leak around the tube or through the mouth. For the average patient, 5 to 7 ml. of air is sufficient.

Oxygen

Compensatory responses to hypoxia, such as increased cardiac output, with hypertension and tachycardia, peripheral sympathetic overactivity, tachypnea (rapid breathing) and hyperventilation, can reach a maximum of usefulness and then the patient's condition deteriorates.

The exact oxygen tension (or partial pressure of oxygen in the arterial blood) at which observable signs of lack of oxygen develop varies among patients. When Pa_{O_2} (partial pressure of oxygen) decreases below the normal of 95 to 100 mm. to about 80, the patient may become tachypneic with a rate of about 25, breathe with his mouth open and be short of breath on walking. With further decrease the patient breathes faster, speaks in short, broken sentences, uses his facial muscles with expiration and may appear dusky. As oxygen tension decreases to dangerous levels, cyanosis, restlessness, hypotension, diaphoresis, and combativeness are likely to be present. Serious cardiac arrhythmias and cardiac arrest can develop quickly.

There is medical controversy regarding optimum and safe levels of oxygen tension. Generally, optimum arterial oxygen tension is maintained between 80 and 120 mm. Hg. An oxygen tension of 70 is of concern and an oxygen level below 60 is dangerous. Recently it has been noted that oxygen toxicity can be as great a problem as hypoxia. Levels of oxygen tension over 120 mm. Hg are unnecessary and may lead to oxygen toxicity. High levels of oxygen depress respiration and also damage the surface membrane of the lung and lead to progressive atelectasis.

If airway clearance and conventional oxygen therapy are not sufficient to maintain adequate oxygenation above 60 mm. Hg and removal of carbon dioxide, a respirator (ventilator) attached to a cuffed endotracheal or tracheostomy tube may be ordered.

The Patient on a Respirator (Ventilator). Ventilators are used to do the work of breathing. Air is forced into the lung to give the patient adequate tidal volume (adequate sized breaths). Small bedside units have replaced the body or tank type respirator, the so-called "iron lung" which was widely used for the respiratory failure of acute poliomyelitis. The patient's respiration can be either assisted (patient cycled) or controlled (machine cycled).

Ventilators are either pressure cycled (pressure limited) or volume cycled (volume limited). Pressure cycled ventilators can be used intermittently for deep breathing exercises or for the delivery of aerosols, or also can be used for continuous cycling of the patient's respirations. For respiratory assist, a valve near the patient connection opens in response to the patient's spontaneous effort. His respiration is then boosted by the machine until a preset inspiratory pressure is exceeded. The inflow valve closes and expiration is into the atmosphere. In many types of machines, after a set period of delay, the machine will trigger a breath if the patient's own effort fails to trigger the machine. For respiratory control, inspiratory flow can be automatically triggered and the machine is used in conjunction with the cuffed tracheostomy or endotracheal tube. Pressure-limited ventilators are small, are driven by compressed air or air-oxygen mixtures rather than electric power, are reasonable in price, but require frequent maintenance. The physician determines inspiratory flow, sensitivity, rate, and expiratory pressure. Maximum pressure is about 40 to 45 cm. of water.

In the volume-cycled respirator, a motor-driven piston pumps air or air-oxygen mixture. The rate of respiration and the volume of air per respiration or stroke (tidal volume) can be varied and are determined by the physician according to the patient's blood gases and predicted tidal volume needs. Volume-cycled machines are always used with a cuffed endotracheal tube if the condition is anticipated to be cleared in a short time, or the tracheostomy tube, for longer periods of treatment. They deliver the predetermined volume regardless of resistance of the lungs. They are more reliable and more expensive then pressure-cycled units.

In controlled ventilation, the inspiration is initiated by the machine at a preset rate. The patient's spontaneous respiratory effort, if any, must be synchronized with the machine. Fighting the respirator, or the patient becoming asynchronous with the respirator, is usually caused by inadequate alveolar ventilation, by hypoxemia, or low cardiac output. The physician may then take certain measures to overcome the patient's spontaneous breathing effort, such as a short period of manually controlled ventilation with an "Ambu" bag and 100 per cent oxygen. If this is unsuccessful, drugs such as morphine or d-tubocurarine (Curare) can be given in small intravenous doses by the physician to depress spontaneous respirations to the point where controlled ventilation can be initiated. The patient who is struggling to breathe on his own has to be convinced that the respiratory care team is concerned and competent to take over, temporarily, the work of breathing for him.

Airway pressure depends on the amount of air delivered and the resistance of the lung to inflation. A safety or "pop-off" valve prevents excessive pressure. Increases or decreases in pressure can be signaled by an alarm built into or attached to the system. An elevation of pressure is an indication of obstruction usually due to retained secretions. A decrease in pressure is usually an indication of a lack of a closed, or airtight, system. The inflation of the cuff of the endotracheal or tracheostomy tube should be checked. Fall in pressure can also indicate a decrease in broncho-constriction and mean progress for the patient. Supplemental oxygen and humidification can be provided with volume-cycled respirators. As with all types of mechanical equipment, precise knowledge of the principles of the instrument and the manufacturer's instructions are essential for all members of the care team who will be involved in its use.

Nursing Care. Some important nursing considerations for the care of the patient on a respirator are:

• One of the major problems leading to intubation and intensive respiratory care is retained secretions. Positive pressure breathing does not adequately ventilate the entire lung parenchyma unless secretions are moved from the distal air passages to the mainstem bronchi and carina, where they can be cleared by suctioning or coughing. This is a nursing responsibility. Pulmonary physiotherapy technics such as gentle vibration and percussion (clapping with cupped hands) over the lung fields from which secretions are to be removed need to be performed at frequent, regular intervals by the knowledgeable nurse or physiotherapist.

• Diffuse atelectasis can develop during constant-volume ventilation. In order to promote ventilation of dependent portions of the lungs, several technics can be employed which simulate the normal sigh mechanism and produce periodic hyperinflation. The pressure of the pressure-cycled machine can be increased 10 to 20 cm. for several breaths every hour or several times an hour. Some volume-controlled machines, such as the Emerson postoperative ventilator, have a built-in sigh mechanism which is automatically activated every seven minutes or longer. Or, the patient's lungs can be inflated for several breaths manually with an anesthesia bag and 100 per cent oxygen.

• The patient must be in synchrony with the ventilator or else he is not getting the proper rate or volume. Notify the physician or therapist if the patient is out of phase.

• Gastric dilatation and paralytic ileus are not uncommon problems of patients on respirator therapy. Gastrointestinal bleeding can also occur. Report abdominal distention promptly to the physician, who can initiate early use of gastric decompression. Vomiting with aspiration spells disaster for these patients. The patient's stools and gastric secretions should be checked for blood, and a fall in the hematocrit should be promptly reported.

• It is convenient to suction the patient at the fixed intervals when the cuff is routinely deflated to avoid necrosis of the tracheal mucosa. Before deflating the cuff, suction the upper airway first so that secretions do not gravitate downward. Suction more frequently if necessary. Note the color, consistency, and odor of secretions. The cuff inflation should not exceed the quantity of air which is just sufficient to prevent the patient from talking or to prevent air escaping from the patient's mouth. For greater safety, 0.5 ml. of air can be removed after reaching the end-point.

• Respiratory alkalosis from hyperventilation can occur in patients on respirators. The patient might complain of chest pain, numbness or tingling of the extremities, vertigo, or lightheadedness, muscle spasm, and may even develop tetany. This can sometimes be avoided in the susceptible patient if the respiratory rate is periodically decreased.

• In order to keep average intrathoracic pressure close to atmospheric and avoid fall in cardiac output for the patient on controlled ventilation, the physician may order that inspiration comprise one-third of each respiration and expiration be twice as long as inspiration, or some other proportion in which the duration of expiration exceeds that of inspiration. Settings on the machines are used to make this kind of adjustment. Report to the physician any signs of decreased cardiac output.

• Patients with tracheostomies may be on oral feedings, but patients with endotracheal tubes receive nothing by mouth.

• Vital signs including blood pressure, pulse, and respiratory rate should be checked hourly.

• Temperature is recorded every four hours.

• The patient on a ventilator *should not be left alone.*

• Check the patient's level of consciousness, color of lips and nailbeds, pupils, and muscle strength every hour.

• Remember that the patient cannot talk, but can hear, and can usually write. A bell should be left with him at all times and a "magic slate" or pad and pencil should be left also. Leave the patient's dominant hand free of intravenous needles, if possible, so that he can write more easily. Avoid discussing frightening aspects of the patient's condition where he may overhear the conversation and become more alarmed.

• Most respirator patients are conscious and alert during the major part of their illness. All are apprehensive; many are depressed, especially if they are victims of recurrent episodes of respiratory failure and between hospitalizations constantly have to fight the battle of breathlessness. Some patients may be bitter, having become acutely ill despite adhering closely to the home regimen prescribed for them. The person under age 65, not covered by Medicare, can incur tremendous debt from his intensive treatment. The patient becomes easily frustrated because of his inability to communicate verbally with physicians, nurses, inhalation therapists, and family. Explanations to the patient must continue, however.

The patient knows that his life is dependent on the competence of people and the mechanics of machines. Accidental disconnection from the respirator, kinking of the tubes, or occlusion of them with a mucus plug can mean immediate asphyxiation. Once an accident occurs, fear of its recurrence can plague a patient and he will expend tremendous energy trying to guard his own life. A manual device such as an "Ambu" bag must be at the bedside of each patient in the event of mechanical breakdown of the ventilator or asynchrony creating an emergency. The patient must have the reassurance that he is under constant, competent supervision. When the patient breathes better, so does the staff!

Weaning the Patient. Considerations employed by the physician to determine that the patient can be gradually removed from respirator support are his vital capacity and blood gas values. Weaning is initiated as soon as possible so that the patient's respiratory muscles can be restored to normal tone more quickly and also because the patient psychologically benefits from control of his own life processes and signs of improvement. Generally, the longer the patient has received artificial ventilation, the slower will be the weaning process. Also, how successfully the patient is weaned from the respirator depends to a large extent on the quality of nursing care he received during the intensive treatment process. Weaning is best initiated early in the morning, the patient's responses closely watched, and the time intervals increased during the day. Patients who were receiving volume-controlled assistance may be switched to a pressure-cycled respirator before weaning is attempted. The sensitivity can be gradually decreased on the pressure-cycled respirator so that more burden is put on the patient to initiate respiration himself.

While off the ventilator, the patient receives humidified oxygen. Some patients may require mild sedation to allay their anxiety. Team efforts are directed towards early mobilization of the patient by having him sit in a chair as soon as possible. All patients require the constant presence of the nurse who observes their tolerance, gives constant support to their own efforts, and is prepared to assist them back to respirator support if they are not up to the task of breathing on their own.

Even when weaning appears complete, the patient should be observed for several days by the specially prepared respiratory staff. This is especially true for the older, debilitated patient.

REFERENCES AND BIBLIOGRAPHY

AYRES, S., *et al.*: Respiratory management of the critically ill patient, *N.Y. State J. Med.* 68:2871, November, 1968.

AYRES, S., and GIANNELLI, S., JR.: *Care of the Critically Ill,* New York, Appleton-Century-Crofts, 1967.

BENDIXEN, H., *et al.*: *Respiratory Care,* St. Louis, Mosby, 1965.

BETSON, C.: The nurse's role in blood gas monitoring, *Cardiovasc. Nurs.* 7:83, November-December, 1971.

Cleaning and Sterilization of Inhalation Equipment, New York, National Tuberculosis and Respiratory Disease Association, 1968.

HARGREAVES, A.: Emotional problems of patients with respiratory disease, *Nurs. Clin. N. Am.* 3:479, September, 1968.

MURPHY, E.: Intensive nursing care in a respiratory unit, *Nurs. Clin. N. Am.* 3:423, September, 1968.

NETT, L., and PETTY, T.: Respirator controls, *Am. J. Nurs.* 67:1852, September, 1967.

————: Acute respiratory failure, *Am. J. Nurs.* 67:1847, September, 1967.

PHIPPS, W., and BARKER, W.: Respiratory insufficiency and failure, *in* MELTZER, L., *et al.*: *Concepts and Practices of Intensive Care for Nurse Specialists,* Philadelphia, The Charles Press, 1969.

Principles of Respiratory Care, New York, National Tuberculosis and Respiratory Disease Association, 1967.

SAFER, P. (ed.): *Respiratory Therapy,* Philadelphia, Davis, 1965.

SECOR, J.: *Patient Care in Respiratory Problems,* Philadelphia, Saunders, 1969.

SOVIE, M., and ISRAEL, J.: Use of the cuffed tracheostomy tube, *Am. J. Nurs.* 67:1854, September, 1967.

TURNER, H.: The anatomy and physiology of normal respiration, *Nurs. Clin. N. Am.* 3:383, September, 1968.

WETMORE, C.: Unusual psychological atmospheres, *Inhalation Therapy* 13:34, June, 1968.

The Patient with Heart Disease: Cardiac Arrhythmias

53

Cardiac Rhythmicity and Its Regulation • Cardiac Arrhythmias
(Dysrhythmias) • Treatment of Cardiac Arrhythmias • Cardiac
Arrest • The Patient with an Artificial Electrical Pacemaker

CARDIAC RHYTHMICITY AND ITS REGULATION

In order to pump blood, the heart must alternately relax and contract, allowing blood to enter its chambers during the relaxation phase and forcing it out during the contraction phase. The alternate contraction and relaxation is provided by an inherent rhythmicity of the cardiac muscle itself.

In the posterior wall of the right atrium is a small area known as the sino-atrial (S-A) node. This node has a rhythmic rate of contraction of muscle fibers at about 72 beats per minute. As one considers the muscle mass of the heart from atria to ventricles, one finds that the tissue retains its capacity to contract rhythmically, but the lower down the pacemaker site, the slower the inherent rate of the pacemaking tissue. An A-V node pacemaker functions at a rate of 40 to 60 times per minute, while a ventricular pacemaker functions around 20 to 40 times per minute. Because the sinus node has a faster inherent rate than the other portions of the heart, impulses originating in the S-A node spread into the atria and ventricles, stimulating these areas so rapidly that they cannot slow down to their natural rates of rhythm. As a result, in health the rhythm of the S-A node is called the pacemaker of the heart.

Cardiac muscle fibers are joined together in a kind of lattice work formation. An electrical impulse arising in any single fiber eventually spreads over the membranes of all of the fibers.

The normal muscle cell has more negative than positive ions inside the cell membrane and the electrical cardiac impulse is caused by sudden transfer of some of these ions through the membrane so that more positive than negative ions then appear on the inside. This process is called *depolarization*. Once depolarization has occurred, another normal cardiac impulse cannot be carried until the ions realign themselves to their original condition. This is called *repolarization*. During this period the cell is said to be *refractory*.

Depolarization and repolarization produce an electrical field. Because of the ease with which body tissues conduct current, this electrical potential can be detected by electrodes placed on the external surface of the body and recorded by a machine known as the electrocardiograph.

A special conduction route known as the *Purkinje* system exists in the ventricles to transmit the cardiac impulses throughout the ventricles as rapidly as possible causing all portions to contract simultaneously and exert a coordinated pumping effort.

Sequentially, the cardiac impulse originates in the S-A node and travels through the atria causing them to contract. A few hundredths of a second after leaving the S-A node the impulse reaches the A-V node where it is delayed a few hundredths of a second while the ventricles fill with blood. The Purkinje system fibers begin in the A-V node, extend through the bundle of His into the ventricular septum, where they divide into major branches, a right bundle branch, and anterior and posterior divisions of a left bundle branch. After the delay at the A-V node, the cardiac impulse spreads rapidly through the Purkinje system, thence to the ventricular musculature, causing both ventricles to contract in full force within the next few hundredths of a second.

The normal heart rhythm can be disturbed in a variety of ways. Some of these are the result of disease. Others are harmless adaptations in normal function. When arrhythmias occur in the absence of heart disease and are noted by the doctor in the course of his examination, he usually does not mention them to the patient.

Each of us has had the sensation of a pounding heart, perhaps in a moment of fright when we are dodging an oncoming car. Most of the time we are not aware that our hearts are beating. Without our conscious awareness, the heart adjusts its work to the changing needs of the body. It can increase the amount of blood that it pumps in two ways: by beating more rapidly and by increasing the volume of blood pumped with each beat. Sudden fright often causes the heart to beat faster and more forcefully, and we become aware of our heartbeat.

These adjustments in heart action are beyond our conscious control. The stimulation of the sympathetic nervous system quickens the heart; the stimulation of the parasympathetic (vagus) system slows it. Both systems constantly affect the heart. In fright usually the stimulation of the sympathetic system causes a temporarily greater effect and, consequently, a faster and a fuller heartbeat.

In some very frightened or shocked people, however, vagal reflexes predominate and heart rate slows, cardiac output falls and the person becomes weak or faint (vasovagal syncope). Assist the patient to a supine position to encourage cerebral blood flow until equilibrium is restored.

CARDIAC ARRHYTHMIAS (DYSRHYTHMIAS)

In disease, the pacemaker of the heart can be too fast or too slow. The myocardial cells can become overly excitable or develop a shortened refractory period, or have a damaged Purkinje system or develop blocks in the conduction system. The cardiac arrhythmias that result can be major, that is, imminently life threatening, or they can be relatively minor. Because of their irregularity, all cardiac arrhythmias affect the rhythmic pumping action of the heart to some degree.

Many ambulatory patients receive treatment for cardiac arrhythmias and are able to live essentially normal lives. When their cardiac reserve, however, becomes overtaxed by coexisting illness, they become subject to more dangerous arrhythmias or more serious consequences of their underlying hemodynamic disturbance.

In recent years it has become evident that "sudden" cardiac arrest is really not so sudden, but is very often heralded by less dangerous warning arrhythmias. In the critically ill patient or the patient with heart disease, even "minor" arrhythmic changes can compromise cardiac function by causing a fall in cardiac output, thereby reducing coronary artery blood flow. Arrhythmias also increase myocardial oxygen need, lead to more dangerous arrhythmic complications, and make treatment of the patient's underlying disease more difficult and complex.

Many clinical states predispose to cardiac arrhythmias. Myocardial ischemia following infarction, disturbances in pH, inadequate ventilation, electrolyte imbalance, anxiety or pain can disturb heart rate, rhythm, or conduction.

Though an arrhythmia can be diagnosed from an electrocardiogram rhythm strip, the effect of the arrhythmia on the patient's cardiac output is the crucial factor. A person with a normal heart who develops a sinus tachycardia (rate over 100) after running up a flight of stairs is showing a normal physiologic response. The patient with an acute myocardial infarction, however, who has a continued sinus tachycardia on bed rest, can add an intolerable workload to his already damaged heart.

A cardiac monitor attached to a patient is useless unless accurate observations are made, interpreted correctly, and acted on appropriately. For example, the nurse may administer a p.r.n. medication, notify the physician, or institute emergency measures required in the interim until the physician arrives.

The development of nursing skill in arrhythmia detection takes considerable study, supervised practice, and time. Only one lead of the ECG is generally necessary to accomplish nursing goals in arrhythmia analysis. The cardiologist reviews the entire 12-lead ECG and in addition to arrhythmia interpretation makes other cardiac diagnoses such as heart enlargement, electrolyte disturbance, ischemic tissue damage, necrosis, or intraventricular conduction delay.

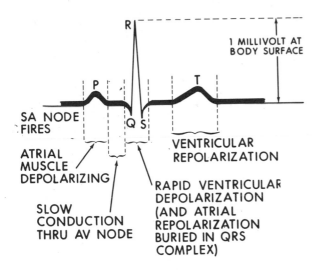

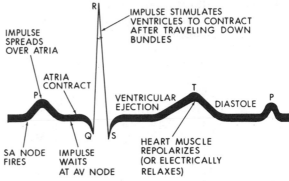

Fig. 53-2. Electrical and mechanical events of basic ECG tracing. (Hewlett-Packard Co., Medical Electronic Division, Palo Alto, Calif.)

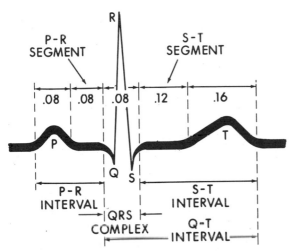

Fig. 53-1. Basic electrocardiographic trace. (Hewlett-Packard Co., Medical Electronic Division, Palo Alto, Calif.)

Arrhythmia Electrocardiography*

The electrocardiographic display of the heart's electrical events (Lead II) is shown in Figure 53-1:

A systematic approach to arrhythmia detection includes knowing certain norms, gathering of data and the comparison of this data with a set of facts characteristic of certain arrhythmias, then gathering data regarding the clinical state of the patient. For example, change in cardiac output can be reflected in blood pressure, pulse

*The arrhythmia ECG tracings which follows are from the Magnetic Tape Recording Library of Physiological Training Company, San Marino, Calif., reproduced on the Brush Instruments Recorder.

volume, skin color and degree of moisture, appearance and orientation of the patient, urinary output, chest pain, and dyspnea.

When looking at the cardiac monitor or rhythm strip, the following steps are recommended:

• Make an overall inspection of the strip. What are the gross abnormalities?

• Measure the atrial rate (P waves).

• Measure the ventricular rate (QRS complexes).

• Is the P-P interval the same as the R-R interval?

• Measure the P-R interval in several complexes.

• Measure the QRS width.

• Observe the configuration of the P wave and QRS.

• Observe the relationship of the P wave to the QRS. Does the P wave consistently precede the QRS? Does it follow the QRS? Are there more or less P waves than QRS's?

• Observe the S-T segment. Though the nurse does not routinely interpret the S-T segment, gross inspection of the strip can reveal changes in the S-T segment which can be referred to the physician for his interpretation. An example of this would be change in S-T segment occurring when the patient experiences chest pain or increases his activity.

• What does the dominant rhythm seem to be?

• What arrhythmias or irregularities are present?

• What is the clinical status of the patient?

• What kinds of therapy might the doctor order?

• What would be the nursing intervention?

Below are illustrations of the normal heart rhythm and some arrhythmias with possible hemodynamic consequences:

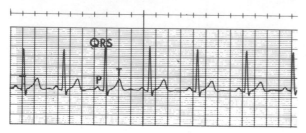

Fig. 53-3. Normal sinus rhythm.

Normal sinus rhythm (NSR) or regular sinus rhythm (RSR). The S-A node is the pacemaker and impulses are conducted normally through the conduction system (see Fig. 53-3).

RATE: 60 to 100
P WAVES: Each has the same configuration and precedes the QRS.
P-R INTERVAL: 0.12 to 0.20 second
QRS: 0.07 to 0.10 second
SIGNIFICANCE: Normal
TREATMENT: None

Sinus Bradycardia. The pacemaker site is the S-A node but the rate is below 60 (see Fig. 53-4). The rhythm is regular. The heart can be slow normally in athletes and laborers who have normally enlarged hearts from regular strenuous exercise and greater than normal stroke volume. Emotional states, such as fear or shock, can result in increased vagal tone and slowing of the heart which can result in syncope. Bradycardia is sometimes seen in patients with increased intracranial pressure, hypothyroidism, or digitalis toxicity. Carotid sinus pressure, the Valsalva maneuver, and eyeball pressure result in vagal stimulation and slowing of the heart. Bradycardia can occur during anesthesia or following administration of morphine.

In acute myocardial infarction, sinus bradycardia is often an ominous sign of reflex vagal mechanisms. The slow rate may not be sufficient to maintain cardiac output in an already damaged heart. In addition, escape ectopic beats or rhythms such as idioventricular rhythm may take over as the primary pacemaker if their inherent rate is faster. This can increase ventricular irritability which is dangerous in myocardial infarction.

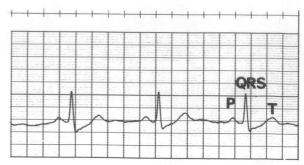

Fig. 53-4. Sinus bradycardia.

RATE: Below 60; a relative bradycardia may exist at a faster rate if it is insufficient to maintain cardiac output.
RHYTHM: Regular
P WAVES: Normal and precede each QRS
P-R INTERVAL: Normal
QRS: Normal
SIGNIFICANCE: Since cardiac output equals stroke volume times heart rate (c.o. = s.v. $\times$ h.r.), slow rate may not be sufficient for adequate cardiac output.
TREATMENT: Atropine sulfate 0.4 mg. I.V. may be ordered to override the vagal stimulus and increase sinus heart rate, thereby suppressing postbradycardia idioventricular beats. Isoproterenol (Isuprel) may be ordered to increase the heart rate by stimulation of the S-A node. An artificial pacemaker may be inserted to keep the heart beating at a minimum rate to maintain cardiac output.

Sinus Tachycardia. Impulses are initiated by the S-A node and the rate is regular, but above 100 beats per minute (see Fig. 53-5). Sinus tachycardia occurs in persons with normal hearts as a physiologic response to strenuous exercise or strong emotion, pain, fever, hyperthyroidism, hemorrhage, shock, or anemia. Cardiac output, coronary blood flow and blood pressure can increase up to the rate of about 150 beats per minute. After that cardiac decompensation can occur. A decrease in vagal tone or an increase in sympathetic tone or both can result in sinus tachycardia. Tachycardia can be the initial evidence of heart failure.

RATE: 100 to 160
RHYTHM: Regular
P WAVES: Normal, but may be obscured in T wave of previous cycle if rate is very fast
P-R INTERVAL: Normal
QRS: Normal
SIGNIFICANCE: Can increase the work of the heart to the point of decompensation
TREATMENT: The underlying disease or the cause of the tachycardia must be treated. For example, anxiety

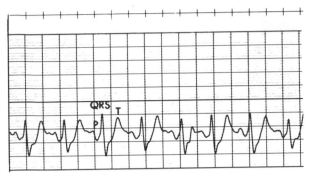

FIG. 53-5. Sinus tachycardia.

is alleviated, fever is reduced, oxygen is given for hypoxia, or digitalis may be ordered for congestive heart failure. Keep the patient to minimum activity until rate decreases to compensated level.

In persons with myocardial infarction or coronary artery disease, coronary insufficiency with chest pain can develop because coronary blood flow cannot keep up with the increased need of the myocardium imposed by the fast rate. With fast rates, diastole is shortened and the heart does not have sufficient time to fill. Congestive heart failure, chest pain or other symptoms of reduced cardiac output can occur.

Atrial Fibrillation. There is totally disorganized rapid atrial activity and the atria quiver rather than contract normally (see Fig. 53-6). The ventricles respond to the atrial stimulus in an irregular fashion depending upon the sensitivity of the A-V node and the conduction system. Some of the ventricular beats are so weak that they are ineffective in opening the aortic valve and propelling blood, and a pulse deficit exists. An apical-radial pulse should be taken.

RATE: 350 to 800 (atrial) Ventricular rate varies but is irregular unless there is also a complete block at the A-V node in which case no atrial impulses are conducted and the lower pacemaker site produces a regular rhythm. In atrial fibrillation which is con-

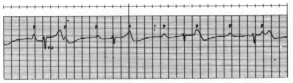

FIG. 53-7. Third degree A-V block (complete heart block).

sidered "controlled" either physiologically or by drugs, the ventricular rate is between 60 to 75 per minute. In uncontrolled atrial fibrillation, the ventricular rate is much faster.

RHYTHM: Irregular

P WAVES: There are no P waves; there is an irregular rapid undulation of the baseline of the ECG; the atrial twitchings are called f waves.

P-R INTERVAL: Since there are no P waves, the P-R interval is not measurable.

QRS: Normal

SIGNIFICANCE: Loss of atrial contraction diminishes cardiac output by about 15 per cent. Irregular ventricular filling and rhythm diminish the pumping efficiency. Decrease in cardiac output can result in congestive heart failure.

TREATMENT: Digitalis may be given to slow the ventricular rate by its action on the A-V node; then, quinidine to convert the atria to normal rhythm. If the patient's condition is potentially deteriorating, electric cardioversion is used.

Complete Heart Block. The atria and ventricles function without any relationship to each other; therefore P waves have no sequential relationship to QRS's though the rhythm of each is regular usually (see Fig. 53-7). The S-A node functions normally; the main pacemaker in the heart is below the block in the A-V node. What might appear to be a P-R interval changes with each complex. However, there is really no P-R interval due to the complete interruption in conduction from atria to ventricles.

RATE: Atrial rate is normal; the ventricular rate is 20 to 40 beats per minute.

RHYTHM: Atrial and ventricular rhythms are regular.

P WAVES: Normal

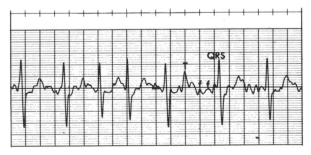

FIG. 53-6. Atrial fibrillation.

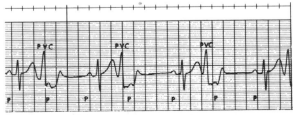

FIG. 53-8. Premature ventricular contractions (ventricular bigeminy).

QRS: Configuration is normal if pacemaker site is in A-V node below block, but widened if pacemaker site is in ventricle.

SIGNIFICANCE: The slow ventricular rate is usually ineffective in maintaining adequate cardiac output; angina, congestive failure, or Stokes-Adams seizures from cerebral hypoxia can occur; ventricular standstill or ventricular fibrillation may ensue.

TREATMENT: Withhold digitalis; isoproterenol (Isuprel) may be ordered. Pacemaker is considered essential; adequate ventilation to correct hypoxia and treatment of other associated clinical conditions is needed.

Premature Ventricular Contractions (PVC's). A PVC is a ventricular ectopic beat which occurs before depolarization of the ventricles by an atrial impulse is due (see Fig. 53-8). Therefore it is not preceded by an atrial impulse and, since it is not dependent on an impulse from above, it is also called an idioventricular beat. A PVC is followed usually by a long pause known as a "compensatory pause." This occurs because the normally occurring atrial impulse finds the ventricle refractory when it arrives because it has not recovered from its depolarization by the PVC. The next normally occurring atrial impulse succeeds in depolarizing the ventricle. If the heart rate is very slow, the ventricles can repolarize after a PVC in sufficient time to receive the atrial stimulus precisely when it is due and there is an extra beat, but the basic rhythm is not interrupted. This is called an *interpolated* PVC.

PVC's are very common; many people experience this at one time or another. It often causes a "flip-flop" sensation in the chest. Some people describe it as a "fluttering of the heart." The symptoms may be associated with pallor, nervousness, sweating and faintness.

PVC's are usually harmless. Some people have them in response to anxiety and stress, and, as it so often happens, the symptoms then make the patient even more tense and fearful. Also, they may be associated with fatigue or excessive use of alcohol or tobacco. Although PVC's usually are unassociated with organic heart disease, the patient who is frequently troubled by them should consult his doctor. A thorough examination is important in making certain that no organic heart disease exists and in assuring the patient that his heart is normal. Once the patient has received his doctor's assurance that nothing is seriously wrong, he will find it easier to ignore the symptoms. This in itself often causes them to occur less frequently and to disappear more quickly.

In the presence of acute heart injury such as after surgery or in acute myocardial infarction, PVC's that occur in certain patterns are indicative of myocardial irritability and are precursors of lethal arrhythmias. These patterns or types are:

- More than six unifocal PVC's per minute. A run of ventricular bigeminy (a normal beat followed by a PVC) could meet this criteria also.
- Runs, bursts, or salvos of PVC's, that is, two or more in a row
- Multifocal PVC's, that is, from more than one location in the ventricle
- A PVC whose R wave falls on the T wave of the preceding complex

RATE: Normal dominant rhythm
RHYTHM: Irregular
P WAVES: Normal, but absent in idioventricular complexes
QRS: Bizarre in configuration; widened above 0.12 second in idioventricular complexes; T wave following PVC usually is opposite in direction to its QRS.
TREATMENT: Notify physician promptly. Digitalis may be withheld; myocardial depressant drug such as Lidocaine is begun promptly if the patient has myocardial infarction to prevent ventricular fibrillation.

TREATMENT OF CARDIAC ARRHYTHMIAS

Methods of treatment for cardiac arrhythmias are aimed at:

1. Cardioversion (reversion) of the disturbed conduction to normal sinus rhythm, if possible
2. Where reversion to sinus rhythm is not possible, to produce maximum physiologic improvement
3. Reduction of the number or severity of arrhythmic episodes or preventing acute life-threatening attacks

Treatment for cardiac arrhythmias includes mechanical, chemical (pharmacologic) and electrical modalities. Mechanical means include physician administered or instituted use of carotid sinus pressure, eyeball pressure, or the Valsalva maneuver which slow the heart, or external cardiac compression.

Drug Therapy

Drugs used in the treatment of cardiac arrhythmias include the following classifications:

1. Drugs acting primarily on tissues within the heart:

   - Myocardial depressants such as lidocaine (Xylocaine), procainamide HCl (Pronestyl) quinidine sulfate, propranolol (Inderal), dilantin sodium, or bretylium tosylate
   - Drugs that increase cardiac rhythmicity and contraction such as epinephrine or isoproterenol (Isuprel).
   - Drugs which depress conduction but increase contractile force, such as digitalis preparations. (Significantly, digitalis toxicity can cause every arrhythmia it is used to treat!)

2. Drugs acting on the autonomic nervous system:

   - Vagolytic or parasympathetic blocking agents to increase heart rate, such as atropine sulfate
   - Vagal stimulants or parasympathomimetic agents which slow the heart such as Tensilon or Prostigmin
   - Alpha and beta adrenergic stimulating drugs such as epinephrine and Isuprel
   - Beta adrenergic blocking agents such as propranolol (Inderal).

Quinidine and procainamide (Pronestyl) are two drugs that are commonly employed to restore normal heart rhythm. Quinidine decreases the irritability and the contractility of the heart muscle. Also, it lengthens the time necessary for the conduction of impulses from the atria to the ventricles, and it lengthens the refractory period of heart muscle (the time between beats when the heart will not respond to another stimulus to contract). Although the mechanism of the action of quinidine in restoring normal heart rhythm is not completely understood, it is believed that these effects of quinidine on the heart are primarily responsible for its usefulness in restoring normal rhythm.

The dosage of quinidine is adjusted according to the patient's response. A usual oral dose would be 0.2 to 0.4 Gm. every four hours. Quinidine also may be given intramuscularly and intravenously. The effective dose may be a toxic one. Watch the patient for faintness, fall in blood pressure, rapid, weak pulse, nausea, vomiting, diarrhea, ringing in the ears, dizziness, headache and visual disturbances. Some patients are allergic to quinidine. The patient might receive a small test dose before therapy is begun and be observed for any allergic reactions. Quinidine blood level can be determined in the laboratory.

Procainamide (Pronestyl) decreases the irritability of the heart muscle. It can be given intravenously and intramuscularly, as well as orally. The oral dose varies from 0.5 Gm. to 1.0 Gm. every four hours. When a rapid effect is required, 100 to 200 mg. diluted in normal saline may be administered slowly, intravenously by the physician while he monitors the patient's electrocardiographic response. Intravenous use may be followed by hypotension. Occasionally, depression of the white blood cells results from repeated use of procainamide. When either drug is given intravenously, resuscitation equipment and drugs should be available.

Lidocaine (Xylocaine), a local anesthetic, depresses ventricular irritability when given intravenously. (The exact mechanism of its electrophysiologic effect is not clear.) It is rapidly metabolized in the liver so that action dissipates within 10 to 20 minutes after intravenous injection. It is given by intravenous drip at a maintenance dose of 1 to 4 mg. per minute or by intravenous bolus dose of 1 mg./Kg. of body weight (usually 50 to 100 mg.). An hourly dose of more than 450 mg. is hazardous.

Lidocaine is contraindicated in the presence of A-V block, A-V nodal and idioventricular rhythm since the last remaining spontaneous pacemaker can be abolished. Untoward reactions include apprehension, disorientation, euphoria, drowsiness, lightheadedness, numbness, sweating, and convulsions. Hypotension is possible.

When myocardial depressants are given, the ECG should be observed for A-V nodal or intraventricular conduction delay. Measure the P-R interval and QRS. Report any widening.

Propranolol (Inderal) blocks beta receptor sites in the myocardium from adrenergic (sympathetic) stimulation, thus producing a *decrease* in all of the following: heart rate (negative chronotropic effect), cardiac output, force of cardiac contraction (negative inotropic effect) and myocardial irritability. Since it is highly specific, the cardiac effects of calcium, digitalis, or the xanthines are not abolished when given simultaneously. It has effects on the conduction system similar to that of quinidine. It is used primarily in the treatment of atrial and ventricular tachyarrhythmias.

Propranolol may be given orally (10 to 30 mg. three or four times daily) or intravenously by a physician. The I.V. dose is 1 to 2 mg. diluted in 50 ml. of fluid infused slowly with constant ECG monitoring. The rate of infusion should not exceed 1 mg. per minute.

Side-effects of propranolol can be bradycardia, heart block, sinus arrest, acute congestive heart failure, shock or asystole. The patient may experience bronchoconstriction and it is therefore potentially hazardous in patients with bronchial asthma or chronic obstructive lung disease. Minor side effects include nausea, diarrhea, mental depression and fatigue.

The drugs most frequently used for brady-arrhythmias are atropine sulfate, isoproterenol (Isuprel), and steroids. Atropine sulfate lessens the effect of the vagus nerve and therefore improves the rhythm of the S-A node and transmission of impulses over the Purkinje system. An emergency dose is 1 mg. (gr. $\frac{1}{60}$) intravenously. Because atropine increases intraocular pressure it is generally not given to patients with known glaucoma. Since patients in the older age group are glaucoma prone, the physician may order one drop of one per cent pilocarpine eye drops in each eye every six hours if the patient requires frequent doses of atropine. Report promptly any blurring or change in vision. Check the pupils for dilatation. Acute urinary retention can result from atropine administration. Check the voiding of patients receiving this drug. Elderly males on bed rest, who may also have some prostatic hypertrophy, are particularly prone to this result of atropine. The patient will probably complain of dry mouth and thirst. Candy lozenges may relieve this.

Isoproterenol (Isuprel) is a very potent drug. In some agencies a physician must be present when it is given. Isuprel is useful for both its chronotropic (rate of contraction) and inotropic (force of contraction) effects. Isuprel enhances conduction by stimulating the S-A and A-V nodes and it accelerates idioventricular pacemakers high in the bundle of His or bundle branches. In high doses or in sensitive patients, Isuprel can cause tachyarrhythmias and ventricular irrita-

bility. The drug is given diluted in an infusion and is titrated using a microdrip set (60 gtts. equals 1 ml. of fluid) to maintain the pulse rate the doctor orders (usually 60 to 65 beats per minute). As the ventricular rate increases, the "piggy-backed" Isuprel infusion is slowed down or turned off and an unmedicated infusion turned on. The Isuprel is also ordered discontinued if dangerous forms of PVC's appear since these are precursors of ventricular fibrillation. Isuprel also increases stroke volume, cardiac output, and cardiac work, as well as heart rate.

Periods of sinus rhythm when Isuprel is turned off are not secure times for the staff because the change from sinus rhythm to complete heart block and low ventricular rate or asystole can occur quite abruptly.

When heart-block is induced by inflammation and edema of or around the atrioventricular conduction system caused by a recent myocardial infarction or by myocarditis, corticosteroid therapy may be given.

There is no agreement regarding the role of the nurse in the administration of intravenous medication. Among the various factors determining this role are institutional policy collaboratively arrived at by nurses, physicians, and hospital administrators and the evolving concept of nurses and physicians and their respective roles. Influencing policy making are state nurse practice acts and medical practice acts, the definition of what constitutes an emergency, as well as opportunities for instruction, guidance, supervision, and continuing education for both physicians and nurses.

Electrical Therapy

Electrical cardioversion can be accomplished by the use of:

- Synchronized electrical cardioversion
- Unsynchronized electrical cardioversion (defibrillation)
- Artificial electrical pacing

Synchronized Electric Cardioversion

Electric synchronous cardioversion is used to terminate rapid cardiac arrhythmias such as atrial flutter, atrial fibrillation, or ventricular tachycardia, all of which compromise cardiac output to some degree. The electric current completely depolarizes the entire myocardium at one time so that the fastest normal pacemaker can regain control of the pacing function. Electric cardioversion avoids the time element and potential side-effects encountered in the use of drug therapy for cardioversion.

In elective electric cardioversion there is time for the physician to explain the procedure to the patient and obtain his consent. Because the patient is generally already anxious as a result of the tachycardia, explanation is limited to what the individual patient is able to comprehend. Where there is sufficient time, the physician may order an anti-arrhythmic drug such as quinidine to be given orally several hours or a day prior to cardioversion so that a blood level of the drug will be achieved sufficient to maintain normal rhythm following cardioversion. Digitalis is sometimes withheld for a period prior to cardioversion because some believe that its presence in myocardial cells increases the incidence of ventricular irritability after cardioversion.

The patient is attached to a cardiac monitor which has an attachment for, or an incorporated cardioverter. An intravenous infusion is started.

Generally the patient is given heavy sedation such as with intravenous diazepam (Valium), 2 to 5 mg. or light general anesthesia. Equipment and drugs used in cardiac arrest are immediately available. The cardioverter is activated and the physician selects the non-vulnerable point of the cycle where the shock will be delivered. Gel is applied to the paddles, or a moist wet saline pad is placed under each paddle in such a position that there is no contact between paddles and the current will traverse the heart. The physician delivers the shock usually in the range of 10 to 200 watt seconds. The patient's cardiac rhythm is observed on the monitor and his vital signs are taken. A nurse remains with the patient until he awakens.

In order to avoid personnel injury from electric shock, the team must be alerted to stand away from the bed and to avoid touching any conducting source when the shock is delivered. To avoid fire hazard, the flow of oxygen is stopped while the shock is delivered.

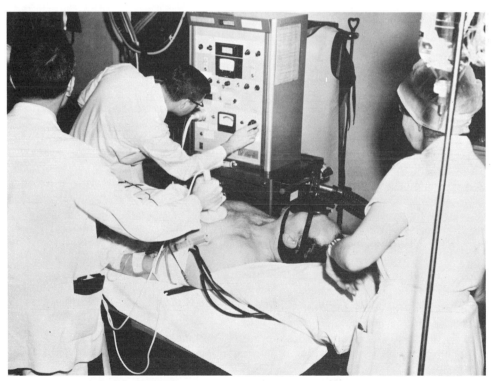

Fig. 53-9. Electric cardioversion. The machine that the doctor is adjusting monitors heart rhythm; also, it can be used as here to apply an electric shock in an attempt to restore normal rhythm. The shock is applied through the electrode held on the patient's anterior chest by the doctor and another electrode positioned against the posterior chest. The anesthetist is prepared to give the patient oxygen. (The Roosevelt Hospital, New York, N.Y.)

Defibrillation (Unsynchronized Electric Cardioversion). The only treatment for ventricular fibrillation is immediate defibrillation. Without it, the patient will die. Cardiorespiratory resuscitation is given immediately before (while awaiting defibrillator) and after the shock and should never be ceased for longer than a period of five seconds since blood flow and blood pressure can drop to zero. Usually a defibrillating shock of 400 watt seconds is delivered.

Ventricular tachycardia which is accompanied by hypotension and loss of consciousness is likewise an extreme emergency. The patient may be defibrillated under these circumstances rather than synchronously cardioverted.

CARDIAC ARREST

Cardiac arrest is the sudden cessation of effective cardiac output. The electrical mechanism of cardiac arrest can be ventricular asystole or bradyarrhythmias, or ventricular tachyarrhythmias (ventricular tachycardia or ventricular fibrillation). An initially slow rhythm can induce myocardial hypoxia which can trigger ventricular fibrillation.

The severity of symptoms of cardiac arrest depends on the duration of the suspension of cardiac output. *Stokes-Adams Syndrome* describes the loss of consciousness due to cerebral ischemia following ineffective ventricular contraction. The duration of loss of effective cardiac output and corresponding signs and symptoms according to Humphries are:

2 to 3 seconds:	palpitations
3 to 5 seconds:	symptoms of cerebral vascular insufficiency with sensations of dizziness and distress
5 to 10 seconds:	syncope with or without seizures (Stokes-Adams syndrome)
30 to 90 seconds:	death usually occurs unless external stimulus reinitiates the circulation

Care of the patient in cardiac arrest should encompass the following stages and maneuvers:

• If patient is on a cardiac monitor, respond to monitor alarm and check electrocardiographic pattern.

• In any situation, note the time. Go to the patient. Clear the *A*, airway. Note the *B*, breathing. Determine *C*, circulation by pulses and pupils. If the patient has neither a carotid pulse (or femoral) or respirations, and is disoriented or unconscious, deliver a sharp blow with the fist over the sternum (precordial blow) unless the patient has a chest injury. This has been shown to be sometimes effective in initiating cardiac action following ventricular asystole and ventricular fibrillation. The patient may be semiconscious and needless to say an explanation will be required after the precordial blow!

• Summon help.

• If necessary and possible the patient should be defibrillated immediately. In a hospital intensive care unit this should be within 30 seconds.

• Observe the following steps (ABCDE's):

1. *Airway* should be established.

2. *Breathing,* using the mouth-to-mouth method or assistive device if available. Give three to four maximal insufflations before initiating circulation so that oxygenated blood will be pumped.

3. *Circulation* should be restored by closed chest cardiac compression. Check the pupils and carotid or femoral pulse.

4. *Definitive therapy* is ordered by the physician, depending on the cause and length of the period of arrest. Sodium bicarbonate, usually 44.0 mEq. for every five to ten minutes in cardiac arrest is given to treat the metabolic acidosis which results from the accumulation of lactic acid as a by-product of anaerobic metabolism.

5. *Evaluation.* Dilation of the pupils starts 45 seconds after cardiac arrest and is complete in one to two minutes. Since the pupil is the best index of brain oxygenation, pupillary response is the best indicator of the effectiveness of heart-lung resuscitation. Adequate oxygenation and good blood flow to the brain is present if the pupil constricts on exposure to flashlight.

Pulses should be present during cardiac compression and the patient's color should improve if he is responding.

The return of a relatively good ECG pattern is not an indication to stop resuscitation efforts. The patient can have sufficient circulation to produce a normal looking ECG, but not enough cardiac output for functional circulation. Restoration of blood pressure and quality of the peripheral pulse are crucial indicators. The carotid pulse is the most reliable pulse and the last to disappear.

Some additional important points about cardiopulmonary resuscitation are:

Airway. A maximum backward tilt of the head is the easiest way to open an airway. Only an experienced person should attempt endotracheal intubation since cardiac massage cannot be halted for more than five seconds. Endotracheal intubation is not essential for an adequate airway. Secretions need to be wiped out or suctioned from the pharynx for an adequate airway. Establishment of an airway may be sufficient to permit spontaneous breathing to resume and restore circulation.

Breathing. One person extends the patient's neck, pulls the lower jaw upward and begins mouth-to-mouth resuscitation. The rescuer blows his breath into the patient's mouth, either directly, by tightly pressing his lips against the patient's mouth, or by means of a small tube.

Mouth-to-mouth breathing done effectively delivers about 18 per cent oxygen to the patient. A self-inflating bag, such as the Ambu bag, used with a face mask or endotracheal tube and oxygen, delivers about 50 per cent oxygen only if used correctly. Three to four maximal insufflations should be given before compression is started so that oxygenated blood will be circulated; then the pulse should be checked again. With two rescuers, one inflation should be interposed after each five compressions without any halting of compression (1:5 ratio or 12 breaths per minute). With one rescuer, two breaths are interposed after each fifteen compressions. The breather should see the chest rise and fall, feel the resistance of the lungs as they expand, and hear the noise of air escaping during exhalation.

Artificial breathing may cause distention of the stomach. This can lead to regurgitation, reduced lung volume, or the initiation of vagal reflexes. The physician may exert moderate pressure between the umbilicus and the rib cage to expel the air. The patient's head should be lowered and turned to one side to avoid aspiration of gastric contents. Mouth-to-nose ventilation can be used if there is difficulty via the mouth-to-mouth route. Mechanical ventilators are also available when prolonged respiratory support is needed.

Artificial ventilation is not accompanied by cardiac compression if cardiac action is spontaneous.

Cardiac Compression. Rhythmic pressure applied over the lower half of the sternum results in compression of the heart and pulsatile arterial

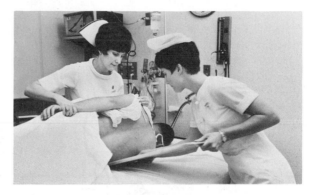

FIG. 53-10. Nurses quickly place cardiac arrest board before initiating cardiac compression. (Photograph taken at Overlook Hospital, Summit, N.J., by Robert Goldstein for *Patient Care* magazine)

circulation. Correctly performed cardiac compression can result in a mean blood pressure of 40 to 50 mm. Hg in the carotid artery and a blood flow of up to 35 per cent of normal.

Lay the patient on his back on a firm surface, such as the floor, the pavement, a bed board, or even a large tray slipped under the patient's chest. (A soft mattress is depressed by pressure and would interfere with the massage.) As part of the emergency equipment, some hospitals keep a board that can be slipped between the patient and the bed. It makes a hard surface from the patient's waist to his shoulders.

The person kneels beside the patient, placing his hands at right angles on the lower sternum (see Fig. 53-11). The hands, one on top of the other, are pressed vertically downward, pushing the sternum inward one and one-half to two inches, thus compressing the heart between the sternum and the spine and forcing the blood out of the heart. Only the heels of the hands are used. The fingers are kept up, out of contact with the patient's ribs.

Manual pressure is released, allowing the heart to fill with blood, and then pressure is reapplied. The cycle is repeated approximately 60 to 80 times per minute with breathing interposed.

Closed cardiac massage is not without its dangers. Hands that are misplaced too close to the diaphragm may rupture the spleen. Hands that are misplaced to one side may break ribs. Considerable force is required to move the chest of an adult two inches.

When prolonged resuscitation or transportation of the patient is required, external cardiac

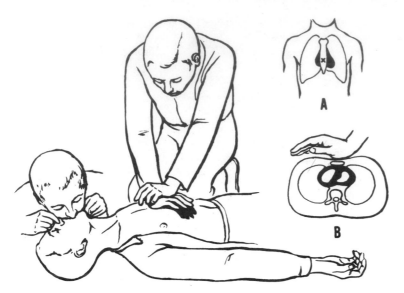

FIG. 53-11. Technic of closed chest cardiac massage. One rescuer gives mouth-to-mouth resuscitation. The other massages the heart by pressing downward on the patient's chest approximately 60 times a minute. (A) X indicates the area where pressure should be applied. (B) Manual pressure on the chest, compressing the heart and forcing blood out of it. (American Heart Association, Inc., New York, N.Y.; adapted from Kouwenhoven, W. B., *et al.*: Heart activation in cardiac arrest, *Modern Concepts of Cardiovascular Diseases* 30[2]:642)

compression machines are commercially available which are more consistent in the application of pressure than would be a number of different team members. The machine must be carefully and continually observed for correct placement and function.

During the resuscitation effort the physician may give an intracardiac injection of epinephrine and an intravenous injection of sodium bicarbonate (to control acidosis). Lidocaine can be ordered to decrease ventricular irritability. Atropine or Isuprel to speed heart rate may be the drug of choice. Calcium chloride to strengthen cardiac contractions also may be administered once heart action starts. Vasopressors may be given intravenously to maintain an adequate blood pressure. The nurse assists in the preparation of the drug and by monitoring the patient's response.

External cardiac compression may be ineffective or contraindicated in such situations as crushing injuries of the chest, internal thoracic injuries or in patients with advanced pulmonary emphysema with enlarged, fixed rib cages. The physician may elect to open the chest and do direct cardiac massage.

After successful cardiac resuscitation the patient needs to be observed closely. Vital signs are taken frequently; the patient will be attached to a monitoring device. Oxygen will be given to reduce the onset of arrhythmias due to hypoxemia. A nasogastric tube may be passed to prevent distention. Shock may have caused renal impairment. Other complications for which the nurse should observe include pneumothorax, hematoma of the liver, brain damage, fractured ribs or sternum, and fat embolism. To minimize the chance of cerebral damage, some physicians may use hypothermia for several days after cardiac arrest.

It is the nurse's responsibility to continue resuscitative efforts until medical help arrives, which is feasible in most areas of this country. A sole rescuer, of course, would continue until exhausted. The decision to terminate resuscitation efforts is a medical one based on the patient's cerebral and cardiorespiratory response.

Who Should be Resuscitated? Involved individuals from each agency should develop policies in response to this broad societal question. Generally speaking, cardiopulmonary resuscitation is a response to sudden, unexpected death. There is a generally agreed upon gap of time between so-called clinical death and actual physiologic death or irreversible cerebral change. The time period of three to four minutes, however, applies to persons with normal circulatory systems. Patients with previous cardiac or respiratory disease or cerebral arteriosclerosis have, of course, less "grace" period. Thus, there must always be a maximal sense of urgency in initiating ECPR and in continuing it because the longer ECPR is necessary, the less likely it is to succeed. ECPR is not indicated when it can be determined with a degree of certainty that cardiac arrest has persisted for more than five or six minutes, or somewhat longer in drowning. Nor is it indicated for patients with terminal cancer or end-stage irreversible disease of the liver, kidneys, heart, or brain. Old age, in itself, is not a contraindication to resuscitation.

Because the nurse is often the one who initiates resuscitation efforts, she should obtain more clear-cut guidelines for individual hospitalized patients through discussion with the patient's physician on admission. These guidelines for the nurse should be written on the chart or other readily available source of information so that all nurses are aware of the situation. This avoids the regrettable situation of a nurse or intern instituting heroic efforts when they are not indicated, such as for the dying cancer patient.

Whether alone at night in a hospital ward in a previously undiscussed situation, on the street, or on the beach the nurse needs to have guidelines for action in her own mind. In such areas of extended nurse activity she does in fact take the legal and moral responsibility for her own decisions and actions, or lack of action. Despite the best heroic efforts, patients do die. Recriminations, blame, and guilt feelings can occur when there are exaggerated expectations of one's own or a team's ability to save a life. Rather than participate in emergency action solely because it is part of a job description, the realistic nurse knowingly takes the risks and can keep in perspective her own gradually improving skills as part of a team, the patient's chances for life, and what can be done for him.

Practice drills are essential so that a team is well prepared for such an emergency as cardiac arrest. After the stress of the emergency is over, an objective evaluation session makes use of various events as opportunities for learning. Without this, inefficiencies can be repeated.

THE PATIENT WITH AN ARTIFICIAL ELECTRICAL PACEMAKER

An artificial cardiac pacemaker is used to maintain the patient's ventricular rate at a minimum level for effective cardiac output. Formerly, an open-chest procedure was necessary to implant electrodes in the myocardium so the use of a pacemaker was limited to "good risk" patients. Today, with the transvenous (or pervenous) technic, a permanent pacemaker can be inserted quickly in most patients under local anesthesia with minimal surgical risk and discomfort.

The most frequent indication for permanent artificial pacing is to eliminate Stokes-Adams attacks associated with a variety of heart diseases, including coronary artery disease, rheumatic heart disease and congenital malformations or as a direct complication of cardiac surgery.

Since pacing increases heart rate, therefore cardiac output, it is also used to increase circulation in patients with slow heart rates with symptoms of right- or left-sided heart failure, angina, renal failure, or slow cerebration.

Formerly drugs such as Ephedrine or Isuprel were used on a long-term basis to treat these conditions, but today pacing is considered to carry less risk than that associated with drug toxicity, changes in metabolic states of the patient, or the human failings associated with self-administration of drugs.

Temporary pacing is indicated in patients with acute myocardial infarction complicated by heart block, or other bradyarrhythmias, in digitalis toxicity with heart block, or in patients with slow heart rate and congestive failure who require digitalis. In most of these situations the pacemaker is removed when the normal sinus rhythm returns. In many patients the temporary pacemaker, though inserted, is not used but is left on "stand-by" as a precautionary measure should complications develop. Should the need arise, the prepared nurse in some hospitals can activate the pacemaker, and some pacing equipment is self-activating, the so-called "demand" pacemaker. Another indication for temporary pacing is to suppress rapid arrhythmias such as recurrent ventricular tachycardia which does not respond to drugs or electric cardioversion.

Since there are many indications for pacing, several kinds of pacemakers, and many still being researched, it is the responsibility of the nurse to know the objectives of the pacing treatment, the precautions and observations of the patient, and to be very familiar with the product literature which describes the individual pacing unit. The doctor determines the rate of the heart beat and the amplitude of the pacing stimulus.

Some common terms used in the field of cardiac pacing are:

External Pacing. A series of shocks of 50 to 150 volts is delivered to the heart through the chest wall via electrodes placed on the chest. It is painful if the patient is conscious and this method of pacing is often ineffective. It can be utilized in asystole or complete heart block, however, while awaiting a more adequate pacing technic or when transporting the patient via ambulance or from one hospital area to another.

Transvenous or Endocardial Pacing. An electrode catheter is passed through a peripheral

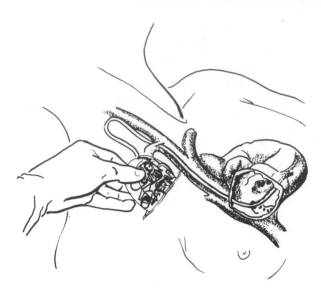

Fig. 53-12. An implanted cardiac pacemaker. The battery and circuitry that make up the pulse generator are placed under the skin below the collarbone. Attached to the pulse generator is an electrode consisting of two encapsulated wires running through a vein to the right ventricle through which the electrical stimulus is carried to the heart.

vein such as the antecubital or external jugular into the right ventricle where it contacts the endocardial surface. The free end of the catheter is attached to an external pulse generating unit for temporary pacing. For permanent pacing, a subcutaneous pocket is prepared in the subclavicular area and the free end of the catheter passed through a tissue tunnel and connected to the pulse generating unit implanted in the pocket.

Asynchronous Pacing. Most pacing is asynchronous because the catheter is placed in the right ventricle, thus ignoring the atrial contribution to cardiac output. The pacer is set to fire at a preset rate and does not change rate in response to increased physiologic needs of the patient. An asynchronous pacing unit can be either a fixed rate or demand pacemaker.

Fixed Rate Pacing. This type is set by the doctor at a heart rate of about 70 beats per minute and fires all the time regardless of what the patient's own conduction mechanism is capable of doing. At times, the patient's own mechanism can compete with that of the pacer and this can be dangerous in the patient with myocardial hypoxia, acidosis, drug toxicity or other states in

which the threshold for ventricular fibrillation is lowered. Ventricular fibrillation is a possibility when electrical stimuli from the pacer fall on or around the summit of the T wave.

Demand Pacing. Competition with the patient's cardiac cycle is avoided with this type pacemaker because of a special sensing circuit that recognizes a QRS complex. In one type of demand pacer, a pulse-blocking circuit prevents the pacer from pulsing when the patient's spontaneous depolarization is detected.

In another type of demand pacing, the pacer issues a pulse when a spontaneous depolarization is sensed rather than withholding one. The pacer stimulus fires into the refractory period of the patient's own QRS and thus is ineffective as a stimulus. If the patient's ventricle fails to depolarize spontaneously after a set period of delay, the pacer issues a pulse which depolarizes the ventricle and causes a ventricular contraction.

Synchronous Pacing. This is the most physiologic type of pacing. A catheter in the atrium detects the patient's own P wave, and it is relayed to an implanted unit where the impulse is delayed similar to the normal delay at the A-V node, then it causes depolarization and contraction of the ventricle via another electrode catheter. Thus the rate can vary according to the patient's need up to a preset maximum, and the booster effect of atrial contraction is maintained. Should the atrial circuit fail, an automatic circuit initiates fixed-rate ventricular pacing. This type of pacemaker is used for younger, more active patients. If the atrial rate exceeds a preset limit of about 150, an automatic 2:1, 3:1 or 4:1 block will be induced. During the change in rate the patient might experience lightheadedness or a fainting feeling. A transthoracic or transvenous approach is used for implantation.

Atrial Pacing. When the A-V node and Purkinje system is intact and the problematic arrhythmia lies in the atria, a pacing electrode can be passed into the atria and attached to a pulse generator. In this way, the atrial boost to cardiac output is conserved.

Nursing Care of the Patient with Bradycardia Requiring a Pacemaker

Patients who are subject to Stokes-Adams seizures are often very apprehensive. They do not know when the next attack will occur and then they have only a few seconds to summon help before they become unconscious. It is not uncommon for patients to be admitted with acute physical injuries such as fractures or lacerations sustained during a Stokes-Adams seizure. Often attacks occur when the patient is away from his own community and he may find himself admitted to a strange hospital under a physician's care who is a stranger to him. Because Stokes-Adams attacks are associated with acute myocardial infarction, a patient with such an attack may be admitted to a cardiac monitoring unit. Since, however, the symptoms are cerebral, the patient may fear that he has a brain tumor or epilepsy or another neurologic condition.

A careful orientation of the patient to the hospital and community environment, close observation at all times, explanation of the cardiac monitor and other happenings, maintaining the patient's privacy and individual preferences, and offering oneself to listen to the patient's fears are nursing measures which can alleviate anxiety. A padded tongue depressor, gauze squares, and an oropharyngeal airway are kept at the bedside and side rails are kept up. A marked decrease in pulse and signs and symptoms of cerebral ischemia is indicative of Stokes-Adams syndrome.

Be prepared for emergency measures. A sharp precordial blow is often sufficient to activate a pacemaker site somewhere in the conduction system or myocardium. If ventricular fibrillation is the mechanism, and the precordial blow is not effective, defibrillation is immediately essential. If the mechanism is sustained ventricular asystole, initiate ECPR until medical help arrives.

Since attacks may be repetitious in acute ischemic conditions of the A-V node, stay with the patient. He often gives clues to the onset by stating that he is getting "whoozy," feeling lightheaded, or going to faint. Explain the reason for the precordial blow in terms that the individual patient can understand. He is often semiconscious and may think he is being abused! For example, assure him that his heart is quite capable of beating, but the signals that help it to beat regularly are temporarily erratic.

While awaiting help, give the patient oxygen and prevent activities that cause vagal stimulation and slowing of the heart. This can happen if the patient strains to lift himself up in bed or to void or defecate. Also, it can occur in response to retching, severe coughing, drinking cold beverages, or during pharyngeal or tracheal suctioning.

While awaiting the preparation of facilities, or if pacemaker facilities are not available, drug therapy (Isuprel or Atropine) is instituted. When the physician decides that a pacemaker is to be inserted he explains this to the patient. A surgical consent is necessary. For most patients, the thought that their heart requires artificial electrical control is anxiety producing. They need time to talk about it and get used to the idea, but often there is very little time for this. The nurse should listen to the surgeon's explanation to the patient, and in her conversation with the patient review, clarify, and correct any misinterpretations that the patient or family might have. Use language that the patient can readily understand.

For emergency temporary pacing, the catheter may be inserted into the right ventricle at the bedside, using electrocardiographic or fluoroscopic control.

If the patient is transported, a portable pulse generator is taken along with the patient to the x-ray department in case of emergency en route. Image-intensifying fluoroscopic control is used to guide the pacing catheter into the ventricle. The implantation room is equipped with a cardiac monitor, a defibrillator and other equipment and drugs needed for cardiac arrest. Ventricular fibrillation can be provoked mechanically by the catheter tip as it enters the ventricle.

For permanent transvenous pacing, local anesthesia is used. The patient may find the procedure tedious and be uncomfortable from the supine position on a hard x-ray table. The patient hears what is going on though his eyes may be shielded. Strict surgical asepsis is essential. Contamination of the catheter or implantable pulse generator can result in infection and failure to pace properly.

The surgeon selects the correct pacing threshold and sets the voltage and rate. An amplitude of 6 mA. and rate of 70 is common.

Eventually the catheter becomes embedded in the right ventricular trabeculae. Immediately after insertion, the electrocardiographic display might show complexes with varying electrical potentials because the tip of the catheter might not touch the ventricle with the same force at first. PVC's are more frequent during the early postimplant period especially in patients who have received Isuprel. The physician may order medication to suppress these. The patient may be returned for several days to an environment where a defibrillator and other emergency equipment and drugs are available.

Postimplantation Care. Patients with newly implanted pacemakers are generally on an electrocardiographic monitor for an evaluation period after insertion. Each pacer has its own characteristic tracing. The electrical artifact or "blip" of the pacing stimulus should appear before the QRS of a ventricular pacer. It is usually identified on the oscilloscope as a thin, straight stroke. Absence of the artifact may mean faulty monitoring equipment, or more seriously, failure to pace due to malposition of the catheter, dislodgement of the catheter, catheter breakage, or rise of the pacing threshold due to tissue reaction to the catheter or to infection. The location of the artifact is particularly important. If the paced rhythm competes with the patient's spontaneous rhythm, the artifact can fall in the vulnerable period of the cardiac cycle.

To assist in determining that each pacing stimulus results in effective ventricular contraction, the patient's pulse should be taken simultaneously with observation of the cardiac monitor.

The small pulse generator of a temporary pacing system should be placed so that it is immovable and there is no tension on the wires. The patient should not be able to manipulate the controls. Because of electrical hazards, wall outlets should never be used as electrical power sources for pacemakers. Remember that when the patient has a temporary pacemaker, a direct route exists from the external exit of the catheter (wire) to the heart. The exposed electrodes at the exit wire can be insulated at their junction with the pulse generator by placing the unit in a rubber glove (Merkel and Sovie). Only grounded electrical equipment should be used in the room and only one machine connected to a wall outlet should be used on the patient at one time. For example, when a 12-lead ECG is to be done, disconnect the single lead cardiac monitor immediately before turning on the ECG machine.

Localized phlebitis and cellulitis can develop around the catheter exit site of a temporary pacemaker. Check the dressing for drainage and report discomfort to the physician.

If the patient develops singultus (hiccups) there can be current leakage across the diaphragm or perforation of the ventricle by the catheter. Report this symptom to the physician.

The extent of nursing care depends on the pacemaker condition of the patient. For example, if the patient developed heart block following acute myocardial infarction he will continue to be on all coronary precautions. The physician will observe the patient after several days with the pacemaker off; if the patient returns to sustained normal sinus rhythm the pacemaker will be removed.

If the pacemaker was implanted permanently because of a gradually progressive bradycardia without acute infarction, he may be discharged after a few days observation and teaching. If the patient had a thoracotomy for myocardial electrode implantation his care will encompass chest drainage and other considerations of such surgery.

The physician should be consulted regarding the initiation of exercise of the shoulder on the side of the catheter insertion. Unless this is mobilized early, the elderly patient is apt to develop "frozen" shoulder.

Predischarge Care. If the patient has a permanent pacemaker, he may be taught to take his pulse for a full minute once or twice a day and is instructed to report rate changes, and episodes of dizziness or unconsciousness.

The patient's prognosis and his activity depend on the adequacy of his myocardium. The pacemaker improves cardiac conduction, but cannot regenerate diseased myocardium. Usually only those activities are restricted which might result in a direct blow to the pulse generator, such as karate. Some patients may needlessly restrict activities such as sexual intercourse because of unfounded fears. The patient and spouse need the opportunity to discuss activities with their doctor and plan life realistically. Meeting a well-adjusted patient with a pacemaker may be a help. The patient who overexerts himself or who gets older and loses cardiac reserve may develop symptoms of angina or congestive failure.

All patients need continuing medical follow-up. The average life of a pacemaker unit is about two and one-half years but this varies with the model. Battery failure is signalized by slight decrease in rate. Other components can fail and result in decrease or increase in rate including the very rapid rate of a "runaway" pacemaker or absence of pacing. Symptoms of weakness or dizziness may be the patient's first clue.

Some pacemakers are sensitive to outside electrical interference. Radiofrequency signals from diathermy, electric shock therapy in the treatment of psychiatric patients, electrocautery treatment, automobile electrical distributors, and the sparkplug of a small one cylinder gasoline engine within a five-foot range have been identified as having the potential to be misinterpreted and cause rapidity or cessation of pacing (Carleton).

In an attempt to detect early pacemaker failure and change the pulse generator before the patient becomes symptomatic, clinics which utilize computer analysis of the waveform of the pacing stimulus are being opened. Some clinics also have associated clubs where patients with pacemakers can gather for social activities.

It is helpful for the patient with a pacemaker to wear a Medic Alert emblem or to carry a card indicating that he has a pacemaker in the event that he needs emergency medical care.

REFERENCES AND BIBLIOGRAPHY

ANDREOLI, K., *et al.*: *Comprehensive Cardiac Care,* St. Louis, Mosby, 1968.

BAIN, BARBARA: Pacemakers and the patients who need them, *Am. J. Nurs.* 71:1582, August, 1971.

CARLETON, R. A., *et al.*: Environmental influence on implantable cardiac pacemakers, *JAMA* 190:938, December, 1964.

CONN, R.: Newer drugs in the treatment of cardiac arrhythmia, *Med. Clin. N. Am.* 51:1223, September, 1967.

CULBERT, PAMELA and ROS, B.: Teaching patients about pacemakers, *Am. J. Nurs.* 71:523, March, 1971.

DRUSS, R., and KORNFELD, D.: The survivors of cardiac arrest (a psychiatric study), *JAMA* 201:75, July, 1967.

FIELDS, SR. M. L.: The C.P.R. team in a medium-sized hospital, *Am. J. Nurs.* 66:87, January, 1966.

GERMAIN, C., and HANLEY, SR. M. P.: Metronome for a music teacher, *Am. J. Nurs.* 68:498, March, 1968.

GREENE, W., and MOSS, A.: Psychosocial factors in the adjustment of patients with permanently implanted cardiac pacemakers, *Ann. Int. Med.* 70:897, May, 1969.

HOCHBERG, HOWARD M.: Effects of electrical current on heart rhythm, *Am. J. Nurs.* 71:1390, July, 1971.

HUMPHRIES, J. O'N.: Treatment of heart block with artificial pacemakers, *Mod. Conc. Cardiovasc. Dis.* 33:857, June, 1964.

HUNN, V.: Cardiac pacemakers, *Am. J. Nurs.* 69:749, April, 1969.

JUDE, J., and ELAM, J.: *Fundamentals of Cardiopulmonary Resuscitation,* Philadelphia, Davis, 1965.

MEEHAN, MARJORIE: EKG primer—a programmed instruction unit, *Am. J. Nurs.* 71:2195, November, 1971.

MERKEL, R., and SOVIE, M.: Electrocution hazards with transvenous pacemaker electrodes, *Am. J. Nurs.* 68:2560, December, 1967.

NATIONAL ACADEMY OF SCIENCE and NATIONAL RESEARCH COUNCIL: Cardiopulmonary resuscitation, *JAMA* 198:372, October, 1966.

Nursing in Cardiovascular Diseases, Contemporary Nursing Series, New York, American Journal of Nursing Company, 1971.

REGAN, W.: The new standing orders and their legal pitfalls, *R.N.* 31:38, April, 1968.

RODMAN, M., and SMITH, D.: Pharmacology and Drug Therapy in Nursing, Philadelphia, Lippincott, 1969.

SHOCKEY, C., and SNOW, S.: Pacemaker to the rescue; its use in the C.C.U., *R.N.* 31:37, December, 1968.

SIDDONS, H., and SOWTON, E.: *Cardiac Pacemakers,* Springfield, Ill., Thomas, 1967.

WINSOR, T.: The electrocardiogram in myocardial infarction, *Ciba Clin. Symp.* 20:107, October-November-December, 1968.

The Patient with Acute Myocardial Infarction

54

Symptoms • First Aid • The Coronary Care Unit • Admitting the Patient • Diagnosis • Pathology • Objectives of Care • Treatment of Complications • Preparation for Transfer • Later Care and Rehabilitation • Prognosis

"Heart attack"—these two words often spell disaster for adults. Regardless of our level of sophistication in knowledge about the condition, as human beings we are all vulnerable to the threat of such a catastrophe or its actual occurrence.

In myocardial infarction the interference with the blood supply to a portion of the muscle of the heart is so severe that necrosis of a part of the heart results. This may be precipitated by the occlusion of a coronary artery from capillary hemorrhage within an atherosclerotic plaque or by the formation of a thrombus on one of the plaques. Myocardial infarction may occur without occlusion of an artery when there is a sudden reduction in the blood supply to the heart—for example, during shock or hemorrhage or during severe physical exertion—whenever, in fact, the need of the heart for blood is increased suddenly beyond that which the atherosclerotic arteries can deliver. Atherosclerosis is almost always the underlying cause of myocardial infarction. The narrowed, roughened vessels are very susceptible to obstruction.

SYMPTOMS

The symptoms of myocardial infarction include sudden, severe pain in the chest, usually precordial or substernal, sometimes radiating to the shoulder and the arm, teeth, jaw or throat, especially on the left side. The pain is more severe and of longer duration than that in angina pectoris, and it is not necessarily related to exertion. Patients sometimes describe it as "grinding" or "crushing" and so severe that every ounce of stamina is needed to endure it. Unlike that of angina pectoris, the pain of myocardial infarction is not relieved by rest or nitroglycerin. It may last several hours or as long as one or two days, and, finally, it becomes a soreness or an ache before it disappears entirely.

In some patients the pain is accompanied by symptoms of shock, pallor, sweating, faintness, a severe drop in blood pressure and rapid, weak pulse brought about by sudden decrease in cardiac output.

It is not unusual for the patient to lose consciousness at the beginning of the attack and, as he regains consciousness, again to become aware of the excruciating pain in his chest. Sometimes the patient is more aware of feeling faint and weak than he is of chest pain. Nausea and vomiting may occur and lead the patient to believe that he has an attack of acute indigestion.

The suddenness and severity of symptoms of acute myocardial infarction have been described as being so stressful that primitive and virtually automatic responses to danger are aroused (Braceland). Fear and restlessness almost invariably occur, unless shock is so profound that the patient is unable to respond emotionally to the situation. Most patients are well aware of the seriousness of chest pain, and they are immediately apprehensive. Symptoms of left-sided heart failure—dyspnea, cyanosis and cough—may appear if the pumping of the left ventricle is sufficiently impaired, and if congestion occurs in the lungs.

FIRST AID

You may be the first person to see a patient who has suffered myocardial infarction, or you may be with him at the time of the attack. A nurse does not make the medical diagnosis; but understanding the possibility of myocardial infarction, knowing what to do, and, especially, what not to do, may save the patient's life. If the patient has had previous attacks of angina, he usually will have taken a nitroglycerin tablet and have stopped whatever he was doing. If these measures fail to relieve the pain within ten minutes, or if he has additional or atypical symptoms, keep him at complete rest in the position most comfortable for him, and call his doctor. If a doctor cannot be reached quickly, as calmly as possible summon an ambulance and direct that the patient be taken to the nearest hospital emergency room. Go with the patient if possible. Cardiac arrest following acute myocardial infarction happens abruptly. The patient needs to be transferred as quickly as possible to a treatment facility where definitive measures such as defibrillation are available. Excessive emotion which results in the release of catecholamines into the blood (epinephrine and norepinephrine) can result in ventricular fibrillation. Because of this, the precautionary reasons for an ambulance ride and emergency room admission need to be explained to the patient in such a manner that he does not become more alarmed.

The majority of deaths from acute myocardial infarction occur in the first four hours after the onset of pain. Studies show that there is an average six- to ten-hour lapse in time between the onset of symptoms and admission to the hospital (A mobile CCU saves lives in New York City, *ICU* 3:12, 1969).

More than two-thirds of the 600,000 Americans who die each year of a myocardial infarction die before reaching a hospital (Lown). Sudden death is attributed in most cases to ventricular fibrillation.

To prevent these out-of-hospital deaths often in young men with "hearts too good to die," a four-pronged approach becomes evident:

1. Prevention of coronary artery disease (see Chap. 31) and identification and treatment of those suspected to be coronary prone.

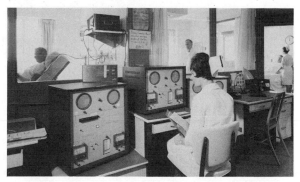

Fig. 54-1. A modern coronary care unit. (Photograph taken at Overlook Hospital, Summit, N.J.)

2. Education of the public to seek medical help promptly after the onset of characteristic symptoms. Preferably, this should be in an emergency room or coronary care unit where electrocardiographic monitoring and arrhythmia prophylaxis are continually available.

3. Bringing medical help to the stricken victim in the community in a fully equipped "mobile" coronary care unit or special ambulance, where, after stabilization of his condition, the victim can be transported under medical supervision to the hospital.

4. Effective rehabilitation after an attack.

Immediate Care. Here are some suggestions for the immediate care of any patient who experiences severe chest pain:

• Keep him at complete rest in the position that is most comfortable for him. Loosen any tight clothing, such as a collar and a belt, so that it does not add to the patient's discomfort or interfere with his breathing. If he has dyspnea, he will be more comfortable with his head elevated. If he has symptoms of shock, keep him flat (provided that he experiences no respiratory distress). A blanket or coat can be used for warmth.

• Call the doctor immediately or, preferably, have someone else do this while you stay with the patient. An immediate call for an ambulance may be indicated.

• Do not let the patient get up and move about, even if he begins to feel better, until the doctor has examined him. Above all, never let him undertake a trip home unattended.

If the patient has not suffered myocardial infarction, nothing will have been lost except a little time and effort. How much better is this kind of mistake than the feeling, "Oh, if I had only known how sick he was!"

• If the patient loses consciousness, go through the ABC's of cardiac arrest (see Chap. 53) immediately instituting cardiopulmonary resuscitative measures as indicated.

THE CORONARY CARE UNIT

Some studies have shown that mortality of patients treated in specialized coronary care units has been reduced by at least one-third compared with traditional hospital care. Approximately 20 per cent of patients die compared with 30 to 35 per cent formerly (Meltzer 1969). Today patients with chest pain or suspicious history of possible myocardial infarction are admitted to such a unit if one is available. Patients with cholecystitis, pericarditis, or pneumothorax may also be admitted with chest pain. Until all of the diagnostic data is available, patients are treated as if they have sustained an infarction. Many will not have this.

The emphasis in a CCU is on the prevention of the need for resuscitative measures by detecting early changes in the patient's condition. Thus all patients receive continuous close observation, including electrocardiographic monitoring for several days. The nursing staff receives specialized education in the early recognition of cardiac arrhythmias and other complications. Prompt reporting of early warning signs enables the physician to institute treatment before complications become serious. Nursing care is directed towards the promotion of rest and healing, the prevention of complications, support of the patient through the experience and the promotion of optimal rehabilitation.

The drama of the coronary care concept most often centers on heroic measures, "aggressive" treatment, and the numbers of lives saved. Just as dramatic and challenging to nursing, though in a different way, is the care of those patients who don't survive. One way to view the present statistics is that despite the current management of the patient in a well operated CCU, one out of every five patients admitted will not live to be discharged from the hospital. Thus, coronary nursing embraces a wide range of intense human situations. The nurse who elects to work in the CCU views her role realistically when she realizes that a sizable aspect of it will be the care of patients and families facing the reality of death. If success is measured only by lives saved then the death of a patient can be viewed as a failure.

This view does not take into account our human limitations. While giving the patient every advantage of knowledgeable and skilled care and hope for his survival, one must come to grips with the fact that our best team efforts will not save all lives. The patient needs our help to die with as much dignity as can be mustered out of the very gross realities of a resuscitation attempt in the event of sudden death; or our sustained, listening, sensitive presence when his course is progressively downhill.

ADMITTING THE PATIENT

The appearance of the patient on admission can vary widely. He may neither look nor feel very ill, or he may be in deep cardiogenic shock. He may have received pain medication in his doctor's office which gave relief, or he may be clutching his chest with muscle splinting of his shoulder and arm indicating severe pain. He may have a tachycardia, a normal response to abruptly leaving one's place of work in an ambulance with flashing lights and siren, or the tachycardia may mean the early onset of heart failure. A bradycardia does not mean that the patient is not excited. Rather this can be an ominous sign of involvement of the S-A or A-V node or marked vagal tone. A slow rate can lead to myocardial hypoxia which fosters lethal cardiac arrhythmias. Vagal slowing of the heart can result from profound fear or drugs, such as morphine or digitalis. Slowing of the rate can mean the patient is in heart block if the A-V node is ischemic from the episode.

One patient may have a large area of muscle damaged; another, a relatively small area. The latter could, though, have more arrhythmic difficulty.

The common denominator of the group is that they all have had a close confrontation with death and are all prime candidates for cardiac arrest. All need a calm, confident, competent admitting nurse who can demonstrate by the way she greets the patient that he is in the best place for him to be under the circumstances. Frenzied activity and hurried or absent greeting or explanation only fosters the patient's feeling of disaster which can promote cardiac arrhythmias, including ventricular fibrillation. Time and speed are important; as is getting the patient on the cardiac monitor to assess his present condition, his response to drugs such as morphine or demerol and to detect lethal arrhythmias early. But ripping the alert patient's clothes apart and jabbing him with needle electrodes without warning or explanation can further activate the autonomic response to fright.

For each patient the admitting nurse has to determine priorities. The life-saving activities always exert priority. Some other areas of nursing concern during the early admission period are:

• Assisting the patient to bed and undressing him with minimal expenditure of effort. A roller placed next to the patient on the stretcher can be used so that the patient does not have to be lifted.

• Giving oxygen. Equipment ready for immediate use is at the bedside. Adequate oxygenation contributes to the relief of pain and the prevention of arrhythmias. Physicians differ in opinion regarding routine oxygen administration. Of course, patients who are dyspneic, tachycardic, or cyanotic are given oxygen as an emergency measure. The danger is that some emergency patients, unknown to the local physician and nursing staff, may have chronic obstructive lung disease. Giving oxygen routinely at high concentration may result in respiratory arrest by depriving the patient of the hypoxic stimulus to respiration. Asking the patient or family promptly on admission if he has lung disease is necessary. Unit policies should offer guidelines for action. For example, oxygen may be given at a lowered concentration and the physician promptly notified. Check the patient's response. If he becomes pink, but increasingly drowsy without drugs, this is an emergency sign!

• Relieving pain. It is imperative to relieve pain which is often severe, crushing, and the source of great fear. Arrhythmias and shock can follow severe pain. Also, arrhythmias and hypotension can follow the administration of a drug such as morphine given to relieve pain. Atropine is sometimes ordered to be given with morphine to prevent bradycardia and other vagal effects.

Watch the patient's response to the pain relieving drug. If he is not relieved in an hour call the doctor back. Often the pain is so severe that the narcotic does not completely relieve it, but makes it less intense and more bearable. Usually, the narcotic is given every three to four hours, as it is necessary, during the period when the pain is severe. Note any depression of respiration, nausea, arrhythmias, and hypotension, particularly when morphine is given. Give the drug as often as it is required and permitted to control the pain. The period during which narcotics are needed usually lasts no more than one or two days; yet it is during this period that rest and the relief of apprehension are especially important. Oxygen should be given also.

• **Observation** of the patient is an on-going process initiated when the nurse first greets the patient, who also observes the nurse. How the nurse confronts the patient during this period can influence the entire course of his illness. He can get from her a message of hope, warm caring, competence, and concern or one that is cold, impersonal, pessimistic, scolding, or panicky.

Using one's sensory apparatus skillfully can quickly give much data:

Eyes. What does the patient look like? What is his color? Is he splinting his shoulder muscles from pain? Is he working hard to breathe (dyspneic)? Does he have a calm or apprehensive look in his eyes? Is he alert or somnolent? Are his neck veins distended? What does the oscilloscope show? What does the sphygmomanometer read?

Ears. What do you hear? Are his respirations wheezing or stertorous? What does the patient have to say? Is he in pain? If talking does not distress him further, what happened that brought him to the hospital? What questions does he have about the unit, the equipment, his condition?

Touch. Is the patient's skin cold and clammy? Warm and dry? Is there good skin turgor? What is the quality of his radial pulse? Full and bounding? Weak and thready? Is his abdomen or bladder distended?

Smell. What odors emanate from the patient? Does his breath smell like alcohol? (The old home remedy for pain and other emergencies) Is there the sweet fruity odor of diabetic acidosis? Is there the odor of perspiration? Of excreta?

• Placing chest electrodes for cardiac monitoring.

The bedside cardiac monitor and a console at the nurses' station or a remote control monitoring system known as telemetry minimally provide for a continuous display on an oscilloscope of one lead of the patient's ECG.

The placement sites of electrodes are chosen so that the best cardiographic tracing appears on the oscilloscope. Care should be taken that electrodes and nonallergenic adhesive tape are so placed that they do not interfere with the taking of the chest leads of the 12-lead ECG or the placement of paddles for defibrillation.

Generally, a high rate and low rate indicator is set on the cardiac monitor for each patient.

Should the patient's pulse rate fall below or exceed these limits on a beat-to-beat basis, an audiovisual alarm system is activated. On some machines, a writeout may be concurrent with that appearing on the oscilloscope or may be written out from a tape or memory-loop with a ten second or longer delay. Hence, the cardiac rhythm immediately before the alarm situation can be identified. After the alarm, the nurse examines the cardiac tracing and observes the patient. Loosening of an electrode or excessive muscular activity can result in false alarms and an irregular monitor pattern. If an arrhythmia is the source of the alarm, the nurse makes a decision regarding nursing intervention.

The alarm system should be ready for use at all times unless the nurse is directly with the patient doing something, such as changing an electrode which would trigger the alarm. The cable that connects the electrodes to the cardiac monitor should be so secured that the patient has sufficient slack when he is moved or turns himself.

The patient and family need to know that a cardiac monitor is neither a dangerous nor a miraculous machine. It simply enables the patient's cardiac conduction to be displayed continuously. Needless apprehension can be built up if the patient fantasizes about this piece of machinery that blinks, beeps, and causes people to jump and take note when an alarm goes off. False alarms frighten patients. Monitors are considered as aids to and not substitutes for nursing care and human contact with the patient.

The patient with a disturbing arrhythmia therefore needs the care of a staff who can recognize early changes and secure prompt medical help, accurately observe the patient's response to treatment, and appropriately manage their own anxiety, which is certain to increase in the presence of life-threatening arrhythmias. A skilled nurse recognizes that her own anxiety can compound the patient's if it is sensed by him. Staying with the patient between the necessary technical duties involved in treatment conveys to the patient that the nurse is not afraid of him or his arrhythmia, but is capable of carrying out necessary emergency treatment should the need arise. This kind of nursing behavior, however, takes a great deal of skill which the nurse needs support to develop.

Observation of the cardiac monitor rhythm must be accompanied by observation of the patient. The advantage of continuous cardiac monitoring of the hospitalized patient is that changes in rhythm or rate can be detected early, reported to the physician and treated promptly, before the clinical condition of the patient deteriorates.

Because of subjective feelings such as palpitations, "jolting" sensations in the chest, or a fluttering feeling, patients are often aware of their arrhythmias. Momentary dizziness or "stoppage of the heart" can be terrifying. These abnormal sensations increase anxiety. Studies have shown that anxiety and other emotional states, in turn, contribute to the onset, severity, persistence, and recurrence of cardiac arrhythmias (Wolf).

• Intravenous Infusion. Because cardiovascular collapse is an always present threat, each myocardial infarction suspect has an intravenous route opened at admission and an infusion started to keep the vein opened. In an emergency, drugs can be quickly given and time is not wasted while the physician attempts to do a cut down on a collapsed vein.

• 12-Lead Electrocardiogram. This can be quickly taken by the nurse during the early admission period. Though the results do not markedly influence nursing care at this point (since all patients are treated with the same precautions) the record serves as a basis for later comparison and immediate arrhythmia treatment.

• Spiritual Care. Generally all patients who are myocardial infarction suspects are listed as "critical." One role of the nurse is to expedite the availability of the patient's spiritual advisor. The suggestion of spiritual help from a clergyman of the patient's religion should be offered. Speak with the family regarding the patient's religious affiliation and usual practices if the patient is too ill to be questioned. Speak with the clergyman regarding the patient's emotional response. A recent study indicated that the suggestion of the reception of the Sacrament of the Sick by the priest to Catholic patients with myocardial infarction was more consoling than frightening (Cassem). The clergyman can also be supportive of the family during this time of crisis.

• Diet. Oral intake is restricted until specific orders are received. Because of the risk of cardiac arrest and aspiration, as well as the increased cardiac workload from digestion, intake for the critical period of the first three days is generally restricted to a full liquid diet. Iced water or iced beverages are contraindicated because they are vagal stimulants. Coffee and tea contain stimulants which may increase heart rate and may also be restricted. Carbonated beverages are not served because they promote gaseous distention.

• Admission Interview. Some specific questions that should be asked the patient or family are:

• What allergies does the patient have? Is he allergic to procaine (or Novocain)? The related drug Xylocaine (lidocaine) may be ordered for him if he has ventricular arrhythmias. Report an affirmative response to the physician.

• Does the patient have glaucoma? (Atropine sulfate, which increases intraocular pressure is a frequently used drug in the coronary care unit.) Does he take eye drops; a diuretic such as Diamox or Diuril?

• Is the patient a diabetic? The diabetic frequently has an atypical response to myocardial infarction. Does he take insulin or an oral hypoglycemic agent? When was the last dose taken? What has he eaten since?

• Has the patient been taking nitroglycerin, digitalis or other cardiac drugs? When was the last dose taken?

• What other drugs has the patient been taking that shouldn't be stopped? Examples are steroids and dilantin for epilepsy. Dilantin is also used as an anti-arrhythmic drug.

Obtaining answers to these questions is a collaborative task of the doctor and nurse.

DIAGNOSIS

A distinctive history is a definite aid in diagnosis. Diabetics frequently have atypical histories. Report any additional data which the patient discloses after the doctor leaves him. If the patient is anxious, which is often the case, he may not recall or may distort events leading up to his admission.

Physical examination includes nonauscultatory modes such as palpation with the fingers for heart size and vibrations (or thrills) as well as inspection of the chest. Auscultation of the heart and chest with the stethoscope can reveal heart murmurs, sounds of valve closure, changes in rhythm and rate, pericardial friction rub, and moist, crackling sounds in the lungs called rales, an early finding in left ventricular failure indicating pulmonary edema. Some nurses may be taught to auscultate the chest for rales at regular intervals so that early treatment for heart failure can be instituted.

Electrocardiogram. Usually, it is ordered promptly as soon as myocardial infarction is suspected, and it may be repeated several times (serial ECG's) in determining the diagnosis and in following the course of the illness.

Laboratory Studies. Necrosis of myocardial tissue results in the release of intracellular enzymes into the circulation. These enzymes are not specific for myocardial tissue alone, but are useful as a diagnostic aid in this as well as other conditions involving tissue damage. The CPK (creatine phosphokinase) and SGOT (serum glutamic oxalacetic transaminase) are especially used as indicators of the severity of tissue damage. Normal values vary according to laboratory methods.

An elevated erythrocyte sedimentation rate and white blood cell count are also evidence of tissue necrosis in myocardial infarction.

Temperature. Fever is common after a day or so. Usually, it is low or moderate, and lasts four or five days. Fever is one of the body's responses to necrosis of tissue. The oral thermometer is most often used. Rectal temperature is most accurate, but is not used in some cardiac units because of the potential harm from vagal stimuli. The use of a well-lubricated rectal thermometer inserted gently with the patient in a comfortable, safe position should prevent harmful vagal stimulation which could result in cardiac slowing and the appearance of arrhythmias.

PATHOLOGY

The location of a myocardial infarction is most frequently in the left ventricle. The area of a myocardial infarction heals by scar tissue. The size of the scar determines the amount of cardiac reserve that is lost. Necrosis can extend through the thickness of the myocardial wall to the subendocardium (transmural infarction), involve part of the myocardium or may just involve the subendocardial area which is furthest from the blood supply. Different terms are used to describe the area of the heart which is affected. For example, in most people the right coronary artery and its branches supply the posterior wall of the ventricle. Occlusion of this artery results in a so-called posterior wall or diaphragmatic infarction. Heart block is more common with this type of infarction because a branch of the right coronary vessel supplies the A-V node. Another branch supplies the S-A node. Because it supplies these vital parts of the conduction system, the right coronary artery is thought to be the artery of sudden death.

The left coronary artery and its branches supply most of the anterior and apical portions of the left ventricle. Infarctions from occlusion of these branches are termed anterior wall, or anteroseptal.

The stages of healing can be correlated with the period of restriction of cardiac workload. From the onset until about the third day, there is acute tissue degeneration and the infarct area is soft, mushy and necrotic. It is dead tissue and therefore electrically inert. Dangerous arrhythmias are most apt to develop during this period, but they are thought to arise from the peri-infarction area which is ischemic and electrically unstable.

From the fourth to seventh days, softening of the infarcted area is greatest and there is danger of aneurysm formation. The weakened area in the ventricular wall may balloon out during systole. About the eighth to tenth day newly formed capillaries develop around the periphery of the infarct, but it is two to three weeks before there is a functionally significant collateral circulation.

Collagen begins to form about the 12th day after the infarction. Rupture of the ventricle is likeliest from onset to the 14th day. It is three to four weeks before the scar begins to grow firm and two to three months before a scar of maximum strength is formed.

OBJECTIVES OF CARE

Most of the time when the myocardial infarction patient arrives at the hospital, the heart damage has been done. The infarction can be extended, however, or other complications can develop. The objectives of care include the reduction of cardiac workload to prevent further damage and promote healing. This is accomplished through a program of optimal rest. Optimal rest includes helping the patient and family to accept and adjust to the experience.

Rest and Activity. Optimal rest is a broad concept. Studies have shown that putting a patient to bed is not synonymous with putting him to rest. Prolonged bed rest favors the development of many complications which at worst can prove fatal, or at best prolong convalescence (Browse; Olson). A program of preventive measures, such as deep breathing and foot or leg exercises, aimed specifically at reducing the hazards of immobility, and a bowel hygiene program is essential if the chief treatment of infarction—rest—is not to become a liability.

Unlike a broken leg which can be immobilized in plaster, the heart can never be immobilized.

It works all the time, even when injured. It rests only during diastole. Therefore, the treatment of cardiac arrhythmias which adversely affect cardiac hemodynamics, or the use of a drug such as digitalis to enhance cardiac systole and the diastolic or resting period of the cardiac cycle affords rest for the heart in the broad sense.

One of the hazards of bedrest is the Valsalva maneuver. This maneuver is accomplished with a forced expiration against a closed glottis. This can occur, for example, while straining to defecate or void, to lift oneself up in bed, during gagging, vomiting, or severe coughing. During the Valsalva maneuver, intrathoracic pressure is increased and blood is trapped in the great veins preventing it from entering the chest and right atrium. The heart actually gets smaller in size and, after an initial decrease in heart rate due to vagal stimulation, the rate accelerates. When the breath is released, blood gushes into the heart and rapidly distends it. This "overshoot" results in increased blood pressure and tachycardia which stimulate pressor receptors in the carotid sinus and aorta. A reflex bradycardia then ensues which can prove fatal for the patient with a damaged heart.

Since it is sometimes physically impossible to move patients precisely when they wish to be moved, patients should be instructed to avoid the Valsalva maneuver by exhaling rather than holding the breath when moving in bed.

Levine and his colleagues who are proponents of the chair rest treatment of myocardial infarction advocate it on the physiologic basis that the heart works less in the sitting position than in the recumbent position. From the first day after infarction the patient is assisted (not lifted) to a chair placed next to the bed where he remains until fatigued. Time in the chair is gradually increased. Only cardiogenic shock, severe pain requiring narcotics which are apt to induce bradycardia, or blood pressure too low for adequate cerebral blood flow are contraindications. The patient is said to benefit from the reduced cardiac workload and reduction of anxiety associated with the hopelessness of long-term confinement to bed. Replication of the original study showed that "chair rest" as a treatment had no adverse effects on cardiovascular function. Hypotension, arrhythmias, vasovagal reactions or other complications were not increased. Measures to prevent the complications of prolonged rest are necessary whether the patient is in a bed or a chair. The patient is permitted no more activity in the chair than he would be if confined to bed (Schmitt).

The type of chair recommended is one with a straight backrest so that the buttocks do not sink down. The thighs should be parallel to the floor, or slanting downward. A slightly angled foot support may be used to allow comfortable extension of the legs (see Fig. 28-2).

Though the physician may order the chair or the bed or both, rest cannot be ordered. Nursing care assists the patient to find rest. The anxious, or fearful, or angry patient, or one under other strong emotion may be pouring out catecholamines (epinephrine or norepinephrine) and subjecting his heart to the vigors of physical exercise though he may be sitting quietly in bed or in a chair.

Whenever you care for a patient with myocardial infarction, find out specifically what the patient may and may not do. Make sure that this information is shared with every member of the nursing staff caring for the patient by approximate notation on the nursing care plan so that one person does not let the patient feed himself at breakfast, and another arrives at lunch time and insists that he be fed.

Certain principles apply to a program of rest, regardless of the exact program of rest that has been prescribed:

• Do not allow the patient to exert himself. Straining at stool is one common example. Find out what the patient's usual bowel routine is and help him to maintain it in the hospital if it does not violate any physiologic principles.

Studies have shown that the use of the bedside commode involves less energy expenditure than getting on and off and using the bedpan (Benton). The risk of inadvertently performing the Valsalva maneuver is minimized. The patient still requires assistance in cleansing himself after defecation.

To avoid straining and bladder distention some physicians permit their male patients to stand at the side of the bed to void. A male orderly is an asset to assist them, especially elderly patients. Sometimes male patients suffer from urinary stream hesitancy if a female nurse is in the room. Give the patient privacy, but stay close by to assist the patient when getting back to bed.

• Place things within easy reach—the glass of water, the radio, the call bell—so that the patient does not have to use effort to reach them.

• If the patient strenuously objects to certain activity restrictions, discuss this with the doctor who may permit more flexibility, or who may be more effectively persuasive than the nurse. Refusal to accept activity restrictions is sometimes a manifestation of denial. Since this is an unconscious defense against anxiety, reasoning with the patient often does not help. Attempting to force restrictions can only increase the patient's anxiety and cardiac workload. The physician may order sedation. The patient needs the nonjudgmental support of the nurse and family during this overwhelming adjustment period. Threatening or scolding increase his need for dangerous defense mechanisms. Supportive listening can gradually assist the patient to begin to acknowledge what has happened.

Observe the patient as well as the cardiac monitor during changes of activity. Physical and emotional strain (such as from an upsetting visitor) can be reflected in cardiac arrhythmias as well as increased pain, pulse rate, dyspnea. The nurse then uses her judgment in slowing down or eliminating the activity temporarily, then discussing it with the physician.

• If care is needed that may tire the patient, do it slowly, and allow for rest periods during care. Giving a bath and changing the bed may be fatiguing if they are undertaken all at once. In a well staffed coronary unit, the bath can be given at any time of the day, according to the need and preference of the patient.

Many physicians believe that the safest, quickest and most effective way of helping the patient to resume activity is to observe meticulously his reaction to slightly increased amounts of activity, and to be guided accordingly in allowing increases in activity. The patient is observed for arrhythmias on the cardiac monitor or irregularity of the pulse, chest pain, excessive fatigue, increased pulse and respiratory rates, and changes in the blood pressure. Such indices are being used increasingly in planning the patient's return to activity instead of regimens of bed rest for a stated number of weeks for every patient who has suffered myocardial infarction (see Chap. 33).

Sedation. Sedatives or tranquilizers are sometimes ordered after narcotics are no longer necessary for pain. These drugs should facilitate the patient's rest and relaxation, but should not make him so somnolent that he no longer initiates deep breathing, leg exercises or moving in bed. Older patients, especially, may have paradoxical reactions to sedative drugs and become hyperactive.

Observation and accurate reporting are essential. Note carefully the location and the intensity of the chest pain, or whether there are any symptoms of dyspnea or cyanosis. Are physical or emotional activity associated with pain and/or arrhythmias? Absence of pain is not necessarily an indication that the patient is recovering. When the affected myocardial tissues die, the nerves in that portion of myocardium can no longer transmit impulses to the brain, and the pain ceases. Sometimes nurses are lulled into a false sense of security when the patient's pain abates or there is normal sinus rhythm. Do not relax your vigilance; patients with myocardial infarction are disposed to sudden changes in their condition.

The patient's T.P.R. and blood pressure are observed carefully. The temperature usually is taken every four hours. Note both the rate and the quality of the pulse. Blood pressure readings usually are ordered every two hours for the first several days. Intake and output are carefully noted for all patients for the first three days and longer if the patient has symptoms of congestive heart failure, or if shock has been severe.

Environment and Emotional Support. A well managed coronary care unit is not a noisy, hectic, place. The principle of the unit is to prevent the drama of resuscitation efforts by close observation and early treatment of complications. There is an element of heightened awareness and periods of sustained tension because changes can occur suddenly. Ideally the hospital area where coronary patients are admitted should be separate from but may be adjacent to the surgical or medical intensive care area.

Though the patient may have a familiarity with the idea of a coronary care unit, coming upon it as he does, abruptly and in the role of patient may make him more bewildered if he notices its difference compared with usual hospital wards. He may ask specific or general questions but due to his anxiety answers may have to be repeated on other occasions. He may initially distort what is in his environment. Some questions need general answers. For example, if the patient asks "How long will I be here?" a general but frank response can be, "I don't know exactly. It depends on how things go for you and also on your doctor's recommendations. The laboratory tests take at least three days."

The patient who suffers a myocardial infarction is beset by many fears. The two that predominate are the fear of death and the fear of living with impending death. The patient must cope with these as well as threats to his physical integrity, change in body image and self-concept, loss of status at work, reduction of income or even loss of the job, loss of prestige in social life, restriction of favorite activities, loss of ability to care for his or her family at least temporarily, and a potentially formidable barrier to the accomplishment of life goals.

Faced with many potential losses, small wonder that patients studied in a coronary care unit were found to experience many disturbing feelings—anxiety, anger, sorrow, depression, bitterness, clingingness, demandingness, and hopelessness (Sobel). This last feeling, intermittent hopelessness, was found to be the most difficult for the patient and for the nursing staff to deal with. An appropriate response by the staff to this feeling was derived from the simple truth that we do not know that a patient's situation is hopeless and that all of our medical knowledge and skills are employed to help him because there is some hope. It was thought that the major part of the struggle with hopelessness remained the patient's task to resolve. Helpful nursing action includes the capacity to confront the patient openly and humanly, to empathize with his situation, to think and feel about it and not turn away from him or rush to intervene in his painful human circumstance over which the nurse has little control. Being able to say to a patient, "The other patient died," rather than "He was transferred," respects the patient's maturity and his capacity to employ defenses against facts which, temporarily, at least, are intolerable to him.

Inevitably some patients will die, many after a predictably downhill course. Assisting the patient to die with dignity is a formidable task in a coronary care unit where resuscitation attempt is a general rule. Visitors and other patients become aware when such an attempt is in progress—from the increase in activity, numbers of personnel, and characteristic sounds. It is well for one staff member to be assigned to visit these people, explain what is happening, discuss what needs to be discussed, and stay with or find someone such as a clergyman to stay with a visitor. Otherwise, a state of heightened anxiety pervades the environment with especially harmful physiologic and psychological consequences on other patients.

TREATMENT OF COMPLICATIONS

Arrythmias. Disturbances of Heat Rate, Rhythm, and Conduction. At least 80 per cent of myocardial infarction patients have some type of arrythmia during the acute phase (Meltzer *et al.,* 1966).

Over half of the deaths from myocardial infarction occur within 72 hours of admission to the hospital (Grace and Soscia). More than half of these deaths result from cardiac arrhythmias. Typically, the abnormal rhythm occurs suddenly within the first three days after the infarction, and it can be fatal within a few minutes. The arrhythmia can represent a transient abnormality in a heart that otherwise is capable of sustaining life and usual activity later. Consequently, prompt, effective treatment of arrhythmia assumes tremendous importance to the life of the patient. If he can be helped to survive the episode of ectopic rhythm, he may not die from myocardial infarction (see Chap. 53).

Venous Thrombosis. This condition arises mostly in the veins of the lower extremities and pelvis. The exact cause is unknown. People who are ambulatory develop venous thrombosis also. Venous stasis, hypercoagulability of the blood, and external pressure against the veins, such as occurs in the side-lying position without a pillow between the legs are thought to be involved. The use of Ace bandages, positioning pillows, and foot and leg exercises on a regularly scheduled basis are measures employed to prevent thrombus formation.

Some doctors treat all patients who have myocardial infarcts, regardless of the severity, with anticoagulants. Others reserve this treatment for patients whose heart damage has been severe, or for those who experience complications. Anticoagulants are given to decrease the likelihood of venous thrombosis and emboli and to prevent further increase in the size of a clot already formed.

Pulmonary Embolism. Most pulmonary emboli arise from venous clots in the lower extremities and pelvis. Many do not cause pulmonary infarction. A lung scan and angiocardiogram would be necessary if embolectomy were contemplated. For the patient with myocardial infarction, however, this is extremely risky. Anticoagulation and vena caval ligation would probably be considered. (See Chap. 32 for further discussion of the problem of pulmonary embolism.)

Arterial Emboli. Anticoagulants are not thought to prevent arterial clot formation. A clot can form in the left ventricular cavity overlying the infarcted area (mural thrombus). Part of it can break off and enter the systemic arterial circulation and cause occlusion of peripheral arteries resulting in a mottled, cold, pulseless extremity, or of arteries in the brain resulting in sudden stroke. Listen carefully to the patient's complaint of extremity pain and check for differences in temperature of the extremities. Arteriotomy and embolectomy may be necessary. Observe for any slight paralysis, slurring of speech, and drooping of a side of the face.

Congestive Heart Failure. See Chapter 28 for nursing care of the patient with congestive heart failure and pulmonary edema.

Cardiogenic Shock. This is a dreaded complication because of the high mortality rate. Eighty per cent of patients with this diagnosis die (Meltzer, 1969). The earlier shock is detected and treatment instituted the better are the patient's chances of survival.

Because some believe that this mortality cannot be reduced further by conventional therapy, and because the size of the infarction is not always related to the extreme degree of shock, research centers are developing and assessing mechanical assistance devices for the failing ventricle following myocardial infarction.

Other complications include ventricular aneurysm, ventricular rupture, and the shoulder-hand syndrome.

Ventricular aneurysm decreases the pumping action of the heart and angina or congestive failure may result. Some ventricular aneurysms can be surgically corrected.

Cardiac rupture occurs when a soft necrotic area gives way. Hemopericardium, cardiac tamponade, and relatively sudden death ensue.

There can also be rupture of the interventricular septum. Dyspnea, rapid right heart failure and shock result and the prognosis is poor though survival is possible.

The shoulder-hand syndrome or periarthritis of the shoulder can develop during the convalescent period. It is characterized by pain, stiffness, and limitation of shoulder motion and sometimes swelling of the hand. The exact cause is unknown but protective disuse of the shoulder during the acute period may be a contributory factor.

PREPARATION FOR TRANSFER

Transfer from the coronary care unit generally means progress for the patient. He has survived one critical period and can go to an area of the hospital where the close observation of the CCU is unavailable but also unnecessary. "Can I get along without my monitor? What happens if I need a nurse right away? What about my chest pain—I still have angina? Can they help me if I have a cardiac arrest?" are questions which the patient probably poses to himself.

Ideally, patients with a myocardial infarction should be transferred to a postcoronary division where specially prepared staff can help the patient through the transition period. Remote control monitoring or telemetry may be available in such an area. This is not always possible. The staff who receives the patient, however, must be aware that despite the fact that the patient may look and feel well and has survived his CCU stay, he is still critically ill and subject to all of the complications of acute myocardial infarction.

The patient should have the opportunity in the CCU to discuss his thoughts and feelings about the transfer. A length of time in the CCU without a cardiac monitor and I.V. (weaning period) gives the patient confidence that he can, in fact, survive without them. A realistic projection of the length of stay in the CCU and visits from the staff of the transfer unit help the patient to make the adjustment when the time comes. That there are adverse and serious cardiovascular effects in patients unprepared for the transfer has been documented (Klein *et al.*).

If possible, nursing visits from the CCU staff should continue after transfer. When all units where coronary patients are cared for are physically adjacent, staff can circulate among units and thus have the opportunity to care for the patient during the various phases of hospitalization. The clinical specialist may be able to follow patients through various hospital areas and stimulate and coordinate continuity of nursing care, including a patient-family education program.

LATER CARE AND REHABILITATION

Of the approximately 80 per cent of patients who survive their first myocardial infarction, some will be troubled by angina or congestive heart failure. Most patients, however, will look and feel well after their transfer from the CCU. They continue to need nursing care, but care at this point involves more of the counseling, teaching, and socializing aspects of the nursing role, rather than technical or mother-surrogate components.

This is the period when the patient hopefully begins to come to grips with some of the changes in life that the infarction has precipitated. This can be a long-term process with much of the "rethinking" coming after discharge. For many, this time is one of profound philosophical dimension.

The nurse helps during this period by offering herself as a listener as the patient attempts to work out his problems; by planning with the patient, family, or volunteer staff for appropriate diversion; and by reviewing with the patient and family those aspects of activity, drugs, diet, or other treatment such as a pacemaker which are part of the postdischarge medical plan.

A family member who might feel foolish or embarrassed to admit difficulty in coping with a situation may need to be encouraged to seek the care of a doctor. Family members who themselves receive support are in a better position to offer support to the patient.

If the patient needs nursing or homemaker assistance at home, or a stay in an intermediate care facility, referrals are instituted early in the postdischarge period.

The nurse also contributes by assisting the patient to get answers to questions which may bother him, but which he may hesitate to ask about. For example, it can be assumed that postcoronary patients will have questions about resumption of sex activity. Many are hesitant to ask questions about this. The nurse can detect clues that the patient may need help with this subject and can assist him and his spouse to formulate the questions and seek the physician's advice. When the limitations are reviewed and understood, the couple is in a better position to make their own decisions. A recent study of postcoronary males showed that conjugal sexual activity subjects the cardiovascular system to no more strain than many other activities of daily living. A conclusion of the study was that the postcoronary patient, without cardiac decompensation can resume conjugal sexual activity when other physical activities are increased usually about the ninth to twelfth weeks (Hellerstein). This, of course, will vary with the individual patient, spouse, and the guidance of the physician.

His arrival at home does not mean that the patient can resume his former activities. Usually, he is instructed to rest for at least two to three months, gradually increasing his activity as prescribed. Strenuous unprescribed physical exertion and emotional strain must be avoided. If all goes well, the patient may be permitted to return to work at the end of two to three months. The doctor may advise working part time, particularly at first. If the patient's work involves heavy responsibilities or considerable physical or emotional exertion, it may be necessary for him to find a less demanding type of work.

There has been a trend in recent years towards a more scientific approach to the prescription of activity for patients after myocardial infarction and the enhancement of their physical fitness.

(See Chapter 33 for rehabilitation of the cardiac patient.)

PROGNOSIS

Although myocardial infarction is a serious event, constituting one of the major causes of death among older people, many patients not only survive the attack but also are able to return to work. Because the underlying condition of atherosclerosis is still present, the patient may have repeated attacks of myocardial infarction, or he may develop angina pectoris. Statistics concerning mortality apply to groups and not to specific individuals within the group. It is difficult to predict what the future holds for the individual patient. Some live comfortably and actively for many years afterward, such as former U.S. presidents Eisenhower and Johnson.

REFERENCES AND BIBLIOGRAPHY

ANDREOLI, K., et al.: Comprehensive Cardiac Care, St. Louis, Mosby, 1968.

ANDREOLI, K.: The cardiac monitor, Am. J. Nurs. 69:1238, June, 1969.

ASPINALL, M.: Nursing intervention for a patient with myocardial infarction, ANA Clinical Sessions, New York, Appleton-Century-Crofts, 1968.

BELAND, I.: Clinical Nursing, New York, Macmillan, 1970.

CARNES, G. D.: Understanding the cardiac patient's behavior, Am. J. Nurs. 71:1187, June, 1971.

CASSEM, N. H., et al.: How coronary patients respond to last rites, Postgrad. Med. 45:147, March, 1969.

DUKE, M.: Bed rest in acute myocardial infarction: a study of physicians' practices, Am. Heart J. 82:486, 1971.

Early care for the acute coronary suspect. Bethesda Conference Report, Am. J. Cardiol. 23:603, April, 1969.

FIELDS, SR. M. L.: The C.P.R. team in a medium-sized hospital, Am. J. Nurs. 66:87, January, 1966.

FOSTER, S., and ANDREOLI, K.: Behavior following acute myocardial infarction, Am. J. Nurs. 70:2344, November, 1970.

GERMAIN, C.: Nursing role variations in coronary care, Hospitals 43:147, September, 1969.

GERMAIN, C., and HANLEY, SR. M. P.: Metronome for a music teacher, Am. J. Nurs. 68:498, March, 1968.

GILMORE, M. E.: Nursing in the coronary care unit, Bedside Nurse 3:11, April, 1970.

GRAHAM, L.: Patients' perceptions in the CCU, Am. J. Nurs. 69:1921, September, 1969.

GREENE, W., and MOSS, A.: Psychosocial factors in the adjustment of patients with permanently implanted cardiac pacemakers, Ann. Int. Med. 70:897, May, 1969.

HAHN, A., and DOLAN, N.: After coronary care—then what? Am. J. Nurs. 70:2350, November, 1970.

HALL, L., and ALFANO, G.: Incapacitation or rehabilitation, Am. J. Nurs. 64:C-20, November, 1964.

HARRISON, T., and REEVES, T.: Principles and Problems of Ischemic Heart Disease, Chicago, Year Book, 1968.

HAZELTINE, L. S.: The weeks of healing, Am. J. Nurs. 64:C-14, November, 1964.

HELLERSTEIN, H.: Sexual activity and the post-coronary patient, Med. Aspects Human Sexuality 3:70, March, 1969.

HUNN, V.: Cardiac pacemakers, Am. J. Nurs. 69:749, April, 1969.

JONES, B.: Inside the coronary care unit: the patient and his responses, Am. J. Nurs. 67:2313, November, 1967.

KINLEIN, M. L.: The critical hours, Am. J. Nurs. 64:C-10, November, 1964.

LOWN, B.: Intensive heart care, Sci. Am. 219:19, July, 1968.

MELTZER, L., PINNEO, R., and KITCHELL, R.: Intensive Coronary Care: A Manual for Nurses, Philadelphia, Charles Press, 2nd ed., 1971.

MELTZER, L., et al.: Acute myocardial infarction, in Concepts and Practices of Intensive Care for Nurse Specialists, Philadelphia, Charles Press, 1969.

MERKEL, R., and SOVIE, M.: Electrocution hazards with transvenous pacemaker electrodes, Am. J. Nurs. 68:2560, December, 1967.

A mobile CCU saves lives in New York City, ICU: A Review of the Literature on Intensive Care, 3:12, 1969.

NARROW, B.: Rest is . . . , Am. J. Nurs. 67:1616, August, 1967.

Nursing in Cardiovascular Diseases, Contemporary Nursing Series, New York, American Journal of Nursing Co., 1971.

OLSON, E. (ed.): The hazards of immobility. A symposium, Am. J. Nurs. 67:780, April, 1967.

PINNEO, R.: Nursing in a coronary care unit, Am. J. Nurs. 65:76, February, 1965.

RAWLINGS, M.: Inside the coronary care unit: trends in therapeutic management, Am. J. Nurs. 67:2321, November, 1967.

REGAN, W.: The new standing orders and their legal pitfalls, R.N. Vol. 38, April, 1968.

SCHMITT, Y., et al.: Armchair treatment in the coronary care unit, Nurs. Res. 18:114, March-April, 1969.

SHOCKEY, C., and SNOW, S.: Pacemaker to the rescue; its use in the C.C.U., R.N. 37, December, 1968.

SISTER ELIZABETH, D. C.: A new dimension in the nursing care of coronary patients, Hosp. Prog. 68:104, 1968.

SOBEL, D.: Personalization on the coronary care unit, Am. J. Nurs. 69:1439, July, 1969.

WINSOR, T.: The electrocardiogram in myocardial infarction, Ciba Clin. Symp. 20:107, October-November-December, 1968.

WOLFF, I. S.: The experience, Am. J. Nurs. 64:C-3, November, 1964.

Cardiac Surgical Nursing

55

Cardiac Valve Replacement • Tissue Transplantation for Valvular Disease • Cardiac Lesions Requiring Corrective Surgery • Surgical Repair of Valvular Heart Disease • Ischemic Heart Disease Ventricular Aneurysm • Tumors of the Heart • Atrial-Septal Defect Traumatic Heart Lesions • Nursing Care of the Cardiac Surgical Patient • Postoperative Nursing Care • General Progression of Patient Care

The patient who has decided to have surgery performed on his heart is taking a calculated risk for a longer and a more healthy life. Patients enter the hospital with varying degrees of emotional readiness to face the operation. The preoperative period can help them to feel secure in the hospital by demonstrating to them the competence and the concern of the doctors and the nurses. If the patient has come to the hospital from some distance, the spiritual advisor connected with the hospital may substitute for the patient's spiritual advisor. There will be time before surgery for them to establish a relationship.

The patient's long illness and perhaps a previous hospitalization that may have prevented his employment, the high cost of past and present hospitalization with the necessary special equipment, drugs and nursing care, may leave the patient drained physically, emotionally, and financially.

One important key to the nursing care of patients undergoing cardiac surgery is to remember that two physiologic systems of the body have been affected, the cardiac and the respiratory. These same systems are directly affected by anxiety and stress-producing situations. The nurse must take this phenomenon into consideration when she is noting physical characteristics as well as vital signs.

As you would with any patient, be alert to the different forms that anxiety may take. Open the door to the expression of fear and anger, remembering that in submitting to cardiac surgery the patient is showing bravery in taking a calculated risk. Refer medical questions to the doctor, and help the patient find answers to those questions which are answerable. Repeated experience has demonstrated that unanswered questions lead to increasing anxiety and lessened confidence in the staff.

Open Heart Surgery or Intracardiac Surgery. A major breakthrough was due to understanding the hemodynamics of cardiopulmonary bypass. This information allowed engineers and biological technicians, as well as many others, to collaborate their efforts and develop the artificial heart-lung machine. The advent of this device provided a means by which the patient's circulation could be rerouted and supported during surgery. Certain drugs, such as concentrated solutions of potassium, can be used to stop the heart beat temporarily (cardioplegia). The surgeon can open the heart, stop the beating, and correct the pathology under direct vision while working in a bloodless field.

Today we are in an era of development of a number of cardiovascular prostheses to repair many congenital and acquired defects.

Researchers are studying the technics for completely replacing the heart by using homotransplantation or by employing a totally mechanical device. Problems in physiologic, biochemical, and ethical values are all being critically reviewed.

CARDIAC VALVE REPLACEMENT

Today severely damaged aortic, mitral, or tricuspid valves can be replaced by artificial valves or by tissue transplantation. Some patients require multiple replacements and as many as two and three damaged valves have been reported as successfully replaced.

While artificial valves differ in design and in the materials from which they are constructed they tend to share a number of common problems. Designs must be perfected in an effort to avoid the recipient's need for long term anticoagulation therapy. A number of valves have a turbulent effect and cause destruction of blood cells. As valves are in use for prolonged periods of time, signs of wearing out, such as changes in the shape and size of the valves as well as strength and elasticity of the material from which they are constructed, are being noted.

TISSUE TRANSPLANTATION FOR VALVULAR DISEASE

This technic is especially popular in England and Europe. Healthy valvular tissue (homografts) may be secured from persons dying from other non-related causes or from animals. The tissue is obtained and processed under sterile conditions and can then be stored until the time a suitable recipient is found.

The possibility of rejection and the long term follow-up of stability of valves are some of the questions being critically reviewed.

CARDIAC LESIONS REQUIRING CORRECTIVE SURGERY

- Congenital heart lesions*

Approximately 1 per cent of adults beyond the second decade of life being considered for cardiac surgery are suffering from congenital pathology (Friedberg).

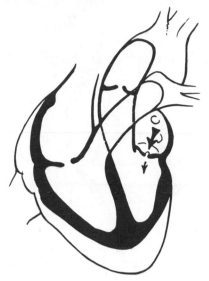

Fig. 55-1. Mitral stenosis. The narrowed valve does not permit blood to flow freely from the left atrium to the left ventricle.

- Acquired heart lesions

Acquired heart disease refers to those pathological processes in the heart or great vessels that were not present at birth but have been incurred since that time:

- Acquired valvular disease due to infectious processes
- Ischemic disease processes
- Tumors of the heart
- Traumatic injuries

Acquired Valvular Diseases of the Heart

Acquired lesions of the valves are most frequently of rheumatic origin. The initial process occurs early in life, usually between 5 and 15 years of age, and only about half of this population can give a definite history of rheumatic fever.

Other causes of acquired valvular diseases may be from subacute or acute bacterial endocarditis which produces an inflammation of the lining of

---

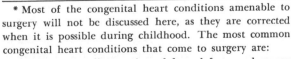

* Most of the congenital heart conditions amenable to surgery will not be discussed here, as they are corrected when it is possible during childhood. The most common congenital heart conditions that come to surgery are:

Tetralogy of Fallot consists of four defects: pulmonary stenosis, intraventricular septal defect, overriding of the aorta, and right ventricular hypertrophy.

Patent ductus arteriosus is a communication between the aorta and the pulmonary artery.

Intra-atrial and intraventricular septal defects are openings in the walls between the chambers of the heart.

Pulmonary stenosis obstructs the flow of blood from the right ventricle.

Coarctation of the aorta, a narrowing of the aorta, may be seen in young adults. It may cause hypertension of the upper extremities and the head, dizziness, retinal or cerebral hemorrhages. It is treated surgically by resection of the part of the aorta that contains the stricture and by anastomosing the aortic ends.

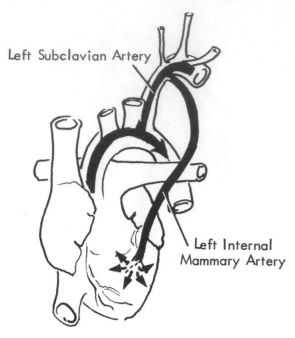

Fig. 55-2. Vineberg revascularization procedure.

the heart including the lining of the valves. As an end result, heart valves, particularly the mitral and aortic valves, can become scarred and function improperly.

Undiagnosed and/or untreated cases of syphilis can also affect the aortic valve. Surgical reconstruction may be necessary for correction.

Pathologic Valve Processes

Stenotic Valves. The valve can become so tightened and narrowed that its lumen is reduced to pencil-point size (stenosis of valve). The scarred valve opens upon cardiac contraction, but the reduced size of the lumen limits the amount of blood that can flow through it.

Insufficient Valves. As a result of the processes of scarring, fusion of the leaflets, and eventual calcification, the valves are no longer capable of closing properly. Blood regurgitates backwards, through the incompetent valve. A damaged heart valve may be either stenotic or insufficient or both. Aortic insufficiency is the most serious of the valvular diseases.

SURGICAL REPAIR OF VALVULAR HEART DISEASE

Closed Repair. The treatment of a stenotic valve used to be limited to closed repair known as commissurotomy. The surgeon felt, rather than saw the abnormal valve thus making this technic useful only to dilate fused valves.

Open Repair. Today the surgeon has the advantage of choosing to dilate, reconstruct (valvuloplasty), or replace the diseased valves. The open heart surgical technic is most frequently chosen. One reason for this is that the preoperative data indicating the degree of valve pliability may be in error and any attempt to correct the damage without replacement would be futile.

Also, the surgeon can control the localization of the obstruction, prevent calcified tissue or an undetected atrial thrombus from dislodging to the bloodstream, and replace the damaged valve.

Mortality has been gradually decreasing. All patients do better if the valvular lesion is corrected before serious secondary involvement of the myocardium and lungs occur.

ISCHEMIC HEART DISEASE

Atherosclerotic heart disease is the leading type of heart disease in the United States. Hence, extensive surgical research technics have been established in an effort to increase the amount of blood reaching the heart muscle and to redirect blood to the ischemic myocardial muscle.

Although more than 2000 revascularization operations are being performed yearly in the United States, this has been assessed as a mere fraction of the total considered necessary to insure adequate care for the countless sufferers from coronary heart disease (Russek).

Indirect Myocardial Revascularization by Closed Technic

A widely used technic to increase the supply of blood to the myocardium is the Vineberg procedure (see Fig. 55-2). The left internal mammary artery is isolated then directly implanted through a surgically created tunnel, into the wall of the left ventricle. The vast network of sinusoids in heart muscle provide open spaces through which the blood supply runs off into the ischemic portion.

Some authorities feel that any significant increase in circulation following a revascularization procedure takes at least nine months to establish. Although the procedures are relatively simple, as they may not require the use of the heart-lung machine, the patient may suffer a difficult postoperative course. The patient is still in a tenuous position, since the trauma of surgery adds to his myocardial workload. The pathology continues to exist until the collateral circulation is established.

Direct Open-Heart Approach

The atherosclerotic deposits or clots obstructing the coronary arteries are frequently confined to a relatively short section of artery. Arterial transplants of blood vessel graft, as well as artificial grafts, have been developed to correct this. The surgical approach is directed at opening the vessel, removing the plaque in the diseased intima (endarterectomy) or replacing the area with an artificial graft or homograft.

VENTRICULAR ANEURYSM

An aneursym of the ventricular wall is the most lethal complication among patients surviving the acute stage of a myocardial infarction (Effler). The frequency of ventricular aneurysms is increased with the presence of high blood pressure and overexertion following a myocardial infarction. The elasticity of the muscle wall is weakened and an outpouching occurs. The diseased area dilates and produces a ballooning of the wall.

Suturing off the weakened area may be required as an emergency treatment as the paradoxical motion of the myocardium may rupture the pouch. If possible the surgical correction is postponed until after the acute stage. The damaged tissue becomes necrotic and cannot tolerate the correction until scar tissue appears. This may take four to eight weeks.

TUMORS OF THE HEART

Primary tumors of the heart are rare. Tumors may be benign or malignant, however. The clinical course usually depends upon the type of tumor and its location within the cardiac system, that is, if it occupies space within the chambers of the heart or is contained within the muscle. Large tumors located on the left side of the heart may produce signs of mitral valve disease.

Surgery, using cardiopulmonary bypass, may be undertaken as cardiac failure may occur and the potential of embolization is often present. Benign tumors may stem from a base of a pedicle and their removal is usually uncomplicated. Malignant tumors are more difficult to remove and the patient's prognosis is extremely poor.

ATRIAL-SEPTAL DEFECT

An *atrial-septal defect* is a hole in the cardiac septum that separates the right and the left atria.

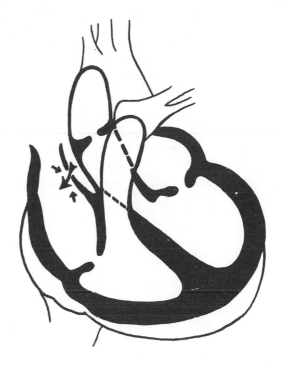

Fig. 55-3. Atrial-septal defect. The abnormal hole in the wall between the right and the left atria at first allows a left-to-right leakage of blood. Later, there may be a right-to-left shunting of blood.

Normally, the pressure within the heart is higher in the left atrium than in the right atrium; therefore, in a heart with an atrial-septal defect, blood flows from the left atrium through the hole to the right atrium. Because this blood already has been through the lungs, it is oxygenated. From the right atrium the blood goes to the right ventricle and back to the lungs. This inefficient functioning puts a strain on the right atrium, which enlarges in response to the extra load of blood. Over a period of time the right ventricle also enlarges and eventually so does the pulmonary artery. If the condition is not corrected, pulmonary vessel resistance may increase, and right-sided pulmonary hypertension occurs. The right ventricle becomes unable fully to empty itself of blood during each contraction because of the increased resistance in the pulmonary vessels. As a consequence, blood is backed up into the right atrium. When the pressure in this chamber grows higher than the pressure in the left atrium, there will be a reversal of the direction of leakage of blood. Now it will go from the right to the left through the defect in the wall. But the blood that goes from the right to the left has *not* been through the lungs; nevertheless it is sent on through the left atrium, the left ventricle and the aorta into the general circulation. Because the oxygen content of the blood being pumped from the left ventricle is lower than normal, the patient at this stage of the pathologic process can develop cyanosis.

Symptoms of right-sided failure include venous distention, ascites and peripheral edema as blood backs up through the venous system network. Patients also may experience bouts of palpitation and tachycardia fatigue and frequent respiratory infections.

Patients who have a small defect may be symptom-free. If the defect is repaired by surgery before a right-to-left shunt develops, there is an excellent chance of complete closure of the defect, followed by a lessening of the secondary pathologic cardiac changes. Usually, surgery is of the open-heart type.

TRAUMATIC HEART LESIONS

A nonpenetrating injury of the chest may include bruising of the heart. For example, a patient who has been crushed against the steering wheel of a car may have some bleeding of the muscle of the heart. Because the heart is in a closed sac, blood will accumulate in the pericardial space and cause tamponade of the heart.

Most often the patient will need to have the fluid in the pericardial sac aspirated. The physician inserts a long needle into the pericardial sac (pericardial paracentesis). During this procedure the patient is usually placed at approximately a 45 degree angle. One aspiration is sufficient in many patients. If the bleeding continues, an open thoracotomy may be indicated to control the bleeding site.

Take the pulse frequently of all patients with compressing chest injuries. There may be inhibition of the vagus nerve, with a slowing pulse, and perhaps cardiac standstill. Keep cardiac and respiratory resuscitation equipment handy and ready for instant use. The pain from a bruised heart may be masked by the pain from other chest injuries.

Direct trauma to the myocardium, such as a stab wound, also may cause leakage of blood into the pericardium; the tear in the pericardium often seals with a clot, while the tear in the myocardium continues to bleed. If the wound is large enough to cause immediate shock from hemorrhage, the patient will be taken to the operating room from the ambulance.

A small wound of the myocardium may lose blood to the pericardium over a longer period of time. Watch for shock and signs of cardiac compression, such as distention of the superficial veins of the neck, cyanosis, dyspnea, hypotension and a paradoxical pulse. Relaxation of the anal sphincter, with fecal incontinence, is a serious sign not found in other types of chest injuries, and it should be reported to the doctor immediately.

Sometimes traumatic tamponade of the heart is treated conservatively, with bed rest and careful observation of the patient. The increased pericardial pressure may serve to stop the leakage of blood and splint the wound. Larger tears will require suturing.

NURSING CARE OF THE CARDIAC SURGICAL PATIENT

The patient who is to have heart surgery is usually hospitalized for one or two weeks prior to the day of operation and is subjected to an extensive and exhausting medical evaluation. A thorough review of all his systems is imperative and a precise anatomic diagnosis of the lesion is desired.

The patient undergoing surgery will be cared for by a large team of people, including surgeons, cardiologists, radiologists, nurses, dieticians and technicians.

Psychological Impact

Disease and the prospect of surgery unavoidably arouse anxiety in most people. Some patients are concerned most about pain; others fear losing their independence.

The patient who is subjected to cardiac surgery may have additional stressful experiences because society has associated the heart with many emotions. The red "heart" shaped valentine suggests joy and love while the expression "my heart in my throat" indicates fear. "I speak from the heart" describes the tendency to believe the heart is the seat of the emotions.

Patients are more informed about medical practices than ever before. Unless physicians and nurses and other members of the cardiac surgical team are prepared to individualize their responses to patients, they may become quite threatened by sophisticated questioning. Few patients enter the hospital for heart surgery without preconceived ideas about the experience.

Preoperative Period

On admission, a nursing history is taken. The nursing care plan for each cardiac surgical patient has similarities but each will differ according to the individual patient. For example:

Mr. A. is a 37-year-old married office worker who states he has never been sick in his life. He goes to work daily, enjoys working around the house and playing with his five-year-old daughter. On weekends he leads a full social life and usually plays golf.

During a recent routine physical by the company doctor a heart murmur, associated with aortic insufficiency was discovered. Past history revealed episodes of light-headedness. A further and more extensive workup was done at his local hospital and revealed a severe case of aortic insufficiency. The patient was told he was "sitting on a time bomb" and needed corrective surgery immediately. The patient was overwhelmed, disbelieved the medical reports and decided to go to a large medical center for another opinion. The original diagnosis was confirmed and the patient is now awaiting surgery.

Across the hall in another bed is Mrs. B. She has had a heart condition since childhood with resulting limitation of physical activity. She attended a special school for the handicapped and was employed in an office for a short time before she married at the age of 20. She soon became pregnant, had a child, but then recalls going on "water and heart pills."

Her exercise tolerance became more and more restricted. She was unable to do much around the house and her family soon took over the cleaning and extra chores. Mrs. B. was medically evaluated at that time and the diagnosis of mitral stenosis was determined. Eight years ago a mitral commissurotomy was performed. The procedure gave her relief from her symptoms for some years. Recently she has begun to get progressively more symptomatic. The constant medical regime of low salt diet, diuretics and digoxin are no longer effective. She has an accumulation of fluid and sleeps upright, supported by three pillows. She is unable to do any housework and cannot walk more than one block.

She has been hospitalized for a possible double valve replacement to correct surgically mitral stenosis and insufficiency and aortic insufficiency.

We can expect the nursing care needs of these two patients to vary widely in many areas, such as the extent of physical care assistance, emotional readiness for the surgical experience, and preparation for postdischarge care.

Diagnosis

During the preoperative period, the patient undergoes many diagnostic studies that determine the capacity of his vital systems, such as cardial catheterization and pulmonary function tests.

The nurse has an obligation to prepare the patient for the test by explaining the importance of it and reviewing some aspects of it. Every effort should be made to ascertain the patient's understanding of the experience and correct any misgivings he may have.

When the procedure is completed the physician evaluates the data and discusses with the patient the findings and the recommended treatment. It is important for the nurse to know what the doctor has explained to the patient. The nurse can learn this either by being present at the explanation or by discussing with the doctor later what he told the patient.

Observations

There are many obvious symptoms that are associated with the pathology of cardiac disease. A patient's color and sitting position may indicate difficulty in breathing. Facial expression may be tense if chest pain exists. Signs of ankle edema may be noted if fluid retention occurs. Distention of the neck veins may indicate signs of increased venous pressure. Slurred speech, unsteady gait, facial paralysis may all be clues to previous embolic pathology. Clubbing of fingers can suggest congenital pathology.

The nurse observes the patient's symptoms when vital signs are taken. A weak, rapid, and/or irregular pulse beat may be felt and its effect on cardiac output reflected in the patient's color, level of alertness, degree of weakness, dyspnea or chest pain. A blood pressure recording can denote hypertension or a reduced cardiac output. The rapid rate of respirations may indicate oxygen need or anxiety.

Vital signs including rectal temperatures are taken and recorded twice daily. They are important as their values serve as a baseline postoperatively.

Environment

One advantage of the waiting period before surgery is to be more certain the patient is free from infection. Persons with cardiac disease and particularly those who have increased pulmonary pressure are prone to lung congestion and frequent upper respiratory tract infections. Patients should be kept away from other patients with contagious diseases. Family or friends with respiratory infections should be encouraged to telephone or send cards rather than visit. An antibiotic may be ordered preoperatively in an effort to prevent postoperative infections.

Preparation of Surgical Site

Careful preparation of the skin over the operative site is important. Bacteria are found on all levels of the skin. A wound infection introduced while performing a thoracotomy could be fatal. It can spread to the sternum, mediastinum and into the circulatory system.

Usually a soap containing hexachlorophene is ordered and scrubs are done twice a day for ten minutes during the week prior to surgery. The patient is taught the correct technic and may assume responsibility for the scrub if he is able to shower himself. The nurse gives whatever assistance is required to those patients whose weakness prevents self-activity. If proper technic is used, hexachlorophene forms a long-lasting bacteriostatic film on the skin and develops suppressive action which is cumulative with routine use. The extensive area to be covered includes front and back, from neck to knees. Special attention is paid to hairy areas, folds and ridges as the bacteria are more protected there. Note the condition of the skin and bring any irritations or allergies to the doctor's attention.

Fluid and Electrolyte Balance

Patients undergoing cardiac surgery are usually on a reduced sodium diet preoperatively. The hospital prepared low sodium diet may not be very palatable to the patient. As he becomes more preoccupied with the thought of surgery he may not feel like eating. Give careful attention to the patient's nutrition so that he receives the necessary carbohydrates, proteins and fats. These play an essential part in the postoperative healing process.

There is a critical need for determining and maintaining fluid and electrolyte balance since most cardiacs have some fluid retention preoperatively and are placed on diuretic therapy and daily weight. Change in weight indicates the daily fluid loss or gain and on the day of surgery serves as a baseline for calculating the volume of fluid needed in the heart-lung machine during surgery. Some diuretics tend to deplete the serum potassium level. Although they are usually discontinued prior to surgery a supplement of potassium may be necessary.

Educational Program

Preoperative preparation for surgery varies with each patient. The nurse begins by trying to ascertain what the patient already knows.

Preoperatively, the nurse should attempt to acquaint the patient and his family with the following:

• Explain the purpose of the intensive care unit, that is, to provide a central, well-equipped and well-staffed facility to provide around the clock care. Explain to the family the time and length of visiting hours.

• Explain the immediate physical preparation that takes place before the patient enters the operating room.

• Explain the function of each of the tubes that may be inserted just before surgery and removed several days afterward. There may be a cutdown, usually in the ankle or the arm (for hydration, drug administration and nutrition); a Foley catheter (for a more accurate measurement of urinary output); one or more chest tubes in the pleural space (for drainage and to help re-expand the lung); and perhaps a nasogastric tube (to prevent postoperative nausea).

• Tell the patient if he will wake from anesthesia with an endotracheal tube and a mechanical respirator which will ease the work load of the heart by making breathing easier for him. A nasal oxygen catheter may be inserted later.

• Have the patient practice deep breathing and coughing which he will use later postoperatively.

• Attempts should be directed toward making general statements rather than specific statements about when tubes are removed, days spent in the intensive care unit and duration of postoperative hospital time. Any deviation from a specific prediction can be interpreted by the patient as a complication or failure of the surgical correction.

• If it is anticipated that the patient will need oxygen administered by a positive-pressure apparatus, preoperative practice with it is indicated until the patient is familiar with how it works and how it feels.

• Before the operation teach the patient the exercises that he will need to employ afterward. Both before and after surgery the patient's condition may warrant only passive exercises.

• Assure the patient that analgesics are available for the control of postoperative pain.

• Most patients are placed on the serious list the evening prior to surgery. Explain this fact to the patient and his family. Also be sure the patient sees a member of the clergy if he so chooses.

POSTOPERATIVE NURSING CARE

Although it is often lifesaving, all cardiac surgery is a severe insult to the body. The patient requires expert care postoperatively. To make significant observations of the patient, the nurse needs to understand the nature of the condition, how the abnormality affected the patient's cardiac function and how the surgery corrected it.

The operating room nurse and the anesthesiologist can briefly provide additional information about the patient's operative experience and the type of procedure done. Any problems during the operative course such as a prolonged pump time, bleeding problems or serious cardiac arrhythmias will alert the intensive care nurses to potential problem areas.

She also needs to learn as much as she can about the equipment used in connection with this new surgery—defibrillators, pacemakers, positive-pressure respirators—know when they are used, how and why. It is up to the nurse to solve the space problem of placing the equipment around the patient, so that it is easily reached when it is needed and yet not in the way.

After the patient is transferred to bed, the nurse notes the rate and quality of the apical and radial pulses and takes the blood pressure, with an arm cuff, as ordered to watch for signs of hypo- or hypertension. Postoperative observations can now be more accurate as they are constantly monitored on a number of devices such as the cardiac monitor. Any change in the electrocardiogram can be noted immediately.

The patient may also have his arterial blood pressure recorded directly and continuously on another channel of the monitoring device. A small polyethylene catheter may have been left in place in the patient's femoral artery following the completion of the cardiopulmonary by-pass. The pressure in this artery is transmitted via the tip of the catheter through rigid plastic tubing to a pressure sensitive device called a transducer or strain gauge. The transducer converts the mechanical energy of pressure changes within the artery to electrical output. This is calibrated and equated to equivalent changes in millimeters of mercury which can be displayed on an oscilloscope or recorder. Small fluctuations in arterial blood pressure can be recorded and are obtainable at times when cuff blood pressures cannot be obtained. The arterial line also serves as a direct means by which blood for gas studies can be obtained.

A central venous pressure reading is also done frequently. This line may also be used for drawing the venous blood samples that are necessary. The normal reading of the central venous pressure in or near the right atrium is estimated around 0 to 4 cm. of water. The numerical value is not as important as the occurrence of a change either increasing or decreasing. Because venous pressure is sensitive to an increased pressure in the respiratory system the patient should be off the ventilator at the time of the recording.

An endotracheal tube or tracheotomy with mechanical ventilation, assisted or controlled, is used initially. A reduction in the patient's lung capacity may be due to the use of anesthetics or other drugs, a prolonged chronic disease process, pain or fear. The selection of the specific type of respirator to be used and the initial setting of the standard is the responsibility of the doctor.

To evaluate the effectiveness of the breathing device and the patient's response the nurse can use a respirometer. Blood gas studies are also done. The color of the patient's nail beds and lips may be a clue to inadequate ventilation. Restlessness, flaring of the nares and a poorly moving chest cage are causes for concern. The prepared nurse can listen to the patient's lungs and note the presence of congestion or diminished breathing sounds. The daily chest x-ray report is also valuable to the doctor.

The type of intravenous solutions that are ordered will depend upon the patient's need for nourishment as well as laboratory reports of serum electrolytes.

The doctor prescribes the total amount that will effect fluid replacement without overloading the cardiovascular system and the approximate hourly rate. This may need to be adjusted because overloading the circulatory system would place an added strain on the vital organs at this time. The same serious state would occur if the amount of fluid volume were decreased as it may contribute to diminished tissue perfusion. Central venous pressure measurement is used as a guide to fluid replacement.

The major reason for the insertion of the Foley catheter is to allow observation of renal function, and especially to enable the early detection of renal shutdown—particularly if a problem with the kidneys is anticipated (for example, if there has been prolonged hypotension). An hourly output of 30 ml. is adequate; output below this should be reported to the doctor. Urinary output upon arrival in the intensive care unit is often elevated due to the osmotic diuretics used when the patient is on bypass. This situation corrects itself in a few hours. The patient may also have hemoglobinuria since lysis of blood cells can occur during prolonged cardiopulmonary bypass.

If the Foley catheter is irrigated to prevent clogging be sure to deduct the irrigating solution from the total output. Specific gravity readings are taken for information about the patient's hydration and how well his kidneys are concentrating the urine.

Drainage from the nasogastric tube also is recorded. Proper functioning of the tube is important as any abdominal distention may exert pressure upon the diaphragm and move it upward, restricting respiratory movement.

The nurse keeps a close watch on the chest tubes, making sure they are not compressed, that there is no leak, and that the drainage flows through them. Unless the connecting tube lies lower than the wound, drainage will not take place. If drainage collects in the coils, the nurse changes the position of the tube so that the drainage flows into the collection bottle. Allowing drainage to remain stationary inside the tube may cause clotting and plugging of the tube. There is need for hourly observation of the amount of drainage. If the drainage is copious, record it more frequently. (This is done at the nurse's initiative; it does not require a doctor's order.) The amount of blood replacement is determined by the loss of blood volume through the tube and the amount of blood drawn for specimens. The usual loss of blood through the chest tube amounts to about 800 ml. in the first 24 hours.

In mitral stenosis there is stasis of blood in the left atrium, and clots may have formed. Any clots observed during surgery are removed, but perhaps one escaped into the general circulation. There is no longer stasis of blood in the left atrium, and the free-flowing blood may push a clot along. Watch for symptoms of emboli in the legs, especially after a commissurotomy. Embolization likewise is a danger after atrial fibrillation, which also allows blood to stay relatively still in the atrium, so that clots may form. After open heart surgery there is danger of air emboli affecting the brain. Neurologic symptoms, such as slurred speech, distortion of facial muscles or the tongue, and hemiparesis, may occur after air or a blood embolus to the brain. Dyspnea, cough, and expectoration of bloody sputum may indicate pulmonary embolism. An embolus to the spleen may cause sudden left flank pain, whereas an embolus to a kidney may result in hematuria and flank pain.

During the early postoperative period the nurse is aware of the patient's color, his pulse and respirations, the rhythm of his heartbeat, his position, the state of his dressing, his blood pressure, the patency of the tubes leaving his body and the steady drip of the infusions and transfusion. She must notice any changes immediately. A sudden but slight drop in blood pressure, central venous pressure, or hourly urine output may suggest a reduced cardiac output. A respiratory rate increase can result from an obstruction such as a mucous plug, improper positioning, splinting from incisional pain or circulatory insufficiency.

Psychological Considerations

If the patient has been on the heart-lung machine, the lightest possible anesthesia was given, and because hypothermia facilitates anesthesia, the patient usually is conscious when he comes to the recovery unit.

As soon as possible he should be told that the surgery is over. He may need to hear this several times. He may or may not be aware of the totality of the room, the people in it and the whole situation. He is aware of his discomfort and the one person with whom he attempts to speak. If the patient complains of pain and the discomfort is not alleviated by positioning and other nursing measures, narcotics are given. The patient's vital signs and the cardiac monitor are checked before a drug is administered and periodically during the time of its effect. The dosage of narcotics given to patients who have had cardiac surgery is frequently less than average because of the danger of respiratory depression. Narcotics are given—only for pain as restlessness is often an indication of hypoxemia.

Some patients develop a psychotic-like reaction after cardiovascular surgery. They are disoriented and have hallucinations. These patients need protection with side rails and the reassurance of a human, caring presence. The cause of this reaction is not known. It may be related to some transient cerebral pathology induced by the surgery, the anesthesia, the drug therapy, or the

ICV environment. The reaction is usually temporary.

Early mobility of patients is encouraged to prevent circulatory stasis and prevent the formation of thrombi. Active leg exercises are begun on the operative day when the patient's position is changed when possible.

GENERAL PROGRESSION OF PATIENT CARE

As the patient's condition stabilizes the respirator is discontinued and the endotracheal tube is removed—usually in 24 to 48 hours. The patient may then be started on nasal oxygen and will be encouraged to use a Bennett or some other intermittent positive pressure respirator for deep breathing and coughing. The Levin tube is usually removed at the same time. The Foley catheter, one intravenous line, the central venous pressure line and the arterial blood pressure line are all discontinued about a day later. The chest tubes may also be removed on the second or third postoperative day depending upon the amount of drainage that has been noted. If the patient has an artificial cardiac valve he is started on anticoagulants at this time. They are not started earlier because additional bleeding from the chest may occur. Digitalis preparations may be restarted. Antibiotics are continued intravenously for another four or five days and then if needed are given orally.

The patient's vital signs are taken every two hours at this stage and he begins progressively to ambulate. A restricted sodium liquid diet is ordered after the endotracheal tube is removed.

The patient who has had an endotracheal tube in place for a day or so will complain of a sore throat and excessive thirst for a few days after it is removed. If the patient is on restricted fluids he will need help in remembering and abiding by this regime. But, careful and consistent explanations from the doctors and nurse plus involving the patient in recording his intake and output gives the patient a chance to participate in his regime, distribute his allotment with some personal choice and understand the reasons for it.

As the patient's course continues to progress he begins to see signs of improvement (for example, ambulation) yet he is still feeling sick and remains in a potentially critical phase. While the need for constant observation and evaluation by the nurse is still important, she must attempt to prepare him for his return to a general medical-surgical unit within the next few days.

The nurse begins to encourage him gradually to become more independent and let him begin to regain assurance in doing things for himself. Gentle encouragement accompanied by support as he tries each new activity can help the patient to pass through the period of extreme dependence on staff to greater independence.

Continuing Care

While the patient is encouraged to progress at his own rate, careful assessment should be made of the patient's response to activity and his attitude towards it.

The expectation of what will happen after surgery can be important in the patient's postoperative adjustment. If he expected a complete cure and has had only partial relief of his symptoms, he may be resentful, and he may refuse to adhere to his low sodium diet or to the restrictions on his activities.

These patient reactions are not unusual. Help the patient to identify what is troubling him and to express what he feels. His family may (or may not) be a comfort to him; perhaps you can perceive this.

The amount of activity the patient can safely tolerate will be determined by the doctor. It will be based upon the severity of his illness preoperatively as well as the nature of his operative procedure and the postoperative course.

It is important to collaborate with the physician in helping the family learn what activities the patient can safely assume after discharge. Often families who have experienced a lifetime of caring both physically and mentally for a patient will try to hold him back as they themselves cannot change their role from one which requires the patient to be dependent on them, or they may expect him to resume a full program of activities. He may or may not be able to do so.

If a patient needs domestic help at home arrangements can be sought with the help of social service. If health supervision and some nursing care are to be given a visiting nurse referral can be initiated several days prior to discharge so that there are no gaps in continuity of care.

Some patients are allowed to return to work six to twelve weeks postoperatively. Others have a more prolonged postoperative course. Most patients can, however, return to a more productive and satisfying way of life.

REFERENCES AND BIBLIOGRAPHY

ALEXANDER, E., et al.: *Care of the Patient in Surgery—Including Techniques,* ed. 4, St. Louis, Mosby, 1967.

Artificial Parts for the Heart and Blood Vessels, Washington, D.C., U.S. Department of Health, Education and Welfare, Public Health Service, 1968.

BELLING, D.: Complications after open heart surgery, *Nurs. Clin. N. Am.* 4:123, March, 1969.

BLACHER, R.: Open-heart surgery patients. 3. Psychological aspects, *RN* 33:51, April, 1970.

Cardiovascular Surgery, Washington, D.C., U.S. Department of Health, Education and Welfare, Public Health Service Publication No. 1701, 1968.

COLEMAN, D.: Surgical alleviation of coronary artery disease, *Am. J. Nurs.* 68:763, April, 1968.

Defusing a coronary—with gas, *Life* 68:75, April, 1970.

EFFLER, D.: Surgery for coronary disease, *Sci. Am.* 219:36, October, 1968.

FERNANDEZ, P.: The insertion of cardiac implants and the nursing care problems involved, *Nurs. Clin. N. Am.* 2:559, September, 1967.

FRIEDBERG, C.: *Diseases of the Heart,* Philadelphia, Saunders, 1966.

ISLER, C.: Open-heart surgery patients. 2. Pre- and post-op nursing care, *RN* 33:44, April, 1970.

JAMES, E.: The nursing care of the open heart patient, *Nurs. Clin. N. Am.* 2:543, September, 1969.

JARVIS, D.: Following open heart surgery, *Am. J. Nurs.* 70:2591, December, 1970.

LAZARUS, R., and WAGENS, H.: Prevention of psychosis following open-heart surgery, *Am. J. Psych.* 124:1190, March, 1968.

LITWAK, R.: Open-heart surgery patients. 1. The surgery, *RN* 33:38, April, 1970.

MACLEAN, D., and FOWLER, E.: Heart transplant; early postoperative care, *Am. J. Nurs.* 68:2124, October, 1968.

Optimal Resources for Cardiac Surgery, Report of Intersociety Commission for Heart Disease Resources, *Circulation* XLIV:A221, September, 1971.

PANSEGRAU, D., et al.: The management of patients with prosthetic heart valves, *Med. Clin. N. Am.* 52:1133, September, 1967.

PITORAK, E.: Open-ended care for the open-heart patient, *Am. J. Nurs.* 67:1452, July, 1967.

POWERS, M., and STORLIE, F.: The apprehensive patient, *Am. J. Nurs.* 67:58, January, 1967.

ROCOZ, B.: Nursing care of the cardiac surgery patient, *Nurs. Clin. N. Am.* 4:631, December, 1969.

The Patient in Renal Failure

56

Etiology • Prevention • Diagnosis, Symptoms, and Pathology
Prognosis and Objectives of Treatment • Treatment and Nursing
Care • Substitutes for Kidney Function • Renal Transplantation

Renal failure, acute or chronic, is a serious inability of the kidneys to carry out the normal functions necessary to maintain fluid and electrolyte balance and to eliminate the end products of metabolism from the body. When kidney function is insufficient and such products as urea, other nonprotein nitrogens, creatinine, and uric acid accumulate in the blood, a state of *azotemia* is present. If unabated, the patient experiences the signs and symptoms of *uremia,* such as lethargy, irritability, and anorexia in the early stage, and progressively more ominous ones as uremia advances.

Fifty thousand people in the United States die from renal failure (uremia) each year. Despite the national "hoopla" about the use of the artificial kidney (hemodialysis) for end stage renal disease, only about 2,500 patients received this type of treatment in 1969 (Hemodialysis—some facts and figures, *Am. J. Nurs.* 70:73). Thus the vast majority of these patients receive conservative treatment; many are in the older age group. The crux of therapy is nursing support of the patient and family through an episode of renal failure which can be completely reversible, an acute death-terminating crisis, or through the many crises precipitated by the physical, emotional, and social changes the patient with progressive renal failure undergoes.

ETIOLOGY

Some conditions markedly decrease the supply of blood to the kidneys, such as shock or thrombosis of the arteries supplying the kidneys. If the ischemia is not immediately remedied, renal failure and uremia can result.

The problem may be within the kidney itself as in acute renal tubular necrosis (lower nephron nephrosis) due, for example, to chemical poisoning from barbiturates, bichloride of mercury, or carbon tetrachloride; or due to transfusion with incompatible blood. In chronic glomerulonephritis and polycystic disease, progressively more nephrons are destroyed which can result in chronic renal insufficiency as well as acute shutdown.

Postrenal problems such as obstruction of the lower urinary tract can cause damage to the kidney parenchyma if not promptly treated.

PREVENTION

Renal failure occurs more frequently when body fluid reserves are depleted. Nurses contribute to its prevention by planning with hospitalized patients a system of oral fluid intake, particularly for those patients who may be too old, too weak, disinterested, or otherwise unable to reach for the water pitcher on the bedside stand.

Lowered cardiac output due to such conditions as cardiac arrhythmias, anaphylactic shock, or accidental blood loss compromises renal blood flow. Careful nursing observation of the patient and prompt reporting of lowered blood pressure to the physician assists him in initiating a course of action which minimizes the threat of renal damage.

The nurse in the teaching role can encourage patients with possible streptococcal infection to seek medical attention promptly to reduce the risk of glomerulonephritis. Alerting the public to the importance of keeping drugs where they cannot be accidentally ingested is important, as some drugs are nephrotoxic. Nurses and physicians, as well as ancillary personnel, must take utmost care to prevent the transfusion of incompatible blood.

DIAGNOSIS, SYMPTOMS, AND PATHOLOGY

Although uremia sometimes has a sudden onset with pronounced initial symptoms, it usually starts so slowly that it is not recognized immediately. The early symptoms may be no more than headaches, easy fatigability, vague gastrointestinal complaints, irritability, and malaise. The patient just does not feel right, and active life becomes increasingly difficult for him.

Urine

Oliguria, or decrease in normal urinary output may be present. However, the quantity of urine can be normal or even increased in volume when the kidneys are failing, but the specific gravity of the urine will be low since waste products appear in less than normal concentration. Total anuria is more indicative of obstruction of the urinary tract (Merrill).

Blood

Examination of the blood may show a gradual increase in the blood urea nitrogen (BUN.) since the kidney's ability to excrete urea, the end product of protein metabolism, is impaired. The BUN. may become markedly elevated before any other symptoms are recognized. Mental clouding, confusion, and disorientation can accompany a rising BUN.

As the condition progresses, more and more products of metabolism—such as creatinine, uric acid, and sulfates—are retained in the blood, causing headaches and nausea. Acidosis appears. Nausea and vomiting, thirst and air hunger are symptoms of acidosis. The deep and rapid respirations are indicative of a respiratory attempt to compensate for the metabolic acidosis.

So much sodium and water may be lost that the patient becomes dehydrated. Anorexia and vomiting intensify the losses. Muscular weakness, more anorexia and overall debility characterize hyponatremia (deficient blood sodium). More rarely, depending on the original pathology causing the uremia, the patient is edematous instead of dehydrated.

In uremia, the blood level of calcium frequently is low because calcium is not reabsorbed in sufficient quantity from the glomerular filtrate.

Early signs of calcium deficiency are numbness and tingling of the fingertips and toes, nose and ears. This can progress to symptoms of tetany, ranging from slight twitching to convulsions. Potassium retention is one of the most critical problems since potassium intoxication causes cardiac failure and pulmonary edema. The nurse observes the patient for excessive coughing, shortness of breath, respiratory wheezing or rales. Severe anemia is a common symptom of advancing renal failure.

Pressure. Hypertension commonly accompanies renal failure. Dimness or blurring of vision, and spots before the eyes may be the result of retinal hemorrhages caused by the hypertension.

Appearance and Skin

The patient with renal insufficiency is usually pale and he may have edema about the eyes and pitting edema of the ankles.

The patient may complain of torturing pruritus (itching of the skin). Since the skin also serves an excretory function, "uremic frost" (a white film composed of waste products excreted by the skin instead of the kidneys) may become visible, especially in dark-skinned patients.

Halitosis is generally marked and ulceration of the oral mucosa due to increased capillary fragility is common. The patient may have a generalized body odor suggestive of urine.

Cerebration

Though some patients remain mentally alert for a long period of time considering their electrolyte imbalance, mental processes are progressively slowed. There may be dizziness and irritability. Behavior can be totally unpredictable and even become psychotic. Cerebral edema can cause projectile vomiting, convulsions and coma.

Gastrointestinal

Ulceration and bleeding of the gastrointestinal tract is a fairly common component of renal failure. The mucous membranes of the mouth often bleed and blood may be found in the feces. Hematemesis (vomiting of blood) is a frequent precursor of death in the patient with uremia. Relentless hiccoughing can also be present.

PROGNOSIS AND OBJECTIVES OF TREATMENT

If the primary cause can be removed or quickly remedied, such as in acute renal tubular necrosis (lower nephron nephrosis) or urinary tract obstruction, renal failure is reversible in about 80 per cent of such patients. The treatment objective is to keep the patient alive and free from complications during the two or three weeks required for regeneration of the damaged epithelium of the renal tubules. Adequate maintenance usually results in diuresis (a 24-hour urine volume of 1000 ml.) during the second week and kidney function gradually returns to normal over a period of several weeks.

Chronic renal diseases such as glomerular nephritis, nephrosis, pyelonephritis and polycystic kidneys progress to deterioration of the nephron involving either the glomeruli or the tubules or both and may finally result in acute renal failure. The onset of oliguria or anuria is ominous. Remissions can occur, however. One objective of treatment is to avoid conditions that increase the workload of the kidneys through control of diet, activity, obesity, and the avoidance of infection. Another is to treat the various symptoms of the uremia itself.

A more aggressive approach is to prevent uremia in acute and chronic renal failure by substitution for kidney function through the use of such modes of therapy as ion exchange resins, hemodialysis (artificial kidney) or peritoneal dialysis.

TREATMENT AND NURSING CARE

General. Report promptly any decrease in urinary output below 500 ml. in a 24-hour period. Remain alert for any symptoms that may indicate renal shutdown or beginning uremia. When the patient who is usually cheerful and pleasant becomes irritable and complains of a headache, it may not be because he has had a disagreeable visit with his family or has experienced some other unpleasant episode. The reverse may be true; his interpersonal relations may suffer because his BUN is elevated.

The patient with uremia is often very ill and may even be comatose. The episodes are long and taxing to both the patient and his family. Encourage members of his family to participate in his care. (For instance, an unpalatable diet fed by a patient's wife may not seem to be quite so depressing.) When the patient is irritable, help the family to understand that his anger is not necessarily directed at them, but that it is rather the result of the accumulated chemicals in his bloodstream.

Fluid Intake. The physician determines how much fluid the patient can have based on exact measurements of intake and output via all routes.

In severe shutdown the patient may be limited to as little as 400 ml. intravenously (artfully regulated to last the 24 hours) and 100 ml. of oral fluid. Some days (depending on the output), tea, ginger ale or water are given with as much sugar or Coca Cola syrup (to increase the caloric intake) as the patient can tolerate. Sucking glucose ice chips made by freezing 20 to 50 per cent glucose in an ice tray can help with the problem of thirst while providing needed calories. Ice chips can extend a small amount of fluid over 24 hours. To count intake accurately the nurse can measure in a graduate the same amount of ice which has been allowed to melt.

Unfortunately most fruit juices contain potassium and since the failing kidney cannot excrete excess potassium, fruit juices are not permitted. Sucking on "sour balls" can increase the carbohydrate intake without adding potassium.

Diet. In severe failure, the demand on the kidneys for the excretion of protein end products is limited by restricting protein foods. Feedings should be spaced so that there are no long periods of fasting. If the patient awakens during the night, for instance, he should be given a high carbohydrate snack or drink.

If the diet is limited to carbohydrate and fat, as for severe kidney shutdown, palatability becomes a problem. A well-chilled equal part mixture of Karo syrup and ginger ale with a drop or two of lemon juice provides a high carbohydrate intake which may be partially tolerated. Patients with edema have severe restriction of their sodium intake.

If the patient with acute renal failure reaches the diuretic phase, nausea and vomiting subside after a few days and appetite returns. Urinary output can be quite large in volume because the patient loses surplus sodium and water previously present as edema. Excess sodium loss may need to be compensated for by encouraging the patient to eat salty foods. On the other hand, because sodium and water balance is unstable, sodium restriction is continued if edema is present. Daily body weight is used as a guide. Do not use salt substitutes containing potassium for seasoning. Rum, vinegar, mint, cloves, brown sugar, or cinnamon probably will be allowed.

Diet is usually low in protein and high in calories until renal function returns to normal.

If the kidneys do not recover and the patient is in a state of chronic renal failure, fluids are forced providing that edema does not develop or urinary output decrease. Forced fluids are necessary because of the kidneys' inability to concentrate solid wastes and more fluid is needed to excrete them. Some physicians recommend diets low in salt and protein to lessen the work of the kidneys already low in reserve. Others believe that the patient should have a liberal choice of foods that appeal to him with a basic balanced diet.

Activity. In the acute stage metabolic demands are kept to a minimum by restricting activity to those measures necessary for preventing the hazards of bed rest. Chronic uremic patients in acute crises may have peripheral neuropathy and require considerable assistance from the nurse or physical therapist who provide passive, then active, assistive exercise to maintain function. Rapid progressive ambulation with the preservation of patient safety is the goal.

Itching. Pruritus can occur with or without frost. Uremic frost can be removed with a weak solution of vinegar (2 tablespoons to a pint of water). The doctor may order an anesthetic ointment to relieve the itching. Cleanliness helps, too: perhaps this patient can have two baths instead of one a day. Although the skin is not efficient for the disposal of such waste chemicals as uric acid, it is all that the body has available when the kidneys are not functioning, and a clean skin is always more efficient and more comfortable.

Anemia, secondary to hematopoietic depression, is common, and may be treated by blood transfusion to maintain the hematocrit above 25. Hematinic drugs are of little value. The anemia contributes to the general weakness and lethargy of the chronic uremic patient.

Prevention of Infection. Infectious processes increase protein catabolism and by increasing the workload of the kidneys hasten the onset or severity of uremia. Pulmonary complications are the most frequent cause of morbidity and mortality in acute renal failure (Muehrcke).

Frequent deep breathing, turning and coughing are indicated.

Patient and Family Support. Many patients with acute renal failure develop it as a complication after some major medical or surgical problem. Thus they have their initial problem plus a serious setback to deal with. Patients with chronic renal insufficiency who develop acute renal failure often are aware that they are approaching end-stage renal disease. For both patient and his close associates, fear of death is present. Added to this is the fear of losing control as the build-up of waste products in the blood affects the sensorium, causing the patient to become restless, confused, belligerent, disoriented, psychotic, or comatose. The nursing staff by their organization and manner can convey to the patient and his associates that they can be depended upon to keep the situation under control even though the patient may not be in control of himself.

SUBSTITUTES FOR KIDNEY FUNCTION

Renal Dialysis (Extracorporeal Hemodialysis)

Hemodialysis is a process designed to bring blood into contact with a semipermeable membrane through which diffusion takes place. By "diffusion" is meant the spontaneous movement of solutes and solvent from areas of high concentration to areas of low concentration until a state of equilibrium is established. Substances which should be removed from the patient's blood, such as urea and creatinine and dangerously high levels of potassium are removed because these are all absent from the dialysate fluid. They move from the patient's blood through the semipermeable membrane to the dialysate fluid. Hemodialysis also permits the replacement of substances that may be low in the blood and present in the dialysate: for example, bicarbonate and calcium.

Technic (Extracorporeal Hemodialysis)

In the many types of artificial kidneys (also called dialyzers) the basic components are cellophane tubing (coil) and dialysate fluid. The cellophane tubing acts as the semipermeable membrane. The dialysate fluid is similar to the electrolyte composition of normal *human plasma.* The composition is ordered by the physician and changed as needed. The patient's blood is removed from an artery, pumped through the coil, and returned to a vein. Water and ions are able to pass through the walls of the membrane, but protein and red blood cells cannot.

Heparin is administered to prevent blood from clotting in the coil. To minimize the risk of systemic bleeding, regional heparinization may be used. This consists of infusing heparin into the blood as the blood passes from patient to coil and protamine sulfate as the blood returns to the patient, to neutralize the heparin. Frequent clotting times are done.

Blood samples taken pre- and postdialysis for urea, creatinine, sodium, potassium, chlorides, CO_2, and hematocrit are indicators of the efficiency of dialysis.

External Arteriovenous Shunt. When a patient is to be hemodialyzed, cannulas (the shunt) are placed surgically in an extremity where blood vessels are available. This allows for repeated treatments without having to cut down on vessels each time. Between treatments, the cannula ends are connected by an external teflon joint and blood is shunted between the artery and vein. To attach the patient to the artificial kidney the joint is opened and the arterial cannula is attached to the inflow tubing of the coil; the venous cannula is attached to the outflow tubing. When the treatment is finished, the joint is reconnected and blood flows through the shunt. (See Fig. 56-1.)

Two cannula clamps (or rubber tipped hemostats) should be close by at all times for use in the event that the cannulas disconnect at the teflon joint.

Internal Arteriovenous Shunt. Instead of an external shunt, some patients on permanent dialysis may have an arteriovenous fistula (internal shunt) formed by way of a surgical anastomosis of an artery and vein lying in close proximity. The vein enlarges and assumes the characteristics of an artery. Venipuncture is performed in a proximal site and is used for the outflow from the coil. A distal needle puncture is used for the inflow to the coil. When dialysis is completed, the needles are removed and pressure dressings applied for several hours. Blood pressures and blood samples should not be taken in the cannulated extremity.

Preparation of Patient for Hemodialysis

The confused, apprehensive uremic patient can become more so when he encounters new faces, new surroundings and new equipment. The seemingly unconscious patient may still be able to hear and attempts should be made to communicate with him.

If the situation is very critical, there may be little time afforded the patient to ask questions or otherwise review the explanation. The dialysis nurse should be informed regarding what explanation was given to the patient and his response so that she can more accurately assess the patient's need for continued support.

If the situation is not too emergent, the nurse's explanation can be enhanced by taking the patient to the dialysis room so that he can see the equipment the nurse describes and observe and talk to other patients as well. The more the patient understands, the less bewildered he is and this reduces his feelings of helplessness. He recognizes that his well-being, his very life, depends upon the machinery, its correct operation and the performance of the dialysis team.

The patient comes to the dialysis room in bed or ambulatory depending on his clinical condition. He need not be fasting. In the dialysis room, emergency equipment and medications are readily available.

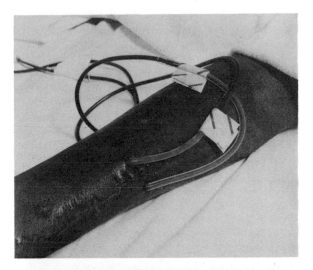

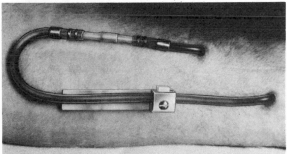

FIG. 56-1. (*Top*) Recently performed arteriovenous shunt of patient undergoing hemodialysis. (*Bottom*) Arteriovenous shunt between periods of use in hemodialysis. (Seattle Artificial Kidney Supply Company, Seattle, Wash.)

A pre- and postdialysis weight is important. A certain weight loss occurs with dialysis, depending upon blood flow rate and duration of dialysis. Fluid removal may be undesirable and a postdialysis weight enables the physician to order fluid replacement if necessary.

Nursing Care During Hemodialysis

Nursing care requirements vary with each patient. The physical needs of chronic dialysis patients are minimal, but there is much opportunity for the professional nurse to function as a teacher or counselor. Nursing measures for the acutely ill patients depend on what their basic medical or surgical condition was as well as the extent of their renal failure, and may include: frequent suctioning of airway to prevent aspiration; tracheostomy care; eye care; skin care for incontinence; cardiac and respiratory monitoring;

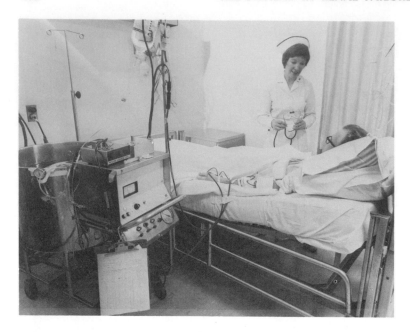

Fig. 56-2. Nurse talks with hospitalized patient while observing his response to hemodialysis. (The New York Hospital, Cornell University Medical Center, New York, N.Y.)

gastric and chest drainage; intravenous feeding; and oxygen therapy.

Some important considerations for all patients are:

Support. During the procedure, especially if it is being done for the first time, a primary aspect of nursing is being there to explain, reassure, and respond to the patient humanly. Once procedures are learned well, the nurse can focus more on the person who is the patient.

Blood Pressure and Pulse. These are recorded predialysis, frequently at the start of dialysis, and depending on the clinical condition of the patient. The dialyzer is adjusted according to the patient's vital signs and symptoms. Arrhythmias may result from potassium removal. Low blood pressure may result from excess fluid removal or a leak in the dialysis circuit.

Positioning. The patient's position should be changed frequently as dialysis is a lengthy procedure. The length of the treatment depends on the condition of the patient as well as the type of dialyzer and can vary from 4 to 8 hours two to three times per week. The patient may be turned, may sit up on the edge of the bed, may keep his head lowered or raised—so long as the dialysis tubing is not kinked or unnecessary tension applied to it. A reclining chair can also be used. A drop in blood pressure may require a flat positioning of the bed temporarily.

Prevention of Complications. Preventive measures and physical care are not interrupted be-cause of dialysis. Diversion and socialization to the extent possible lessen boredom.

Mentation. An unconscious patient may become aware and coherent during dialysis, or vice versa. Restlessness frequently occurs. Any change in the mental status of the patient should be reported to the doctor.

Hemorrhage. Because of the administration of heparin, regionally or systemically, frequent observations should be made for bleeding, including inspection of dressings, stool specimens and gastric drainage. Epistaxis and bleeding from gums are not uncommon.

Complications. Headache, muscle cramps, nausea and vomiting, fever, diaphoresis, anxiety and/or chest pain may reflect serious complications occurring during hemodialysis.

Mechanical Problems. Membrane ruptures, clotting in coil or shunt, and reduced blood flow through the dialyzer may necessitate termination of hemodialysis. The nurse needs to be so well prepared technically that should such problems arise, she can promptly identify them, take the precise corrective steps, and promptly also attend to the patient's response. Breaking or other mishaps with this equipment, while relatively routine to the nurse, can be very frightening to the patient, whose life depends on it. The difficulty and the remedial steps are explained to the patient and particular effort is made to remain with the patient more frequently right after the occurrence. Although this supportive action is crucial for all patients, these events are viewed as critical incidents in learning for the patient and relative in a training program for home dialysis who may face a similar situation in the absence of professional help.

Teaching and Counseling. A patient with end-stage renal disease anticipating chronic dialysis or renal transplant needs a nurse who recognizes that listening to his expression of thoughts and feelings as he contemplates his future is an important dimension of the nursing role. Some trials and tribulations for patient and family in a home dialysis training program are described in an interesting article by Schlotter.

Care After Hemodialysis

Vital signs are taken frequently. The nurse continues to observe the patient for bleeding. No intramuscular injections are given for two to four hours postdialysis because, due to the administration of heparin, bleeding may occur at the injection site. Daily care is given to the external shunt and it is observed for patency.

Fluid and dietary restrictions are regulated according to the degree of recovery of renal function and the patient's clinical condition.

Chronic dialysis patients continue on fluid restrictions based on urinary output. The potassium and sodium content of the diet may be restricted. A normal protein diet may be allowed.

The long-term treatment of patients with end-stage renal disease by hemodialysis is not only a medical, nursing, and family problem. The large number of patients, the high monetary cost, the limited number of specialized facilities and personnel make this a social and ethical problem for the community and the nation.

Peritoneal Dialysis

The simplicity of peritoneal dialysis and the availability of the equipment for this procedure are in sharp contrast to the complexity of the technic and equipment used in extracorporeal hemodialysis. The latter is limited to hospitals that have the equipment and the personnel trained to use it; peritoneal dialysis can be performed in any hospital. Peritoneal dialysis, however, provides only a fraction of the plasma clearance that the artificial kidney can provide.

Procedure

In peritoneal dialysis, a bathing solution (dialysate) is made to flow into and out of the peri-

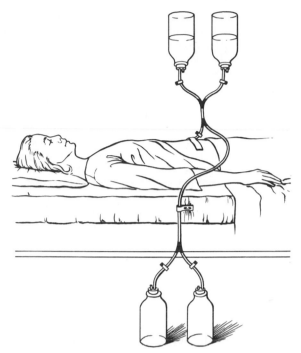

Fig. 56-3. Peritoneal dialysis. After the solution flows into the patient it is allowed to remain in situ for the period of time ordered by the physician. During this time, dialysis takes place. Then the clamps on the lower bottles are opened and the solution is drained off.

toneal cavity. The peritonium acts as the semipermeable membrane. The dialysate causes urea, electrolytes and dialyzable poisons to pass through the peritoneum and carries them out of the body.

The patient is weighed, the bladder emptied and a small incision is made in the midline of the abdomen. A catheter with many perforations is inserted by the physician so that the end lies free in the peritoneal cavity. The catheter is sutured in place and a dressing applied. Blood pressure, pulse and respirations are recorded.

The bottles of dialysate are set up and their administration tubing (inflow tube) is attached to the catheter in the patient. The outflow tubing leading to a closed drainage system is clamped off.

Instillation Period. Two liters of dialysate should run into the peritoneal cavity in 10 to 15 minutes by gravity. If the drip is slow, the doctor may need to reposition the catheter. When the bottles are empty, but the tubing is still filled with dialysate to prevent entrance of air, the inflow tube should be clamped. The nurse records instillation time, the volume and type of dialysate, plus any medications added.

Equilibration Period. The solution is left in the abdomen the length of time ordered by the physician (usually 30–35 minutes).

Drainage Period. The outflow tube is unclamped and the dialysate drains into a closed sterile drainage system. Gravity drainage, facilitated by raising bed-height or changing the patient's position, should take no longer than 10 to 15 minutes. If it does, the doctor may need to irrigate the catheter to remove plugs, or he may need to reposition or replace the catheter.

The time of the start and finish of the drainage period should be recorded. Note should be taken of the appearance of the fluid removed. It may be blood-tinged because of bleeding due to heparin, or cloudy from protein loss. The differences between the volume instilled and the volume removed is recorded. The physician should be notified of excessive fluid retained or removed from the patient ($\pm$ 500 ml.).

Commercially manufactured automatic cycling machines for peritoneal dialysis are available. A pumping system delivers the dialysate to the patient from a large reservoir. The patient's response is observed, particularly pain in the outflow cycle. Volume and timing are set and adjusted by the physician.

The number of exchanges performed in peritoneal dialysis is ordered by the doctor. When dialysis is completed, the doctor removes the catheter and applies a dry sterile dressing. A purse string suture may be necessary. A bacteriologic culture is obtained from the catheter tip as well as from the last dialysate drained. A postdialysis weight is obtained.

Several prostheses are available which provide ready access to the peritoneal cavity. These can be plugged when not in use.

Observations

Blood pressure and pulse are taken frequently, usually at the end of each drainage period. A drop in blood pressure and increased pulse rate may occur when fluid removal is too rapid, especially when the dialysate has a high concentration of dextrose. The patient may need to be weighed after completion of drainage and before starting another exchange, if the doctor so orders. Pain in the left shoulder may be due to diaphragmatic irritation caused by the high concentration of dextrose when present in the dialysate.

Abdominal pain present at the end of the drainage period may be relieved by the next instillation or by procaine.

The procedure is tedious and the patient may become bored and restless. It is not sufficient for the nurse to appear only when she has some task to do such as hanging bottles or measuring drainage. This conveys to the patient that the equipment is the major concern, not him, though he may recognize too that the technical aspects are important. Listening to the patient's reactions, providing physical comfort measures, or offering some tolerable diversion assists the pa-

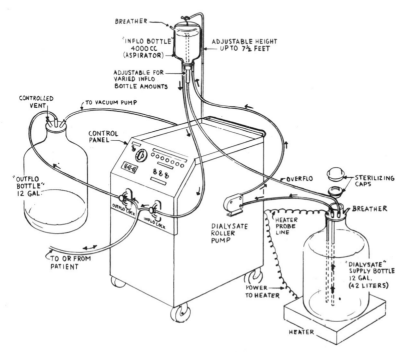

Fig. 56-4. Automatic administration equipment for peritoneal dialysis. (Seattle Artificial Kidney Supply Company, Seattle, Wash.)

tient through the procedure. A relative may sit quietly by or sedation may be given.

The patient's position should be changed frequently and individual supportive nursing measures carried out. The patient undergoing peritoneal dialysis may eat and drink as permitted. His state of mentation should be observed.

Peritonitis (chemical or bacterial) is a major complication of peritoneal dialysis.

RENAL TRANSPLANTATION

In some patients with chronic, progressive renal disease (end-stage renal disease) that threatens life from kidney failure, a kidney transplant may be considered. This procedure, though still within the realm of research, is fast becoming less so. These patients are usually sent to special transplant units for surgery and treatment.

REFERENCES AND BIBLIOGRAPHY

BOIS, M., et al.: Nursing care of patients having kidney transplants, Am. J. Nurs. 68:1238, June, 1968.

CUMMINGS, J.: Hemodialysis—The pressures and how patients respond, Am. J. Nurs. 70:70, January, 1970.

FELIX, K.: Total patient care—the team approach to (renal) transplantation, Nurs. Clin. N. Am. 4:451, September, 1969.

Hemodialysis—some facts and figures, Am. J. Nurs. 70:73, January, 1970.

HINCKLEY, B.: The changing role of the dialysis nurse, Nurs. Clin. N. Am. 4:395, September, 1969.

JUZWIAK, M.: Nursing the kidney-transplant patient, RN 31:34, May, 1968.

KOSSORIS, P.: Family therapy: an adjunct to hemodialysis and transplantation, Am. J. Nurs. 70:1730, August, 1970.

LENNON, E.: The surgical dialysis patient, Nurs. Clin. N. Am. 4:443, September, 1969.

LEOPOLD, A.: Psychological problems in hemodialysis, RN 31:42, May, 1968.

MARTIN, A.: Renal transplantation: surgical technique and complications, Am. J. Nurs. 68:1240, June, 1968.

SCHLOTTER, L.: Learning to be a home dialysis patient, Nurs. Clin. N. Am. 4:419, September, 1969.

SHOCKLEY, D., and STIEHL, R.: Hemodialysis in a community hospital, Nurs. Clin. N. Am. 4:409, September, 1969.

STEWART, B.: Hemodialysis in the home, Nurs. Clin. N. Am. 4:431, September, 1969.

TOPOR, M.: Nursing the renal transplantation patient, Nurs. Clin. N. Am. 4:461, September, 1969.

WINTER, C., and ROEHM, M.: Sawyer's Nursing Care of Patients with Urologic Diseases, ed. 2, St. Louis, Mosby, 1968.

The Burned Patient

57

Types of Burns • Prognosis • First Aid • Shock Phase (First 48 Hours Postburn) • Skin Treatment • Turning Point (2 to 5 Days) Recovery and Convalescence

Suddenly a well person sustains serious burns, and is confronted with problems resulting from pain, mutilation, fear of death, disfigurement, separation, immobilization, helplessness, and possible abandonment. Together with his own injuries and problems he may be grieving over the death of others involved in the accident such as spouse or children or co-workers. He may experience guilt over the cause of the accident to others and anger that this catastrophe should have happened to him. If he lives he has a long battle with prevention of infection, continuing pain from dressing changes, and surgery, scarring, malnutrition, finances, social relationships, among other problems.

Everything said about the severely burned patient in this chapter can apply also, with modification, to the patient with a milder or less extensive burn. A patient with a 1 per cent burn is not likely to go into shock, but the basic pathology remains the same. Infection, contractures and emotional disturbances can occur with a ½ per cent burn as with a 32 per cent burn.

TYPES OF BURNS

A *first-degree burn* is characterized by erythema. It does not blister. There may be a small amount of edema in and under the burn. Only the corium layer of the epidermis is involved. There is no necrosis of skin, and systemic derangement is minimal. It peels in three to six days.

A *second-degree burn* is characterized by a blister that contains water and electrolytes in ratios similar to those in plasma. The fluid comes from local vessels (lymphatics and capillaries) and cells. It is carried away by the lymphatics, but not so rapidly as it accumulates. The interstitial spaces soon are flooded. Most or all of the epithelial layers are involved, but the deepest layers of skin are not burned, and therefore re-epithelization can occur. A second-degree burn heals without scarring in 10 to 14 days.

A *third-degree burn* destroys the entire dermis down to the subcutaneous fat. Massive edema is present, collected deep in the wounded tissue, but there is no blister. There is necrosis of tissue. This is the kind of burn that causes scarring.

In a *fourth-degree burn* not only is the full thickness of skin destroyed, but also tissue underneath the skin. This may include subcutaneous tissue, fascia, muscle, tendon, and bone.

Burns caused by *electricity* are characteristically deep, involving not only the skin, but also blood vessels, muscles, tendons and bones.

The diagnosis of the depth of a burn often is difficult. There may be a combination of all degrees of burn. Both locally and systemically, the deeper the burn, the greater the damage.

The second measure of damage is the extent of the area: the larger the burn area, the greater is the damage to the body. Severe sunburn (first-degree) over 85 per cent of the body will cause a much greater disturbance of fluid and electrolyte regulation than a third-degree burn on the tip of a forefinger. Since doctors base their prescriptions for fluid replacement therapy both on the degree and the extent of the body surface injured, the diagnosis includes both these factors. The "Rule of Nines" (Fig. 57-1) is one method of estimating how much of the patient's skin surface is involved.

PROGNOSIS

In recent years such large strides have been made in the treatment of burn shock that patients are saved today who would have died several years ago. This is especially true of patients who are not very young or very old, and who have no pre-existing disease. However, those patients saved from dying in shock may later succumb to other complications, such as septicemia and renal failure. The prevention of infection, which has always been an important nursing consideration in the care of the burned patient, now assumes even more urgent proportions.

FIRST AID

If the clothes are flaming, the first thing to do is to put out the fire. A blanket, a coat or a loose rug can be used. Outdoors, if there is nothing of the sort to smother the flames, slowly roll the person on the ground. Avoid using sand or dirt to cover him; this can lead to infection.

If the burn is due to a chemical, it should be diluted by flushing the area with copious quantities of clean, cool water as quickly as possible. The longer the chemical is on the skin, the more it burns. Ideally, the water should be sterile, but chances are sterile water will not be available. Use whatever liquid is at hand, so long as it is not hot.

Any clothing that does not adhere to the skin should be removed. Rings, bracelets and wrist watches are taken off before edema forms and causes constriction. If the patient has to be transported, the burned area should be covered with the cleanest dressing obtainable, or the patient can be wrapped in a clean sheet. No two body surfaces should be wrapped together; fingers are bandaged separately, and a pad is placed between the arms and the trunk. No oil, ointment or any other medication should be put on the burns, since it would have to be removed after the patient enters the hospital, adding to the trauma that the skin already has received. If the face has been burned, the eyes should be rinsed in large amounts of clean, cool water, and a drop of mineral or liquid petrolatum oil should be instilled in each to protect the cornea from specks of dust and dirt.

If there will be delay before the patient is seen by a doctor (as might happen in a large-scale disaster, such as an explosion aboard ship or in an enemy attack), and if the patient is conscious, give a mixture of one teaspoon of table salt and half a teaspoon of soda bicarbonate (or baking

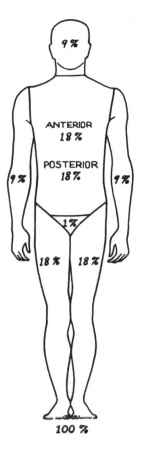

FIG. 57-1. The "Rule of Nines," a simplified method for estimating the per cent of the body surface covered by burns. According to this method, the entire head is 9% of the body surface area; each entire arm is 9%; each entire leg is 18%; the genital region is 1%; the front torso is 18%; and the back torso is 18%. Doctors often sketch the area burned on a diagram such as this to facilitate the calculation of the per cent of the body burned.

soda) mixed in a quart of water. The salt provides some of the sodium lost to the body as it is poured into the edematous tissues, and the baking soda is a base to help to correct the acidosis of burns.

SHOCK PHASE
(FIRST 48 HOURS POSTBURN)

As soon as the body suffers a burn, the burned area is flooded with fluid containing electrolytes and protein. Edema results from increased capillary permeability, increased osmotic pressure, and vasodilation. Protein molecules, which usually are too large to pass through the capillary walls, in this instance move freely from the bloodstream into the injured skin through damaged capillary walls, pulling even more water with them. Some areas swell more than others. For instance, the hands and the face become more edematous than the middle of the back. The amount of fluid lost to the body as a result of the burn is large.

The water that goes from the bloodstream into the wounds causes a fall in the volume of blood in the normal paths and avenues of the circula-

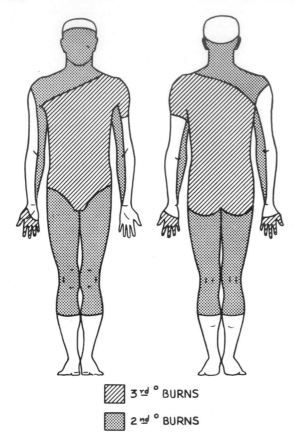

☒ 3ʳᵈ ° BURNS

▨ 2ⁿᵈ ° BURNS

Fig. 57-2. Diagram used to calculate the per cent of burns: 2nd-degree, 48½%; 3rd-degree, 31%; total 79½%.

tory system. The blood thickens as a consequence. Blood pressure drops, and the kidneys may receive insufficient blood to process urine. Less blood is available to maintain circulation. The heart beats faster and harder to push the sludge along. The result of this process is shock.

These fluid shifts proceed rapidly for the first eight hours after the accident, and they continue for about two days. Then the process slowly tapers off. The amount of fluid and electrolytes lost is related to the extent and the depth of the burn, and the resulting shock may be fatal. Timing is vital. Replacement therapy with fluids and electrolytes needs to be started soon after the burn, because the fluid shifts rapidly. Starting replacement therapy before irreversible shock has set in may make the difference between life and death.

Not all those who have been burned go into shock; it depends on the extent and the degree of the burn, the age and the general physical condition of the patient. An 80-year-old woman with hypertension may go into shock with a 10 per cent burn, which might not put a younger, healthier person into shock.

Treatment and Nursing Care

A lot needs to be done within the first hour of a severely burned patient's admission. Because the patient needs such complex and intensive medical attention, it is usual for a team of doctors to care for him. One doctor may perform the tracheostomy, another computes the patient's fluid and electrolyte requirements, and a third cares for the wounds. Ideally, the team includes several nurses, but in practice only one nurse may be available. She has a double role: to assist the doctors and to render direct care to the patient. She also has a role in comforting the family and helping them to understand what care is being given and in what ways they can help. For example, some family members may donate blood.

Tetanus prophylaxis should be ordered at the time of admission for all patients.

Equipment. Any hospital unit to which burned patients are admitted needs to have the equipment necessary for the emergency collected and in readiness for immediate use. Sterile goods should be periodically checked to make sure that they are not outdated. Some hospitals keep the necessary equipment on a burn cart that can be rolled to a patient's room.

While emergency treatment is being carried out, a bed can be prepared for the patient. The arrangement of draw sheets allows wet linen to be changed with minimal handling of the patient. A bed cradle is kept in readiness to place over the patient.

Since the introduction of topical antibacterial agents in skin care of burns, some hospitals use regularly cleaned linen instead of sterile sheets and gowns with no apparent risk to the patient. Reverse isolation is used by staff and visitors who wear a clean gown or scrub dress and mask to protect the patient from organisms which they carry.

Some hospitals have burn units, including the ventilation system, isolated from the rest of the hospital so that exposure to microorganisms is minimized (Potter).

Intake and Output. If there is no respiratory distress, the severely burned patient's most urgent need is the replacement of the fluid lost, so that an adequate blood volume is maintained, and irreversible shock is avoided. To determine the amount and the type of fluid to give, the physician estimates the extent of the burn and its severity. He usually draws a diagram of the burn area (such as that in Fig. 57-2), and he may use the "Rule of Nines" as a basis of his calculations. Several burn and fluid replacement formulas are available (Winkley).

In the emergency room a cutdown may be done or an intracath is inserted and intravenous fluid started. Blood is sent to the laboratory for typing and crossmatching, hematocrit, serum protein, complete blood count (CBC), blood urea nitrogen (BUN.), sodium, chloride, potassium, sugar, and CO_2 combining power. Blood gas studies may be done.

A Foley catheter is inserted and the volume of urine is measured every hour. Inspect the urine for any visible abnormalities such as blood or purulence.

The amount of urine excreted is an indication as to whether the patient's fluid requirements are being met. Urine should be produced in at least the rate of 30 to 50 ml. an hour (Larson). Too little urine means either renal shutdown or inadequate fluids; too much urine may mean an overload of fluids. Either situation is serious and demands immediate medical attention. A central venous pressure catheter may also be inserted to guide fluid administration. A rising CVP (above 15 cm.) heralds pulmonary edema.

Restlessness in a patient who has been quiet may be an indication that fluid replacement has not kept pace with fluid loss, and it should be reported immediately to the doctor. Not all patients in burn shock are unconscious. A patient may be extremely thirsty, and this thirst can be relieved by replacement of the lost fluids. In the hospital the nurse awaits the doctor's orders before she gives any patient anything to drink. No cracked ice, milk, fruit juice, or anything else is given. Unlimited tap water, if it is tolerated, would lead to water intoxication. If the patient is given anything to drink, an electrolyte solution probably will be ordered in preference to plain water. Even though the patient finds the salty solution highly palatable, the nurse should be careful to give him only sips at first, and she should not give any more than 200 ml. an hour unless the doctor orders a different amount. Citrus fruit juices (and other potassium containing fluids) are not given to the patient during the first few days postburn, unless specifically ordered

by the doctor. Many burned patients develop gastric distention, which leads to vomiting. Vomiting is to be avoided, if it can be, because of the danger of aspiration, and because more valuable fluids and electrolytes are lost. A Levin tube may be passed.

Medications. To relieve the pain of the burns, the doctor may give morphine intravenously. It is not given subcutaneously or intramuscularly to a patient in shock; the sluggish circulation would hinder its absorption. However, because morphine is a respiratory depressant, it may not be used at all, especially in a patient with burns of the head and the neck. Instead, intravenous barbiturates may be used for sedation. When medication for pain is ordered, the nurse should prepare it promptly. Subsequently, p.r.n. orders for medication to relieve pain should be given only when the patient is actually in pain (not, for example, for restlessness), since depressants are dangerous.

Intramuscular antibiotics usually are given. Cortisone is not generally used because it masks symptoms of infection.

Airway. The nurse makes continuous, careful observations for respiratory difficulty, especially in patients with burns of the face and the neck. Patients who breathe in fumes of the fire will have respiratory tract damage, even in the absence of burns of the face. If any respiratory difficulty, hoarseness or cyanosis occurs, she reports it promptly to the physician. Blood-tinged or smoke-stained sputum is an ominous sign.

A constant inhalation of warm mist from an ultrasonic or other nebulizer keeps tracheal secretions liquefied and easier to cough up (Crews). Intermittent medicated positive pressure breathing may be ordered or the patient may require assisted or controlled mechanical respiration (see Chap. 52).

The care of a tracheostomy in a burned patient is different from that of a patient whose respiratory passages have not been burned. As the tracheostomy wound easily becomes infected, suctioning should be done using aseptic technic, with sterile glove and fresh sterile catheter for each suctioning. Suctioning must be very prompt but very gentle to avoid starting small hemorrhages or causing an increase in edema that would lead to further obstruction. Unlike the suctioning of patients whose respiratory passages have not been burned, suctioning should be turned off whenever the catheter is moved. After the physician has done tracheobronchial suctioning, the nurse helps the patient in deep breathing, which is important to reinflate any alveoli that have been caused to collapse, leading to atelectasis. Regular deep breathing (when possible) and turning the patient (when possible) may help to minimize respiratory complications.

SKIN TREATMENT

After an immediate, life-saving treatment has been instituted, the patient's wounds are cleansed by washing with a suitable antibacterial detergent and saline solution under sterile conditions. Devitalized skin that is loosely adherent is debrided and blisters are excised. The object of skin care is to keep the wound as clean and as free from microorganisms as possible. The introduction of several new topical germicidal agents has resulted in a definite decrease in the mortality rate in serious burns. Included among these effective topical germicidal agents are Mafenide hydrochloride or Acetate (sulfamylon hydrochloride or acetate), 0.5 per cent silver nitrate solution, and gentamycin sulfate ointment (Garamycin ointment).

Sulfamylon is a cream-based sulfa drug. After cleansing of the burn wound, the ointment is applied to all burned surfaces in a fairly thick layer using the gloved hand or a spatula. Thereafter, the patient's wounds are cleansed daily, preferably by immersion in a Hubbard tank. After thorough washing, the sulfamylon ointment is reapplied. If a Hubbard tank is not available, cleansing may also be performed in a bathtub or shower.

Silver nitrate solution, 0.5 per cent, has also proved to be a highly effective topical antibacterial agent. After initial cleansing of the burn wound, occlusive dressings of coarse mesh gauze without a filler are applied to the wounds and the dressings are kept constantly saturated with the silver nitrate solution. Dressings are then changed at specified intervals, from every 12 hours to three to five days. Disadvantages of the use of the 0.5 per cent silver nitrate solution include staining, hyponatremia, and hypokalemia.

A third effective topical antibacterial agent is Gentamycin ointment or cream. Gauze impregnated with the Gentamycin ointment is applied to the burn wound after cleansing as described above, and an occlusive dressing is applied over the gauze.

The exposure method of treatment or the occlusive dressings technic currently are utilized in the majority of patients with major burns, in combination with the use of one of the topical antibacterial agents.

Debridement is performed at the time of each dressing change or wound cleansing until wound healing has occurred or a suitable granulating bed has developed. Skin grafting to obtain permanent wound closure is begun as early as possible by the surgeon. (See p. 698)

Exposure Method. In some hospitals the burned patient is put to bed inside of a germ-free plastic tent (Kress). Patients treated by the exposure method find every draft painful, and therefore a draft should be avoided. The patient is especially likely to feel cold because, due to the injury of these tissues, the superficial vascular bed cannot contract to retain body heat and because no covering is placed on him. The regulation of room temperature is therefore especially important. If the patient becomes cold, his discomfort is increased; if too warm, further vasodilation occurs with additional loss of fluids by perspiration. If an electric thermometer is available, rectal temperature readings can be taken frequently without disturbing the patient. In the absence of an electrical thermometer, his temperature has to be taken very carefully at frequent intervals. When direct care is not being given to the patient, a sterile blanket stretched across the top of the side rails and securely pinned there may help to keep him warm or the blanket can be pinned over a cradle which contains an electric light for warmth. Another method for providing warmth to the burned patient is by the use of ordinary portable home hair dryers. The warm air produced by the dryer can be directed on the patient.

Occlusive Dressings. Because bandaging immobilizes the part, good alignment and proper splinting are necessary to help to prevent deformities. The hands should be bandaged in the position of function with the injured hand grasping a roll of gauze; the wrist should be straight. If the hands are bandaged, they may be suspended on I.V. poles or the limbs may be splinted (in the position of function) for immobilization. The leg should not be in outward rotation; nor should the foot be pronated. No two skin surfaces should be touching. Medicated gauze is placed between the fingers, the folds of the genitalia, the arm and the trunk, and the ear and the scalp. Uniform pressure is important; tight uneven constriction, especially around the limb, may interfere with circulation. The doctor may leave an unburned finger or a toe out of the bandage so that the color can be checked as a test for the adequacy of circulation. Drainage is to be expected. When the bandage becomes wet from exudate, it is changed. A wet bandage forms an easy avenue of access for microorganisms to invade the burned tissue. Sterile waterproof material should be used to protect dressings around the perineum from contamination when the patient urinates or defecates.

Homografts. In third-degree burns an early grafting procedure may be done to protect large denuded areas. Frequently skin must be donated to the patient from another person, because the patient with extensive burns does not have sufficient unburned skin left to cover the burned areas. Such grafts are called homografts. They act as temporary physiologic dressings. They are used to alleviate pain, lessen fluid loss, and hasten the reduction of partial infection in the burned area. They are replaced after no longer than five days by other homografts until the site is ready for autografting (Winkley).

Position. Although immobilization of the skin is important, the patient must breathe deeply at frequent intervals as a precaution against hypostatic pneumonia. Also his position must be changed at intervals. If he is burned front and back, the air must be able to reach both sides. The patient may be placed in a Stryker frame or CircOlectric bed to facilitate turning. If he is not on a Stryker frame, he may prefer to move unaided because touching him causes pain. Flotation therapy, or the use of a nylon fish net stretched and secured tightly to a Bradford frame are other methods which allow air circulation and prevent pressure maceration (Noonan; Crews).

In any circumstance, be careful not to jar the bed, to hurry the patient, or to be rough in any way. The less he is touched, the better. When he is turned, hands should be placed only on the unburned skin even though sterile rubber gloves are worn.

TURNING POINT (2 TO 5 DAYS)

Pathology

For about two days after the burn, edema accumulates, and fluid seeps out through the wounds. Some time between the second and the fourth day the fluid that has gone to the burned tissues and has not left the body moves to the bloodstream. This is the period of diuresis, in which urinary output suddenly changes from a

trickle to a flood. (One patient put out 11,000 ml. on the third day.) For this reason the doctors restrict intake, especially intravenously. The patient looks thinner, and actually he is losing weight. Daily weights are taken when possible to keep careful track of the loss. The great outpouring of fluid into the bloodstream swells the volume of circulating fluid, and it may tax the heart with resultant pulmonary edema. Observe carefully for any respiratory distress and especially for the sound of moist rales.

This is the period when the patient's body is changing from its emergency response to the burn injury to repairing the damage. There is spontaneous nitrogen balance (which will aid in rebuilding proteins), and local re-epithelization has started. The patient is beginning to recover.

Intake. Unless specifically ordered otherwise, start any type of oral feedings very slowly—not more than 500 ml. the first day. If the patient tolerates this well, slowly increase the intake up to 2,500 ml. or the amount that was ordered. Observe the patient for distention, vomiting and diarrhea. Early oral fluids may be an electrolyte solution or a salty broth; later they may be changed gradually to a protein drink. Patients with severe burns rarely can tolerate solid foods until the beginning of the second week. Continue to maintain accurate records of intake.

Urinary Output. Once diuresis is well established, the hourly recording of urinary output probably will be replaced by measurement and recording q. 8 h. As long as the patient has an indwelling catheter in place, irrigation every four or six hours may be ordered.

Position. Contractures due to poor positioning are easily acquired because the patient finds comfort in the nonfunctional position. The patient needs the nurse to help him keep long-term goals in mind and prevent additional complication (Crews). Portions of the patient that are not burned should be exercised regularly to maintain muscle tone.

Skin Care. Prevent the exposed patient from picking at his scabs. If the patient is irrational or otherwise cannot resist the temptation, ask the doctor if you may wrap his hands during the periods when the patient is alone. A single layer of fine mesh gauze may cover the wound to avoid picking.

If wet dressings are ordered, they usually are changed by the nurse every four hours, and she keeps them wet as long as they are in place. The three most important nursing points in caring for wet dressings are:

1. To maintain the sterility of the dressings
2. To keep them wet
3. To change the dressings very slowly to avoid pain, bleeding, and further damage to the skin. In spite of the moisture some of the tissue may adhere to the dressing, and pulling the dressing away quickly will also detach skin. Use more sterile saline, and pull very gently and slowly. The doctor may order pHisoHex tub baths to soak the dressings off.

Emotional Response. By the turning-point period the patient barely has had time to begin to adjust. Although he probably is no longer in constant pain, he still is uncomfortable. He is probably still too ill to talk much about how he feels.

Family members may be shocked at the rapid changes in the patient's appearance. The burn itself may be seen as ugly and disfiguring, and the change from marked edema to leanness in a few days is startling. Questions about scarring can be referred to the doctor. It is well to know what the doctor has said to the family on the subject.

RECOVERY AND CONVALESCENCE

When the emergency is over, the body must repair itself. The energy that was required to meet the emergency was greatly in excess of normal. Because large areas of fat deposits have been used, and the caloric intake over the past five days has been low, patients often are emaciated. As much as 20 pounds may be lost, even if the loss of edema is not considered. The debilitation is dangerous, because it reduces the patient's resistance to infection, it delays the healing of the skin, and it impedes the growth of new granulation tissue and the progress of new skin grafts. Accordingly, the nurse does everything possible to improve the patient's nutrition.

The drying of the skin wounds becomes evident early in this phase, starting about the fifth or the sixth day and continuing until the dead skin sloughs away, about two to three weeks after the burn occurred. The convalescent period can be said to start about three weeks after the accident.

Treatment and Nursing Care

Nutrition. Nutrition may make the difference between an uncomplicated recovery and progressive emaciation. The patient's physiologic need for food usually is greater than his appetite. He still is sick, and he feels weak and not equal to eating the high caloric, high protein diet that he needs.

Gradually, his diet is increased to 3,000 to 6,000 calories and 2 to 3 Gm. of protein per kilogram of body weight per day. Vitamins are given. This large intake is essential, but it is a problem for the patient and the nurse alike. Protein-enriched drinks help to fulfill the protein requirement without excess bulk, and they should be served in any way that the patient can ingest them (warm, iced, at bedtime, etc.). The patient on such a large intake needs to be observed carefully for distention, diarrhea and vomiting. The intake may have to be reduced, slowing the patient's nutritional recovery. Oral hygiene is essential to promote appetite.

Solid foods are begun cautiously about the second week (or sooner, if possible), and they are increased rapidly if the patient tolerates them. Conferences between patient, dietitian, and nurse will help the patient to feel that he is contributing to his recovery by participating in his treatment. The nurse can point out to the patient that every mouthful he swallows is another building brick for a patch of skin. During this period patients usually are weighed twice a week. The patient can be encouraged to keep a record of his progress.

Skin Care. *Exposure.* By about the third week, or longer with local antibacterial treatment, the crusts of second-degree burns spontaneously separate, leaving pink, thin, new skin. Now immobilization of the burned parts is replaced by exercise and physiotherapy to recondition muscles and to encourage circulation and healing. In third-degree burns the crust cracks, and it is at this time that grafting may be done.

Bandages. Dressings may be changed about once a week. Frequently, these changes are so painful that anesthesia is needed. Dressings on third-degree burns may be changed daily until the skin is grafted.

Grafting. (See p. 605 for a discussion of the problems of disfigurement, and Chap. 49 for a discussion of plastic surgery.) After the recovery period, grafts may be used to improve appearance or function when scar tissues limit motion. Corrective grafting may take the form of split-thickness, full-thickness, or pinch grafts. The skin for them is taken from the patient's own body (*autografts*). They are permanent, and usually they take about two weeks to heal. The patient should expect pain for a day or two. Full-thickness skin loss requires complete skin replacement. Grafting may be done every 10 to 12 days until coverage is complete. Hospitalization is long and the procedures are multiple. The maintenance of the patient's nutrition and his morale is important. Diversional therapy is a help.

Complications. This is a phase all too frequently plagued by complications. Although patients usually receive ample attention while they are in shock, it is harder to continue to give them the concentrated care that they need over a period of months.

Infection. Wound infection and septicemia are responsible for a large number of the deaths of burned patients who survive the shock period. Besides the overall lowered resistance of the burned patient, edema and thrombosis in the traumatized subcutaneous tissue obstruct bacterial-fighting mechanisms. There always is some infection in third-degree burns.

An increase in temperature may be the first indication of infection, and it characteristically mounts rapidly, rarely below 102° F. The pulse is rapid and yet regular. The odor or the appearance of the burn (if it is exposed) may change. Smell the burned area at least once a day. The odor of infection is different from that of burn exudate. On the other hand, a dry-appearing crust may harbor copious amounts of pus beneath its surface. By her close and frequent contact with the patient the nurse is in an excellent position to be the first observer of infection, and she should remain alert to its possible existence.

Treatment may include continuous saline soaks and antibiotics as Coly-Mycin for Pseudomonas and Staphcillin (sodium methicillin) for Staphylococcus. The doctor may order dressing changes by the nurse every four hours with removal of the dead tissue loosened by the soaks. The saline should be warmed to normal body temperature before it is applied to the dressings.

Septicemia may result in oliguria, hypotension, tachypnea, paralytic ileus, disorientation (related to the degree of the fever) and cardiac failure. The patient may need oxygen, nasogastric suction, and blood; and intravenous fluid therapy may have to be resumed or increased.

Aspirin and sponging of the unburned areas may be ordered for the fever. Sponge only those portions of his body that are covered by unbroken skin. If there is a high fever the patient may be placed on a hypothermic blanket.

Kidney Failure. Some studies report that this complication of burns is second only to infection as a cause of death of those patients who survive the shock phase (Crews). Oliguria or anuria are usual symptoms, but occasionally there is diuresis. If this complication is going to occur, it usually does so by the 10th to the 12th day postburn (McAninch).

Curling's Ulcer. For unknown reasons, burned patients sometimes develop a gastrointestinal ulcer. Ulcers are more common in patients with extensive burns, but may be seen in any burned patient. The symptom most suggestive of an ulcer is onset of, or increase in, anorexia, associated with abdominal distention due to gastric dilatation. As the patient recovers physiologic balance from the widespread disturbances caused by the burn, his appetite should slowly improve. If there is reversal of this trend, it should be reported to the doctor. Also watch for blood in the stool and in the nasogastric tube or hematemesis. Some patients have no symptoms until there is sudden gastrointestinal hemorrhage. The peak incidence of onset of a Curling's ulcer is at the end of the first week postburn (Moncrief).

Gastrointestinal Disturbances. Dilatation of the stomach may occur, characterized by regurgitation of fluid, discomfort, anorexia and nausea. The patient may be dyspneic, because the bloated stomach is pressing on the diaphragm, interfering with respiration. Also, fecal impaction may follow paralytic ileus.

Anemia. A number of factors contribute to the burned patient's anemia. Heat causes red blood cell destruction or makes them abnormally fragile which shortens their life. Red blood cells are trapped in dilated capillaries. Infection depresses the function of hematopoietic tissue. Blood is lost from granulating wounds at dressing changes. The treatment is blood transfusions, a high protein and iron-rich diet, with iron supplements.

Contractures. Due to the pull of tightening scar tissue, patients with third-degree burns may develop contractures that are both disfiguring and crippling. For example, a healed third-degree burn of the right side of the neck can twist and hold the head in a permanently fixed position. To minimize contractures, parts with third-degree burns sometimes can be held in extension during the period of immobilization with splints, sandbags or casts. As soon as healing has advanced sufficiently so that movement will not crack the eschar, a program of physical therapy is started—perhaps whirlpool baths, and under water and then dry exercises, both passive and active. If contractures develop nonetheless, plastic surgery is indicated.

Decubitus Ulcers. Conditions are ripe for this complication. The patient has lost much body protein. He is immobilized for a time; therefore some areas of his body are compressed between the hard bed and an even harder bone. Frequent turning and good skin care to unburned areas help to prevent decubiti.

Respiratory Problems. Pneumonia also can follow immobilization and debilitation. A patient with burns of the chest finds it painful to cough up secretions, but he should be encouraged to do so anyway. Atelectasis may be caused by the aspiration of gastric contents following Levin-tube feedings or vomiting, as well as by mucus plugs retained in the respiratory passages.

Emotional Considerations. Any questions that can be answered need answering. Some can be answered immediately, some may be referred to the doctor, and the unknowns can be shared with a good listener.

Diversion may help the patient to keep from prolonged brooding. Can any of his special interests be tapped? Talk it over with him. A patient who is flat on his back and isolated in a tepee of sterile sheets may be able to watch television or the hall through a prism lens or by a strategically placed mirror. Initially, with mirrors, the patient may become frightened by his appearance. The patient's bed can be placed where he cannot easily see himself in the mirror until the edema phase is over, and until he has had a chance to see his chest or his arms start to heal. The patient's concept of his appearance can be a vital factor in restoring relations with his family and his friends. "How do I look?" and "Will people be repelled by my appearance?" may worry the patient. Also, he may worry about work in the future. Community resources can offer help after he leaves the hospital such as the Visiting Nurse Service or the State Vocational Rehabilitation Agency.

REFERENCES AND BIBLIOGRAPHY

AKEY, D. T.: Catastrophe: the employee with critical burns, *Am. Ass. Indus. Nurs. J.* 16:17, October, 1968.

ARTZ, C. P., and MONCRIEF, J.: *The Treatment of Burns,* ed. 2, Philadelphia, Saunders, 1968.

CHUTZ, SR. A., D.C.: *The Development of a Nursing Categorization of Burn Patients and a Burn Patient Nursing Care Index.* The League Exchange No. 88, New York, National League for Nursing, 1969.

CREWS, E.: *A Practical Manual for the Treatment of Burns,* ed. 2, Springfield, Ill., Thomas, 1967.

KRESS, B. R., et al.: Isolated in a life-island, *Canad. Nurse* 64:48, May, 1968.

LARSON, D., et al.: Current trends in the care of burned patients, *Am. J. Nurs.* 67:319, February, 1967.

MCANINCH, J., et al.: Renal patho-physiology in severe burns: 5-year review of kidney pathology in fatal burns, *Texas Rep. Biol. Med.* 22:348, 1964.

MAXWELL, P., et al.: Silver nitrate treatment of burns. Routines on the burn ward, *Am. J. Nurs.* 66:522, March, 1966.

MILNER, C.: Nursing care of severely burned patients, *Am. J. Nurs.* 54:456, 1954.

MONCRIEF, J. A., et al.: Curling's ulcer, *J. Trauma* 4:481, 1964.

MOYER, C. A., et al.: Treatment of large human burns with 0.5% silver nitrate solution, *Arch. Surg.* 90:812, June, 1965.

NOONAN, J., et al.: Two burned patients in flotation therapy, *Am. J. Nurs.* 68:316, February, 1968.

PHILLIPS, A. W., et al.: Burn therapy. IV. Respiratory tract damage (an account of the clinical, x-ray, and postmortem findings) and the meaning of restlessness, *Ann. Surg.* 158:799, 1963.

POTTER, B.: Even the air is isolated in this burn unit, *Mod. Hosp.* 110:95, March, 1968.

PRICE, W., and WOOD, M.: Operating room care of burned patients treated with silver nitrate. *Am. J. Nurs.* 68:1705, August, 1968.

SCHLICHTMANN, K.: Adaptive mechanisms in a selected group of burned patients, *ANA Clinical Sessions 1968,* p. 259, New York, Appleton-Century-Crofts, 1969.

SHAW, B.: Current therapy for burns, *R.N.* 34:33, March, 1971.

SHERMAN, R.: Burn fluid management, *Nurs. Forum* 4:93, 1965.

SISTER MARY CLAUDIA: TLC and Sulfamylon for burned children, *Am. J. Nurs.* 69:755, April, 1969.

STRATHIE, A., et al.: Silver nitrate treatment of burns, problems in one patient's care, *Am. J. Nurs.* 66:524, March, 1966.

SULLIVAN, M., and DIMICK, A.: Management of the burn patient in a general hospital, *Surg. Clin. N. Am.* 48:79, August, 1968.

WINKLEY, J., et al.: Topical treatment of burns, *Surg. Clin. N. Am.* 48:1365, December, 1968.

WOOD, M., et al.: Silver nitrate treatment of burns. Technique and controlling principles, *Am. J. Nurs.* 66:518, March, 1966.

WOOD-SMITH, D., and POROWSKI, P. (eds.): *Nursing Care of the Plastic Surgery Patient,* St. Louis, Mosby, 1967.

The Patient with Neurologic Disease

58

Increased Intracranial Pressure • Brain Injuries • Brain Tumors

INCREASED INTRACRANIAL PRESSURE

The brain is enclosed in a sealed bony vault, the skull. Cerebrospinal fluid, produced in the ventricles, passes down into the spinal subarachnoid space, then up through the basilar cisterns and over the cerebral hemispheres to the region of the dural venous sinuses, where most of the absorption takes place. A tumor, a hematoma or an abscess may increase intracranial pressure because of the added bulk within the rigid confines of the skull, as well as by obstruction of the cerebrospinal fluid pathways. A mass, such as a tumor, presses on and displaces the adjacent brain tissue, perhaps causing compression of the midbrain and displacement of the cerebellar tonsils through the foramen magnum, with compression of the medulla.

The underlying pathology of increased intracranial pressure is basically constant, even though the etiology may vary. The most crucial pathologic change is anoxia of the brain cells, or edema of white matter. Permanent brain damage may result.

Signs and Symptoms

There are three cardinal signs and symptoms of increased intracranial pressure with an intracranial mass:

Headache. The pain usually is intermittent. Constant headache usually indicates that the patient's prognosis is grave. Anything that increases intracranial pressure, such as coughing, sneezing or straining at stool, increases the headache. Lying quietly in bed—especially if the head of the bed is elevated—tends to reduce the intracranial pressure and thus helps to relieve the headache.

Vomiting. This usually occurs without the forewarning of nausea and without any relation to eating. Frequently, vomiting occurs before breakfast. It may be projectile.

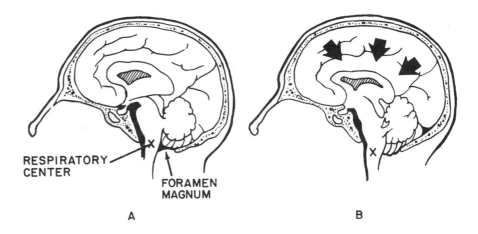

FIG. 58-1. (A) The normal brain. (B) Herniation of the lower portion of the brain stem (medulla) through the foramen magnum, caused by increased intracranial pressure. Note the position of the respiratory center.

RESPIRATORY CENTER

FORAMEN MAGNUM

A

B

TABLE 58-1. COMPARISON OF SIGNS AND SYMPTOMS OF INCREASED INTRACRANIAL
PRESSURE WITH THOSE OF SHOCK

INCREASED INTRACRANIAL PRESSURE	SHOCK
1. The pulse rate is increased initially; later, it is slow and bounding, 40–60 beats per minute. If hypoxia develops, the pulse becomes rapid again.	1. The pulse rate is rapid, weak and thready, 100–160 beats per minute.
2. Widening pulse pressure, i.e., the difference between the systolic and the diastolic blood pressure becomes greater than normal—example, 180/90.	2. Both the systolic and the diastolic blood pressures drop.
3. The respirations are irregular.	3. The respirations are rapid and shallow; they may be as high as 40–50 per minute.
4. The skin is dry and warm. The color may be pink or red.	4. The skin is cold, clammy and moist; there is pallor due to peripheral vasoconstriction.
5. The pupils may be unequal or unreactive.	5. There is no pupillary change.
6. There are decreasing levels of consciousness, progressing to coma.	6. The patient usually is stuporous.
7. There is increasing loss of motor power, such as hemiparesis.	7. Loss of motor power is present only as it is related to low blood pressure.

Papilledema. This edema of the optic nerve at the point at which it enters the eyeball is caused by obstruction of venous drainage from the globe by the increased intracranial pressure.

The other symptoms of increased intracranial pressure, and their comparison with symptoms of shock, are summarized in Table 58-1.

Treatment

The treatment may be medical or surgical, depending on the etiology. When possible, the underlying cause is removed: the infection is cured, the hematoma is drained, or the tumor is excised.

Cerebral edema may be treated with corticosteroids in high doses or with a hypertonic intravenous solution, such as mannitol or Urevert (intravenous urea). Hypertonic solutions may be given by rectum as well as intravenously. When patients have been given mannitol or Urevert, the urinary output is recorded every hour, and observation of the vital signs and the level of consciousness is made frequently to assess the effects of the drug. The urinary output is expected to increase.

Some typical orders given by the physician when the patient may have increased intracranial pressure are:

- Check vital signs every 30 minutes.
- Check levels of consciousness, pupillary reaction, and any areas of paralysis, every 30 minutes.
- Give nothing by mouth.
- Elevate head of bed 30° and maintain the patient's head to one side.
- Give Dilantin 100 mg. I.M. stat.

These orders of the doctor represent the classic management of the patient with possible increased intracranial pressure for any reason. They aid in both the recognition and the prevention of this important symptom. And they have important implications for the nurse.

- *Vital signs q. 30 minutes.* As with all disease conditions, the vital signs tell a story to the observer. A rapid increase in the pulse rate usually occurs initially. The rate may vary as much as 10 to 20 beats from the original reading; then, there is usually a drop. If the pulse becomes less than 60 beats per minute and bounding, the physician should be notified immediately. Accompanying this change in pulse rate is an increase in the pulse pressure, and respirations may be variable. As the pressure on the cerebrum increases, there is usually an associated hypoxia. In order to compensate for this, the heart again beats faster.

- *Check the levels of consciousness and pupillary reaction.* The brain stem has a great deal to do with the maintenance of the conscious state. Any direct trauma or associated pressure on the brain stem will cause a change in the level of consciousness. If a person is hit on the back of the head, he is likely to lose consciousness much more quickly than if he is hit on the forehead;

however, if there is edema, hemorrhage or increased production of cerebrospinal fluid, the brain substance itself will press down on the pons and cause progressive stupor.

If the temporal lobe is displaced medially by a mass, it may press on the 3rd cranial (oculomotor) nerve, with the result that the muscles of the eye become paralyzed, and the corresponding pupil dilates and no longer reacts to a beam of light, such as that from a flashlight. Damage to the nuclei in the brainstem may result in constricted pupils, which also are unreactive.

• *Check for paralysis.* Loss of motor function is another valuable yardstick in ascertaining the amount of increased intracranial pressure. On admission of the patient, the physician and the nurse will determine whether or not he can move all four extremities. If the patient is asked to move his arm or hand, the nurse can determine not only the amount, the kind and the type of motion but also whether the patient understands and responds to requests. If the patient is semicomatose, he will respond only to a pinch or other painful stimuli. If he is able to move initially and later begins to lose this ability, the physician should be called immediately.

• *Nothing by mouth.* The previous three orders have been concerned with the recognition of increased intracranial pressure. This order is directed toward its prevention. If the patient is given food or fluid by mouth, he runs the risk of vomiting. Vomiting, sneezing, coughing and hiccoughing cause an increase in pressure. This must be guarded against, since any sudden increase in the pressure may precipitate herniation of the cerebellar tonsils through the foramen magnum, with medullary compression. The vital cardiopulmonary center is contained in the medulla. Pressure on this center will cause irregular respirations or apnea. An unconscious patient is never given fluids by mouth, because he may aspirate them.

Although intake is prohibited by mouth, fluids are given intravenously. If the patient has been perspiring profusely, vomiting or bleeding, additional fluid will be given. When there is marked increase in intracranial pressure, the fluid intake may be restricted. Overhydration or an infusion run too rapidly can increase intracranial pressure. The fluid should be administered at approximately 40 drops per minute.

• *Elevate the head of the bed 30°, and maintain the patient's head to the side.* Patients with cerebral lesions are usually positioned with the head of the bed elevated to promote the return of venous drainage of blood and cerebrospinal fluid. The doctor orders the degree to which he wishes the bed elevated. Patients with basal skull fractures may be kept flat. In no instance should the patient's head be allowed to rest below the level of the rest of his body.

Turning the patient on his side does not automatically result in a patent airway. He also may need suctioning. The principles of positioning of the patient with any cerebral lesion are (a) maintaining a patent airway, (b) avoiding increasing cerebral pressure by promoting or at least not inhibiting venous return from the brain, (c) preventing pressure sores, and (d) preventing deformities. Herein lie some of the real skills of the neurologic nurse.

If positioning and suctioning do not result in an airway clear of secretions, a tracheostomy may be performed. Oxygen is used frequently to combat the hypoxia associated with increased intracranial pressure.

Always have an emergency oxygen mask, nasal oxygen equipment, a suction machine and an emergency tracheostomy tray at the bedside for any patient who has an acute cerebral lesion of any type.

• *Dilantin 100 mg. I.M. stat. and q. 8 hours.* Dilantin sodium is one of the anticonvulsants in widespread use. It is superior to phenobarbital in that it produces no drowsiness. This medication, used in the treatment of epilepsy, has come to be used also as a precautionary measure against seizures following brain surgery or trauma. Bleeding, edema and infection as well as tumors impinging on the corticospinal tracts may cause seizures. Seizures increase intracranial pressure.

The usual dose of Dilantin is between 60 and 400 mg. It may be given in conjunction with phenobarbital. When seizures have been uncontrollable and relaxation is needed, this combination has been found to be superior.

Patients admitted to the hospital with traumatic brain pathology often have multiple injuries. Basal skull fractures may be fatal because of their close proximity to the brainstem, which houses the vital centers of respiration and circulation. There may be direct bleeding into this area or edema in or around the medulla, which may precipitate respiratory or circulatory collapse. Bleeding into the meninges will irritate them and cause a stiff neck.

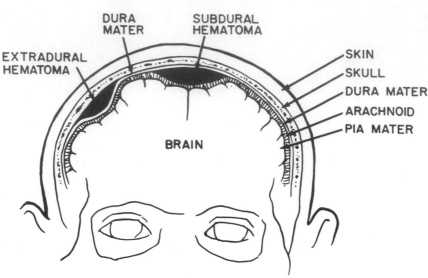

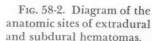

FIG. 58-2. Diagram of the anatomic sites of extradural and subdural hematomas.

Bleeding from the ears most often occurs when the patient has a basal skull fracture. The seepage of clear drainage indicates the loss of cerebrospinal fluid and is of serious consequence. Bleeding from the ears or the nose is advantageous in one respect: intracranial pressure is lessened. However, large quantities of bright red blood from this area may indicate rupture of a major vessel. Unobstructed drainage from the ears is desirable; the auditory canal is not packed with gauze or cotton. Cleaning or swabbing may introduce bacteria and result in meningitis.

When possible, opiates and sedatives are avoided, because they tend to depress the level of consciousness, to mask the symptoms of increased intracranial pressure and to depress respirations; lowered respirations increase intracranial pressure. The nurse should evaluate pain before administering any drug. Suppose, for example, that a patient has an order for aspirin which was written for a headache after a lumbar puncture. After being free of pain for several days, the patient suddenly develops a severe headache. The nurse should call the doctor instead of giving the aspirin. This pain represents a new neurologic symptom, which should be assessed by the doctor.

Retention of urine may coexist with incontinence. The patient may dribble urine but not empty the bladder fully. Distention of the bladder can cause restlessness in a stuporous patient. The nurse observes for retention even when the patient is incontinent and urinating frequently.

BRAIN INJURIES

The bony casing of the skull protects the brain. Slight injuries do not affect the brain, because of the skull. However, a severe blow to the head, such as that sustained in some automobile accidents, can cause lacerations, bruises, hemorrhage and edema. When the moving head is brought to an abrupt stop by hitting a solid object, such as the roof of a car, the brain tissue continues to move until it is stopped short by the skull bones. This action can injure the brain.

Trauma can cause the following conditions:

Concussion. Concussion results from violent jarring of the brain, and it is often associated with a loss of consciousness. It may be followed by headache, irritability, dizzy spells, confusion and an unsteady gait, but complete recovery is usual. However, recovery at times takes many months, particularly in older people.

Cerebral Laceration and Contusion. These are more severe than a concussion and are the most common serious brain injuries. Permanent damage may result, causing impaired intellect, speech difficulties, epilepsy, paralysis, impaired gait and continuing stupor.

Epidural (Extradural) Hematoma. An epidural hematoma is caused usually by arterial bleeding and occurs on top of the dura ("Epi" means "above"). This is a true surgical emergency. The bleeding occurs very rapidly, separating the dura from the cranium. Unless the increased intracranial pressure produced is relieved immediately destruction of brain substance will take place. Characteristically, the patient will have a momentary lapse of consciousness. He may appear perfectly alert and clear after the injury and carry on a lucid conversation. Within an hour or so he may state that he feels drowsy. This is one of the first signs of increasing intracranial pressure due to arterial bleeding. The patient becomes comatose. Patients usually are detained in the hospital for 24 hours after a significant head injury. Vital signs may be taken as often as every 15 minutes. Also, watch for decreasing consciousness, dilated pupils, asymmetry of the pupils, convulsions and hemiparesis. Observation for change in these neurologic symptoms is even more important than observation for change in the vital signs.

Subdural Hematoma. This condition occurs as a result of venous bleeding in the space below the dura. The patient may appear to have recovered completely from the blow on the head, because the bleeding is more in the nature of oozing than gushing. There may be no symptoms for as long as two months. The clot that gradually forms is walled off. Often the clot is absorbed by the body, and no treatment is necessary. When absorption fails to occur, the patient experiences symptoms of compression of the brain. These may include periodic episodes of memory lapse, confusion, drowsiness or personality change. Burr holes are made into the cranium, and the hematoma is aspirated.

Depressed Skull Fracture with Brain Injury. The broken bone is pushed in on the brain and injures it. The symptoms depend on what area of the brain is being crushed. For example, a bone fragment pressing on the motor area may cause hemiplegia. Characteristically, symptoms are not progressive, but they tend to remain static until the bone is elevated, and the pressure is relieved. Epilepsy is a common late complication.

Other Skull Fractures. Most skull fractures are in themselves of little clinical importance. They cause no symptoms, and they tend to heal without trouble. However, this characteristic is not true of fractures of the base of the skull. Trauma to this area may cause edema of the brain near the origin of the spinal cord (foramen magnum) and interfere with the circulation of cerebrospinal fluid, or it may injure nerves passing into the spinal cord, or it may cause a communication between the brain and the middle ear that may result in meningitis.

Nursing Care

All patients who have received trauma to the head should be considered to have had a fracture, and they should be watched for the development of signs of increased intracranial pressure—until it is proved otherwise. Very slight trauma, especially in patients who bleed easily (such as poorly nourished patients and those with arteriosclerosis), can cause the slow-growing subdural hematoma. Sometimes the blow to the head is so slight that the patient has paid no heed to it and makes no connection between it and later symptoms of recurrent headache, drowsiness or personality change. Such patients should be urged to seek medical attention.

One of the essentials of nursing a patient with a head injury is to keep him quiet. His room should be free of confusion, noise, sudden jarring of the bed and other such stimuli. Although he has to be disturbed frequently for observation of levels of consciousness, he should be aroused gently and slowly. Mechanical restraints should be used only when they are required for the patient's safety, because they may make a restless patient more irritable. When the patient is first admitted, his need for quiet is greater than his need for cleanliness. If his condition is serious, do not disturb him with a bath even if he needs one. It is better to use scotch tape to hold the dressing, because it is less painful to remove from hair than is adhesive. Look at it frequently, and note the drainage. Later, blood can be removed from the hair with hydrogen peroxide. Secure the hair out of the way of the drainage and the bandage. Leave the blood-pressure cuff in place on the patient's arm, so that he is not disturbed by having it replaced every 15 or 30 minutes.

Because the nurse is constantly with the severely injured patient and frequently with the mildly injured patient, she is in an excellent position to observe changes in his signs and symptoms. Is he harder to arouse at 4 A.M. than he was at 3:30 A.M.? Is there a slight facial weakness starting on either side? Does the pulse seem to be more bounding? The recognition of small changes may bring the physician to the bedside before serious brain damage has occurred.

Because the patient is unconscious in both sleep and coma, the only way to differentiate between the two is to try to rouse him. The doctor usually determines the frequency of awakening. If there is no such order, and if there is

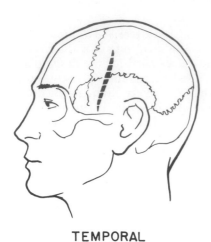

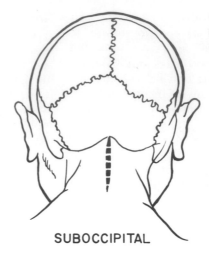

FIG. 58-3. Common cranial incisions.

TEMPORAL   SUBOCCIPITAL

a possibility that the patient is comatose, the nurse should try to arouse him periodically. Awakening the well-oriented but tired patient every half-hour to differentiate sleep from coma may make him angry, but an explanation of the importance of how this seemingly cruel practice protects a patient may help him to accept it. Intoxication may be one factor that led to the accident, and the nurse needs to differentiate between behavior due to intoxication and a change in behavior due to increasing intracranial pressure. The nurse should note and report whether there is an odor of alcohol on the patient's breath.

Besides vital signs the nurse also notes the size and the symmetry of the pupils. Reaction to light, deepening coma, motion and power of the limbs, weakness anywhere in the body, tremors, rigidity and convulsions, headache, dizziness, periorbital edema, deafness, blindness and drainage from any orifice of the head also are observed. Diplopia is a frequent complaint in subdural hematoma.

BRAIN TUMORS

Neoplasms of the central nervous system occur more frequently than tumors of the stomach and less frequently than tumors of the breast. Although they do not tend to metastasize, even a benign tumor, when untreated, can kill the patient, because, as it expands within the narrow confines of the skull, it encroaches on brain tissue that is vital for life. Some tumors are extracerebral, that is, they are situated outside the brain but within the cranium. These tumors, such as meningiomas (tumors of the meninges), press on the brain tissue from without. About 4 per cent

of brain tumors are metastases from the other sites.

Brain tumors are seen in all age groups. Some are more common under 20 years, whereas others more frequently strike older people. Approximately half of brain tumors are gliomas.

Symptoms

Because tumors take up space, and because they may block the flow and thus the absorption of cerebrospinal fluid, symptoms of increased intracranial pressure result. The classic triad of headache, vomiting and papilledema is common. Headache is most common early in the morning, when the patient gets out of bed, and it becomes increasingly severe and frequent as the tumor grows. The pain may be relieved by putting the patient to bed. Vomiting occurs without nausea or warning. Convulsions may be the first symptom. Sixty to 90 per cent of the patients have papilledema.

In addition to symptoms of generalized cerebral irritation and increased intracranial pressure, there may be other symptoms of disturbed bodily function. The symptoms depend on where the tumor is exerting pressure.

When the intracranial pressure is such that the brainstem is forced through the foramen magnum, the patient is in grave danger, since the vital centers are compressed, stretched and become ischemic (see Fig. 58-1). Respirations become embarrassed: deeper, labored and noisy, and then slow and only periodic. Unless the condition is relieved, the patient dies of respiratory failure. In the early stages there is bradycardia; tachycardia appears near the end. Blood pressure may remain relatively stable, but hyperthermia

Fig. 58-4. Facial sling for patients with muscular weakness. The rubber bands should not be so tight that the patient cannot easily open his mouth, or so slack that they give no support. The adhesive tape continues under the patient's chin.

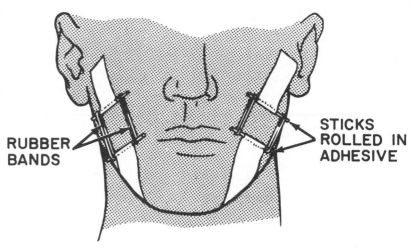

RUBBER BANDS

STICKS ROLLED IN ADHESIVE

may occur as the temperature-regulating center in the brain is affected. Coma becomes progressively deepened.

A characteristic of brain tumors is progression of symptoms. As the tumor grows and exerts increasing pressure, symptoms intensify.

Treatment

Some brain tumors are easily removed without damage to nearby brain tissue; others can be excised only with the result of residual, permanent brain damage; and some cannot be reached at all without killing the patient. If healthy brain tissue has to be cut to reach the tumor, some of the patient's postoperative symptoms will be determined by the location and the function of the damaged tissue. Brain tissue does not regenerate.

The surgery performed is a craniotomy (incision through the skull) or craniectomy (excision of part of the skull). A bone flap may be made by sawing the skull in order to get to the brain. After the tumor is removed, the dura is reapproximated (the cut edges are lined up and sewn together), the bone flap is replaced, and the skin is sutured. On occasion the bone fragment is not reinserted, but the space is left free, so that the brain has room to expand. This procedure may be followed when increasing intracranial pressure is expected, as in cases in which the tumor is found to be inoperable. When the patient's condition allows it, the bone flap can be replaced weeks later, or the area may be covered with a Vitallium plate.

When an inoperable tumor obstructs the flow of cerebrospinal fluid, sometimes the fluid is shunted out of the cranial cavity. A polyethylene tube may be placed in the lateral ventricle and the other end inserted into the spinal cord, a large vein or into the pleural cavity to allow an outlet for the fluid that is continuously produced. When the tube is placed so that it lies outside the skull but under the skin, care must be taken not to allow the patient to lie on that side of his head and to occlude the tube. The head of the bed usually is kept in an elevated position to facilitate drainage.

Postoperative Nursing Care

The postoperative bed is made with the head at the foot for easy access to the patient's dressing. The room should be equipped with a mouth gag, side boards on the bed, a ventricular puncture tray, an airway, a tracheostomy tray, a tray with emergency drugs (including stimulants and depressants), syringes and needles, and suction apparatus.

Observation of vital signs and levels of consciousness are ordered frequently for the postoperative patient. All patients—and especially those who have had surgery on or near the brainstem—should be watched for respiratory collapse, which may be caused by the pressure of edema on the respiratory center. Watch for decreasing pulse rate and increasing blood pressure—a sign that increasing intracranial pressure may be compressing vital areas in the brain.

• If all the bone is not replaced under the flap at the end of the operation, the brain will be covered only by the scalp and possibly the temporal muscle. If intracranial pressure is increased, the flap then will bulge. As time passes, swelling and edema becomes less, the bulge diminishes, and eventually the flap may become

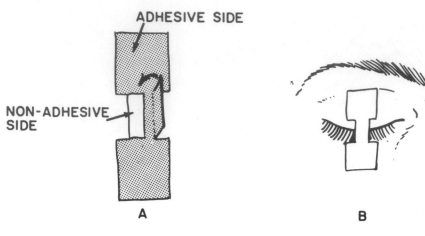

ADHESIVE SIDE

NON-ADHESIVE SIDE

A   B

Fig. 58-5. A butterfly bandage to keep the eye closed. (A) Shows the side that goes on the patient. (B) Applied to the eye.

concave. Increased intracranial pressure may be indicated by other symptoms, such as vomiting. Vomiting is dangerous, because its very act increases intracranial pressure. Prevent it when you can. To help to prevent nausea, keep the room free from odor, and protect the patient from cigarette smell on the breath and the clothing of vistors and those who care for him. Do not encourage fluids until the patient can tolerate them without vomiting.

• Meningitis and the associated fever may increase intracranial pressure and cause bulging of the flap, headache, and a stiff neck.

• Disturbance of motor function may be a symptom of injury to the pyramidal tract. Look for weakness of one side of the body, evidenced by a weakening hand grip or progressive impairment in movement of a lower limb. Increased flaccidity or spasticity also should be reported.

• Tremors and convulsions should be observed in minute detail. Report where the condition started, what (if anything) seemed to precipitate it, whether it was fine or gross movement, if it spread and where, how long it lasted, the position of the eyes, and any other accompanying symptoms, such as vomiting, loss of consciousness or cyanosis.

• Urinary output is important. A Foley catheter may be inserted if the patient has retention of urine. Watch especially the amount voided by the patient who has had a pituitary tumor, because damage to the gland may impair its manufacture of vasopressin, which regulates the amount of urine excreted. Postoperatively, the patient usually will be incontinent of urine and feces for one or two days, due to the depression of the voluntary cortical centers that control bladder and bowel habits.

• Edema may be present in the face, especially around the eyes. Ice compresses may be allowed. If the patient's face looks swollen and has ecchymotic areas, forewarn his family. Before they see him, tell them that the swelling and the black-and-blue spots are both expected and temporary.

• Watch the eyes. The patient may suffer a loss of the corneal reflex and keep his eyes open without blinking. Because blinking keeps the eye moist and free from specks of dust, the unblinking eye becomes dry and prone to corneal ulcers.

Position. The neurosurgeon will prescribe the position in which the patient is to be placed postoperatively, depending on the surgery performed, the amount of cerebral edema and his preference. In general, the heads of patients who have had craniotomies are kept elevated, often to 35° or 50°. If there is considerable edema, the doctor may order that the head of the bed be kept at a 90° angle. Patients usually are not kept flat, because this position increases the blood supply to the brain and may start venous bleeding. However, when a patient is in shock, the physician may order that he be kept flat.

When the postoperative neurologic patient is helpless, he is positioned as carefully as is any patient who cannot move himself. Special attention is given to placing the limbs in positions of function, so that even the patient whose prognosis is unfavorable will get as much use of his limbs as possible.

Fluid and Food. After the patient has recovered from anesthesia, his intake is determined by his condition, which may necessitate intravenous feedings, gastric lavage or a soft diet. Intravenous fluids should run no faster than 40 drops a minute. Cerebral edema may cause the doctor to order restricted fluids. Some postoperative patients who are otherwise able to eat may not be able to swallow well. They should be fed slowly and carefully to avoid aspiration of food or fluids, which may start a fatal pneumonia.

Rehabilitation. As soon as the patient returns from the operating room, his rehabilitation begins. Even the patient who is not expected to return to full activity should be given every chance and encouragement for as full a return of function as is possible. Proper positioning is the first step. Then passive exercises are done until the patient can move himself. At this point he is supervised in active exercises.

REFERENCES AND BIBLIOGRAPHY

BROOKS, H. L.: The Golden Rule for the unconscious patient, *Nurs. Forum* 4:12, 1965.

BUTTS, C., and CANNEY, V.: The unresponsive patient, *Am. J. Nurs.* 67:1886, September, 1967.

CARINI, E., and OWENS, G.: *Neurological and Neurosurgical Nursing*, ed. 5, St. Louis, Mosby, 1970.

GARDNER, E.: *Fundamentals of Neurology*, ed. 5, Philadelphia, Saunders, 1968.

GARDNER, M. A.: Responsiveness as a measure of consciousness, *Am. J. Nurs.* 68:1034, May, 1968.

HILKEMEYER, R., *et al.*: Nursing care of patients with brain tumors, *Am. J. Nurs.* 64:81, March, 1964.

LEAVENS, M. E.: Brain tumors, *Am. J. Nurs.* 64:78, March, 1964.

LUESSENHOP, A. J.: Care of the unconscious patient, *Nurs. Forum* 4:6, 1965.

McLAURIN, R. L., and FORD, L. E.: Extradural hematoma, *J. Neurosurg.* 21:364, 1964.

MERRITT, H. H.: *Textbook of Neurology*, ed. 4, Philadelphia, Lea, 1967.

OLSON, E. V., *et al.*: The hazards of immobility, *Am. J. Nurs.* 67:779, April, 1967.

TATE, G., *et al.*: Correct use of electric thermometers, *Am. J. Nurs.* 70:1898, September, 1970.

Index

Abdomen, distention of, 137
surgery of, urinary retention following, 137
Abortion, nursing care in, 562
treatment in, 562
types of, 561
Abscess, breast, 594, *594*
inflammation of, 69, *69*
lung, 319
rupture of, 70
Accident(s), cerebrovascular. *See* Cerebrovascular accident
fractures in. *See* Fracture(s)
reporting of, 113
to nurses, safety checklist in, 111
Acetazolamide, in epilepsy, 221
in glaucoma, 264
Acetone, 535
in urine, tests to measure, 535
Acetylcholine, related to stress, 56
Acetylsalicylic acid. *See* Aspirin
Acids, stomach, in peptic ulcer, 431
neutralization of, 432
Acidemia, and alkalemia, 635
Acidosis, and alkalosis, 635
and diabetes, 534
Acne, 609
steroid induced, 186
Acromegaly, 532
ACTH. *See* Adrenocorticotropic hormone
Acthar, in arthritis, 185
Actinomycin D, for cancer, 149
Acute, definition of, 59
Adaptation, diseases of, 57
Adaptation syndrome, 56
Adaptive response, limitations upon, 57
support of, by nurse, 58
Addison's disease, diagnosis of, 529
nursing care in, 529
symptoms of, 528
treatment of, 529
Adenocarcinoma, 143
renal, 513
Addiction, alcohol. *See* Alcohol, addiction to
drug. *See* Drugs, addiction to
Admitting record, operation permit with, 123
prior to surgery, 123
Adolescence, sexual adjustment in, 2
Adolescent(s). *See also* Adult, young
female, and menstrual cycle, 548
hospitalization of, 10
privacy of, 10

Adrenal cortex, hormonal activity of, as body defense, 66
hyperfunction of. *See* Cushing's syndrome
hypofunction of. *See* Addison's disease
Adrenal glands, 528
Adrenal medulla, tumor involving, 531
Adrenal-pituitary system, adaptive hormones of, 57
Adrenal shock, 529
Adrenal steroid hormones, for cancer, 150
Adrenalectomy, bilateral, 593
in Cushing's syndrome, 531
Adrenalin, related to stress, 56
secretion of, as body defense, 66
Adrenergic agents, in allergy, 75
in shock, 632
Adrenocortical crisis, acute, 528
Adrenocorticotropic hormone, for cancer, 150
in arthritis, 185
in nephrosis, 513
in purpura, 344
in ulcerative colitis, 429
overproduction of, 530, 531
secretion of, and stress, 56
side effects of, 186
underproduction of, 528, 529
Adult(s), aged. *See* Elderly patient; Patient, geriatric
development of, 1-4
intangibles in, 4
sensitivity of nurse to, 2
developmental tasks of, 1-4
cultural determination of, 3
elderly. *See* Elderly patient; Patient; Geriatric
in middle life, aging in, 1
alcoholism in, 92
caring for, 12-19
demands upon, 15
dependence upon, by aged, 15
development of, implications of, 17
developmental tasks of, 14
summary of, 17
exercise by, 13
eyesight of, 13
hearing in, 14
height and weight of, 12
illness in, 17
increase in numbers of, *18*
independence in children of, 14
menopause in, 13

Adult(s), in middle life (*Cont.*)
pace of, 13
physical changes in, 12
satisfactions of, 16
sexual vigor of, 13
single, problems of, 15
strength of, 12
uncooperative, attitude of nurse toward, 51
young. *See also* Adolescent(s)
aging of, 1
and hospital rules, 6
caring for, 5-11
counseling of, by nurse, 9
development of, implications for nursing in, 9
developmental tasks of, 8
effects of hospitalization upon, 6
encouragement of, by nurse, 9
hearing changes in, 8
idealism of, 7
identification with, by nurse, 7
independence of, from parents, 8
nutritional requirements of, 10
parents of, working with, 10
physical changes in, 7
position sense in, 8
privacy of, 10
restlessness of, 5
self-esteem in, 8
speed of reaction in, 8
visual accommodation in, 7
Age, hearing loss as sign of, 8
relationship of, to physical work, *3*
Aging, osteoarthritis as symptom of, 190
patterns of, 25
physiologic changes in, 23
rates of, 1
signs of, 12
visual accommodation as, 7, *8*
Agranulocytosis, 345
Air hunger, 534
Airborne infection, combating, 326
Airway, maintenance of, following surgery, 133
maintenance of, in coma, 211
in respiratory failure, 637
oropharyngeal, following surgery, 133
pharyngeal, *132*
Albumin, tests of, 474
Alcohol, addiction to. *See also* Alcoholism
economic aspects of, 91

Alcohol, addiction to (*Cont.*)
    incidence of, 91, 92
    treatment of, 91
    dependence upon, ambivalence toward, 91
    and tolerance, 91
    onset of, 91
    drugs and tobacco, abuse of, 90-106
    in diabetic diet, 537
    in trigeminal neuralgia, 225
    ingestion of, physiologic effect of, 93
Alcoholics Anonymous, 96
Alcoholism. *See also* Alcohol, addiction to
    effect upon family, 94
    effect upon liver, 93
    etiology of, 92
    incidence of, 92
    malnutrition in, 93
    patterns of consumption in, 94
    physiologic aspects of, 93
    rehabilitation in, 96
    symptoms of, 93
      delirium tremens as, 94
    treatment of, 95
      drugs in, 95
Aldosterone, overproduction of, 531
Alienation, of young adult, 6
Alkalemia, and acidemia, 635
Alkaline phosphatase, 474
Alkalosis, and acidosis, 635
Alkylating agents, for cancer, 149
Allergen, avoidance of, 74
    definition of, 72
Allergic reactions, in heart disease, 355
    in skin, 611
Allergic rhinitis, 305
    treatment of, 306
Allergy(ies), 71-76
    anaphylactic shock in, 75
    complicating use of ostomy appliance, 451
    definition of, 71
    diagnosis of, 73
    drug, 72
    etiology of, 72
    incidence of, 72
    treatment of, 74
      antihistamines in, 75
      desensitization in, 74
      nurse's role in, 73
Aluminum hydroxide gel, in peptic ulcer, 432
Ambulation, following cerebrovascular accident, 238
    following surgery, 140
Amenorrhea, 551
Amino acid solutions, 64
Aminophylline, in bronchial asthma, 309
    in pulmonary edema, 365
Ammonia, odor of, in incontinence, 503
Amnesia, in alcoholism, 94
Amphetamines, addiction to, 98
Ampicillin, in pneumonia, 298

Amputation, 195-204
    breast. *See* Mastectomy
    casts in, 198
    causes of, 196
    closed, 199
    complications of, 202
    emotional adjustment to, 195
    lower extremity, 198
    management of, bandaging in, 202
      bed positioning in, 199
      contractures in, 200
      hemorrhage in, 199
      phantom limb in, 197, 202
      postoperative, 199
        complications during, 202
      preoperative, 196
      surgical, 198
    open, 199
    phantom limb in, 197, 202
    prostheses in, temporary, 200
      training with, 203
      upper extremity, 201
    stump in, care of, 203
    Syme's, 198
Amyl nitrite, in angina pectoris, 383
Anal sphincter, dilatation of, 138
Analgesic(s), addiction to, 100
    to relieve pain, 86
    following surgery, 135
Analgesic ointments, 87
Anaphylactic shock, 75
Anaplasia, definition of, 143
Androgen, in metastatic cancer, 593
Anemia, 336
    aplastic, 339
    Cooley's, 339
    due to blood loss, 339
    due to destruction of red cells, 339
    hemolytic, acquired, 339
    in renal failure, 686
    iron deficiency, 337
    pernicious, 338
    regenerative, 339
    sickle cell, 339
Anesthesia, surgical, recovery following, 132, 133
Aneurysms, 405, *406*
    of blood vessels of brain, 234
    ventricular, 675
Anger, associated with casts, 169
    physical symptoms of, 77
    reaction toward, 38
Angina pectoris, 382
Angiocardiogram, in heart disease, 355
Angiography, cerebral, 209
Animal bites, first aid in, 117
Ankylosis, fibrous, 182
    of stapes, 273
      surgery of, 274
    osseous, 182
Anoscopy, 419
Anorexia, and nausea, 425
Anoxia, 60
Antabuse, in alcoholism, 96
Antacids, in peptic ulcer, 432

Antibiotics, in bronchial asthma, 310
    in bronchitis, 312
    in chronic bronchitis, 313
    in endocarditis, 377
    in pneumonia, 297
    in tuberculosis, 330
    in ulcerative colitis, 430
Antibodies, definition of, 71
Anticoagulant therapy, in cerebrovascular accident, 233
Anticonvulsants, in epilepsy, 220
Antidiuretic hormone, 532
Antigen(s), definition of, 71
    desensitization with, 74
Antihistamines, in allergy, 75
    in Parkinson's disease, 215
Antimalarials, in arthritis, 185
Antimetabolites, in cancer, 149
    in leukemia, 341
Antipruritics, 606
Antithyroid drugs, in hyperthyroidism, 521
Antitoxins, definition of, 71
Antrotomy, 282
Anus, hemorrhoids involving, 470, *470*
Anxiety, Addison's disease associated with, 530
    alleviation of, 38
    and drug dependence, 100
    in bronchial asthma, 309
    levels of, 39
    of nurse, 40
    pain augmented by, 85
    physical symptoms related to, 77
    preoperative, 126
    relief of, through alcohol, 92
    vs. fear, 38
Aortic insufficiency, 373
Aortic stenosis, 373, *373*
Aortogram, in heart disease, 355
Appendicitis, diagnosis of, 461, *461*
    nursing care in, 462
    treatment of, 462
Aqueous humor, and glaucoma, 263
Arachnoid, 212
Arabinosylcytosine, in leukemia, 341
Aramine, in shock, 631
Arm, fracture of, cast in, 170
      windows in, 168
    Volkmann's contracture with, 168
Arrhythmias, and dysrhythmias, 644
    electrocardiography in, 645
    in myocardial infarction, 669
    treatment of, 648
Arterial blood pressure, 386
Arterial clamp, in cerebrovascular accident, 234
Arterial pressure, physiologic control of, 386
Arteriograms, in heart disease, 355
Arteriosclerosis, 358
Artery(ies), aneurysms of, 405
    coronary. *See* Coronary artery disease.
    ischemia involving, 392
    of leg, *407*

Artery(ies) (*Cont.*)
  radial, Volkmann's contracture associated with, 167
  Raynaud's disease of, 398
Arteriography, hepatic, 475
  renal, 493
Arteriosclerosis, 228, 393
  definition of, 393
  in diabetes, 542
  symptoms of, 229, 394
  treatment of, 394
Arthritis, 181. *See also* Osteoarthritis
  infectious, 181
  means of living with, 189
  related to stress, 57
  rheumatoid, 182, *182, 183*
    diet in, 184
    etiology of, 183
    incidence of, 182
    pathology of, 182
    symptoms of, 183
    treatment of, 184
      cold in, 188
      drug therapy in, 184
      equipment in, 188
      exercise in, 187
      heat in, 188
      nursing care in, 186
      rest in, 187
      surgery in, 189
  types of, 181
Arthroplasty, in rheumatoid arthritis, 189
Asepto syringe, *290*
Asphyxiation, dangers of, in coma, 211
Aspirin, adverse effects of, 184
  allergy to, 72
  in arthritis, 184
  in common cold, 303
Asthma, bronchial, 306
  anxiety during, 309
  attacks of, prolonged, 311
  causes of, inhalants as, 310
  incidence and course of, 307
  symptoms of, 307
  treatment of, 307
    bronchodilators in, 308
    drug therapy in, 308
    long-term, 310
    nursing care in, 311
  definitions in, 306
  extrinsic, 307
  psychosomatic, 80
  stress related, 77
Astigmatism, 261
Atabrine, in arthritis, 185
Atelectasis, postoperative, 138
Atheromas, treatment of, surgical, 234
Atherosclerosis, 228, 358, 406
  and coronary artery disease, 381
  definition of, 392, 393
  symptoms of, 394
  treatment of, 394
Athlete's foot, 615
Atrial fibrillation, 647
Atrial septal defect, 675

Atrophy, definition of, 65
Atropine, in Parkinson's disease, 215
  prior to surgery, 127
Auditory canal, disorders of, 277
  insects in, 277
  straightening of, 278
Azoospermia, permanent, 582

Bacille Calmette Guerin, 334
Bacilli, tubercle, characteristics of, 325
  in sputum, 330
  transmission of, 327
Back, care of, 173
Bacteremia, transient, and endocarditis, 375
Bacterial endocarditis. *See* Endocarditis, bacterial
Bacterial infection, of brain, 213
Bandage, elastic, application of, 139, *139*
Banthine, in hypermotility, 432
Barbiturates, addiction to, 100
  prescription of, nursing considerations in, 100
  prior to surgery, 127
  withdrawal symptoms in, 100
Barium, in gastrointestinal roentgenography, 418
Barium esophagogram, 475
Bathing, in paraplegia, *253*
  of patient in traction, 173
Bathtubs, grab bars for, *31*
BCG, in tuberculosis prophylaxis, 334
Bed, CircOlectric, in paraplegia, 248, *249*
  hi-lo, use of, by elderly, 33
    safety precautions in, 111
  oscillating, in peripheral vascular disease, 394
  safety factors involving, 111, 112, 113
  side rails of, 111
Bed cradle, in peripheral vascular disease, 396
Bed rest, in spinal cord impairment, 244
Bedpan, with spica cast, 168
Bees, first aid against, 120
Belching, and heartburn, 425
Belladonna, in hypermotility, 432
  in Parkinson's disease, 215
Belts, ileostomy, 452
Benadryl, in Parkinson's disease, 215
Benedict's test, 535
Benemid, in gout, 192
Benzalkonium chloride, in animal bites, 117
Benzedrine, addiction to, 98
Bergonie and Tribondeau, law of, 155
Beta adrenergic stimulator, in shock, 632
Bicarbonate of soda, in shock, 116
Bile, formation of, 483
Biliary system. *See* Gallbladder
Bilirubin, total serum, 474
Bilirubin concentration, in jaundice, 475

Biopsy, aspiration, of breast, 587
  cervical, 560
  endometrial, in infertility, 553
  of breast, 587
  of liver, 475
  of thyroid gland, 525
  testicular, in infertility, 553
Birth control, religious attitudes toward, 553
Birthmarks, 618
Bites, and infestations, 615
  first aid in, 117
  snakes, 116, *116*
Blackouts, in alcoholism, 94
Bladder. *See also* Urinary tract; Kidneys, etc.
  bulging of, into vagina, 572
  calculi involving, 507
  cystoscopy of, 493
    care following, 494
  definition of, 489
  drainage of, catheters in, 499, *500*
  emptying of, prior to surgery, 129
  inflammation of, 509
  pyelography of, retrograde, 493
  spasm of, with prostatectomy, 578
  surgery of, 514
  tumors of, 514
Bladder rehabilitation, in paraplegia, 252
Blanching, following surgery, 133
Blanching sign, in fracture treatment observation, 167
Bleeding. *See* Hemorrhage
Blepharoplasty, 620
Blepharospasm, in Parkinson's disease, 215
Blindness, aid in, 260
  courtesies and attitudes in, 261
  definition of, legal, 258
  in diabetes, 543
  misconceptions in, 259
  night, and vitamin A, 257
  self-care in, 259
Blood, cells of, and anemia, 337, 339
  capillary fragility test of, 336
  chemistry of, and urine, 490
  cholesterol in, in hyperthyroidism, 521
  circulating, volume of, in pulmonary edema, 365
  circulation of, and healing, 68
    and heart anatomy, 351, *351*
    decrease in, 60
    in elderly, 31
    measurement of, 360
  clotting of, and leukemia, 340
    emboli associated with. *See* Embolism
  coagulation defects of, in jaundice, 476
  coagulation time of, 340
  disorders of, 335-346
    diagnosis of, 335
      sternal puncture in, 336
  glucose in, 533

Blood (*Cont.*)
  hemoglobin in, and blood dyscrasias, 336
    and etiology of anemia, 337, 339
  in renal failure, 684
  ketone bodies in, in diabetes, 533
  leukocytes in, and leukemia, 340
  loss of, anemia due to, 339
  oxygenation of, and hypoxia, 135
  precautions involving, in hepatitis, 482
  sugar in, measurement of, 535
  supply of, lack of, ischemia as, 392
    measures to increase, 393
  thrombocytes in, and leukemia, 340
  transfusion of, in leukemia, 344
  whole, in replacement therapy, 63
Blood dyscrasias, 335
Blood-gas studies, in chronic obstructive pulmonary disease, 315
Blood pressure, arterial, 386
  in shock, 629
  diastolic, 386
    and primary hypertension, 387
  drop in, and cerebrovascular disease, 229
  in heart disease, 353
  in heart failure, 359
  in urologic disorders, 495
  recording of, prior to surgery, 131
  systolic, 386
Blood tests, in diabetes, 535
Blood urea nitrogen, 490
Blood vessels. *See also* Veins; Intravenous
  aneurysms of, 405
  diseases of. *See* Vascular disease, peripheral
  emboli of. *See* Embolism
  inflammation of, 399
  of brain, aneurysms of, 234
  surgical conditions of, 405, *406*
  thrombosis of. *See* Thrombosis
  trauma to, 406
Body, interaction of, with mind, 77-83
Body defenses, 65
  and tissue repair, 67
  internal, 66
  source of, 65
Body response, to infection, 69, *69, 70*
Body tissues, repair of, 67
Boils. *See* Furuncles
Bone(s), diseases of, 181-194. *See also* Joints and specific conditions.
  fracture of. *See* Fracture(s)
  grafts of, in treatment of fractures, 175
    material from, 175
  infection of. *See* Osteomyelitis
  infection of, amputation in, 196
  joints of. *See* Joints.
  lesions of, radiotherapy in treatment of, 154
  necrosis of, following fixation, 177
  repair of, physiology of, 161
  tumors of, 192

Bone marrow, depression of, in leukemia, 342
  in radiotherapy, 157
  specimens of, in diagnosis of blood dyscrasias, 336
Bone marrow failure, 339
Botulism, first aid in, 117
Bowel(s), ostomies involving, 446-460
Bowel habits, and diarrhea and constipation, 426
Bowel movement, following hemorrhoidectomy, 471
  following prostatectomy, 579
  in coma, 211
  prior to surgery, 129
Bowel rehabilitation, in paraplegia, 251
Bowman's capsule, *490*
Braces, in rheumatoid arthritis, 188
Bradycardia, pacemakers in, 656
  sinus, 646
Braille, 260, *260*
Brain. *See also* Cerebral; Cerebro-; Neurologic
  blood vessels of, aneurysms of, 234
  effect of shock upon, 630
  electrical impulses of, 210
  injuries to, 704
    nursing care in, 705
    intracranial pressure of, 701
  lesions of, visualization of, 208
  structures of, *206*
  transport of blood to, related to cerebrovascular disease, 228
  tumors of, 706
    shifts in, 209
    treatment of, 707
Brain scanning, 210
Breast, abscess of, 594, *594*
  cancer of, metastases of, 593
    treatment of, 150
  diseases of, 584-595
    cystic, 587
      incidence of, 584
  disease of, diagnosis of, 584
    incidence of, 584
    signs and symptoms of, 585
  examination of, 585
    biopsy in, 587
    by physician, 586
    emotional factors in, 586
  mastectomy of. *See* Mastectomy
  physiology of, 584
  surgery of, 587. *See also* Mastectomy
    complications of, 592
    preoperative care in, 587
Breath, shortness of. *See* Asthma
Breathing. *See also* Respiration
  in cardiac arrest, 653
  mouth-to-mouth, 115
  positive pressure, in pulmonary edema, 366
Breathing exercises, to improve respiratory function, 317
Bright's disease, 511
Bromsulphthalein time, 474
Bronchiectasis, 319

Bronchitis, acute, 312
  chronic, 312
    diagnosis of, 313
    diet in, 313
    etiology of, 312
    prognosis in, 314
    treatment of, 313
  effect of tobacco upon, 102
Bronchodilators, in bronchial asthma, 308
Bronchography, 293
Bronchoscopy, 292
  complications of, 293
BSP test, 474
Buboes, 599
Buck's extension, as simple traction, 173
Buerger-Allen exercises, 394
Buerger's disease, 399
Burns, convalescence in, 698
  emotional considerations in, 700
  infection in, 699
  nursing care in, 694
  nutrition in, 698
  prognosis of, 693
  recovery from, 698
  shock phase in, 693
  treatment of, 692-700
    and skin, 696
    complications in, 699
  turning point in, 697
  types of, 692
Busulfan, in leukemia, 342
Butazolidin, in arthritis, 185
  in gout, 192

Calcium, and hyperparathyroidism, 527
  and hypoparathyroidism, 528
  concentration of, in body fluid, 62
Calcium carbamide, in alcoholism, 96
Calculi. *See also* Lithiasis; Stones
  etiology of, 505
  in renal pelvis, 507
  involving bladder, 507
  prevention of, 507
  symptoms of, 506
  treatment of, 506
  urinary, 505
Callus, in pathology of fracture, 161
Caloric requirements, of young adults, 10
Calycectomy, 507
Cancer, 143-153. *See also* Neoplasia; Sarcoma ; Tumor (s)
  as intestinal obstruction, 467
  cells of, 143
  control of, 150
  cytologic test for, 559
  definition of, 61, 143
  diagnosis of, 146
  "Pap" smears in, 146
    patient's reaction to, 150
  epidemiology of, 143
  etiology of, 145
  incidence of, by site and sex, *145*
  metastatic, involving breast, 593

Cancer (*Cont.*)
  of cervix, 145, 568
  of colon, 443, *443*
  of esophagus, 440
    treatment of, 441
  of fundus, 569
  of gastrointestinal tract, 437-445
    conditions associated with, 438
    symptoms of, 437
    treatment of, 438
  of larynx. *See* Larynx, cancer of
  of lung. *See* Lung, cancer of
  of mouth, 438
    complications of, 440
    problems in, 439
  of prostate, 149, 579
    treatment of, 580
  of rectum, 443
  of skin, 145
  of stomach, 145, 442
  of testes, 582
  of uterus, 568
  of vulva, 569
  pathology of, 143
  prevention of, 150
  radiotherapy in. *See* Radiotherapy
  sites of, primary, 144
  spread of, routes of, 144
  squamous cell, 143, 619
  symptoms of, 146
    warning signals as, 146
  thyroid, 525
    radioactive iodine in, 159
  treatment of, 147
    antineoplastic agents in, 148
    chemotherapy in, 149
      dosages of, 149
    hormones in, 149, 593
    radiation therapy in, 147
    role of nurse in, 151
    surgical, 147
Candida albicans, causing vaginitis, 564
Cannabis, 99
Capillary fragility test, 336
Carbohydrate, in insulin shock, 542
Carbon dioxide combining power, 536
  and diabetic coma, 541
  and respiratory failure, 636
Carbon tetrachloride, toxicity of, 452
Carbuncles, 614
  in diabetes, 544
Carcinoma. *See* Cancer
Cardiac. *See also* Cardio-; Heart
Cardiac arrest, 652
  breathing in, 653
  resuscitation in, 654
Cardiac arrhythmias. *See* Arrhythmias
Cardiac catheterization, 356
Cardiac chair, 362, *362*
Cardiac compression, in cardiac arrest, 653
Cardiac disease, valvular, acquired, 673
Cardiac lesions, requiring surgery, 673
Cardiac orifice, 431
Cardiac output, in elderly, 24

Cardiac rhythmicity, and regulation, 643
Cardiac septum, atrial-septal defect involving, 675
Cardiac surgery, continuing care in, 681
  education program in, 678
  fluid and electrolyte balance in, 678
  lesions requiring, 673
  myocardial revascularization in, 674
  nursing in, 672-682
  postoperative period in, 679
  preoperative period in, 677
  psychological considerations in, 676, 680
Cardiac valve, diseases, acquired, 673
  surgical repair in, 674
  replacement of, 673
  tissue transplantation in, 673
Cardio-. *See also* Heart
Cardiopulmonary system, anatomy of, 351, *351*
Cardiovascular deaths, causes of, *350*
Caseation, in tuberculosis, 328
Castration, fear of, in young adult, 10
Casts, bivalved, in rheumatoid arthritis, 188
  for fractures. *See* Fractures, casts for
  in amputation, 198
  spica, in lumbar laminectomy, 246
Cataracts, 262
  treatment of, 263
Catheterization, cardiac, 356
  of female patients, 547
  postoperative, 137
  preoperative, 129
Catheters, in prostatectomy, 577
  in urinary incontinence, 502
  maintenance of, 134
  urologic. *See* Urologic disorders, catheters in
Catholicism, and birth control, 554
CCC, in alcoholism, 96
Cecostomy, 459
Celiac disease, 470
Cells, cancer, 143
  concentration of particles in, *62*
  damage to, and inflammatory response, 66
  fluid components of, 61
  membranes of, and fluid exchange, 62
  radiation of, 155
  Reed-Sternberg, 346
  spinal cord, 242
Cephalin flocculation, 475
Cephalothin, in pneumonia, 298
Cerebral. *See also* Brain; Cerebro-; Neurologic
Cerebral edema, 702
Cerebral embolism, 229
Cerebral hemorrhage, 229
Cerebral insufficiency, 234
Cerebral ischemia, 230
  treatment of, 234
Cerebral laceration, 704
Cerebral thrombosis, 229, *229*

Cerebritis, 213
Cerebro-. *See also* Brain; Cerebral; Neurologic
Cerebrospinal fluid, lumbar puncture to obtain, 206
  pressure of, measurement of, 207, *207*
Cerebrovascular accident, aphasia in, 233
  consciousness in, 236
  diagnosis of, 233
  hemiplegia in, 232
  recovery from, ambulation in, 238
    exercise in, 238, *235-238*
  symptoms of, 232
    care of affected arm in, 239
    long-term, 239
    medical, 233
    nursing care in, 235, *235*, 236, *236*
      and family visits, 236
    rehabilitation following, 239
    speech rehabilitation in, 240
    surgical, 234
Cerebrovascular disease, 228-241
  and hypertension, 229
  death rates from, 228
  memory deterioration associated with, 230
  pathophysiology of, 228
  patient behavior in, complexity of, 230
  patients with, dependence of, 231
    families of, 231
    mental status of, evaluation of, 231
    orientation of, 231
  special problems in, 230
Cerumen, impacted, treatment of, 277
Cervical biopsy, 560
Cervical disk, rupture of, 244
Cervical spine, injury to, 246
Cervicitis, 565
Cervix, cancer of, 145, 568
  dilatation of, and curettage of uterus, 560
  inflammation of, 565
Chalazion, 266
Chancre, of syphilis, 598, *598*
Chancroid, 599
Charcot joint, 599
Chemical hepatitis, 483
Chemotherapy. *See* Drug therapy
Chest, injuries to, 303
  roentgenography of, in respiratory disorders, 292
  surgery of, postoperative care in, 320
Chest drainage, 321
  effect upon patient, 322
Cheyne-Stokes respiration, in heart failure, 359
Chills, as sign of infection, 70
  nursing care in, 71
Chloral hydrate, prior to surgery, 128
Chlorambucil, in leukemia, 341
Chloramphenicol, in pneumonia, 298
Chloromycetin, for pneumonia, 298

Chloride concentrations, in body fluid, 62
Chloroquine, in arthritis, 185
Cholecystectomy, 484
  Penrose drain following, 484
Cholecystitis, 483
  acute, 484
  treatment of, 484
Choledocholithiasis, 485
Cholelithiasis, 483
  treatment of, 484
Cholesteatoma, and perforation of eardrum, 275
Cholesterol, in atherosclerosis, 393
  serum, 475
Chordotomy, percutaneous, 89
  to relieve pain, 88
Choriocarcinoma, treatment of, 149
Chronic, definition of, 59
Circulation, of blood. See Blood, circulation of
Cirrhosis, 476
  fluid retention in, 478
  Laennec's, 476
  treatment of, 477
Claudication, intermittent, 392
Clavicle, fracture of, 179
Cleanliness, in coma, 212
  involving colostomy, 456
  of skin, 603
  patient, attitude of nurse toward, 48
  prior to surgery, 129
Climacteric, and menopause, 549
Clinistix, in diagnosis of diabetes, 535
Clostridium botulinum, food poisoning by, 117
Clostridium perfringens, food poisoning by, 117
Clothing, preoperative disposition of, 130
Cobalt therapy, 158. See also Radiotherapy
  nursing care in, 160
Codeine, in pneumonia, 299
Colchicine, in gout, 192
Cold, common, 303
  in rheumatoid arthritis, 188
  overexposure to, 119
Cold sores, 614
Colic, renal, 506
  ureteral, 506
Colitis, stress-related, 77
  ulcerative. See Ulcerative colitis
Colon, cancer of, 443, 443
  diverticula of, 468, 468
  inflammation of. See Ulcerative colitis
  irritable, 426
  polyps involving, 469
  volvulus of, 467, 467
Colostomy, clothing with, 459
  diet with, 459
  double-barreled, 455
  irrigation with, 457
    scheduling of, 458
    types of, 456

Colostomy (Cont.)
  management of, cleanliness in, 456
    methods in, 456
  or ileostomy, 446. See also Ostomy
  single-barreled, 455
  stoma of, 454
    covering of, 458
    maturation of, 450
  types of, 454, 455
Colporrhaphy, 572
Coma, and diabetic ketosis, 534, 540
  as level of consciousness, 211
  bowel movements during, 212
  cleanliness during, 212
  diabetes, 534, 540
    symptoms of, 543
    treatment of, 541
  hepatic, in cirrhosis, 477, 478
  in cerebrovascular accident, 232
  nursing care in, 51, 211
Combined system disease, and pernicious anemia, 338
Common cold, 303
Complaints, by patient, 49
Compresses, for inflammation, 67
Concussion, 704
Conflict, between patient and nurse, 42
Confusion, in delirium, 81
  of elderly, 33
Congenital defects, range of, 59
Conization, in cervicitis, 565
Conjunctivitis, 266
Connective tissue, inflammation of. See Arthritis, rheumatoid
Consciousness levels of, 210
Constipation, and diarrhea, 425
Contact lenses, dangers of, 255
Contracture, associated with amputation, 200
  in burns, 699
  Volkmann's, 167
Convulsions, epileptic, 219
  clonic phase of, 218
  nursing care in, 219
Cornea, infection of, 255
Coronary artery disease, 380. See also Heart disease
  and angina pectoris, 382
  epidemiology in, 381
  pathophysiology of, 382
  treatment of, drugs in, 383
  surgery in, 384
Coronary care unit, 662
Coronary circulation, 380, 380
Coronary occlusion, 382
Corpus luteum, 548
Corticosteroids. See also Steroids
  Addison's disease associated with, 528
  in allergy, 75
  in arthritis, 185
  in tuberculosis, 331
  side effects of, 186
Corticotropin, in arthritis, 185

Cortisol, related to stress, 56
Cortisone, in cancer, 150
  in Addison's disease, 529
  in purpura, 344
  in ulcerative colitis, 429
  secretion of, related to stress, 56
Cosmetic surgery, and functional improvement, 620
Coumadin, in cerebrovascular accident, 234
Counseling, of young adults, 9
Cranial nerves, neuralgia involving, 225
Cranium, pressure in, increase in, 701
Creams, skin, allergy to, 451
Crutch palsy, 177
Crutch walking, 177
Crutchfield clamp, with carotid artery, 234
Crutchfield tongs, 178
  in cervical spine injury, 246
  in traction, 171, 172
Crying, by patient, 42
  attitude of nurse toward, 47
Cryosurgery, 263
Cryptorchidism, 581
Cultural determination, of developmental tasks, 3
Curettage. See Dilatation and curettage
Cushing's syndrome, 530
  diagnosis of, 530
  treatment of, 531
Cyanosis, following surgery, 133
Cyclophosphamide, in leukemia, 342
Cycloserine, in tuberculosis, 331
Cystic disease, of breast, 587
  incidence of, 584
Cystitis, 509
Cystocele, 572
Cystoscope, 492
Cystoscopy, of bladder, 493
  care following, 494
Cystourethrography, 493
Cysts, ovarian, 568
  sebaceous, 615
Cytologic test, for cancer, 559

Dandruff, 604
  treatment of, 610
Death, attitudes toward, 107
  of family, 109
  of nurse, 107, 109
  of patient, 108
  care of patient prior to, 107-110
  causes of, 59
Decubitus ulcers. See Ulcers, decubitus
Defects, congenital. See Congenital defects
Defibrillation, 652
Deficiency diseases, 60
Dehiscence, of surgical wounds, 140
Dehydration, in diabetes, 534
Delerious patient, 81
  nursing care of, 82

Delirium tremens, in alcoholism, 94
in cirrhosis, 477
Demerol, in pulmonary edema, 364
postoperative, 135
preoperative, 127
Dentures. *See also* Prostheses
of elderly, care of, 31
Deodorants, following ostomy, 453
Dependency, in coma, 212
of elderly patient, 26
Depression, emotional. *See* Emotional
depression
Dermabrasion, 621
Dermatitis, seborrheic, 610
Dermatitis venenata, 613
Dermatologic conditions, 603-619. *See
also* Skin and specific conditions
description of, 609
disfigurement caused by, 605
nursing in, 604, 607
symptoms of, systemic, *617, 618*
treatment of, 606
nursing care in, 604, 607
Dermatophytosis, 615
Desensitization, and allergy, 74
Desoxycorticosterone, in Addison's disease, 529
Detached retina. *See* Retina, detached
Dexedrine, addiction to, 98
Dextran, in replacement therapy, 63
Dextroamphetamine, addiction to, 98
Diabetes, coma in. *See* Coma, diabetic
complications of, 540
diagnosis of, tests in, 535
diet in, 537
etiology of, 533
exercise in, 540
hypoglycemic reaction in, 541
infection in, 544
insulin shock in, 541
symptoms of, 543
ketosis in, 534, 540
neuropathy in, 543
pathology of, 533
patients in, uncooperative, 52
prognosis of, 544
social aspects of, 544
symptoms of, 533
training in, self-care, 58
treatment of, 536
diet in, 537
hypoglycemic agents in, 540
insulin in, 538
vascular disturbances in, 542
vision problems in, 543
Diabetes insipidus, 532
Diabetes mellitus, 533-544
Diabetic ketosis, and coma, 534, 540
Diacetylmorphine, addiction to, 101
Dialysis, peritoneal, 689
Diaphragm, wall of, defects in, 466
Diarrhea, and constipation, 425
in ulcerative colitis, 428
stress-related, 77
Diazepam, in epilepsy, 221
Dibucaine, in hemorrhoids, 471

Dicumarol, in cerebrovascular accident, 233
Diet, and feeding, in coma, 211
and fluids, following surgery, 136
in radiotherapy, 157
in chronic bronchitis, 313
in congestive heart failure, 362
in diabetes, 537
in gout, 192
in peptic ulcer, 432
in pneumonia, 300
in rheumatoid arthritis, 184
in ulcerative colitis, 429
low sodium, 362
potassium in, 363
purine-free, 192
Dietary deficiency, diseases caused by, 60
Dietary excesses, 60
Dietetic products, 537
Digestive tract. *See* Gastrointestinal tract
Digitalis, in congestive heart failure, 363
Digitalis intoxication, 363
Digitalization, 364
Dilantin, in epilepsy, 221
in increased intracranial pressure, 703
Dilatation, and curettage, 560
bath following, 561
nursing care in, 546
Diphenylhydantoin sodium, in epilepsy, 220
Diplococcus pneumoniae, 296
Diplopia, in Parkinson's disease, 215
Disease. *See also* Illness and specific diseases
adaptational, 57
congenital, range of, 59
deficiency, 60
etiology of, nonbiological factors in, 57
terminology in, 59
Disfigurement, conditions causing. *See* specific conditions
skin, 605
Disk, cervical, rupture of, treatment of, 244
intervertebral, herniated, *243*
and spinal cord impairment, 242
treatment of, conservative, 244
surgical, 245
lumbar, herniated, 244
Dislocations, and sprains, 179
Disorientation, following eye surgery, 269
of elderly, 33, 34
Disulfiram, in alcoholism, 96
Diuretics, in congestive heart failure, 361
Diverticulitis, 468, *468*
Diverticulosis, 468
Douching, of female patients, 547
precautions in, 554

Drainage, chest, 321
effect upon patient, 322
postoperative, 134
postural, 316, *317*
Dressings, in pruritus, 608
Drinking, of alcoholic beverages. *See* Alcohol; Alcoholism
Drug allergy, 72
Drug poisoning, 118
Drug therapy. *See also* Drug(s); Narcotics
in alcoholism, 95
in allergy, 74
in arthritis, 184
in bronchial asthma, toxic effect of, 312
in cancer, 149
metastatic, 594
in cardiac arrhythmias, 649
in congestive heart failure, 363
in glaucoma, 264
in pain, 86
in Parkinson's disease, 215
in peptic ulcer, 432
in pneumonia, 298
in tuberculosis, 330
in ulcerative colitis, 429
Drug(s). *See also* Drug therapy; Narcotics
abuse of, 90 106
addiction to, 90
drugs associated with, 98
economic aspects of, 91
incidence of, 91
treatment of, 91
antihypertensive, *389, 389*
antithyroid, in hyperthyroidism, 521
bronchodilating, 308
dependence upon, 97-102
ambivalence toward, 91
and tolerance, 91
characteristics of persons in, 97
drugs associated with, 98
nursing aspects of, 97
onset of, 91
prevention of, 102
relevance to nursing, 97
treatment of, 101
withdrawal sickness in, 101
habituation to, 90
in cancer, 148, 149
in congestive heart failure, 363
in psychosomatic illness, 79
in shock, 631
mood-elevating, 98
narcotic, nursing aspects of, 102
poisoning by, 213
psychotomimetic, 99
thyrourea, 521
uricosuric, 191
Dumping syndrome, and peptic ulcer, 434
Duodenum, and peptic ulcer, *430,* 431
perforation of, 436
Dura mater, 212 ·

Dust, and allergy, 74
  causing lung disease, 319
Dying. *See* Death
Dysmenorrhea, 550
Dyspareunia, 565
Dysphagia, in diverticulosis, 468
Dyspnea, in chronic obstructive pul-
  monary disease, 315
Dysrhythmias, and arrhythmias, 644

Ear, auditory canal of, disorders of,
    277
    insects in, 277
    straightening of, 278
  disorders of. *See* Hearing impair-
    ment
  inner, 278
  irrigation of, 279
  labyrinth, 278
  middle, 273
    infections of, 274
  ringing in, 273
  structures of, *271*
Eardrops, 278
Eardrum, incision of, 275
  puncture of, 275
Ectopic pregnancy, 563
Ectropion, 266
Eczema, 611
  stress-related, 77
  treatment of, 612
Edema, angioneurotic, 611
  causing obstruction of sinus drain-
    age, 282, *282*
  cerebral, 702
  in heart disease, 354
  pitting, of feet, *359*
  pulmonary, in shock, 630
    treatment of, oxygen in, 365
      positive pressure breathing in,
        366
      tourniquets in, 365, *366, 367*
Elastic bandage, application of, 139,
  139
Elderly patient. *See also* Adult(s);
    Patient, geriatric
  advantages in life of, 29
  aging of, patterns of, 25
  amputations in, 197
  and epidemiology of heart disease,
    350
  attitude toward, by nurse, 30
  care of, 20-35
    implication for nursing, 30
    myths in, 20
    nutrition in, 23
    senility in, 22
  dentures of, 31
  developmental tasks of, 26
    summary of, 29
  diabetes in, 536, 537, 538
  disengagement of, from family, 22
  disorientation in, 33, 34
  elimination problems of, 32
  employment of, 26

Elderly patient (*Cont.*)
  falls of, 24
    prevention of, *31*
  feet of, 31
  female, vaginal discharge of, 32
  fractures in, 24
    treatment of, 175, 176
  hobbies of, 28
  hospital care of, 33
  housing of, 28
  income of, 26
  incontinence in, 47, 501
  institutionalization of, 20, 29
  intellectual development of, 24
  learning ability of, 25
  loneliness of, 28
  marriage and, 22
  medical expenses of, 27
    Medicare and, 27
  night-time confusion in, 33
  personal hygiene of, 30
  physical care of, 30
  physical changes in, 23, 24
  physiological changes in, 23
  position sense of, 23
  posture of, 32
  siderails for beds of, 111
  skin of, 24
    lubrication of, 31
  sleep required by, 33
  speed of reactions of, 23
  susceptibility of, to temperature
    change, 24
  teeth of, 24
  time sense of, 32
  weight loss of, 23
Electric shock, first aid in, 116
Electrical potentials, in body fluid, 62
Electrical therapy, in arrhythmias, 650
Electrocardiogram, in heart disease,
    354
  in myocardial infarction, 665
  monitoring of, 411
Electrocardiography, arrhythmia, 645
Electroencephalography, 210
  in epilepsy, *217*
Electrolyte. *See also* Fluids
  and water regulation, 61
Electrolyte solutions, in replacement
    therapy, 64
  in shock, 116
Elephantiasis, 403
Elimination. *See also* Bowels
  in paraplegia, 249
  prior to surgery, 129
  problems of, in elderly, 32
Embolism, and thrombosis, 391-408
  cerebral. *See* Cerebral embolism
  definition of, 392
  in veins of legs, 139
  nursing care in, 404
  pulmonary, 405
    in myocardial infarction, 669
  surgery in, 404
  symptoms of, 404

Emergencies, first aid in, 114
    general principles of, 113
  hospital nursing involving, 120
  minor, first aid in, 119
  nursing in, 111-122
    legal aspects of, 121
    principles of, 121
    recognition of, 121
Emergency nursing, hospital, 120
Emergency wards, in hospitals, 120
Emollients, in skin disease, 606
Emotional dependence, in cerebrovas-
    cular disease, 231
Emotional depression, amphetamines
    in, 98
  guarding against suicide in, 48
  signs of, 48
Emotional factors, in etiology of can-
    cer, 146
  in gastrointestinal disorders, 424
  in gynecologic disorders, 545
Emotional problems, anxiety as, 38
  in gastrointestinal function, 415
Emotional reactions. *See also* Stress
  in menopause, 549
  to surgery, 126
Emotional support, of patients, 36, 43
  during physical examination, 45
Emphysema, effect of tobacco upon,
    102
  etiology of, 314
  pathology of, 314
  symptoms of, 315
  treatment of, 315
    breathing exercises in, 317, *317*
    nursing care in, 316
    postural drainage in, 317, *318*
Employment, of elderly, 26
Empyema, 302, 319
  complicating pneumonia, 301
Encephalitis, treatment of, 213
Encephalopathy, 213
Endocarditis, 371
  bacterial, etiology of, 375
    prognosis in, 377
    treatment of, 376
  signs and symptoms of, 376
Endocrine disorders, 519-532
Endocrine gland, ablation of, 593
  secretions of, as body defenses, 66
Endocrine system, related to stress, 56
Endolymph, 278
Endometrial biopsy, in infertility, 553
Endometriosis, 567
Endometrium, 548
Endoscopy, 419
Endotracheal intubation, in respira-
    tory failure, 637
Enemas, in paraplegia, 252
  prior to surgery, 129
Enteritis, regional, 469
Entropion, 266
Enucleation, of eye, 266
Ephedrine, in bronchial asthma, 309
Epididymitis, bilateral, 582
Epididymoorchitis, 581

Epilepsy, 216, *217*
  causes of, 217
  convulsions in, 219
  diagnosis of, 219
  electroencephalogram in, *217*
  seizures in, depression of tongue
    during, 219
    grand mal, 218
    Jacksonian, 219
    petit mal, 218
    psychomotor attacks as, 219
    types of, 218
  social and emotional implications
    of, 221
  status epilepticus in, 218
  treatment of, 220
    anticonvulsants in, 220
    relapse in, 221
Epileptic equivalent, 219
Epinephrine. *See also* Adrenalin
  in bronchial asthma, 308
  in gastric analysis, 417
  in nosebleed, 284
  in shock, 632
  secretion of, 531
Epistaxis, 284
Epitheliomas, 618
Ergometer, in heart disease rehabili-
  tation, 410
Erythromycin, in pneumonia, 298
Escherichia coli, urinary infection
  caused by, 508
Esophageal hiatus hernia, 466, *466*
Esophageal speech, 286
Esophageal varices, bleeding, 479
Esophagoscopy, 475
Esophagus, cancer of, 440
    treatment of, 441
  diverticula of, 468
Estrogen, and the menstrual cycle, 548
  in metastatic cancer, 593
Ethambutol, in tuberculosis, 331
Ether, vomiting following, 136
Ethionamide, in tuberculosis, 331
Ethosuximide, in epilepsy, 221
Eustachian tube, obstruction of, 275
Evisceration, of eye, 267
  of surgical wounds, postoperative,
    140
Excretion, in pneumonia, 300
Exercise, breathing, prior to surgery,
    127
    to improve respiratory function,
    317
    Buerger-Allen, 394
    following fracture, 168
    in coma, 212
    in middle life, 13
    in treatment of arthritis, 187
    postoperative, 139
Exercise test, in heart disease, 410
Exophthalmos, in hyperthyroidism,
  523
Expectorants, in bronchial asthma, 309
Extracellular compartment, 61
Etiology, idiopathic, 61

Eye (s). *See also* Vision; Visual
  adjustments of, to distance, 7, *8*
  aqueous humor of, and glaucoma,
    263
  care of, in coma, 211
    daily, 257
  disorders of, cataracts as, 262
    detached retina, 265
    glasses in, 262
    glaucoma as, 263, *264*
      iridectomy in, 264
    refractive, 261, *262*
  enucleation of, 266
  first aid of, 257
  foreign bodies in, 257
  iris of, glaucoma affecting, 263
  lens of, conditions affecting, 262
  refractive media of, disorders of, 261
  removal of, 266
  retina of, detached, 265
  rolling of, in Parkinson's disease,
    215
  sclera of, operation involving, 265
  structures of, *256*
  vitreous humor of, and detached
    retina, 265
    loss of, 263
Eyeball, pressure in, measurement of,
  256, *256*
Eyedrops, use of, 255, 268, *268*

"Face lifting," 620
Face masks, protective, 326
Facial nerve, injury to, in ear surgery,
  276
Fainting, first aid in, 119
Fallopian tubes, inflammation of, 566
Falls, by elderly patient, 24
  prevention of, 112
Family(ies), attitude toward elderly, 20
  attitude toward nurse, 53
  counseling of, with amputation, 196
  developmental tasks of, 9
  economic burden upon, and Medi-
    care, 27
  effect of alcoholism upon, 94
  elderly in, 21
    disengagement by, 22
  in cerebrovascular accident, atti-
    tudes of, 239
  of comatose patient, 212
  of dying patients, 109
  of patients with cerebrovascular dis-
    ease, 231
Families, of patients with ostomies,
  447
  prior to surgery, 127
Farsightedness, 261
Fat(s), emulsified, in replacement therapy, 64
  metabolization of, and diabetes, 534
Fear, accompanying inflammation, 67
  alleviation of, 38
  of castration, in young adult, 10
  of loneliness, 3

Fear (*Cont.*)
  of surgery, 126
  vs. anxiety, 38
Feathers, allergy to, 74
Fecal urobilinogen, 474
Fecalith, complicating appendicitis,
  461
Feces, odors and gas associated with,
  following ostomy, 453
Feeding. *See also* Diet
  in coma, 211
  Levin tube, 290
Feet. *See also* Foot
  care of, in elderly, 31
  pitting edema of, 359
Femur, fracture of, *163*
    internal fixation of, 174, *175*
Fenestration, in otosclerosis, 274
Fentanyl, as anesthetic, 134
Fertility, and infertility, 551
Fever, as sign of infection, 70
  of influenza, 303
  of viral pneumonia, 297
  rheumatic. *See* Rheumatic fever
  typhoid, chloramphenicol in treat-
    ment of, 298
Fibroids, of uterus, 567
Fibroblasts, and tissue repair, 67
Fire, safety precautions during, 112
First aid, for burns, 693
  for eyes, 257
  general principles of, 113
  in cessation of respiration, 115
  in emergencies, 114
    minor, 119
  in exposure to temperature ex-
    tremes, 118
  in fractures, 162. *See also* Fractures,
    treatment of
  in paraplegia, 248
  in poisoning, 117
  in shock, 115
  in snake and animal bites, 116, 117
  in tracheostomy, 288
  in wounds, 116
Fistula, vaginal, 571, *571*
Fit. *See* Epilepsy
Flatus, accumulation of, postoperative,
  137
Fluid(s). *See also* Electrolyte; Water
  administration of, 63
  and diet, following surgery, 136
    in paraplegia, 249
    in radiotherapy, 157
    prior to surgery, 130
  and electrolyte balance, 61
    in cardiac surgery, 678
  body requirements of, 62
  in pneumonia, 299
  in renal failure, 685
  in urologic disorders, 495
  intracellular, *62*
  intravenous, following surgery, 134
  loss of, insensible, 62

Fluid(s) (*Cont.*)
retention of, in cirrhosis, 478
weight taking to determine, 63
Fluoroscopic image amplifier, in cardiac catheterization, 356
Fluoroscopy, gastrointestinal, 418
in heart disease, 355
in respiratory disorders, 292
Foaming at the mouth, in epilepsy, 218
Foley catheter, *498*, 499
Folic acid antagonists, for cancer, 149
Follicle stimulating hormone, 548
Fomites, and protective measures against tuberculosis, 327
Food, and fluids, in paraplegia, 249
prior to surgery, 130
Food poisoning, 117
Foot. *See also* Feet
care of, in peripheral vascular disease, 397
footdrop involving, 174
in hemiplegia, exercise of, 236, *236*
Footdrop, in paraplegia, 248
in traction, prevention of, 174
Foreign bodies, in eyes, removal of, 257
Foster frame, in cervical spine injury, 246
Foster homes, for aged, 15
Fracture(s), 161-180
bleeding in, 162
bone grafts in, 175
casts for. *See* Fracture(s), treatment of, casts in
causing osteomyelitis, 193
closed, 161
comminuted, 161
complete, 161
complicated, 161
complications of, 163, 164
osteomyelitis as, 193
crutch walking in, 177
displaced, 161
evaluation of, 162
exercise following, 168
first aid in, 162
greenstick, definition of, 161
hip, 175, *175*
impacted, definition of, 161
in elderly patients, 24
incidence of, 162
infection of, 163
internal fixation of, 174
muscles associated with, changes in, 161
nonunion of, 161
of arm, casts in, care of, 170
windows in, 168
Volkmann's contracture associated with, 168
of clavicle, 179
of femur, *163*
internal fixation of, 174, *175*
of mandible, 179
of rib, 179, 303

Fracture(s) (*Cont.*)
of skull, and brain injury, 705
of spine, 178
of tibia, splinting of, 163
open, blood loss in, 162
definition of, 161
first aid of, 163
infection of, 163
pathologic, definition of, 161
pathology of, 161
pulse-taking following, 162, 163
splinting of, 162, 163
symptoms of, 162
treatment of, casts in, application of, 165, *165*
bivalve, 171
care of, 166
by patient, 170
compression caused by, 167
drying and finishing of, 166, *167*
edges of, 166, *167*
exercise with, 168
itching associated with, 168
maneuvering problems in, 168
observations of, 166
psychological problems of, 169
removal of, 170
spica, 166, *167*
use of bedpan with, 168
windows in, 168
wristdrop caused by compression of, *167*
elevation of limb in, 166
first aid, 163
tourniquets in, 164
hospital, 164
internal fixation in, 174
necrosis of bone following, 177
traction following, 176
reduction in, 164
open, 165
traction in, 163, 171
associated with splinting, 163
care of patient in, 173
bathing and back care of, 173
Crutchfield tongs in, 171, *172*
deep breathing in, 174
patient apprehension of, 172
pillows with, 173
placing of patient in, 172
pneumonia associated with, 174
postoperative care in, 175
prevention of footdrop with, 174
removal of, 174
Russell, 172
ulcers with, 174
types of, 161, 178
Frostbite, first aid in, 119
Fundus, cancer of, 569
Fungicide, in vaginitis, 564
Furuncles, 614
definition of, 69
in auditory canal, 277
in diabetes, 544
Furunculosis, 614

Gait, in Parkinson's disease, 215
Gallbladder, inflammation of, 483
removal of, 484
Gallstones, 483
treatment of, 484
Gangrene, definition of, 60
in diabetes, 542
Garamycin, in pneumonia, 299
Gas, accumulation of, postoperative, 137
poisoning by, 118
Gastrectomy, subtotal, 433
total, 442
Gastric. *See* Stomach
Gastric analysis, 417
Gastric aspiration, in diagnosis of tuberculosis, 330
Gastric balloon tube, 480, *480*
Gastric distress, with steroid therapy, 186
Gastric hypothermia, and peptic ulcer, 435
Gastric juice, and physiologic aspects of peptic ulcer, 431
Gastric resection, subtotal, 433
Gastric surgery, complications of, 434
Gastroenterostomy, 433
Gastrointestinal decompression, 420
in cancer of rectum, 444
mouth care in, 423
patient support in, 423
problem of swallowing in, 423
tubes in, 421, *421*, *422*
irrigation of, 424
withdrawing of, 424
Gastrointestinal disorders, diagnostic tests in, 415-427
emotional aspects of, 415, 424
irritable colon associated with, 426
nutrition in, 415
psychological aspects of, 424
"G.I. series," 418
in diagnosis of peptic ulcer, 431
Gastrointestinal tract, and interaction of psychological and physical, 424
cancer of, 437-445. *See also* Cancer, of gastrointestinal tract
diagram of, *416*
Gastroscopy, 419
Gastrostomy, 441
Genetic limitation, upon adaptive responses, 57
Genetics, in diabetes, 533
Genitalia. *See* Reproductive system
Genitourinary tract, *576*. *See also* Reproductive system
Gentamycin, in pneumonia, 299
Geriatric. *See also* Adult(s); Elderly patient; Patient
Geriatric case, and preservation of family ties, 15
Geriatric patient, dependence of, 14
Geriatrics, foster homes for, 15
guilt with institutionalization of, 15
Gigantism, 532

Glands. *See* specific glands
hormones secreted by. *See* Hormones
Glasses, visual accommodation with, 262
Glaucoma, 263, *264*
chronic, 264
control of, 265
tests for, 256, *256*
treatment of, 264
drugs in, 264
Globulin level, 475
Glomerular filtrate, kidney formation of, 62
Glomerulonephritis, acute, 511
chronic, 512
Glomerulosclerosis, in diabetes, 543
Glucocorticoids, secretion of, related to stress, 56
Glucose, and diabetes, 535
in blood, and hypoglycemic reaction, 541
in urine, 534
tests to measure, 535
in water, in replacement therapy, 63
levels of, excessive, 534
in blood, 533
Glucose tolerance test, 535
Glutamic pyruvic transaminase, 474
Gluten, ingestion of, 470
Glycosuria, 534
Goiter, nontoxic, 525
Gold, radioactive, in liver tests, 475
nursing care in, 159
Gold salts, soluble, in arthritis, 185
Gold sodium thiosulfate, in arthritis, 185
Goldmann tonometer, use of, *256*
Gonorrhea, 596
and urethritis, 510
incidence of, 601
symptoms of, 596
treatment of, 596
Gout, 190
diet in, 192
symptoms of, 191
treatment of, 191
Gowns, patient, for surgical procedures, 130
protective, 326
Grab bars, to prevent falls, *31*
Grand mal seizures, in epilepsy, 218
Granulation tissue, and tissue repair, 68
in traumatic wound, *69*
Granuloma inguinale, 600
Graves' disease, 519
Grief, expression of, stages of, 42
Guillotine operation, 199
Guilt, associated with institutionalized geriatrics, 15
Gumco machine, in gastrointestinal decompression, 421
Gunshot wounds, 69, *69*

Gynecologic examination, 557
doctor's role in, 558
nursing care in, 559
Papanicolaou test in, 559
positions in, *557, 558*
Gynecologic patients, the nurse and, 545
Gynecologic problems, anatomy and physiology in, 547
teaching patient, 547
Gynecologic tumors, 567
general care in, 570
inoperable, 571

Hair, and nails, care of, prior to surgery, 130
facial, in elderly women, 32
shaving of, prior to surgery, 129
Hallucinations, 81
in delirium tremens, 94
LSD-induced, 99
Hand, spastic, use of, 235, *235*
Hand washing, protective, 327
Headache, 224
in lumbar puncture, 208
in pneumoencephalography, 208
Healing, and blood flow, 68
"by first intention," 67, *68*
Health, and illness, processes of, 56-76. *See also* specific processes
Hearing, in middle life, 14
in young adults, 8
Hearing aids, 272
Hearing impairment, and visual impairment, 255-282. *See also* specific conditions
conditions of middle ear causing, 273
disorders of the external auditory canal causing, 277
disorders of inner ear as, 278
infections as, 276
infections causing, 274
otitis media as, 275, 276
lip reading in, 272
mastoiditis as, 279
Meniere's disease causing, 278
otitis media as, 275
otosclerosis as, 273
rehabilitation in, 272
speech reading in, 272
tinnitus as, 273
treatment of, 278
eardrops in, 278
fenestration operation in, 274
hearing aids in, 272
irrigation in, 279
nursing procedures in, 278
surgical, 276
Hearing loss, communication problems in, 271
conductive, 270
demonstration of, *272*
sensorineural, 270

Heart. *See also* Cardiac; Cardio-
anatomy of, 351
aortic valve of, stenosis of, 373, *373*
effect of shock upon, 630
inflammatory disease of, 368-382
lesions of, traumatic, 676
mitral valve of, conditions involving, 372
myocardium of, ischemia of, 382
pacemakers for, electrical, 655
tumors of, 675
valvular disease of, 368-382
ventricles of, aneurysms of, 675
Heart block, complete, 647
Heart disease, 357-367. *See also* Coronary artery disease and other diseases
allergic reactions in, 355
anatomical factors in, 349-356
and anatomy of cardiopulmonary system, 351, *351*
blood pressure in, 353
diagnosis of, 349
tests in, 354
edema in, 354
epidemiology of, 350
fever associated with, 352
functional, 385
ischemic, 674
patients with, classification of, 410
energy expenditure of, 410
functional capacity of, 410
pulse in, 352
rehabilitation following, 409-414
classification in, 410
nursing implications in, 413
principles in, 412
respirations in, 353
rheumatic. *See* Rheumatic heart disease
signs and symptoms of, 352
temperature in, 352
venous pressure in, 350
Heart failure, blood pressure, 359
congestive, 352, 357
causes of, 357
diagnosis of, 359
diet in, 362
nurse teaching in, 362
process of, 358
recovery from, 362
symptoms of, 358
treatment of, 360
drugs in, 363
edema in, 359, *359*
nursing care in, 360
pacemakers in, 655
Heartburn, and belching, 425
Heat, application to, in distention, 138
to increase blood supply, 393
in arthritis, 188
in herniated disk, 244
in rheumatoid arthritis, 188
vasodilating effect of, 399
Heat exhaustion, 118
Heatstroke, first aid in, 118

Headache, stress-related, 77
Hematemesis, in peptic ulcer, 434
Hematoma, epidural, 704
    subdural, 705
Hemicorporectomy, 199
Hemigastrectomy, 433
Hemipelvectomy, 198, 199
Hemiplegia, 232, *243*
    exercises in, 236, *236*
Hemodialysis, care following, 689
    extracorporeal, 686
    nursing care during, 687
Hemoglobin, and etiology of anemia,
    337, 339
    as factor in blood dyscrasias, 336
Hemolysis, and etiology of anemia,
    337, 339
Hemophilia, 345
Hemophilus ducreyi, 599
Hemoptysis, in tuberculosis, 332
Hemorrhage, control of, 114, *114,* 115
    as postoperative complication, 134
    cerebral, 229
        changes in cerebrospinal fluid as-
            sociated with, 207
    complicating peptic ulcer, 434
    first aid in, 114, 115, *115*
    following prostatectomy, 578
    in cancer of the mouth, 440
    in cataract removal, 263
    in ocular surgery, 269
    in tuberculosis, 332
    in urologic surgery, 497
    of fractures, 162
    tourniquet in, 115
Hemorrhoidectomy, 471
Hemorrhoids, 470, *470*
    treatment of, 471
Hemothorax, 304
Hemovac, Snyder, 176, *176*
Henylbutazone, in arthritis, 185
Heparin, in cerebrovascular accident,
    233
Hepatic. *See also* Liver
Hepatic arteriography, 475
Hepatic coma, in cirrhosis, 477, 478
Hepatitis, noninfectious, 483
    viral, 481
        nursing care in, 482
        signs and symptoms of, 481
        treatment of, 482
Hereditary conditions, 59
Hernia, 464, *464*
    complications of, 465
    esophageal hiatus, 466, *466*
    nursing care of, 465
    strangulation of, 465, 467
    treatment of, 465
    types of, 464
Herniated disk, *243*
    and spinal cord impairment, 242
    treatment of, conservative, 244
        surgical, 245
Herniorrhaphy, 465

Heroin, addiction to, 101
    onset of, 91
    methadone in treatment of, 101
Herpes simplex, 614
Herpes zoster, 614
Hexachlorophene, cleansing with, 129
Hiccups, 120
Hip, disarticulation of, 198
    fractures of, 175, *175*
Hives, 611
Hoarseness, in laryngitis, 285
Hobbies, for elderly patient, 28
Hodgkin's disease, 346
    treatment of, 347
        radiotherapy in, 155
Homan's sign, 402
Homeostasis, 56
    in elderly, 24
Hordeolum, 266
Hormonal therapy, in arthritis, 185
    in cancer, 149
        metastatic, 593
Hormone(s), antidiuretic, 532
    as body defense, 66
    glands producing, *520*
    growth, 532
    secretion of, related to stress, 57
    thyroid, 519
        deficiencies of, 525
Hornets, first aid against, 120
Hospital, admission to, care of valu-
        ables upon, 130
    for eye disorders, 267
    prior to surgery, 124
    care of elderly in, 33
    effect of, upon young adults, 6
    infections in, airborne, 326
        prevention of, 71
    intensive care units in, 625, *626*
    rules in, and young adults, 6
    safety in, 111
    tuberculosis treatment in, 333
    visiting hours in, 6
Humidification, in bronchial asthma,
    309
Hydration, in radiotherapy, 157
Hydrocele, 582
Hydrochloric, in etiology of peptic
    ulcer, 431
Hydrochloric acid, neutralization of,
    432
Hydrocortisone, as body defense, 66
    in Addison's disease, 529
Hydronephrosis, *504, 505*
Hygiene, following prostatectomy, 579
    personal, 30
    preoperative, 124
    prior to surgery, 124
Hyperaldosteronism, 531
Hypercapnia, 635
Hyperemia, 261
Hypermotility, of stomach, 432
Hyperparathyroidism, 527
Hyperplasia, 65
Hyperpnea, and arthritis, 184

Hypertension, 386-390
    associated with cerebrovascular acci-
        dent, 229, 239
    malignant, 388
    portal, 479
    prevention of, 388
    primary, 387
    related to anger, 77
    related to stress, 57
    secondary, 387
    symptoms of, 387
    treatment of, 389
        drugs in, 389, *389*
        nursing measures in, 389
Hypertensive disease, categories of, 387
Hyperthermia. *See* Fever
Hyperthyroidism, 519
    diagnosis of, 520
    exophthalmos in, 523
    symptoms of, 519
    treatment of, 521
        radioactive iodine in, 159
        surgery in, 522
Hypertrophy, definition of, 65
Hypnotics, addiction to, 100
Hypocapnia, 635
Hypoglycemia, in Addison's disease,
    528
    treatment of, 530
Hypoglycemic agents, in diabetes, 540
Hypoglycemic reaction, symptoms of,
    541
    treatment of, 542
Hypokalemia, 363
Hypoparathyroidism, 527
    treatment of, 528
Hypophysectomy, 593
Hypophysis, 532
Hypothermia, gastric, 435
Hypothyroidism, 525
    diagnosis of, 526
    treatment of, 526
Hypovolemia, 339
Hypoxemia, 635
Hypoxia, 60, 635
    postoperative, 135
Hysterectomy, 556
    complications of, 570
    general care in, 570
Hysterosalpingography, in infertility,
    553

I^{131} rose bengal, 474
I^{131} urine excretion test, 531
Icterus. *See* Jaundice
Idiopathic etiology, 61
Ileal conduit, 516
Ileostomy, 446-460
    appliance for, 451, *451*
        allergies complicating use of, 451
        cement for, 452
        changing of, 453
        Karaya gum ring used with, 451
        solvent for, 452
    bag for, permanent, 451, *451*
        temporary, 450

Ileostomy (*Cont.*)
  belts used with, 452
  blockage of, 454
  care of skin in, 453
  control of odor and gas in, 453
  dressing of, 450
  indications for, 449
  management of, 449
  prolapse of, 454
  stoma of, bags for, 451
    dressing for, 450
    maturation of, 450
Ileum, and peptic ulcer, 431
  resection of, in ureteral transplants, 516
Ileus, paralytic, 138, 462
Illness. *See also* Disease and specific illnesses
  and health, processes of, 56-76. *See also* specific processes
  and self-concern, attitude of nurse toward, 17
  reactions to, at various ages, 4
Illusion, definition of, 81
Immune bodies, 71
Immunity, 71
Immunogen, definition of, 72
Immunologic reactivity, and allergy, 72
Impetigo contagiosa, 613
Impotence, in paraplegia, 250
Incisional hernia, 464
Income, of elderly, 26
Incontinence, 501. *See also* Urinary incontinence
  attitude toward, 47
  in coma, 211
  in paraplegia, 250
Indigestion, and peptic ulcer, 431
Indocyanine green, 474
Indomethacin, in arthritis, 185
Infarction, myocardial. *See* Myocardial infarction
Infection, airborne, 326
  and burns, 699
  and immunity, 71
  bacterial, 212, 213
  body response to, 69, *69*, *70*
    lymph nodes in, *70*
  chills as sign of, 70
  classification of, 328
  complicating peripheral vascular disease, 395
  definition of, 61
  ear, 274
  fever as sign of, 70
  in diabetes, 544
  localized, 69
    bacterial, 70
  mechanism of, 61
  of bone. *See* Osteomyelitis
  of female reproductive system, 563
  of open fracture, 163
  prevention of, in hospitals, 71
  puerperal, 566
  respiratory. *See* Respiratory

Infection (*Cont.*)
  staphylococcal, 70
  streptococcal, *69*
  urinary, 508
    in urinalysis, 490
    prevention of, 496
    with calculi, 506
  venereal. *See* Venereal
  viral. *See* Viruses
  wound, postoperative, 140
Infectious hepatitis, 481
Infarction, definition of, 60
Infectious mononucleosis, 347
Infertility, and fertility, 551
  diagnosis of, 552
  treatment of, 553
Infestations, and bites, 615
Inflammation, as response to infection, 69, *69*
  fear accompanying, 67
  of blood vessels, 399
  of colon. *See* Ulcerative colitis
  of gallbladder, 483
  of intestine, 469
  of joints. *See* Arthritis
  of larynx, 284
  of lungs, pneumonia as, 295
  of peritoneum, 462
  of pleura, 301
  of sinuses, 280
  of veins, 402
  symptoms of, 66
  tissue repair following, 67
  urinary, 508, 509, 510
Inflammatory disease, pelvic, 566
  of heart, 368-382
Inflammatory response, 66
Influenza, 302
  symptoms of, 302
  treatment of, 303
Inguinal hernia, 464, *464*
Inhalants, causing asthma, 310
Innovar, as anesthetic, 134
Insects, in auditory canal, 277
Institutions, mental, elderly in, 29
Insulin, and Addison's disease, 529
  forms of, 538
  in diabetes, 538
  injection of, 538
  insufficiency of. *See* Diabetes
Insulin clearance, of kidneys, 491
Insulin shock, 541
  symptoms of, 543
Intellectual development, of elderly patient, 24
Intensive care, 625
  following surgery, 132
Internal fixation, of fractures, 174, *175*, *176*
Intestinal decompression, tubes in, *421*, *422*, *422*
Intestinal disorders, patients with, 461-472. *See also* specific disorders
Intestinal obstruction, cancer as, 467
  mechanical, 467, *467*

Intestinal tube, in gastrointestinal decompression, 423
Intestine(s), absorption by, disorder of, 469
  break in, and peritonitis, 462
  decompression of, 420
  large, colostomy involving. *See* Colostomy
  obstruction of, mechanical, 467
  paralysis of, 462
  perforation of, in appendicitis, 461
  protrusion of. *See* Hernia
  small, inflammation of, 469
Intracellular fluid, 61
Intracranial pressure, increased, 701
  increase in, 702
Intraocular pressure, measurement of, 256
Intravenous therapy, 63
  cautions in, 64
  infusion bottle for, 64, *65*
  needle used in, 64
  procedure for, 64
  transfusion reactions in, 64
Intubation, endotracheal, in respiratory failure, 637
Involucrum, in osteomyelitis, 193
Iodine[131], in liver tests, 475
Iodine, in goiter, 525
  in hyperthyroidism, 522
    nursing care in, 159
  protein-bound, in hyperthyroidism, 520
Ions, concentrations of, 62
Iridectomy, 264
Iron deficiency anemia, 337
Irrigation, and suction, in gastrointestinal decompression, 423
Ischemia, 60, 392
  cerebral, 230
  myocardial, 382
Isoniazid, in tuberculosis, 331, 334
Isoproterenol, in arrhythmias, 650
Isotopes, radioactive, in brain scanning, 210
  in cancer, 159, 160
Isuprel, in shock, 632
Itching, associated with fracture casts, 169
  lotions to relieve, 606
  treatment of, 607
I.V.P., involving kidneys, 492

Jacksonian seizures, 219
Jaundice, 475
  as diagnostic sign, evaluation of, 474
  signs and symptoms of, 476
Jejunum, and peptic ulcer, 431
Jewelry, disposition of, prior to surgery, 130
Joints, diseases of, 181-194. *See also* Bone(s) and specific conditions
  diseases of, degenerative. *See* Osteoarthritis
  dislocations and sprains involving, 179

Joints (*Cont.*)
inflammation of. *See* Arthritis
Judaism, and birth control, 553

Kanamycin, in tuberculosis, 331
Kaopectate, for irritable colon, 426
Karaya gum rings, 452
with ileostomy appliance, 451
Keloid formation, 57
Keratitis, 266
Keratoses, senile, 618
Ketone bodies, 534
Kidneys. *See also* Bladder; Urinary
tract
arteriography of, 493
damage to, in nephritis, 511
diagnostic tests associated with, 489
drainage of, catheters in, 499
effect of shock upon, 630
function of, 62, 488
substitutes for, 686
hydronephrosis involving, *504*, 505
interior of, 489, *489*
plasma clearance of, 491
polycystic disease of, 517
pyelogram of, intravenous, 492
transplantation of, 514
tumors of, 513
Kidney shutdown, in radiotherapy,
157
Korsakoff's psychosis, 93
Kyphosis, in ankylosing spondylitis,
190

Labyrinthitis, complicating otitis
media, 275
Lactic dehydrogenase, 474
Laennec's cirrhosis, 476
Laminectomy, 245
postoperative care in, 245
to relieve pain, 88
with spinal fusion, 246
Laryngectomy, 285
recovery following, 290
sedation in, 290
Laryngectomy tube, 286, *287*, *289*
Laryngofissure, 285
Laryngospasm, following surgery, 133
Laryngitis, 284
Larynx, anatomy of, 284
cancer of, 285
symptoms of, 285
tracheostomy for, 286, *287*, *289*
treatment of, 285
nursing aspects of, 285
postoperative, 289
late, 291
preoperative, 285
L-dopa, in Parkinson's disease, 216
Learning ability, of elderly patient, 25
Leg, arteries of, *407*
ischemia involving, 392
thrombophlebitis affecting, 139
ulcers of, in peripheral vascular disease, 395

Leg (*Cont.*)
venous stasis in, avoidance of, 402
Legal rights, of patients, 52
Lens(es), contact, 255
of eye, conditions affecting, 262
Lethargy, as level of consciousness, 210
Leukemia, acute, 340
treatment of, 341
characteristics of, 144
chronic, 341
treatment of, 341
radiotherapy in, 155
splenomegaly in, 341
treatment of, bleeding in, 343
disorientation in, 343
nursing care in, 342
physical care in, 343
toxic drug effects in, 344
transfusions in, 344
Leukocytes, and leukemia, 340
Leukopenia, 340
in radiotherapy, 157
Leukoplakia, 618
and cancer of the gastrointestinal
tract, 438
Levarterenol, intravenous, effect upon
skin, 64
Levin tube, 290
in peptic ulcer, 433
Levophed, in shock, 631
Lidocaine, in arrhythmias, 649
Lifting, in spinal cord impairment,
247
Ligation and stripping, in varicose
veins, 400
Limb, phantom, 197
upper extremity, 202
Lip reading, 272
Liposarcoma, 143
Lithiasis, 505. *See also* Calculi; Stones
Litholapaxy, 507
Liver. *See also* Hepatic
anatomy of, 473, *479*
biopsy of, 475
cirrhosis of, 476
disease of, diagnosis of, 474
nursing care in, 475
disorders of, 473-483. *See also* specific disorders
cirrhosis as, 476
coma with, 477, 478
jaundice as, 475
patients with, 473
viral hepatitis as, 481
effect of alcohol upon, 93
function tests of, 474
portal vein of, 479
Liver scan, 475
Lobeline, to stop smoking, 104
Locomotor ataxia, 599
Loneliness, fear of, 3
of elderly patient, 28
LSD, addiction to, 97, 99
Lugol's solution, in hyperthyroidism,
522

Lumbar disks, herniated, 244
Lumbar laminectomy, 245
Lumbar puncture, 206, *207*
nursing care in, 207
Lumps, in breast, 585
Lungs. *See also* Pulmonary
abscess of, 319
accumulation of fluid in, postoperative, 138
cancer of, 145, 320
incidence of, 145
related to smoking, 102, *103*
disorders of, caused by dust, 319
dysfunction of, 635
function of, 634
injury to, as cause of pulmonary
edema, 364
pneumonia in, 295
Lymph disorders, 346
Lymph nodes, effect of radiotherapy
upon, 155
enlargement of, 346
metastatic cancer involving, 593
in response to infection, *70*
spread of cancer by, 143
swelling of, 70
Lymphadenitis, 70
Lymphedema, 403
Lymphogranuloma inguinale, 599
Lymphomas, effect of radiotherapy
upon, 155
Lymphopathia venereum, 599
Lymphosarcoma, 346
Lysergic acid diethylamide, 97, 99

Maalox, in peptic ulcer, 432
Magnesium concentrations, in body
fluid, 62
Magnesium trisilicate, in peptic ulcer,
432
Makeup, prior to surgery, 130
Malabsorption syndrome, 469
Malingering, vs. psychosomatic illness,
78
Malnutrition, and alcoholism, 93
Mammography, 586
Mammoplasty, 621
Mandible, fracture of, 179
Mantoux test, 329, *329*
Marihuana, addiction to, 99
Marriage, in later years, 22
Mastectomy, attitude toward, 590
dressing for, 589
exercises following, 590
operative phase of, 588
postoperative care in, 588
radical, 587, *591*
prosthesis for, 591
simple, 587
Mastitis, cystic, 587
Mastoiditis, 279
Maxillary sinus. *See* Sinus
McBurney's point, and appendicitis,
461
Medical expenses, increase of, with
age, 27

Medical-surgical patients. *See* Patient(s)
Medicare, 27
Medication. *See also* types of medication
administration of, and allergic response, 72
for apprehension prior to surgery, 127
preoperative, 127
Melanomas, 619
malignant, 143
Memory, deterioration of, in cerebrovascular disease, 230
in alcoholism, 93, 94
Menarche, 548
Meniere's disease, 278
Meningitis, 212
bacterial, 213
changes in cerebrospinal fluid in, 207
symptoms of, 213
treatment of, 213
Menopause, 13, 549
accompanied by illness, 17
physiology of, 549
treatment in, 550
Menorrhagia, 551
Menstrual cycle, 548
instruction in, 548
normal, *547*
Menstruation, disorders of, 550
Mental institutions, elderly in, 29
Meperidine, postoperative, 135
Mephobarbital, in epilepsy, 220
Meprobamate, prior to surgery, 127
Metabolic rate, basal, in hyperthyroidism, 520
slowing of, in middle life, 12
Metastases, definition of, 61
in cancer, 144
involving breast, 593
Methadone, in treatment of drug dependence, 101
Methamphetamine, addiction to, 98
Methedrine, addiction to, 98
Methicillin, in pneumonia, 298
Methotrexate, in cancer, 149
Methsuximide, 221
Methyl phenylethylhydantoin, in epilepsy, 221
Methyltestosterone, in Addison's disease, 529
Metrorrhagia, 551
Migraine, 225
Mind, interaction of, with body, 77-83
Miotics, in glaucoma, 264
Mitral insufficiency, 372, *373*
Mitral stenosis, 372
Mononucleosis, infectious, 347
Morbidity, definition of, 59
Morphine, addiction to, 101
in pulmonary edema, 364
postoperative, 136
preoperative, 127
Mortality, definition of, 59

Mouth, cancer of, 438
complications of, 440
problems in, 439
care of, in gastrointestinal decompression, 423
prior to surgery, 130
dryness of, in urologic disorders, 496
Mouth-to-mouth resuscitation, 115
Multiple sclerosis, 222
complications of, 224
prognosis in, 224
symptoms of, 223
treatment of, 223
Muscles, spasm of, in grand mal seizures, 218
Muscle contracture, in amputation, prevention of, 200
Mycoplasma pneumoniae, causing pneumonia, 296
Mycobacterium tuberculosis, 325
Mydriatics, administration of, technique of, 268
Myelin, destruction to, in multiple sclerosis, 223
Myelography, 210
Myocardial infarction, 382, 660-671
age at time of, 381
care in, objectives of, 666
complications of, 669
coronary care unit in, 662
diagnosis of, 665
first aid in, 661
pathology of, 665
patients in, admitting of, 662
prognosis of, 671
rehabilitation in, 670
symptoms of, 660
treatment of, 666
Myocardial ischemia, 382
Myocardial revascularization, 674
Myomas, of uterus, 567
Myopia, 261
Myringotomy, 275
Myxedema, 526

Nails, and hair, care of, 130
Narcotics. *See also* Drug Therapy; Drugs
addiction to, 90
administration of, postoperative, 135
for apprehension, 127
postoperative, 135
prescription of, nursing aspects of, 102
to relieve pain, 88
Narcotic analgesics, addiction to, 100
Nasal mucosa, swelling, in allergic rhinitis, 306
Nasogastric tube feeding, 290
Nausea, and vomiting, 425
Nearsightedness, 261
Nebulizers, in epinephrine administration, 308
Neck, lymph nodes of, 70
Necrosis, tissue, 60
Needles, for intravenous therapy, 64

Neisseria gonorrhoeae, 596
Neo-karaya, 452
Neoplasia, 60. *See also* Cancer; Sarcoma; Tumors
Neostigmine, in distention of abdomen, 138
Neo-synephrine, in sinusitis, 281
Nephrectomy, 507
care following, 513
Nephritis, related to stress, 57
Nephrolithotomy, 507
Nephron, 490, *490*
Nephropathy, in diabetes, 543
Nephrosis, 512
related to stress, 57
Nephrotic syndrome, 512
Nephrotomogram, 493
Nephrotomy, in treatment of calculi, 507
Nerve(s)
cells of, cerebral, oxygen lack of, 228
cranial, neuralgia involving, 225
facial, injury to, in ear surgery, 276
myelin covering of, and multiple sclerosis, 223
trigeminal, neuralgia involving, 225, *226*
vagus, division of, 433
Nerve root, spinal, compression of, 242
Nervous system, autonomic, 65
Nervousness, and anorexia, 425
Neurectomy, to relieve pain, 88
Neurodermatitis, 611, 612
Neurologic. *See also* Brain; Cerebro-; Cerebral
Neurologic disease, 701-709
Neurologic disorders. *See also* specific disorders
tests for, 207
Neurologic examination, 205
electroencephalography as, 210
tests in, 206
brain scanning as, 210
cerebral angiography as, 209
lumbar puncture as, 206, *207*
myelography as, 210
pneumoencephalography as, 208
ventriculography as, 209
Neuropathy, in diabetes, 543
Nevi, 618
Night blindness, and vitamin A, 257
Nipple discharge, 585
Nitrogen mustard, in cancer, 149
in leukemia, 341
Nitroglycerin, in angina pectoris, 383
Norepinephrine, increased secretion of, 531
Nose, disorders of, 280-291. *See also* specific disorders
polyps in, 283
septum of, deviated, 283
structures of, *281*
submucous resection of, 283
Nosebleed. *See* Epistaxis
Nosedrops, in sinusitis, 281

Nurse, anxiety of, 40
  attitude of, toward elderly, 30
    toward stress, 57
  care by, of elderly, 30
  counseling of young adults by, 9
  sensitivity of, to adult adjustments, 2
Nurse-patient relationships, 36-55
  and demanding patients, 46
  and factor of suicide, 48
  and patient's family, 53
  and unattractiveness of patient, 49
  and visitors, 53
  anxiety in, 40
    anxiety of patient, 38
  basic concepts in, 36, 38
  brief, 43
  collaboration with physician as factor in, 44
  conflict in, 42
  emotional support as factor in, 36
  frustration of, dealing with, 40
  grief in, stages of, 42
  guidelines in, 37
  observation of patient reactions in, 45
  patient complaints as factor in, 49
  patient familiarity in, 48
  physician as factor in, 44
  prior to surgery, 128
  reactions in, unconscious, 41
  "self-care" patients in, 50
  support of patient as factor in, 44
  sustained, 46
  when patient is unconscious, 51
Nurse-physician collaboration, 44
Nursing, in emergencies, 111-112. *See also* Emergencies and specific situations
  intensive, 625
Nursing homes, elderly in, 20
Nutrition, and overeating, 425
  in burned patient, 698
  in gastrointestinal disorders, 415
  of elderly patient, 23
  of young adults, 10
Nystatin, in vaginitis, 564

Oculist, definition of, 255
Oculogyric crises, in Parkinson's disease, 215
Oxyphenbutazone, in arthritis, 185
Odor, and gas, ileostomy, 453
  with urinary incontinence, 503
Oliguria, in renal failure, 684
Oophorectomy, 556
  bilateral, 588
Operating room, safety hazards of, 113
  transportation of patient to, 131
Operation. *See* Surgery; Surgical and specific operations
Operative permit, prior to surgery, 123
Ophthalmia, sympathetic, 266
Ophthalmologist, 255
Ophthalmoscope, 255
Optician, 255

Optometrist, 255
Orchitis, 582
Osmotic pressure, 62
Osteoarthritis. *See also* Arthritis
  pathology of, 190
  treatment of, 190
Osteomyelitis, 193
  chronic, following amputation, 202
  complicating open fracture, 164
  complications in, 194
  treatment of, 193
  with open fracture, 165
Osteotomy, in rheumatoid arthritis, 189
Ostomy (ies). *See also* Colostomy; Ileostomy; Stoma
  appliances for, allergies complicating use of, 451
    cement for, 452
    solvent for, 452
  attitude toward, 447
  clothing with, 459
  description of, 446
  diet in, 459
  explanation of, to patient, 448
  organization of persons having, 449
  patient care with, planning of, 446
  stoma of, adjustments in use of, 447
    bags for, 450, 451, *451*
      application of, 451
    covering of, 458
    dressing of, 450
    explanation of, 448
    maturation of, 450
Otitis media, chronic, 276
  purulent, 275
  serous, 275
Otosclerosis, 273
  fenestration in, 274
Otrivin, in sinusitis, 281
Ovarian follicle, maturation of, 548
Ovariectomy, 556
Ovaries, cysts of, 568
  inflammation of, 566
  tumors of, 568
Overeating, 425
Ovulation, 548
  cessation of, 549
  occurrence of, 552
Oxacillin, in pneumonia, 298
Oxygen, administration of, in pulmonary edema, 365
  and respiratory disorders, 292
  blood levels of, 155
  hyperbaric, in cancer, 149
  in bronchial asthma, 307
  in obstructive pulmonary disease, 315
  in respiratory failure, 639
  insufficiency of, 60
    and cerebrovascular disease, 228
  precautions in use of, 112
  traced from nose to alveoli, *294*
Oxygenation of blood, and hypoxia, 135

Pace, in middle life, 13
Pacemakers, artificial electrical, 655
  nursing care with, 656
Pain, 84-89, *84*
  herniated disk, 244
  in breast, 585
  in fractures, 162
  in myocardial ischemia, 382
  in osteomyelitis, 193
  in peptic ulcer, 431
  in peripheral vascular disease, 391, 392, 395
  in rheumatoid arthritis, 184
  in shock, 629
  in urologic disorders, 496
  intractable, 87
  narcotics to relieve, nursing aspects of, 102
  nursing care in, 85
  observations in, 85
  phantom limb, 197
  postoperative, 135
  preoperative explanation of, 127
  psychological reaction to, 85
  sources of, 84
  treatment of, drugs in, 86
    narcotic, 88
    surgery in, 88
Palsy, crutch, 177
  shaking, 214
Pancreas, 485
Pancreatitis, acute, 486
  chronic, 486
  nursing care in, 487
Panhypopituitarism, 532
"Pap" smears, in diagnosis of cancer, 146
Papanicolaou test, for cancer, 559
Papilledema, 702
Para-aminosalicylic acid, in tuberculosis, 331
Paracentesis, 275
Paraldehyde, in alcoholism, 95
Paralysis, footdrop as, 174
  of hand, 235, *235*
  of intestines, 462
Paralysis agitans, 214
Paralytic ileus, 138, 462
Paramethadione, in epilepsy, 221
Paraplegia, *243. See also* Quadriplegia
  complications of, 248
  crutch walking in, 177, *177*
  due to multiple sclerosis, 222
  elimination in, 249
  environment of patient with, 253
  first aid in, 248
  food and fluids in, 249
  impotence in, 250
  incontinence in, 250
  injections in, 248
  psychological problems in, 249
  rehabilitation in, 250
    bathing in, *253*
    bowel and bladder, 251, 252
    nursing guidelines in, 252
    positioning in, 251

Paraplegia, rehabilitation in (*Cont.*)
  wheelchair in, 252, *252*
  treatment of, beds in, *252*
    early, 248
Parathyroid glands, 527
Parents, care of, by children, 15
  independence from, of young
    adults, 8
  working with, 10
Parkinson's disease, 214, *214*
  physical therapy in, 216
  symptoms of, 214
  treatment of, 215
    surgery in, 216
Paste boot, Unna's, 402
Patch tests, 73, 329
Pathogen, definition of, 61
Pathophysiology, processes of, 56-76.
  See also specific processes
Patients, adult, grief expressed by, 42
  anesthetized, incontinence of, 501
    anger in, 38
    anxiety in, 38
    cleanliness of, 48
  comatose, 211
  complaints by, 49
  delirious, 81
  demanding, 46, 51
  dying, care of, 107-110
  emotional problems in, 38
  emotional requirements of, 46
  emotional support of, 36
  familiarity with, cautions in, 48
  fear in, 38
  incontinent, 47
  long-term, 46
  poise of, 36
  "self-care," 50
  shock affecting, 627-633
  surgical, 123-142. *See also* Surgical
    patient and Surgery
  turning of, in coma, 212
  unattractive, 49
  unconscious, incontinence of, 501
  relationship of nurse to, 51
  uncooperative, 52
  with heart disease, rehabilitation of,
    409-414
Pediculous corporis, 615
Pediculous pubis, 618
Pelvic exenteration, 570
Pelvic inflammatory disease, 566
Pelvic muscles, relaxed, 572
Penicillin, in pneumonia, 298
  in rheumatic fever, 370, 374
  in venereal disease, 599
Penis, rubber urinal adapted to, *502,*
  503
Penrose drain, following cholecystec-
  tomy, 485, *485*
Penrose drain, in prostatectomy, 577
Pepsin, in peptic ulcer, 431
Peptic ulcers. *See* Ulcer(s), peptic
Percutaneous cordotomy, 89

Pericarditis, 377, *378*
  acute, 378
  chronic constrictive, 378
Perilymph, 278
Perineal care, in D & C, 560, 561
Perineal pruritus, 565
Perineorrhaphy, 572
Peripheral vascular disease, 391-408.
  See Vascular disease, peripheral
Peristalsis, stimulation of, postopera-
  tive, 138
Peritoneum, inflammation of, 462
Peritoneal dialysis, 689
Peritonitis, complicating peptic ulcer,
  436
  diagnosis of, 462
  nursing care of, 463
  treatment of, 463
Pessary, ring, *573*
Petechiae, and blood dyscrasias, 336
Petit mal seizures, in epilepsy, 218
Phantom limb, 197
  upper extremity, 202
Pharyngeal airway, *132*
Phenacemide, in epilepsy, 221
Phenobarbital, in alcoholism, 95
  in epilepsy, 220
  prior to surgery, 127
Phenolsulfonphthalein test, 491
Phenothiazine, in alcoholism, 95
Phensuximide, in epilepsy, 221
Phenylbutazone, in gout, 192
Pheochromocytoma, 531
Phlebothrombosis, 402
  postoperative, 139
Phlebotomy, in polycythemia, 345
  in pulmonary edema, 365
Phosphate concentrations, in body
  fluid, 62
Phosphorus, radioactive, 160
Phosphorus-calcium balance, in hyper-
  parathyroidism, 527
Physical therapy, in amputation, 200
  in chronic obstructive pulmonary
    disease, 317, *317*
  in hemiplegia, 235, 236, 237, *235-
    237,* 238
  in herniated disk, 244
  in Parkinson's disease, 216
Physical work, relationship of, to
  age, *3*
Physician, collaboration with, by
  nurse, 44
Physiological processes, in health and
  illness, 56-76. *See also* specific processes
Pia mater, 212
Pillows, with traction apparatus, 173
Pilonidal sinus, 471
  nursing care in, 472
Pinkeye, 266
Pituitary gland, 532
  removal of, 593
  secretions of, as body defense, 66
Pituitary-adrenal system, adaptive
  hormones of, 57

Placebo, in psychosomatic illness, 80
Plaquenil, in arthritis, 185
Plasma clearance, of kidneys, 491
Plasma expanders, in replacement
  therapy, 63
Plaster of Paris, for casts, 166
Plastic surgery, nursing care in, 623
  patients undergoing, 620-624
Pleural space, blood in, 304
Pleurisy, 301
  complicating pneumonia, 301
  pathology of, 301
Pleurisy, treatment of, 302
Pneumococcus, 296
Pneumoconiosis, 319
Pneumoencephalography, 208
Pneumonia, 295
  associated with coma, 211
  bacterial, symptoms of, 297
  complicating multiple sclerosis, 224
  complications of, 301
  convalescence from, 301
  diagnosis of, 297
  etiology of, 296
  hypostatic, 138
    associated with traction, 174
  lobar, *295,* 296
  pathology of, 295
  postoperative, 138
  prevention of, 301
  staphylococcal, 300
  symptoms of, 297
  treatment of, 297
    diet in, 300
    drug therapy in, 298
    nursing care in, 299
    supportive, 299
  viral, 297
Pneumoperitoneum, in hernia, 466
Pneumothorax, 304
  spontaneous, 332
Poisoning, by gas, 118
  drug, 118
    encephalopathies as, 213
  first aid in, 117
  food, 117
Pollution, causing chronic bronchitis,
  312
Polyarthritis, migratory, 370
Polycystic disease, of kidney, 517
Polycythemia, 345
Polydipsia, in diabetes, 534
Polyphagia, 534
Polyposis, 469
Polyps, 283
  complicating allergic rhinitis, 306
Polyuria, in diabetes, 534
Pomeroy syringe, *277*
Portal hypertension, 479
Portocaval shunt, 480
Position sense, of elderly patient, 23
Positioning, of patient, in peripheral
  vascular disease, 392
Postpericardiotomy syndrome, 378
Posture, in elderly, correction of, 32

Postural drainage, in emphysema, 317, 318
Potassium, in body fluid, 62
  intravenous administration of, 64
Potassium iodide, in bronchial asthma, 309
Pott's disease, 245
Powder, Karaya gum, 452
Pregnancy, complications in, 598
  ectopic, 563
Presbycusis, onset of, 14
Presbyopia, 262
  onset of, 14
Primidone, in epilepsy, 221
Privacy, of young adult, respect for, 10
Probenecid, in gout, 192
Procainamide, in arrhythmias, 649
Proctoscopy, 419
  knee-chest position for, 420
Proparacaine, in eye examination, 256
Propranolol, in arrhythmias, 649
Prostate, cancer of, 149, 579
  treatment of, 580
  hypertrophy of, 575
    diagnosis of, 576
    in elderly males, 32
    treatment of, 576
      complications following, 578
      surgical, 577
Prostatectomy, 577
  bleeding following, 578
  drainage and irrigation in, 578
  nursing care following, 577
Prostheses. See also Dentures and types of prostheses
  amputation, temporary, 200
    training with, 203
    upper extremity, 201
  breast, 591
  care of, prior to surgery, 130
Prostigmin in distention of abdomen, 138
Protein-bound iodine, in hyperthyroidism, 520
  in infertility, 552
Protein derivative, purified, in Mantoux test, 329
Proteins, liver, tests involving, 475
Protestantism, and birth control, 554
Prothrombin time, 474
Pruritus, in cancer of vulva, 569
  in jaundice, 476
  in renal failure, 686
  in urologic disorders, 496
  perineal, 565
  treatment of, 607
Psoriasis, 613
P.S.P. test, 491
Psychic reactions, to pain, 85
Psychological adaptation, genetic limitations upon, 57
Psychological equilibrium, and stress, 56
Psychological factors, in gastrointestinal disorders, 424

Psychological problems, associated with casts for fractures, 169
  in paraplegia, 249
Psychomotor attacks, in epilepsy, 219
Psychosis, Korsakoff's, 93
  toxic, amphetamine-related, 98
Psychosomatic illness, concept of, 77
  reality of, 78
  treatment of, 79
    drugs in, 79
    nursing considerations in, 80
    placebos in, 80
    suggestibility in, 81
Psychotherapy, in ulcerative colitis, 430
Psychotomimetic drugs, 99
Ptosis, 266
Puberty, in female patient, 548
  physical changes beyond, 7
Pubic area, infestation of, 618
Puerperal infection, 566
Puinidine, in arrhythmias, 649
Pulmonary. See also Lungs
Pulmonary disease, chronic obstructive, chronic bronchitis as, 312
  emphysema as, 314
    treatment of, 315
      oxygen in, 316
      postural drainage in, 317, 318
Pulmonary embolism, in myocardial infarction, 669
Pulmonary edema. See Edema, pulmonary
Pulmonary embolism, 405
Pulmonary emphysema. See Emphysema
Pulmonary tuberculosis. See Tuberculosis, pulmonary
Pulse, in shock, 629
  relationship of, to degree of work, 412
  taking of, following fracture, 162, 163
Pulse deficit, in heart disease, 352
Pulse pressure, 386
Purines, metabolism of, associated with gout, 191, 192
Purpura, idiopathic thrombocytopenic, 344
Pus, definition of, 69
  in pleural space, 302
  in thoracic cavity, 319
  in urine, 506
Pyelogram, intravenous, 492
Pyelography, retrograde, of bladder, 493
Pyelolithotomy, 507
Pyelonephritis, 509
Pyloric orifice, 431
Pyrazinamide, in tuberculosis, 331
Pyuria, 506

Quadriplegia, 243. See also Paraplegia
Queckenstedt's sign, 207

Radiation, protection from, 157
  shielding in, 158
  reactions to, 156
  sensitivity of tissues to, 155
Radiation sickness, 156
  emotional aspects of, 157
Radioactive gold, 159
Radioactive iodine, 159
  uptake test with, 521
Radioactive phosphorus, 160
Radiography, of brain, cerebral angiography as, 209
  pneumoencephalography as, 208
  of spinal canal, myelography as, 210
Radioisotopes, 158
Radiotherapy. See also Cobalt Therapy; X-Ray Therapy
  applicators in, precautions with, 159
  avoidance of temperature extremes in, 157
  clinical applications of, 154
  exposures in, 157
  external beam, 155
  fluids and diet during, 157
  follow-up care in, 157
  for cancer, 147
  hydration in, 155, 157
  hyperbaric, 155
  in laryngofissure, 285
  in metastatic cancer, 594
  kidney function in, 157
  leukopenia in, 157
  nausea and vomiting in, 156
  nursing management in, 154-160
    hydration of patient in, 155
    prophylactic, 157
    protection against radiation in, 158
    protection of skin in, 156
    radiation sickness in, 156
      emotional aspects of, 157
    reactions to, individual, 155
Raynaud's disease, 398
Reactions, speed of, in elderly patient, 23
Recovery room, 132
Rectal disorders, 461-472. See also specific disorders
Rectocele, 572
Rectum, accumulation of gas in, postoperative, 138
  cancer of, 443
  hemorrhoids involving, 470, 470
  herniation of, into vagina, 572
  polyps involving, 469
Reed-Sternberg cells, 346
Regitine test, 531
Rehabilitation, in heart disease, 409-414
  cardiac work evaluation units in, 411
  classification of, 410
  nursing implications in, 413
  principles in, 412
  in paraplegia, 250
Relatives. See Family(ies)

Religious attitudes, and death, 108
    toward birth control, 55
Renal. *See also* Kidneys
Renal dialysis, 686
Renal failure, diagnosis of, 684
    etiology of, 683
    patient in, 683-691
    prevention of, 683
    prognosis of, 684
    treatment of, 685
Renal parenchyma, infection of, 509
Renal pelvis, calculi in, 507
Renal transplantation, 691
Renal tubules, nephrosis involving,
    512
Replacement therapy, 63
    in shock, 630
Reproduction, physiology of, 551, *552*
Reproductive pattern, female, 545-555
    and birth control, 553
    fertility and infertility in, 551
    menopause in, 549
    menstruation in, disorders of, 550
    puberty in, 548
    summary of, 554
Reproductive system. *Sell also* Geni-
        tourinary tract
    female, anatomy of, *546*
    dilatation and curettage in, 560
    disorders of, 556-574. *See also* spe-
        cific disorders
    diagnostic procedures in, 557
    examination of, 557, *557*, 558
    infection of, 563
    male, disorders of, 575-583. *See also*
        specific disorders
    involving prostate, 575, 579
    involving testes, 581
Respiration, cessation of, first aid in,
    115
    Cheyne-Stokes, 359
    depressed, postoperative, 135
    in shock, 629
Respirator, patients on, 639
Respiratory disorder, 292-304. *See also*
        specific disorders
    chronic, 305-323
    patient's attitude toward, 322
    treatment of, 322
    common cold as, 303
    death rates in, *305*
    diagnostic tests in, 292
    emphysema as, 302
    examination of sputum in, 294
    function tests in, 294
    influenza as, 302
    injuries to chest as, 303
    pleurisy as, 301
    pneumonia as, 295
Respiratory failure, acute, 636
    treatment of, 637
    nursing care in, 640
Respiratory function, exercises to im-
    prove, *317*
    tests in, 294
Respiratory infections, upper, and
    bronchitis, 312

Respiratory insufficiency, and failure,
    634-642
Respiratory obstruction, in surgery of
    the mouth, 440
Respiratory problems, following sur-
    gery, 133
Respiratory secretions, during surgery,
    127
Respiratory tract, diagram of, 293
Rest, in myocardial infarction, 666
    in rheumatoid arthritis, 187
Restlessness, in pneumonia, 300
    in shock, 629
Resuscitation, mouth-to-mouth, 115
Retina, detached, treatment of, 265
Retinopexy, 266
Retirement communities, 28
Retirement policies, 26
Rheumatic fever, active phase of, 369
    nursing care in, 371
    symptoms in, 369
    treatment in, 370
    causes of, 368
    diagnosis of, 369
    prevention of, 374
    prognosis of, 374
    rehabilitation in, 374
Rheumatic heart disease, 368, 371
Rheumatoid arthritis. *See* Arthritis,
    rheumatoid
Rheumatoid spondylitis. *See* Spondy-
    litis, ankylosing
Rhinitis, allergic, 305
    treatment of, 306
Rhinoplasty, 621
Rhizotomy, to relieve pain, 88
Rhythm, sinus, 646
Ribs, fractured, 179, 303
Roentgenography, gastrointestinal,
    418
    in respiratory disorders, 292
    in tuberculosis, 329
Rosacea, 613
Rubin test, in infertility, 553
Rubber, allergy to, 451
Rupture, intestinal. *See* Hernia
Russell traction, 172

Safety, first aid in, 113, 114
    in hospital, 111
    and reports, 113
Safety checklist, 111
Safety devices, grab bars as, to, *31*
Salicylates, in ankylosing spondylitis,
    190
    in arthritis, 184
    in rheumatic fever, 370
Saline, in sinusitis, 281
    with eyes, 257
Salmonella, food poisoning by, 117
Salpingectomy, 556
Salt, diets low in, 362
Sarcoma. *See also* Cancer; Neoplasia;
        Tumors
    definition of, 143
    osteogenic, 143
Scar tissue, and tissue repair, 67

Schiotz tonometer, 256
Scleral buckling, care following, 266
    in detached retina, 265
Sclerosis, multiple. *See* Multiple scle-
    rosis
Scorpions, first aid against, 120
Scratch test, 329
Scurvy, 60
Sebaceous cysts, 615
Seborrheic dermatitis, 610
Sedative(s), addiction to, 100
    in bronchial asthma, 309
    in eye disorders, 267
    in psychosomatic illness, 79
    postoperative, 136
    preoperative, 128
Seizures, epileptic, 218
Self-concern, during illness, 17
Self-esteem, in young adults, 8
Selverstone clamp, use with carotid
    artery, 234
Selye's theory, of stress, 56
Semen, examination of, 553
    physiology of, 551
Semicoma, as level of consciousness,
    210
Sengstaken-Blakemore balloon tube,
    480, *480*
Senility, 22
    and cerebrovascular disease, 228
Sensation, abnormalities of, in neuro-
    logic examination, 205
Septicemia, definition of, 70
Septum, deviated, 283
Sequestrum, in osteomyelitis, 193
Serum albumin, 475
    in brain scanning, 210
Serum ammonia, 475
Serum bilirubin, 474
Serum cholesterol, 475
Serum glutamic oxaloacetic transami-
    nase, 474
Serum hepatitis, 481
Serum values, in urologic disorders,
    496
Sex. *See* Reproductive pattern; Re-
    productive system
Sexual adjustment, at various ages, 2.
Sexual anxieties, of urologic patient,
    488
Sexual function, in paraplegia, 250
Sexual intercourse, painful, 565
Sexual vigor, in middle life, 13
Shaking palsy, 214
Shaving, of hair prior to surgery, 129
Shingles, 614
Shock, 627-633
    anaphylactic, 75
    effect upon vital organs, 630
    electric, 116
    first aid in, 115
    in cirrhosis, 478
    in increased intracranial pressure,
    702
    in myocardial infarction, 669
    insulin, 541
    symptoms of, 543

Shock (*Cont.*)
  kinds of, 627
  position in, 632
  postoperative, 134
  prevention of, 628
  prognosis in, 633
  signs of, 628
  symptoms of, 628
  treatment of, 630
Showers, in hygiene of elderly, 31
Sight. *See* Visual
Sigmoidoscopy, 419
Simmonds' disease, 532
Sims-Huhner test, 553
Single persons, aging of, 16
Singultus, 120
Sinus(es), disorders of, 280
  drainage of, *282*
  frontal, 280
  maxillary, inflammation of, 280
    treatment of, 281
  paranasal, 280
Sinus bradycardia, 646
Sinus rhythm, 646
Sinus tachycardia, 646
Sinusitis, 280
  treatment of, 281
Sitz baths, in urologic disorders, 496
Skin. *See also* Dermatologic
  allergic reactions involving, 611
  as body defense, 66
  bites of, 615
  burned, treatment of, 696, 698
  cancer of, 145
  care of, in coma, 212
    in mastectomy, 590
    with ileostomy, 453
  characteristics of, in cirrhosis, 476
  cleanliness of, 603
  creams for, allergy to, 451
  diseases of, 605
    dressings for, 608
    nursing care in, 607
    treatment of, 606
  dryness of, 603
  of elderly, 24
    lubrication of, 31
  grafts of, 621
  in renal failure, 684
  in shock, 628
  infestations of, 615
  injury to, 605
  itching of, 607
  lesions of, malignant, 616
  preparation of, in reduction of open
      fracture, 165
    prior to surgery, 125, *125*, 129
  problems involving, in urologic dis-
      orders, 496, 498
  radiated, 156
  sloughing of, in intravenous ther-
      apy, 64
  sunlight affecting, 604
  transplants of, 621
Skin tests, in allergy, 73, *73*
Skull fracture, depressed, 705

Sleep, requirements, of elderly, 33
Sleeplessness, prior to surgery, 127
Smoking, and peripheral vascular dis-
    ease, 399
  causing chronic bronchitis, 312
  discontinuance of, irritability fol-
      lowing, 104
    Lobeline in, 104
    methods to achieve, 104
    nursing aspects of, 103
  habituation to, 102
  lung cancer associated with, 102, *103*
  physical effects of tobacco in, 102
  prevention of, 105
  safety precautions involving, 112
  withdrawal from, effect of, 103
Snakebite, first aid in, 116, *116*
Snyder hemovac, 176, *176*
Sodium chloride, diets providing, 362
  in replacement therapy, 63
Sodium concentrations, in body fluid,
    62
Sodium ethocrynate, in congestive
    heart failure, 361
Sodium pentobarbital, prior to sur-
    gery, 127
Sodium urate, associated with gout,
    191
Solvents, ostomy appliance, 452
Somatropin, 532
Somnolence, as level of consciousness,
    210
Sores, cold, 614
Spastic patients, nursing care of, 235,
    235, 236, *236*
Speculum, bivalve, *558*
Speech, esophageal, 286
Speech reading, 272
Speech rehabilitation, following cere-
    brovascular accident, 240
Sperm, physiology of, 551
Spermatic cord, torsion of, 582
Sphincter, anal, dilatation of, 138
  urinary, incontinence involving, 501
Spica casts, in lumbar laminectomy,
    246
Spiders, poisonous, 120
Spinal canal, radiography of, myelog-
      raphy as, 210
  impairment of, treatment of, 245
  normal, 243
Spinal cord, compression of, 242
  function of, 242
  fusion of, 245
    lifting following, 247
  impairment of, bed rest in, 244
  causes of, 242
    paraplegia as, 248. *See also* Para-
        plegia
    patient with, 242-254
    surgery of, 245
    treatment of, conservative, 244
      laminectomy in, 245
        with spinal fusion, 246
      lifting following, 247
      spinal fusion as, 246, 247

Spinal cord (*Cont.*)
  surgery of, to relieve pain, 88
  tumors of, surgery of, 245
Spinal nerve root, compression of, 242
Spinal sclerosis, syphilitic, 599
Spine, ankylosing spondylitis involv-
      ing, 189
  cervical, injury to, 246
  fracture of, 178
  thoracic, injury to, 247
  tuberculosis of, 245
Splenomegaly, in leukemia, 341
Splenorenal shunt, 480
Splinting, of fractures, 162, 163
Splints, in rheumatoid arthritis, 188
  Thomas, *163*
  with traction, 173
Spondylitis, ankylosing, 189
  pathology of, 189
  symptoms of, 190
  treatment of, 190
Sprains, and dislocations, 179
Sputum, disposal of, in pulmonary tu-
      berculosis, 327
  examination of, 294
    in pulmonary tuberculosis, 330
    in pneumonia, 297
Stapes, ankylosis of, 273
  surgery of, 274
Staphylococcus aureus, food poison-
      ing by, 117
  pneumonia caused by, 298
Staphylococcal infections, 70
  and arthritis, 181
Status asthmaticus, 311
Status epilepticus, 218
Stenosis, aortic, 373, *373*
  mitral, 372
Stereotactic, in Parkinson's disease, 216
Sternal puncture, in blood disorders,
    336
Steroids. *See also* Corticosteroids
  adrenal, for cancer, 150
  in arthritis, 185
  in bronchial asthma, 310
  in shock, 632
  peptic ulcers caused by, 186
  side effects of, 186
  supplements to, 186
  weight gain associated with, 186
Stoma. *See also* Colostomy; Ileostomy;
    Ostomy
  description of, 446
Stomach. *See also* Gastric
  acids in, decrease of, therapeutic,
      432
    in physiology of peptic ulcer, 431
    neutralization of, 432
  bleeding in, from aspirin, 184
  cancer of, 442
    incidence of, 145
  contents of, analysis of, 295
  gastric juice of, 431
  hypermotility of, reduction of, 432
  obstruction of, complicating peptic
      ulcer, 435

Stomach (*Cont.*)
  peptic ulcer involving, 431. *See also* Peptic ulcer
  tissues of, perforation of, 436
Stones, urinary, 505. *See also* Calculi
Stool, evaluation of, 416
  specimens in, 418
Strength, of adult in middle life, 12
Streptococcal infection, *69*
  and arthritis, 181
  and endocarditis, 375
  and rheumatic fever, 368
Streptomycin, in pneumonia, 298
  in tuberculosis, 330
Stress, ability to withstand, 150
  and nursing, 57
  concept of, 56
  definition of, 56
  illness related to, 77
  necessity of, 58
  modification of, 57
  prior to surgery, 126
Stretchers, safety precautions with, 112
Stripping, and ligation, in varicose veins, 400
Stryker frame, in cervical spine injury, 246, *247*
Stupor, as level of consciousness, 210
Sty, 266
Submucous resection, 283
Suction, and irrigation, in gastrointestinal decompression, 423
  in gastrointestinal decompression, 421
Suicide, guarding against, 48
Sunburn, first aid in, 119
Sunlight, effect of, upon skin, 604
Sunstroke, first aid in, 118
Suppositories, in colostomy irrigation, 457
  prior to surgery, 130
Surgery, abdominal, urinary retention following, 137
  ambulation following, 140
  apprehension prior to, 127
  cardiac. *See* Cardiac surgery
  complications in, 134
  cosmetic, and functional improvement, 620
  elective, preparation for, 126
  elimination prior to, 129
  exercises prior to, 127
  foods and fluids prior to, 130
  for cancer, 147
  for varicose veins, 400, *400, 401*
  gastric, 439, 441, 443
    complications of, 434
  in coronary artery disease, 384
  in embolism, 404
  in ear disorders, 276
  in eye disorders, preoperative care in, 267
  in Parkinson's disease, 216
  in peptic ulcer, 433

Surgery (*Cont.*)
  in rheumatoid arthritis, 189
  in ulcerative colitis, 430
Surgery, intracardiac, 672. *See also* Cardiac surgery
  laryngeal, 285
  of bladder, 514
  of blood vessels, 405, *406*
  of chest, 320
  of urinary tract, 497
  open heart, 672. *See also* Cardiac surgery
  patients in. *See* Surgical patient
  permission for, 123
  plastic, 620-624
    nursing care in, 623
  postoperative phase of, 132
    abdominal distention in, 137
    atelectasis in, 138
    complications in, 134
    drainage in, 134
    exercise in, 140
    fluids and diet in, 136
    pain in, 135
    pneumonia in, 138
    respiratory considerations in, 133
    responsibilities of nurse in, 133
    thrombophlebitis in, 139, *139*
    urinary retention in, 137
    visitors in, 140
    vomiting in, 136
    wound infection in, 140
  preoperative phase of, 123
    food and fluids in, 130
    preparation of patient in, 131
      immediate, 125
    preparation of skin in, 125, *125, 129, 130*
  respiratory secretions during, 127
  stapes, 274
  tests prior to, 124
    role of nurse in, 128
  thoracic, postoperative care in, 320
  to relieve pain, 88
Surgical patient, 123, 142
  admission of, to nursing unit, 124
  apprehension of, 126, 127
  diet of, 136
  elimination, 129
  family of, 128
  gowns for, 130
  medication for, 127
  pain in, postoperative, 136
    preoperative, 127
  post-anesthesia recovery of, 132
  postoperative care of, 132
    fluids in, 134
    respiratory considerations in, 133
  personal hygiene of, 124
  preoperative care of, 123
    and hospital procedures, 128
    checklist in, 125, 131
    immediate, 128
    medication in, 127

Surgical patient (*Cont.*)
  transportation of, to operating room, 131
  valuables of, 130
Surgical wounds, drainage of, 176, *176*
Swallowing, difficulty in, 468
  mechanism of, *282*
Syme's amputation, 198
Sympathectomy, in Raynaud's disease, 399
Syndrome. *See* specific syndromes
Synovitis, in rheumatoid arthritis, 182
Syphilis, chancre of, 598, *598*
  complications of, 598, *598*
    neural, 599
  diagnosis of, 597
  symptoms of, 597
  treatment of, 599
Syringe, Asepto, *290*
  Pomeroy, 277
Systemic disease, dermatologic symptoms of, *617, 618*

Tachycardia, sinus, 646
Tarantulas, first aid against, 120
Tattooing, 621
Teaching, by nurse, of elderly patient, 24
Teenager. *See* Adult, young
Teeth. *See also* Dentures
  of elderly patient, 24
Teletherapy, 156, *156*. *See also* Radiotherapy
Temperature, atmospheric, changes in, 24
    extremes of, first aid in, 118
    in infective states, 70, 71
    in radiotherapy, 156
    in trigeminal neuralgia, 225
  basal body, and ovulation, 552
  in shock, 629
Temposil, in alcoholism, 96
Tenderness, rebound, in appendicitis, 461
Teratoma, definition of, 143
Terminal, definition of, 59
Terminology, disease, 59
Tests. *See also* specific tests
  BSP, 474
  capillary fragility, 336
  concentration and dilution, of urine, 491
  cytologic, in cancer, 148, 559
  diagnostic, 50
    gastrointestinal, 415-427
  in diabetes, 535
  in venereal disease, 597
  neurologic, 206
  of functional capacity, 410
  of liver function, 474
  phenolsulfonphthalein, 491
  pigment, of liver disorders, 474
  prior to surgery, 128
  Queckenstedt's, 207
  respiratory function, 294
  skin, in allergy, 73, *73*

Tests (*Cont.*)
support of patient during, 44
thyroid, 520, 521
tuberculin, 328
urea clearance, 491
Tes-Tape, in diagnosis of diabetes, 535
Testes, biopsy of, in infertility, 553
cancer of, 582
disorders of, 581
hidden, 581
torsion of, 582
Testosterone, in endometriosis, 567
in metastatic cancer, 593
Tetany, complicating thyroidectomy, 524
in hypoparathyroidism, 528
Tetracycline, in chronic obstructive pulmonary disease, 315
in pneumonia, 298
Thalassemia, 339
Thephorin, in Parkinson's disease, 215
Therapy. *See* Treatment
Thermography, in examination of breast, 587
Thomas splint, with traction, 173
Thoracic cavity, drainage from, 321
Thoracic spine, injury to, 247
Thoracic surgery, postoperative care in, 320
Throat, diseases of, 280-291. *See also* specific diseases
structures of, *281*
swallowing in, mechanism of, 282
Thromboangiitis obliterans, *398, 399*
Thrombophlebitis, complicating hysterectomy, 570
postoperative, 139, *139*
Thrombocytes, and leukemia, 340
Thrombocytopenia, 340
Thrombosis, and embolism, 391-408
cerebral. *See* Cerebral thrombosis
definition of, 392
nursing care in, 404
surgery in, 404
Thrombophlebitis, 402
Thymol turbidity, 475
Thyroid cancer, 525
radioactive iodine in, 159
Thyroid crisis, 524
Thyroid gland, disorders of, 519
enlargement of, 525
hypothyroidism involving, 525
surgery of, 522
Thyroid scanning, in hyperthyroidism, 521
Thyroid suppression test, 521
Thyroidectomy, complications of, 524
postoperative care in, 523, *523*, 524
subtotal, 522
Thyrotoxicosis, treatment of, 522
Thyrotropin, production of, 519
Thyrourea drugs, 521
Tibia, fracture of, splinting of, 163
Tic douloureux, 225

Ticks, first aid against, 120
Time, attitude toward, 16, 32
Tinnitus, 273
Tissue, granulation, 68
repair of, 67
and blood flow, 68
scar, 67
Tobacco, drugs and alcohol, abuse of, 90-106
habituation to, 102
need for, 90
physical effects of, 102
withdrawal from, 103
Toe, gangrene of, in diabetes, 542
Toenails, care of, 31
Tongs, Crutchfield, 178
in cervical spine injury, 246
in traction, 171, *172*
Tongue, depression of, during seizures, 219
Tongs, Vince, in traction, 171
Tonometer, use of, *256*
Tourniquet, first aid in, 115
in fractures, 164
in snakebite, 117
rotating, in pulmonary edema, 365, 366, *367*
Toxic hepatitis, 483
Toxins, definition of, 61
Tracheal dilator, *287*
Tracheobronchial tree, irritation of, 314
Tracheobronchitis, 312
Tracheostomy, care of, 286, *287, 289*
in respiratory failure, 638
obstruction of airway in, 288
tube feeding with, 290
Traction, Buck's extension, in herniated disk, 244
in amputation, 199
in first aid of fractures, 163
in herniated disk, 244
Tractotomy, to relieve pain, 88
Tranquilizers, in bronchial asthma, 309
in psychosomatic illness, 79
in therapy for alcoholism, 95
minor, addiction to, 100
prescription of, nursing considerations in, 100
Transfusion, in leukemia, 344
Transfusion reactions, 64
Transplantation, for valvular disease, 673
renal, 691
skin, 621
ureteral, 514, 517
Trauma. *See also* Wounds, traumatic
causing spinal cord impairment, 242
definition of, 60
to blood vessels, 406
to urinary tract, 517
Treadmill, in heart disease rehabilitation, 410

Treatment, refusal of, attitude of nurse toward, 51
legal aspect of, 52
support of patient during, 44
Tremors, in Parkinson's disease, 214, 215
Treponema pallidum, 597
Trigeminal nerve, neuralgia involving, 225, *226*
Trigeminal neuralgia, 225
nursing care in, 225
postoperative, 226
Trimethadione, in epilepsy, 221
Trocar, use of, 281
TSH, production of, 519
in hypothyroidism, 525
Tubercle bacilli, characteristics of, 325
in sputum, 330
transmission of, 327
Tuberculin, in Mantoux test, 329, *329*
Tuberculin tests, 328
Tuberculosis, attitude toward, 325
miliary, 328
mortality rates in, 324
of spine, 245
pulmonary, 324-334
caseation in, 328
complications of, 332
control of, 333
diagnosis of, 328
examination of sputum in, 330
gastric aspiration in, 330
roentgenography in, 329
tests in, 328, 329, *329*, 330
disposal of sputum in, 327
etiology of, 325
hemorrhage in, 332
pathology of, 327
prophylactic measures in, 334
rehabilitation from, 333
signs and symptoms of, 328
spontaneous pneumothorax in, 332
treatment of, 330
chemotherapy in, 330
in general hospitals, 333
protection of personnel during, 326
surgical, 332
untreated, and arthritis, 181
urinary infection with, 509
Tubes, Cantor, 422, *422*
endotracheal, in respiratory failure, 637, 638, *638*
for gastrointestinal decompression, 420, *421, 422*
care of, 423
irrigation of, 424
withdrawing of, 424
gastric balloon, 480, *480*
intestinal, 423
Levin, 421, *421*
in peptic ulcer, 433
Miller-Abbott, *421*, 422
nasogastric, 421, *421*

Tumor(s). *See also* Cancer; Neoplasia; Sarcoma
  benign, characteristics of, 144
    definition of, 60
    of uterus, 567
  cardiac, 675
  causing spinal cord impairment, 244
  gynecologic, 567
    general care in, 570
    inoperable, 571
  malignant, categories of, 143
    definition of, 61
  of brain, 706
    treatment of, 707
  of bladder, 514
  of bone, 192
  of brain, shifts in, 209
  of kidney, 513
  of pituitary gland, 532
  of urinary tract, 513
  ovarian, 568
  spinal cord, surgery of, 245
Tunica vaginalis, 582
Tympanoplasty, 276
Typhoid fever, chloramphenicol in treatment of, 298

Ulcer(s), Curling's, 699
  decubitus, complicating multiple sclerosis, 224
    in elderly, 32
    with traction, 171
  of leg, 395
  peptic, caused by steroids, 186
    complications of, 434
    diet in, 432
    dumping syndrome in, 434
    duodenal, *430*
    management of, 428-436
    related to stress, 57, 77
    symptoms of, 431
    treatment of, drugs in, 432
      medical, 432
      neutralization of acid in, 432
      rest and relaxation in, 433
      surgical, 433
  varicose, 401
Ulcerative colitis, management of, 428-436
  symptoms of, 428
  treatment of, 429
    drugs in, 429
    nursing care in, 430
    psychotherapy in, 430
    surgery in, 430
Unconscious patient, 51
Unna's paste boot, 402
Urea clearance test, 491
Urea nitrogen, levels of, 490
Ureteral calculi, 505
Ureteral dilator, *492*
Ureteral transplants, 514
  nursing points in, 517
Ureterosigmoidostomy, 514
Ureterostomy, cutaneous, 515

Ureters, definition of, 489
Urethra, definition of, 489
  and catheterization, *498*, 499, 547
Urethral obstruction, 505
Urethral strictures, 508
Urethritis, 510
Urethroplasty, in urethral stricture, 508
Urethrostomy, in urethral stricture, 508
Uric acid, associated with gout, 191
Urinalysis, 489
  prior to surgery, 128
Urinary incontinence, 501. *See also* Incontinence
  home care in, 504
  in ambulatory patients, 503
  in bed patients, 503
  nursing care in, 502
  odor associated with, 503
  rehabilitation in, 502
Urinary infection, 508
  with calculi, 506
Urinary obstructions, *504*, 505
Urinary output, in pneumonia, 300
Urinary retention, postoperative, 137
Urinary sphincter, incontinence involving, 501
Urinary tract, 488, 489. *See also* Kidneys; Bladder, etc.
  blockage of. *See* Urinary obstruction
  diagnostic procedures involving, 489
  infection of, prevention of, 496
  inflammations of, 508, 509, 510
  nephritis involving, 511
  nephrosis involving, 512
  observation of, 494
  surgery of, 497
  tumors of, 513
  trauma to, 517
Urination, problems involving, 32
Urine, analysis of, in Cushing's syndrome, 530
  blood chemistry of, 490
  calculi formed in, 505
  characteristics of, 489
  concentration and dilution tests of, 491
  drainage of, catheters in, *498*, 499
  excessive, in diabetes, 534
  excretion of, in hyperthyroidism, 521
  measurement of, 63
  formation of, 62
  glucose in, 534
  in diabetes insipidus, 532
  in renal failure, 684
  observation of, 495
  pus in, 506
  specimens of, 535
Urine bilirubin, 474
Urine tests, in diabetes, 535
Urobilinogen, fecal, 474
  urine, 474

Urologic disorders, blood pressure in, 495
  catheters in, bleeding associated with, 497
    changing of, 500
    drainage and irrigation of, 501
    patients with, 498
    types of, *498*, 499, *500*
  fluid intake in, 495
  observations in, 494
  odor associated with, 496
  pain in, 496
  patients with, comfort of, 496
    infection of, 496
  serum values in, 495
  sexual concerns of, 488
  surgery of, bleeding in, 497
    care following, 497
    care prior to, 497
    protection of skin in, 498
Urologic patient, 488-518
Urticaria, 611
Uterine displacement, 573
Uterus, cancer of, 568
  curettage of, 560
  displacement of, 572
  prolapse of, 572
  tumors of, benign, 567
Urinal, rubber, *502*, 503
Uveitis, 266

Vagina, and prolapse of uterus, 572
  examinations of, 557, *557*, 558
  irrigation of, 547
Vaginal fistula, 571, *571*
Vaginal mucous membrane, in elderly, 32
Vaginitis, 563
  treatment of, 564
Vagotomy, 433
Valium, in epilepsy, 221
Valuables, care of, prior to surgery, 130
Valve, cardiac. *See* Cardiac valve
Varicele, 582
Varicose ulcers, 401
Varicose veins, 399, *400, 401*
  hemorrhoids as, 470, *470*
Vascular dilatation, following inflammation, 67
Vascular disease, cerebral. *See* Cerebrovascular disease
  peripheral, 391-408
    leg ulcers in, 395
    pain in, 391
    pain in, 395
    patient instruction in, 397
    treatment of, positioning of patient in, 392
Vascular disturbances, in diabetes, 542
Vascular insufficiency, peripheral, amputation in, 196
Vasoconstriction, avoidance of, 393
  measures to lessen, 394

Vasodilator, heat as, 399
  to increase blood supply, 393
Vasopressin, 532
Vectorcardiogram, in heart disease, 354
Veins. *See also* Blood vessels; Intravenous
  inflammation of, 402
  ligation and stripping of, 400
Veins, varicose, 399, *400, 401*
  hemorrhoids as, 470, *470*
Venereal infection, 596-602. *See also* specific infections
  nursing care in, 600
Venography, portal, 475
Venous pressure, central, in shock, 629
  measuring of, 359
Venous stasis, avoidance of, 402
  postoperative, 139
Venous thrombosis, in myocardial infarction, 669
Ventilation, tests to determine, 294
Ventilator, patient on, 639
Ventricular contractions, premature, 648
Ventriculography, 209
Vertebrae, cervical. *See also* Spinal cord injury to, 242
Vertigo, following ear surgery, 277
  in Meniere's disease, 278
Vinblastine, for cancer, 149
Vince, tongs, in traction, 171
Vincristine, for cancer, 149
  in leukemia, 341
Viomycin, in tuberculosis, 331
Viral hepatitis. *See* Hepatitis, viral
Virus(es), causing bronchitis, 312
  causing encephalopathies, 213
Vision. *See also* Visual
  normal, 258
  partial, 258
  problems associated with, in diabetes, 543

Visitors, attitude of nurse toward, 53
  following surgery, 141
Visual. *See also* Eyes; Vision
Visual accommodation, 261
  in young adults, 7
Visual disorders, assessment of, instruments in, 255
  treatment of, eyedrop technic in, 268, *268*
  first aid, 257
  sedation in, 267
Visual impairment, and hearing impairment, 255-282. *See also* specific conditions
  detached retina as, 265
  sympathetic ophthalmia as, 266
  treatment of, nursing considerations in, 267
  surgery in, enema prior to, 268
  postoperative care in, 269
  preoperative care in, 267
  prevention of hemorrhage in, 269
Visually handicapped, 258
Vital capacity, tests to determine, 294
Vitamins, malabsorption of, 470
Vitamin A, and night blindness, 257
Vitamin B, in therapy for alcoholism, 95
Vitamin B_{12}, and cancer of stomach, 442
  and pernicious anemia, 338
Vitamin C, lack of, 60
Vitamin D, in hypoparathyroidism, 527
Vitreous humor, and detached retina, 265
  loss of, 263
Voice box. *See* Larynx
Volkmann's contracture, 167
Volvulus, of colon, 467, *467*
Vomiting, and nausea, 425
  following surgery, factors associated with, 126

Vomiting (*Cont.*)
  induction of, in drug poisoning, 118
  of blood, in peptic ulcer, 434
  postoperative, 136
Vulva, cancer of, 569
Vulvectomy, 569

Wakefullness, as level of consciousness, 210
Walking, crutch, 177
Wasps, first aid against, 120
Water. *See also* Electrolyte(s); Fluid(s)
  sterile, administration of, 65
  and electrolyte regulation, 61
    nursing care in, 62
    replacement therapy and, 63
    weight-taking in, 63
Weight, loss of, in elderly, 23
  of adult in middle life, 12
Weight-taking, to determine fluid retention, 63
Wheelchair, in paraplegia, 252
Whole blood, in replacement therapy, 63
Withdrawal sickness, in drug abuse, 101
Wounds. *See* Trauma
Wound, disruption of, postoperative, 140
  first aid in, 116
  infections of, postoperative, 140
  penetrating, of chest, 304
  surgical, drainage of, 176, *176*
  traumatic, *69*
    inflammation associated with, 66
    repair of, 67
Wristdrop, caused by cast compression, *167*

X-ray, gallbladder series, 484
  in heart disease, 355
X-ray therapy. *See also* Radiotherapy

Zollinger-Ellison syndrome, 417